MW00640313

THE COMPLETE ENCYCLOPEDIA OF MEDICINE & HEALTH

THE COMPLETE ENCYCLOPEDIA

OF MEDICINE & HEALTH

FOREIGN MEDIA
BOOKS

The records of illustrations, photographs, graphic arts etc. have been deposited with Continental Copyrights AG and Concord Publishing AG.
Jacket design by DPS Design & Prepress Services Amsterdam

ISBN 1-60136-001-0
ISBN 9781601360014
Library of Congress Control Number: 2006932428

EDITOR-IN-CHIEF

Johannes P. Schadé, M.D., Ph.D. D.Sc.hc

CONTRIBUTORS AND ADVISORS

Prof. A. Agrawal, M.D., Ph.D., K. Barbier, M.D., Prof. E. Blechschmidt, M.D., Ph.D., Prof. J. Bossy, M.D., Prof. Eric Chipman, M.D., Ph.D., Prof. Donald L. DeVincenzi, M.D., Ph.D., Prof. Th. A. Doxiades, M.D., Ph.D., Bevan M. French, M.D., Prof. David Gilman, M.D., Ph.D. Prof. G. Gondony, M.D., Prof. A. Hanley, Ph.D., Prof. H.J. Jongkind, M.D., Prof. K. Heinkel, M.D., Ph.D., Prof. A.P. Heinz, M.D., Ph.D., Prof. M. Hyodo, M.D., Ph.D., Prof. J.P. Johnson, M.D., Ph.D., Prof. Hirotake Kakehi, M.D., T. Loftas, M.D., Stephen P. Maran, Ph.D., Prof. S. Obrador, M.D., Ph.D., Prof. C. Omura, M.D., Ph.D., Prof. I G. Sanio, M.D., Ph.D., Prof. A. Stacher, M.D., Prof. P. C. Sylvester-Bradley, M.D., W.E. Taylor, M.D., Prof. D. Turk, M.D., Ph.D., Prof. S. Ullberg, M.D., Ph.D., Prof. W. Umbach, M.D., Ph.D., Prof. A. Vermeulen, M.D.

TECHNICAL STAFF

Joyce Isaak (Head DTP), Hedi von Banniseht, Harriet Zuidervaart, John Ingleson, Peter Holloway

INSTITUTIONS AND ORGANIZATIONS

During the compilation of the encyclopedia over a period of 4 years the editorial staff have benefitted from the co-operation of the following agencies, university institutions, and foundations.
National Institutes of Health, Bethesda, USA
National Cancer Institute, Washington, USA
World Health Organization, Geneva, Switzerland
Medical Library Foundation, Zürich, Switzerland
Health Education Council, London, UK
International Society of Alternative Medicine
Department of Agriculture, US Government
Department of Health and Social Security, London, UK
Department of Medicine, University of New York, NY
Department of Pathology, Univ. of San Francisco, USA
Department of Internal Medicine, Univ. College, London
School of TropicaL Medicine, Liverpool, UK

PREFACE

■ This encyclopedia aims to meet the growing demand of the general public for highly detailed, complete, authoritative medical information.

■ This information includes anatomy, function, diagnostic tests, and medical procedures. Medical terms are defined, so that people better understand their doctors.

■ No book can replace the expertise and advice of health care professionals who have direct contact with the patient. This encyclopedia is meant to supplement that relationship, not replace it.

■ This encyclopedia is not meant for self-diagnosis and self-treatment. Rather it is a source of accurate, reliable information that should stimulate better communication between patients and their doctors and other health care professionals.

■ The information in this encyclopedia is true and complete to the best of our knowledge. The book is intended only as a guide to better understand your body and illnesses.

■ It is not intended as a replacement for sound medical advice from a doctor. Only a doctor can include variables of an individual's age, gender and past medical history needed for wise treatment and drug prescription.

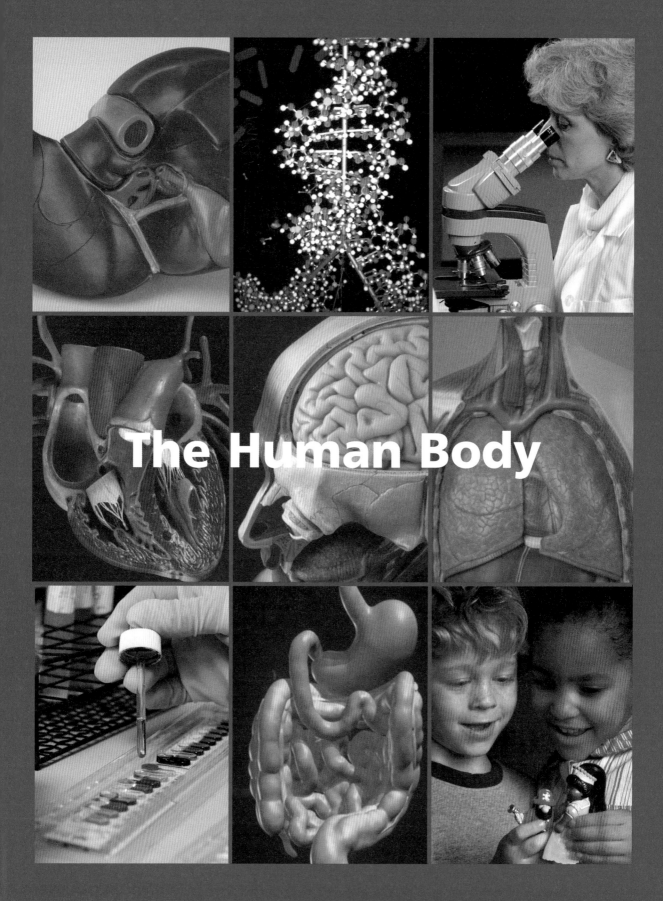

The Human Body

1 Introduction

Evolution of mankind

The evolution of mankind is a fascinating story. Evolution is defined as the process by which living organisms have changed since the origin of life. The formulation of the theory of evolution by natural selection is credited to Charles Darwin, whose observations after setting sail around the world on HMS Beagle in 1831, when taken together with elements from the population theory of Thomas Malthus, led him to the concept of natural selection. Darwin defined the mechanism of natural selection on the basis of three series of observations:

▲ That animals and plants produced far more offspring than were required to maintain the size of their population;

▲ that the size of any natural population remained more or less stable over long periods;

▲ that the members of any one generation varied from each other.

From the first two, he argued that in any generation there was a high mortality rate, and from the third that, under certain circumstances some of the variants had a greater chance of survival than did others.

Comparative anatomy

Today, the evidence for evolution is overwhelming and comes from many branches of biology. For instance, the comparative anatomy of the human arm, the foreleg of a horse, the wing of a bat and the flipper of a seal reveals that these superficially different organs have a very similar internal structure, this being taken to indicate a common ancestor. The study of the embryos of mammals and birds also reveals that, at some stages, they are virtually indistinguishable and they have common ancestors. Again, vestigial organs such as the appendix of a human and the wing of the ostrich are of no use to these mammals, but in related species such as herbivores (e.g. cows) and flying birds, they clearly are of vital importance.

Upright position

The bipedal (upright) posture and habit of moving of humans and certain primates were established in the early Pliocene era, some 12 million years ago, and it seems certain that these were fully developed in human ancestral individuals for well over one million years ago. Such limb bones as exist of ancestors who lived 500,000 years ago indicate clearly that erect standing and walking were well-established, continuing features of humans' descent at that distant time. If, then, bipedalism has been evolving and becoming more efficient over such a long period, it is difficult to imagine circumstances in which many of the physical defects attributed to the evolution of an upright posture could have persisted in the gene pool from which the modern human population had emerged.

Such features as abdominal hernias, prolapsed uteruses, intervertebral disk lesions (s-called slipped disks) and varicose veins in the legs would appear to be susceptible to extinction by natural selection.

Natural selection

When assessing any factor in natural selection, one has to consider whether its possession will interfere with breeding. Adverse factors that appear in individuals only after they have produced and reared their family have little or no influence in future evolution. In human ancestors, the shortening, broadening and fixation of the pelvis necessary for bipedalism restricted the size of the skull after birth and meant that birth had to

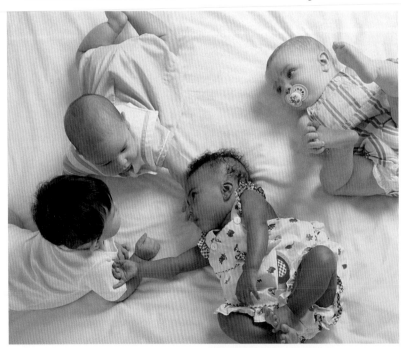

occur before fully independent existence could be established by the newborn.

This, exaggerated by the increase in brain and head size that followed the adoption of an upright posture, has led to the human nursing and rearing period being far longer than that of any other mammalian species. Even so, the existence of disproportion between fetal head and maternal pelvis is common, and labour in women verges on the extreme of natural mechanical processes.

Since prolapses of the uterus and bladder occur in young women following a difficult labour, one can perceive a balance between the opposing selective forces of the need for as late a birth of the fetus as possible and reduction of the pelvic cavity for efficient bipedal locomotion.

Skeleton fossils

Our knowledge about human evolution is largely based on the study of fossils of the skeleton. The study of early humans is hampered by the difficulty of distinguishing between what was to become Homo sapiens and the ancestors of our modern apes. The actual point of the two strains - the "missing link" - is so long ago, probably before either bore any resemblance to their modern descendants, that it is unlikely ever to be discovered.

The earliest known form of human is *Ramapithecus*, though there is still debate as to whether it should be classed as of the Hominidae (human family) or of the Pongidae (anthropoid-ape family).

Only small fragments of *Ramapithecus* fossil skeleton exist, the earliest of these dating from some 14 million years ago, the latest from some 10 million years.

The next earliest human fossil skeleton dates from about three million years ago and is tentatively designed Australopithecus africanus, once again only fragments exists. In 1972, the anthropologist Richard Leakey discovered a skull, known as Skull

1476, which dates from 2.6 million years ago and which shows strong resemblance to modern man.

It is now thought that the humans of Skull 1476 type evolved over a period of more than 2 million years into our recent ancestors, Neanderthaler Man and Cro-Magnon Man, although there is as yet no fossil evidence to show this evolution.

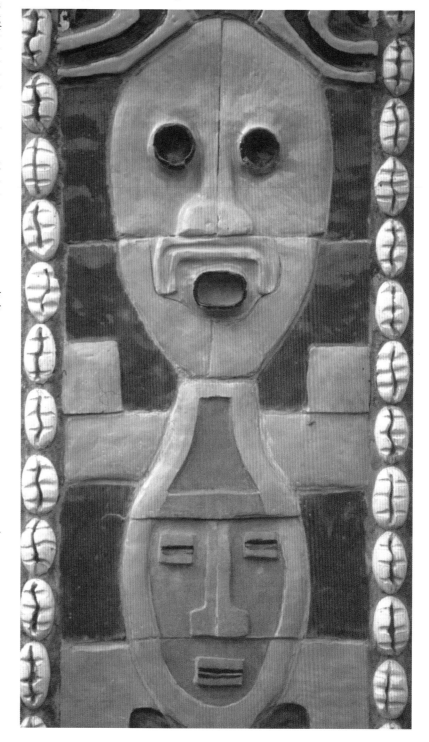

Man and woman (Zambia, 1980).

11

2 Cells and Genes

Introduction

The cell is the fundamental component of all living organisms, from orchids and earthworms to human beings. Obviously, there are major differences among cell types. Muscle cells, which can contract, have to be quite different from liver or bone cells. Nerve cells have long, thin fibers that, in humans, might extend more than 3 feet from the spinal cord to the toes, while blood cells have no projecting fibers at all. Plant cells have a unique ability to use light for energy.

Then what do all these cells have in common? Discovering their shared properties was difficult. At first, scientists thought that the cell was just a blob of jelly, or some primordial soup enclosed in a bag. They named the jelly "protoplasm." For a long time they could not find anything in the protoplasm, which later became known as "cytoplasm."

Part of the difficulty in studying cells, of course, is due to their extremely small size. The cells of multicellular organism are impossible to see with the unaided eye. Microscopes are therefore an important tool for studying cells.

Microscopic research

A microscope - even one with perfect lenses and perfect illumination - simply cannot be used to distinguish objects that are smaller than one-half the wavelength of light.

White light has an average wavelength of 0.55 micrometers, half of which is 0.27 micrometers. One micrometer is a thousandth of a millimetre, and there are about 25,000 micrometers to an inch. Micrometers are also called microns.

Any two lines that are closer together than 0.27 micrometers will be seen as a single line, and any object with a diameter smaller than 0.27 micrometer will be invisible - or, at best, show up as a blur.

Although the nucleus of a typical human cell is relatively large (about 7 micrometers in diameter), most organelles vary from a width of only 1 micrometer to structures so fine that they must be measured in nanometres (which are 1,000 times smaller than micrometers), or even in angstrom units (10 times smaller than nanometres).

To see such tiny particles under a microscope, scientists must bypass light altogether and use a different sort of "illumination," one with a shorter wavelength. The invention of the electron microscope made it possible to see much smaller objects than with the light microscope. If pushed to the limit, electron microscopes can resolve objects as small as the diameter of an atom.

Uniformity of life

All cells - whether from a bacterium, plant, mouse, or human - are made of the same basic materials: nucleic acids, proteins, carbohydrates, water, fats, and salts. The genetic material in all these cells is deoxyribonucleic acid (DNA), a large molecule that directs the making of duplicate cells.

DNA also directs the building of proteins according to a complex code. Even the simplest living cells - the mycoplasma - contain a relatively large amount of DNA, enough to code for up to a thousand different proteins.

Representation of the interior of a cell. The quantity of water represents the fluid content - about 40 to 45%. All chemical reactions than take place in a watery medium.
1. Cell nucleus with chromosomes and nuclear body (nucleolus)
2. Endoplasmic reticulum
3. Golgi apparatus
4. Mitochondria
5. Lysosome
6. Fibrils
All higher creatures consist of an accumulation of elementary units, and these basic elements of living matter are the cells. Each human has about one hundred thousand million million cells - an almost unimaginable number: 100,000,000,000,000,000.

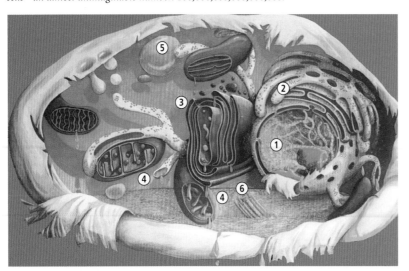

Every human cell has about six feet of very tightly wound DNA strands contained within its nucleus, and every adult carries about 100 billion miles of ultrathin DNA strands in his or her body - a distance greater than the diameter of the solar system.

Each cell is separated from the rest of the world by a membrane so thin that it cannot be seen under a light microscope. Despite its ethereal nature, the surface membrane is extremely powerful, controlling everything that goes into and out of the cell and relaying vital messages. Similar membranes enclose or make up a large number of the cell's organelles.

Nucleus

The nucleus is the biggest, densest, most obvious structure in the cell. For many years, nobody knew what the nucleus did. In the 19th century, several researchers noted that before a cell divided, the nucleus divided.

But it was not until the beginning of the 20th century that scientists grasped the connection between the rodlike chromosomes (tightly packed bundles of DNA and protein) that had been observed in the nucleus and the transmission of hereditary traits. At that point, the importance of the nucleus became clear.

The nucleus is the cell's command center. The chromosomes contain the genes (made of DNA) that give directions for everything the cell is and will be, and thus control the cell's reproduction and heredity.

The nucleus, where the genetic material is stored, is the cell's largest organelle. It is surrounded by a double membrane that is permeated with "gates" called nuclear pores, which may be the routes by which genetic messages pass into the cytoplasm. A small round organelle inside the nucleus - the nucleolus - is the site of ribosome manufacture.

Ribosomes

Ribosomes are extremely tiny - less than 30 nanometres in diameter. However, due to their crucial role in protein manufacture, ribosomes can

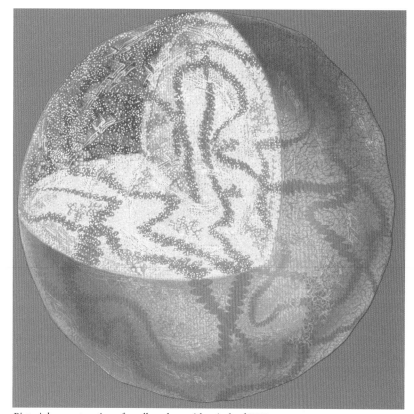

Pictorial reconstruction of a cell nucleus with spirals of DNA.

be extremely numerous. Each ribosome is made of two unequally sized subunits, which are composed of at least 40 different proteins and a form of RNA called ribosomal RNA.

Ribosomes work very quickly to connect the required amino acids into a protein. Each ribosome in a single bacterium, for example, can link 15 amino acids in a second. The speed and efficiency of translation means that each gene is capable of directing the manufacture of very large quantities of protein.

For example, in each cell of a silk worm's silk gland there is a single gene that codes for the protein fibroin, the chief component of silk. Each time it is activated, the gene can make 10,000 copies of a specific RNA and each copy of this molecule can direct the synthesis of 100,000 molecules of fibroin. In 4 days, a silk gland cell can manufacture a billion molecules of fibroin.

Ribosomes fall into two categories: those that are free in the cytoplasm and those that are bound to membranes. The two kinds of ribosomes play similar roles in the manufacture of proteins. But while the free ribosomes leave the proteins equally free to float in the cytoplasm, the bound ribosomes transfer their finished proteins into a large, cobwebby organelle - the endoplasmic reticulum.

Ribozymes

Ribozymes are RNA molecules with enzymatic activity, particularly the ability to cleave the normally unreactive phosphodiester bonds that link the nucleotides in RNA strands. Enzymatic reactions occur at certain base pairs that are formed as RNA folds back on itself, and most naturally occurring ribozymes cleave the RNA strands of which they are part. By analogy with enzymatic reactions involving proteins, the oligonucleotide that is cleaved is called the substrate.

Like their protein counterparts, RNA enzymes are highly specific with respect to the substrates they act on

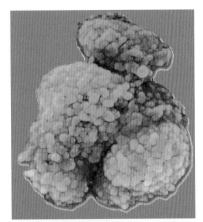

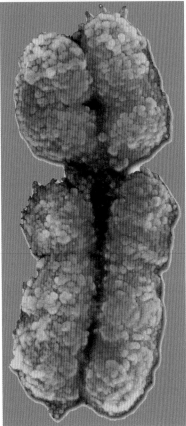

Human cells contain 23 pairs of chromosomes. Molecular structure of the human sex chromosomes. Upper figure: X-chromosome; lower figure: Y-chromosome.

and the products they produce. In spite of their evident therapeutic potential against viral RNA's or deleterious gene transcripts, ribozymes have been slow to move from experimental cell-free systems to cell lines or

animal models. Difficulties include instability of the synthesized molecules in the presence of nucleases and accessibility to RNA whose three-dimensional structure is not known.

The endoplasmic reticulum

The endoplasmic reticulum is a vast network of channels bounded by membranes in the cytoplasm of cells. At times this network looked like the concentric circles of a slice of onion. This network was called endoplasmic reticulum because it is more concentrated in the inner (endoplasmic) region of the cell than in the peripheral (ectoplasmic) region.

The membranes of this endoplasmic reticulum all interconnect, forming a system of tubes and flattened sacs that is continuous with the nuclear membrane. In effect, this system divides the cytoplasm into two main regions, one enclosed within the "plumbing" and the other forming the outer region, or cytoplasmic matrix.

Some parts of this membrane look smooth, while others appear "rough" because they are dotted with ribosomes that form granules on their outer surfaces. These ribosomes deposit newly formed proteins into the lumen, or inner space, of the endoplasmic reticulum.

The endoplasmic reticulum then segregates the proteins into those that will be needed in the cytoplasm and those that will be transported to other organelles or secreted from the cell. The amount of rough endoplasmic reticulum in a cell corresponds closely to the quantity of protein the cell exports.

Those white blood cells that produce infection-fighting immune system proteins called antibodies have highly developed rough endoplasmic reticula, for instance. These antibodies are found mainly in cellular storage areas, from which they go forth to combat infections.

The smooth endoplasmic reticulum, on the other hand, is particularly well developed in cells where it takes on some extra function - for example, in liver cells, where it breaks down drugs by making them water soluble. In addition to its role in protein segrega-

tion, the endoplasmic reticulum is the cell's membrane factory. Phospholipids and cholesterol, the main components of membranes throughout the cells, are synthesized in the smooth portion of the endoplasmic reticulum.

These compounds form the coating of protein-filled sacs, called vesicles, that "bud off" from the endoplasmic reticulum, migrate to another organelle, fuse with it, and then deposit the protein cargo. Most of the proteins leaving the endoplasmic reticulum are still not mature; they must undergo further processing in another organelle, the Golgi apparatus, before they are ready to perform their functions within or outside the cell.

Golgi apparatus

Each Golgi apparatus consists of a stack of flat, membranous sacs that are piled one on top of the other like dinner plates. The stack is composed of at least three chemically distinct regions, and each sac in the organelle contains enzymes that modify proteins as they pass through. The sacs closest to the nucleus receive vesicles filled with protein molecules from the endoplasmic reticulum. The proteins must pass through all the sacs in sequence to be processed correctly.

Why does the cell go to such elaborate lengths to modify and sort proteins? The compartmental organization of the Golgi apparatus is crucial to the functioning of the cell, because without it thousands of enzymes would be randomly mixed, resulting in a chaotic splay of biochemical activity.

The Golgi apparatus controls the chaos by packaging proteins into vesicles as they pass through the organelle. The protein-filled vesicles migrate to another organelle or to the cell's surface, where they fuse with the cell's outer membrane and release their contents. This is how cells secrete hormones, enzymes, and other types of proteins as needed.

Inside the Golgi apparatus, proteins are modified depending upon their ultimate destinations. For example, proteins bound for the cell's surface membrane are modified in one way, while proteins that will eventually move to the cell's "digestive" organelles undergo a different series of changes.

Lysosomes

When a white blood cell engulfs a bacterium and destroys it, the white cell's lysosomes do most of the work. They fuse with the vesicles of engulfed material and release digestive enzymes to break up the material. Similarly, when a cell takes in large molecules of food, enzymes in the lysosomes break the food down into smaller and simpler products that the cell can use. These products diffuse through the lysosomes' membranes and go into the rest of the cell, where they serve as building blocks for various structures, until nothing is left inside the lysosomes but indigestible material and the lysosomes become what are called residual bodies. In some cells, the residual bodies then migrate to the cell surface and eject the undigested material into the external environment.

Lysosomes in health and disease

Lysosomes are known to contain over 40 different enzymes that can digest almost anything in the cell, including proteins, RNA, DNA, and carbohydrates. These enzymes work best in environments more acidic than that found in cytoplasm, and lysosomes are specially equipped to provide this acidic environment. As corrosive as these enzymes are, they do not ordinarily damage the cell because the lysosomal membrane remains intact. When cells are programmed to die in some normal process of embryonic development, however - for example,

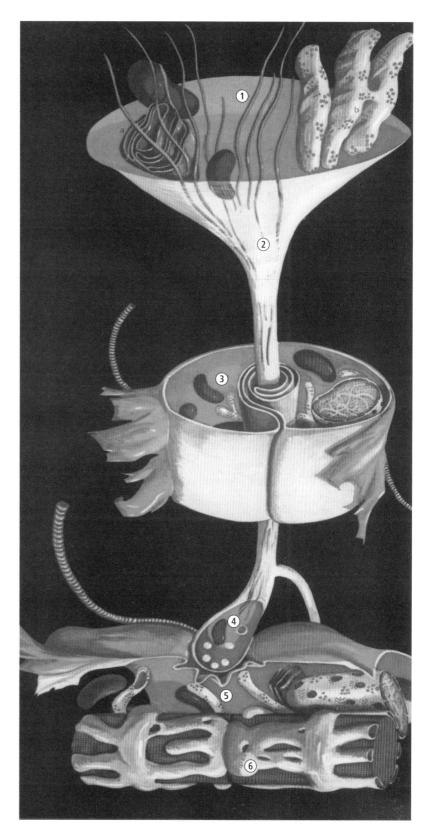

Reconstruction of part of a nerve cell, showing the connection with the muscle fiber.
1. Cell body of the nerve cell with various organelles, such as (a) Golgi apparatus, (b) endoplasmic reticulum.
2. Nerve fiber
3. Myelin sheath of nerve fiber
4. Nerve fiber where it meets the muscle fiber
5. Synapse between nerve fiber and muscle fiber
6. Muscle fiber surrounded by connective tissue

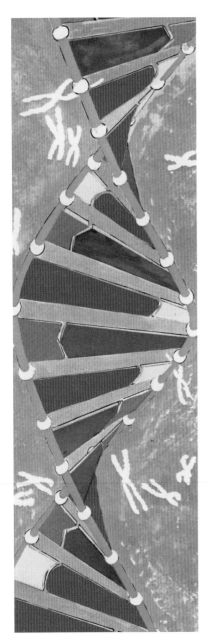

Schematic drawing of the molecular structure of DNA. The DNA molecule is a long, coiled double helix that resembles a spiral staircase. In it, two strands, composed of sugar (deoxyribose) and phosphate molecules, are connected by pairs of four molecules called bases, which form the steps of the staircase. In the steps, adenine is paired with thymine, and guanine with cytosine. Each pair of bases is held together by a hydrogen bond. Thus, a gene consists of a sequence of bases, each sequence of three bases coding for one amino acid (amino acids are the building blocks of proteins).

DNA

Description

DNA is the widely used abbreviation for deoxyribonucleic acid. Living cells in the human body contain two basic types of informational molecules: DNA and ribonucleic acid (RNA). These molecules contain and transmit the genetic information of the cell. In terms of informational content, they are the most important elements in living organisms.

The instructions contained by the nucleic acids are finally expressed by another group of molecules called proteins. Proteins form many of the structural and mechanical components of living systems.

Some of them, the enzymes, play very important roles as chemical catalysts. The chemical activities of the cell are thus controlled indirectly by DNA and RNA, which direct the synthesis of proteins. These in turn regulate the metabolic activities of the cell.

Structure of DNA

The deoxyribonucleic acid molecule is an extremely long chemical thread made up of two strands. Unlike most threads, however, the strands are not wound round one another but are held as a pair that is wound round an imaginary central core to form a spiral or double helix. This arrangement means that the gross structure of the helix looks like a long screw from the side; but if it is examined from one end, a hole can be seen passing from one end to the other, up the center of the helix. Each strand of the double helix consists of a long chain of the sugar deoxyribose and phosphate residues. These chains are formed by the loss of two water molecules to condense a phosphoric acid residue with two deoxyribose molecules. Each of these deoxyribose molecules is, in turn, connected to further phosphate residues, and so the chain is built up. Two purines - adenine and guanine - and two pyrimidines - thymine and cytosine - are also commonly found in DNA. Although no intrinsic pattern seems to emerge when the order of the bases along the strand is examined, the bases on one strand are clearly related to the bases on the strand opposite. In the DNA double-helical thread, the purine and pyrimidine bases of the two strands lie opposite one another in the structure and the pattern is always one in which a thymine on one strand is faced by an adenine, and a guanine by a cytosine. Thus thymine and adenine are said to be a complementary base pair, as are guanine and cytosine. The presence of an adenine opposite a thymine and a guanine opposite a cytosine means that, in DNA, there is always one molecule of adenine to every molecule of thymine and one guanine for every cytosine. This arrangement is largely responsible for holding the two strands in their close position in the double-helical thread. The very precise alignment of base pairs on the double-stranded molecule of DNA leads to a structure of great regularity, whatever the ratio of $(A+T)/(G+C)$. There are about ten base pairs per turn, and these, being virtually in planes, are stacked on top of one another like a pile of pennies. Their interaction with the other atoms of the helix ensures that they are spaced at regular intervals. Although the overall structural features of the DNA molecule are now clear, little is yet known about the order of bases along the deoxyribose strands in any piece of DNA of biological importance.

However, in the process of protein synthesis, it is known that the order of the amino acids in the strand-like polypeptide chain of a protein is determined by the order of purine and pyrimidine bases on one of the strands of the DNA double helix.

Since four different purine and pyrimidine bases are found in DNA, 64 different base triplets are possible, if it is assumed that the base order can only be read in one direction along the DNA strand and that the triplets do not overlap. Since only 20 amino acids are found in proteins under natural conditions, more than one triplet is available for each type of amino acid.

DNA

The genetic code

Carrying and replicating information is one feature, but expressing information is something completely different and is a far more complex project. One millimeter of DNA contains about five million base pairs. If you wanted to print the genetic code of such a piece of DNA in a book, you would need a volume of about 2,000 pages, with 5,000 letters to the page. The DNA of a human cell is about two meters long.

It would thus take 1,000 of these huge 2,000-page volumes to describe a single human cell in the same four-letter code. Such an encyclopedia would contain all the information needed to make a human being.

How has nature organized the system for expressing genetic information? In the early evolutionary phase of development, various systems probably competed with each other to see which would be the most effective in expressing information. This evolutionary lottery was won by the amino acids that can polymerize to make proteins. The amino acids are fairly simple molecules, but they have a number of different side-chains and these introduce important variations. The side-chains can be hydrophillic or hydrophobic - that is, water-loving or water-repelling - and they can be either positively or negatively charged. There are 20 different kinds of amino acids that are used in contemporary biological systems, and with them a great variety of micro-environments can be created on the surface of protein molecules, which can perform the kind of catalysis that is needed to regulate the chemical reactions inside living cells. DNA may be regarded as the master blueprint. The cell must make copies of that blueprint for use in the workshop, and these will be destroyed after they have been used.

During the copying process, the same opening up or separation of the two strands of the DNA double helix occurs that is used in replication; however, only one of the strands is copied. Messenger RNA (mRNA) contains a set of information for assembling amino acids in the correct sequence for the formation of different proteins.

The sequence of amino acids in a protein tells you what kind of protein is being formed and defines the nature of its chemical reactivity. But how does the right amino acid find a particular triplet of nucleotides? For this purpose, there is a molecule that interacts with mRNA at one end and with a particular amino acid on the other. This molecule is called transfer RNA (tRNA).

Transfer ribonucleic acid

Transfer RNAs play a central role in the transfer of genetic information. They stand at the crossroads of information encoded in nucleic acids and information encoded in the polypeptide chain.

At one end they interact with messenger RNA through hydrogen bonding of three bases, called the anticodon, to three bases on the messenger RNA codon. At the other end of the molecule, they are conveniently linked to a polypep-tide chain that grows continuously as the ribosome works its way down the messenger RNA strand. These molecules are called transfer RNAs because they are active in transferring free amino acids into polypeptide chains. Associated with the 20 amino acids that are used in forming proteins in present-day biological systems are 20 different families of transfer RNA molecules, each of which will accept a particular amino acid.

Genes and genome

Genes are the hereditary determinant of a specvifies difference between individualsa. Molecular analysis has shown that a specific sequence oif parets of a sequence of DNA can be identified with the classical gene. The human cells contain some 30,000 active genes. The genome is defined as the totality of the DNA sequences of an organism.

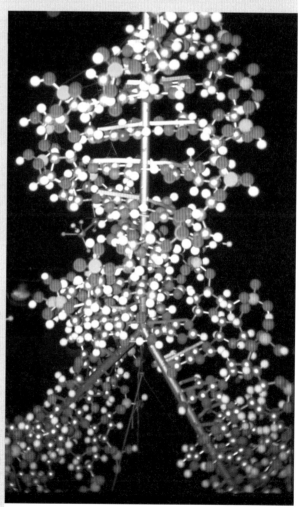

Model of RNA.

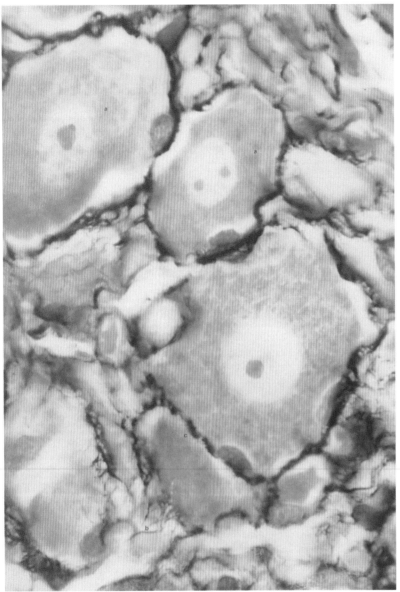

Microscopic picture of a group of nerve cells. The surface membrane of nerve cells contain numerous receptors for synapses.

in the metamorphosis of insects - the membranes of the lysosomes become permeable and release their enzymes to digest the cells from within.

In very old cells, too, the lysosomes may release their contents, which destroy the cell. A more limited form of "autodigestion" can also occur in cells that have been injured by lack of oxygen, an excess of vitamin A, exposure to certain cancer-causing agents or starvation.

Mitochondria

One and a half billion years ago, scientists believe, cells derived the energy they needed through a variety of relatively inefficient processes, none of which required oxygen. Oxygen, a waste product of some of these processes, gradually began to accumulate in the atmosphere.

It was at this time, scientists hypothesize, that one primitive cell engulfed

another primitive cell that had somehow acquired the ability to use oxygen to produce large quantities of energy. Over the millions of years, a symbiotic relationship evolved between the cells, and today all plant and animal cells have organelles that are the descendants of the primordial energy producers. In animal cells, these organelles are called mitochondria, while the energy-producing organelles in green plants are called chloroplasts.

The surface membrane

A cell's outer membrane is often thought of as a boundary that defines the living cell from its surroundings. And indeed, surface membranes are crucial in keeping cells intact. Moreover, the internal membranes that wrap around many organelles separate the cytoplasm into discrete regions, somewhat like the walls that form rooms in a house.

These inner membranes enable the cell to perform many biochemical activities simultaneously, thereby greatly increasing the cell's efficiency. Yet despite its barrier function, the cell membrane - which is often less than 0.01 micrometer thick - is not impassive.

Rather, it is exclusively sensitive to its surroundings and selectively allows certain substances to enter and leave the cell while barring others. It takes in nutrients and excretes wastes. It sends and receives chemical and electrical messages, including signals for the cell to manufacture proteins or to divide. In multicellular organisms, it joins with other cells to form tissues.

These myriad abilities are due to the membrane's composition. Although surface membranes differ in their precise composition depending on the cell's type, and although a membrane's configuration changes from moment to moment, all membranes are composed of two basic kinds of molecules - proteins and lipids (fats).

Stem cells

A stem cell is a generalized cell whose descendants specialize, often in different directions. Stem cells can replicate indefinitely and can also give rise to more specialized tissue cells when exposed to appropriate chemical cues. Embryonic stem cells, which are derived from the earliest developmental stages of an embryo and can spawn almost all types of cells in the body, can now be cultured from human tissue.

The most impressive findings have come from animal work on neural stem cells, which are derived from the fetal brain and seem likely to exist in the adult brain, too. They grow readily in culture - unlike some other specialized stem cells - and can form all the types of cells normally found in the brain.

Thus they may be able to repair damage caused by Parkinson's disease and other neurological conditions. Scientists from Harvard Medical School have demonstrated that human neural stem cells respond appropriately to developmental cues when introduced into the brains of mice; they engraft, migrate and differentiate the way mouse cells do.

Moreover, they can produce proteins in a recipient brain in response to genes that are artificially introduced into the donor cells. Neural stem cells also seem to have a previously unsuspected developmental flexibility. It has been shown that neural stem cells can form blood if they are placed in bone marrow.

Embryonic stem cells could be the most powerful ones of all, but only a small group of investigators is working with them. Medical applications of embryonic stem cells will probably require cells that are genetically matched to the patient, as to avoid rejection. Nuclear transfer, the central technology of cloning, could in principle provide matched cells, because a cloned embryo derived from a patient's cell sample could yield embryonic stem cells.

Yet there could still be show-stoppers. It may turn out that embryonic stem cells derived from cloned embryos lack the full potential of those from natural embryos, for example. Indeed, many embryos resulting from nuclear transfer have defects, possibly because gene expression is abnormal in embryos that lack two genetic parents.

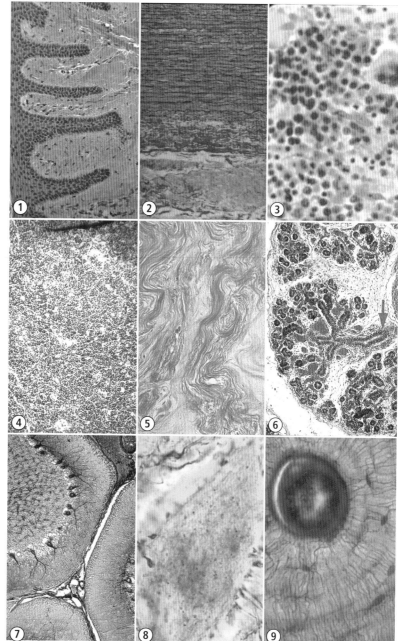

Microscopic pictures of cells and tissues. Related cells joined together are collectively referred to as a tissue. The cells in a tissue are not identical, but they work together to accomplish specific functions. The body is composed of four kinds or primary tissues: epithelial, connective, muscle, and nerve. Connective tissue is so named because it constitutes the connective and supporting element of the body. Connective tissue has various forms, such as fibrous bands, fat, blood, and bone.

1. Epithelial tissue (skin)
2. Connective tissue and endothelium (blood vessel)
3. Blood cells
4. Glandular tissue (thymus)
5. Connective tissue
5. Glandular tissue (exocrine gland)
7. Nerve cells
8. Motor neurons and synapses
9. Bone

3 Digestion

The digestive tract

The organ system involved in the digestion of food consists of a specialized canal (digestive tract or alimentary canal) which begins in the oral cavity and ends at the anal opening (anus). A large number of organs form this system and they fulfil a series of functions:
- ingestion of food;
- mechanical processing and chemical digestion;
- transport of digested food through the intestinal walls for absorption in the blood and lymphatic vessels;
- expulsion of the undigested residue.

Other organs (liver, gallbladder, pancreas) are connected by ducts with the alimentary canal; the substances produced by these organs aid the digestive process. Functionally the whole system is made up of three parts:
- ▲ *Upper section* (oral cavity and throat, stomach and duodenum): the mechanical and chemical processing of the food components takes place;
- ▲ *Middle section* (the small intestine): the transportation of the small, digested food particles through the intestinal wall takes place;

- ▲ *Last section* (large intestine, rectum and anus): the indigestible remainder is stored, transported and expelled from the body. A dehydration process, in which much water is withdrawn from the contents of the large intestine also takes place.

On its way from the oral cavity to the anus, the food passes the following components of the digestive tract:
- oral cavity with tongue and palate (roof of the mouth), teeth and salivary glands;
- esophagus;
- stomach;
- small intestine:
- duodenum;
- jejunum;
- ileum;
- large intestine:
- caecum;
- appendix;
- colon;
- rectum and anal opening.

Oral cavity and esophagus

In the oral cavity the food is finely ground, with the help of the teeth and tongue, and mixed with saliva. The tongue is composed of intrinsic and extrinsic muscles, which allow it great mobility. This organ, covered by mucous membrane, serves for sucking, chewing and swallowing of food, and for speech.

The oral cavity is bordered on both sides by two palatal arches. Between the arches lie the palatine tonsils. The throat (pharynx) is the area in the back of the oral cavity and nose; below, it extends into the esophagus and, via the voice box (larynx), into the windpipe (trachea). Food passage (oral cavity - esophagus) and air passage (nasal cavity - larynx) are sepa-

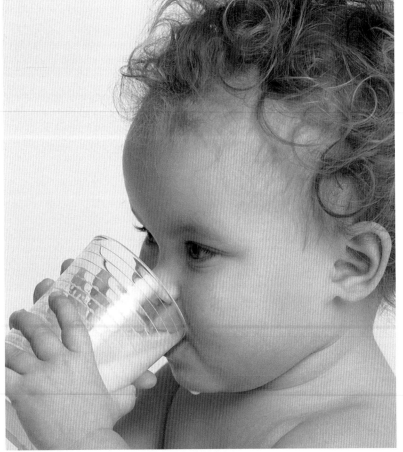

The first phase of the digestive process.

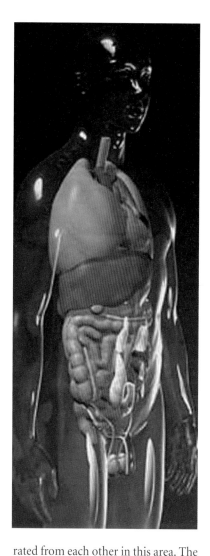

Internal organs
The thoracic and abdominal cavities contain a number of organs, which regulate many essential life functions. The left illustration shows the human body from the front, the right illustration from the back.

Thoracic cavity
The thoracic cavity contains the organs concerned with respiration and blood circulation, and parts of other systems such as the esophagus. These vulnerable organs are protected by a bony structure, consisting of the ribs, the breast bone, and part of the spine. This area is separated from the abdominal cavity by the muscular diaphragm.

Abdominal cavity
The abdominal cavity contains the organs of digestion and secretion. Also present are the liver, gallbladder and spleen, and a number of glands, e.g., the pancreas and the adrenals. In the lowest part of the abdominal cavity (pelvic region) the bladder, a portion of the intestinal system, and an important part of the sexual apparatus are located.

rated from each other in this area. The food is brought to the esophagus by the tongue and the muscles in the wall of the pharynx; swallowing is a reflex action.

The esophagus, with a length of approximately 25 cm and a width of approximately 2 cm, has a strong, smooth muscle wall which transports food to the stomach by means of peristaltic movements. Directly under the diaphragm, the esophagus has an outlet into the entrance (cardia) of the stomach.

Stomach

The stomach is a dilated, sac-like, distensible portion of the alimentary canal or digestive system below the

esophagus and below the diaphragm. The organ is usually pear-shaped, divisible into a more expanded upper portion comprising about two-third of the volume and a narrower lower one-third that curves toward the right. The junction of the two portions is referred to as gastric angle. At the upper end is the cardia, the aperture communicating with the esophagus. At the lower end is the pylorus, the aperture leading into the duodenum. The stomach has two borders and two surfaces. The right border forms the lesser curvature, which is concave and directly continuous with the right border of the esophagus. The left border forms the greater curvature. It is convex and gives attachment to the greater omentum. This is a double layer of lining of the abdom-

inal organs and wall - peritoneum attached to the stomach and connecting it with certain of the abdominal organs. The dilated portion of the stomach to the left and above the level of the cardia is the fundus. The fundus is continuous below with the body or corpus of the stomach. The third and narrower part of the stomach extends from the gastric angle to the pylorus and is designated as the pyloric portion. This portion presents a variable dilation to the right of the gastric angle, the pyloric antrum. It is succeeded by a short constricted pyloric canal. When nearly empty, the stomach presents throughout a narrow, tubular form, except in the region of the fundus. This region, which contains the gas bubble, remains somewhat dis-

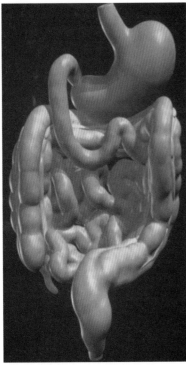

Stomach, duodenum, small intestines and large intestine.

tended even when the remainder of the stomach is empty and contracted. When food is introduced, it fills successively the various portions of the stomach, the body (corpus) and pyloric antrum being filled first and the pyloric canal usually last.

The J-shape is the most common form in the upright posture. In contrast to this type is the "cow-horn" stomach, a form that is rare in the upright, but common in the supine position. Here the greater curvature moves upward and the contents gather mainly in the fundus that becomes distended and displaced to the left.

Functions of the stomach

The stomach receives the softened mass of food, the bolus, that has been masticated and mixed with saliva in the mouth and delivered by way of the pharynx (throat) and esophagus. The muscular wall of the stomach must complete the physical breakdown of large bits of food that the teeth failed to grind up.

The glands of the stomach produce hydrochloric acid and enzymes which are thoroughly mixed with the food converting the bolus in time into a semifluid mass called chyme. The enzymes can work in an acid medium. The chyme is then delivered to the small intestine, while solid particles are retained in the stomach until they too are converted to chyme. Practically no absorption of food takes place in the stomach. Each anatomical area of the stomach has a different type of mucosa and contributes different secretions to the gastric juice.

Intestines

The intestines are defined as the part of the alimentary canal extending from the pylorus of the stomach to the anus. It is approximately 7.5 meters long and is divided into the small and large intestine, or colon.

Small intestine

This has a total length of approximately 3 meters. It begins with the duodenum (20-25 cm), which receives the food mass from the stomach through the pylorus, bile from the liver and gallbladder, and pancreatic juice from the pancreas.

It connects with the jejunum, about 2.5 meters long. This, in turn, joins the ileum that is about 3.7 meters long, and is attached to the large intestine by the ileocecal, or colic, valve that controls passage of food into the large intestine. In the wall of the small intestine are found Bruner's glands (which secrete protective mucus), intestinal glands called the crypts of Lieberkuehn (which secrete digestive enzymes and alkaline juice to neutralize stomach acid), blood and lymph vessels (lacteals) and lymphatic tissue in the form of solitary nodules or aggregated nodules (Peyer's patches).

The inner surface of the small intestine is folded to give a greater amount of surface estimated to be 800 square meter - and it is entirely lined by minute finger-like villi through which the products of digestion - simple sugars, amino acids, and fatty acids and glycerol - are absorbed.

The villi are from 0.5 to 1.5 mm long and there are 10 to 40 to each square millimetre of intestinal mucosa, making the total number of villi to exceed 5 billion. A mucous layer protects and lubricates the wall of the intestines. The mucus is increased from globet cells interspersed among the columnar epithelial cells in the intestine.

Secretion of mucus is increased by local irritation caused by foods and cathartics. The mucus is more viscous in the upper part of the small intestine than in the large intestine and forms a protective physical barrier to the intestinal lining, reducing contact with irritating substances and bacteria. The alkalinity of the mucus contributes further to the protection of the intestinal lining by neutralizing acidic dietary and bacterial products.

Large intestine

The large intestine extends from the ileum to the anus, and consists of the caecum (which includes the vermiform appendix), colon and rectum. The mucous coat lining the colon is much smoother than that of the small intestine, and produces much more mucus.

The caecum is a blind pouch to which is attached the vermiform appendix, which is about 1.5 to 10 cm long. This is a relict left over from the time when humans ate grass. It has no significance now except that it can become seriously infected.

The colon is approximately 1.5 m in length. The first portion or the ascending colon extends from the caecum to the undersurface of the liver where, at the hepatic flexure, it turns to the left and becomes the transverse colon.

This passes horizontally to the left to the region of the spleen where, at the splenic flexure, it turns downward to become the descending colon. This continues downward on the left side of the abdomen until it reaches the pelvic brim and curves like the letter S in front of the sacrum until it becomes the rectum.

This S-shaped section is known as the sigmoid colon. The rectum - about 23-25 cm long - passes downward to terminate in the lower opening of the tract, the anus or anal opening.

The circular muscle layer of the colon is thickened at the anus to form a sphincter muscle (internal sphincter). A striated muscle (external sphincter), which forms part of the floor of the pelvis, is under voluntary control and regulates the opening and closing of the anal orifice.

Digestion of food

The chemical break-down of food in the alimentary canal is called hydrolysis (Greek, hydro = water, lysis = loosening), because water is essential for the process. The rate of most chemical reactions can be speeded up by substances called catalysts, and the catalysts that are produced by living organisms are called enzymes.

Enzymes
In industrial chemistry, catalysts work at high temperatures or pressure. An enzyme, on the other hand, promotes reactions at body temperature and ordinary atmospheric pressure. Enzymes consist of large protein molecules whose surfaces are the site of intense chemical activity.
Scientists have learned much about enzymes in the past two decades, but less is known what happens to the substance (substrate) that the enzyme works on. Each enzyme has a unique surface with a particular spot where the substrate molecule can work on. For this reason the enzyme-substrate complex is often compared to a lock and key, where the substrate is the lock and the enzyme the key.
Nearly all the chemical reactions in the body - syntheses, break-downs and slight alterations to molecules - are catalyzed by enzymes. A special feature of enzymes in the alimentary canal, is that although they are made inside the cells they work outside.

Absorption of molecules
By the action of various digestive juices saliva, stomach and pancreatic juices, succus entericus, and bile - the food materials have eventually been reduced to their final state ready for absorption through the cell lining of the remaining part of the small intestine (usually 5.5 meter). The starch and sugars have been changed to glu-

cose, the proteins to amino acids and the fats to fatty acids and glycerol.
The epithelium of the small intestine consists of billions of villi. The villus is the point of entry of digested food into the body. Within each villus is a network of blood capillaries into which pass amino acids, glucose, and some fat; these are carried by veins to the liver.
Each villus also carries a short tube called a lacteal, which accepts other fats; these drain through the lymphatic system and finally empty into the great veins near the heart. Normal intestinal motility and peristalsis are maintained by smooth muscles and intrinsic nerves.
The parasympathetic part of the autonomic nervous system stimulates motility of the intestines; while the sympathetic part inhibits intestinal motility and secretion.
The extrinsic autonomic innervation influences the strength and frequency of these movements and mediates reflexes by which activity in one part of the intestine influences another.

Function of colon
Water recovery is the main function of the colon. About every four hours the contents of the small intestine are dis-

charged into the large intestine through a valve. Food stays a long time in the large intestine; peristalsis is very slow and this gives enough time for the water to return to the blood stream by osmosis.
The residue that is left behind is called the faeces. It consists of 70 per cent water, worn-out and discarded epithelial cells, indigestible cellulose (fibers), salts, and many bacteria. The presence of bacteria illustrates an interesting relationship between higher and lower organisms. The bacteria live in a safe and stable environment with a plentiful supply of food.
They suppress moulds that have survived the digestive juices and are also instrumental in the production of essential substances such as vitamins. Finally, the accumulated faeces are passed to the last 12 cm of the large intestine, or rectum, which ends at the anus.
This transfer occurs by a remote-control reflex whenever food
Normal bowel movement, or defalcation, begins with the stimulation of stretch receptors in the rectum by faeces. Peristaltic waves propel the faeces to the anal canal where the voluntarily controlled external anal sphincter regulates defalcation.

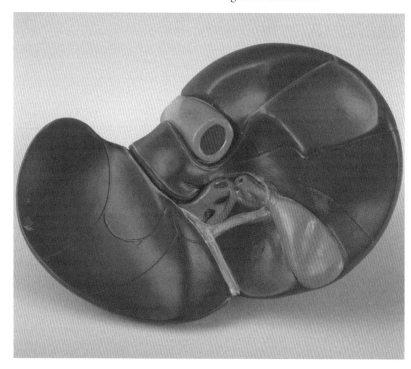

Topography of the liver and gallbladder. View from below.

4 Respiration

Introduction

The respiratory tract or system consists of the organs and structures associated with breathing, gaseous exchange, and the entrance of air into the body.

It includes organs and structures of the upper respiratory tract: the nasal cavity (nose), pharynx (throat), larynx (voice box), and trachea (windpipe), and those of the lower respiratory tract: bronchi, bronchioles (small branches of the bronchial system), alveoli and associated muscles.

Nose

The nose is a reparatory organ. As a passageway for airflow into and out of the lungs, it humidifies and warms inspired air and filters inhaled particles. Several anatomical features facilitate the performance of these functions. The nasal cavity is divided by a central septum and finger-like projections (turbinates) that extend into the cavity, increasing the nasal surface area.

The nasal passageway surface is coated with a continuous thin layer of mucous, a moderately viscous, muco-proteinaceous (consisting of mucus and proteins) liquid secreted continuously by the mucous glands. Under normal conditions, foreign bodies such as dust, bacteria, powder, and oil droplets are trapped in the film and carried out of the nose into the nasopharynx (region of the throat behind the nose).

The epithelium of the nasal passageways is beset with cilia (ciliated). The constant beating of the cilia causes the mucus film to be moved continually toward the nasopharynx, carrying with it trapped particles to be expec-

Auscultation of the organs in the chest. The main purpose of listening to the lungs with a stethoscope is to hear how the air moves in and out of the chest. When the bronchial tubes are unobstructed and free of disease, your breathing has a distinct, clear sound.

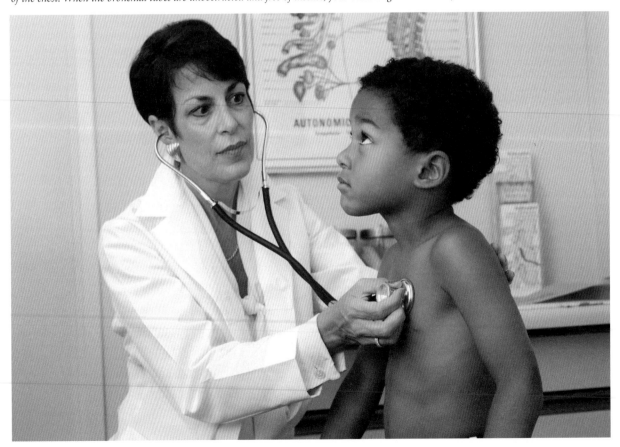

torated or swallowed. Because this ciliary movement is one of the body's main mechanisms, care should be taken to avoid agents that impair this movement.

Pharynx, larynx, trachea

The pharynx (throat) is the muscular tube extending from the base of the skull to the esophagus (foodpipe) that serves as a passageway for food from the mouth to the esophagus and for air from the nose and mouth to the larynx. It is divided into the nasopharynx (part behind the nose), oropharynx (part behind the mouth), and laryngopharynx (part connected to the voice box).

The larynx or voice box connects the pharynx to the windpipe. It is here that the vocal cords are found and where speech is made possible. The whole organ is made up of a number of bones, cartilages, and muscles, which are connected to each other in a complicated manner and which can be moved with respect to each other. The thyroid cartilage and below it the ring-shaped cartilage are the most important.

The entrance to the larynx is closed by the epiglottis, which moves upward when swallowing takes place, closing off this area, so that no food can enter the windpipe. Between the thyroid cartilage and the cup-shaped cartilage, the elastic vocal cords are stretched and can vibrate when air is expired. These cords run horizontally in a front-to-back direction.

Between them is a slitlike opening, the glottis, located. The opening can be narrowed or widened by muscular contraction and relaxation. Chest, lips, tongue and palate (roof of the

Topography of the lungs, the trachea and the primary bronchi. The lungs are concerned with respiration (breathing), the absorption of oxygen from and release of carbon dioxide into atmospheric air. The right lung has three lobes, and the left has two lobes. The lung surfaces are separated from the chest wall by two layers of membrane called the pleura. The small amount of fluid between them allows free movement of the lungs and enables the forced expansion of the chest and diaphragm to fill them with air.

mouth) also play important roles in sound (voice) production.

The trachea or windpipe is the tube extending from the larynx to the bronchi that conveys air to the lungs. It is about 11 centimetres long, covered in front by the isthmus of the thyroid gland, and is in contact in the back with the esophagus. The trachea has a pseudostratified ciliated columnar epithelium with so-called globet cells and numerous mucous and serous glands with duct openings through the epithelium. The mucous secretions provide a sticky slimy layer which traps the particles; the mucus and its contents are moved upwards by the action of the cilia, pass through the larynx and are swallowed.

Chest cavity and pleura

The thoracic (chest) cavity is the term used to denote the space within the walls of the chest and occupied by various large organs. These are, on each side, the lung and the pleura with its cavity; and in the middle the thymus gland or its remains (for it shrinks as we grow older); the peri-

cardium (heart sac) and heart, large blood vessels, nerves, trachea, thoracic duct (a large lymphatic vessel) and esophagus (foodpipe or gullet).

The limits of the thoracic space are set by the skeletal parts of the chest (thorax) together with the ligaments involved in the joints and muscles interposed between the bones. The arched diaphragm forms the lower boundary and the barrier presented by the scalene muscles (which connect the spine to the ribs) determines the upper limit.

The shape of the internal thoracic space differs from the external contour of the chest chiefly through the projection into it of the ridge made by the spine, and by the presence on either side of the latter of a broad, deep lung groove. On account of these features, a cross-section of the thoracic space is somewhat heart-shaped, but much compressed in the front-to-back direction.

Pleura

The pleura is the smooth, transparent membrane that, as a closed sac, covers nearly the whole surface of each lung, forming the pulmonary pleura, and in

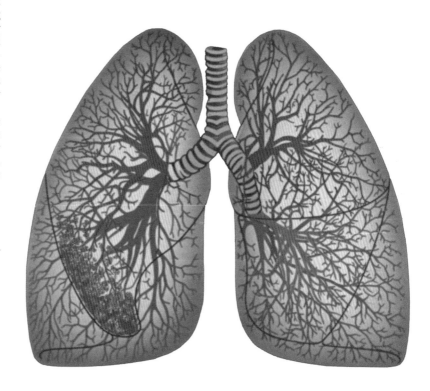

large measure, lines the inner surface of the chest walls, forming the parietal pleura.

The walls of the sacs enclose paired spaces, or cavities, known as the pleural cavities, which in the normal state are merely spaces containing a small amount of fluid for the lubrication of the surfaces of the pulmonary and parietal pleura where they come into contact.

The lungs

The lungs are two largely air-filled organs in the chest, or thoracic cavity, concerned with respiration (breathing), the absorption of oxygen from and release of carbon dioxide into atmospheric air. The right lung has three lobes, and the left has two.

The lung surfaces are separated from the chest wall by two layers of membrane called pleura. The small amount of fluid between them allows free movement of the lungs and enables the forced expansion of the chest and diaphragm to fill them with air.

Air is drawn into the trachea via the mouth or nose; the trachea divides into the bronchi (airways) which divide repeatedly until the terminal air sacs, or alveoli, are reached. In the alveoli, air is brought into close contact with deoxygenated blood (i.e. blood from which the oxygen has been extracted in the cells) in the smallest blood vessels capillaries - in the lungs.

The blood circulation through these comes from the right ventricle of the heart via the pulmonary (lung) artery, and returns to the heart's left atrium via the pulmonary (lung) veins. Ventilation of the lungs is the first step in the supply of oxygen in the excretion of carbon dioxide. The oxygen stores of the body are very small, and lung ventilation must supply the body's needs from minute to minute if life is to continue.

Ventilation

As an organ of excretion, the lung is of great importance: it eliminates as carbon dioxide more than 50 times as much acid as the kidneys. These functions entail, in a person at rest, a daily ventilation of 8000-12,000 litres of air,

from which about 360 litres of oxygen are taken into the body and to which about 300 litres of carbon dioxide are added from the blood and then expelled in the breath. All these figures must be doubled for a heavy worker.

Not all the inspired air takes part in the respiratory exchange, for some of it travels no further than the airways at each respiration. This wasted volume is called "respiratory dead space." About 20-30 per cent of the respiratory air is expanded in ventilating the nose, mouse, pharynx (throat), larynx (voice box), trachea (windpipe) and large- and medium-sized bronchi. The rest ventilates the alveolar units and exchanges oxygen for carbon dioxide with the capillary blood of the lungs. This is the alveolar ventilation.

Chemical mediators and mast cells

Although the major role of the lungs is respiratory, they have other diverse and complex activities. For example, the lungs produce surfactant, an agent that lines the alveoli and prevents them from collapsing; a lack of surfactant is thought to be one of the factors in respiratory distress syndrome in premature babies.

Apart from this the lungs participate in the production of several vaso-active substances (i.e. substances that affect the diameter of blood vessels and so the rate of blood flow). Lung tissue also contains a high concentration of prostaglandins, which it synthesizes; these are complex chemicals that act on many parts of the body such as causing the uterus to contract, etc.

Mast cells are plentiful and the lungs are the richest source of histamine in the body; they are, therefore, greatly affected by allergic reactions. Most of the serotonin (a substance intimately involved in blood clotting and the working of the brain) in the blood is contained within platelets, and the lungs are an important store of megakaryocytes, the large cells that manufacture platelets.

In addition, over 90 per cent of this vaso-active substance can be removed by the lungs in one respiration. The presence of mast cells makes the lungs the richest source of heparin (a substance that delays clotting), and thus,

with the added presence of serotonin, the lungs play a significant role in blood clotting.

Finally, the lung can synthesize fatty acids, hydrolyse triglycerides and form phospholipids, functions that are probably carried out mainly in the large alveolar cells.

Oxygen and carbon dioxide

These chemically bound gases move in the body by diffusion, but only across concentration gradients. The exchange of oxygen and carbon dioxide that occurs in the alveoli and at the individual cells takes place simultaneously.

Oxygen

The air that fills the alveoli contains an ample supply of oxygen, but the blood passing through the alveolar capillaries has just completed a circuit through the body and has lost much of its oxygen. Thus there is a gradient between the alveolar oxygen and the blood oxygen; consequently oxygen diffuses into the capillaries.

Once inside the capillaries it combines with the hemoglobin (colouring protein complex) in the red blood cells (erythrocytes). When the blood reaches the tissue capillaries the gas gradient is reversed.

The oxygen pressure in the erythrocytes is higher than that in the tissue cells outside the capillaries so that there is a natural tendency for oxygen to leave the capillaries and to diffuse into the tissue cells. At this stage an interesting mechanism comes into play. The degree to which hemoglobin binds oxygen depends on the amount of carbon dioxide and acid present. When the pressure of carbon dioxide is high, oxygen is more readily liberated. This is appropriate, because the existence of a high concentration of carbon dioxide and acid means that oxygen previously present has been used up, so that there is an urgent demand for further supplies.

Carbon dioxide

The concentration of carbon dioxide (a waste product of metabolism) in the cells of organs and tissues is higher than in blood. Carbon dioxide therefore diffuses from the cells into the blood. The transport of carbon dioxide in the blood is not, however, as straightforward as it is with oxygen. For example, this gas is toxic and unlike oxygen in that it combines chemically with water.

So the problem is how to transport it from the cells to the lungs without harming the body on its way. Carbon dioxide dissolves readily in the watery blood plasma to form carbonic acid. Like all acids, this dissociates into ions, one of which is the acidic hydrogen ion.

Respiratory mechanisms

The ventilation of the alveoli necessary for gas exchange is brought about by a rhythmic alternation of inspiration (breathing in) and expiration (breathing out). The air movements during inspiration and expiration result from the alternating expansion and diminution of the chest cavity. Two events cause expansion of the chest volume:

▲ elevation of the ribs and
▲ flattening of the diaphragm.

The diaphragm forms the lower boundary of the chest cavity. It consists of a central tendon and the muscle fibers radiating out from it on all sides and attached at their other ends to the lower chest opening. Normally the diaphragm is dome-shaped, curving up into the chest cavity. In the expiration position it lies against the inner wall of the chest over about three ribs. During inspiration the muscles of the diaphragm contract and flatten it, pulling the sheet of muscle away from the inner chest wall. Depending on whether the chest expansion during normal breathing results chiefly from elevation of the ribs or more from depression of the diaphragm, the respiration is of the thoracic (chest) type or the abdominal type.

In thoracic respiration the work of breathing is done primarily by the muscles between the ribs (intercostal musculature), the diaphragm tending to follow passively the pressure changes within the chest. In abdominal respiration the stronger contraction of the diaphragm muscle displaces the

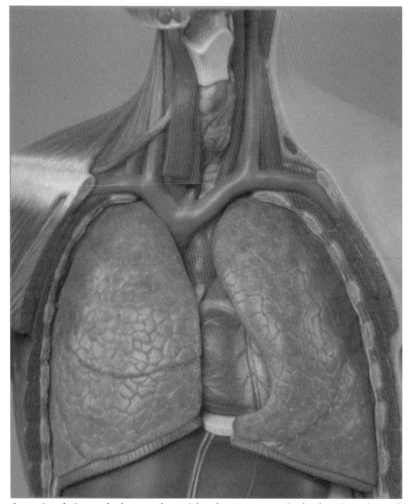

Lungs in relation to the heart and arterial and venous system in the thoracic cavity. Red: aorta; blue: superior cava vein and jugular veins.

abdominal internal organs to a greater extent, so that during inspiration the abdomen bulges outward.

Control of respiration

Control of breathing can be defined very generally as the adjustment of external respiration to meet the needs of the organism as a whole. The rhythmic sequence of inspiration and expiration is brought about by alternating series of signals from the inspiratory and expiratory nerve cells in the respiration center of the brain stem.

During the phase in which the inspiratory nerve cells are activated the expiratory nerve cells do not discharge, and conversely. Complex circuits and networks of nerve brain stem are responsible for this mechanism. Signals from receptors located in or near the lungs have a stabilizing influence on this mechanism.

There is also a chemical control of respiration, exerted by the partial pressures of oxygen and carbon dioxide in the arteries. An increase in the partial pressure of carbon dioxide in the arteries causes an increase in the amount of air displaced (minute volume).

When the partial pressure of oxygen in the arterial blood falls, ventilation is increased. The chemical control of respiration thus contributes to homeostasis and ensures that breathing is adjusted to the organism's metabolic rate.

5 Circulation

Introduction

The blood circulation is the transport system of the human body: it delivers food and oxygen to every organ. At the same time, all metabolic waste materials produced in the body are collected by the circulating blood and delivered to their respective destinations. The circulatory blood also contains antibodies, hormones, vitamins, etc.

To fulfil its transport function, blood circulation must be continuous throughout the whole body. Blood passes through a closed system of vessels, propelled by the contractile activity of the heart.

The powerfully developed muscle wall of the left ventricle drives the blood into the large or systemic circuit of the body, while the thinner walled muscle of the right ventricle propels the blood into the shorter circuit through the lungs. A considerable portion (2000 to 3000 litres per day) of the fluid content of the thin walled capillaries located between arteries and veins diffuses from these vessels into the tissue spaces, where its composition changes and it is later reabsorbed into the circulation.

Another function of the circulation is to transport the heat produced by the muscles to the rest of the body. Together with the skin, our circulation is, to a large extent, responsible for the temperature regulation of the body.

Structure of the heart

The heart is a hollow, muscular organ, situated in the chest between the lungs and above the central depression of the diaphragm. It is about the size of the closed fist, shaped like a blunt cone with the broader end, or base, directed upward, backward and to the right. The pointed end, or apex, points downward, forward and to the left. As placed in the body, it has an oblique position, and the right side is almost in front of the left.

The impact of the heart during contractions is felt against the chest wall in the space between the fifth and sixth ribs, a little below the left nipple, and about 8 cm (3 in) to the left of the median line. The wall of the heart is composed of:
- an outer layer, the pericard;
- an inner layer, the endocard;
- a middle layer, the myocard.

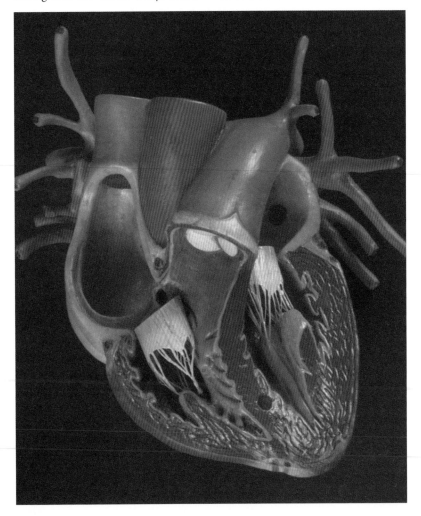

Heart cut open to show the four chambers and related structures. The heart is divided into left and right sides by a septum; reach side has an upper atrium (auricle) and lower ventricle. Under outer epicardium membranes, the heart wall - myocardium - consists of cardiac muscle; the innermost layer - endocardium - is continuous with the lining of the blood vessels.

Two types of valves occur in the heart, one type is represented by valves of the pulmonary artery and aorta, the semilunar valves, while the other type is represented by the atrioventricular valves.

Topography of the heart.
Left: Anterior view of the heart with aorta (red) and caval veins (blue)
Right: Lateral view of the heart with large systemic arteries and veins and arteries of the lungs.
The powerfully developed muscle wall of the left ventricle drives the blood into the large or systemic circuit of the body, while the thinner walled muscle of the right ventricle propels the blood into the shorter circuit of the lungs.

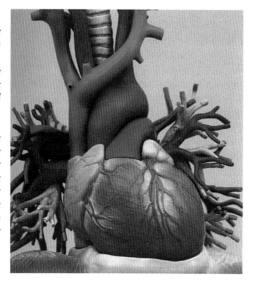
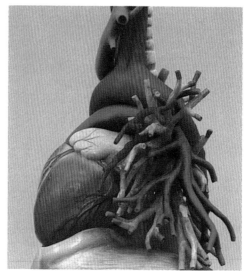

Left: Posterior view of the heart and trachea (windpipe).
Right: Lateral view with large arteries and lung vessels. The largest artery of the body (aorta) has a diameter of over 1 inch. All systemic arteries take their origin from the aorta. To fulfill its transport function properly, blood circulation must be continuous throughout the whole body.

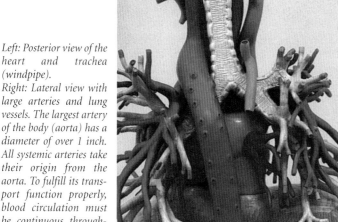
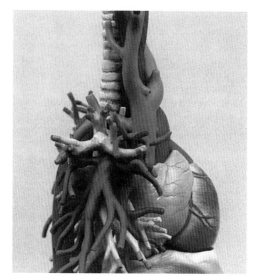

Myocardium

The main substance of the heart is cardiac muscle, called myocardium. This tissue includes the muscle bundles of:
- the atria
- the ventricles
- the atrioventricular bundle (bundle of His)

The principal muscle bundles of the atria radiate from the area that surrounds the orifice (opening) of the superior vena cava. One, the interatrial bundle, connects the anterior surfaces of the two atria. The other atrial muscle bundles are confined to their respective atria, though they merge to some extent.

The muscle bundles of the ventricles begin in the atrioventricular fibrous rings. They form U-shaped bundles with the apex of the U toward the apex of the heart. There are many of these bundles, but for general description they may be divided into four groups.

One group begins at the left atrioventricular ring, passes towards the right and the apex, where it forms whorls, and then ends either in the left ventricular wall, the papillary muscles, or the septum and the right ventricular wall.

A second bundle repeats this path except that it starts at the right ventricular ring, passes to the left in the anterior wall of the heart, and ends in the same structures as above. These two groups form an outer layer that ends around both ventricles. Under these is a third group of muscle bundles that again wind around both ventricles.

There is a fourth group of muscle bundles that wind around the left ventricle. Thus the left ventricle has a much thicker wall than the right. During contraction the squeeze of the spirally arranged muscle bundles forces blood out of the ventricles.

The muscular tissue of the atria is not continuous with that of the ventricles. The walls are connected by fibrous tissue and the atrioventricular bundle of

The left ventricle ejects blood into the body's extensive circulatory system under much higher pressure than is required of the right ventricle for ejecting blood into the relatively short pulmonary circulation (i.e. in the lungs).

The structural arrangement of cardiac muscle fibers provides for the thicker muscle required in this pumping action. Both the right and left sides of the heart contract and relax almost simultaneously.

Muscular columns project from the inner surface of the ventricles. They are of three kinds: the first are attached along their entire length and form ridges, or columns. The second is a rounded bundle; the moderator band projects from the base of the anterior papillary muscle to the ventricular septum, and is formed largely of specialized fibers concerned with the conducting of electrical impulses. Third are the papillary muscles, which are continuous with the wall of each ventricle at its base. The apexes of the papillary muscles give rise to fibrous cords, which are attached to the cusps of the atrioventricular valves. These muscles contract when the ventricular walls contract.

Valves of the heart

Between each atrium and ventricle there is a somewhat constricted opening, the atrioventricular orifice, which is strengthened by fibrous rings and protected by valves. The openings into the aorta and pulmonary artery are also guarded by valves.

Tricuspid valve

This valve lies between the right atrium and right ventricle. It is composed of three irregular-shaped flaps, or cusps, hence its name. The flaps are formed mainly of fibrous tissue covered by endocardium. At their bases, they are continuous with one another and form a ring-shaped membrane around the margin of the atrial openings. Their pointed ends project into the ventricle and are attached by the chordae tendinae, thin cords of muscle, to small muscular pillars, the papillary muscles, in the interior of the ventricles.

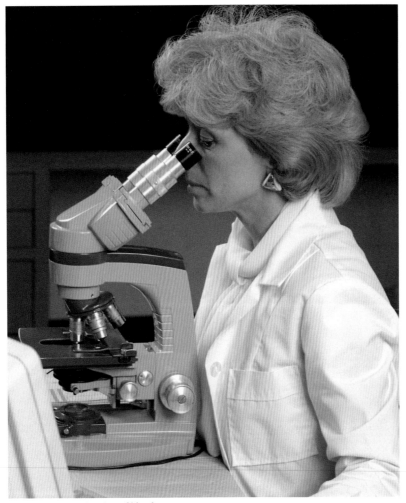

Microscopic examination of blood.

modified muscle cells. This bundle arises in connection with the atrioventricular (AV) node, which lies near the opening of the coronary sinus in the right atrium.

From this node the atrioventricular bundle passes forward to the membranous septum between the ventricles, where it divides into right and left bundles, one for each ventricle. In the muscular septum between the ventricles, each bundle divides into numerous strands that spread over the internal surface just under the endocardium.

The greater part of the atrioventricular bundle consists of spindle-shaped muscle cells. Inflammation of the myocardium is known as myocarditis.

Cavities of the heart

The heart is divided into right and left halves (frequently called the "right heart" and the "left heart") by a muscular partition, the ventricular septum, which extends from the base of the ventricles to the apex of the heart and the atrial septum, between the two atria, which is relatively thin. The two sides of the heart have no communication with each other after birth.

The right side of the heart contains venous (deoxygenated) and the left side arterial (oxygenated) blood. Each half is subdivided into two cavities: the upper, called the atrium, and the lower, called the ventricle.

Bicuspid (mitral) valve

This valve lies between the left atrium and left ventricle. It consists of two flaps, or cusps, and so is named the bicuspid, or mitral, valve. It is attached in the same manner as the tricuspid valve, which it closely resembles in structure except that it is much stronger and thicker in all its parts. Chordae tendinae are attached to the cusps and papillary muscles in the same way as on the right side; they are less numerous but thicker and stronger.

Semilunar valves

The orifice between the right ventricle and the pulmonary artery is guarded by the pulmonary valve, and the orifice between the left ventricle and the aorta is guarded by the aortic valve. These two valves are called semilunar valves and consist of three half-moon-shaped cusps, each cusp being attached by its convex margin to the inside of the artery where it joins the ventricle, while its free border projects into the vessel. Small nodular bodies are attached to the center of the free edge of each pocket.

The aortic valve is larger and stronger and the nodular bodies are thicker and more evident. Between the cusps of the valve and the aortic wall, these are slight dilatations called the aortic sinuses of Valsalva. The coronary arteries have their origin from two of these sinuses.

Function of the heart

The muscles of the atria and ventricles are so arranged that, when they contract, they lessen the capacity of the chambers that they enclose. The contracting chambers drive the blood through the heart to the arteries.

Wave of contraction

If an electrical stimulus is applied to one end of a muscle, a wave of contraction sweeps over the entire tissue. It is therefore easy to conceive how a wave of contraction - begun by the heart's natural pacemaker, the sinu-atrial (SA) node - can sweep over the muscular tissue of the atria, which is practically continuous. The question is: how is this wave transmitted to the

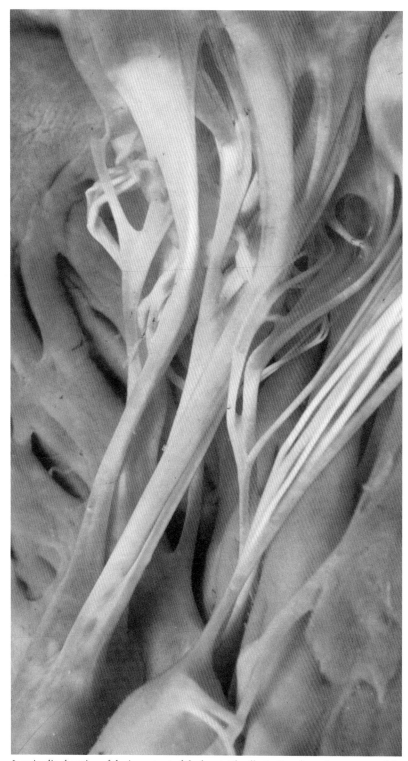

Longitudinal section of the inner part of the heart. The illustration shows the structure of the tricuspid valve, located between the left atrium and left ventricle. The tricuspid valve, guarding the right atrioventricular opening, is so called because it consists of three irregularly shaped flaps (or cusps) formed mainly of fibrous tissue covered by endocardium.

muscular tissue of the ventricles, which, in humans, is not continuous with that of the atria? The connecting pathway is furnished by the atrioventricular (AV) node, which transmits the nerve impulses by means of the AV bundle - also called the bundle of His - and causes the wave of contraction to spread from the atrioventricular openings, over the ventricles to the mouths of the pulmonary artery and the aorta.

Cardiac output
At each systole (contraction), about 80 ml of blood (for an adult male at rest) moves from the left ventricle into the aorta. This is known as the stroke volume.

A similar amount is forced from the right ventricle into the pulmonary artery. The total cardiac output per beat is, therefore, 160 ml. Taking a pulse rate of 70 beats per minute, 5.6 litres (just under 10 pints) - that is, 70 x 80 ml - of blood leave both the left and right ventricles every minute. This is known as the minute volume. With an increase or decrease in stroke volume, in pulse rate or in both, the total output per minute would be increased or decreased. During exercise, the total cardiac output may be doubled. The heart muscle receives 10 per cent of cardiac output; the brain, 20 per cent; the liver, stomach and intestines, 25 per cent; the kidneys, 15 per cent; and the rest of the body, 25 per cent.

Blood supply to the brain is the most constantly maintained. In other organs the supply varies directly with activity - for example, during digestion the stomach and intestines receive far more blood than when at rest.

Heart sounds and murmurs
If the ear is applied over the heart or one listens with the stethoscope, certain sounds are heard that recur with great regularity. Two chief sounds can be heard during each cardiac cycle: the first is a comparatively long, booming sound; the second, a short, sharp one; the two sounds resembling the syllables lubb-dup.

Heart sounds are caused by acceleration or deceleration of blood and turbulence developing during rapid blood flow. The first sound occurs at the onset of ventricular contraction: blood is accelerating and surging towards the tricuspid and bicuspid (mitral) valves. The acceleration occurs just before the valves are completely closed and taut, and at this time, vibrations of the first heart sound are heard.

The second sound is heard towards the end of systole (contraction) when blood decelerates, and ventricular and arterial pressures fall. Blood in the pulmonary artery and in the root of the aorta rushes back towards the ventricular chambers, but the flow is abruptly arrested by the closing of the semilunar valves. This causes much turbulence of the blood, and the second sound is heard.

In certain diseases of the heart these sounds become changed and are called murmurs. These are often due to failure of the valves to close properly, thus allowing a back flow of blood into the heart.

Heartbeat
The cause of the heartbeat is still unknown. General belief favours the myogenic theory - that is, the theory that the function of the nerve tissue in the heart is regulatory, that the contractions are due to the inherent power of contraction possessed by the muscle cells of the heart themselves.

It is believed that inorganic ions, neurohumoural substances and other factors still unknown are responsible for the innate rhythmic contractions of the heart muscle, but the exact role of each remains to be determined. Three ions are especially important - namely, calcium, potassium and sodium, which are always present in blood. There is a well-marked antagonism between the effects of calcium and the effects of potassium and sodium.

Calcium has a direct stimulating effect and promotes contraction; potassium and sodium promote relaxation. Heart muscle becomes flaccid and heart rate slows in the presence of excess potassium ions in extracellular fluids.

The heart is not in a state of continuous contraction because of the long "refractory phase" of the cardiac muscle. From the time just before the contraction process begins in response to a stimulus until some time after relaxation begins, the heart muscle is unable to be further stimulated. Once the heart muscle begins to contract, it must relax (partially or completely) before it will contract again.

Automaticity and nervous control
The most remarkable power of cardiac muscle is its automaticity. By this is meant that the stimuli that excite it to activity arise within the tissue itself. The degree of automatic power possessed by different regions of the heart varies: some parts beat faster than others. The most rapidly contracting part is the SA node.

The heart is supplied with two sets of motor nerve fibers. One set reaches the heart through the vagus nerve of the craniosacral system. Nerve impulses over these fibers have a tendency to slow or stop the heart-beat and are called inhibitory. The other set comprises the visceral branches of the first five thoracic nerves, which have their cells of origin in the lateral column of grey matter in the spinal cord. These fibers terminate in the sympathetic ganglia, forming the superior, middle and inferior cardiac nerves. The postganglionic fibers pass to the heart where they quicken and augment the heartbeat, and are called accelerators. The vagus nerve has its origin in a nucleus in the medulla, or brain stem. The accelerator nerves also have connections in the medulla, and through these centers either set of nerves may be stimulated.

In addition, the heart is supplied with afferent nerve fibers: one set from the aortic arch, called depressor fibers; the other set from the right side of the heart, called pressor fibers. Both sets of afferent fibers run within the sheath of the vagus nerves to the cardiac center in the medulla. Impulses over the depressor fibers bring about reflex inhibition of the heart - aortic reflex. Impulses over the pressor (sympathetic) fibers bring about reflex acceleration of the heart - right heart reflex.

Although the heart contracts automatically and rhythmically, the continuously changing frequency and volume of the heart are controlled by the two sets of nerve fibers that enter the cardiac plexus. The sympathetic

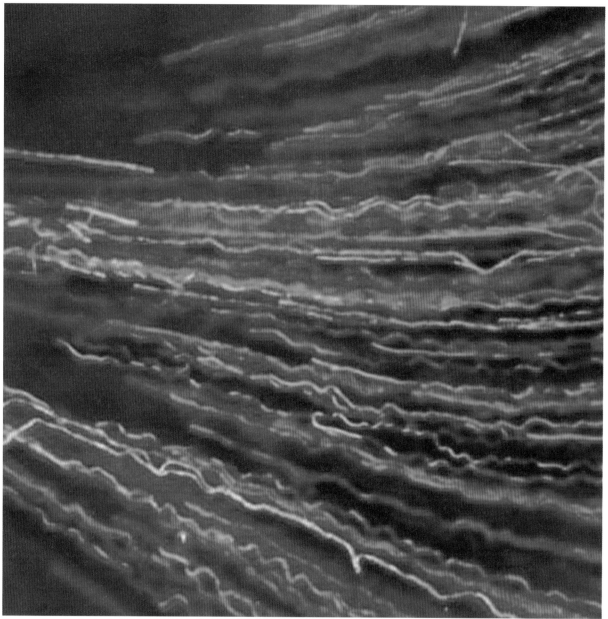

System of capillaries in the kidney. Capillaries are the smallest blood vessels in the body, formed of endothelial cells with an external basement membrane. The total length of capillaries in the human body amounts to approximately 2,000 miles.

fibers follow along the coronary blood vessels and innervate all areas of both atria and ventricles.

In general, stimulation of the sympathetic system increases the activity of the heart by increasing both force and rate of heartbeat, thereby increasing the effectiveness of the heart as a pump. The vagus nerves chiefly innervate the atria and decrease the activity of the heart. At the SA node the chemical transmitter acetylcholine is secreted at the vagal endings, and this decreases the rate and rhythm of the node. It also decreases excitability of the AV junctional fibers between the muscles of the atria and the Purkinje system, thereby slowing transmission of impulses. This means that the heartbeat is controlled by two antago-nistic influences: one tending to slow the heart action and the other to quicken it. If the inhibitory center is stimulated to greater activity, the heart is slowed still further; if the activity of this center is depressed, the heart rate is increased, because the inhibitory action is removed. Stimulation of the accelerator nerves results in a quickened heartbeat.

6 Excretion

Introduction

The organs forming the urinary apparatus are the kidneys that produce the urine; the ureters that convey the urine to the bladder; the urinary bladder that serves as a reservoir for the urine and from which a single duct, the urethra, the urine is carried to the exterior.

The kidneys control the volume, composition and pressure of body fluids by regulating the excretion of water and dissolved substances. Through hormonal mechanisms they also influence the transformation of vitamin D into its active form, certain aspects of the formation of red blood cells, and blood pressure.

Urine is formed in the kidneys as an aqueous solution containing waste products of the metabolism, foreign substances and water-soluble constituents of the body.

The kidneys

The kidneys are paired organs in the back part of the abdomen, on each side of the vertebral column (spine) immediately behind the peritoneum (serious membrane that covers the abdominal wall and envelops most of the abdominal organs).

The right kidney is normally lower than the left, probably because of the presence of the liver on the right side. Each kidney is somewhat bean-shaped and is slightly tilted. The upper extremity of the kidney is usually larger than the lower extremity, and is about 1 cm nearer to the spine.

The part of the kidney nearest the side of the trunk (lateral border) is narrow and convex, while the part closest to the spine (medial border) is concave and, within its middle third, has a slit-like aperture, the hilus.

This is the orifice of a cavity called renal sinus that is about 2.5 cm in depth and is occupied by the pelvis and calyces (sing. = calyx) of the kidney, by the blood vessels and nerves, and by small amounts of fat tissue.

Except for the sinus, the kidneys are solid organs, moderately elastic and, because of the high number of blood vessels, of a dark, reddish-brown colour.

The length of the kidney in the adult male averages 10 to 12 cm, its breath about 5 to 6 cm, and its thickness 3 to 4 cm. Its average weight is 160-170 g.

In the child, the organ is relatively large, the combined weight of both kidneys in relationship to the entire body weight being 1 to 140. The ratio of 1 to 170 is usually attained by the age of 10 and maintained throughout adult life.

Pelvis of the kidney

The pelvis of the kidney is a small reservoir that collects, and in which is

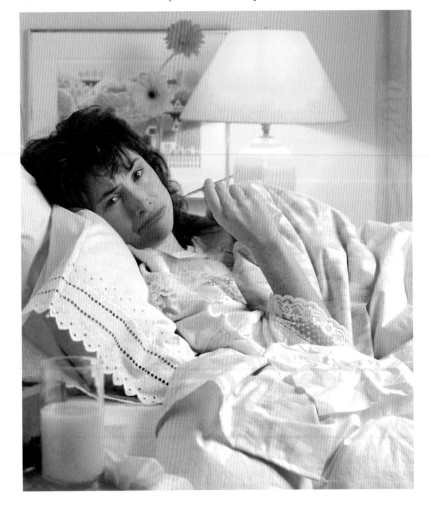

Patient with a disease of the kidneys. Disorders and malfunctioning of the kidneys often require a stay in the hospital for thorough examination of the urinary apparatus.

mixed, the urine from all parts of the kidney. It is funnel-shaped, the broad portion lying within the renal sinus while the narrow end passes out through the hilus to unite with the ureter.

Within the sinus, the pelvis usually splits into two main divisions: the major calyces divide into the minor calyces, each of which terminates in one, two or sometimes three papillae. The papillae, protruding into the ends of the calyces, give to the latter a characteristic cup-shaped appearance.

At the summits of the papillae are a number of small openings, through which the urine enters the calyces. Not only is there considerable variation in the number of calyces and the shape of the pelvis, but there is also marked variation in the position of the pelvis. Thus the pelvis may lie almost entirely within the sinus, or its main portion may be a dilated sac and lie outside the kidney itself.

Microstructure

A cross-section through the kidney shows its substance to be composed of an internal medulla (marrow) and an external cortex (bark).

The medulla consists of a variable number (8 to 18) of conical segments called pyramids, the tops of which project into the bottom or sides of the sinus of the kidney and are received into the various minor calyces of the pelvis, while their bases are turned towards the surface, but are separated from it and from each other by the cortex.

The pyramids are smooth and somewhat glistening in cross-section and are marked with delicate stripes that converge from the base to the apex and indicate the course of the tubules of the kidney.

The microscopic architecture of the kidney is due to the arrangement of these tubules, which constitute the essential units of the kidney.

Principally, the basic functional unit of the kidney is the nephron, a long tubular structure made up of successive segments of diverse structure and transport functions.

Functions of the kidney

The kidneys are concerned in a number of activities, which include:
- the removal of nitrogenous waste, mostly in the form of urea;
- the maintenance of electrolyte balance;
- the maintenance of water balance;
- the regulation of the acid-base balance.

In addition, a number of chemical substances (acting as hormones) are released into the blood. Urine is formed in the kidneys as an aqueous solution containing metabolic waste products, foreign substances and

Side view of the lower part of the abdominal cavity and pelvis. Topography of the male (left) and female (right) bladder and urethra.

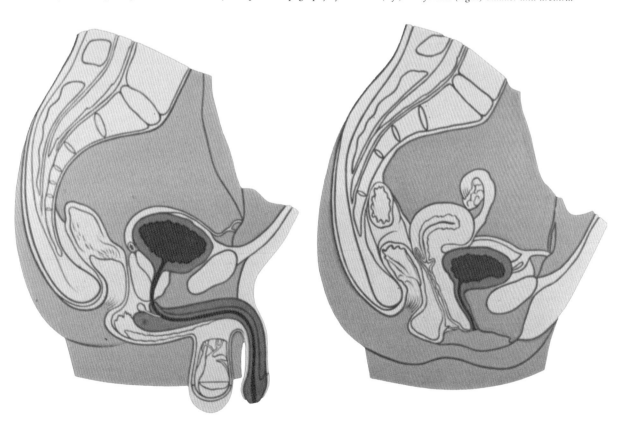

water-soluble constituents of the body in quantities depending upon homeostatic needs - that is, the balance of water and other essential substances in the body.

Studies of kidney function in humans tend to fall into two categories: acute observations lasting for a few hours, and prolonged studies of several days' duration during which all the urine excreted during each 24-hour period is pooled for analysis.

If, however, the urine is collected at three- to four-hourly intervals for a period of several days, rhythmical changes in volume and composition can be detected. When the rate of excretion of substances such as sodium, potassium, chloride and phosphate are plotted against time, a cyclical pattern with a mean period of 24 hours emerges.

This phenomenon has been named the circadian or diurnal rhythm, and its existence has been recognized for more than 100 years, but the factors controlling the cyclical changes in kidney function are still by no means clear.

Present concepts about how the kidney manufactures urine from blood plasma may be summarized as follows. A large volume of blood plasma is filtered by the glomerulus. As this "ultrafiltrate" passes from the capsule along the proximal convoluted tubule, most of the salt and water is reabsorbed, and some other substances are reabsorbed completely and others only partially.

Thus, this part of the tubule roughly separates the substances that must be conserved from those that are to be rejected in the urine. Thereafter, Henle's loop, the distal convoluted tubule and the collecting ducts are concerned mainly with the fine regulation of water, electrolyte (for instance, sodium, potassium, calcium, bicarbonate) and hydrogen ion balance.

The processes involved in tubular reabsorption and secretion are chemical and physical and are under control of hormones.

Function of the glomerulus

The glomerulus acts as an ultrafilter, allowing passage of water, electrolytes and small organic molecules such as glucose out of its semi-permeable membrane, but not blood cells and large protein molecules.

The ultrafiltrate produced by the glomeruli of both kidneys amounts to about 170 litres per day; this rate is termed the glomerular filtration rate. About 99 per cent of the glomerular filtrate is reabsorbed during passage through the tubules, with most of the reabsorption taking place in the proximal tubules.

Function of the tubules

Transport or movement of solutes and water across the cells of the tubules is one of the principal activities of the kidney tubules. Transport is called reabsorption when it is moved from within the tubules out to the interstitial fluid surrounding the cells, and secretion when it proceeds in the reverse direction.

Many solutes are transported in both directions simultaneously, but one direction usually dominates and the resultant is called net transport. Transport is energy-dependent, and transport across the tubular cells is classified according to the energy source used in the transfer process - that is, either active or passive transport.

Active transport is the movement of a substance against a gradient of electrical potential or chemical concentration. Passive transport, or diffusion, is the migration of a substance across an electrochemical gradient that is usually generated by the active transport of another solute.

Fine adjustment of water and solute excretion takes place in the distal tubule (convolutions and collecting ducts). Transport in the distal tubule differs from that in the proximal tubule in the former's capacity to reabsorb and secrete against large gradients.

Furthermore, the distal tubule is the only segment of the nephron that responds to both antidiuretic hormone (ADH) secreted by the pituitary body, and aldosterone secreted by the adrenal glands. ADH enhances water reabsorption, while aldosterone enhances the transport capacity for reabsorption of sodium with reciprocal secretion of potassium and hydrogen ions.

Reabsorption

Since glucose is found in the capsule and in healthy bodies is absent from urine, it must be reabsorbed somewhere in the nephron. The volume of urine is always far less than the volume of filtrate, so water is also reabsorbed.

In addition, many dissolved substances present in capsular fluid are partly reabsorbed and, since the degree of concentration varies for different substances and is independent of the water removed, there must be a number of reabsorptive mechanisms. Some information on where and how these processes occur has been provided by microchemical and microphysical methods. From this, it is known that most of the glucose has disappeared halfway along the proximal tubule, and has virtually all gone by the end. Also in the proximal tubule, large amounts of sodium, chloride, bicarbonate, about 80-85 per cent of the water and a variety of other substances are reabsorbed.

Secretion

This differs from reabsorption only in the direction of movement. The transport may be active or passive and is subject to the same limitations as reabsorption. Potassium and hydrogen are substances whose clearance is higher than the glomerular filtration rate.

A number of transport mechanisms can be distinguished in the tubular cells. One transport system carries organic acids such as glucuronides and creatinine, both of which are metabolic products, and also foreign chemicals.

The other system carries organic bases such as histamine and choline, and a number of foreign substances, many of which are medicines used for medical reasons.

Ureters and urethra

The ureters are hollow ducts, 25 to 35 cm in length, which arise in the pelvis of the kidney, run beside the vertebral column along the back part of the abdominal wall, and then takes an oblique direction along the side wall of the pelvis to enter the back surface of the wall of the bladder.

Several layers of smooth muscle fibers in the wall of the ureter move the urine to the bladder by peristalsis. The urethra is shorter in the woman than in the man. The female urethra follows a straight course and discharges from the vaginal vestibule.

The male urethra has a double bend and serves not only in the transportation of urine but also of sperm. The urethra perforates the floor of the pelvis, a complex of membranes and muscles which close off the pelvic exit.

Urinary bladder

The urinary bladder is a membranous sac serving as receptacle for the collection and secretion of urine. The organ is connected to the outside of the body by the urethra.

The urinary bladder, which is generally referred to simply as the bladder, is a hollow organ lying behind the junction of the pubic bones (symphysis) and in front of the rectum, and is surrounded by peritoneum. The empty bladder is the size of an orange, with a very thick wall and practically no central cavity.

Both kidneys secrete a steady stream of urine droplets and these are stored in the reservoir of the bladder. The capacity of the bladder is so great that, under normal conditions, it needs only be emptied once or twice every 24 hours.

Depending upon age, its maximum capacity ranges from 200 to 900 mL, but when the bladder contains about 400 mL in adults, all the sensory nerves in the area are stimulated, and this brings about contraction of the bladder muscles so that urination can take place.

The inner lining of the bladder consists of a layer of mucous membrane which, when the bladder is empty, falls into many folds. Next there are three layers of smooth muscle fibers that enable the bladder to adapt itself to the varying content.

At the outlet of the bladder, this muscular tissue forms a ring or sphincter, which is regulated by the voluntary nervous system. The sphincter, which consists partly of smooth and

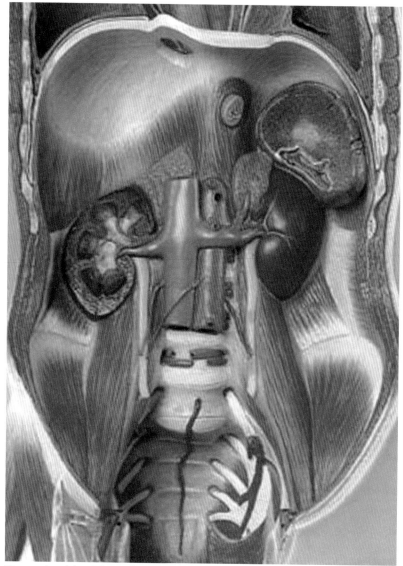

Topography of the abdominal cavity. The major organs for digestion (e.g., liver, gallbladder, intestines, stomach) have been removed to show the localization of the kidneys in the upper part of the abdominal cavity. The kidneys are bean-shaped organs lying behind the parietal peritoneum against the muscles of the posterior abdominal wall, just above the waistline. The right kidney is cut open to show the marrow and cortex.

partly of striated muscle tissue, serves to regulate the discharge of urine from the bladder. The tension (tone) of the muscles of the bladder wall and that of the sphincter muscles are mutually adjusted. Thus, when the bladder is extremely full, tension is high in the wall muscles, and in the striated muscle of the sphincter, up until the moment when a signal from the brain opens it to allow urine to

pass. The emptying of the bladder is brought about by an intricate system of nerve signals. In infants there is only one reflex: when the bladder wall is stretched to a certain point, urination occurs.

During the second year of life, conscious control of the bladder function generally takes over, and as a result, children become capable of controlling their urination voluntarily.

7 Reproduction

Introduction

Sexual activity is a physical activity that depends upon anatomical and physiological characteristics. A thorough understanding of the functions of the male and female reproductive systems helps sexually mature people derive pleasure and satisfaction form their sexual relationships.

Reproductive systems

The male and female reproductive systems differ in fundamental ways.

Male reproductive system

The male sexual organs consist of a sperm-generating and a sperm-discharging portion. Sperm are found in the two testes, two egg-shaped organs which, surrounded by membranes, hang below the groin in the scrotum, so situated because human temperature is too high for proper sperm formation. Sperm are stored in the epididymis, just above the testes.

During sex the sperm move through tubes and are mixed with secretions from the prostate and Cowper's gland, both ducted glands. Semen exits the body through a tube in the penis called the urethra, which is otherwise used for the excretion of urine.

The penis has a double function: the transportation of the urine and the transfer of sperm in copulation. The quantity of sperm at one ejaculation is approximately 2 to 4 cc, which may contain 400 to 500 million sperm cells.

Female reproductive system

The female sex organs consist of the internal organs (ovaries, Fallopian tubes, womb, and vagina) and the external organs (labia, clitoris, and mons pubis).

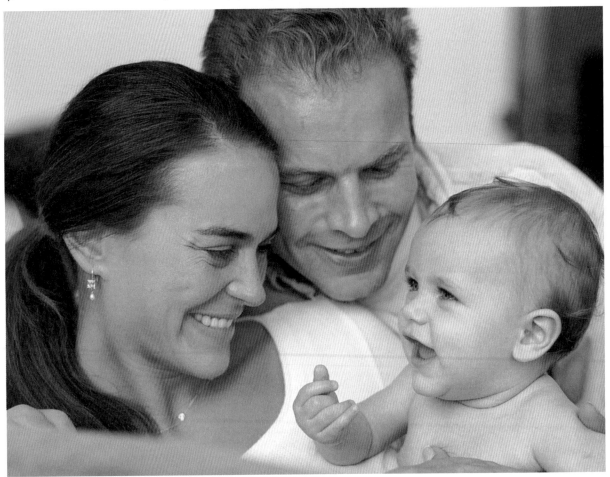

Schematic drawing of the molecular processes involved in conception. The four phases of the penetration of a sperm through the wall of the ovum are shown on the left.

Form top to bottom:

1. Sperm cells (spermatozoa) approach an ovum (egg cell). The spermatozoa are attracted to the membrane of the ovum by a specific chemical substance secreted by the ovum.

2. When the sperm reaches the ovum, it releases acrosomal enzymes, and a proteolytic enzyme utilized in penetrating the membrane of the ovum. The ovum itself also releases receptor enzymes to facilitate the process of penetration.

3. The various specific chemical (proteins and enzymes) interact with each other.

4. As soon as the penetration has occurred, the sperm sheds its tail and the chromosomal material forms the male pronucleus. Simultaneously, the ovum becomes impenetrable to other spermatozoa and prevents fertilization by several sperm.

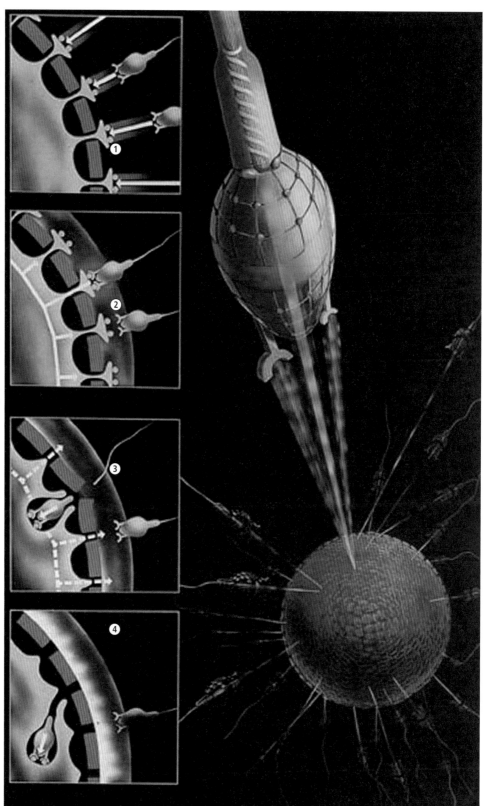

Corresponding to the testes in males, the ovaries produce eggs (also known as ova).

The contents of the ovaries, with the exception of connective tissue, blood vessels, etc., consists of eggs of different size, representing different stages of development.

Unlike sperm, eggs can be produced at human body temperature, allowing for the ovaries and related organs to be located inside the pelvis. The fertilized egg reaches full development in the womb (uterus).

Eggs pass through the Fallopian tubes to the womb, which is sealed at the other end of the cervix. On the other side of the cervix is a muscular tube called the vagina, or birth canal.

The womb is a pear-shaped organ, 3 to 4 inches (8 to 10 cm) long, with a thick wall and a cavity in the form of a triangular cleft. It is situated in the middle of the pelvis and is attached to its walls by means of a fold of the peritoneum.

If a fertilized egg develops fully, the wall of the womb is very much stretched and contractions of the muscle wall (birth pains) force the expulsion of the child through the vagina. If fertilization has not taken place, the egg degenerates and is eliminated from the womb, together with some mucous membrane from the womb during menstruation (monthly bleeding).

Menstrual cycle

The ovarian and uterine cycles are key factors in human reproduction. Both are governed by a delicate system of hormonal interplay. Controlling the process of both cycles are the pituitary gland, located at the base of the brain, the hypothalamus, also located within the brain, and the ovaries.

All three of these endocrine glands secrete hormones that act as chemical messengers among them. Hormonal levels within the bloodstream act as the trigger mechanism for release and regulation of the various hormones involved in the female reproductive cycle.

The menstrual cycle occurs in three distinct phases that are characterized by different hormonal secretions. The length of the cycle varies with individuals, with 28 days used as a point of reference to explanation the cycle. The first day of menstrual bleeding is called the first day of the cycle.

Estrogens

Hormones called estrogens are produced in the ovaries. In addition to regulating the reproductive cycle, estrogens also assist in the development of secondary sex characteristics such as breasts, fat deposits on hips, higher voice, and fine-textured skin and body hair.

When estrogen levels drop below a certain point, as during menstruation, the hypothalamus releases another hormone called gonadotrophin-releasing hormone. This function in turn signals the pituitary to release a follicle-stimulating hormone (FSH).

The release of these hormones moves the body into the second phase of the cycle, the proliferative phase. During this stage, FSH stimulates the maturation process of from 10 to 20 ovarian follicles (egg sacks). In turn, the follicles secrete estrogens. At the same time, the lining of the uterus, the

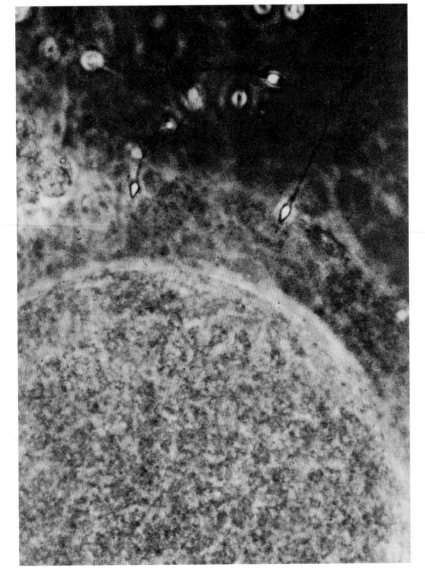

Microscopic view of sperm cells moving into the direction of the outer all of the ovum.

endometrium, begins to grow in response to hormonal secretions from the developing follicles. The inner walls of the uterus become coated with a thick spongy lining composed of blood and mucus. In the event of fertilization, the endometrial tissue will serve as a nesting phase for the developing embryo.

Progestogen

Of all the follicles maturing in the ovaries, only one each month normally reaches complete maturity (the others disintegrate gradually but continue to secrete vital estrogens). At about the fourteenth day of the proliferatory phase, the one egg destined to mature bursts from the ovary in a process called ovulation. Just prior to ovulation, the mature egg's follicle secretes a hormone called progestogen, the first function of which is to add further nutrients to the developing endometrium.

After ovulation, the ovarian follicle - the corpus luteum, or yellow body - continues to secrete estrogen and progestogen, but in decreasing amounts. In addition, FSH also falls back to its preproliferatory levels. Essentially, the woman's body is waiting to see if fertilization will occur. During this time after ovulation, LH declines, and progestogen levels begin to rise slightly, causing additional tissue growth in the endometrium. This phase of the cycle is called the secretory phase.

Fertilization

If fertilization takes place, the developing embryo releases a hormone, called human chorionic gonadotrophin (HCG). Chemically identical to LH, HCG is also similar in function; it produces increased levels of progestogen secretion.

When fertilization does not occur, the egg gradually disintegrates within approximately 72 hours. The corpus luteum gradually becomes nonfunctional, causing levels of progestogen and estrogen to decline.

As hormonal levels decline, the endometrial lining of the uterus loses its nourishment, dies, and is sloughed off as menstrual flow. Menstruation is the third phase of the reproductive cycle.

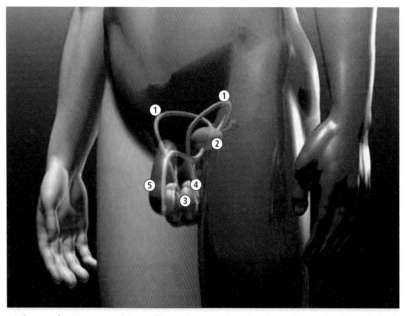

Male reproductive organs (Upper illustration: anterior view; lower illustration: lateral view).
1. Sperm duct
2. Prostate gland
3. Scrotum
4. Epididymis.
5. Penis

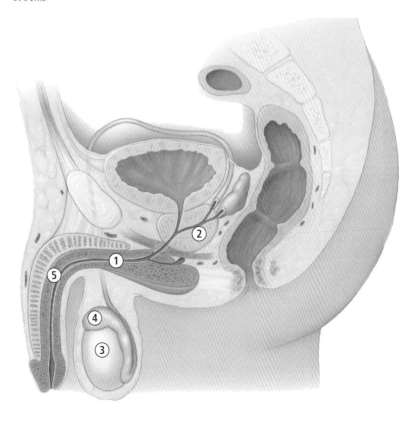

Behavior or beliefs of sexually mature people

- Sexually mature people understand and accept the mental, physical, spiritual, and social aspects of human sexuality.

- Sexually mature behavior is based upon a set of carefully explored and continually examined personal values.

- Sexually mature people are able to discuss sexuality with little or no embarrassment.

- Sexually mature people are able to discuss sexual concerns tactfully and sensitively with their partners.

- Sexually mature people do not use sexual behavior to manipulate or injure other human beings.

- Sexual maturity involves acceptance of responsibility for the consequences of sexual activity, including the prevention of unwanted pregnancies and procedures to prevent the spread of sexually transmitted diseases.

- Sexually mature people are able to recognize and seek help for sexually related problems.

- Sexually mature people assume active responsibility for their reproductive health.

- Sexually mature people are able to integrate their choice of sexual expression into their lives.

- Sexually mature people do not allow their desires for sexual gratification to rule their lives. Rather, they balance sexual gratification with other pleasures, values, and rewards.

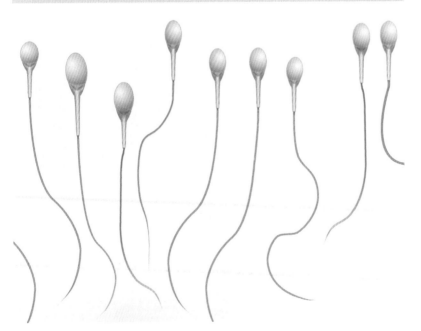

Sexual identity

Although we are born as sexual creatures with the potential to reproduce, we are not born with our sexual identities. The development of our sexual identity - a composite of biological gender, social gender role, sexual preference, body image, and sexual script - begins at birth.

Our sexual identities develop just as do our family, social, religious, political, professional, and ethnic identities. Like others, our sexual identities reflect many influences: our parents' attitudes toward sex; our gender, personal and cultural definitions of masculinity and femininity; sexual preference; personal body image; previous and present sexual experiences; and the meanings, implications, and effects of sexual relationships in our lives.

Sexual maturity
Part of our sexual identity is also reflected in our sexual maturity. Sexual maturity goes far beyond the capacity to reproduce. Unlike physical maturity, sexual maturity is not something we automatically achieve. Rather, the process of achieving sexual maturity, although loosely linked to physical age (we need to be physically capable of reproduction in order to manage our sexual growth process), involves intentional effort on the part of the individual. We must desire to grow up sexually in order to begin the process. Sexual growth follows a different timetable for each person. Achieving sexual maturity is not limited to one group of people: heterosexuals, bisexuals, and homosexuals are all capable of sexual maturity.

Sexually mature people exhibit the following behavior or beliefs.

The journey to sexual maturity begins at birth and continues into our adult lives. It is a long process that involves pitfalls, heartbreaks, alternate setbacks and successes, positive self-examination, problem resolution, and the desire for personal growth.

As men and women move through their late teen years, sexual activity becomes more important in their lives. Confusion about whether or not

Spermatozoa.

to engage in sexual relations, either casually or in the context of some type of committed relationship, is typical among men and women recently liberated from home and high school.

Human sexual response

Sexual response is a physiological process that involves different stages. The biological goal of the response process is the reproduction of the species. Because of the intense pleasure involved in sexual relations, sexual activity transcendends procreation. As emotional and spiritual creatures, human beings find the sexual experience to be a powerful factor in bonding one person to another.

Human psychological traits greatly influence sexual response and sexual desire. Thus, we may find relationships with one partner vastly different from those we might experience with other partners. Sexual response generally follows a pattern. Laboratory research has delineated four or five stages within the response cycle, and researchers agree that each individual has a personal response that may or may not conform to the stages observed in experimental research.

Both males and females exhibit four common stages:
- excitement/arousal stage;
- plateau stage;
- orgasm;
- resolution stage.

In addition, some males experience a fifth stage, the refractory stage. Identification of these stages was achieved in laboratory situations in which genital response was carefully measures using specifically designed instruments. The response stages occur during masturbation, heterosexual activity, and homosexual activity.

Sexual pleasure and satisfaction are possible without orgasm of intercourse. Achieving sexual maturity includes learning that sex is not a context with a real or imaginary opponent. The sexually mature person enjoys sexual activity whether or not orgasm occurs. Expressing love and sexual feelings for another person involves many pleasurable activities, of which intercourse and orgasm are only a part.

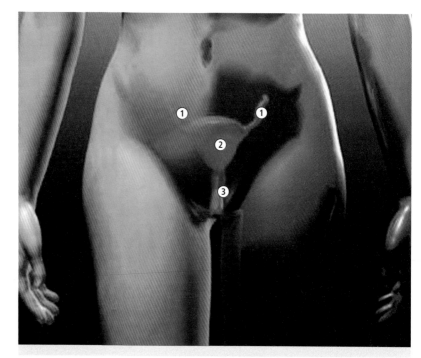

Female reproductive organs (Upper illustration: anterior view; lower illustration: lateral view).
1. Uterine tube
2. Uterus
3. Vagina
4. Ovary

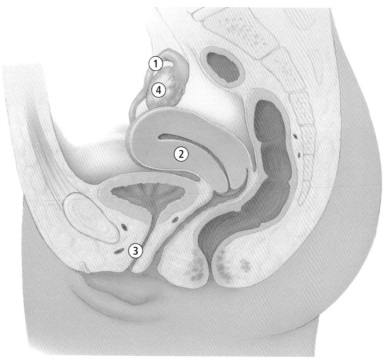

8 Sense Organs

Introduction

If man is to survive he must have some means of keeping tract of what is going on both inside and outside his body. He needs a continuous news service that sends reports on his bodily condition to the central control.

Some of these reports concern the position of his limbs, his blood pressure, temperature, and so on; others convey information about the world outside.

We take our own actions so much for granted that it is hard to realize that we are constantly in situations that could become dangerous if we failed to take the right action. For instance, we must be able to detect food from non-food.

The decision to eat the hamburger and not the plate is a very real and important one; we take it without a moment's hesitation, yet behind that decision there is a stream of information arriving at the brain. And during the meal a great variety of cells called receptors is at work.

Receptors

The receptors are specialized cells whose sole job is to react to change. They are connected to sensory nerve endings so that when the cell has anything to report the nerve carries its impulses to the central nervous system.

Receptors are to be found all over the body. Those that register internal conditions we call proprioceptors. Much of the work that they do passes completely unnoticed, but it is none the less important in keeping the body in good trim and ready for action.

Other receptors detect changes at the body's surface, and the work these do is something that we are usually more conscious of. This is logical because the information that they supply is about the world around us; they steer us away from danger and toward the things we want.

The skin

The part of the body that makes direct contact with objects around us is the skin. This layer, naturally enough, contains a vast number of receptors that register touch, heat, cold, and pain.

The sense of touch is very complex; if we shut our eyes and reach out to pick up a hammer we can instantly tell whether we have grasped the wooden handle or the steel head, even if they are both highly polished. When we touch the wood, very little heat flows from our fingers, but if we take hold of the steel, which is a much better heat conductor, more heat flows from the fingers.

We also obtain information regarding roughness, sharpness, texture, and wetness and these modalities involve the use of several types of receptors, and it is left to the brain to interpret the different combinations.

Differentiated skin receptors

Many types of receptors have been identified in the skin, but it is not always possible to say which sensation corresponds to which type. Sometimes the sensations of touch, temperature, and pain can be registered by a single receptor.

The special senses are located in the head: vision, hearing, equilibrium, taste, olfaction.

Also, under extreme conditions, receptors give the wrong response. Anyone who has been rash enough to touch metal with bare hands at subzero temperatures knows that the metal feels as if it were red hot.

The mechanisms of skin sensation are in fact not well understood and this is especially true of pain, even though it is the most vivid sensation of all.

Adaptation

There is one merciful feature of sensory reception, called adaptation; certain unimportant sensations become reduced with time, thus saving the conscious mind from being bombarded continuously with unimportant information.

For instance, we feel the clothes against the skin disappear very soon after dressing. One region in the brain that helps suppress unwanted stimuli is the reticular formation of the brain stem.

But the receptors also play their part; they appear to become tired of reporting something about which no action needs to be taken.

The eye

Many of the skin receptors provide us with general information about our closest surroundings. But we also need to perceive the dangerous and desirable at a distance.

It is not enough to know in what direction something lies; we must also decide how far away it is and what it looks like. For this purpose man has a pair of special sense organs - the eyes.

Very simply, the eye consists of a transparent part at the front that focuses images on to a light-sensitive layer at

Eyeglasses for correction of myopia. People who are farsighted (hyperopic) have trouble seeing anything close, and those who are nearsighted (myopic) have trouble focusing on distant objects.

Everyone should have regular eye examinations, by a family doctor, ophthalmologist, or optometrist. The eyes are tested together and individually. Vision testing usually also includes assessments unrelated to refractive error, such as a test of the ability to see colours.

the back. Several comparisons can be made with the camera to make the eye easier to understand; for instance, the transparent part corresponds to the lens and the light-sensitive part, or retina, corresponds to the film.

Cornea

The front of the eye bends, or refracts, light on to the retina. In a camera the image must be carefully focused and the same is true of the eye.

The refractive part of the eye, however, is not quite the same as that of a camera. Whereas there is only one refractive part to a camera (the lens), there is a second one in the eye, called the cornea; this curved and transparent part lies in front of the lens proper, and it is here that most of the refraction of light takes place.

The cornea forms the delicate front surface of the eye, and we find several safe-guards. It is protected from dust particles by being continuously washed by antiseptic tears that drain into the nose at the inner edge of the eye. At the same time the upper eyelid

passes up and down over the font of the eye, acting like a windscreen wiper. But the greatest protection of all is the fact that the front of the cornea consists of a transparent membrane called the conjunctiva, consisting of self-repairing stratified epithelium.

The cornea is fixed and it focuses images roughly somewhere near the retina; the image, in other words, may lie either in front of or behind that layer. It is left to the lens to act as a fine adjuster and to bring the image accurately on to the retina. It does this by means of muscles that cause the lens to alter its shape according to the distance of the image.

The refractive parts of the eye are like any other organ; they must be fed. But they are transparent, so it is out of the question to provide nourishment through a network of capillaries. Instead, the refractive parts are nourished by transparent fluids that themselves exchange nutrients and gases with the capillaries of the eyeball. These fluids also maintain a constant pressure against the inside of the eye-

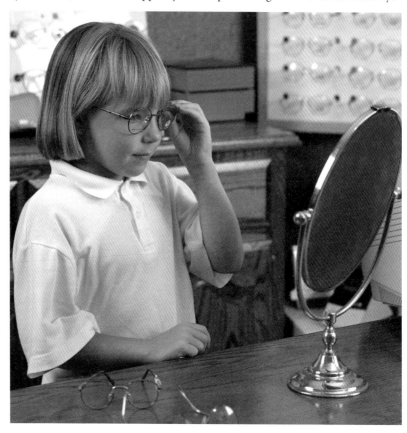

ball, to keep it rounded to its proper shape and also exert a necessary pressure on the nerve cells of the retina. In both the eye and the camera there is an optimum intensity of light at which images can clearly imprint themselves on the light-sensitive surface. By reducing excess light entering a camera, the sharpness of the photo is increased, and exactly the same is true of the eye.

But the eye is more vulnerable than a film because excessive stimulation could damage or even burn the retina. Therefore light intensity is regulated by an automatic diaphragm called the iris.

In the eye the iris is placed between the lens and the cornea and its center is an opening called the pupil. In bright light the pupil narrows and in dim light it dilates.

Retina

The retina consists of over 100 million receptors of two kinds - rods and cones. The rods are used when the light intensity is low and they give a picture in varying shades of grey.

They are most densely crowded at the front of the retina so that weak light entering from in front. It is thus easier to see a star by looking to one side of it. The rods are like other receptors in that they turn a stimulus - in this case, light - into a volley of electrical impulses that travel along sensory nerves to the brain. It is not quite certain how the rods do this but we do know that, to some extent, they use the same principle as a camera.

A photographic film carries a layer of silver salts that are sensitive to light; when these salts absorb light energy they break down, and the degree of breakdown is proportional to the strength of the light.

The retina also has a pigment, called rhodopsin, that slowly breaks down when it absorbs light of low intensity. When this happens, there is a release of energy that triggers off nerve impulses. But rhodopsin can rebuild itself so that it is ready to receive new impulses.

The other type of receptor in the retina - the cone - is used in daylight vision and is also responsible for our appreciation of colour. The cones also use complex chemical systems to transform the various types of light energies representing colours into trains of nerve impulses.

The rods and cones are not the only types of nervous tissue in the retina; both types of receptor are connected to two layers of nerve cells. These run over the surface of the retina so that light has to travel through them before reaching the receptors. Perhaps this seems inefficient; nevertheless the rods are so sensitive that on a very clear dark night they can detect a candle flame more than 10 miles away. At this distance the eye receives less than one hundred-million-millionth part of the original light, and the rods could hardly be more sensitive. The receptors and their nerve cells are joined to each other in a complex way. In some parts one receptor is joined to many nerve cells; in other parts many receptors are joined to one nerve cell. The arrangement is similar to that found in the brain, which is not surprising because the retina itself is an extension of the brain. Thus the nerve cells do more than merely pass light signals to the brain; they also process information before sending it to the visual cortex.

How our brain interprets visual images is still a mystery, but we do know that different groups of cells in the visual area of the cortex deal with a definite part of the retina and with images of a particular shape.

The ear

By day man keeps in touch with his position mainly by using his eyes; in the dark, however, he relies mainly on his ears. Each ear is two distinct organs, one for hearing and one for balance. The visible part of the ear is called the outer ear; it helps to collect and guide sound to the eardrum, or tympanic membrane.

Vibrations set up in this membrane travel along three linked bones in the middle ear to another membrane called the oval window. These bones form a system of levers which magnify pressure changes in the tympanum. In addition, the oval window is very small so that it vibrates more forcibly than the larger tympanum.

The middle ear contains muscles that prevent the bones transmitting excessive noise; the bones also form a sort of ratchet mechanism that slips when the ear is assailed by very loud noise and so prevents damage to the window. If the tympanum is to vibrate efficiently there must be an equal atmospheric pressure on both its sides. We realize the importance of this when we quickly change altitude in a lift or airplane; at such times it is often difficult to hear.

A ventilation shaft (the eustachian tube) links the middle ear with the nasopharynx so that, when we swallow, air passes into or out of the middle ear to equalize the pressure.

Hearing

The organ for hearing, in the inner ear, is a spirally wound tune called the cochlea, lined with groups of sensory cells mounted on a membrane. Vibrations of the oval window pass first through fluid surrounding the cochlea and then through fluid inside it, finally spreading along the membrane. Much of the membrane vibrates to all frequencies, but a particular note makes one part vibrate more strongly than the rest. When the membrane vibrates it deforms the hair-like sense cells; impulses set up in all the sense cells transmit information along about 30,000 nerve filers.

This, however, is apparently only one factor in the complex process of hearing. Both the ear and the brain must further analyze the sound, but how this is done is still obscure.

Balance

The part of the inner ear concerned with balance is connected to the cochlea, but we must remember that hearing and balance are two quite distinct senses. The part that responds to changes of motion - that is, to acceleration and deceleration - are called the semicircular canals.

These canals lie in three different planes at 90 degrees to each other; each canal is swollen at its base and contains hair-like sense cells. When the head or body moves, the canals move as well, but the fluid inside them is momentarily left behind so that it presses on the receptors. As the canals are in three different planes, a movement in any direction will stimulate

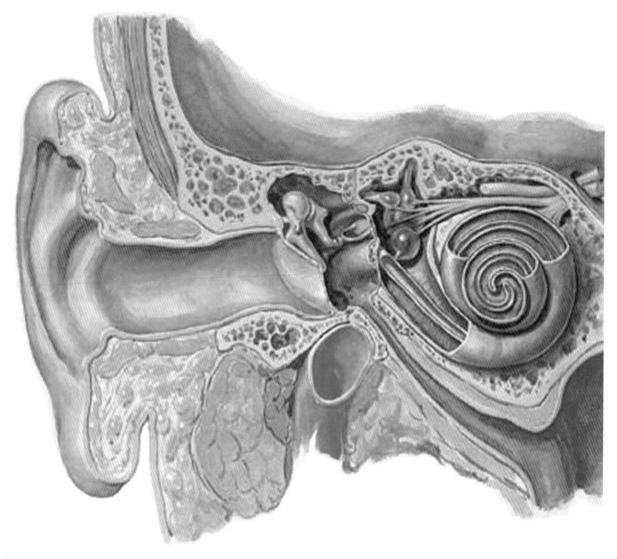

Frontal section through the outer, middle and inner ear.
Outer ear (left): pinna, external acoustic meatus, mastoid cells, and tympanic membrane.
Middle ear (middle): tympanic cavity. auditory ossicles (hammer, anvil and stirrup)
Inner ear (right): bony and membranous labyrinths. The bony labyrinth consists of the cochlea, containing the organ of hearing, and the vestibule and semicircular canals, containing the organs of equilibrium. The membranous labyrinth consists of the cochlear duct and the semicircular ducts.

the hairs in one or more of the canals; the quicker the body accelerates or slows down, the faster do the receptors send impulses to the brain.

The semicircular canals lead into two connected sacs, each containing groups of hair-like sense cells on which rest particles of chalk. This is the part of the inner ear that senses the body's position in space.

As the position of the body and head alters, the pressure of the particles on the receptors varies. The more the body tilts away from its normal vertical position, the faster do impulses travel to the brain.

The nose

Man's face is characterized by hairs, a projecting nose and chin, and moving lips. The frontal nasal opening has the shape of an inverted heart. It is bordered by the nasal bones and the upper jaw. The nasal septum is formed by the ethmoid bone and the vomer.

The roof consists of the ethmoid bone and the floor is composed of the palatine bone and the upper jaw. The inner (and largest) section of the nose consists of two cavities, separated by

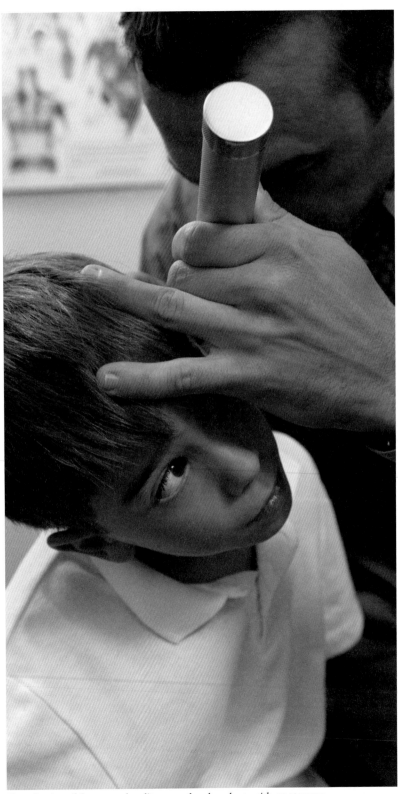

Examination of the external auditory canal and eardrum with an otoscope.

the body septum. On the outer walls of this area three nasal conchae lie one above the other.

The nasal cavity is connected to a number of other cavities or sinuses (frontal, sphenoid, maxillary, and ethmoid). The three bony folds (conchae) of each nasal cavity are covered by a mucous membrane, in which the olfactory sensory receptors are localized.

The olfactory epithelium in man is no larger than 5 square centimetres. The branches of the olfactory nerve arise in this area and the thin, small bundles of nerves perforate the cribriform plate of the ethmoid bone. The stimuli are carried to the central nervous system via the olfactory tract. Olfactory perception is determined by receptor cells of the olfactory mucous membrane and the concentration and quality of the substance to be perceived.

Our perception of olfactory stimuli is highly developed. Thus, we can perceive 0.000,000,000,002 g of valeric acid in 1 litre of air.

The tongue

The gustatory sensory or taste receptor cells are located primarily in the mucous membrane of the tongue and occasionally in the throat and palate. On the tongue, four kinds of papillae are found.

The mushroom-shaped papillae contain the taste buds with the gustatory sensory cells. They are concentrated on the border of the anterior two-thirds and the posterior end of the tongue.

The qualities of taste are distributed over the tongue in a specific manner:
- sweet at the tip;
- salty on the edge of the frontal section;
- bitter at the back of the tongue.

The perception of taste stimuli is supported to a large degree by the sense of smell.

The sense of taste tells us nothing about the chemical composition of a substance and is strongly dependent on the concentration; thus 0.02 per cent potassium bromide tastes bitter sweet and 0.2 per cent, on the other hand, tastes salty.

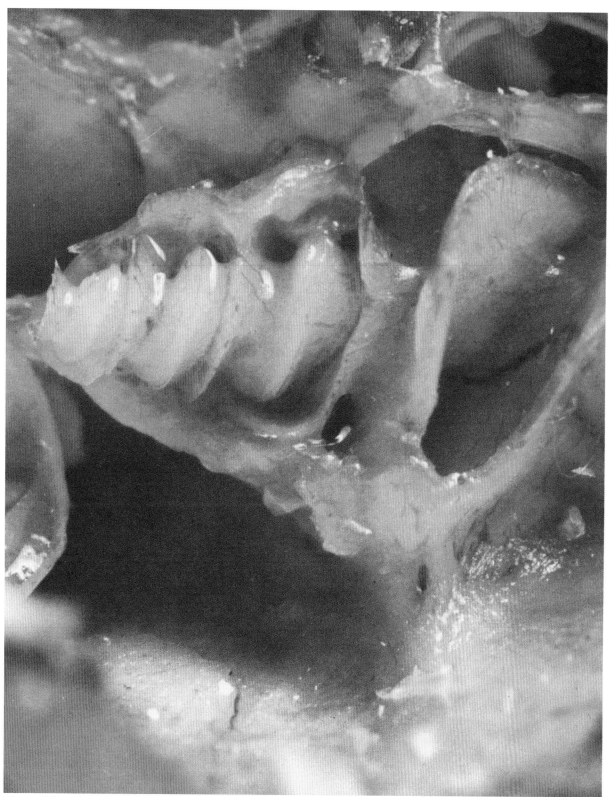

Picture of the cochlea in the inner ear. The cochlea is coiled two and one-half times in the shape of a snail shell about a central axis of bone.

9 Nervous System

Introduction

For descriptive purposes the nervous system can be divided into the central nervous system, consisting of the brain and the spinal cord, and the peripheral nervous system, consisting of the nerves which run throughout the body.

The entire nervous system functions as a single unit, receiving and processing information.

From sensory receptors it receives many millions of signals, processes these and sends back thousands of signals to the body, such as the muscles and glands.

The main functions of the nervous system fall into three groups:

- ▲ It efficiently integrates the performance of diverse organs, each directed to its own function, in a much faster way that would be possible through transportation of substances via the blood vessels. As a result, organ function is integrated to serve a higher order: that of the entire organism.
- ▲ The individual can react in an efficient and rapid manner to changes in the external environment. The ability to adapt to environmental changes contributes to the preservation of the species.
- ▲ Specific parts of the human nervous system must be regarded as the places where, in a manner yet unknown, the connection is made between mind and body, and where functions such as abstract thinking and consciousness are localized.

Basic brain functions

The brain is a complex organ that, together with the spinal cord, comprises the central nervous system and coordinates all nerve-cell activities. In humans, the brain is dominated by the highly developed cerebral cortex, the outer bark of the cerebral hemispheres.

The brain is composed of some 100 billion interconnecting nerve cells and many more supporting cells (neuroglia).

All the bodily systems are necessary to the support of life, but the nervous system is the most important among them for it governs and coordinates the operations of all tissues and organs.

The beating of the heart, the secretion of glands, breathing, the processes of digestion, for example, are all triggered, monitored and adjusted by nervous signals. And the nervous system is of primary importance in another way: it is the physical basis of all the mental activities and properties without which human life would be of no interest: consciousness, sensation, thought, speech, memory, emotion, character and skill.

The nervous system has a certain gross similarity to a telephone system: it works electrically, it carries information in the form of electrical signals, and all the nervous pathways converge upon the brain and spinal cord, just as all the telephone lines in an area converge upon a central system or exchange.

The *central exchange*, the brain and spinal cord, is known as the central nervous system (often abbreviated as CNS); the remaining outlying pathways of nervous fibers constitute the peripheral nervous system (PNS).

The analogy with a telephone system must not, however, be pressed too far. For one thing, nervous pathways are not continuous like wires, but are made up of separate units - nerve cells known as neurons. For another thing, the speed of propagation of a charge in a wire is about one million times faster than it is in a nerve pathway.

Thirdly, whereas a telephone system has one central power supply, the power supply of the nervous system is spread throughout; each nerve cell is, in effect, its own booster battery.

Finally, although a line connecting one telephone to the exchange is able to carry information in both directions, nerve fibers conduct in one direction only; those that carry information from the sensory organs to the brain and spinal cord are called afferent or sensory pathways. Those that carry impulses outwards from the brain and spinal cord to the muscles and glands which they activate are called efferent or motor pathways.

Divisions of the brain

For convenience of description the full-grown brain can be divided into three parts:

- brainstem;
- cerebellum;
- cerebrum.

The brainstem is, in the main, a relay station for nervous pathways between the higher parts of the brain and the rest of the body; consequently, if it is damaged, sensory and motor functions are greatly impaired. But the brainstem is also responsible for sub-voluntary activities - for example, digestion and respiration.

Both the cerebellum and cerebrum are divided into two hemispheres each, one on either side of the head. The cerebellum is responsible for the coordination of voluntary muscular movements and for posture.

Cerebral hemispheres

In the adult, the cerebral hemispheres become divided into frontal, occipital, parietal and temporal lobes. Each of these subdivisions becomes further subdivided by grooves into smaller raised areas.

A fifth lobe may be described that include parts of the frontal, parietal and temporal lobes. This is the limbic lobe which is a C-shaped structure extending completely around the diencephalon (interbrain).

A small area of cortex remains that may not be considered as being part of any particular lobe. This is the insular cortex that is overgrown by the frontal, temporal and parietal lobes and lies in the deep lateral sulcus (groove) on the lateral surface of the brain.

It appears to be somewhat concerned with the organs of e chest and abdomen. The cortex overlying the insular cortex is frequently called the operculum.

Frontal lobe

The major functions of the frontal lobe are:

▲ voluntary motor function;
▲ the organization of the motor units necessary for speech;
▲ some contribution towards what may be called original thinking;
▲ evaluation of ideas.

The location of these functions on the cortex may be more precisely stated. Thus, the cortex of the precentral gyrus (convolution) (area 4) forms a primary motor area with a relatively specific separation into smaller areas for different regions of the body.

The face is represented on the lower third of the gyrus, with an upright orientation; the hand, with a large proportion of the cortex concerned with thumb movements, occupies the middle third, followed by the trunk and hips in the upper third.

A premotor area, which exists just in front of the primary motor area, occupies the back part of three horizontally oriented frontal gyri (area 6). Associated with this is a so-called frontal eye field (area 8).

Stimulation of various areas of the motor cortex produces movement in specific structures usually in the opposite side of the body; for example, stimulation of the frontal eye field on one side of the cortex induces eye- and head-turning movements on the opposite side of the body. A cortical area more in front of the premotor cortex has been considered by some to be involved with processes relating to original thought, though how one defines thought has been subject to considerable disagreement.

Another region of interest is located in the inferior frontal gyrus. This is the pars opercularis (area 44), which in the left hemisphere (in right-handed persons) appears concerned with the organization of the motor units involved in speech. Stimulation of this region may induce vocalization, but not true speech.

Parietal lobe

This lobe is mainly concerned with the reception of body sensations and memory in regard to language and learning. The region has also a role in spatial organization. The areas 1, 2 and 3 comprise the primary sensory cortex. The location of functions comparable to that observed in the motor cortex has been mapped, largely by direct stimulation of the exposed cortex during brain surgery.

The remainder of the parietal lobe may be divided into a superior and inferior parietal lobule. Areas 5 and 7 in the superior lobule appear to be concerned with the correlation of different types of sensory information to provide for conscious appraisal of the weight, texture, size and contour of an object. The ability to recognize these types of sensation would appear related to the less closely defined function of "hand dexterity" that has been applied to this region.

The inferior parietal lobule appears closely related to speech mechanisms, in that disease or injury in the left hemisphere (in right-handed individuals) in this area lead to speech disturbances.

The role of the parietal lobe in spatial organization has been less extensively studied. However, there does appear to be a defect in spatial judgement in patients with right parietal lobe lesions.

A similar defect may occur with lesions of the left parietal lobe, but the speech defect that occurs is of such a magnitude as to make any evaluation impractical.

Temporal lobe

This lobe serves several functions:

▲ reception of auditory sensations (the sense of hearing);

Side view of a model of the head. Skull cut open to show the localization of the brain.

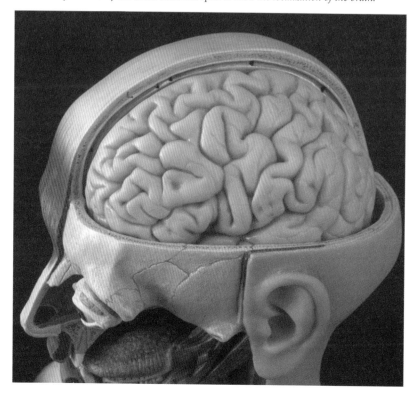

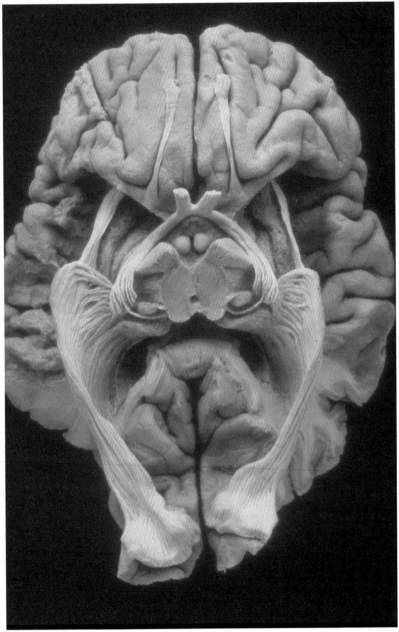

Bottom view of the brain with a number of cranial nerves.

as lesions in this region result in individuals who are unable to comprehend the spoken word. They act as if they are unable to monitor the words they hear or speak.

There is also some evidence that the temporal lobe is associated with balance since stimulation of some part of the superior temporal gyrus in conscious patients induces vertigo and a sensation of rotation.

Deep lesions in the temporal lobes often involve the lowest fibers of nerve cells involved in sight, arising from the lateral geniculate body, and this produces visual defects. This should not be related to the function of the temporal lobe, however. The temporal lobe has also been variously claimed to be concerned with memory and dreams.

Occipital lobe

The lobe in the back of the head is the primary center for vision. A primary visual cortex (area 17) is recognized. Adjacent to it is a "psychic" or interpretive visual area (18) which is believed to assemble the signals received by area 17 into an image.

Patients with lesions in area 18 see but do not recognize objects. Area 19 surrounds area 18 and blends with the adjacent parietal cortex. It is at this level in the visual cortex that the significance of what is seen appears to be appreciated. Stimulation of this area triggers hallucinations and dreamlike images.

The so-called *psychic* areas (5, 7, 19, 22) all have an interpretive or associational role in comprehending information.

Thus, it is perhaps not too difficult to understand why left hemisphere lesions (in right-handed individuals) in the center of this confluence of psychic cortical areas have such a global effect in the understanding of those symbols used in communication.

Limbic lobe

The function of this lobe, which contains components of the frontal, parietal and temporal lobes, is more complex. It involves behavioral reactions of the individual toward the external environment as a result of receiving information through all of the senso-

▲ participation in speech through auditory monitoring;
▲ some role in spatial organization;
▲ a memory mechanism.

The transverse temporal gyrus (area 41) has long been recognized as the primary hearing center. A small area (42) surrounding this gyrus has been described as a psychic or interpretive auditory area.

Stimulation of most of the temporal lobe, particularly along the middle temporal gyrus, induces a sensation as if the person has heard something. A patient with lesions in the temporal lobe in the "psychic area" may lose appreciation of tones.

Area 22 in the left hemisphere (in right-handed individuals) has also been associated with speech inasmuch

ry areas of the brain.

In addition, the response may be influenced by the internal environment, which may alter the excitability of the nervous system. It seems to operate in preserving the individual (feeding, fleeing or fighting) or the species (reproduction). A major part of the limbic lobe is concerned with all psycho-affective functions (aggression, hate, fear, anxiety, sexual responses, etc.).

General cerebral functions

The deep nuclear masses (caudate nucleus, etc.) are a part of what might be termed the primitive or older sensory-motor system. This system appears to be associated with stereotypes of instinctual behavior. It also coordinates all motor systems related to posture.

The corpus callosum is a large white bundle of fibers that connects the two cerebral hemispheres to each other. Only recently have experiments demonstrated that the function of this large bundle appears concerned with the transfer of learning from one hemisphere to another.

Roger Sperry, professor of psychobiology at the California Institute of Technology who, in l981, received the Nobel Prize for his outstanding research, performed a series of remarkable experiments, on what he and his co-workers have called the *split-brain* preparation.

Brains of cats and monkeys were divided surgically by cutting the corpus callosum and other connecting structures, so that the performance of each half could be tested separately. There is sufficient evidence that cats and monkeys with split brains can hardly be distinguished from normal animals in most of their activities.

However, in various types of learning and training experiments, it appeared that learning in one hemisphere is usually inaccessible to the other hemisphere if the connections between them are missing.

The obvious conclusion is that the corpus callosum has the important function of allowing the two hemispheres to share learning and memory.

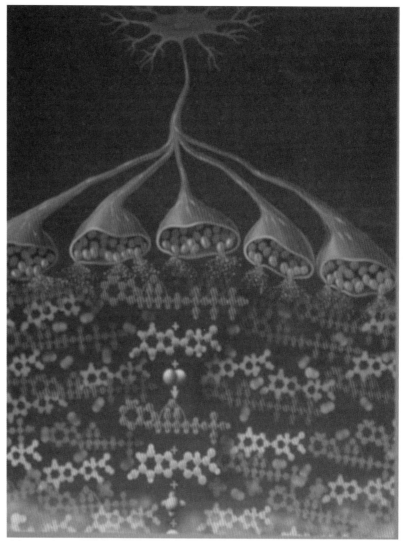

Schema of nerve endings and synapses. The chemical structure of a number of neurotransmitters - chemical messenger molecules - are indicated.

Autonomic nervous system

The use of the term "autonomic" to describe certain sections of the brain, spinal cord and nerve pathways often gives rise to mis-understanding. In this context, the descrip-tion autonomic means that this part of the nervous system is in charge of the activity of a number of organs, and makes them func-tion more or less without us willing or being conscious of it.

Specifically, these are the organs of the chest (heart and lung-s), the abdomen (stomach, intestine, liver, etc.) and of the pelvis, and many other organs and tissues of the body inclu-ding the blood vessels and skin.

"Autono-mic," therefore, does not mean that this part of the nervous system works indepen-dently of the rest of the brain and the spinal cord.

Somatic nervous system

The nervous system can be divided into a somatic and an autonomic part. The somatic nervous system comprises those parts of the brain, spinal cord and nerve pathways that keep us in touch with our environment. The term "somatic" means "bodily," but we should add "reacting to external stimuli." This response is achieved by the sensory organs, the sensory and motor nerves and the stria-ted (striped, voluntary or skeletal) muscles. By means of these organs, we are brou-ght into contact with our environment so that we can react to environmental changes.

The somatic nervous system can therefore be conside-red that organic system that handles all information from the external world. Stimuli enter us through the many hundreds of thousands of receptor cells on and in our bodies. The stimuli are processed in the brain and spinal cord, and information out-put occurs in the form of nerve impulses and hormones.

Maintenance of the individual and species

The autonomic nervous system, on the other hand, governs all the processes that serve to maintain the individual and the spe-cies. In particular, these are meta-bolism, growth, reproducti-on, respiration, nutrition and digestion, the functioning of the heart and blood vessels, the excretion of waste products, temperature control, etc.

The differences between the autonomic and somatic nervous systems rest on a number of factors of structure and function. One real-ly needs to appreciate that the autonomic nervous system, as a subdivision of the brain, spinal cord and perip-heral nervous system, is not merely in charge of the regu-lati-on of the function of less interesting organs such as the stomach, liver, kidneys or intestines.

It also plays a funda-mental part in our relationship with the outside world because an important part of the world of our emotional experience finds expression mostly via the autonomic nervous system.

Thus, emotions can give rise to, among other things, quicke-ning of the heartbeat, changes in breathing patterns, increa-sed secretion of gastric acid in the stomach, and alterations in the secretory pattern of the gallb-ladder.

All these processes are under the control of the central and peripheral parts of the autonomic nervous system, and malfunc-tion of this system can easily lead to, or be the originating factor in, serious disturbances in the functioning of an organ.

Often the occurrence of a stomach ache is ascribable to the malfunction of one of the subsystems of the autonomic nervous system. Furthermo-re, an intricate system of nuclei and nerve pathways in the brain is in control of the joint and individual adjustment of the many functions of the various organs.

Organization of the autonomic nervous system

These areas lie in a subdivision of the cerebrum, the limbic system, and in a part of the diencep-halon, the hypotha-lamus, in the forebrain. In the hypothalamus lie dozens of nuclei and pathways that exert a controlling influence over many basic life functions such as ea-ting and drinking behavior, temperature regulation, the percentage of sugars, fats and water in the blood, and other mecha-nisms.

The autonomic nervous system can be divi-ded into two more or less separate parts according to position and function: these are the sympathetic and the parasympathetic systems, which in general produce opposite effects on various organs.

The nerve pathw-ays invariably consist of two consecutive nerve cells. The cell body and the short axons (nerve fibers) of the first nerve cell lie in the brainstem or the spinal cord.

The long axons leave the central nervous system and run out in the spinal cord or, further still, to various parts of the body. The second nerve cell begins close to the spinal cord (in the case of the sympathetic nervous system) or close to the organ concerned (in the case of the parasympathetic nervous system).

Thus groups of nerve cell bodies are formed outside the brain and spinal cord. A ganglion is a massed group of nerve cell bodies with their short axons and con-tact points.

Parasympathetic nervous system

The nerves of the system are made up from axons that originate from cells situated in the brainstem, and from nerve cells which lie in the lower part of the spinal cord. The most important parasympathetic nerve is the tenth cranial nerve - the nervus vagus. The Latin word vagus means wandering; there-fore, the nerve is called the vagus nerve because of its wandering path through the body.

It supplies most of the internal organs. From its nerve cell body in the brain stem, the vagus nerve leaves the cranial cavity through a hole in the base of the skull, extends, branching out, through the area at the back of the neck, and then runs along the upper surface of the gullet.

Many branches lead off to the heart and lungs from about here. The vagus nerve and the esophagus pierce the diaphragm and form an extensive network around the anterior and posterior walls of the stomach.

Further branches run to the other abdominal organs, such as the liver, spleen, pancreas and most of the intestinal system, up to the left-h-and bend of the large intestine, which lies close to the stomach. The ganglia (groups of nerve cells) of this parasympathetic part of the autonomic nervous system lie close to, or even in, the walls of the organs concerned.

As already mentioned, sympathetic and parasympathetic pathways consist of two nerve cells that make contact with each other in a ganglion situated outside the brain. The first nerve cell arises from the brain or spinal cord and runs to the appropriate ganglion - a pre-ganglionic fiber. The cell body of the second nerve cell lies in the ganglion - a post-ganglionic nerve cell. As a rule, in the parasympathetic nervous system the fibers of the first nerve cell are long and those of the second nerve cell short. In the sympathetic nervous system the rever-se situation applies: here the first (pre-ganglionic) fibers are short, and the se-cond (post-ganglionic) are long.

The parasympathetic nerve fibers that accompany other crani-al nerves apart from the tenth serve, for example, the pupil of the eye and the various glands of the head such as the tear and salivary glands.

From the lowermost part of the spinal cord, the sacral region, come a number of parasympa-thetic nerves that

Parasympathetic nervous system

The nerve cells from which the nerves of the parasympathetic system originate lie in a number of nuclei in the brainstem and in the lower part of the spinal cord. The fibers to the ganglia are shown as solid lines, those from the ganglia to the target organs as broken lines.

Four ganglia are located in the brain.

1. The eye ganglion.
2. The sphenopalatine ganglion.
3. The ear ganglion.
4. The lower jaw ganglion.

Nerve fibers run out from these, for example, to the eye muscles (5), the lacrimal (tear) glands (6), the salivary glands (7) and a number of glands in the upper and lower jaws (8).

The other parasympathetic ganglia lie close to or even in the walls of the organs served by these nerves.

9. Nerve fibers to the lungs.
10. Nerve fibers to the heart and aorta.
11. Nerve fibers to the stomach.
12. Nerve fibers to the liver, gallbladder and pancreas.
13. Nerve fibers to the abdominal aorta.
14. Nerve fibers to the kidneys.
15. Nerve fibers to the ascending part of the colon.
16. Nerve fibers to the descending part of the colon and bladder.
17. Nerve fibers to the genital organs.
18-29. Abdominal ganglia.

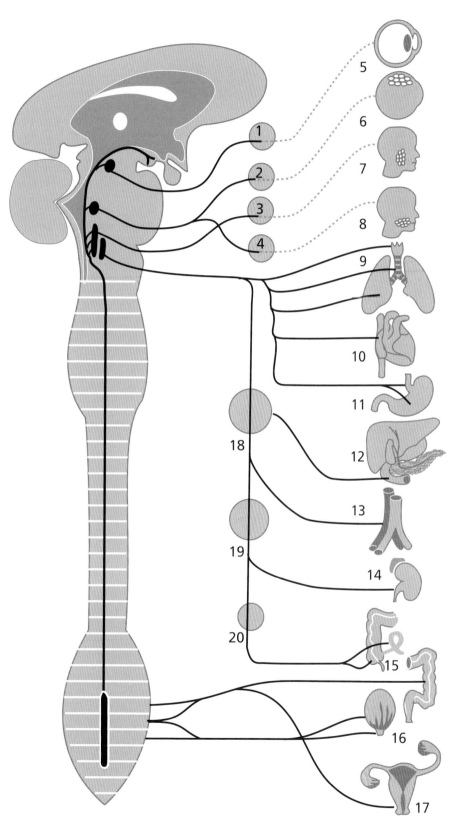

run together as one tra-ct, the pelvic nerve, supplying the or-gans in the pelvis as well as the lowest part of the large intestine. These nerves form a number of networks or plexi, such as the vesicular plexus and the uterovaginal plexus of the female reproductive organs.

Sympathetic nervous system

The cell bodies of the nerve fibers lie alongside the spinal cord from the level of the top of the shoulders to the pelvis. The fibers themselves leave the cord in the anterior root. They then go on to form the paravertebral chain. The connecting link between a spinal cord nerve and the paraver-tebral chain is formed by a white connecting branch.

The axons of the first nerve cell in the spinal cord can make contact with the second nerve cell in various ways. They may run directly to the first gan-glion of the paravertebral chain, and make contact, after which the axon of the second cell accompa-nies the nerve fibers of the somatic ner-vous system.

The connecting link between the par-avertebral chain and the voluntary nerve is a gray connecting branch. In the white branch connecting the spinal cord and perip-heral chain run nerves ensheathed in a fatty insulating layer, while the nerve axons without a similar layer run in the gray connect-ing branch.

The axons run either up or down the para-vertebral chain for a certain dis-tance, then make connection in a higher- or lower-lying ganglion. This explains the difference in length between the paravertebral chain and the extent of spinal cord in which the cell bodies of the first nerve cells lie, for the paravertebral chain lies next to the entire vertebral column.

A third possibility is that the axon of the first nerve cell passes out through the paravertebral chain without mak-ing a connec-tion, and then makes contact with cell bo-dies of second nerve cells in one of the ganglia that lies in front of the vertebral column by the source of the large abdominal arte-ries; they are also named after these arteries.

There are, accordingly, right and left abdominal arterial ganglia lying next to the root of the abdominal artery, which supplies the stomach, liver and spleen with blood.

The second ganglion lies next to the root of the upper mesenteric artery; the third ganglion lies next to the root of he lower mesenteric artery. The axons of the second spinal cord nerve cells start from these ganglia; they accompany the arteries and supply the same areas.

Functions of the autonomic nervous system

If we are to understand the function of the autonomic nervous system, and therefore how the sympathetic and parasympathetic nerves control and modulate the action of many organs, it is important to realize that almost all the organs of the body are doubly innervated.

This means that nerves of both the sympathetic and the parasympathetic nervous systems terminate in the walls of organs to supply the smooth muscles, etc. Only a few organs in the body have a single nerve supply. These are the core (medulla) of the adrenal glands, the sweat glands and most of the blood vessels, particularly those of the skin and muscles.

This means that, in the case of the most important organs, one can therefore speak of antagonistic action (action in opposite directions).

This difference in function is made possible by the fact that different chemical transmitters are secreted at the terminals of the sympathetic and parasympathe-tic nerves, acetyl-choline being the one discharged at the terminals of the parasym-pathetic fibers and noradrenaline at the termi-nals of the sympathetic fibers.

For the transmission of stimulation, it is also important that, in the ganglion, the acetyl-choline employed for trans-mission between the first and second nerve cells is used up. The nerves that secrete acetylcholine are called cholin-ergic, and those that secrete noradren-aline are adrenergic.

Besides this double innervation, a dis-tinction can still be drawn between an anta-gonistic and a synergistic twin innerva-tion. Antagonistic twin innervation has both an activating and inhibiting effect.

This me-chanism plays a part in the innerva-tion of such organs as the heart, lungs, stomach and intesti-ne. In the case of synergistic twin inner-vation, both parts of the autonomic nervous system, i.e. both sympathetic and parasympathetic nerves, have an activating effect on the organ.

This is the case in the salivary glands, for example, where stimula-tion of either the sympathetic or parasympa-thetic nerves increases the secretion; but the composition of the saliva that is secre-ted changes accordingly.

Although the sympathetic nervous system is capable of affec-ting the var-ious organs individually, it should be realized that it has a tendency to affect a number of organs at the same time. This function can be defi-ned as the mobilization (making available) and utilization of energy. To achieve this the metabolism must be speeded up. The blood supply of active organs such as the muscles is increased by the widening of blood ves-sels (to increase blood flow) and a quicke-ning of the heart rate. If possible, the action of a number of other organs, such as the stomach and intestines, is simultaneous-ly inhibited.

In general, the sympathetic mecha-nism or reaction pattern is activated in situations in which the body must act, in what have been called "flight or fight" situations. Another good description of the whole complex is given by the term stress.

The sympathetic nervous system is mainly activated when increased mus-cle activity is necessary. Apart from such situations, the sympathetic reac-tion pattern also plays a part in excite-ment, pain, exposure to cold, etc.

The parasympathetic nervous system, on the other hand, has the opposite function, whi-ch, to put it in the same terms, is to redu-ce activity and save energy. Stimulation of the para-sym-pathetic nerves gives rise to a slacken-ing of the heart rhythm and rates of breathing, while the organs that are concerned with the taking up and digestion of food (stomach, intestine) are restored to their normal function. Those parts of the parasympathetic nervous system that origina-te from the lower area of the spinal cord have a particular evacuating function: their activation leads to contraction of the large intestine, rectum and bladder.

Sympathetic nervous system

The nerve cells from which the nerves of the sympathetic system originate lie in the thoracic and upper two lumbar segments of the spinal cord. The fibers to the ganglia in the paravertebral chain are shown as solid lines, those from the ganglia to the target organs as broken lines.

Four ganglia are located in the brain.

1. The eye ganglion.
2. The sphenopalatine ganglion.
3. The ear ganglion.
4. The lower jaw ganglion.

Nerve fibers run out from these, for example, to the eye muscles (5), the lacrimal (tear) glands (6), the salivary glands (7) and a number of glands in the upper and lower jaws (8).

The other sympathetic ganglia lie in the paravertebral chain.

9. Nerve fibers to the lungs.
10. Nerve fibers to the heart and aorta.
11. Nerve fibers to the stomach.
12. Nerve fibers to the liver, gall-bladder and pancreas.
13. Nerve fibers to the abdominal aorta.
14. Nerve fibers to the kidneys.
15. Nerve fibers to the ascending part of the colon.
16. Nerve fibers to the descending part of the colon and bladder.
17. Nerve fibers to the genital organs.
18-29. Abdominal ganglia.

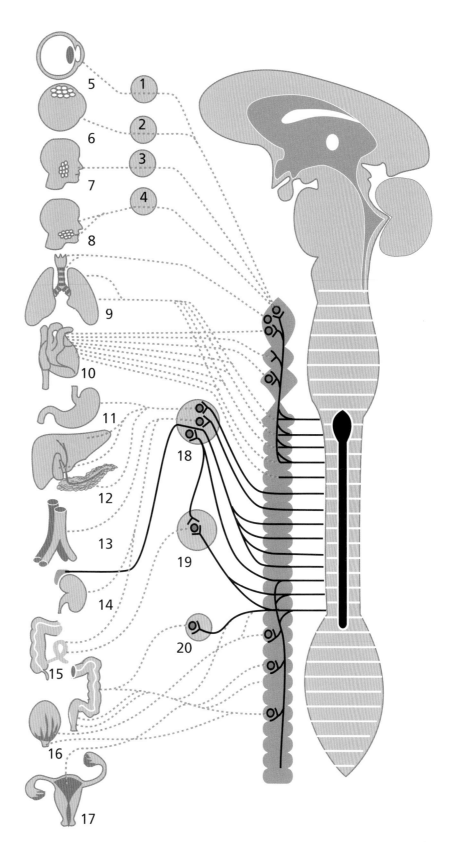

10 Glands and Hormones

Introduction

A gland is a cell or tissue that removes specific substances from the blood, alters or concentrates them, and then either releases them for further use within or on the body or eliminates them.

Typically, a gland consists of either cuboidal or columnar epithelium resting on a basement membrane, and is surrounded by a plexus, or meshwork, of blood vessels.

Endocrine or ductless glands (e.g., pituitary, thyroid, adrenal) produce substances known as hormones directly into the bloodstream rather than through ducts. Exocrine glands (e.g., salivary, sweat, digestive) discharge their products through ducts.

Exocrine glands

The structure and function of exocrine glands will be illustrated by

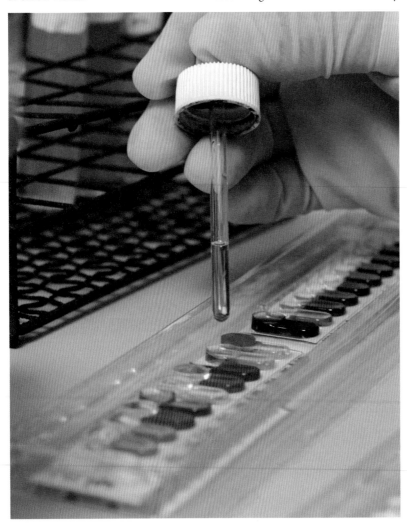

the glands in the skin, which are the most numerous of all exocrine glands in the body.

Sebaceous glands

These occur everywhere over the skin surface with the exception of the palms of the hands and the soles of the feet. They are abundant in the scalp and face and are numerous around the apertures of the nose, mouth, external ears, and anus.

Each gland is composed of a number of epithelial cells and is filled with larger cells containing fat. These cells are cast off bodily, their detritus forms the secretion, and new cells are continuously formed.

Occasionally, the ducts open upon the surface of the skin, or more frequently they open into the hair follicles. In the latter case, the secretion from the gland passes out to the skin along the air. Their size is not regulated by the length of the hair.

The largest sebaceous glands are found on the nose and other parts of the face, where they may become enlarged with accumulated secretion. This retained secretion often becomes discoloured, giving rise to the condition commonly known as blackheads. It also provides a medium for the growth of pus-producing organisms and consequently is a common source of pimples and boils.

Sebum is the secretion of the sebaceous glands. In contains fats, soaps, cholesterol, albuminous material, remnants of epithelial cells, and inorganic salts. It serves to protect the hairs from becoming too dry and brittle, as well as from becoming too easily saturated with moisture.

Upon the surface of the skin sebum forms a thin protective layer, which serves to prevent undue absorption or evaporation of water from the skin.

Microchemical analysis of the molecular structure of hormones.

This secretion keeps the skin soft and pliable. An accumulation of this sebaceous matter upon the skin of the fetus furnishes the thick, cheesy, oily substance called the cervix caseosa.

Sweat glands

Sudoriferous, or sweat, glands are abundant over the whole skin but are largest and most numerous in the axillae, the palms of the hands, the soles of the feet, and the forehead.

Each gland consists of a single tube, with a blind, coiled end which is lodged in the subcutaneous tissue. From the coiled end, the tube is continued as the excretory duct of the gland up through the corium and epidermis and finally opens on the surface of a pore.

Each tube is lined with secreting epithelium. The coiled end is closely invested by capillaries, and the blood in the capillaries is separated from the cavity of the glandular tube by a thin membranes which form their respective walls.

Under ordinary circumstances, the perspiration that the body is continually throwing off evaporates from the surface of the body without one's becoming aware of it and is called insensible perspiration.

When more sweat is poured upon the surface of the body than can be removed at once by evaporation, it appears on the skin in the form of drops and is then spoken of as sensible perspiration.

Ceruminous glands

The skin lining the external auditory canal contains modified sweat glands called ceruminous glands. They secrete a yellow, pasty substance resembling wax, which is called cerumen. An accumulation of cerumen deep in the auditory canal may interfere with hearing.

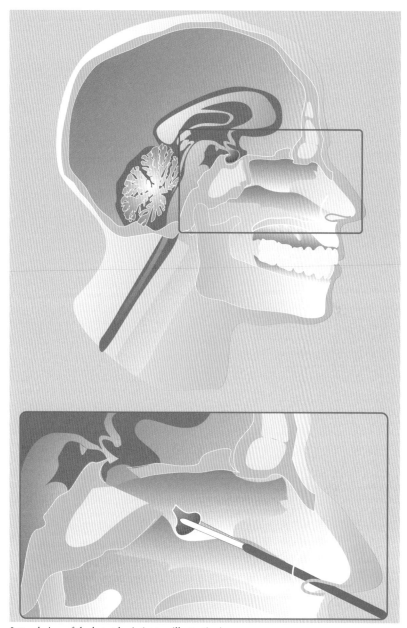

Lateral view of the hypophysis (upper illustration).
The lower figure shows schematically the approach of a tumor in the hypophysis through the nose.

Endocrine glands

The endocrine system consists of glands or parts of glands whose secretions (called hormones) are distributed in the human body by means of the bloodstream rather than being discharged through ducts. The glandular tissues of the endocrine system have in common that they secrete into the bloodstream "chemical messengers" that regulate and integrate body functions. One of the characteristics of the endocrine glands is their wanderlust, their tendency to leave their source and look for work elsewhere. The human embryo develops gills like those of primitive fishes, but parts of these turn into endocrine glands and leave their birthplace at the sides of the throat in the course of their embryonic development. The pituitary gland, the thyroid, the parathyroids and the thymus develop in part from these primitive gills.

The two adrenal glands do not migrate far. They form in the peritoneum of the abdomen and then settle on top of the kidneys. A group of

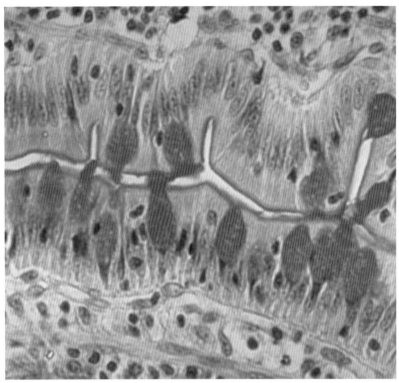

Microscopic section of epithelium showing various endocrine glands.

Hormones

A hormone is a complex chemical product produced and secreted by endocrine (ductless) glands that ravels through the bloodstream and controls and regulates the activity of another organs or groups of cells - its target organ.

For instance, growth hormone released by the pituitary body controls the growth of long bones in the body.

Hormones are produced and released by the endocrine system. This is a network of endocrine glands of the following organs:
-   pituitary gland or body;
-   hypothalamus;
-   thyroid;
-   thymus
-   parathyroids;
-   adrenal medulla;
-   adrenal cortex;
-   islets of Langerhans in the pancreas;
-   gonads;
-   thymus;
-   pineal gland or epiphysis;
-   groups of cells in the stomach and intestines.

Along with the nervous system, the endocrine system coordinates and regulates many of the activities in the body, including growth, metabolism, sexual development, and reproduction.

The rhythm of hormone secretions

Unlike the heart or skin or stomach, the hormonal glands do not work in the same way from the birth of the body to its death.

The life of man has three divisions. The first part is childhood, during which he grows; in this period the growth hormone from the pituitary is particularly active, while the gonads or sex glands are at rest.

Then comes puberty, so called from the pubes, the hair around the genitals. This hair appears only after the gonads begin to work, and they start only after the growth hormone is slowing down and the body has grown to a certain size.

In the third division of life, some thirty to forty years after the onset of the function of the gonads, these latter glands usually begin to wither. A

cells from the neighbouring sympathetic nervous system migrates into the adrenal glands and forms a core there. Thus the adrenal glands become double organs, with a nervous core or marrow and a glandular cortex or bark. The cortex produces a series of steroids, the corticosteroids, which have wide-ranging effects. The core functions in conjunction with the sympathetic nervous system, regulating the blood pressure, the heart action and other activities of the body, through the secretion of adrenalin and noradrenaline.

Another double organ is the pancreas. Its ordinary glandular tissue produces the various digestive enzymes that serve to open the molecular chains of proteins, carbohydrates, and fats. In this digestive gland there settled an endocrine gland in the form of little islands of tissue that fabricate the hormones insulin and glucagon.

Similar double organs are the sex glands. These produce the germinating cells, the sperm cells in the man and the egg cells (ova) in a woman; they also produce sex hormones that

flow through the blood and give rise to such secondary traits as the beard of the male and the breasts of the female. One gland, the pituitary or hypophysis, hangs under the brain like a fire bell, serving to regulate all the endocrine glands.

An outstanding example of the transformation of an old organ is the pineal body or epiphysis. Among the ancestors of man there must have been a reptile that spent its days lying lazy in the mud of primordial swamps, looking toward the sky through a third eye that developed out of the midbrain.

Only some reptiles of an almost vanished prehistoric past around Australia still possess faint remnants of such an eye. In man this remnant has been transformed into a small cone-shaped body on the roof of the brain, the pineal body.

Its function in man is unknown; some believe it is merely investigial while others believe that it is an endocrine gland whose secretions affect the gonads either directly or via the anterior part of the pituitary gland.

woman's menstruation ends and with it her fertility; the man may loose part of his potency.

The endocrine glands and their hormones determine part of the fate of man.

A child with an underactive thyroid gland remains stunted physiologically, a cretin is mentally and sluggish in temperament. The endocrine glands may well be called the glands of our destiny.

The hormone concept

The difficulty in formulating a precise definition of the term *hormone* is particularly well illustrated by the catecholamines noradrenaline and adrenalin.

When their production in and release from the adrenal medulla is being considered adrenalin and noradrenaline are usually called hormones, but in their role as signal mediators at the sympathetic nerve endings they are called *transmitter substances.*

The hormone concept has become even more vague since it has been realized that the so-called regulatory hypothalamic hormones - a group of peptides that includes the enkephalins and endorphins as well as the neurohormones ADH (antidiuretic hormone, or vasopressin) and oxytocin as the releasing hormones - act not only as hormones in the strict sense but also have what appears to be a transmitter function or a modulating influence on the function of other transmitter systems.

Basic functions of hormones

The hormones perform three basic functions:

▲ hormones enable and promote physical, sexual and mental development;

▲ hormones enable and promote the adjustment of performance level; the ability of organs and organ systems to modify their activity to meet the demands made upon them is lost in the absence of certain hormones;

▲ hormones are necessary to keep certain physiological parameters constant (e.g., osmotic pressure and the blood glucose level). These hormones have a homeostatic function.

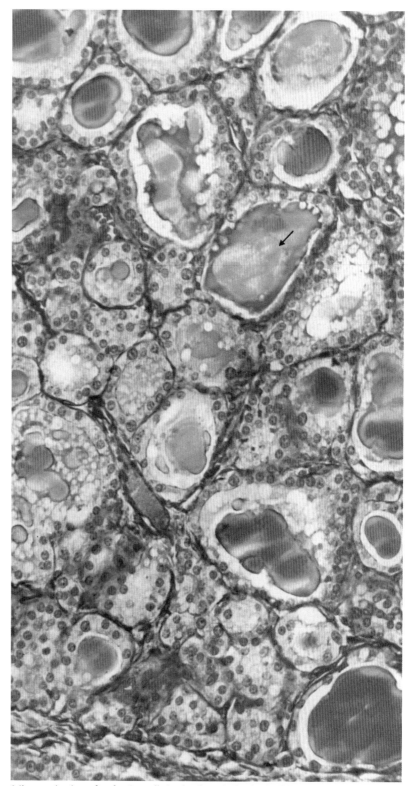

Microscopic view of endocrine cells in the thyroid gland. The follicles (arrow) contain hormones bound to proteins.

Making of a family

Models of relationships

We want to be close to other people - to matter to them, to know that thy will be there when we need them, to feel safe, loving and loved - this closeness is essential to our well-being. Most men and women seek to fulfil much of this need for closeness through intimate sexual relationships with women or men. As we grew up, we learned one pattern or model for these relationships: our families and communities expected women to marry and have children; men would earn the most money.

When two people meet, there are actually six selves present simultaneously. There is myself as I perceive me, as the other perceives me and as I actually am. Then there is the other person as she/he perceives herself/himself, as I perceive her/him and as she/he actually is.

How we develop and perceive ourselves is obviously very tricky and complex, but it is all the more complicated when others are involved. Not only do we all cover up our real selves to others, but we hide parts of our "selves" from ourself. In order to live a happy life, we must have a positive self-concept. Sometimes we tell ourselves as good-looking, intelligent or having a good singing voice, for example. Usually we are put on the tract of accurate perception by the cues of others around us, particularly close friends and relatives, people whose judgment we trust and have confidence in. These cues may be vary direct or subtle. Sometimes we pick up on them; at other times we may choose to ignore them.

At times, though, we are unable to be our real selves for a variety of reasons. Consider the boy who is afraid of animals and cries when approached by a barking dog. His father or mother may comment that men are not afraid of such small animals. What a quandary! The developing and evolving self and self-concept are dependent upon what others will or will not allow us to be. Reactions of others, however, are not always responses to what we are doing as much as they are responses to how they are handling the situation. A dying person, for example., is usually very angry but may not know how to express the anger or at whom to direct it. Frequently, the nurse, being the most available person, may bear the brunt of this emotional expression. Each of us wears many masks or roles that we move into and out of. Certainly, we maintain a certain set of roles, and other persons expect us to act consistently within these roles. But occasionally we act out of character, and that can present problems for everyone. Nevertheless, we have a constant, ongoing need to alter our roles or try new ones. The growing individual continually probes his or her potentials, including all the possible functioning roles. Usually these changes are minor, involving such things as hair style, clothing, or friends.

Roles and social environment

The hardest part of the task of venturing into different roles is that our social environment fosters getting and keeping a fixed role. We are forced into

At every stage along the line of growth and development, your actions, your attitude, your love affect the emotional outlook and behavior of the child.

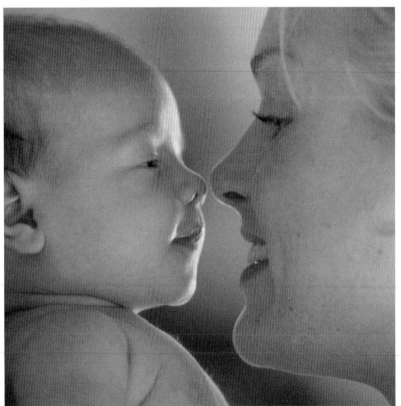

a certain identity, beginning with the expectations of basic sexual and cultural roles and moving quickly into employment oles.

The usual first question when meting a person is: What do you do? This necessitates a role answer - I am a student, doctor, dancer, salesperson - with all the accompanying stereotypes. Even the answer "nothing" conjures up stereotypical images such as a loafer, hippie, unambitious, incompetent and the like.

People are simultaneously part of many larger groups. Others see us as having sexual, racial, and religious roles; living in a certain geographical area; working at a particular job; being married or not; and so on.

It is impossible to be so objective that we can immediately put all biases aside and see the real persons we encounter. Perhaps one of the most difficult tasks of the helping professions is enabling persons to overcome the stifling aspects of role playing and to focus on true identity or self-concept.

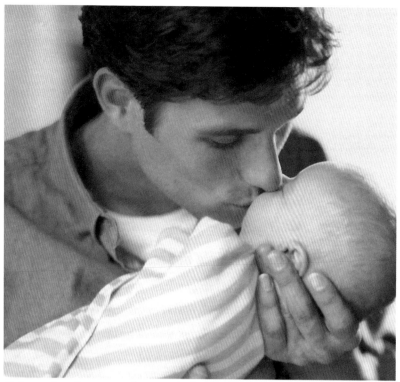

Fathers and mothers are equal partners in the education of their children.

Parent, adult or child

We interact with others in the role of parent, adult or child. Being in the role of parent is to act as your parent did in the past in terms of oral and body language and feelings.

Since everyone has had a parent or parent substitute, we have all observed how to act as parent, how to set rules, protect and teach. The parent role may be played directly, as our own parents acted, or indirectly, as parents generally influence children.

Everyone likewise plays an adult role, which begins during the first years of life, in that we are all capable of some independent, autonomous thinking and self-determinant actions. This is the part of ourselves that must be present for survival. It takes in external data, processes it and makes decisions leading to correct, objective responses. The adult role also has the function of balancing or regulating the parent and child activities.

The child role is also present in each of us. We were all cared for during early life and are still cared for in var-ious ways from time to time, even if it is a simple thing like being served in a restaurant.

Whereas the adult processes external data, the child records internal records to external stimuli. The child may then respond either naturally (creatively) or simply as the parents direct. How any role exhibits itself is dependent upon the many complex factors that make up personality, as well as the specific situation.

Changing and growing

Throughout life, each person continues to change. These changes may be significant and observable or minor and hardly noticeable. It is all part of the evolutionary process, progressing perhaps at the proverbial snail's pace but always proceeding.

It is hoped that this change will be largely in a positive meaningful direction, which then fulfils our definition of growth. healthy growth is that which is allowed to develop with freedom, leading to independence, progress and maturity. It is a matter of reaching forward, toward achievement of potential, and in time further expanding that potential.

Growing involves acting from healthy spontaneity rather than from fear of the repercussions, whether physical or psychological, of one's behavior. Change, however, is not easily accomplished, for it must be accepted not only by oneself but also by other people - particularly, significant others. They must allow these changes to take place. Otherwise, they may invalidate these new aspects of self.

Many people may resist changing and growing because of the pressures put on them to stay the same. This may be particularly true in a marriage relationship when one partner moves into different areas of interest. If the marriage is to remain intact, one partner must accept the change or grow with the other. A long-term satisfactory marriage involves, among other things, a continuous process of moving and catching up. of changing, adjusting, changing again and readjusting.

Maturation

A significant term to characterize a person who is changing, growing and becoming is "maturing." Probably the most important part of the word maturing is the suffix -ing; which implies an ongoing process. It begins, perhaps, with the idea that the human mind at birth is like a tabula rasa, or smooth tablet, with no impressions on it, to be etched or moulded throughout life. The mind is therefore never completed or "mature."

In addition, there are many dimensions of maturity. We mature professionally, physically, psychologically, sexually, socially and philosophically, as a speaker, writer, mover, lover, parent or child. We also mature within the cultural criteria of maturity.

Maturation is a time-consuming process that is based upon undergoing experiences, both positive and negative. We must be involved in a variety of situations and must try out various tactics or behaviors for ourselves before we can meet any criterion for maturity.

The truism "there is no substitute for experience" bears repeating. No amount of reading or simulation can ever truly replace involvement, although obviously, many situations are too dangerous or too involving to experience firsthand. We cannot experience with all kinds of relationships (heterosexual, homosexual, group sex, community living, etc.), for example, in order to know their effects upon our personality.

We cannot experiment with all types of drugs, for example, in order to know their effects upon our organs or brain. We need to depend upon others for information about them. Likewise, we may safely sit in a drive simulator to practice reacting to emergency traffic situations. Even so, the process of doing is an irreplaceable necessity to becoming a mature individual.

Although some experiences may be painful, we ought to approach new experiences with an attitude of challenge and enjoyment, for they promote growth and sustain the process of becoming. Seeking growth experiences involves taking risks, more or less so depending on set and setting. Image a hurdle racer, who is quite advanced in this racing skill. When running at top speed, the hurdler is in a state of controlled, forward-leaning unbalance.

Each hurdle will seemingly come up to the hurdler, rather than the hurdler running up to it. The successful hurdler need only lift the forward leg, and momentum will carry him or her over each barrier, as opposed to having jump over.

If we are in control of our psychological growth and development, we meet each experience as the capable hurdler meets each hurdle. Running at a high speed may increase the consequences of a spill, but significantly reduces the possibilities of falling and simultaneously increases the satisfaction of more fully achieving potential. Likewise, we add to meaning in life by seeking new experiences.

All these experiences involve restructuring or evaluation of previously held beliefs and values. That is risky to both of us and those around us because their consequences may involve such changes as leaving old friends and acquaintances, living in new environments and, most important, altering life styles.

Prof. T. Holmes and Dr. Richard Rahe hypothesize on the basis of American and European data that large or significant alterations in life styles can contribute to physical and mental illness. They have developed a social readjustment rating scale, which compares changes in an individual's life with disabling conditions. Their findings show that a correlation exists between change and illness.

Such events as divorce, death of a sig-

Regardless of culture, climate or background, all children need low and affection to provide a stable environment in which they can mature.

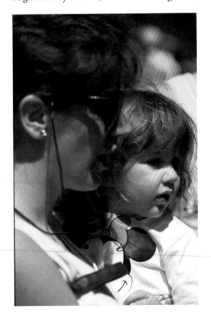
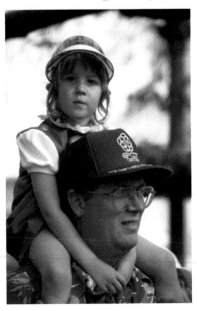
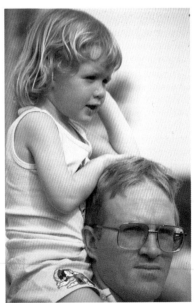

nificant other, change of jobs an moving, alone or in combination, may be stress enough to produce actual physical illness. Among the first ten life events six have to do with relationships, stressing the importance of inter-human contacts in our daily life.

Love and trust

Love is described as:
- a strong feeling of affection
- devoted attachment to a person
- especially, devoted attachment to a person of the opposite sex
- courtship (as in the phrase to make love to, that is, to court).

Love is risky and scary, but not as scary as the alternative - not loving. To love truly and without qualification involves deep commitment, a basic trust and authentic caring for another person. It is reciprocal that we are lovable as well as loving.

Love almost defies definition, since its meaning needs to be qualified over and again.
- To whom or what is love limited?
- What are its conditions?
- How must it be transferred or communicated?
- Are there exceptions to any of the criteria that make up this definition?

Perhaps the best discussion if love is presented by Erich Fromm in his book *The Art of Loving*. He says that "love is the only satisfactory answer to the problem of human existence." Nearly every definition of the mentally healthy individual contains love as one of its criteria.

One of the most useful concepts put forth by Fromm is that there are five basic kinds of love or objects of love:
- brotherly love
- motherly love
- erotic love
- self-love
- love of God

Brotherly love

The first, and most fundamental kind of love is brotherly love - a love of the world. It is the loving feeling we get when we are together with a mass of people and our skin tingles from being with others. This love of all human beings is a love of equals in

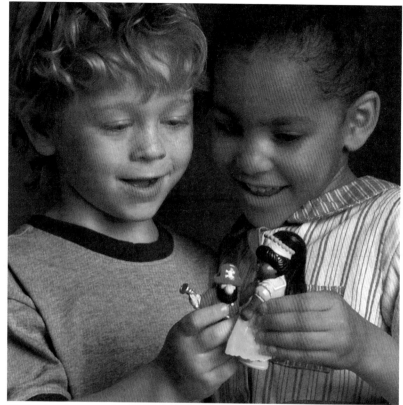

Playing is so important for children that it takes up a large part of the first six-year period of growth.

that we are all people and share a common humanity.

Motherly love

Motherly love is an unconditional affirmation of a person's life. I exist, therefore I am loved. It is in one sense passive, since the child need not to do anything overtly to earn this love. A love that must be earned by deed is tenuous and unstable, since it may disappear whenever the desired behavior is withdrawn.

As a child grows, this more or less one-way love becomes reciprocal, beginning at about age eight to ten years. Unlike brotherly love, this relationship is based on inequality, in which one fulfils the other's need.

A difficulty in motherly love occurs when the child passes infancy, and parents expect the child to show a reciprocating appreciation. If the child does not respond as the parent expects, all kinds of conflict arises that may or may not be satisfactorily

resolved. Eventually, this love should grow into a mature motherly/fatherly love, transferring not only to the father but to others as well. As an adult, the person that develops a motherly or fatherly conscience.

Erotic love

Erotic love involves the desire for complete union with another person. Unlike motherly or brotherly love, it is not universal in nature but is aimed at completing a relationship physically as well as "spiritually" with another.

It is a sexual fulfilment that extends beyond immediate gratification. Although erotic love is exclusive, involving two people, there may also be present an element of brotherly lover, since it is a love involving equals.

Self-love

To love others as human beings is to love oneself as a human being. Thus, self-love and love of others are sepa-

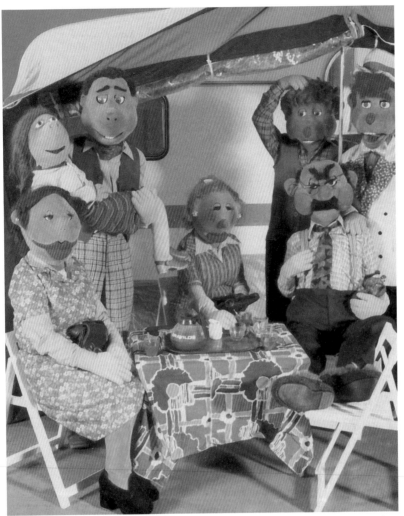

All children move along the upward ladder of growth according to their own inner development. Children love to make a show and perform.

we may feel both erotic and brotherly love for the same person; and different people may love us in many ways. One important characteristic of love between two people is that each fits into the life space of the other.

Man and wife may have equal and reciprocal needs that each other can fulfil, and the meeting of these needs, or wants, forms the basis of a loving relationship, although it is certainly not enough for a lasting, mature love. A relationship of only meeting wants (for instance, a simple motherly love relationship), would be only temporary and not unconditional.

There is a distinction between a symbiotic union, in which each partner feeds the wands and needs of the other, and mature love, in which a desired union occurs simultaneously while preserving individual identity.

The symbiotic union may be passive, in which one partner submits to the dominance of the other. In clinical psychological terms, this is a masochistic role in that the subdominant person copes with separateness by becoming part of the other person's personality. There is also an active role, which is the antithesis of the passive type. It is the dominant partner who makes the "weaker" one part of himself or herself.

Mature love

Mature love requires a high degree of giving and taking. it is virtually impossible in a practical sese for both partners to be constantly and completely equal. Dominance may swing from one person to the other. Each may have a set of strengths and weaknesses; each may have greater or lesser desires and motivation in particular realms of interest.

Mature love beings with it a fusion of two strong and equal but complementary individual personalities. Both must be able to give as well as to receive. Love mst also incorporate the elements of care, responsibility, respect and knowledge. Care is the genuine concern for the life and well-being of those we truly love.

Responsibility is a completely voluntary readiness to act in the best interests of another. Respect is the ability

rately connected. It has been a normal value that to love oneself is sinful, but self-love is not synonymous with selfishness.

A selfish person is incapable of loving himself or herself and therefore is unable to love others. A common fear is that narcissism may be carried to extreme so that love of self becomes an obsession. It is normal and healthy, however, to go through the narcissistic stage; it is only when someone returns to it later in life that it can interfere with functioning.

Love of God

Love of God is the realization of that which "God" represents to oneself. It is dependent upon the individual's spiritual perceptions of what is best for that person, and is not universal for all people.

It emanates from the desire to overcome a separateness and find union within the universe. In the Western religions, love of God is through experience, but for Eastern religions, love of God is a feeling of oneness.

Loving relationship

Merely describing love objects does not say anything about the quality of a loving relationship or the complexity of various kinds of love. For example, to see loves ones as unique individuals and to allow them to grow and develop at their pace ad style.

Knowledge is the accurate perception of the partner's individual density aside from oneself. All these elements constitute the prerequisite to mature love.

Love as a basic human need

Another way of distinguishing between what is and is not mature love has been developed by Prof. Abraham Maslow. Love is one of the basic human needs; if not met, the individual is, of course, deficient and must strive to overcome this deficit.

Maslow calls this love need D-love, or deficiency love, which is selfish love. On the other hand, the person (child or adult) whose love need is being fulfilled has B-love, or love for the being of others, which is an unselfish and giving love.

B-love is enjoyed completely for itself rather than as a means to achieve some goal. It is an en in itself and yet has no ending, since it continually grows. B-lovers are less demanding, feel less threatened or jealous, and act more independently and autonomously than D-lovers.

B-love is open; partners disclose more of themselves, drop their defences, act with spontaneity and need not depend upon living a role to protect themselves.

This may seem to involve a higher degree of risk-taking, but there is actually more security in the relationship. B-love is obviously a more complete, richer, worthwhile and enhancing experience. It allows the optimum development for each person.

I-You relationship

Similar to Maslow's B-love is Martin Buber's I-You relationship. I-You is not two single words, but a word pair; thus, it described not two beings but the relationship of one to the other.

This relationship must involve the sphere of nature, other human beings or spiritual beings. Buber uses another word pair, I-IT, to describe our attitude toward another person or an object. The I of I-It is different from the I and I-you, just as the I-You rela-

tionship differs from the I-It attitude. I-You centers on people (including ourselves) and things as part of the whole. They are not objects to be experiences or explained. It is like a song that we experience in its entirety, rather than listening to one note at a time. I-IT analyzes ad perceives each note of the song as a separate entity. I-It encounters and sees objects. I-You is an association.

We react on the world on two levels. On the one hand, we meet everything and everyone as being and becoming. This is a cosmic existence that defies measurement. On the other hand, we perceive our physical boundaries, we see things and record them in terms of time and space.

This is an orderly and logical world, which is relatively reliable, has definable physical properties, and constitutes what we know to be tested truths. In practical terms related to the process of living the best life., we each need to reach a happy medium of I-You and I-It perceptions and relationships.

This is not to say that everyone has to achieve the same absolute balance of I-You and I-It, but both are necessary for optimal functioning. Not with everyone we meet can we establish strong I-You connections, although there are some who mistakingly think they are able to do this on the personal level.

The I-You love situation is only occasionally effectuated, and these peak experiences, in order to happen, must be tempered with I-=It perceptions. The I-It world sets up the I-You relationships and makes it possible.

An I-You relationship is the goal of loving. It is the implicit trust that allows and leads to the communication (or co-union) of two people as one. Lovers may be parent-child, brother-sister, man-woman or any two people. Communion between two people can take an infinite number of symbolic and actual forms.

Committed relationships

Feelings of love or sexual attraction do not always equate with commit-

"Oral activity" is an important tool in exploring the world. Children will put everything in their mouth.

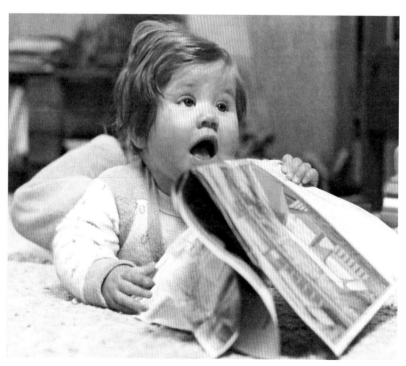

ment in relationships. There can be love without commitment and there can be sex without commitment. The concept of commitment in a relationship with another person means there is an intent to act over time in a way that perpetuates the well-being of the other person, yourself, and the relationship. A committed relationship involves tremendous diligence on the part of both partners. Over the years, partners learn one another and constantly adjust the direction of their relationship. The amount of work creating a successful relationship may intimidate the uncommitted person. It should be remembered that very few people have the skills and tools at the beginning of the relationship to sustain it. What separates committed from uncommitted relationships is the willingness of committed partners to dedicate themselves toward acquiring and using the skills that will ensure a lasting relationship. Data from polls in various Western countries show that more than 90%of the population strives to develop a committed relationship.

Marriage

Marriage is the traditional committed relationship in our society. When a couple marries, they enter into a legal agreement that includes shared financial plans, property, and responsibility in raising children. For religious people, marriage is also a sacrament stressing the spirituality, rights, and obligations of each person.

As with all relationships, there are marriages that work and bring much satisfaction to the partners, and there are marriages that are not healthy for the people involved. A good marriage can yield much support and stability not only for the couple but also those involved in the couple's life. Because marriage is socially sanctioned and highly celebrated in our culture, there are numerous incentives to stay together and improve the relationship. Large weddings, elaborate wedding gifts, and the honeymoon are just the beginning of the social sanctions that reinforce marriage. Behavioral scientists agree that couples who make some type of formal commitment are more likely to stay together and develop the fulfilling relationship they initially sought than those who do not commit.

Because marriage is the most traditional and socially accepted form of committed relationship, it has both the advantage and disadvantage of carrying with it certain expectations.

Cohabitation

For various reasons, many people prefer to live together without the bonds of matrimony. Commonly called cohabitation, this type of relationship is defined as two people who have an intimate connection with each other living together in the same household. The relationship can be very stable with the highest level of commitment between the partners.

The disadvantage of cohabitation lies in the lack of societal validation for the relationship and, in some cases, the societal is approval of living together without being married. The couple usually does not experience the social incentives to stay together that they would if they were married. If they decide to separate, however, they also do not experience the legal problems of going through a divorce.

Lesbian couples

In estimated 6.5% of all women in our country are involved in intimate relationships with other women. Lesbians are socialized like other women in the culture and tend to place high values on relationships. Lesbians seek the same things in their primary relationships as do heterosexual partners: communication, validation, companionship. and a sense of stability.

Some lesbians to achieve long-term., and even life-long relationships. General statements concerning the frequency of these relationships are difficult to make. We do not know that because of social, legal, and some religious restrictions against homosexual people it is more difficult for lesbian couples to create and maintain a balanced, long-lasting relationship than for heterosexual couples.

Homosexual male couples

Media attention given to gay men often centers around their sexual behavior. especially since the AID epidemic. Although it is true that young homosexual men generally have more sexual partners than heterosexual men and women, it is also true that gay men form committed, long-lasting relationships.

As with the data for lesbian couples, reports on numbers of partners and length of relationships are varied. The literature indicate that some male homosexuals enter life-long, monogamous relationships whereas others have many sexual partners.

Among both homosexuals and heterosexuals, younger men express a greater need for independence and freedom from a partner, whereas older man place more emphasis on companionship and commitment. Gay men who form partnerships in their thirties or forties tend to stay together for many years or for a lifetime.

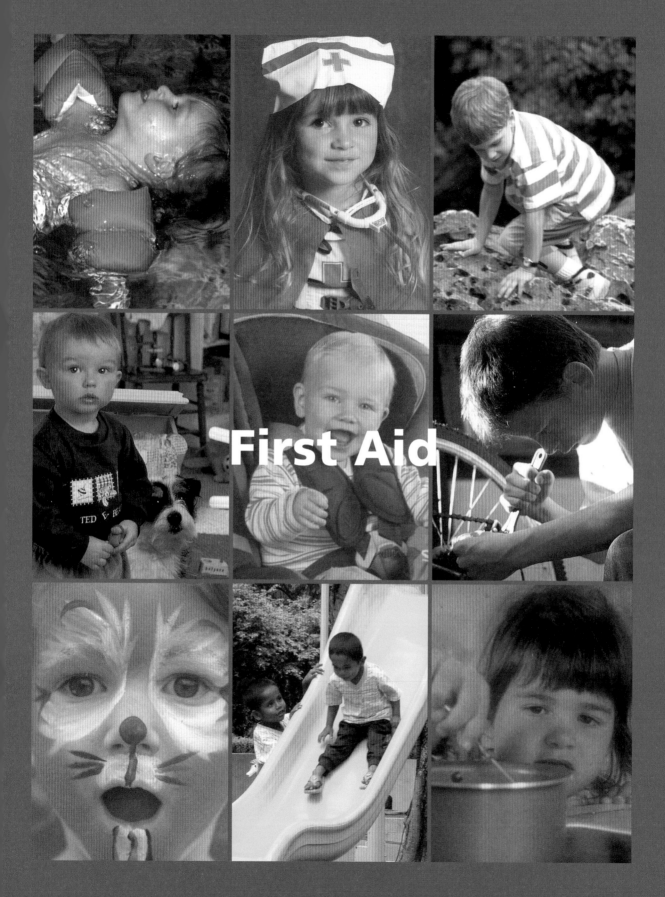

First Aid

General principles

First aid is the immediate care given to a person who is injured or suddenly becomes ill. First aid includes recognizing life-threatening conditions and taking action to keep the injured or ill person alive and in the best possible condition until medical treatment can be obtained.

First aid does not replace the physician. One of the first principles of first aid is to obtain medical assistance in all cases of serious injury. The principal aims of first aid are as follows:
- To care for life-threatening injuries and complications.
- To minimize infection.
- To make the victim as comfortable as possible to conserve strength.
- To transport the victim to medical facilities, when necessary, in such a manner as not to complicate the injury or subject the victim to unnecessary discomfort.

First-aiders should know how to supply artificial ventilation and circulation, control bleeding, protect injuries from infection and other complications. When first aid is properly administered, the victim's chances of recovery are greatly increased.

First-aiders must be able to take charge of a situation, keep calm while working under pressure, and organize others to do likewise. By demonstrating competence and using well-selected words of encouragement, first-aiders should win the confidence of others nearby and do everything possible to reassure the apprehensive victim.

When a person is injured, someone must
- take charge;
- administer first aid;
- arrange for medical assistance.

First-aiders should take charge with full recognition of their own limitations and, while caring for life-threatening conditions, direct others briefly and clearly as to exactly what they should do and how to secure assistance.

Primary survey

Several conditions are considered life-threatening, but three in particular require immediate action:
- Respiratory arrest
- Circulatory failure
- Severe bleeding

Respiratory arrest and/or circulatory failure can set off a chain of events that will lead to death. Severe and uncontrolled bleeding can lead to an irreversible state of shock in which death is inevitable. Death may occur in a very few minutes if an attempt is not made to help the victim in these situations.

The first-aider should perform the primary survey to determine the extent of the problem as soon as the victim is reached, and if any of the life-threatening conditions are found, begin first aid procedures without delay. In checking for adequate breathing, an open airway must be established and maintained. If there are no signs of breathing, artificial ventilation must immediately be

General First Aid Principles

The following procedures are generally applicable:
- Take charge: instruct someone to obtain medical help and others to assist as directed.
- Make a primary survey of the victim.
- Care for life-threatening conditions.
- Care for all injuries in order of need.
- If several people have been injured, decide upon priorities in caring for each victim.
- Keep the injured person lying down.
- Loosen restricting clothing from the victim.
- When necessary, improvise first aid materials using the most appropriate material available.
- Cover all wounds completely.
- Use a tourniquet only as necessary.
- Exclude air from burned surfaces as quickly as possible by using a suitable dressing.
- Remove small, loose foreign objects from a wound by brushing away from the wound with a piece of sterile gauze.
- Do not attempt to remove embedded objects.
- Place a bandage compress and a bandage over an open fracture without undue pressure before applying splints.
- Support and immobilize fractures and dislocations.
- Leave the reduction of fractures or dislocations to a doctor except lower jaw dislocations when help is delayed.
- Never move a victim, unless absolutely necessary, until fractures have been immobilized.
- Test a stretcher before use, and carefully place an injured person on the stretcher.
- Carry the victim on a stretcher without any unnecessary rough movements.

First Aid Kit

To make a complete home set of emergency supplies, the following additional items should be added.
- a three- or four-inch-wide elastic bandage
- two slings - pieces of cotton material about 36 inches square
- scissors with rounded tips
- tweezers
- large and small safety pins
- syrup of ipecac (to induce vomiting)
- acetaminophen or aspirin
- antihistamine
- petroleum jelly
- rubbing (isopropyl) alcohol (used to relieve itching and to clean skin)
- calamine lotion (used to relieve itching)
- two thermometers (one oral, one rectal)
- cotton swabs
- cotton balls
- ce bag
- hot-water bottle or heating pad
- a first-aid manual

given. If a victim experiences circulatory failure, a person trained in cardiopulmonary resuscitation (CPR) should check for a pulse, and, if none is detected, start CPR at once. A careful and thorough check must be made for any severe bleeding, Serious bleeding must be controlled by proper methods.

In making the primary survey, the first-aider must be careful not to move the victim any more than is necessary to support life. Rough handling or any unnecessary movement might cause additional pain and aggravate serious injuries that have not yet been detected.

Secondary survey

When the life-threatening conditions have been controlled, the secondary survey should begin. The secondary survey is head-to-toe examination to check carefully for any additional unseen injuries that can cause serious complications.

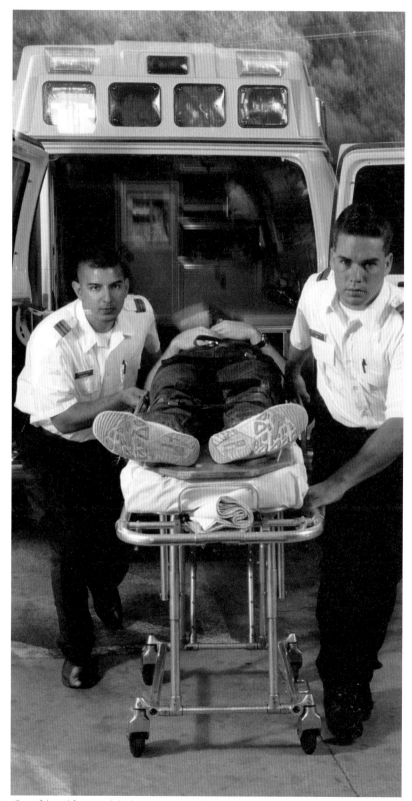

Casualties with severe injuries require immediate action and urgent transport to hospital.

2 Scalds and burns

A burn is an injury that results from contact with heat, chemical agents, electricity, or radiation. Burns vary in depth, size, and degree of severity. The problems most often associated with burns are the following:

▲ Loss of body fluids contributing to shock.
▲ Pain contributing to shock.
▲ Anxiety contributing to shock.
▲ Swelling.
▲ Infection due to destruction of skin tissue.
▲ Airway or respiratory difficulties.

Classification of burns

Burns may be classified according to cause. The four major types of burns by cause are as follows: thermal, chemical, electrical, and radiation. Burns may also be classified according to extent and depth of damage:

▲ First degree burns
- The burned area is painful.
- The outer skin is reddened.
- Slight swelling is present.
▲ Second degree burns
- The burned area is painful.
- The underskin is affected.
- Blisters may be formed.
- The area may have a wet, shiny appearance because of exposed tissue.
▲ Third degree burns
- Insensitive due to the destruction of nerve endings.
- Skin is destroyed.
- Muscle tissues and bone underneath may be damaged.
- The area may be charred, white, or greyish in colour.

Determining the Severity of Burns

The "Rule of Nines" can be used to quickly calculate the amount of skin surface that has received burns. Most areas of the adult body can be divided into portions of 9 per cent or multiples of 9 per cent. The hand can be used as a good reference, as it represents about one percent of the body. For determining the severity of burns in children and infants, the same percentage as used in adults may be used, with the exception of the head and legs.

The severity of the burn can be determined when the degree of the burn and the amount of body surface burned have been determined. Burns are classified by severity: critical (severe), moderate, or minor.

Critical burns

The following conditions constitute critical burns:

▲ Second degree burns over more than 25 percent of the body.
▲ Third degree burns over more than 10 percent of the body.
▲ Third degree burns involving critical areas (face, hands, feet, or groin).
▲ All burns complicated by respiratory problems, major wounds, or fractures.
▲ All burns that encircle a joint, which may lead to loss of the joint's mobility.

Moderate burns

The following conditions constitute moderate burns:

▲ First degree burns involving most of the body.
▲ Second degree burns between 15 percent to 25 percent of the body.
▲ Third degree burns between 2 and 10 percent of the body (excluding face, hand, and feet).

Minor Burns

The following conditions constitute minor burns:

▲ First degree burns.
▲ Second degree burns over less than 15 per cent of the body.
▲ Third degree burns over less than 2 per cent of the body. (excluding face, hands, and feet).

First Aid Care for Burns

The first aid care rendered to the burn victim largely depends on the cause of the burn and the degree of severity. Regardless of the severity of the burn, however, infection can be serious problem.

Certain principles need to be kept in mind when dealing with any burn victim:

▲ Remove the victim from burn source.
▲ Maintain airway and monitor respiration.
▲ Control any bleeding.
▲ Treat for shock and maintain body heat.
▲ When a burn and soft tissue wound are in the same area, treat as if a burn only.
▲ Remove clothing and loose debris, unless they are sticking to the burned surface.
▲ *Do not* try to clean the burn.
▲ Separate burned surfaces from contact with one another.
▲ Never use ointments, lotions or sprays unless recommended by a physician.
▲ Never use industrial grease or oil, butter, or similar cooking fats on burns.
▲ Do not break blisters.
▲ Splint fractures.
▲ If the victim can receive medical attention within one hour, do not administer fluids orally, as this could induce vomiting.
▲ For the victim of critical or moderate burns, if competent medical help is not available for one hour or more and the victim is conscious and not vomiting.

▲ Give the victim a weak solution of salt and soda (two pinches of slat and one pinch of baking soda to each 8 to 10-ounce glass of water).

▲ Recommend that victim check on tetanus immunization (needed every 5 years).

▲ Transport to a medical facility as soon as possible.

How to prevent accidents

Kettles and teapots
- Keep kettles and teapots out of children's reach, well away from the edges of tables or worktops.
- Remember too that the water in a kettle or teapot can still scald up to half an hour after it has boiled.
- Make sure that your kettle fix is short and out of reach so that children can't tug at it.
- Never keep a kettle simmering. Steam can bald badly.

Hot drinks
- Don't drink anything hot with a child on your lap.
- Don't carry hot drinks over a child's head.
- Don't use table cloths that children can pull.
- Keep hot drinks away from the edges of tables. And remember that a mug is safer than a cup with a narrow base.

Bath time
- Children have died in baths of very hot water. So always put cold water in the bath first and don't have your hot water thermostat set too high.
- Always test the temperature of the water before you put your child in the bath. It should be comfortable warm but not hot. Water doesn't have to be very hot to scald a small child.
- Never leave a baby or toddler alone in the bath.

Cookers
- Toddlers are quite likely to pull at any pan handles they can reach. A good answer is to fit a safetly guard round the cooker top. And turn pan handles away from the edges of the cooker or worktop.

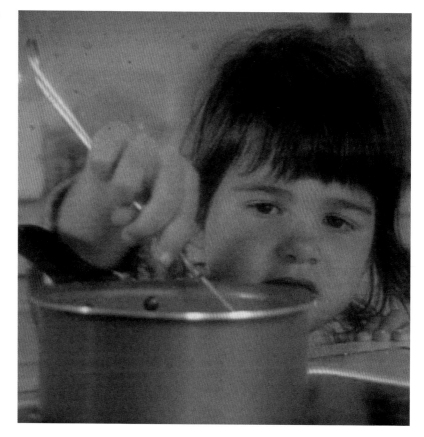

- When you're cooking, or boiling nappies, put your baby in a playpen away from where you are cooking.
- It's best if your cooker is not too near a door and doesn't have cupboards fitted above it. Running through the door, or climbing up to reach something in the cupboard, a child could easily knock over a pan on the cooker.
- It is a good idea to have worktops on both sides of the cooker so that you don't have to carry hot pans across the kitchen.

Around the house
- Switch the iron immediately you finish ironing and put it out children's reach. Remember too that children might pull at the iron flex.
- Keep matches and lighters well out of the reach of children.
- Never take off the guards that are fitted to gas or electric fires. Remember that crawling babies will try to grab hold of anything they can reach, such as a glowing fire element.

- Use special safety fireguards in front of all fires. These should have a cover on top and should be fixed to the fireplace or wall. Use them even before your baby starts to crawl. You never know when your baby will make that first dangerous journey.
- Don't lean anything against, or hang anything on, fireguards.
- Don't use movable electric fires in the bathroom.
- Don't hang a mirror on the wall above a fire. Anybody going close to look in the mirror may be burnt.
- Keep petrol and paraffin away from children and don't store in large quantities.
- When you buy children's night clothes or dressing gowns, try to make sure they are flame-resistant. For derssing gowns and other clothes, remember that flimsy cotton is the most dangerous material.

73

3 Choking and suffocation

Causes

Accidents that cause choking and suffocation can happen all too easily, especially when your children are left alone with something that might be dangerous. So it is important to know what the dangers are and how to avoid them.
Babies are most in danger of choking or suffocation. But older cildren can be at risk when they are playing on their own.

How to prevent accidents

- Beware of polythene bags. They can suffocate if children pull them over their heads.
- Don't use a pillow for babies. Pillows can suffocate.
- Make sure that your baby's cot, and other nursery equipment, are made to an approved design.
- A dummy on a long string or ribbon can get caught or twisted and strangle a baby. If your baby has a dummy, pin it on with a safety pin

and a short ribbon.
- Never leave a baby alone when feeding. A baby left alone with a propped up bottle can easily choke.
- Beware of open-weave nylon cardigans and cardigans with cords or ribbons threaded through the neck. They can catch on a hook or knob in a pram or cot and pull tightly round the baby's neck.
- Babies learn by putting things in their mouths. So remember they can easily choke on small things like buttons, coins, tiny toys and any loose parts of toys like glass eyes.
- Don't give peanuts to young cildren. They are a very common cause of choking.

What to do in an emergency

Choking
- Don't waste time trying to pick the object out with your fingers unless

it is easy to get hold off. Probably it will be too far back and too slippery.
- Hold the baby upside down by the legs. Slap the baby's back smartly between the shoulder blades. If the object doesn't come out, do it again.
- If after several times this hasn't worked, as a last resort give the baby's tummy a short sharp squeeze. This should push the object out of the baby's windpipe.

Suffocation
- Quickly take away whatever is causing the suffocation.
- If the child has stopped breathing, give mouth-to-mouth resuscitation (artificial ventilation).

Artificial ventilation

Artificial ventilation is the process for causing air flow into and from the lungs when natural breathing has ceased or when it is very irregular or inadequate.
The first thing to do when coming upon an unconscious person is to establish unresponsiveness by tapping on the shoulder and asking "Are you OK?" The victim should then be placed on his or her back. All foreign objects, such as loose dentures, tobacco, gum, and any loose material should be very quickly removed from the victim's mouth.
Then check for breathing by tilting the head and looking at the chest for movement, listing for air movement, and feeling chest movement. Afterwards, if no air movement is detected, lift under the neck and tilt the crown of the head downwards.
Another way to open the airway is to tilt the head and pull the lower jaw so that the chin points straight up. This pulls the tongue forward so that the air passage is open. Sometimes the victim will resume the breathing. If

Transportation of a heart attack victim in a cardiolance.

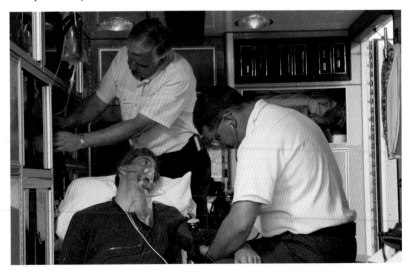

the victim is still not breathing, start resuscitation at once. Any delay may prove fatal.

Traditionally, four methods of artificial ventilation have been taught for us on a victim of respiratory arrest:

- mouth-to-mouth or mouth-to-nose ventilation;
- Holger-Nielsen (back pressure, arm lift);
- Shafer (prone pressure);
- Silvester.

Mouth-to-mouth ventilation

Mouth-to-mouth ventilation is by far the most effective means of artificial ventilation. Although the other manual methods work, they are not nearly as efficient.

They do not provide as much air and it is more difficult to maintain an open airway. Unless there are special circumstances, such as severe facial injuries, that require the use of another method, mouth-to-mouth ventilation should be used.

The most important principle in mouth-to-mouth ventilation is to keep the victim's head and neck properly extended to allow adequate passage in the throat for air to enter the lungs.

- Pinch the nostrils together to prevent loss of air through the nose.
- Inhale deeply.
- Place your mouth over the victim's mouth (over mouth and nose with children) making sure of a tight seal. Blow into the air passage until the victim's chest rises.
- Keep the victim's head extended at all times.
- Remove your mouth and let the victim exhale.
- Feel and listen for the return flow of air, and look for a fall of the victim's chest.
- Repeat this operation 12 times a minute for an adult and 20 times a minute for a small child.

Mouth-to-nose Ventilation

In certain cases, mouth-to-nose ventilation may be required.

The mouth-to-nose technique is similar to mouth-to-mouth except that the lips are sealed by pushing the lower jaw against the upper jaw and air is then

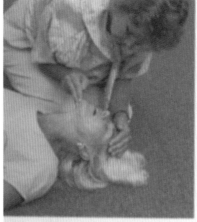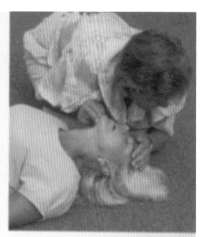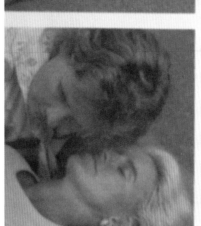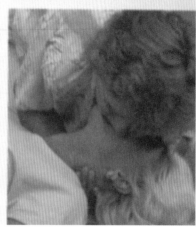

Cardiopulmonary resuscitation (CPR)

Skill in CPR is best obtained through a training course. The American Heart Association, American Red Cross and many local hospitals offer CPR training courses. Because procedures may change over time, it is important to stay up to date on training and to repeat courses as recommended

To begin CPR, the rescuer lays the person on his back, rolling the head, body, and limbs at the same time. The rescuer tilts the person's head back slightly (upper left photograph) and lifts the chin, which sometimes opens a blocked airway.

If breathing does not resume, the rescuer covers the person's mouth with his own and begins artificial respiration (mouth-to-mouth resuscitation or ventilation) by slowly exhaling air into the person's lungs (bottom right).

forced into the victim by way of the nose.

Holger-Nielsen (Back Pressure, Arm Lift) Method

The Holger-Nielsen (back pressure, arm lift) method lies on manual pressures to imitate the natural breathing process.

- Place the victim face down, with the victim's elbows bent and the victim's hands placed one upon the other, under the head.

- Turn the victim's head slightly to one side, so the cheek rests on the victim's hand.
- Kneel on one or both knees at the victim's head.
- Place your hands on the victim's back just below an imaginary line between the armpits; the tips of the thumbs should be just touching and the fingers spread downward and outward.
- Rock forward and press on the victim's back until your arms are

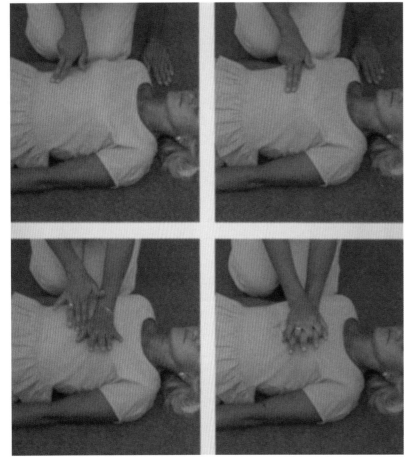

Cardiopulmonary resuscitation (CPR)
Failure of the chest to rise after artificial respiration indicates that the person's airway is blocked. If the chest rises, the rescuer gives two deep, slow breaths.
Next, chest compressions are performed. The rescuer kneels to one side (upper left photograph) and places both hands (bottom right), on the lower part of the breastbone. The rescuer compresses the chest to a depth of 1½ to 3 inches in an adult, less deeply in a child. For an infant, the rescuer uses two fingers to compress the infant's breastbone just below the nipples to a depth of ½ to 1 inch.
CPR can be performed by one person (who, alternately performs artificial respiration and chest compression) or by two people (one to perform artificial respiration and one to perform chest compressions. Breaths are given about 15 to 20 times per minute, and chest compressions are performed about 80 to 100 times per minute.

Cardiopulmonary re-suscitation

Cardiopulmonary resuscitation (CPR) involves the use of artificial ventilation (mouth-to-mouth breathing) and external heart compression (rhythmic pressure on the breastbone). These techniques can only be learned through training and supervised practice. Incorrect application of external heart compressions may result in complications such as damage to internal organs, fracture or ribs or sternum, or separation of cartilage from ribs. (Rib fractures may occur when compression are being correctly performed but this is not an indication to stop compression). Application of cardiopulmonary resuscitation when not required could result in cardiac arrest. It should be emphasized that when CPR is *properly applied*, the likelihood of complications is minimal and acceptable in comparison with the alternative-death.

Recognizing the problem
The person who initiates emergency heart-lung resuscitation has two responsibilities:
▲ To apply emergency measures to prevent irreversible changes to the vital centres of the body.
▲ To be sure the victim receives definitive medical care; this requires hospitalization.

When sudden death occurs, the rescuer must act immediately upon recognition of heart failure. In order to prevent biological death, the rescuer must be able to do the following:
▲ Recognize rapidly the apparent stoppage of heart action and respiration.
▲ Provide artificial ventilation to the lungs.
▲ Provide artificial circulation of the blood.
In addition to performing CPR, the rescuer must summon help in order that an ambulance and/or physician may be called to the scene.

Step by step procedure
The CPR procedures should be learned and practised on a training

approximately vertical.
▲ Allow the weight of the upper body exert slow, steady, even pressure upon the hands. Keep the elbows straight, and exert pressure almost directly downward on the victim's back.
▲ Release the pressure, avoiding a final thrust.
▲ Grasp the victim's elbows an pull them toward you by rocking backward slowly. Apply enough lift to feel resistance and tension in the victim's shoulders.
▲ Keep your own elbows straight while rocking backward, and draw the victim's elbows up and towards you as natural part of sitting back.
▲ Lower the victim's elbows to the ground.
▲ Replace your arms at the starting position and repeat the cycle at a rate of 12 times per minute.

manikin under the guidance of a qualified instructor. The step by step procedure for cardiopulmonary resuscitation is as follows:

- ▲ Establish unresponsiveness. Shake the victim's shoulder and shout, "Are you O.K?" The individual's response will indicate to the rescuer if the victim is just sleeping or if he/she is unconscious.
- ▲ Call for help. The rescuer will need help, either to assist in performing CPR or to call for medical help.
- ▲ Position the victim. If the victim found in a crumb led up and face down, the rescuer must roll the victim over; this is done while calling for help.
- ▲ When rolling the victim over, care must be taken that broken bones are not further complicated by improper handling. The victim is rolled as a unit so that the head and shoulders move simultaneously with no twisting.
- ▲ Kneel beside the victim, a few inches to the side.
- ▲ The arm nearest the rescuer should be raised above the victim's head.
- ▲ The victim's legs should be as straight as possible.
- ▲ The rescuer's hand closest to the victim's head should be placed on the victim's head and neck to prevent them from twisting.
- ▲ The rescuer should use his other hand to grasp under the victim's arm furthest from him. This will be the point at which the rescuer exerts the pull in rolling the body over.
- ▲ Pull carefully under the arm, and the hips and torso will follow the shoulders with minimal twisting.
- ▲ Be sure to watch the neck and keep it in line with the rest of the body.
- ▲ The victim should now be flat on his or her back.
- ▲ Open the airway. The most common cause of a airway obstruction is an unconscious victim is the tongue. The tongue is attached to the lower jaw; moving the jaw forward, lifts the tongue away from the back of the throat and opens the airway.
- ▲ Kneel at the victim's side with the

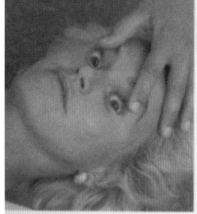
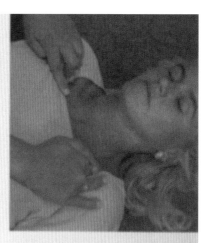
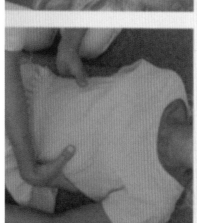
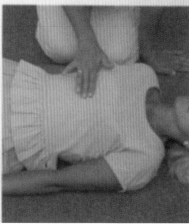

Cardiopulmonary resuscitation (CPR)
Cardiac arrest is what happens when a person dies; the heart does not beat and breathing ceases, which starves the body of oxygen. Sometimes a person can be revived during the first several minutes after suffering cardiac arrest, However, the more time that passes, the less likely it is that the person can be revived and, if revived, the more likely it is that he will have brain damage.
A person in cardiac arrest lies motionless without breathing and does not respond to questions or to stimulation, such as shaking (upper left). A rescuer who encounters someone who fits this description first determines whether the person is conscious by loudly asking: "Are you OK?". If there is no response, the rescuer uses the "look, listen, and feel approach" (upper right) to determine whether breathing has stopped. Looking to see whether the chest moves up and down (upper right), listening for sounds of breathing, and feeling for air movement. If the person is not breathing he or she will start CPR (lower right).

knee nearest the head opposite the victim's shoulders.
- ▲ Place one hand under the neck and lift the other hand is placed on the victim's forehead and pushed downward to tilt the head.
- ▲ Establish breathlessness. The airway must be open to determine breathlessness.
- ▲ Turn your head toward the victim's feet with your cheek ear close

over the victim's mouth.
- ▲ *Look* for a rise and fall in the victim's chest.
- ▲ *Listen* for air exchange at the mouth and nose.
- ▲ *Feel* for the flow of air.
- ▲ Watch for signs of cyanosis; bluish or greyish colour in the lips, tongue, ear lobes, nailbeds, and skin due to deficiency of oxygen in the blood.

4 Bleeding and shock

Bleeding

Hemorrhage or bleeding is a flow of blood from an artery, vein, or capillary. In severe bleeding, place the patient in such a position that he or she will be least affected by the loss of blood. Lay the victim down and elevate the victim's legs in a semi-flexed position. This prevents aggravation of spinal injury or breathing impairment. Control the bleeding. Maintain an open airway and give the victim plenty of fresh air. Prevent the loss of body heat by putting blankets under and over the victim. The victim should be kept at rest, as movement will increase heart action, which causing the blood to flow faster, and perhaps interfering with clot formation of dislodging a clot already formed.

▲ Bleeding from an artery
When bright red blood spurts from a wound, an artery has been cut. The blood in the arteries comes directly form the heart, and spurts at each contraction. Having received a fresh supply of oxygen, the blood is bright red.

▲ Bleeding from a vein
When dark red blood flows from a wound in steady stream, a vein has been cut. The blood, having given up its oxygen and received carbon dioxide and waste products in return, is dark red.

▲ Bleeding from capillaries
When blood oozes from the wound, capillaries have been cut.

Myocardial infarction. Defibrillation with an apparatus that arrests ventricular fibrillation (irregular heart beat) and restores normal rhythm of the heart muscle.

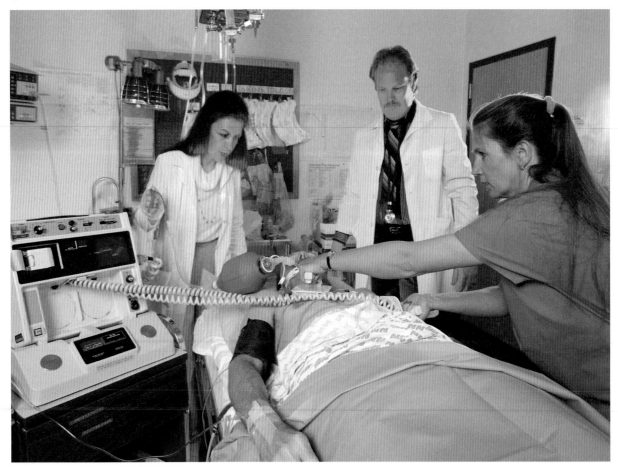

There is usually no cause for alarm, relatively little blood can be lost. Usually direct pressure with a compress applied over the wound will cause the formation of a clot. Where large skin surface is involved, the threat of infection may be more serious than the loss of blood.

Methods of controlling bleeding

Bleeding control is often very simple. Most external bleeding can be controlled by applying direct pressure to the open wound. Direct pressure permits normal blood clotting to occur. In cases of severe bleeding, the first aider may be upset by the appearance of the wound and the emotional state of the victim. It is important for the first aider to keep calm.

▲ Direct pressure

The best all around method of controlling bleeding is applying pressure directly to the wound. This is best done by placing gauze or the cleanest material available against the bleeding point and applying firm pressure with the hand until a bandage can be applied. The bandage knot should be tied over the wound unless otherwise indicated. The bandage supplies direct pressure and should not be removed until the victim is examined by a physician. When air splints or pressure bandages are available, they may be used over the heavy layer of gauze to supply direct pressure. If bleeding continues after the bandage has been put on, this indicates that not enough pressure has been applied. Use the hand to put more pressure on the wound through the gauze, or tighten the bandage. Either method should control the bleeding. In severe bleeding, if gauze or other suitable material is not available, the bare hand should be used to apply direct pressure immediately.

▲ Elevation

Elevating the bleeding part of the body above the level of the heart will slow the flow of blood and speed clotting. Elevation should be used together with direct pressure when there are no unsplintable fractures and it will

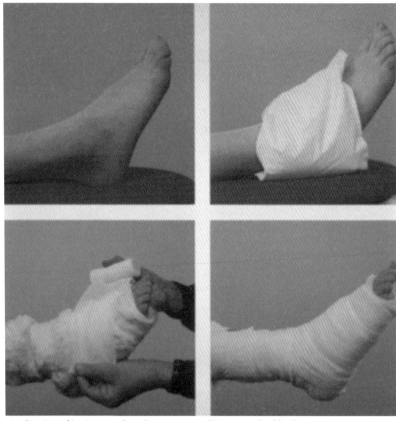

Application of ice in case of a subcutaneous and intracapsular bleeding.

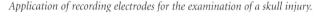

Application of recording electrodes for the examination of a skull injury.

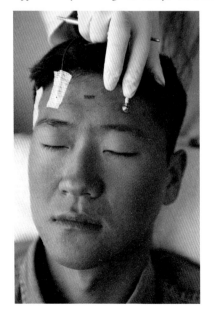
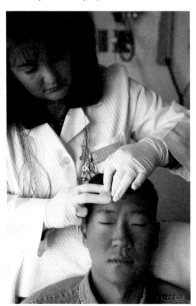

cause no pain or aggravation to the injury.

▲ Indirect pressure
Arterial bleeding can be controlled by digital thumb or finger pressure applied at pressure points. Pressure points are places over a bone where arteries are close to the skin. Pressing the artery against the underlying bone can control the flow of blood to the injury. There are some twenty pressure points on the body - 13 on each side - situated along main arteries. In cases of severe bleeding where direct pressure is not controlling the bleeding, digital pressure must be used. Pressure points should be used with caution, as indirect pressure may cause damage to the limb as a result of an inadequate flow of blood. When the use of indirect pressure at a pressure point is necessary, indirect pressure should not be substituted for direct pressure; both kinds of pressure should be used. The pressure point should be held only as long as necessary to stop the bleeding. Indirect pressure should be reapplied if bleeding recurs.
Pressure points on the arms (brachial pressure point) and in the groin (femoral pressure point) are the ones most often used in first aid. These pressure points should be thoroughly understood.

▲ Brachial artery
Pressure on the brachial artery is used to control severe bleeding from an open wound on the upper extremity. This pressure point is located in a groove on the inside of the arm and the elbow. To apply pressure, grasp the middle of the victim's arm with the thumb on the outside of the arm and the fingers on the inside. Press the fingers toward the thumb. Use the flat, inside surface of the fingers, not the fingertips. This inward pressure closes the artery by pressing it against the arm bone.

▲ Femoral artery
The femoral artery is used to control severe bleeding from a wound on the lower extremity. The pressure point is located on the front, center part of the crease in the groin area. This is where the artery crosses the pelvic basin on the way into the lower extremity. To apply pressure, position the victim flat on his or her back, if possible.
Kneeling on the opposite side from the wounded limb, place the heel of one hand directly on the pressure point and lean forward to apply the small amount of pressure needed to the close artery.
If bleeding is not controlled, it may be necessary to press directly over the artery with the flat surface of the fingertips and apply additional pressure on the fingertips and apply additional pressure on the fingertips with the heel of the other hand.

Shock

The signs and symptoms of shock are both physical and emotional. The first-aider should become familiar with these. Some of the reactions known to take place within the body in cases of shock bear directly on the symptoms presented. The most important reaction that occurs in shock is a decided drop in normal blood flow, believed to be caused by voluntary nervous system losing control over certain small blood vessels. This is one of the reasons the victim is nauseous.
The removal of blood from general circulation causes the blood pressure to fall, decreases the volume of blood passing through heart and lungs, and causes the vessels to dilate.
As a large amount of blood fills the dilated vessels within the body, the circulation near the surface is decreased, causing the skin to become pale, cold, and clammy. Other areas suffer as a result of the drop in circulation; the eyes are dull and lacklustre and pupils may be dilated.
With the fall in blood pressure and the unusual amount of blood that goes to fill the dilated blood vessels within the body, less blood returns to the heart for recirculation. In an effort to overcome the decreased volume and still send blood to all parts of the body, the heart pumps faster but pumps a much lower quantity of blood per beat. Thus, pulse is rapid and weak.

The blood suffers from this decreased blood supply and does not function normally; the victim's powers of reasoning, thinking, and expression are dulled.

First aid care of shock

Shock is a serious condition, but it is nor irreversible if it is recognized quickly and treated effectively. Proper first aid care means caring for the whole victim, not just one or two of the victim's problems.
First aid care for the victim of physical shock is as follows:

▲ Keep the person lying down. Make sure that the head is at least level with the body, if the person is on the ground.

▲ Elevate the lower extremities if the injury will not be aggravated and there are no abdominal or head injuries.

▲ It may be necessary to raise the head and shoulders if a person is suffering from a head injury, sunstroke, apoplexy, heart attack or shortness of breath due to a chest or throat injury.

▲ It should be noted that if an accident was severe enough to produce a head injury there may also be spinal damage. If in doubt keep the victim flat.

▲ Control for bleeding.

▲ Always assure adequate breathing, as in all emergencies. If the victim is breathing, maintain an open airway. If the victim is not breathing, start artificial ventilation, or CPR if necessary.

▲ Remove all foreign bodies from the victim's mouth, such as loose false teeth, tobacco, or gum, and cleans the mouth of mucus or phlegm.

▲ Permit the victim to have plenty of fresh air. If possible administer oxygen. Oxygen deficiency results from the poor circulation, in cases of shock.

▲ Loosen tight clothing at the neck, chest, and waist, in order to make breathing and circulation easier.

▲ Handle the victim as gently as possible, and minimize movement.

▲ Keep the victim warm and dry by

wrapping in blankets, clothing, or other available material. These coverings should be placed under as well as over the victim to reduce the loss of body heat.

▲ Keep the victim warm enough to be comfortable. The objective is to maintain as near normal body temperature as possible not to add heat.

▲ The victim should not be given anything by mouth.

▲ The victim's emotional well-being is just as important as his or her physical well-being. Calm and reassure the victim.

▲ Never talk to the victim about his or her injuries. Keep onlookers away from the victim as their conversation regarding the victim's injuries may be upsetting.

How to prevent accidents

• If you have large or dangerous areas of glass in your house, especially doors or windows with glass in the lower part, the best thing you can do is fit safety glass. This is glass that is specially laminated or toughened and, like wired glass, it is much safer than ordinary glass.

• You can also get special film to cover glass in doors and windows and this too makes it much safer.

• At least mark the dangerous glass by sticking on colored strips, or board up the glass in low doors and windows. Remember, frosted or patterned glass is unlikely to be safety glass.

• Don't let a toddler walk around holding anything made of glass like a tumbler or milk bottle.

• If your child wears glasses, ask the optician or at the clinic about splinter-proof or plastic lenses.

• Keep all sharp things away from toddlers. Teach older children how to use sharp tools safely.

• Make sure toys have no sharp edges or points.

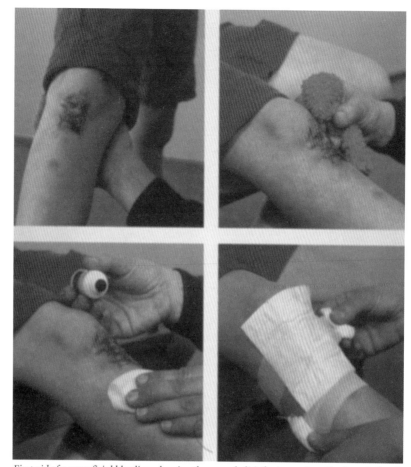

First aid of a superficial bleeding: cleaning the wound, disinfection and application of a bandage.

What to do in an emergency

▲ If there is severe bleeding, press firmly on the wound using a pad of clean cloth if available, or your fingers.

▲ Keep pressing until the bleeding stops. This may take 10 minutes or more. If it is a large wound, try to press the edges of the wound together.

▲ Don't use a tourniqwuet or tie anything so tightly that it stops the circulation.

▲ If possible, lay the child down and raise the injured limb. This helps to stop the bleeding. But don't do this if you think the limb is broken.

▲ Cover the wound with a clean dressing.

▲ Then call an ambulance or take the child to hospital.

▲ If the wound is dirty, or the accident happened outside, ask your doctor about a tetanus shot.

5 Fractures and dislocations

Fractures

A fracture is a broken of cracked bone. Fractures are caused in several ways:

- ▲ Direct blow
  The bone is broken at the point of impact. For example, a person is hit in the leg by a piece of flying rock and the bone is broken at the point where the rock hit the leg.
- ▲ Indirect blow
  The bone is broken by forces travelling along the bone from the point of impact. Form example, a person who falls and lands on the hands may suffer a broken arm.
- ▲ Twisting forces
  A severe twisting force can result in a fracture. For example, a person playing football or skiing is susceptible to this type of injury.
- ▲ Muscle contractions
  Violent muscle contractions can result in fracture. For example, a person who receives an electrical shock can experience muscle contractions so as to cause fractures.
- ▲ Pathological conditions
  Localized disease or aging can weaken bones to the point that the slightest stress may result in a fracture.

Broken bones, especially the long bones of the upper ad lower extremities, often have sharp, sawtooth edges; even slight movement may cause the sharp edges to cut into the blood vessels, nerves, or muscles, and perhaps through the skin. Careless or improper handling can convert a simple fracture into a compound fracture, and damage the surrounding blood vessels or nerves can make the injury much more serious.

A person handling a fracture should always bear this in mind. Damage due to careless handling of a simple fracture may greatly increase pain and shock, cause complications that will prolong the period of disability, and endanger life through hemorrhage of surrounding blood vessels.

The general signs and symptoms of a fracture are as follows:

- pain or tenderness in the region of the fracture;
- deformity or irregularity of the fracture;
- loss of function (disability) of the affected areas;
- moderate or severe swelling;
- discoloration;
- victim's information, if conscious.

Types of fractures

Fractures are nearly always the result of external forces but occasionally from violent muscular contractions as in tetanus and grand mal epilepsy. A closed fracture is one which does not communicate with the surface of the body. In a compound fractures, the broken bone pierces the skin and leaves an open wound.

The distinction is sometimes drawn between the fracture which is compound from without, i.e. the open wound results from the external violence, and one which is compound from within, i.e. a sharp spike of the fractured bone punctures the skin. The difference is of little importance as both are potentially infected and should be treated as any other open wound. Spiral, transverse, oblique fractures are self-explanatory descriptive terms applied to the direction of the fracture. The pattern of fractures depends on the direction of the force applied and on the internal structure of the bone at the site of fracture.

In the long bones, the axial orientation of osteones make sharp transverse fractures rare. A broken bone, like a broken stick, and for similar reasons, usually splinters and shows minor irregularities in the fracture line; by their arrangement thy can contribute greatly to the stability of a reduction. Otherwise oblique and spiral fractures tend to override due to

Application of an arm sling for a wrist injury.

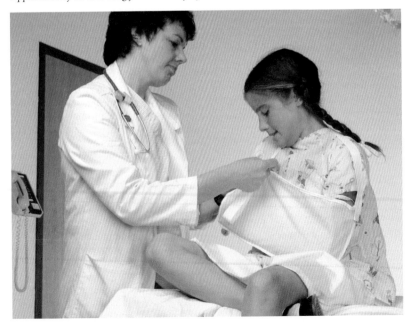

First Aid Kit

A basic kit usually contains rolls of two- and three-inch-wide gauze bandages, a dozen two- and four-inch-square gauge pads, adhesive tape, and assorted sizes of adhesive-strip bandages. To make a complete home set of emergency supplies, the following additional items should be added.

- a three- or four-inch-wide elastic bandage
- two slings - pieces of cotton material about 36 inches square
- scissors with rounded tips
- tweezers
- large and small safety pins
- syrup of ipecac (to induce vomiting)
- acetaminophen or aspirin
- antihistamine
- petroleum jelly
- rubbing (isopropyl) alcohol (used to relieve itching and to clean skin)
- calamine lotion (used to relieve itching)
- two thermometers (one oral, one rectal)
- cotton swabs
- cotton balls
- ice bag
- hot-water bottle or heating pad
- a first-aid manual

the pull of soft tissues. Segmental and comminuted fractures, where the bone is broken in two or more places, mat heal slowly because of the poor blood supply of the smaller fragments. A compression fracture is a compaction of cancellous bone, as mar occur in the vertebral bodies. A greenstick fracture is an incomplete break occurring in tot pliable bones of a growing child.

An epiphyseal fracture separation, also confined to the growing period, takes place through the hypertrophic zone of epiphyseal cartilage which is a site of structural weakness. The cartilage plate retains its attachment to the epiphysis from which it gains its nutrition, and its growth is consequently not interrupted. Avulsion fractures detach small fragments of bone at the sites of muscle insertions. In the growing period the entire epiphysis may become detached. A stress fracture is an undisplaced crack arising in a bone which has been subjected to repeated stresses, any one of which would be insufficient to produce a fracture.

The march fracture of the metatarsal bones in army recruits is an example. These fractures may not be visible on the initial radiograph but may be recognized by a surrounding cuff of callus after a few days.

Pathological fractures occur in bone which is weakened by disease. Common underlying causes are osteoporosis, primary and secondary bone tumors and bone cysts.

Dislocations

Where two or more bones come together, they form a joint. The bones forming a joint are held in place by bands of strong, fibrous tissue known as ligaments.

There are three varieties of joints:
- immovable joints;
- joints with limited motion;
- freely movable joints.

A dislocation is the slipping out of normal position of one or more of the bones forming a joint. Dislocation happens most often in freely movable joints. Violence past the point the point of ligament rupture may result in displacement of bony relationships of the joint, producing a dislocation which is characterized by:
- severe pain;
- loss of mobility;
- usually an obvious deformity.

X-ray confirmation is necessary because of the possibility of associated fractures. Following reduction, a period of immobilization is necessary to allow the inevitable capsular and ligamentous damage to heal, so minimizing the chance of recurrence.

The complications of dislocation are similar to those of fractures. Associated damage to major vessels or nerves may occur. Recurrent dislocation is most common after shoulder dislocations in young people, because in the shoulder joint stability is sacrificed to mobility. Recurrence is rare in other joints with a greater degree of

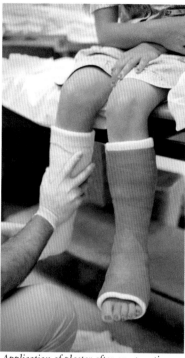

Application of plaster after an operation on both legs for a congenital bone deformity.

congruence. Recurrent dislocations require surgical reconstruction and reinforcement of the damaged ligaments and capsule.

Signs and symptoms

Dislocation of a joint may result from the following:
- force applied at or near the joint;
- sudden muscular contractions;
- twisting strains on joint ligaments;
- falls were the force of landing is transferred to joint.

Some general symptoms of dislocation are as follows:
- rigidity and loss of function;
- deformity;
- pain;
- swelling;
- tenderness;
- discoloration.

Reducing dislocations requires skill in manipulating the parts so as not to damage further the joint ligaments and the numerous blood vessels and nerves found close to joints. Only a physician should reduce dislocations. Because of the pain involved, one exception may be a dislocated jaw.

BANDAGES

Roller bandages are made of flannel, linen, crepe, muslin or highly absorbent gauze. The bandage must be applied to fit neatly, neither too tight nor too loose, so that it cannot shift position.

Always begin and end with a circular turn, if possible working from left to right, holding the roll towards the upper side. Each new turn should cover two-thirds of the underlying one, so that the finished bandage is three layers thick.

If the bandage must be lengthened, fasten one end of the new roll with some adhesive tape some way above the end of the one already in place, so that you can roll the two together for a few turns.

When the bandage is in place, fasten the end with adhesive tape, safety pins or bandage clips, or cut the last portion of the bandage lengthwise into two, twist the ends around in opposite directions and tie them up in a knot.

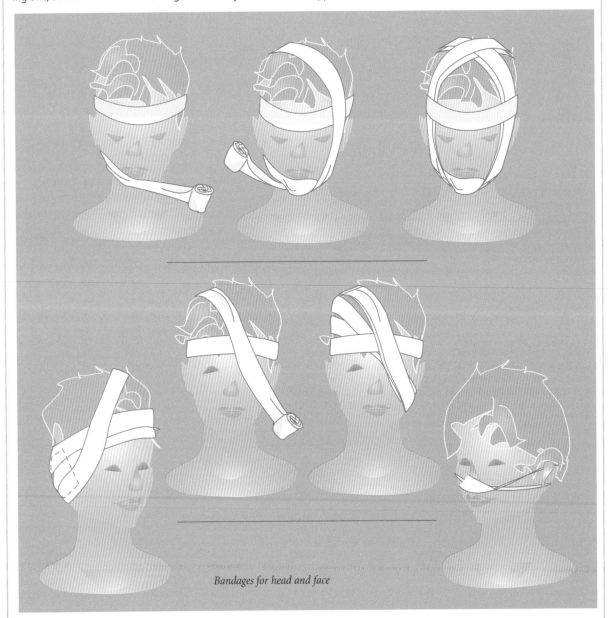

Bandages for head and face

BANDAGES

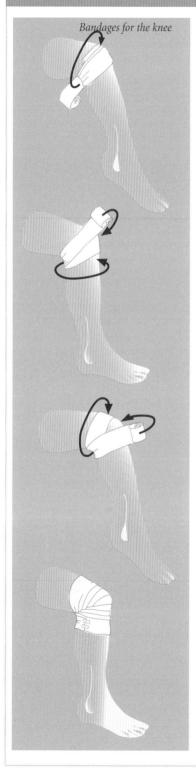

Bandages for the knee

Bandage for head and face

Such a bandage is used to hold in place a dressing over a wound (sterile gauze covered with cotton wool). Roll the bandage in a circle around the forehead and the back of the head, lead it down at the back under the right ear, along the chin and up again behind the head. Now roll it form the right side of the back of the head diagonally across the top of the head and downwards in front of the left ear and under the chin, going upward again in front of the right ear and diagonally across the top of the head. Repeat the crown-to-chin rolls. To finish, roll the bandage around the forehead and back of the head and fasten.

Bandage for eye

The first circle of the bandage passes horizontally from forehead to the rear of the head in the direction of the injured eye. The next turn goes diagonally over the skull, descends across the middle of the forehead, over the injured eye and under the ear to the nape of the neck. Repeat these diagonal turns as many times as seems necessary. To finish, make a circle around the forehead.

Ear bandage

Apply in the same manner as the eye bandage, but cover the ear and one side of the head.

Bandage for nose

This is used for covering and compressing the nose and for keeping nose plugs in place. The ends of a broad roller bandage are cut down the middle, and the nose inserted into the broad, uncut middle portion. On each side, cross the cut ends of the bandage and take them under and above the ear, respectively, tying the top and bottom pairs together with a knot at the nape of the neck.

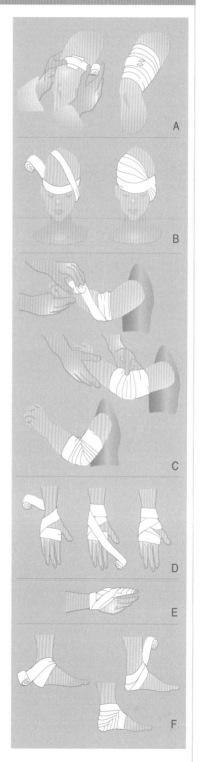

A. Bandages for leg
B. Bandage for head
C. Elbow bandage
D. Hand bandage
E. Finger bandage
F. Bandage for foot

6 Wounds

An open wound is any break in the skin. When the skin is unbroken, it affords protection from most bacteria or germs. However, germs may enter through even a small break in the skin, and an infection may develop.

An open wound should receive prompt medical attention. If germs have been carried into an open wound by an object causing the break in the skin, the flow of blood will sometimes wash out the germs; but some types of wounds do not bleed freely. Breaks in the skin range from pin punctures or scratches to extensive cuts, tears, or gashes.

An open wound may be the only surface evidence of a more serious injury such as a fracture, particularly in the case of head injuries involving fracture of the skull. In first aid, open wounds are divided into five classifications:
- abrasions;
- avulsions;
- incisions;
- lacerations;
- punctures.

Abrasions

Abrasions are caused by rubbing or scraping. These wounds are seldom deep, but a portion of the skin has been removed, leaving a raw, bleeding surface. The bleeding in most abrasions is from the capillaries. Abrasions are easily infected in proportion to the amount of underskin surface exposed.

Avulsions

An avulsion is an injury that tears a whole piece of skin and tissue loose or leaves it hanging as a flap. This type of wound usually results when tissue is forcibly separated or torn from the victim's body. Body parts that have been wholly or partly torn off may sometimes be successfully re-attached by a surgeon.

Incisions

Wounds produced by a sharp cutting edge such as a knife, a piece of glass or metal, or a sharp edge of rock are referred to as incised wounds. The edges of such wounds are smooth without bruising or tearing. If such a wound is deep, large blood vessels and nerves may be severed. Incised wounds bleed freely, and are often difficult to control.

Lacerations

Lacerated wounds are those with edges. The flesh has been torned or mashed by blunt instruments, machinery, or rough surfaces. These wounds may not bleed as freely as incised wounds.

The ragged and torn tissues, with the foreign matter that is often forced or ground into the wound, make the danger of infection greater than in incised wounds.

Punctures

Puncture wounds are produced by pointed instruments such as needles, splinters, nails, or pieces of wire. Such wounds usually are small in surface area, but they may be very deep. Often, the articles causing puncture wounds are soiled, and may cause infection.

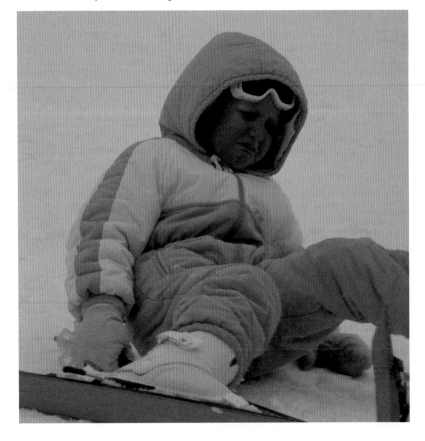

The small openings in puncture wounds and the small number of blood vessels cut can prevent free bleeding. The danger of infection in puncture wounds is far greater than in any other type of open wound because of this poor drainage.

How to prevent accidents

- Children can easily climb and fall out of windows. Look at your windows and see if you can make sure they can't be opened too wide. This can be a simple do-it-yourself job.
- Always check the windows for safety when you move house.
- Try not to put chairs, or anything a child might climb on, near to windows.
- It is a good idea to fit safety catches on your upstairs windows. Then make sure they're used.
- If you think that a window is very dangerous, especially in a child's bedroom, then fit window bars. It is important that the bars can be removed in case of fire. Some types have keys for this, so keep the keys safely.
- Stairs are tempting for climbing on, both up and down. So use a movable safety gate. Make sure that there's no room for a child to crawl under the bannisters at the top of the stairs.
- Board up horizontal bannisters so that they can't be used like ladders for climbing up.
- Balconies can be dangerous for young children. If you have a private balcony, keep the door to it locked so that your child can't go out onto the balcony alone.
- Horizontal balcony railings are very dangerous because they're so easy to climb. Board them up, or fit wire-netting guards.
- Never put anything a child can climb on near balcony railings.
- Never leave a small baby where it might roll off the edge of something and fall.
- Don't put your baby in a bouncing cradle on a table or worktop.
- If your baby's high chair or pushchair has a harness, make sure you use it.

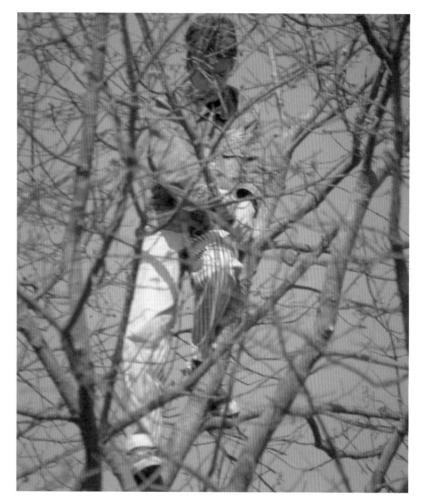

- Try to teach older children to take risks sensibly. Try to teach them how to decide whether what they want to do is too dangerous or not.
- If your children like adventure sports, such as rock-climbing, make sure they are properly taught and have the right equipment.

What to do in an emergency

- If the child has stopped breathing, give mouth-to-mouth resuscitation (rescue breathing) immediately.
- If the injury looks at all serious, or you don't know what's wrong, then call an ambulance.
- If you think there may be broken bones or internal injuries, don't move the child unless you have to.
- If the child is breathing but unconscious, gently place in the recovery position.
- If you think the child has a broken bone; don't move the child unless you have to. This is especially important if you think the child may have injured his/her spine or neck.
- If the child has to be moved, be very gentle as you may cause further damage. If it is a leg that is broken, tie it gently but firmly to the uninjured leg before you move the child. Put some padding in between the leg.
- It it is the arm that is injured and if it can be moven, put it in a sling or support. Be very gentle and comfort the child.

BANDAGES

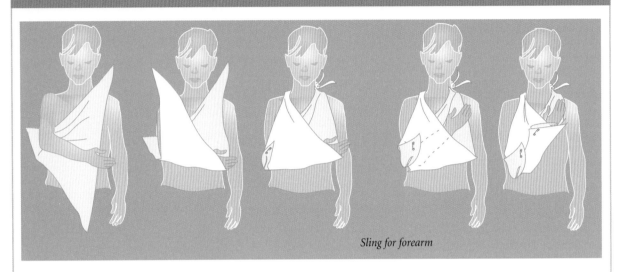

Sling for forearm

Forearm bandage

For a good fit, the roller bandage must be applied in spirals with reserves. The bandage is fixed to the arm by a few turns around the wrist, and is then conducted diagonally upward. Keeping your thumb on the bandage, roll it diagonally in the opposite direction on top of your thumb and then pull tight; repeat this until the bandage comes close to the elbow, finishing with a circle around the arm. This is also the method to be used to bandage the upper arm, thigh or lower leg.

Elbow bandage

This is often used for compression. The first turn is made around the middle of the elbow, which is held in a slightly bent position. The rest of the turns are made above and below the original turns, winding the bandage in a figure-of-eight.

Hand bandage

Take the bandage round the back and palm of the hand a few times to secure it. Then take it from the side of the hand, across the back to the top of the thumb. Take it completely round the wrist 1_ times and then down across the back of the hand to below the thumb. Repeat these crossings and circles round the wrist, and finish with a circle around the wrist.

Finger bandage

Take a narrow bandage along the top of the finger, over the tip and down along the underside. take the bandage between the fingers and up over the top of the injured finger, then round the wrist and back to the top. Next, make enough spirals to cover the finger, and spiral back to its base. Again take the bandage round the hand on both sides, and finish off with a circle round the wrist.

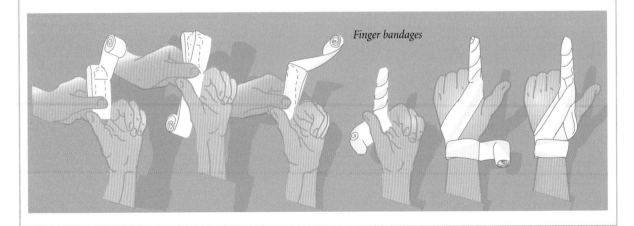

Finger bandages

BANDAGES

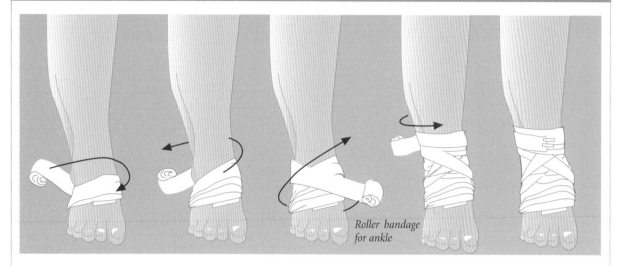

Roller bandage
for ankle

Bandage for an open hand

The hand is laid in the middle of an open triangle, with the fingers pointed towards its point. The point is then folded over the fingers and the back of the hand, and up over the wrist. The ends are folded and crossed over the back of the hand and the wrist, carried round it twice and tied on the upper side of the wrist.

Bandage for hip

Tie a narrow bandage around the waist with the knot on the uninjured side. Lay an open triangle over the injured hip with the point at the waist. Pull this point through under the narrow bandage, fold it over and pin it. Fold the base of the open triangle around the leg and back to the outside, and tie.

Bandage for knee

A triangle that has been folded into a broad bandage is laid around the slightly bent knee. The ends are crossed in front, carried round the leg, crossed again in front, carried around the thigh and ties on the inside. This is used as a covering and compression bandage, and is similar to that used for the elbow.

Bandage for foot

The foot is laid in the middle of an open triangle, with the toes pointed towards its point. The point is then folded over the toes and the back of the foot, and up over the ankles. The ends are folded and crossed over the back of the foot and the ankles, carried round it twice and tied on the upper side of the foot.

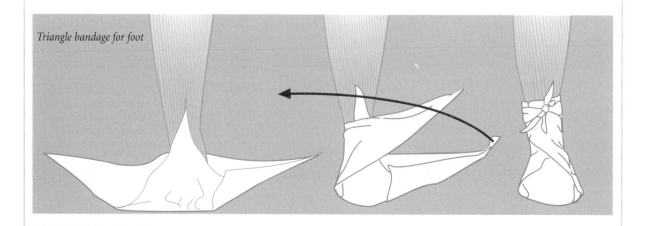

Triangle bandage for foot

7 Heat and Cold Disorders

Heat stroke

Heat stroke is a sudden attack of illness from exposure to the direct rays of the sun or from high temperature without exposure to the sun. Physical exertion is definitely a contributing factor, and heat stroke is more likely to occur in high humidity than in low.

The most important characteristic of heat stroke is the high body temperature which is caused by a disturbance in the heat regulating mechanism. The person can no longer sweat, and this causes a rise in body temperature.

This illness is more common in persons over age 40. Males are more vulnerable to heat stroke than females. Alcoholics are very susceptible to heat stroke.

The signs and symptoms of heat stroke are as follows:

- The skin is flushed, very hot and very dry.
- Perspiration is absent.
- The pulse is strong and rapid.
- The body temperature can reach 106°F to 112°F degrees.
- The victim rapidly becomes unconscious.

Care should be centered around lowering the body temperature as quickly as possible. Failure to do this may result in permanent brain damage or death. The first-aid care for heat stroke is as follows:

- Maintain an open airway.
- Move the victim to a cool environment.
- Remove as much clothing as possible.
- Use cold applications on the head and the body.
- Immerse in cool bath if possible.
- Wrap in a cool sheet; use a fan if available.
- Get the victim to medical help as quickly as possible.
- Watch the individual for relapse and repeated elevated temperatures.

Heat exhaustion

Heat exhaustion occurs in individuals working in hot environments. It is brought about by the pooling of blood in the vessels under the skin. The blood brings the heat from the interior of the body to the surface in an attempt to cool the body. This increase in blood flow to the surface causes a decrease in the amount of circulating blood and may lead to an inadequate return to the heart and brain and eventually to physical collapse. This illness occurs most commonly to persons not accustomed to hot weather, those who are overweight, and those who perspire excessively. Women are generally more susceptible to heat exhaustion than men. The signs and symptoms of heat exhaustion are as follows:

- Pale and clammy skin.
- Profuse perspiration.
- Rapid and shallow breathing.
- Weakness.
- Dizziness.
- Headache.
- In some cases, faintness.

First aid care for heat exhaustion is as follows:

- Move the victim to as cool and comfortable a place as possible, but do not allow chilling.
- Loosen the victim's clothing.
- If fainting seems likely, have the victim lie down with feet elevated 8 to 12 inches.
- If the victim is conscious, give sips of salt water (1 teaspoonful of salt per quart of water). Sugar should be added if possible.
- Treat the victim the same as for shock.

Heat Cramps

Heat cramps affect people who work in a hot environment and perspire. The perspiration causes a loss of slat from the body and if there is inadequate replacement, the body will then suffer from cramps. Heat cramps may also result from drinking iced water or other cold drinks in too large quantities or too quickly.

Signs and symptoms of heat cramps:

- Muscle cramps or spasms in the leg or abdomen which may be painful.
- Faintness.
- Profuse perspiration.

First-aid care for heat cramps is as follows:

- Move the victim to a cool environment.
- If the victim is conscious, give sips of cool salt and sugar water (1 teaspoon of salt plus as much sugar as the person can stand, per quart of water).
- Massage the cramped areas.

Frostbite

Frostbite results from exposure to severe cold. It is more likely to occur when the wind is blowing, taking heat from the body rapidly. The nose, cheeks, ears, toes, and fingers are the body parts most frequently frostbitten. As a result of exposure to cold, the blood vessels constrict. Thus the blood supply to the chilled parts decrease and the tissues do not get the warmth they need.

The signs and symptoms of frostbite are not always apparent to the victim. Since frostbite has a numbing effect, the victim may not be aware of it until told by someone. Frostbite goes through the following stages:

- First the skin becomes red.
- As exposure continues, the skin becomes grey or blotchy white.
- The exposed surface becomes numb due to reduced circulation.
- If frostbite or freezing is allowed to continue, all sensation is lost and the skin becomes a "dead" white.

First aid care for frostbite is as follows:
- Wrap and keep the victim as warm and dry as possible until brought indoors.
- Lower the affected part to increase circulation.
- Place gauze pads between the fingers and toes if affected.
- Bring the victim indoors.
- Place frostbitten extremities in warm water (102°F to 105°F) and make sure the water remains warm. Test the warmth of the water by pouring some on the inner surface of the forearm.
- Apply warm cloths to areas that cannot be submerged.
- Allow the victim to drink hot, stimulating fluids such as coffee or tea.
- Never thaw frostbitten areas if the person will have to go outdoors into the cold again, as this will refreeze thawed areas.
- Do not rub, chafe, or manipulate frostbitten parts.
- Do not use hot water bottles or heat lamps.
- Do not place the victim near a stove of fire, because excessive heat can cause further tissue damage.
- Discourage the victim from smoking, because tobacco constricts the blood vessels.
- Do not allow the victim to walk if the feet are frostbitten.
- Once thawed, have the victim gently exercise the frostbitten areas to stimulate the return of the circulation.
- For serious frostbite, seek medical aid for thawing, because the pain will be intense and tissue damage extensive.

Hypothermia

Hypothermia is a general cooling of the entire body. The inner core of the body is chilled so the body cannot generate heat to stay warm. This condition can be produced by exposure to low temperatures or the temperatures between 30 and 50 F with wind and rain. Also contributing to hypothermia are fatigue, hunger, and poor physical condition.
Exposure begins when the body loses

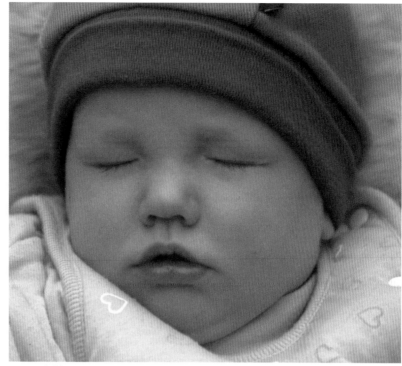

Young children can easily suffer from heat stroke when exposed to high temperatures in the surrounding.

heat faster that it can be produced. When the body is chilled, it passes through several stages:
- The initial response of a person exposed to cold is to voluntarily exercise in order to stay warm.
- As the body tissue is cooled, the person begins to shiver as a result of an involuntary adjustment by the body to preserve normal temperature in the vital organs. Up to this point the person can foresee and take steps to prevent hypothermia. However, these responses drain the body's energy reserves.

If exposure continues until the victim's energy reserves are exhausted, the following symptoms appear:
- Cold reaches the brain and deprives the victim of judgment and reasoning powers.
- The victim experiences feeling of apathy, listlessness, and indifference.
- The victim does not realize what is happening.
- The victim loses control of the hands.

Cooling becomes more rapid as the internal body temperature is lowered. Eventually hypothermia will result in stupor, collapse, and even death. The victim of hypothermia may not recognize the symptoms and deny that medical attention is needed. Therefore, it is important to judge the symptoms rather than what the victim says. Even mild symptoms of hypothermia need immediate medical care.

First aid care for a victim of hypothermia is as follows:
- Get the victim out of the elements (wind, rain, snow, cold, etc.)
- Remove all wet clothing.
- Get the victim into dry clothing or wrap the victim in warm blankets.
- Provide external heat by any possible means such as hot water bottles or even body heat from rescuers. Be careful that any external source of heat does not burn the victim.
- If the victim is conscious, give something warm to drink. (Never give alcoholic beverages).
- If the victim is conscious, try to keep the victim awake.

8 Drowning

Causes

Children love playing with water. Whether it's in the bath at bedtime or in the nearest pond or stream, water is fun. But it is also dangerous. A baby or toddler can drown in very shallow water - far less than you put in the bath. And every year young children do drown in places like ponds and streams, canals, water troughs, garden ponds and swimming pools.

Young children who wander off alone to explore can be in real danger. Older cildren too get into difficulties in sports like sailing or canoeing. So they need to be taught how to cope.

How to prevent accident

- Don't leave young children alone when playing with or in water.
- Never leave a baby or young todd-ler alone in a bath or basin for one second. If the front door bell or telephone rings, lift your baby out of the bath.
- Keep a close eye on young children when they're paddling. At the sea-side, make sure they wear inflat-able arm bands.
- Cover the garden pond with strong wire mesh or fence it off.
- Make sure your children learn to swim as early as possible, and that

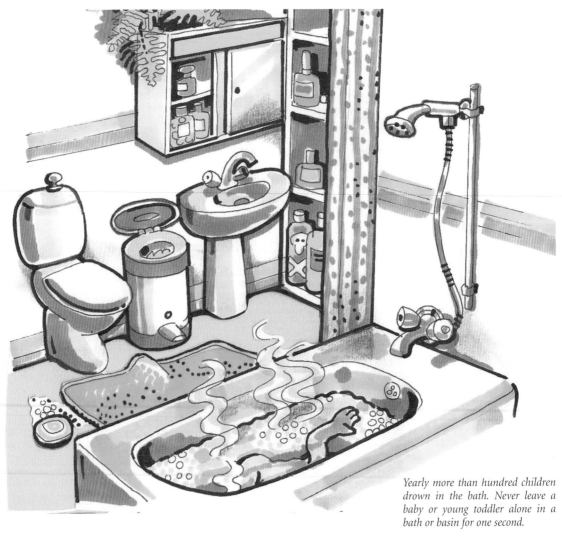

Yearly more than hundred children drown in the bath. Never leave a baby or young toddler alone in a bath or basin for one second.

they learn about water safety.

- Don't let children play by themselves with inflatable mattresses or dinghies at the seaside because they can easily drift out to sea.
- If your children want to do water sports lime sailing or canoeing, they must be properly taught. Make sure they always wear life-jackets.
- Beware of the dangers of thin ice on ponds.

What to do in an emergency

- ▲ If the child is not breathing, give mouth-to-mouth resuscitation (rescue breathing) immediately. Don't give up too soon. Breathing can start again up to an hour after it has stopped so long as you keep on with resuscitation.
- ▲ If the heart has stopped, give heartmassage (CPR).
- ▲ If the child is unconscious but still breathing, place in the recovery position.

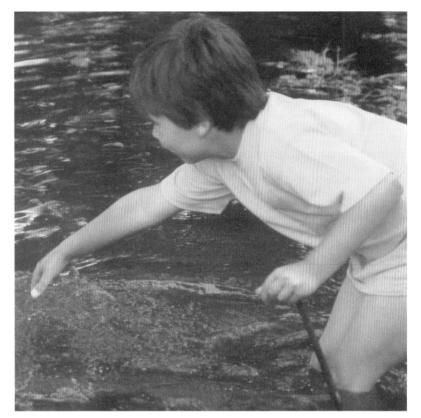

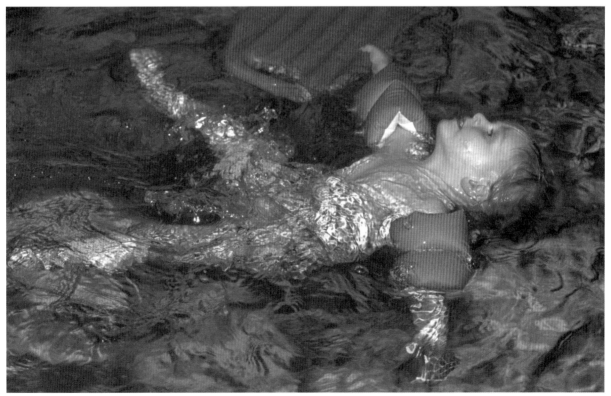

19 Poisoning

Causes

Every year thousands of children swallow poisonous things in and around the home. Many have to go into hospital and some even die.

Very often these accidents happen because medicines, or dangerous household or garden products, have been left where children can find them. To small children, these things don't seem dangerous. Pills can look just like sweets. Medicine, or a bottle of bleach, can look like something to drink. And children will even try anything, just out of curiosity.

How to prevent accidents

- Keep medicines out of children's reach. Use a cupboard that locks,

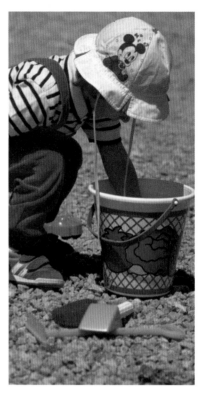

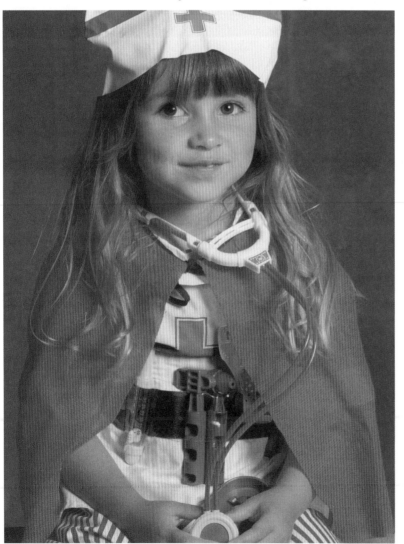

and keep it locked. Keep all your pills and medicines in the cupboard. Don't be tempted to keep the old bottle out just for convenience.

- Be especially careful when your child goes to visit grandparents or other people's houses, or when a grandparent or friend comes to stay. A lot of people still have dangerous medicines in easy-to-open bottles and they forget to keep them away from children.

- Ask your chemist to give you your pills in child-resistant containers and always close the contrainers properly after use. Blister or strip packs also make it kmore difficult for a child to swallow a lot of pills at once.

- Keep dangerous household and garden chemicals in a safe place. A locked cupboard is best, or a very high cupboard - but remember that children climb to places you would never have thought they could reach.

- Keep all dangerous chemicals in their original containers. For

example, never put paraffin or weed killer into a lemonade or squash bottle.
- Don't use bleach and lavatory cleaner together. The mixture can give off dangerous fumes.
- Check were you keep those dangerous chemicals:
  Caustic soda
  Bleach
  Lavatory cleaner
  Disinfectant
  Weed killer
  Slug pellets
  Insecticides
  Petrol
  Battery acid
  Paraffin
  White spirit or turps
  Paint stripper
  Methylated spirit
  Rat poison
- Discourage children from eating any plants or fungi. Some are poisonous.

What to do in an emergency

Pills and medicines
- ▲ If you're not sure whether your child has swallowed something, spend a minute or two looking for the missing pills. Check they haven't rolled under a chair, for example.
- ▲ If you think something has been swallowed, take your child straight away to your doctor or hospital - whichever is quickest.
- ▲ If possible, take with you the container and a sample of whatever you think has been swallowed.
- ▲ Don't give salt and water to make your child sick. Salt can be very dangerous in large amounts.

Household and garden chemicals - turps, petrol, paraffin, acids, caustics, etc.
- ▲ Gently give the child a glass of milk to drink. If there's no milk, give water instead. This dilutes the poison.
- ▲ Then quickly take the child to hospital.
- ▲ If possible take with you the container and a sample of whatever you think has been swallowed.

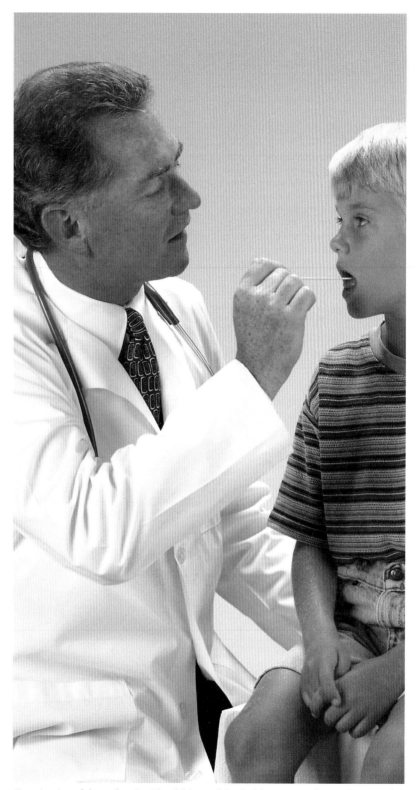

Examination of the oral cavity. The child complained of throat pain after swallowing a foreign body.

Children on the roads

Traffic is probably the most compli-cated and dangerous everyday thing children have to cope with. Crossing a road is far from easy. It means being able to judge the speeds and distances of traffic accurately.

It means being able to react quickly. And young children simply can't man-age it. Unfortunately, a lot of parents think that they can and let their chil-dren cross roads alone long before they can do it safely. Many parents also think that accidents only happen on busy roads. So it's worth remem-bering that a great many of the chil-dren killed on the roads are killed within a few hundred yards of their own homes.

How to prevent accidents

Don't let very young children out on the roads by themselves. They don't understand the dangers. When you go out, talk to your child about the roads and traffic and explain what the dan-gers are.

- For toddlers, use walking reins when you're out near roads.
- Teach your child a special traffic code. Go through the code every time your child cross the road until your child really knows it. Then get your child to cross quiet roads while you watch. But even when they know the code, don't let young children out alone where the traffic is busy or fast.

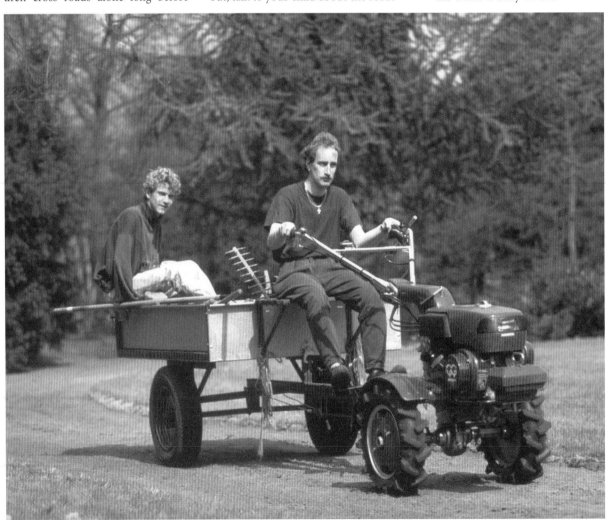

Car seat

We all know that the injuries caused in car accidents can be serious ones. Yet we don't give much thought to the safety of children in cars. Perhaps we think "it won't happen to me." But sadly, it does happen. In the US and Europe every year more than 100,000 child passengers are injured in car accidents, and some 1,100 children are killed.

How to prevent accidcents
- Never hold a baby in your arms in the front seat. Even if you are wearing a seat belt, you won't be able to keep hold of the baby in a crash. The baby will probably be crushed between you and the dashboard.
- Never let a young child stand, or sit, without a restraint, in the back seat. Never let a child stand on the back seat.
- Always make sure your child is safely restrained in the car. If you do, you can dramatically cut down the risk of serious injury in a crash. Remember too that if children are restrained, they are less likely to distract the driver.
- Babies under one year old should be in a carrycot fastened by a restraint in the back of the car. Use a cot cover, net or bedclothes so that your baby can't be thrown out.
- Toddlers aged one to four should be belted into a child safety seat properly fastened in the back of the car.

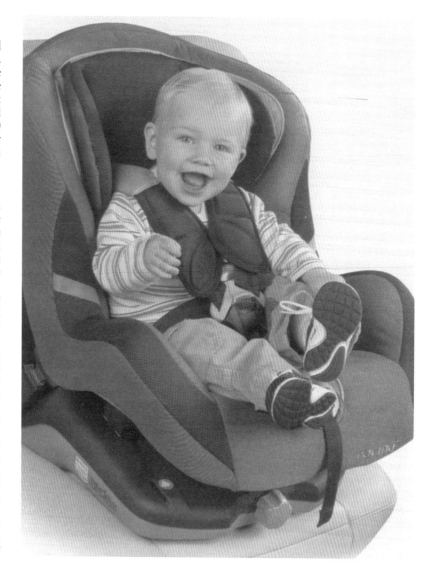

Code for crossing roads

1. First find a safe place to cross, then stop.
2. Stand on the pavement near the curb.
3. Look all round for traffic and listen.
4. If traffic is coming, let is pass. Look all around again.
5. When there is no traffic near, walk straight across the road.
6. Keep looking and listening for traffic while you cross.

- Young, school-age children should sit in child harnesses in the back of the car. In cars, where there is no child restraint fitted, your child should use an adult seat belt.
- Older children about 10 years old and over can use an adult seat belt in the front or back of the car.

Children on bikes

Cycling accidents often happen because children are allowed out on the roads before they're really ready. After all, it takes time to learn to ride a bike safely, and riding safely means much more than just staying on.

For example, a child must be able to turn and look behind, and do hand signals without wobbling. And at the same time as handling the bike safely, the child must be able to cope with the roads and traffic.

How to prevent accidents
- Make sur that your child's bike has the right size of frame and that the saddle and handbars are correctly adjusted. When sitting on the saddle, a child's feet should comfortable touch the ground and hands must be able to work the brake levers.
- Make sure children can ride safely and can cope with roads and traf-

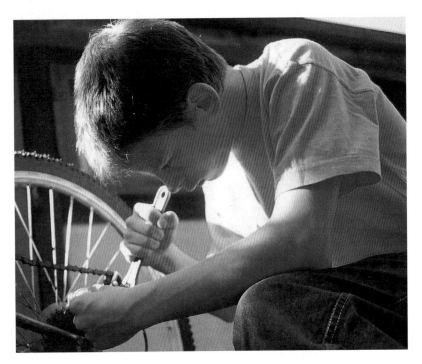

Riding off the pavement onto the road without looking
Roundabouts
Passing parked cars
Motorists coming out of side roads

- Teach children to ride in single file on narrow roads or in traffic. Show them how to plan routes to avoid busy roads or tricky junctions.
- Teach your child that it is dangerous to show off on a bike by riding with "no hands."
- It is safer for young children on tricycles or small bikes to cycle on the pavement. Teach them to be careful of people walking on the pavement.
- Make sure that your child wears reflective clothing when out on a bike, especially in the dark or in bad weather. For night-time riding, lights must be working and reflectors must be clean.
- Bicycle maintenance can be life-saving. It is up to parents to check their children's bikes regularly and get repairs done properly. Teach your child, too, to check brakes and lights regularly.

fic before you let them out alone. As a general rule, children under nine years old should never be allowed out on the roads on a bike alone. An adult should always be with them.

- Make sure that your child understands road signs. Explain, for example, that "cross roads" does not mean "cross the roads."
- Teach your child the dangers of: Turning left

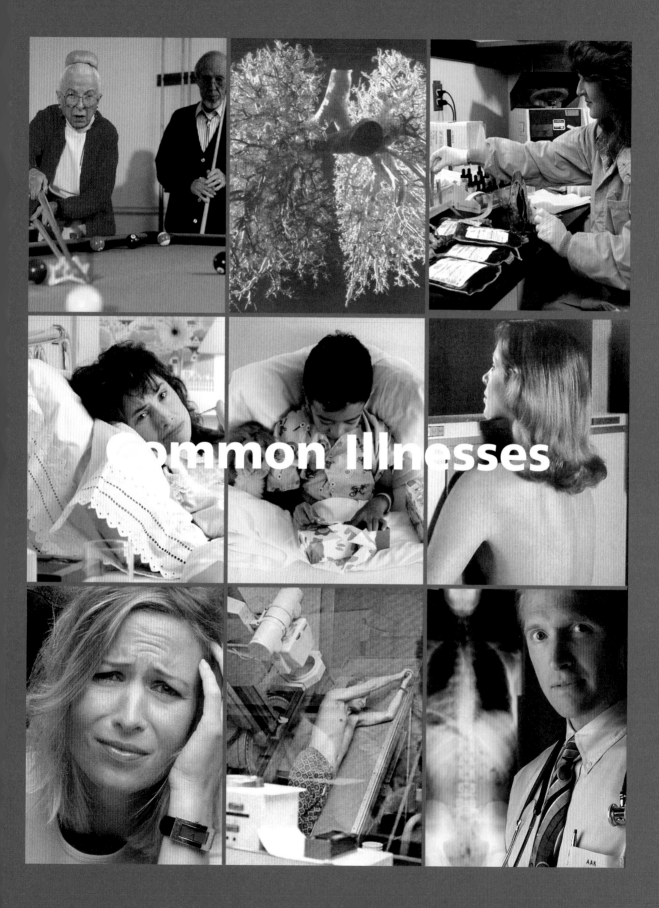

Common Illnesses

ABDOMINAL DISORDERS

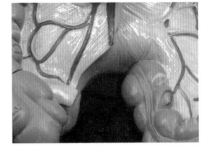

Introduction

Description and causes

The abdomen is that part of the body lying between the thorax (chest) end the pelvis, and containing the abdominal cavity and viscera.

The abdominal cavity contains the organs of digestion and excretion. Also present are the liver, gallbladder and spleen, and a number of glands, e.g., the pancreas and the adrenals.

In the lowest part of the abdominal cavity (pelvic region) the bladder, a portion of the intestinal system, and an important part of the sexual apparatus are located. The organs of the upper abdomen are partly protected by the ribs, and those in the lower abdomen are protected by the pelvic bones. The greater part of the abdominal cavity is covered by a number of abdominal muscles running in various directions. On the posterior or dorsal side of the body the vertebral column or spin provides a flexible but extremely strong support. The abdominal wall is lined, as is the outer surface of the digestive organs, by a membrane called the peritoneum.

■ *Liver and gallbladder*

Most of the liver lies in the upper right part of the abdominal cavity and is protected by the thoracic cage.

The lower margin of the liver is most easily palpated when the patient inspires deeply and the diaphragm contracts and pushes down the liver. Because of the relatively large size of the liver in the child, its lower margin is found at a lower level in children. Below the liver and attached to it, lies the gallbladder.

■ *Stomach and spleen*

Although fixed at both ends, the stomach - located in the upper left part of the abdominal cavity - shows considerable variation in size, shape, and position, depending on the individual, degree of filling, and subject's posture, and respiration.

The stomach serves mainly as a storage center for food prior to passage into the duodenum (the first part of the small intestine), but it permits some digestion.

The spleen is a soft, vascular, oval body, 5 inches long and 3 inches wide. It lies in the left upper abdomen beneath the diaphragm and behind the lower ribs and costal cartilages.

■ *Pancreas and intestines*

The pancreas is a large, lobulated gland resembling the salivary glands in structure. The pancreas has topographically a close relationship to the duodenum. The duodenum receives pancreatic enzymes from the pancreas and bile from the liver and gallbladder.

It is important to be able to distinguish between the large and small intestines by external examination;

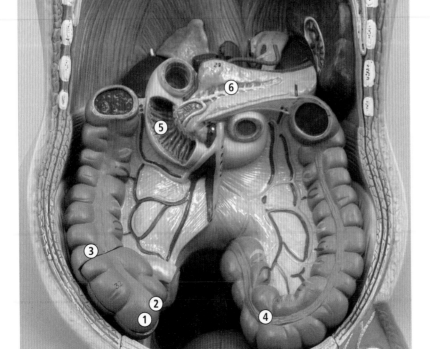

Abdominal cavity and some of the major abdominal organs.
1. *Ileocolic transition*
2. *Appendix*
3. *Ascending colon*
4. *Sigmoid*
5. *Duodenum*
6. *Pancreas*

the small intestine (with the exception of the duodenum) is mobile, with the ascending an descending parts of the colon are fixed. The small intestine had no fatty tags attached to its wall; the large intestine does have fatty tags. The wall of the small intestine is smooth, whereas that of the large intestine is sacculated.

The small intestine extends from the distal end of the stomach to the first portion of the large intestine. It is approximately 18 feet in length and is divided into three portions: the duodenum, jejunum and ileum.

The cecum, or first portion of the large intestine, is an elongated pouch situated in the right lower portion of the abdomen. The ascending colon extends upward from the cecum on the right posterior abdominal wall to the undersurface of the liver just in front of the right kidney. The transverse colon overlies the coils of the small intestine and crosses the abdominal cavity from right to left below the stomach.

The descending colon begins near the spleen, passing downward on the left side of the abdomen to the iliac crest to become the pelvic colon. The pelvic, or sigmoid, colon is so called because of its S-shaped course within the abdominal cavity.

The rectum (anatomically the lower end of the large intestine) lies on the anterior surface of the sacrum and terminates in the narrow anal canal, which opens to the exterior of at the anus.

Abdominal mass

Description

An abdominal mass is a lump or an area of swelling in the abdominal region. Among young children, an abdominal mass os often associated with the kidneys, but it can also appear in the abdominal tract, adrenal glands, genital organs, liver, or spleen. Abdominal masses are unusual occurrences. They can appear at any age. Often a parent is the first to notice the mass, while a child is at play of taking a bath. Or a newborn may have a mass which is obvious to a physician during the first physical examination. More often, a mass becomes apparent only

if pain occurs or a vital bodily function is affected.

Occasionally an abdominal mass may go unnoticed even during routine physical examination if the lump is not large enough to be obvious on sight or to be felt when a hand is run over the surface of the child's body.

An abdominal mass may appear as a slight swelling above the surface of the body or as a substantial bulge, sometimes the size of a golf ball or even a tennis ball.

Conversely, it may be obvious only when the skin of the abdomen is pressed with the fingers. Sometimes the location of a mass is to deep as to be unapparent to either sight or touch, but there is pain.

Cause

Abdominal masses are either abnormal growths, unusual extensions of a body structure, or the result of an injury. Masses can be abnormal growth on

- a kidney
- the genital organs
- the small intestine
- the large intestine
- the adrenal glands
- the liver
- the spleen
- the bile duct

Each kind of mass must be treated differently, according to its size, its location, the type of tissue involved, and the general health of the child.

Abnormal masses in newborns are commonly the result of conditions or abnormalities present at birth (congenital), requiring immediate treatment. Occasionally, especially among newborns, abdominal masses can be the cause or the result of an obstruction which must have emergency corrective treatment. Rapidly growing abdominal masses often need immediate attention because their rate of increasing size may indicate a malignant, or cancerous, condition.

More that half of tall abdominal

Incision and drainage of abscess. Preliminary aspiration (A); incision (B); introducing the tip of a pair of forceps to improve drainage (C); breaking down loculi with a finger (D); further incision (E); trimming the corners of the cruciate incision to deroof the cavity (F).

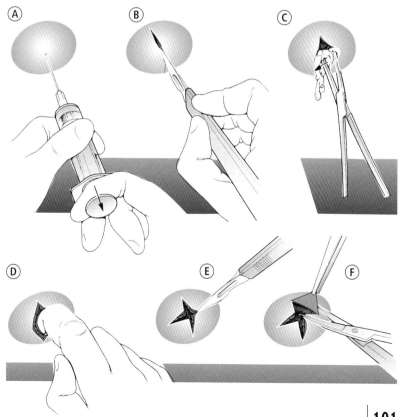

A

masses affecting newborns are associated with the kidneys. Almost half of these masses are caused by hydronephrosis, a condition in which urine cannot escape from the kidney. Other common kidney-associated masses stem from kidney malfunction caused by the development of cysts (encapsulated collections of fluid or semisolid matter) inside or on the surface of the kidney.

The rarest kidney-related mass affecting newborns is a cancerous growth (a mass of abnormal rapidly dividing cells), such as Wilms's tumor.

Diagnosis

An abdominal mass is difficult to diagnose until it is large enough to be felt. However, if a newborn or an infant cries and cannot be comforted, even in the absence of any abdominal mass or swelling, a physician should be notified. If an older child, adolescent or adult complains of pain in the abdomen and reacts with distress when any part of the abdomen is touched, a physician should examine the child adolescent or adult.

Initially, a physician performs a thorough examination. A child's medical history may help identify any prior instances of abdominal distress of illness. Blood and urine tests may be performed.

The process of identifying and defining abdominal masses relies heavily on tests performed in radiology departments. All these tests are performed under the supervision of a radiologist.

A CT- or MRI-scan can provide highly detailed pictures. Ultrasound is a pain-free procedure that outlines abdominal structures on a monitor by using sound waves. Ultrasound and high-definition scans (CT or MRI) are particularly helpful in distinguishing fluid-filled masses from solid ones.

Treatment

Specific treatment depends upon the underlying cause, the organ involved, and the location of the abdominal mass. If an abdominal mass causes partial or total obstruction of the affected organ or system, surgery may be necessary, possibly on an emergency basis. Regardless of the kind of treatment necessary, abdominal masses often require hospitalization.

Abdominal abscess

Description

An abdominal abscess is a pocket of pus, usually caused by a bacterial infection. Abdominal abscesses may form below the diaphragm, in the middle of the abdomen, in the pelvis, or behind the abdominal cavity. Abscesses may also form in or around any abdominal organ such as: kidneys, spleen, pancreas, liver Often, abdominal masses are caused by injury, infection or rupture of the intestine, or infection of another abdominal organ.

Causes and symptoms

An abdominal abscess may form when infected fluid, for example, from a ruptured appendix, accumulates in a cavity. Abscesses may also result from a ruptured intestine, or an abdominal wound. The abdomen is usually painful in the area of the abscess. Abscesses behind the abdominal cavity (called retroperitoneal abscesses) lie behind the peritoneum, the membrane that lines the abdominal cavity and organs. The causes, which are similar to those of abscesses in the abdomen, include inflammation and infection of the appendix and of the pancreas. Pain, usually in the lower back, worsens when the person moves the leg at the hip. Liver abscesses may be caused by bacteria or amebas. Bacteria can reach the liver from an infected gallbladder; a penetrating or blunt wound; an infection in the abdomen, such as a nearby abscess; or an infection carried by the bloodstream from elsewhere in the body.

Diagnosis and treatment

Doctors can easily misdiagnose an abscess, because the symptoms are commonly caused by less serious problems. When a person has an abscess, blood tests often reveal an abnormal number of white blood cells. Radiological tests (X-rays or scans), ultrasound scanning, can be used to distinguish an abscess from other problems (for example, tumors of cysts), as well as to determine the size and position of the abscess once it has been diagnosed.

In nearly all people with an abdominal abscess, the pus must be drained, either by surgery or by a needle inserted through the skin. To guide the placement of the needle, a doctor uses CT or ultrasound scanning.

Antibiotics are usually given in conjunction with drainage to prevent the infection from spreading and to help completely eliminate the infection.

Abdominal pain

Description and causes

A pain in the belly (abdomen) is a very common symptom, and disorders of any of the organs (liver, spleen, intestine, bladder, uterus, ovaries, pancreas), glands, lymph nodes, arteries, veins or nerves may be responsible, as well as the structures around the area such as the muscles, ligaments, skin or the vertebrae in the back. The doctor may make a diagnosis depending on the nature of the pain (sharp, ache, dull), whether it is constant or intermittent, if it is affected by eating or passing urine or faeces, if it starts in one area then, moves to another, what tends to make the pain better or worse, and the presence of associated symptom s such as vomiting, diarrhea, constipation, loss of appetite, fever, pain on passing urine and menstrual period problems. Investigations to further aid a doctor may include blood tests, X-rays, CT scans, ultrasound scans, endoscopy, and as a last resort, surgery. A very large number of conditions may be responsible for pain in the belly. These include:

- constipation
- colic in children
- inflammation or infection of the gall bladder
- tear of muscle in the belly wall
- gastric or intestinal disorders
- infections of the liver
- cancer of the colon
- appendicitis
- irritable bowel syndrome
- adhesions after surgery to the abdomen
- diverticulitis
- infections of the bladder
- disorders of the internal female genital organs
- peritonitis

Diagnosis

Diagnosis varies according to the age and sex of the patient, location and kind of pain, and when the pain began, and how long it has lasted.

A patient's physical and emotional condition are also important as is information about fever, nausea, vomiting, or changes in defecation or urination.

An examining physician takes a detailed history, noting prior conditions - an accident, chronic disease, and previous operations.

Physical examination focuses upon the painful area and the overall effects of pain upon the patient. The abdomen is checked carefully and an internal rectal examination is performed.

Blood and urine samples are analyzed. Further tests, including X-ray examination, ultrasound imaging and CT- or MRI scans may be postponed until initial tests can be evaluated along with the medical history and results of the physical examination.

Complications

Complications depend upon the cause of pain, the organ or system involved, and the speed with which diagnosis can be made and treatment begun.

If a child is in the care of experienced medical personnel, especially in a hospital emergency room, the threat of serious complications and long-term aftereffects is reduced significantly. Life-threatening complications may develop if diagnosis is delayed or inappropriate treatment is begun.

Treatment

Treatment depends upon diagnosis of the cause of acute pain. Surgery may be necessary. In certain situations, such as acute appendicitis, surgery is almost always chosen.

In the case of appendicitis, an infected appendix could burst, causing, perhaps, a serious infection in the abdominal cavity (peritonitis).

In others, where a choice exists between surgery and medical management, the physician discusses with the parent (and child if appropriately) alternative methods of treatment and any risks that may be involved. Then medical and surgical treatment begins.

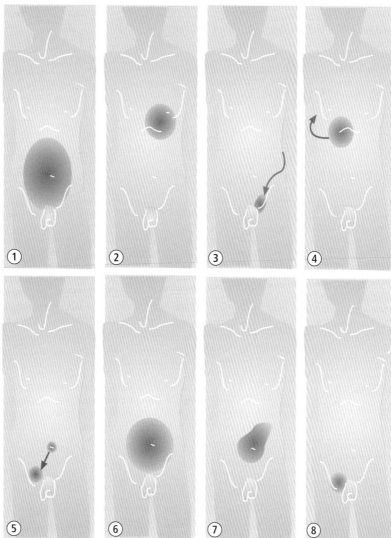

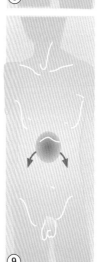

Abdominal pain in men. Acute abdomen is an acute intra-abdominal condition of abrupt onset, usually associated with pain due to inflammation, perforation, obstruction, infarction, or rupture of abdominal organs, and usually requiring emergency surgical intervention.

The localization of the pain, as indicated by the patient, is important for the differential diagnosis.

Some common sites of abdominal pain are indicated.

1. Colic of the small intestine.
2. Acute indigestion.
3. Kidney colic, usually due to the presence of stones.
4. Colic of the gallbladder, usually due to the presence of stones.
5. Appendicitis.
6. Peritonitis (inflammatory process of the peritoneum).
7. Intestinal obstruction.
8. Incarcerated hernia.
9. Perforation of the stomach wall due to a peptic ulcer.

ACNE

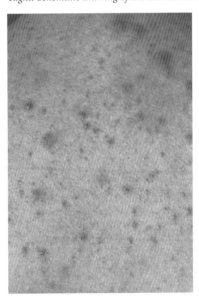

Introduction

Acne or acne vulgaris is a common skin disease of pimples on the face and upper trunk, and is most prominent in adolescence. Blackheads may also become inflamed, and this is due either to local production of irritant fatty acids by bacteria or to bacterial infection; because sufferers may pick these spots, scarring may occur. The onset of acne is most frequent between the ages of 14 and 19 years, but cases up to 40 years may occur.

Causes

The sebaceous glands secrete sebum, a fatty substance which lubricates and protects the skin. These glands are under endocrine (hormonal) control, especially by androgens, the male sex hormones produced by the testes and adrenals, and there is a relationship between the severity of patients' acne and the greasiness of their skin.

This increased production by the sebaceous glands - seborrhoea - could be due to an increase of circulating androgens, but many patients show no such abnormality, suggesting that the abnormality is a over-reaction of the sebaceous glands to androgens in the blood circulation.

There is evidence that an inflamed acne lesion is preceded by a non-inflamed lesion - a whitehead or blackhead (medically called a comedo) which is a plugged sebaceous gland - but how these lesions form is uncertain. Certain constituents of the sebum may produce comedones, and it is possible to induce comedones (whiteheads or blackheads) in man. A closed comedo, or whitehead, occurs when the sebum plug becomes enclosed in a cellular sac. This sac keeps its contents from being exposed to the air, so the plug remains white. Whiteheads can mature into blackheads - or can mark the first stage of inflammatory acne.

The two main types of bacteria on the acne-prone skin and in the follicular ducts (the tiny tubes leading from the sebaceous glands at the base of hair follicles) are the *Staphylococcus epidermidis* and the *Propionibacteria acnes*. Clinically, only a few follicles out of many thousands are affected at any time. The bacteria grow only under certain conditions, when they may produce biological active products that may cause inflammation; this may explain why one follicular duct develops acne and another does not. If the whitehead's sac ruptures, the sebum mixture spills into the surrounding skin tissue, causing it to become inflamed. The red bump that results is called an inflamed papule - the medical term for a pimple. White blood cells (the body's infection fighters) rush to the area to clear up this material, causing pus to form. As a result, the pimple gets a yellow cap; at this stage, it's called a pustule.

In severe cases of acne, the entire inflammation can become encapsulated within a thickened cell wall, forming a cyst. If left untreated, cysts can eventually cause skin to become permanently scarred.

Treatment

Patients with mild acne will only need topical therapy, such as the application to the skin of a preparation containing either retinoic acid (a deriva-

Left: Magnification of the skin area with acne.
Right: Schematic drawing of the distribution of acne on the body.

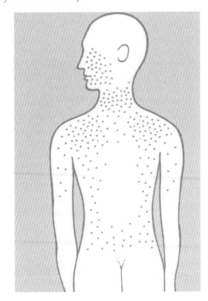

A

tive of vitamin A) or benzoyl peroxide. Patients with more severe acne
require drugs as well as topical treatment, and the most commonly used
oral antibiotics are tetracycline and
erythromycin.

There have been many medical
reports on the treatment of acne for a
few weeks only, but acne is a disorder
which requires long-term treatment, a
minimum of six months being recommended. In patients with severe
acne, the dose of the antibiotic may be
reduced after three months to a twice-
daily dosage. If the patient is responding well after six months, the doctor
may then decrease the antibiotic to a
once-daily regime and stop the drug
entirely at seven months. On this
regime, improvement is seen in 60 per
cent of patients.

Although topical therapy is continued, relapses occur in 40 per cent of
patients by the end of a further five
months. However, as the drug therapy
is safe, repeated courses can be given.
Some patients respond less well than
others; for example, young people
aged 14 to 17 do less well than other
age groups - no doubt due to the fact
that in this age group acne is usually
worse. Such patients are given doses of
antibiotic larger than that which is
commensurate for the degree of acne.

Self-treatment tips

In most cases of acne, specialized
medical care is not necessary. A consistent self-treatment program may be
a helpful and important first step
toward clear skin. This program consists of eight points.

■ *Analyze your skin*
Is your skin dry, moderately oily or
very oily?
Do you have a light, medium or dark
complexion?
Is your acne problem mild, moderate
or severe?
You can estimate the severity of your
acne by counting the pimples on your
face. If you have ten or fewer pimples,
your acne is mild. Ten to 30 pimples
signifies a moderate problem. If you
have more than 30 pimples -or one or
more large cysts - your acne problem
is severe.

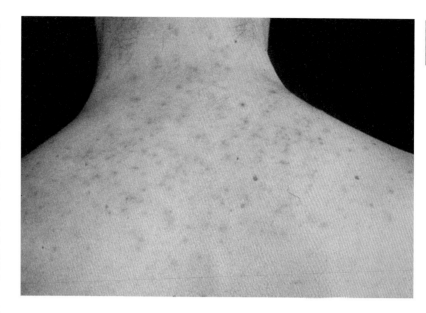

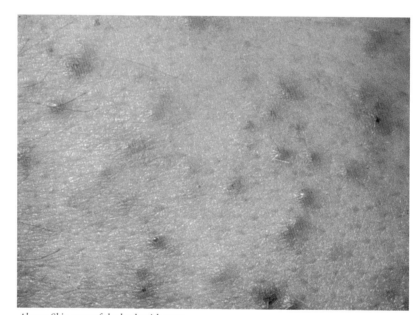

Above: Skin area of the back with acne.
Below: Magnification of the skin area with acne.

■ *Plan a skin care regimen*
How frequently you wash your face
and the strength of acne medication
you choose depends on the factors
listed above. For example, if you have
a medium complexion, a moderate
acne problem and moderate oiliness,
you could wash your face three times
a day and use a mild acne medicine -
or wash once a day and use a moder-
ate-strength acne preparation.

With dry, fair skin and mild acne, a
once-a-day wash and use of a mild
preparation may be sufficient. If you
have dark, very oily skin plus a severe
acne problem, you might try washing
three times a day and using a strong
acne preparation.

You may have to experiment a little to
hit on an effective combination - just

Acne   Questions & Answers

What is acne vulgaris?
Acne vulgaris is a chronic skin condition characterized mainly by comedones (whiteheads and blackheads) and papules (a small, firm raised skin lesion). In severe cases, inflammation, pustules (small, pus-containing elevations on the skin), cysts, and scaring may occur. Acne occurs most commonly on the face, back, and chest. Although it does not pose a severe physical threat, acne should not be ignored since it may cause a great deal of emotional stress and anguish.

When does acne vulgaris occur?
The condition occurs most often in adolescence, a period in which many physiologic, social, and psychological adjustments are made and when self-image and peer acceptance are extremely important.

What are the causes of excess sebum formation?
Acne vulgaris has its origin in the pilosebaceous units in the skin (dermis). These units, consisting of a hair follicle and the associated sebaceous glands, are connected to the skin surface by a duct through which the hair shaft passes. On the smooth skin of the body, the hairs may be very fine or entirely absent. Because the sebaceous glands are most common on the face, back, and chest, acne tends to occur most common in these areas. The sebaceous glands produce sebum, which passes to the skin surface and then spreads over the skin surface to retard water loss. At puberty here is an increase in the production of androgenic hormones in both sexes..

What is the relation of androgens and sebaceous glands?
Androgens are the major stimulus to sebaceous gland development and sebum secretion. However, patients with acne do not necessarily have higher androgen levels. It is theorized that acne-prone patients have increased end-organ sensitivity to normal levels of androgens, facilitating the excessive formation of sebum.

What is the cause of steroid acne?
Exogenous sources of corticosteroids, both systemic and topical (prescription and nonprescription), may also induce the hypertrophic changes by sensitizing the follicle and producing 'steroid acne'. These lesions are characterized by uniform red papules succeeded by closed comedones and finally open comedones. Oral contraceptives with high androgenic activity also have been implicated in the production of acne.

What is the cause of noninflammatory acne?
The cause of acne is an increased activity of the sebaceous gland and of the epithelial lining: the infundibulum. This increase is induced by the greater production of hormones, especially androgenic hormones, as puberty approaches. Sebum exists of free and esterized fatty acids as well as unsaponifiable lipid components. The glands produce more sebum, causing increased skin oiliness.

What is a microcomedo?
The so-called impaction plugs and distends the follicle to form a microcomedo. As more cells and sebum are added, the microcomedo enlarges and becomes visible (whitehead) and is called a closed comedo (its contents do not reach the surface of the skin).

be careful not to overdo it, since some treatments can dry out the skin.

■ Choose an acne medication
Over-the-counter acne preparations from a chemist do work if you choose the right one for your skin and use it properly and regularly. Effective acne preparations work by getting down into the follicular ducts and breaking apart the plugs of dead cells and sebum, allowing them to flow out of the ducts.

When used properly, acne medications will cause mild surface drying and peeling of the skin (which is why these are called DP - drying and peeling - agents).

This drying and peeling, however, is not harmful to your skin. The best preparations will usually contain a benzoyl peroxide solution in cream or gel form.

However, some people (about 1 per cent of all users) find that they are allergic to this substance. If your skin becomes red, itchy or blotchy after you use a benzoyl peroxide product, you may be experiencing an allergic reaction.

Use either your hands or a flannel. If you have mild acne, any soap will do, but stay away from oily cleansing soaps and creams.

If your acne is more severe, a special acne cleanser can help. After washing it is suggested that you rub the DP agent not just on existing pimples, but on to all breakout-prone areas. Be careful to avoid the sensitive areas around the eyes and the corners of the mouth.

■ Avoid beauty products
Oil-based make-up can make your skin oilier, so if you use it while trying to control acne, you may be sabotaging your entire treatment. Instead, use oil-free, water-based make-up.

■ Give trouble spots extra attention
If your forehead breaks out more than your cheeks, for instance, apply more of the DP agent to that area, or use a stronger one. You can also apply a DP agent directly to back or chest acne without washing every time - although if you have severe acne in these areas, a shower or bath twice a day is essential.

■ *Stick to your skin care plan*

The aim of your treatment program is to prevent new pimples from forming; it may take some time for existing ones to clear up. In some cases, there is noticeable improvement within a week, but for most people, progress is gradual. Improvement and control (that is, getting no new pimples) can be expected in three to eight weeks of daily skin care. However, if self-care isn't working after about two months, consult your family physician or a dermatologist.

Diet

Dietary treatment of acne has taken some new directions. Many foods, once strictly forbidden, are now considered possible preventives.

Breakfast
▲ 170 ml (6 fl. oz) of any of the following unsweetened juices: orange, grapefruit, pineapple, or tomato
▲ 225 g (8 oz) high-protein cereal with 115 ml (4 fl. oz) skim milk
▲ 1 cup regular or decaffeinated coffee or tea with 1 teaspoon honey

Mid-morning
▲ 1200 mg lecithin capsule
▲ 25,000-unit vitamin A capsule
▲ 500 mg vitamin C tablet
▲ 50 mg zinc gluconate tablet

Lunch
▲ Tuna and chopped celery salad
▲ 1 thin toasted slice whole-grain bread with natural peanut butter, spread very thinly
▲ 1 slice pineapple with a generous sprinkling of mint, if desired
▲ 1 cup of herb tea with a squirt of fresh lemon juice and a teaspoon of honey

Dinner
▲ Dairy foods: cottage cheese, eggs, low-fat hard cheese, whole or skim milk and low-fat yogurt
▲ Fish: almost all varieties are included these days; even the fattier varieties - salmon, trout, tuna - are now acceptable. The natural fish oils are good for the skin.
▲ Fowl: chicken, turkey, even duckling, are regarded as anti-acne

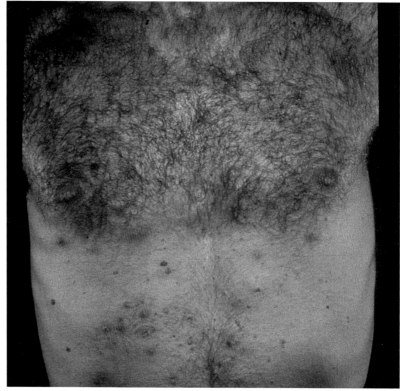
Severe form of acne involving the hairy skin.

foods. The preferred methods of cooking are broiling and roasting.
▲ Fruits: apples and pears; all berries, but especially cranberries; the entire melon family; pineapple and all citrus fruits are recommended daily for acne sufferers.
▲ Meat: lean beef is good in modest quantities, as are lamb and veal.
▲ Vegetables: almost unlimited: asparagus, lettuce, broccoli and all leafy green vegetables except spinach; carrots, courgettes, green beans, okra, potatoes, tomatoes, turnips, water chestnut and yams are excellent for the skin.
▲ Beverages: almost any fruit or vegetable juice is permitted; also regular or decaffeinated coffee and tea (especially the herbal varieties). Additionally, be sure to drink large daily quantities of plain water.

■ *What not to eat or drink*
Some of the most marvellous foods from a nutritional standpoint are so loaded with androgens that for the acne victim to experiment with them is a chancy affair. High on the list are shellfish and offal. Most soft drinks are heavy with brominated vegetable oil, a substance to be avoided by the person with troubled skin. Avoid mixers or juices laced with so-called "blushing" seasonings. The most common of these are cayenne, chili peppers and curry powder, and alcoholic beverages are also "blushers." In fact, anything that dilates the blood vessels is bad news for the acne-prone person.

Acne scars

If you have extensive scars due to acne, there are several ways you can be helped. These include dermabrasion, chemical peeling, cryotherapy and surgery.

■ *Dermabrasion*
This is a procedure performed on the face, involving numbing the skin with a freezing aerosol spray, then removing the top layers of the skin with a

A

Acne   Questions & Answers

What factors are responsible for the occurrence of acne?

Acne (or acne vulgaris) occurs at puberty and is commoner in boys than girls. The tendency to acne often runs in families. The spots, which can be very disfiguring, occur mainly on the face but also on the back of the neck, the shoulders, and the chest.

Acne affects appearance, not physical health, but it can be severe enough to cause mental anguish by making a young person feel ugly at the very age when it is becoming important for him, or her, to feel attractive. Parents and doctors must, therefore, take the child's worries seriously and do more than advise patience.

The cause of acne is the excessive greasiness of the skin that occurs at puberty. Under the influence of hormones circulating during puberty, the sebaceous glands in the skin become especially active and produce extra amounts of the normal grease (sebum) that lubricates the skin.

So much is produced that the mouths of the skin pores through which the sebum has to pass to get out become blocked. These are very liable to become inflamed, causing pimples and boils, which can leave scars. It is now known that this inflammation is due not to infection but is the result of chemical changes in the sebum.

Can the physician prescribe an efficient remedy for acne?

Acne stops soon after puberty is completed and the associated chemical changes have settled down. Treatment to reduce the greasiness of the skin and to clear the blocked sebaceous glands does a great deal to keep the condition down until a natural cure occurs with the end of adolescence.

The face should be washed with soap in very hot water as often as possible; washing should be vigorous, and it is a good idea even to use a scrubbing brush. This helps to get rid of the blackheads. Squeezing blackheads is usually discouraged on the ground it increases the risk of secondary infection.

However, some skin specialists now feel that the risk of secondary infection has been exaggerated and that, since the inflammation in acne is chemical, it is safe for blackheads to be removed by hand after a thorough washing. A drying lotion, such as calamine and 3 percent sulphur, which you can get from the pharmacist without prescription, should be applied.

This is rubbed in when the face has dried in order to encourage peeling of the skin and cleaning of the blocked pore. The lotion can be used during the daytime because once it has been rubbed in it is not obvious. The slight color from the lotion may camouflage the spots without making a boy look made up.

Only in the case of a serious infectious complication, a prescription for antibiotics from a physician is needed.

Is ultraviolet light or an antibiotic effective for acne?

Ultraviolet light also helps to dry the skin and encourage peeling. Children with acne should therefore spend as much time as possible out in the sun. Their hair should be cut in such a way that it does not stop the sun from reaching the face.

Fringes may hide spots on the forehead but they also screen off the sunlight, so that the spots remain. Ultraviolet light can also be obtained from a special lamp, but the length of exposure must be strictly controlled. The eyes should be covered while the lamp is being used.

If acne is severe your doctor may also give antibiotic treatment for a long period. The antibiotics used do not act in their usual way, by destroying germs, but alter the chemical composition of the sebum.

Whatever line of treatment your doctor recommends, the aim is also reassurance. Sometimes the spots are not half as noticeable as your child images.

Benzyl peroxide is probably the most effective local treatment for acne and is sometimes prescribed in combination with tretinoin. Local treatment must be applied to the back and chest, as well as to the face, if they are involved. It must be emphasized that treatment is lengthy, lasting for a minimum of six months.

I repeatedly get cold sores or herpes simplex on my lips, especially when I get tense, or nervous. The sores often go into the skin surrounding my lips. Is there a way to keep them from doing that?

As soon as you feel the sore forming, become aware of it and leave it alone. Do not touch it with either your tongue or your fingers. The touching with your fingers may transfer the germs and bacteria and make it harder for your body to deal with the initial problem.

The touching or "caressing" with your tongue will irritate the sore and cause it to multiply. Instead of keeping your lips moist with your own saliva, use a clear lipstick (you can buy special ones for herpes) either alone or under a colored one.

---

high-speed rotating wheel so that new skin will form, minus the scars.

Deep scars may need several treatments before much improvement is made. Dermabrasion is not a good idea for those with a black or very dark skin, because the darker your skin, the more likely it is that you will have excess scar tissue, called keloids.

■ *Chemical peeling*

The doctor uses a chemical solution to burn off the upper layers of skin. A mild chemical peel can make lesions look better by opening them up and allowing drainage.

■ *Cryotherapy*

This method involves peeling the skin by freezing its surface with a roll-on or spray-on liquid nitrogen.

Drugs used to treat acne

Drugs that kill bacteria (applied topically)

Clindamycin
- Selected side effects
  Diarrhea

Erythromycin
- Selected side effects
  No side effects

Benzoyl peroxide
- Especially effective when combined with erythromycin
  - Selected side effects
    Dries the skin
    May discolor clothing
    May discolor hair

Drugs that kill bacteria (taken by mouth)

Tetracycline
- Inexpensive and safe
- Must be taken by itself or with tretionin
- Should be used cautiously in people with dark skin
  - Selected side effects
    Sensitizes skin to sunlioght

Doxycycline
- Protective clothing should be worn during sun exposure
  - Selected side effects
    Sensitizes skin to sunlight

Minocycline
- Most effective antibiotic
  - Selected side effects
    Head\iscoloration

Drugs that unlog pores (applied topically)

Tretinoin
- May take 3 to 4 weeks to notice any improvement
- Protective clothing should be worn during sun exposure
- Sunscreen is important
  - Selected side effects
    Skin irritation
    Sensitizes skin to sunlight

Tazarotene
- May take 3 to 4 weeks to notice any improvement
- Protective clothing should be worn during sun exposure
- Sunscreen is important
  - Selected side effects
    Skin irritation
    Sensitizes skin to sunlight

Adapalene
- As effective as tretinoin
- Minimally irritating
- Protective clothing should be worn during sun exposure
- Skin-lightening effects may occur
  - Selected side effects
    Some redness
    Burning
    Increased sun sentitivity

Azelaic acid
- May be used by itself or with tretinoin
- Should be used cautiously in people with dark skin
  - Selected side effects
    May lighten skin

Drugs that unlog pores (taken by mouth)

Isotretinoin
- Should not be used by pregnant women
- Blood tests are necessary to test for side effects
  - Selected side effects
    Can harm a developing fetus
    Can affect blood cells
    Dry eyes
    Drying of mucous membranes
    Pain or stiffness of large joints
    Has been associated with depression

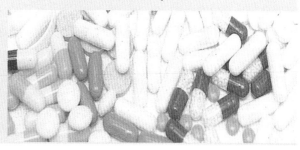

■ *Surgery*

Surgical methods involve cutting out scars. In addition, dermatologists will sometimes raise a crater-like scar to skin level with a liquid filler made of either silicone or collagen. This is called injection therapy, a treatment that is especially helpful if you are not a good candidate for dermabrasion.

In the past, young people afflicted with acne really had no choice; they had to learn to live with their bumps and blemishes - and hope the acne would disappear at the end of their teen years without leaving them with too many scars. But with the proper treatment, there is no reason why you cannot get your acne problem under control.

ADHD *Attention deficit/hyperactivity syndrome*

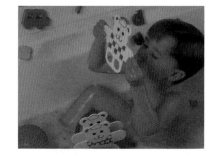

Description

The attention deficit/hyperactivity syndrome is defined as poor or short attention span and impulsiveness, inappropriate for the child's age; some

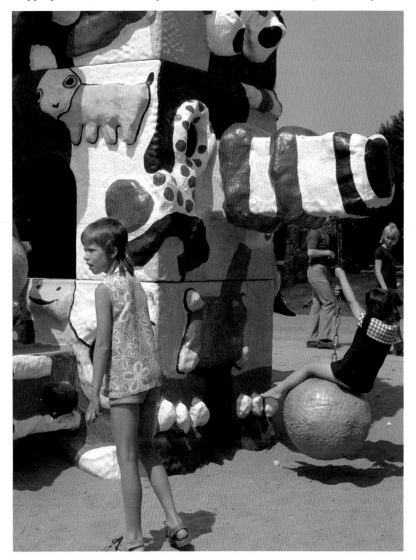

children also manifest hyperactivity. Virtually all children appear hyperactive at one time or another in the eyes of their parents. A small child who seems impatient during an adult social occasion may, for example, be

considered hyperactive. Hyperactivity is often accompanied by attention problems, such as an ability to concentrate and by impulsiveness (a tendency to begin an activity without thinking about its merits or drawbacks). Other attention problems that tend to affect such children include:
- excitability;
- restlessness;
- tendency to deny mistakes and blame others;
- failure to finish things;
- childishness or immaturity;
- distractability;
- quick mood changes;
- drastic mood changes;
- tendency to become frustrated easily.

An affected child may also have behavioral problems, such as frequent temper tantrums.

Because those parts of the brain that control attention and filter out unwanted stimuli seem to be impaired, physicians call this syndrome attention-deficit disorder (ADD) or attention deficit/hyperactivity syndrome (ADHD). About 5 per cent of all children have an attention deficit/hyperactivity syndrome, and it is one of the behavioral problems most frequently brought to the attention of pediatricians. Boys are affected at least 4 times as often as girls. Although hyperactivity frequently accompanies ADD, it is not necessarily a part of the syndrome. Some children with ADD are not hyperactive, and those who are hyperactive often become less so as they get older.

Children with ADHD have a hard time paying attention and are easily distracted from play. They do not want to do things that require ongoing mental effort.

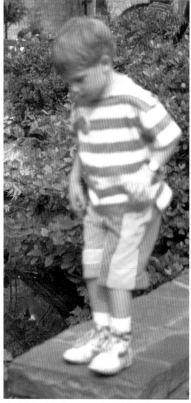 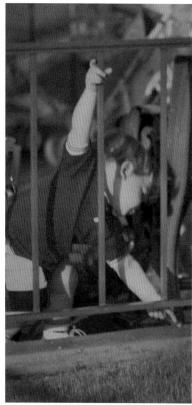 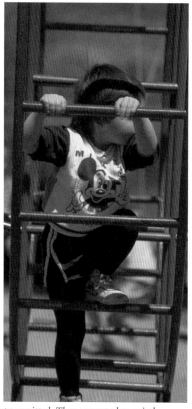

A child with the attention deficit/hyperactivity syndrome runs, jumps, and climbs when this is not permitted. They cannot play quietly.

Cause

The exact cause of attention deficit/hyperactivity syndrome is unclear because little is yet known definitely about how the brain controls attention. Medical experts believe they have identified a brain mechanism, called the reticular activating system, that enables a person to screen out certain noises and sights at will.

When a person decides to concentrate on something, chemicals (neurotransmitters) may be released by the brain in the reticular activating system. For instance, this mechanism may help a person to speak and listen to someone in a crowd while blocking out other conversations. One theory is that people with attention deficit/hyperactivity syndrome do not release enough neurotransmitters. Another contributing factor to the problem among growing children may simply be the immaturity of frontal brain systems.

Heredity may play a role in some cases of ADHD. Specialists believe that some parents pass along to their children a tendency toward slow maturation of certain parts of the brain - including the part that controls attention. Other major causes of ADHD are thought to include:
- improper fetal development;
- injury at birth;
- deprivation of oxygen at birth;
- other birth complications.

Signs and symptoms

How a child with the specific symptoms may behave:

Inattention
- ▲ Has a hard time paying attention, daydreams
- ▲ Does not seem to listen
- ▲ Is easily distracted from work or play
- ▲ Does not seem to care about details
- ▲ Does not follow through on instructions or finish tasks
- ▲ Is disorganised
- ▲ Loses a lot of important things
- ▲ Forget things
- ▲ Does not want to do things that require ongoing mental effort

Hyperactivity
- ▲ Is in constant motion
- ▲ Cannot stay seated
- ▲ Squirms and fidgets
- ▲ Talks too much
- ▲ Runs, jumps, and climbs when this is not permitted
- ▲ Cannot play quietly

Impulsivity
- ▲ Acts and speaks without thinking
- ▲ May run into the street without looking for traffic first
- ▲ Has trouble taking turns
- ▲ Cannot wait for things
- ▲ Calls out answers before the question is complete
- ▲ Interrupts others

A

ADHD   Questions & Answers

What is ADHD?
ADHD - attention deficit/hyperactivity disorder is a syndrome characterized by poor or short attention span and impulsiveness inappropriate for the child's age; some children also manifest hyperactivity.

What are the major characteristics of ADHD?
ADHD is a condition in which a child's level of activity interferes significantly with home, school, and social life. A hyperkinetic or hyperactive child typically seems to in constant motion and always full of energy.

Although actual diagnosis of ADHD is not simple, hyperkinetic or hyperactive children have several characteristics in common; hyperactivity is just one of the symptoms and may or may not be present.

The children tend to behave inappropriately in many situations. They are unable to control their actions and seem to have much difficulty in learning self-control. They usually have a short attention span, and are easily distracted or frustrated.

Their behavior is often described as fidgety, restless, impulsive, and quarrelsome. They may have emotional problems and specific learning difficulties.

What causes ADHD?
The exact origin of ADHD is unknown - no single cause has been established. The disorder has been described as the result of genetic, biological, physiological, social, and environmental factors.

Although there are many theories about the causes, hard evidence is scarce. For example, there is little evidence to support the theory of brain damage as a major cause. Since research has shown that the parents of some hyperactive children were themselves hyperactive, it may be that certain children inherit a predisposition for hyperactivity. Other possible causes cited by various investigators include food additives, lead poisoning, vitamin deficiencies, and complications of pregnancy, including premature birth.

What are the major signs of inattention in children with ADHD?
The major signs of inattention are:
- ▲ The child often fails to pay close attention to details.
- ▲ Has difficulty sustaining attention in work and play.
- ▲ Does not seem to listen when spoken to directly.
- ▲ Often does not follow through on instructions and fails to finish tasks.
- ▲ Often avoids, dislikes, or is reluctant to engage in tasks that require sustained mental effort.
- ▲ Often loses things and is often forgetful.
- ▲ Is early distracted by extraneous stimuli.

Is there a medical treatment for children with ADHD?
There is really no "cure" for ADHD. While research continues to seek an understanding of the underlying causes, treatments have been developed to provide relief of the symptoms. Management of the condition may involve a variety of methods (medicines, play therapy, psychotherapy, etc).

The most effective medications, to date, are the stimulants. Administered properly, these drugs produce favorable therapeutic results in 70 to 80 percent of children with hyperkinesis or hyperactivity.

It was previously believed that the stimulants had a "paradoxical" effect in children, i.e., the drugs stimulate adults and calm children.

Recent research has shown that, given equivalent dosages, normal adults and hyperactive children respond in much the same way; both exhibit improved attention spans and task performance. With medication, the child, no longer driven by his impulses, is more able to control his behavior.

Diagnosis

Although signs and symptoms are evident as early as infancy, most children with attention and hyperctivity disorders are not diagnosed until they begin school.

Many teachers are trained or otherwise experienced in recognizing hyperactive behavior and disorders of attention span. A teacher may recommend that a child suspected of having the problem see a professional, in which case a physician - preferably one familiar with a child's medical history - should be consulted.

Physicians base a diagnosis of attention deficit/hyperactivity syndrome on a child's symptoms and medical history. No specific tests exists to detect hyperactivity, although evidence of neurological immaturity, obtained from sophisticated neurological tests, may suggest ADHD.

Nonetheless, it is crucial for physicians to test for possible causes of hyperactivity and/or attention disorders. A physician can be expected to perform vision and hearing tests as well as psychological and physical examination. The physician initially consulted may refer a child to a psychiatrist or neurologist for further tests or treatment.

Because a physician's office usually contains fewer distractions that a classroom, a hyperactive child may be fairly calm during the examination procedure. For this reason, parents should be prepared to report in detail their own and teachers' observations of a child's behavior.

With parental consent, a physician may request intelligence test scores and other academic measurements from a child's teacher. It may also be helpful for a physician to sprak directly with a teacher about a child's classroom behavior.

Historically, the label of hyperactivity has been incorrectly applied to any child who seems "abnormally" active. Mistaken labels of hyperactivity have been applied to children who simply were too active for rigid or fussy teachers or parents. This mistake has caused problems for many children whose true maladies are stress, anxiety, other emotional disorders, or auditory-perception problems.

Complications

The most common complications affecting hyperactive children are psychological problems stemming from other people's reactions to their behavior. A child may develop anything from a poor self-image to periodic depression to severe friendship and social problems. In the absence of proper diagnosis and treatment, such complications are likely to develop.

Treatment

The goal of treatment is to minimize the ill effects of a child's ADHD and related problems by providing a small, structured, supportive environment that is conducive to improved attention.

Any treatment plan should be administered with much love and understanding. Success should be measured by how comfortable a child becomes and not by any arbitrary standards.

Treatment for ADHD may involve:
- medication (for instance, Concerta or Ritalin);
- behavior modifications;
- psychotherapy;
- special diets.

The exact treatment approach used varies from child to child, but almost all children benefit from a tailor-made combination of several methods. Even if some symptoms disappear, treatment may be necessary throughout childhood. Many children with attention deficit/hyperactivity syndrome benefit from medication. Although it seems to parents that an affected child needs tranquilizers, such drugs tend to aggravate a child's hyperactivity without improving behavior.

Prevention

Some cases of hyperactivity and ADHD may not be preventable. However, reduction of environmental lead, control of alcohol intake by mothers during pregnancy, and improvements in prenatal care and birth (delivery) procedures may well prevent a considerable number of cases of children with attention deficit/hyperactivity syndrome.

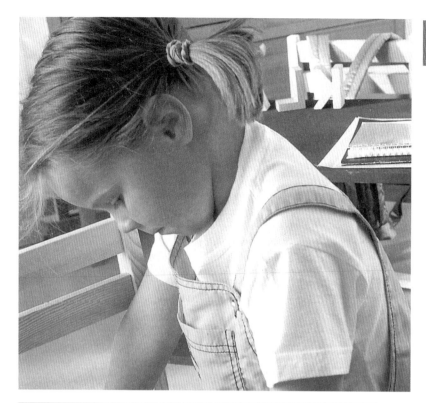

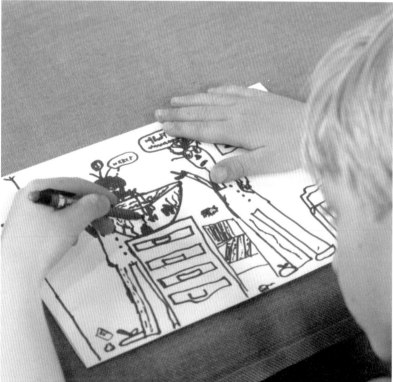

The goal of treatment is to minimize the ill effects of the child's ADHD by providing a small, structured, supportive environment.

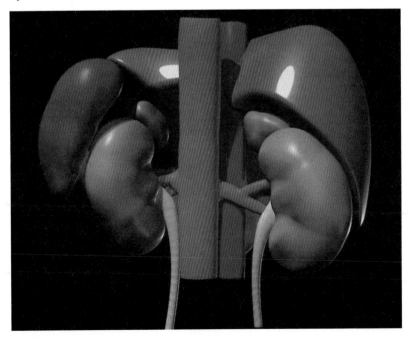

ADRENAL GLAND DISORDERS

Description

The adrenal glands belong to the endocrine system of glands, whose secretions (called hormones) are distributed in the human body by means of the bloodstream rather than being discharged through ducts.

The glandular tissues of the endocrine system have in common that they secrete into the bloodstream 'chemical messengers' that regulate and integrate body functions. One of the characteristics of the endocrine glands is their wanderlust, their tendency to leave their source and look for work elsewhere.

The human embryo develops gills like those of primitive fishes, but parts of these turn into endocrine glands and leave their birthplace at the sides of the throat in the course of their embryonic development.

The pituitary gland, the thyroid, the parathyroids and the thymus develop in part from these primitive gills. The two adrenal glands do not migrate far. They form in the peritoneum of the abdomen and then settle on top of the kidneys.

A group of cells from the neighbouring sympathetic nervous system migrates into the adrenal glands and forms a core there. Thus the adrenal glands become double organs, with a nervous core or marrow and a glandular cortex or bark. The cortex produces a series of steroids, the corticosteroids, which have wide-ranging effects.

The core functions in conjunction with the sympathetic nervous system, regulating the blood pressure, the heart action and other activities of the body, through the secretion of adrenalin and noradrenaline.

The suprarenal or adrenal glands, each perched over one of the kidneys, are double glands. The yellow-brown triangular glands lie close to the upper end of the kidneys alongside the vertebral column (spine). Like all endocrine glands they have a rich blood supply. A microscopic section shows that the cortex is made up of lightly stained cells containing much fat, arranged in three zones. Outside is a zone where the cells are in rounded groups, and beneath there is a layer of cell columns running at right angles to the surface and an innermost irregular layer.

Adrenal medulla

The hormone-producing cells of the adrenal glands contain innumerable granules which stain with potassium bichromate, hence the term 'chromaffin cells.' The core, or medulla, manufactures adrenalin, noradrenaline and a small amount of dopamine. These are also produced by the nerve endings of the sympathetic nervous system.

Anger or fear stimulates this gland and secrete adrenalin and noradrenaline into the bloodstream. As a result, the heart beats faster, the liver sends sugar into the blood, the blood supply to the intestines is reduced and digestion stops, the blood supply to the muscles is increased, and the body burns sugar faster. In short, adrenalin makes it possible to meet an emer-

The adrenal glands lie close to the upper end of the kidneys alongside the vertebral colon (spine).

gency by flight and fight.

Adrenalin and noradrenaline have slightly different effects, and they are probably produced by two different sorts of cells. Thus of the two, adrenalin has much stronger inhibitory actions (for example, on the bladder and intestines), while noradrenaline is more powerful in raising blood pressure and constricting arterioles.

■ *Disorders of the adrenal medulla*
No functional abnormalities result from insufficiency of the adrenal medulla, the continuing production of these hormones by the sympathetic nerve cells being sufficient to maintain adequate levels in the body.

In the absence of any recognizable deficiency state the gland owes its clinical importance to tumors which may arise from the medullary cells. The best-known is the phaeochromocytoma, a tumor of chromaffin cells that secrete catecholamines (for instance, adrenalin, noradrenaline, dopamine), causing high blood pressure.

The tumor appears equally in both sexes, are on both sides in ten percent of cases (twenty percent in children) and are usually benign (95 percent). Although these tumors occur at any age, the maximum incidence is between the third and fifth decades.

The tumors vary in size but average only 2 inches in diameter. They usually weigh 50 to 200 g. but tumors weighing several pounds have been reported. The most prominent features are sudden attacks of high blood pressure or a continuous elevated blood pressure.

The following symptoms may also be found:
- increased heart rate;
- increased breathing rate;
- flushing;
- cold and clammy skin;
- severe headache;
- angina pectoris;
- palpitations;
- nausea and vomiting;
- visual disturbances;
- constipation;
- a sense of impending doom.

The diagnosis can be established by tests for catecholamines in the urine and provocative tests; the tumor is being localized by radiographic pro-

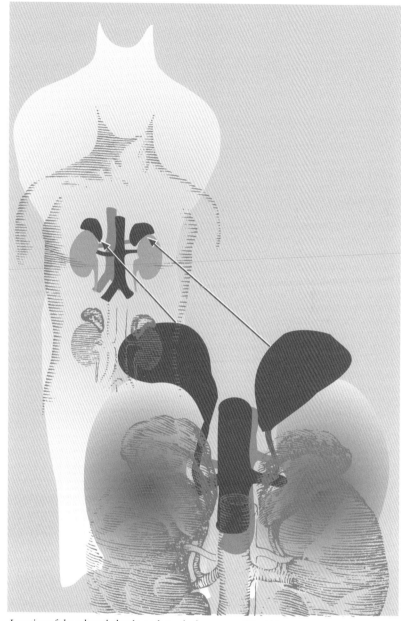

Location of the adrenal glands, each perched over one of the kidneys.

cedures. Surgical removal of the tumor is the treatment of choice.

Adrenal cortex

The adrenal cortex secretes hormones called the corticosteroids. One such hormone is cortisone. It affects the storage of starch glycogen, thus of sugar in the liver, and it combats inflamma-

tion as well. The latter explains why cortisone and its derivatives are used to treat a number of ailments.

■ *Disorders of the adrenal cortex*
Total removal of the adrenal glands in animals leads to a disorder of function so severe as to be incompatible with survival under these circumstances. A similar condition in human is known as Addison's disease, named after the

A Adrenal glands disorders   Questions & Answers

What are the adrenal glands?
The suprarenal or adrenal glands, each perched over one of the kidneys, are double glands. The yellow-brown triangular glands lie close to the upper end of the kidneys alongside the vertebral column (spine). Like all endocrine glands they have a rich blood supply.
A microscopic section shows that the cortex is made up of lightly stained cells containing much fat, arranged in three zones. Outside is a zone where the cells are in rounded groups, and beneath there is a layer of cell columns running at right angles to the surface and an innermost irregular layer.

What is the function of the adrenal medulla?
The hormone-producing cells of the adrenal glands contain innumerable granules which stain with potassium bichromate, hence the term 'chromaffin cells.'
The core, or medulla, manufactures adrenalin, noradrenaline and a small amount of dopamine. These are also produced by the nerve endings of the sympathetic nervous system.
Anger or fear stimulates this gland and secrete adrenalin and noradrenaline into the bloodstream. As a result, the heart beats faster, the liver sends sugar into the blood, the blood supply to the intestines is reduced and digestion stops, the blood supply to the muscles is increased, and the body burns sugar faster.

What are the effects of adrenaline and noradrenaline?
Adrenaline and noradrenaline have slightly different effects, and they are probably produced by two different sorts of cells. Thus of the two, adrenaline has much stronger inhibitory actions (for example, on the bladder and intestines), while noradrenaline is more powerful in raising blood pressure and constricting arterioles.

What are the major disorders of the adrenal medulla?
No functional abnormalities result from insufficiency of the adrenal medulla, the continuing production of these hormones by the sympathetic nerve cells being sufficient to maintain adequate levels in the body.
In the absence of any recognizable deficiency state the gland owes its clinical importance to tumors which may arise from the medullary cells.

What is a phaeochromocytoma?
A phaeochromocytoma is a tumor of chromaffin cells that secrete catecholamines (for instance, adrenalin, noradrenaline, dopamine), causing high blood pressure. The tumor appears equally in both sexes, are on both sides in ten percent of cases (twenty per cent in children) and are usually benign (95 per cent).
Although these tumors occur at any age, the maximum incidence is between the third and fifth decades. The tumors vary in size but average only 2 inches in diameter. The most prominent features are sudden attacks of high blood pressure or a continuous elevated blood pressure.

What are the symptoms of a phaeochromocytoma?
The following symptoms may be found:
▲ attacks of high blood pressure;
▲ increased heart rate;
▲ increased breathing rate;
▲ flushing;
▲ cold and clammy skin;
▲ severe headache;
▲ angina pectoris;
▲ palpitations;
▲ nausea and vomiting;
▲ visual disturbances;
▲ constipation;
▲ a sense of impending doom.

How is the diagnosis made of a phaeochromocytoma?
The diagnosis can be established by tests for catecholamines in the urine and provocative tests; the tumor is being localized by radiographic procedures.

What is the best treatment of a phaeochromocytoma?
Surgical removal of the tumor is the treatment of choice. It is usually possible to delay operation until the patient is in optimal physical condition by the use of special medicines.

What is the function of the adrenal cortex?
The adrenal cortex secretes hormones called the corticosteroids. One such hormone is cortisone. It affects the storage of starch glycogen, thus of sugar in the liver, and it combats inflammation as well. The latter explains why cortisone and its derivatives are used to treat a number of ailments.

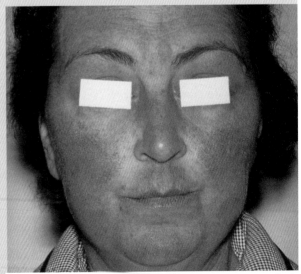

Cushing-syndrome; the person shows a large, round face (moon face). The skin becomes thin, bruises easily and heals poorly when bruised or cut.

English physician Thomas Addison, beginning of the 19th century.

The illness is characterized by weakness and muscle wasting, and the patient's skin nearly always turns dark. Until modern therapy was available, the patient went slowly downhill and died. This was due to the lack of corticosteroids, the physiologically active substances of the adrenal cortex.

Disorders of the adrenal cortex may be due to either defective or excessive secretion of hormones. The two most important deficiency syndromes are:

▲ Acute adrenal insufficiency (adrenal crisis) due to failure of cortisol secretion. This can be a life-threatening complication of an infection with meningococci.

▲ Chronic adrenal insufficiency (Addison's disease) in which secretions of both cortisol and aldosterone are defective.

Since with modern pharmaceutical techniques all adrenal hormones can be synthesized insufficiency of the gland can now be treated with supplementary treatment with hormones.

Cushing's syndrome

There are a number of clinical syndromes resulting from oversecretion of adrenal hormones of which Cushing's syndrome is the most important one.

Clinical manifestations include:
- moonlike appearance of the face;
- obesity of the trunk;
- muscle wasting;
- weakness;
- the skin is thin and atrophic and shows 'pregnancy streaks;'
- poor wound healing.

Cessation of linearly growth is characteristic in children. Females usually have menstrual irregularities. An increased production of androgens may lead to excessive hair growth, temporal balding, and other signs of virilism in the female. Cushing's syndrome may be caused in several ways:
- an ACTH-secreting tumor in the pituitary;
- a hormone-secreting tumor in the adrenal gland;
- oversecretion of the cortex;
- overdosage of corticosteroids.

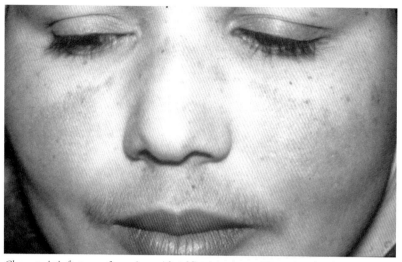

Characteristic features of a patient with Addison-syndrome. The patient developed patches of dark skin (upper figure); appearing like tanning. but it appears on areas not even opposed to the sun.
The other figure shows typical changes of the subcutaneous tissue due to a disturbance of the balance of water, sodium, and potassium in the body

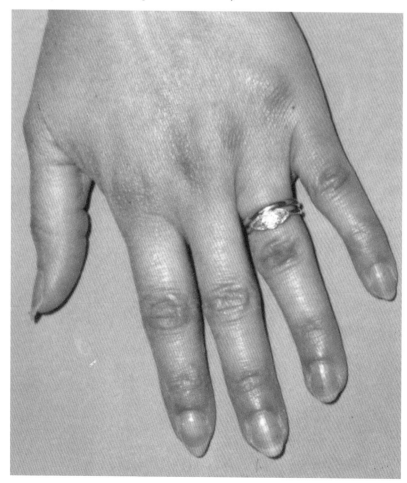

AGING

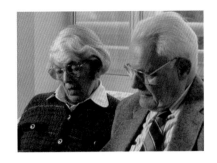

Introduction

Biologists usually divide the life span into three segments. First, there is growth and maturation, including increases in body functions and culminating in reproductive capability. Then, during adolescence, physical maturity is attained; and during young adulthood, social and psychological maturity hopefully is reached. The third segment of the life span is referred to as senescence. The onset of senescence is marked by the decline of body functions and is the period of biological aging in which the individual becomes more susceptible to disease and death and less able to withstand stress than during other times throughout the life span.

It has long been assumed that, in physical and some behavioral terms, human life is a discouragingly steady downhill slope from about the age of 30 onward. Standard graphs based on studies of thousands of persons of all ages show a steady decline from the 30s in such things as hand-grip strength, kidney function, breathing capacity and heart rate.

Each declines at its own rate, but they all go in the same direction. Accordingly, a group of 30-year-olds will out-perform any comparable group of octogenarians. But recent findings of a longitudinal study at Oxford University (2003) have shown that individuals do not always behave like the hypothetical "average person": some people simply do not decline in

the simple straight-line fashion that the standard graphs show, and for many years, some show no decline at all.

The study has documented this lack of decline for two important signs of the ravages of time: kidney function and problem-solving ability. Kidney function has been holding steady in a certain percentage of people, sometimes for many years. On tests of problem-solving ability, too, people seem to be able at least to hold their own against age.

These tend to be those for whom problem-solving has been a way of life for years. The new behavioral evidence reinforces the truism that functions that are continually exercised are less likely to grow rusty even with age

There is no specific age at which a person becomes "elderly". Traditionally, age 65 has been so designated because it is the age at which people in industrialized societies generally leave the work force, though this is changing.
These people have passed the age of 75, but they do not regard themselves as elderly.

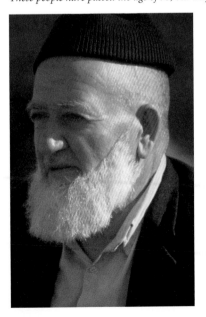

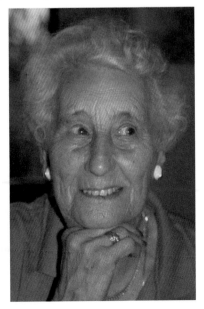

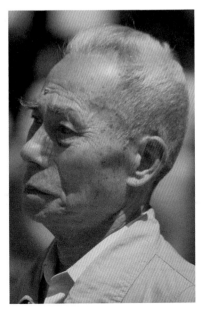

or, more succinctly, "use it or lose it." Many scientists have made an effort to try to understand what aging is all about. One theory holds that there may be some specific internal chemistry at work to produce aging effects. What would happen, then, if the blood circulation of an old individual could be connected to that of one who is young? These experiments have been performed on laboratory animals, but only one specific effect could be found: the immune defense system did not age in the same way as the other organs.

Physical changes

A common sign that someone is getting old is the appearance of wrinkled skin. Wrinkles are caused by the loss of subcutaneous (under the skin) fat, along with the decrease in elasticity of the skin's connective tissue. The degree of wrinkled skin is also influenced by the amount of exposure to harsh weather conditions.

Another common association with aging is grey hair. This is caused by the decline in the cells that produce melanin, the pigment that colours our hair and skin, and heredity is also a factor. Some people's hair starts turning grey in their 20s, and usually we find that their relatives have had the same condition.

Another common condition of old age is loss of teeth. This occurs because, in the preceding years, the person did not take care of their teeth. Not brushing the teeth and, particularly, the gums properly leads to hardened calculus lodging in the area between tooth and gum; this loosens teeth and they may eventually fall out. Chewing food well is especially important in old age because the production of enzymes and other processes important for digestion may be slowed down and not as efficient.

Sensory impairment also may accompany aging, although the degree of impairment varies. The eye ages from infancy onward and becomes less elastic, thereby making it increasingly difficult for the lens to focus and for the pupil to adjust to light input. Hearing loss is a gradual process and it may go unnoticed as long as everyday

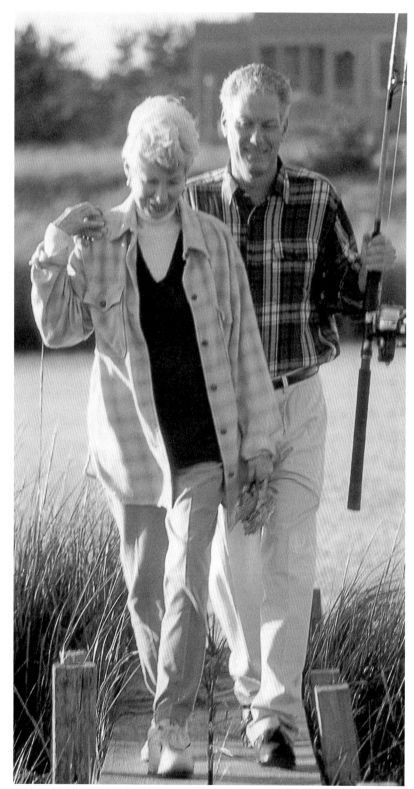

An example of successful (healthy aging). This refers to a process by which aging is not accompanied by debilitating disease and disability.

A

Aging   Questions & Answers

Do nutritional needs change with age?
As you age, you may need fewer calories, but you will still need the same amount of, or more, protein, vitamins, and minerals to stay healthy.

What kinds of food should I eat?
Make plant-based foods the foundation of your diet. Eat a variety of whole grains, fresh fruits, fresh vegetables, and legumes - beans, peas, nuts, and seeds. They contain fiber, which can keep you regular, and important vitamins and minerals. They can also lower your cholesterol and blood sugar. Include foods such as milk, yoghurt, cheese, meat, poultry, fish, and eggs in your diet as well.

What should I limit?
Watch the number of calories you take in. One of the best ways to reduce calories is to increase your consumption of fruit, vegetables, and whole grains - they make you full with fewer calories. Limit your fat intake, especially saturated fat, as it can raise your risk of heart disease. Choose low-fat dairy products and lean cuts of meat, fish, or poultry with the skin removed. Be careful with the salt, as well. Too much can cause high blood pressure.

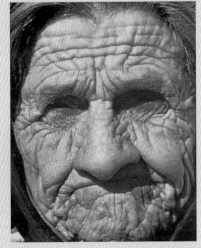

What should I increase?
Drink water. Drink six to eight 8-ounce glasses of water each day. Your cells and organs depend on water to function. Don't wait until you feel thirsty to start drinking. With age, you may lose some of your sense of thirst.

Food doesn't taste the same as it once did. Why?
With age, sense of taste and smell may change. Food may seem to have lost flavor. Some medicines can also change your sense of taste or make you feel less hungry. Ask your physician about alternatives. Try adding herbs and spices to your food.

Do nutritional needs change with age?
Some conditions, such as tooth pain, loose dentures, dry mouth, and mouth and lip sores can make it difficult and painful to chew and swallow. Softer foods can make a big difference: low-fat cottage cheese and yoghurt, for instance. Chopping or grinding foods can make chewing easier. Hot oatmeal is an easy way to get your whole grains.

I am bound to slow down as I age, so why bother to do exercises?
Many people believe that physical decline is an inevitable consequence of aging, but that's generally not true. Much of the physical frailty that we attribute to aging is actually the

result of inactivity, disease, or poor nutrition. Many people aged 90 and older who have become physically frail from inactivity can more than double their strength through simple exercises.

How can exercise benefit me?
Exercise can help prevent or delay some diseases and disabilities associated with aging. It can also improve the health of people who are already frail or who have chronic diseases and disabilities.
A balanced, moderate plan of exercise can build stamina and strength, improve your state of mind, and enable you to do this on your own, such as climbing stairs or grocery shopping. It can delay or prevent health problems such as diabetes, colon cancer, heart disease, stroke, and osteoporosis. It can improve balance and flexibility and prevent falls and the disability that often results from them. Simply put, exercise can mean the difference between independence and dependence.

What kind of exercises should I do?
A balanced program should include three types of exercise:
- strength training
- aerobic training
- flexibility exercises
A warm-up period before and a cool-down period afterwards is of great importance.

Do I need to join a gym?
No. Many exercises can be done with little or no equipment. And exercise can include activities that you already engage in, such as walking briskly, dancing, and gardening.

How much exercise should I do?
Research has found that you don't have to do strenuous exercise to gain health benefits. Just 20 to 30 minutes of moderate activity each day can produce significant benefits.

What precautions should I take?
To avoid injuring your muscles, begin an exercise program slowly and gradually work up to greater levels of exertion. If you have a chronic or serious condition, chest pain, or shortness of breath, see your physician before you begin an exercise program. Use common sense and listen to your body's warning signs. If you experience pain or uncomfortable symptoms, stop and see your doctor.

How can I stay motivated to exercise?
Find exercises that you enjoy. Work with a partner if you wish. Once you begin feeling the improved well-being that exercise brings, you'll want to keep doing it.

A

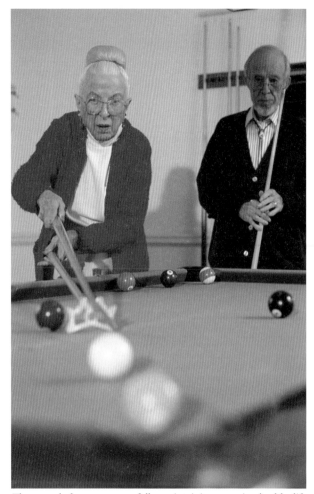
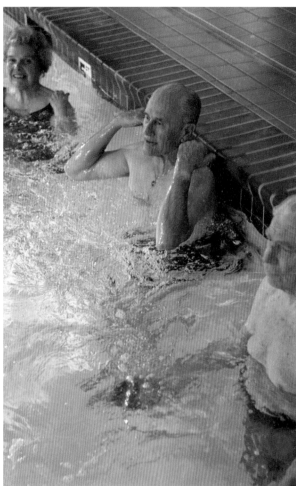

These people face ages successfully, maintaining an active, healthy life, not experiencing many of the unwanted features of aging.

encounters do not demand sensitive ears. Hearing loss is greater for higher tones than for lower ones, and is usually more common in men than women.

Several changes in the circulatory system come with age. The blood vessels' function is to carry blood to and from the heart. As a person ages, there is generally a hardening of the arteries due to fibro-fatty deposits. As a result, arteries become more rigid and narrower; thus it becomes more difficult for the blood to reach the organs and tissues of the body. This condition causes the heart to work much harder and may lead to high blood pressure. Poor circulation may cause strokes and heart attacks.

A common ailment of aging - arthritis - is not a single disease but rather has many different expressions and causes. Wrinkled skin, grey hair, loss of teeth, sensory impairment, circulatory malfunctioning and arthritis are some of the numerous changes that can take place as part of the aging process. In general, there is an overall slowing down of the systems of the body.

Mental changes

The mental changes in old age are many and complex. There is a reduction in the capacity to learn new principles, resulting in a progressive dependency on principles and ideas learned in the past.

Older people tend to be more rigid in their thinking, less able to adapt themselves readily to new ideas and experiences.

There is a demonstrable reduction in the capacity to handle information and less can be held at any one time. Retention of information in the short term is also easily disturbed by any other activity going on at the same time. These changes result in a tendency for older people to be slower in grasping ideas, poor in concentration and unreliable in their memory for recent events.

Social changes

The social changes in old age reflect in large measure the role which society offers to its older citizens. Normally retirement from work occurs at the

A

Aging - Coping with the Changes

Old age does not have to mean illness and endless health problems. You can still lead ann active, comfortable life by taking proper care of yourself.

Bladder control
- Perform pelvic floor exercises (also known as Kegel exercises) to improve bladder control.
- If you cannot control your bladder, see your doctor to find out the cause and types of treatment available.

Bones
- Osteoporosis or bone-thinning can lead to broken bones. It affects mainly women. The cause is unknown but low hormone levels, not enough calcium in the diet, and lack of exercise may all play a role.
- Get enough calcium in your diet from
  - low-fat or skim milk
  - yoghurt and cheese
  - sardines and salmon
  - dried peas and beans
  - beancurd and soya bean milk
  - leafy green vegetables and seaweed
- Women at menopause should check with their doctor if they need a hormone supplement.

Eyesight
- See an eye doctor if your eyesight is poor. You may need new spectacles.
- You should also see an eye doctor every 2 to 3 years to check for cataracts and glaucoma and to examine the inside of your eyes.
- Use bright lights for reading. Light bulbs are better than fluorescent tubes for older people.

Hair
- Use a mild shampoo to wash your hair every 3 to 4 days.
- Use cold or lukewarm water. Hot water loosens hair roots.
- If white hair bothers you, dye it when necessary.

Hearing
- Avoid exposure to loud music or machine noise.
- If you have problems with your hearing, see your doctor for a check-up.
- Wear a hearing aid if your doctor recommends it.

Joints
- Keep your joints supple with stretching exercises
  - rotate shoulders, wrists and ankles
  - bend elbows and knees
  - bend body forwards, backwards and sideways
  - raise legs up in front, to the side and to the back
  - play an imaginary piano with your fingers
- Take up yoga of taiji. They keep your joints supple as well as help you maintain good balance top avoid falls.

- Keep your hands and feet under a thin blanket at night to prevent stiffness.

Mind
- Keep up with current events by listening to the radio, watching TV and by reading newspapers, magazines and books.
- Discuss and exchange views with your family and friends.
- Play games with and read stories to your grandchildren.
- Learn new skills, games or languages.
- Offer your services to charitable organisations and be active in your community.

Muscles and Heart
- Exercise strengthens your heart and lungs. However, if you have not been active or have a medical condition, ask your doctor for advice on suitable exercises.
- Brisk walking, cycling and swimming are good aerobic exercises for older people.
- Build up slowly until you can do 20 to 60 minutes of continuous exercise, including warm-up and cool-down, 3 to 5 times a week.

Sex
- Older people are able to lead a normal sex life. Men and women do not lose their ability to have an orgasm although they may have a slightly slower response.
- For women with dry vaginas, use a water-soluble surgical jelly for lubrication.
- Men may need slightly longer stimulation to have an erection.

Skin
- Apply a moisturiser like lanolin after bathing to prevent dry skin or too much wrinkling.
- Use an umbrella and apply sunblock lotion when you go out into the sun.
- To prevent dryness of hands, wear rubber gloves when washing dishes or using strong cleaning agents.

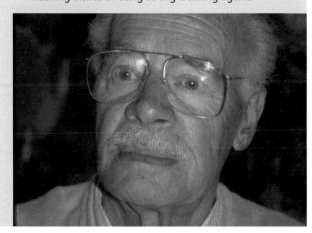

ages of 60 or 65 although today people may have many years of life ahead. Early retirement is often encouraged because of high unemployment rates. It is not until retirement that many people realize how dependent they have been on their work, even though their job may have been uncongenial or dull. Retirement may involve separation from familiar surroundings and friends and, most important, a negation of the lifelong pride of being an independent being contributing to society.

It may demand an abrupt change in established habits at a time when new adjustments may be difficult to make. By being denied a viable functioning role, the older person may be made to feel he or she is a social liability rather than an asset.

It is impossible to estimate how many of the less fortunate changes and physical and mental disorders associated with aging are a direct and avoidable result of the social vacuum in which many elderly people are placed. In societies where the elderly are still given a clearly defined and useful social role, there tends to be a lower incidence in the mental and emotional disturbances of old age. A special research group, set up in l995 by the World Health Organization, is studying this problem.

Life expectancy

In 1900 the life expectancy for a person born in western Europe was 48 years. At mid-century, things started to stir. In a single year, subtle improvements in medical care caused the 48-year figure to jump 2 per cent. The next year it jumped another 2 per cent; then another. The average life expectancy rose from 71.5 years in 1970 to more than 78 years today.

Cell damage

In the same way that the modern era of genetics research began in 1953 when the DNA double helix was identified, the modern era of aging research is thought to have begun in 1961, when anatomist Leonard Hayflick has been troubled by the question of where aging begins. Is it the cells themselves that falter, drag-

Longevity

If you are serious about fighting the aging process - and a regimen of exercise and low-fat food is not doing it for you - plenty of self-styled remedies mat be available by prescription or at health-food stores, depending on where you live. None of them will make you younger. Some should be taken only under a doctor's care. Some might actually do some good.

Human-growth hormone
■ Promise
Responsible for growth spurts in teenagers, human-growth hormone also restores lost muscle mass and redistributes fat cells in the elderly.

■ Reality check
Human-growth hormone is expensive - at least $ 10.000 for a year's supply - and has been shown to trigger such serious side effects as diabetes and heart disease.

DHEA
■ Promise
DHEA is a precursor to sex hormones. The theory is that by boosting levels of this precursor to the sex hormone estrogen and testosterone - levels of which fall off with age - you can reset your body's internal clock and fool it into thinking it is decades younger. Enthusiasts claim DHEA gives them more energy, restores muscle tone, boosts their cognitive abilities and perks up their libido.

■ Reality check
No evidence exists that the hormone slows aging or reverses it. Mice treated with DHEA do tend to act younger and friskier, but it is hard to extrapolate these results to humans. And there is a theoretical danger that taking DHEA could confer a greater risk for developing prostate or breast cancer.

Melatonin
■ Promise
A proved natural antidote for insomnia, this hormone is also being investigated as a stress reducer and anticancer agent.

■ Reality check
Take too much melatonin (more than 0,5mg) and you could feel groggy the next day. The hormone may lessen the side effects of standard chemotherapy, but the jury is still out on that.

Antioxidants hormone
■ Promise
By scooping up free radicals before they can damage cells in the body, antioxidants like beta-carotene could help stave off cancer, heart disease and other age-related illnesses.

■ Reality check
Clinical trials have produced conflicting results. One study showed that beta-carotene supplements can actually increase the risk of cancer and heart disease for some people.

A

Aging · Major characteristics

We start to age from the moment we are born. But most of us only become aware of it when we reach our 40s. We do not all age the same way. Some people may look and act old at 60 while others may still be active at 80. Even different parts of the body may age at different rates. The face may be wrinkled while the body remains agile. But there are some changes that, in varying degrees, do come to everyone.

Physical changes

Changes appearing in the 40s
• smile lines
• white or thinning hair
• stiffer joints
• farsightedness - when we have to hold things further away to see them clearly

Changes appearing in the 50s
• skin may become dry, less elastic and have brown spots
• muscles weaken
• bones become thin and brittle
• women stop menstruating and can no longer have babies
• men continue to produce sperms but may take longer to get an erection

Changes appearing in the 70s
• eyesight becomes poorer
• hearing, particularly of high-pitched sounds, may be less sharp
• ability to taste and smell may lessen
• reaction time is slower
• digestion is slower
• arteries become harder and less elastic
• the heart pumps less efficiently

Changes appearing in the 80s
• bladder control may be weaker
• memory, particularly of recent events, becomes poorer
• mild confusion may be present

Mental changes

Intelligence does not change. If intelligence does decline, it is usually caused by disease and not buy aging. We can keep on learning if we want to, although perhaps at a slower rate. With age, abstract reasoning (e.g. solving puzzles) may decline but problem-solving abilities based on judgement and experience actually improve.

somewhere in the microcosmos of each cell there was an actual hourglass that gave it only so much time to live and no more. If the clock could be found - and more important, reset - both the cells and the larger corpus that gave rise to them might be made immortal.

In the years since then, senescence scientists have taken two approaches to achieving this goal. The first idea researchers have explored is broadly thought of as the cellular-damage model of aging. Like all organisms, cell produce waste as the metabolize energy. One of the most troublesome by-products of this process is a species of oxygen molecule known as a free radical - essentially an ordinary molecule with an extra electron.

This addition creates an electrical imbalance that the molecule seeks to rectify by careening about, trying to bond with other molecules or structures, including DNA. A lifetime of this can lead to a lot of damaged cells, which may lead to a range of disorders, including cancer and the more generalized symptoms of aging like wrinkles and arthritis.

Disposable soma theory

Another theory is called the disposable soma theory. For any complex system - whether it is made of inorganic metal or protoplasmic goo - the process of wearing out begins as soon as the hardware starts operating. Damage is the inevitable consequence of interaction between an organism and its environment.

Aging is, in fact, rare in the animal kingdom because death usually occurs early, from accident, disease or predators. Depending on the safety of their environment then, organisms evolved to specialize in either reproduction (the most short-lived creatures are the most prolific procreators) or bodily maintenance (the longest-lived creatures have the best DNA repair kits).

The disposable soma theory suggests that there is no built-in biological aging clock as Hayflick thought. Senescence has more to do with a network of damaging agents in the form of environmental hazards and a network of cellular defences.

ging the whole human organism down with them? Or could cells live on indefinitely were it not for some age-related deterioration in the higher tissues they make up?

To find out, Hayflick harvested cells from fetal tissue and transferred them to a Petri dish. Freed from the responsibility of doing anything to keep a larger organism alive, the cells did the only other thing they knew how to do: divide. Shortly after they were placed in culture, they doubled. The cycle repeated itself about 100 times, until all at once it stopped.

Form then on, the cells did something a lot like aging. They consumed less food; their membranes deteriorated; and the culture as a whole languished. Hayflick repeated the experiment but this time used cells from a 70-year-old, and found that the cellular aging began a lot earlier, after 20 to 30 doublings. Clearly, it seemed, the cells from the older human were older themselves. It was concluded that

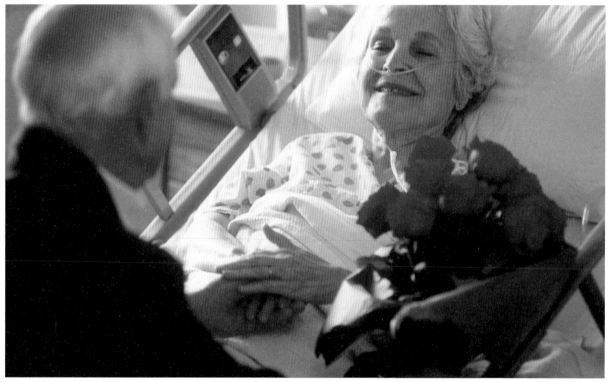

Acute illness that were one likely to result in death for older people, such as heart attacks, is now often treatable and controllable.

Chromosomes

Scientists are also trying to understand the role of telomerase, an enzyme that regulates growth at the ends of chromosomes.

At the tip of every chromosome is a chunk of DNA that experts long assumed to be superfluous, since it gets lost in replication. Now they think that piece of DNA may be critical in aging, and some speculate that the key to preserving it may lie in preventing the shrinkage of the telomeres that protect chromosome tips from deteriorating.

Many rehabilitation devices help people with disabilities function more independently. Commonly used assistive devices are canes, grab bars, raised bath seats, wheelchairs, etc.

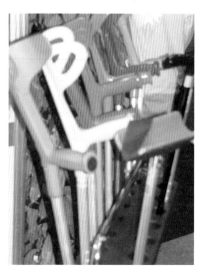
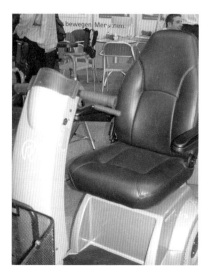
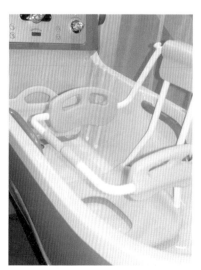

AIDS

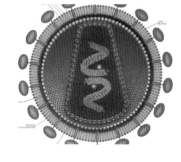

Description

AIDS or *acquired immune deficiency syndrome* is a serious and mostly fatal condition in which the immune system breaks down and does not respond normally to infection.
AIDS is an internationally recognized lethal disease first identified in 1981. It is characterized by a severe, progressive breakdown in the immune system caused by infection with a retrovirus, human immunodeficiency virus (HIV).
By 2000 more than 37,500,000 have

been reported by the World Health Organization to be infected with HIV. Adults and children newly infected with HIV in 2005 amount to more than 7 million.

Pathogenesis and infection

Two major types of HIV have been recognized. HIV-1 and HIV-2. HIV-1 is the dominant type worldwide, HIV-2 is found principally in West Africa but cases have been reported from East Africa, Europe, Asia, and Latin

America.
There are at least 10 different genetic subtypes of HIV-1, but their biological and epidemiological significance is unclear at present. Both HIV-1 and HIV-2 are transmitted in the same way.
When HIV infects a cell, it combines with that cell's genetic material and mnay lie inactive for years. Most people infected with HIV are still healthy and can live for years with no symptoms or only minor illnesses.
HIV is lymphotrophic, binding primarily to T4 (helper) lymphocytes (alsom named CD4+) and macrophages. There is a progressive decline in immunocompetence secondary to decreased number and function of T helper lymphocytes. This decrease in cell-mediated immunity appears to result in susceptibility to the infections and malignant disease's that are the common manifestations of AIDS.
Additionally, there are significant abnormalities in B lymphocyte function, with a generalized increase in production of functionally ineffective immunoglobin. HIV breaks down the immune system, the body's shield against disease. People with HIV develop infections that don't usually harm people with healthy immune systems. These infections are called opportunistic infections. A number of unusual cancers also develop more commonly in people with HIV.
The disease was initially recognized in previously healthy homosexual men and intravenous drug users and these two groups still have the highest risk of HIV infection in the United states, although the relative number of patients who are drug abusers is rising. The virus is transmitted by sexual contact, via contaminated blood or blood products, or through contami-

To educate young people various methods are being used.

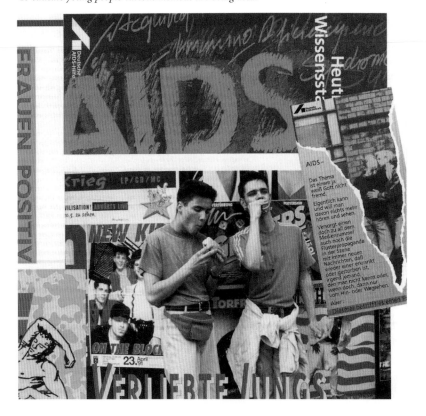

nated intravenous drug equipment. It can also be transmitted from mother to infant via the placenta or the birth canal.

The virus is not transmitted by casual contact, and transmission to health care workers in the work place is quite rare. Seroconversion has occurred in only 0.3 per cent of needle stick exposures in health care workers followed longitudinally.

Infection with HIV

The virus that can cause AIDS is hard to catch, unless you take unnecessary risks. The virus can get into the body in the following ways:
▲ having vaginal, anal, or oral intercourse with someone who has the virus;
▲ sharing needles or syringes with someone who has the virus;
▲ getting transfusions of blood or blood products donated by someone who has the virus;
▲ getting blood, semen, or vaginal secretions infected with the virus into open wounds or sores;
▲ receiving organs transplanted from a donor with the virus;
▲ having artificial insemination using sperm of a man with the virus;
▲ becoming accidentally punctured or cut with a needle or surgical instrument contaminated with the virus.

A woman may give the virus to her fetus during pregnancy or birth. Breast-feeding also may pass the virus to an infant. Contrary to common believe, there are numerous conditions that do not cause a HIV infection after being into contact with an AIDS-patient. In this respect the following general rules are applicable:
▲ It is not possible to get HIV by visiting, socializing, working, or going to school with someone who has it.
▲ It is not possible to get HIV by being sneezed on, coughed on, or breathed on by someone who has it.
▲ It is not possible to get HIV by crying with, laughing with, sweating with, kissing, or hugging people with AIDS or HIV.

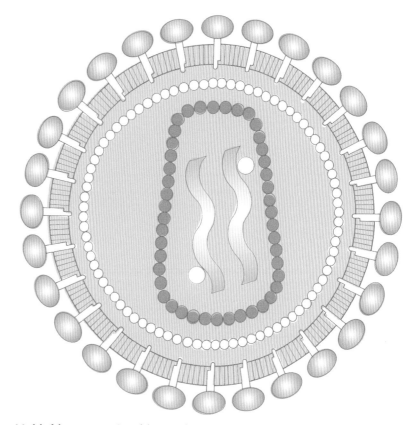

Model of the reconstruction of the HIV, the virus causing AIDS. The reconstruction was made on the basis of molecular and electron microscopic data.

▲ It is not possible to get HIV from mosquitos, or other insects.
▲ It is not possible to get HIV by touching or sharing things that a person with HIV has touched; for instance, doorknobs, bed linens, clothing, towels, toilets, telephones, showers, swimming pools, eating utensils, drinking glasses. None of these have been found to transmit HIV.

Stages of HIV infection

There are several stages of HIV disease.
(1) It usually takes a person with HIV three to six months to develop detectable antibodies. Some people have symptoms during this time that usually are not severe. Slight fever, headaches, fatigue, muscle aches, and swollen glands may last for a few weeks.

(2) There usually is a long period without symptoms after antibodies develop. This period may last many years; the average is about 10. Although there are no symptoms, the immune system and various bloody tissues become damaged during this time.
(3) People with HIV often have swelling of the lymph glands in the throat, armpits, and groin. This may be the only symptom of HIV infection for a number of years. This is called 'persistent generalized lymphadenopathy.'
(4) When HIV seriously damages the immune system, symptoms include:
▲ yeast infection causing a white coating of the vagina, mouth, and throat (thrush);
▲ viral infections that affect the skin and mucous membranes of the anus or genital area;

A

AIDS   Questions & Answers

What is AIDS?
Acquired immune deficiency syndrome (AIDS) is a disease in which the body's natural immune system breaks down, leaving it unable to fight off infections. A person with AIDS gets illnesses that are little or no threat to someone with a healthy immune system.

What causes AIDS?
AIDS is caused by a virus called human immunodeficiency virus (HIV). HIV is a sexually transmitted and blood-borne virus.

Do all HIV infected people have AIDS?
No. It can take years for illness to appear. Most people infected with HIV may have initial flu-like symptoms for a few days, and then go for years without any symptoms. People may not even know they are infected. Illness may then develop, varying in severity from mild to extremely serious. AIDS is the most severe result of HIV infection.

Is there a cure for AIDS?
There is still no cure for AIDS, but early diagnosis of HIV infection and treatment with new medications can help HIV-infected people stay healthy longer.

How is HIV transmitted?
HIV is not an easily transmitted virus. HIV is spread by direct contact with infected blood or body fluids, including semen, vaginal secretions and breast milk. There is no evidence that the virus can be transmitted through air, water, food or casual body contacts.

How infectious is HIV?
Unlike most viral infections - colds, flu, measles, etc. - HIV is not transmitted through sneezing, coughing, eating or drinking from common utensils or merely being around an infected person. Casual contact with HIV infected people does not place others at risk. No cases have ever been found where HIV has been transmitted through casual (nonsexual) contact with a household member, relative, co-worker, etc.

What kind of behavior increases the risk of HIV infection?
Behaviors that may put an individual at increased risk for HIV infection include:

- sharing IV (intravenous) drug needles and works;

- having unprotected sexual intercourse (vaginal, oral, anal) with a person whose past history or current health status is unknown;

- HIV-infected women can also pass the virus to their children during pregnancy and through breast-feeding.

Who can become infected with HIV?
Anyone who engages in high risk behaviors can become infected with HIV and develop AIDS. Most cases of AIDS are linked with sexual activity and intravenous drug use. More than 90 per cent of all cases have occurred among the following groups of people:

- about 50 per cent: homosexuals or bisexual men, 5 per cent of whom have used IV drugs;

- about 40 per cent: male and female heterosexual IV drug users;

- 3 per cent: heterosexual partners of HIV infected people;

- 2 per cent: children who became infected at birth from infected mothers;

- 1 per cent: people who received transfusions of infected blood or blood products.

Why have many homosexual and bisexual men developed AIDS?
Cases of AIDS among homosexual and bisexual men are linked with sexual contact, particularly anal intercourse and other sexual practices that result in semen-to-blood or blood-to-blood contact. Anyone who engages in anal sex is at increased risk for HIV infection, whether the person is homosexual or heterosexual.

Why is IV drug use a high risk behavior for AIDS?
IV drug users often share needles, syringes, cookers and other equipment for injecting drugs. Small amounts of blood from an HIV-infected person may remain on the equipment and be injected into the bloodstream of the next person who uses the equipment.

Why have many hemophiliacs developed AIDS?
People with hemophilia receive frequent transfusion of blood plasma concentrates that must be prepared from several hundred to thousands of donations. Cases of AIDS among hemophiliacs have been linked with receipt of blood products from HIV infected donors prior to mid-1985 when blood screening and heat treatment of plasma products were implemented.

▲ severe and frequent infections like herpes zoster or pelvic inflammatory disease.

AIDS is the final stage of HIV disease. It may take 10 or more years after HIV infection for AIDS symptoms to develop. Some conditions associated with HIV disease, including those associated with opportunistic infections, are:

(1) a thick, whitish coating of the tongue or mouth (thrush), caused by a yeast infection and sometimes accompanied by a sore throat;

(2) severe or recurring vaginal yeast infections;

(3) chronic pelvic inflammatory disease;

(4) periods of extreme and unexplained fatigue that may be combined with headaches, lightheadedness, and/or dizziness;

(5) rapid loss of more than 10 pounds of weight that is not due to increased physical exercise or dieting;

(6) bruising more easily than normal;

(7) long-lasting occurrences of diarrhea;

(8) recurring fevers and/or night sweats;

(9) swelling or hardening of glands located in the throat, groin, or armpit;

(10) periods of continued, deep, dry coughing that are not due to other illnesses or to smoking;

(11) increasing shortness of breath;

(12) the appearance of discoloured or purplish growths on the skin or inside the mouth;

(13) unexplained bleeding from growths on the skin, from mucous membranes, or from any opening in the body;

(14) recurring or unusual skin rashes;

(15) severe numbness or pain in the hands or feet, the loss of muscle control and reflex, paralysis or loss of muscular strength;

(16) an altered state of consciousness, personality change, or mental deterioration.

Such symptoms are often unrelated to HIV disease. In fact, when symptoms of HIV disease appear in women, they are easily mistaken for the symptoms of less serious conditions.

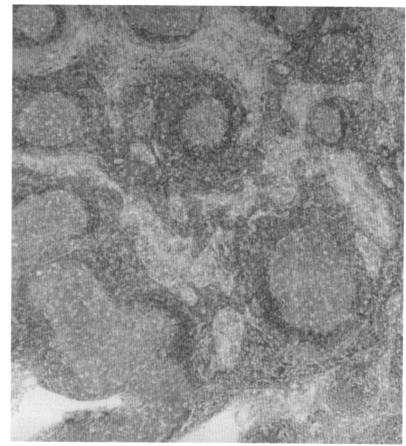
Biopsy of a lymph node, showing the presence of viral particles.

Signs, symptoms and clinical manifestations

The diagnosis of AIDS is based on clinical findings indicative of a moderate or severe defect in cellular immunity or neurologic function. The Centers for Disease Control (CDC) surveillance definition is summarized below:

A complete analysis and examination of a patient expected to have a HIV infection should comprise of:
- history;
- physical examination;
- skin testing;
- laboratory studies;
- blood (serological) studies.

■ *History*
The initial evaluation should include a complete history, including previous sexually transmitted diseases, exposure to tuberculosis, intestinal parasites, or thrush. The patient will be questioned about fever, diarrhea, fatigue, night sweats, unintentional weight loss, enlarged lymph nodes, or neurologic problems.

■ *Physical examination*
A thorough physical examination will be performed, with emphasis on the neurologic symptoms, skin, perirectal area, oral cavity, and lymph nodes.

■ *Skin testing*
This will be done for delayed hypersensitivity and a number of control antigens.

■ *Laboratory testing*
Various tests for body fluids will be performed. Various factors associated with an increased risk of progression to AIDS will be tested.

A

AIDS · Surveillance definition

Indicator Diseases: CDC AIDS

- Candidiasis of the esophagus, trachea, bronchi, or lungs.
- Cryptococcus, extrapulmonary.
- Cryptosporidosis, with diarrhea persisting longer than 1 month.
- Cytomegalovirus, mucocutaneous ulcer persisting longer than 1 month, or bronchitis, pneumonia, or esophagitis.
- Kaposi's sarcoma.
- Lymphoma, primary of the brain.
- Lymphoid interstitial pneumonia in a child under age 13 years.
- Mycobacterium avium complex
- Pneumocystis carinii pneumonia.
- Progressive multifocal leukoencephalopathy.
- Toxoplasmosis of the brain.

With laboratory evidence of HIV infection

- Bacterial infections, multiple or recurrent in child under age 13 years.
- Coccidiomycosis, disseminated.
- HIV encephalopathy.
- Histoplasmosis, disseminated.
- Isopsoriasis with diarrhea persisting longer than 1 month.
- Non-Hodgkin's lymphoma.
- Tuberculosis, extrapulmonary.
- Salmonella septicemia, recurrent.
- HIV wasting syndrome.

■ *Serological (blood) studies*

The enzyme-linked immunosorbent assay (ELISA) is commonly used to screen for HIV infection by detection of antibody to the virus.

The sensitivity and specificity of the various commercial tests vary from greater than 95 per cent to 99 per cent. Since the predictive value of the ELISA is dependent up[on the prevalence of the infection in the population tested, a positive test must be confirmed with a Western blot or other specific test.

The p24 antigen (core protein) can be detected early after the start of infection before the production of antibodies, but is generally undetectable during the period of asymptomatic infection.

Specific syndromes of HIV infection

There are a number of specific syndromes associated with HIV infection:
- acute infection syndrome;
- AIDS-related complex (ARC);
- AIDS.

■ *Acute HIV infection syndrome*

Acute HIV infection usually occurs 1-6 weeks following exposure to the virus. It may be asymptomatic or may be an influenza-like or mononucleosis-like syndrome with the following characteristics:
- rash;
- fever;
- myalgias;
- arthalgias;
- pharyngitis;
- diarrhea.

HIV antibody tests are generally negative at the time of this acute syndrome, but seroconversion occurs within 6-12 weeks in most patients. HIV antigen is usually present during acute HIV infection.

■ *AIDS-Related complex (ARC)*

ARC is a poorly defined entity referring to persons manifesting symptoms related to HIV infection but not meeting the criteria for true AIDS.

Symptoms may be the following:
- fever;
- fatigue;
- diarrhea;
- weight loss.

Laboratory abnormalities such as anemia, lymphopenia, or thrombocytopenia may also be present. Generalized lymphadenopathy may be present but is not predictive of progression to AIDS.

Oral candidiasis (thrush) is strongly predictive for development of AIDS in an HIV-positive person not taking corticosteroids.

■ *Full-blown AIDS*

In addition to the symptoms and signs described above, the following neoplastic and opportunistic infectious diseases are common in full-blown AIDS:
- Kaposi's sarcoma;
- lymphoma;
- pulmonary infection;
- gastrointestinal infection;
- neurologic infection;
- dermatologic disease;
- multisystem infections such as tuberculosis.

Test for HIV

Blood tests for HIV infection are available from most physicians, health clinics, and Planned Parenthood centers, as well as local, state and federal health departments. Blood tests also are available from special HIV counselling and testing sites.

The tests detect antibodies to HIV. HIV antibody tests are very accurate, but it usually takes from three to six months for antibodies to develop. People with HIV and people who risk HIV infection should not donate blood, plasma, sperm, body organs, or other tissues.

One should receive counselling before and after testing, if one chooses to be tested.

You can be tested 'confidentially' or 'anonymously.' 'Confidential testing' means your name and HIV test result will be put in a confidential medical record. Your name ism not used with 'anonymous testing.'

Treatment

In the treatment of HIV and AIDS three groups of disorders has to be distinguished:
- opportunistic infections;
- malignant disease;
- HIV infection.

Opportunistic infections

These infections are often less responsive to conventional courses of therapy than in other hosts, and most require life-long maintenance treatment to prevent progression or suppressive therapy to prevent recurrences.

Therapy is further complicated by the high incidence of side effects with many drugs in AIDS patients.

Malignant disease

Since most patients with Kaposi's sarcoma die of opportunistic infection rather than directly from the tumor, the objective of therapy is to reduce the illness associated with the disease, which may include edema secondary to lymphatic involvement, pain due to large skin lesions or oropharyngeal disease, or respiratory compromise.

Radiation therapy is used for localized disease and chemotherapy for more diffuse disease. Alpha-interferon may induce remission in some patients without the toxicity of traditional chemotherapy.

HIV infection

The drugs currently available that have proven to slow down the infection are zidovudine (AZT, Retrovir) and analogous compounds. Usually these drugs are given as a so-called cocktail, a mixture of three or four drugs.

Patients treated with a cocktail containing zidovudine and other drugs have fewer opportunistic infections. The drug causes significant suppression of red and white blood cell counts in approximately 25 per cent of patients.

Recent studies in asymptomatic patients with HIV infection showed that patients with less than 500 T helper lymphocytes were less likely to progress to AIDS or advanced AIDS-related complex if treated with AZT and similar medicines.

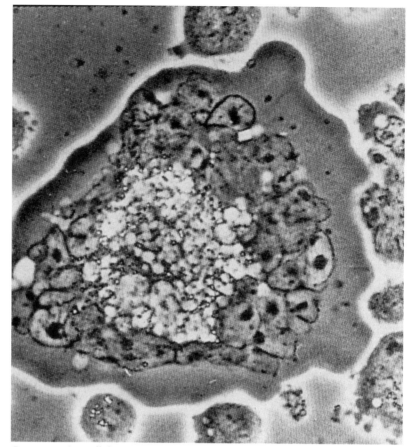

Damage to giant cells by HIV (AIDS-virus).

Although it appears that for symptomatic patients, AZT and similar medicines prolong life and improve its quality, the patients ultimately die because the drug does not eliminate the virus from infected cells.

Prevention and vaccines

With no cure at present, prudence could save thousands of people who have yet to be exposed to the virus. Use of condoms lessens the possibility of transmission as does the elimination of sharing hypodermic needles.

The fate of many will depend less on science than on the ability of large numbers of human beings to change their behavior in the face of growing danger. New drugs and tests have given researchers renewed optimism in treating AIDS. As of January 2000, four dozen preventive HIV vaccines were being tested in small-scale clinical trials around the world. In the summer of 1998, the first AIDS vaccine trials began in the United States. Five thousand volunteers are involved in this trial, and the study will last three years. For those already infected, powerful drug combinations are able to decrease the amount of HIV virus in the blood to undetectable levels.

Infection control in health care workers

The Centers for Disease Control has issued precautions regarding transmission of HIV infection in the medical setting, including universal precautions for health care workers exposed to body fluids. Gloves, masks, goggles, and gowns should be used appropriately.

ALCOHOLISM

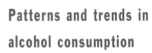

Introduction

Compulsive drinking in excess is one of the most serious problems in modern society. Many people drink for relaxation and can stop drinking without ill effects, but alcoholics cannot give up drinking without great discomfort.

They are dependent on alcohol, both physically and psychologically. Alcohol is a depressant that acts initially by reducing activity in the higher centers of the brain.

The consumption of alcohol has long been a social custom in Western countries. Although everybody is familiar with the terrible consequences of drinking to excess, the general public fails to recognize that alcohol is a potent addictive drug that affects the mind.

Alcohol is relatively special among potent drugs in that moderate, self-induced levels of intoxication are likely to be socially acceptable. Because alcohol is so readily available and its use is so generally accepted, alcohol remains by far the most serious drug problem in our country.

In economic terms, if we count the loss of production, the cost of medical care and the amount of crime, delinquency and accidents caused by the abuse of alcohol, the total burden in the Western countries is estimated at more than 110 billion dollars yearly.

The cost in human misery cannot be measured; it includes not only the suffering imposed upon the afflicted and those around them but also unfulfilled human potential. Alcoholism may be defined as a chronic, progressive and often fatal disease of major prevalence, but one that is treatable.

Experience has shown that proper treatment will produce significant long-term improvement in up to 75 percent of cases.

One might suppose that the general public and the medical profession would want to apply all the resources and ingenuity possible to combat alcoholism, but, on the contrary, the public is often apathetic.

There are a number of reasons for this curious social attitude. Alcoholics are often regarded as morally delinquent, as though they had chosen to be afflicted with the disease.

Also, many problem drinkers will deny that they are alcoholics because they don't want to face the fact. There is much confusion as to what actually constitutes alcohol excess, alcoholism or alcohol addiction.

Patterns and trends in alcohol consumption

Considerable variation is found from one society to another in habits and patterns of drinking, which may differ in terms of frequency, beverage choice, amount consumed, location, social setting and occasion.

In recent years, certain changes in drinking patterns have been noted. There is now far less difference in the beverages drunk in different countries and cultures, and drinking habits, too, are becoming similar.

Alcohol is consumed in new and more diverse situations, and these new types of consumption have, in many instances, simply overlaid traditional drinking patterns rather than replacing them. Another important development has been the recruitment of new groups to the drinking population. Abstinence among women has decreased dramatically, and in a number of settings, young people have also increased their drinking.

A study in 2004 of 6000 students in secondary schools in a number of cities in the mid-West of the United States indicated that more than 70 per

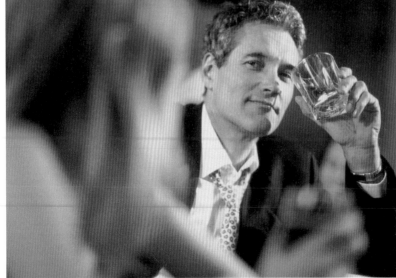

cent of those 16 to 19 years-old drank to some extent, and that 12 percent seemed to be problem drinkers.

The study asked such questions as:

▲ Do you have more than five drinks at a time?

▲ Do you drink before or during school?

▲ Did you got drunk more than three times in the last year?

▲ Do you experience blackouts?

The increasing consumption of alcohol should not looked upon in isolation from its social context. There has been an increased availability of alcohol through a drop in real cost, a weakening of restrictions and the substitution of industrial technologies of production for traditional methods of brewing.

Range and extent of alcohol problems

Until recently, there has been a widespread tendency to lump together the whole gamut of alcohol problems as all part of an underlying alcoholism. Undoubtedly a wide variety of problems are related to the development of the "alcohol dependence syndrome." One criterion for diagnosing this syndrome is an individual's changed behavior that includes, in addition to an alteration in openly drinking, a continuation of drinking in a way not approved of, despite painful direct consequences, such as physical illness. It should be pointed out, however, that there are many physical, mental and social problems that are not necessarily related to dependence. Alcohol dependence, while prevalent and in itself a matter for serious concern, constitutes only a small part of the total of alcohol-related problems.

Classification of alcohol problems

Alcohol problems may be classified:

▲ According to whether they are primarily physical, mental or social in nature;

▲ According to whether they principally affect the individual drinker, the drinker's family or the general community;

▲ According to whether they are consequences of acute episodes of

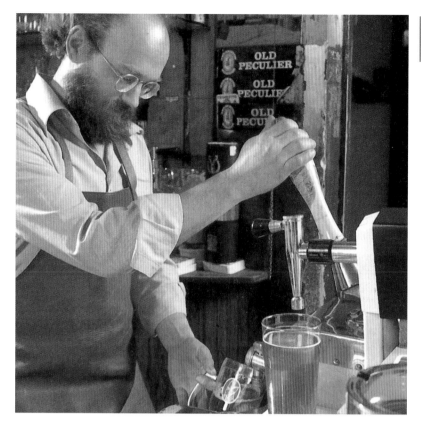

drinking or consequences of prolonged drinking.

Thus, acute episodes of heavy drinking are likely to bring about short-term impairment of functioning and control of the individual drinker, possibly leading to violence, accidents, physical disorders as a consequence of exposure to climatic conditions, or arrest for drunkenness.

Prolonged heavy drinking may result in liver cirrhosis, aggravation of other physical disorders and malnutrition, more prolonged impairment or functioning and control, leading again to accidents and impairment of working capacity, and perhaps, finally, to the alcohol dependence syndrome or alcoholic psychosis. These problems may possibly be accompanied by loss of friends, family, self-esteem, occupation, means of support and even liberty.

Whether or not they reach the level of the alcohol dependence syndrome, there may be a variety of repercussions on the family, including marital discord, family disruption, poverty, child neglect and child development difficulties.

Both individual and family problems may have consequences for the wider community, such as public disorder and property damage, increased expenditure on health, welfare and law-enforcement services, as well as financial losses, not only in industry and agriculture output, but also with respect to administrative and professional responsibilities.

Tolerance and threshold

Chronic use of alcohol brings a tolerance for it - that is, progressively higher levels of blood alcohol concentrations are required to produce intoxication. However, there is no particular amount of alcohol that can be called the lethal dose - a dangerously low level of breathing may be reached in chronic alcoholic intoxication at any time.

A sober alcoholic can combine alcohol, general anesthetics and sedative-hypnotic drugs such as barbiturates, tranquillizers and sleeping pills without serious effects. At high levels of

Alcoholism   Questions & Answers

A

How can I tell if I have an alcohol problem?

It is not always easy to spot a drinking problem, especially in yourself. An alcohol problem cannot be measured by how many drinks you have each day, how many years you have been drinking heavily, where you drink, or how much you can hold. Nor does it have anything to do with the kind of alcohol you typically use: the 'strictly beer' drinker can have an alcohol problem as surely as the person who favours wine and hard liquor.

Ask yourself, how and why you drink, and what alcohol is doing to you.

- If you sometimes get drunk when you fully intend to stay sober.
- If you no longer get as much pleasure from drinking as you once did.
- If your reliance on drinking has become progressively greater.

Are many people suffering from alcoholism?

If drinking has become a problem to you, you have lots of company. Alcoholism is an illness suffered by millions of people, and it does not discriminate by age, sex, race, or income. But, most importantly, it is a treatable disease, with recovery possible regardless of the severity of the symptoms. Like most illnesses, however, the sooner you get help, the better your chances for recovery and the easier it will be.

How does alcohol work in the body?

Unlike other 'food' alcohol does not have to be digested. When you drink an alcoholic beverage, 20 per cent of the alcohol in it is absorbed immediately in the bloodstream through the stomach walls. The other 80 per cent of the alcohol enters the blood stream very quickly after being processed through the gastrointestinal tract.

Moments after it is consumed, alcohol can be found in all tissues, organs and secretions of the body, and it eventually acts on certain brain areas to slow down or depress brain activity.

Is there a difference between low and high levels of blood alcohol?

A low level of alcohol in the blood, such as would result from sipping one drink - for example a 350 ml can of beer - has a mild tranquiLlizing effect on most people. Although basically a sedative, alcohol seems to act temporarily as a stimulant for many after they first start drinking.

This is because alcohol's initial effects are on those parts of the brain affecting learned behavior patterns such as self-control. After a drink or two, this learned behavior may temporarily disappear, making you loose your inhibitions, talk more freely, or feel like the 'life or the party.'

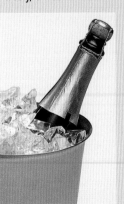

On the other hand, you may feel aggressive or depressed. Higher blood alcohol levels depress brain activity to the point where memory, as well as muscle coordination and balance, may be temporarily impaired. A still larger alcohol intake within a relatively short period of time depresses deeper parts of the brain, severely affecting judgment and dulling the senses.

Alcoholism; how fast does alcohol take effect?

The rapidity with which alcohol enters the bloodstream and exerts its effects on the brain and body depends on several factors:

- How fast you drink.
- Whether your stomach is empty or full.
- What you drink.
- How much you weigh.
- Your mood or expectations.

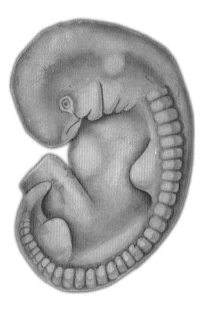

Alcohol abuse by the mother during pregnancy may cause severe damage to the young fetus.

blood alcohol, however, the depressant effect of such drugs is added to that of the alcohol and thus increases the danger of a lethal effect such as respiratory arrest, and alcohol may interfere with many other drugs.

Risks

The individual risk of experiencing adverse effects of drinking can be broken down into two elements, exposure and vulnerability. Exposure to alcohol can be said to exist on two levels, physical and social.

Physical exposure refers to the individual intake of alcohol, and social exposure to the availability of alcohol as indicated by the extent of its presence, its use by other people and their attitude towards it. Vulnerability may exist on a physical, psychological or social level.

Physical vulnerability has been shown to be clearly related to sex, females running a considerably higher risk than males of suffering from various health ailments (liver cirrhosis, for instance) by drinking the same amount of alcohol. In addition, undernourished persons may be more vulnerable than those with an adequate diet.

Psychological vulnerability refers to the fact that, under similar conditions of social exposure to alcohol, certain individuals are especially prone to excessive drinking because of their personalities, beliefs, values or attitudes.

People who have experienced a series of traumatic life events may also be more vulnerable to alcohol problems than those who have not.

Social vulnerability is related to different expectations of normal behavior as well as different life experiences. Depending on the sex, age and social position of the individual, similar drinking behaviors are met with varying degrees of social disapproval and negative reactions.

Drinking is also more likely to produce adverse effects if it is done in certain situations. For example, the consequences of drinking are more likely to be of a serious nature in work and traffic situations than in leisure situations.

It is important to bear in mind that exposure and vulnerability often work in opposite directions. Young people drink on average considerably less alcohol than adults but may be more vulnerable both because of physical factors and because of differing degrees of social censure; the same is true for females compared to males.

Because of the interplay between exposure and vulnerability, these cultural values may be at work in the defining of certain population groups as high-risk groups.

Prevention of alcohol problems

The objective is to reduce the incidence of new alcohol problems - that is, to prevent their occurrence in the first place.

Requirements are:

▲ identification of the factors responsible for the development of alcohol problems;

▲ intervention to reduce or eliminate them.

Efforts to accomplish these objectives may be directed at any of the three

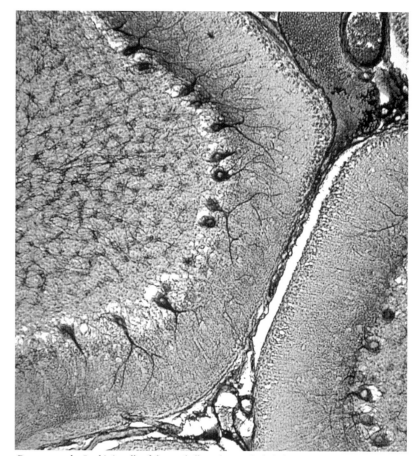

Damage to the Purkinje cells of the cerebellum due to alcohol abuse.

Severe damage to the liver in a case of alcohol intoxication.

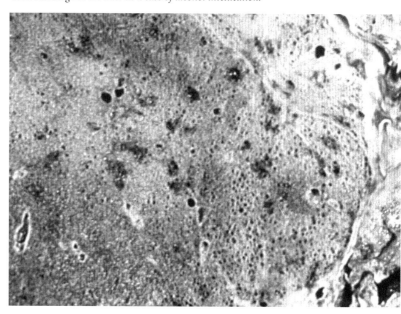

A

Alcoholism   Questions & Answers

Why do people drink?
People drink for a variety of social, cultural, religious or medical reasons. They drink at parties and celebrations with friends and relatives. They drink at religious ceremonies. Some drink wine to complement the taste of their dinners. Some drink to relax. Some drink to increase their appetites. The drinking of most people is 'integrative' drinking, that is, the use of alcohol is an adjunct to other activities, such as meals, family and religious feasts, or an evening with friends. There are, however, large numbers of people, who drink for reasons that are not social, cultural, religious or medical. They use alcohol to forget their worries, to escape from reality or to gather courage to face the stresses of life. They are using alcohol as a drug and are in danger of becoming dependent upon it.

What is drunkenness?
Drunkenness is characterized by a temporary loss of control over physical and mental powers caused by excessive alcohol intake. Symptoms of drunkenness vary, but they can include:
• impaired vision;
• thick speech;
• bad coordination.
The ability to solve problems is reduced, emotions and moods become unpredictable, memory is impaired and judgment becomes poor.

When is a person drunk?
A person is drunk when he or she has a 0.10-0.15 per cent (or more) blood alcohol level. This means, in the case of 0.10 per cent, that one part in every 1,000 parts of a person's blood is presently composed of pure alcohol. Such a situation generally results when a person weighing 75 kg has had about seven drinks within two hours of eating.
A person will reach this stage with fewer drinks if body weight is less than 75 kg, and with more drinks if weight exceeds this figure. It takes a specific amount of time for the body to burn up a quantity of alcohol, generally at a rate of 7 g of pure alcohol per hour. The effect of drinking alcohol can be varied only by controlling the rate and concentration by which it is drunk. Once alcohol is in the bloodstream nothing can be done about its effects except to wait until it is metabolized by the body.

What is a hangover?
A hangover is the body's reaction to excessive drinking. The associated miseries of nausea, gastritis (stomach upset), anxiety and headache vary from case to case, but

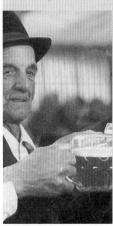

there is always extreme fatigue. No scientific evidence supports the curative claims for coffee, raw eggs, oysters, chili peppers, vitamins or other drugs. Doctors usually prescribe aspirin, rest and plenty of liquids. If you choose to drink, the best way to avoid a hangover is to avoid drunkenness. .

When do I have an alcohol problem?
If any of the symptoms in the previous question apply to your own drinking, you may well have an alcohol problem. This is a time to be absolutely honest with yourself. Sometimes only you can know how seriously alcohol is affecting your life. Often others close to you can recognize your problems as well, but they may be embarrassed to bring it up. If they do, you have all the more reason to take a hard look at what your drinking is doing to you.

components of the public health model for prevention:
▲ the agent (alcohol);
▲ the host (the drinker);
▲ the environment (the immediate setting or the broader social context).
A reduction in alcohol consumption might be achieved, for example, by lowering the alcohol content of beverages (agent), or by changing the habits of the drinker (host), or by changing the context in which drinking is expected or permitted (the environment).
The incorporation of all these efforts within a framework of the health promotion of individuals and of society at large permits prevention to be seen as oriented toward goals that are inherently positive and worthwhile.
Reducing the demand for alcohol entails the provision of information about the health risks of alcohol, of education about the types of things that restrain socially irresponsible behavior, and of leisure activities as alternatives to those that involve drinking, as well as a concern for improving the more general social conditions that may instigate the abuse of alcohol.
Alcohol is enjoyed by so many people in such a wide diversity of situations, and has come to play a crucial role in so many everyday pleasures and celebrations, that the imposition of restrictive legislation would at best be resented and at worst lead to defiance of the laws in question.
Limiting the availability of alcohol by restricting the times of sale of alcoholic beverages and the number, types and location of premises permitted to sell them has been practised in this country.
The evidence suggests that changes in closing hours have a significant impact on the pattern of consumption, though not necessarily on total consumption or the frequency of excessive consumption.
Health education is likely to be more successful in inducing behavior change if geared to selected target groups:
- schoolchildren
- pregnant women
- drivers
- alcoholics and their families

- supervisory and management personnel
- students undergoing professional training
- religious groups

Management of alcohol problems

The range of psychiatric, neurological, gastro-intestinal, heart, liver and blood disorders to which the consumption of alcoholic beverages may give rise is so wide that it would be impossible to consider them all without writing a medical textbook.

The range of social ills directly or indirectly attributable to alcohol consumption is equally broad. In this context the following major issues will be discussed:

▲ the treatment of heavy drinkers, including those who have become dependent on alcohol;
▲ the handling of the repercussions in the family;
s@inspring driehoek:s the management of alcohol problems in the work situation;

■ *Treatment of the individual drinker*
In recent years the treatment of people identified as 'alcoholics' has been the main focus of attempts to combat alcohol problems.

A wide variety of treatments have been offered by different organizations, ranging from compulsory hospitalization and subsequent work therapy to spiritual guidance.

Even medical regimes have shown great diversity, some being based on individual or group psychotherapy, others on the use of sedative and antidepressant drugs to relieve the anxiety or depression assumed to underlie the excessive drinking, or on drugs such as disulfiram (Antabuse) which produce highly unpleasant symptoms if alcohol is consumed.

There are also specialized units for treatment.

The more lavishly endowed of these have a multidisciplinary staff of psychiatrists, clinical psychologists, neurologists, nurses, social workers, occupational therapists and sometimes former alcoholics as well, and use

some form of group or individual psychotherapy as a main therapeutic tool.

There has been an increasing emphasis on quite simple forms of treatment, perhaps amounting to little more than firm advice to stop drinking or to drink less, coupled with the provision of information about the consequences of continued heavy drinking, the adoption of simple strategies for reducing consumption and the monitoring of progress.

■ *The drinker's family*
Although a significant proportion of excessive drinkers are isolated from their families, the majority are not and the drinking habits of these men and women almost always have profoundly harmful consequences for other family members.

The catalogue is all too familiar:

▲ loss of income or unemployment;
▲ loss of friends;
▲ financial hardship and sometimes outright poverty;
▲ progressive breakdown of affectionate, trusting relationships;
▲ emotional problems with children;
▲ recurrent episodes of unpredictable violence.

Because alcohol dependence usually has such far-reaching consequences for the family, most forms of treatment for the individual drinker aspire to involve at least the spouse in the treatment process, and sometimes other family members as well.

Alcoholism treatment units run on psychotherapeutic lines often involve both husband and wife in some form of marital therapy. In several clinical studies of alcoholics, up to 50 per cent of the subjects themselves have been the offspring of alcoholic parents.

Although genetic factors may play some part in this sequence, it is generally assumed that social and other environmental influences are primarily responsible.

In theory this ought to provide possibilities for intervening in such a way as to break the cycle, but in practice there has been so far little attempt to assess whether this can be done on any major scale, either by economic or by psychotherapeutic interventions at a family level.

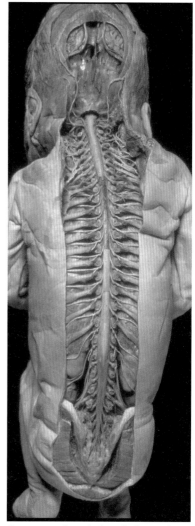

Damage to the spinal cord of a newborn. The mother was an alcoholic.

■ *Problems in the work situation*
The work-place is a convenient setting in which to achieve many of the objectives referred to earlier, such as early identification and the development of low-cost approaches to the management of alcohol problems.

Some trade unions have taken the initiative in promoting joint programs of assistance in a broader context of general behavioral problems that impair job performance.

The advantage of such programs is that they tend to encourage voluntary requests for help and increase the participation of female employees and younger workers.

ALLERGY

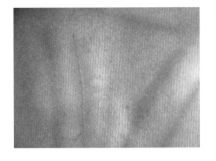

Description

An allergy is an abnormal reaction to an ordinarily harmless substance. It is a state of abnormal sensitivity to foreign material - called an allergen - in susceptible individuals. It is essentially the inappropriate reaction of antibody and antigen defense responses to environmental substances. Susceptibility is often inherited and manifestations vary with age. For instance, to the average person, pollen is simply a substance necessary for the propagation of plants, but to the hay-fever, sufferer it is an allergen that can make life miserable. The body is equipped with an immune or defense system that produces antibodies to fight harmful invaders. The allergy sufferer also produces another type of antibody that combines with antigens that are inhaled, swallowed, injected or absorbed through the skin.

When the allergic antibody and the allergen (such as ragwort pollen) meet, they cause certain chemicals to be released that produce allergy symptoms. One of the most well-known of these chemicals is histamine, released from mast cells in the tissues.

Inflammation follows, with local irritation, redness and swelling. In the skin, this appears as eczema or urticaria (nettle rash); in the nose and eyes, hay fever results; and in the gastrointestinal tract, diarrhea may occur. In the lungs, the release of a specific chemical - slow-reacting substance of anaphylaxis - leads to spasm of the bronchi or airways, which gives rise to the wheezing and breathlessness of asthma.

In most cases, the route of the allergen's entry determines the site of the response, but skin rashes may occur regardless of route (when they are called 'atopic') and asthma may follow eating allergenic material. Localized allergic reactions in skin following exposure to chemicals (for instance, nickel and stinging nettles) are the basis of contact dermatitis.

Common allergens include:
- ▲ drugs (penicillin, aspirin);
- ▲ foods (shellfish);
- ▲ plant pollens;
- ▲ animal furs or feathers;
- ▲ insect stings and the house dust mite.

Contact allergy due to a plant.

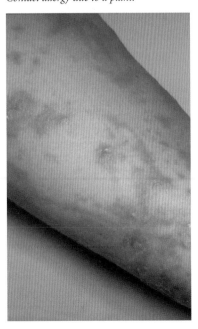

Allergic dermatitis due to sun light.

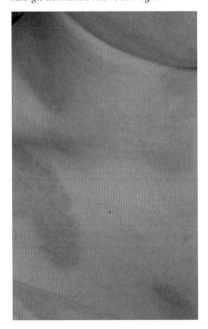

Tissue reaction to a chronic infectious process.

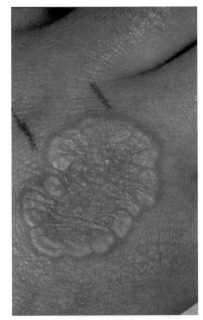

Self-treatment

A total cure for allergies may be a long way off, but there are steps you can take to reduce the risk of allergic reactions.

- If you have already had allergies or respond positively to skin tests for allergy, you should be particularly careful not to smoke or drink during pregnancy and to eat a sensible diet which is low in dairy products and in stimulants such as tea and coffee. A baby can be sensitized before birth by the food, drink and drugs the mother takes.
- Breastfeed your baby for at least six months and don't introduce solids before the infant is four months old. When you do introduce solids, make sure you offer fruit and vegetable meals, not milk, eggs, wheat and fish, which are potent allergens.
- Do not allow contact with animals in early infancy. The sooner a baby is exposed to animal fur, the more likely he or she is to become allergic.
- Smoking, overeating and excessive drinking may increase your own risk of developing allergy.

If you have allergies, you can usually blame your parents - and their parents - because allergies tend to be inherited. Exactly which members of your family will get allergies cannot be determined, and not everyone who inherits the tendency to get allergies will suffer from the symptoms.

Likewise, you may not be allergic to the same things your mother is. For example, your mother may have skin allergy eczema, while you sneeze your way through the pollen season.

What you become allergic to depends a great deal on what you are most frequently exposed to. Your allergy might be more likely to manifest itself as hay fever if you live in a ragwort-dense region, for example.

Your body must produce a sufficient number of antibodies before an allergic reaction occurs. You may not experience symptoms the first time you eat a certain food, pet a cat or

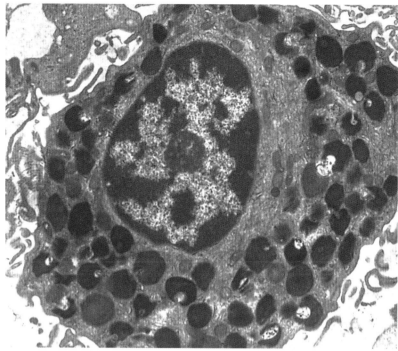

Microscopic view of a mast cell. These cells in tissues release histamine and other substances involved in allergic reactions

Microscopic view of macrophages. These cells develop from a type of white blood cells called monocytes after monocytes move from the bloodstream to the tissues. Macrophages ingest bacteria and other foreign cells.

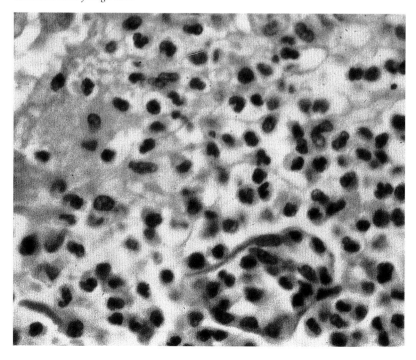

A

Allergy   Questions & Answers

What are allergies?
An allergy is a reaction to something normal in the environment. For example, pollens can cause an allergic reaction called hay fever. Exposure to cats, dogs, and dust mites can cause allergic nasal symptoms, sneezing, tearing, and in some cases, asthma. An allergic reaction to medicines can cause a rash and fever. Allergic reactions to foods can cause hives and swelling.

What causes an allergic reaction?
The substance which causes an allergic reaction is called an allergen. It may be either obvious or difficult to detect. When exposure to an allergen occurs, certain cells in the body, called mast cells, release histamine, which is responsible for the tearing, itching, runny nose, sneezing, and hives that signal an allergy attack.

I am sneezing all day; my doctor tells me I have an allergy to pollens. Which pollens are allergenic?
Pollens are the small, spherical or egg-shaped grains which, as the male germ cells of plants, are necessary for plant fertilization. While pollen allergy usually occurs first during childhood or young adulthood, it may develop at any age. At least two seasons of exposure to a pollen are generally necessary.
Not all pollens cause allergy. People often think that pollens of colourful, scented flowers such as roses are the source of their allergy. This is true for people like gardeners or florists, who spend a lot of time close to these flowers, but in general, tree, grass and weed pollens are the most frequent causes of pollen allergy.
Pollens may be divided into two types: those carried by insects and those borne on the wind. Most flowers have large and waxy pollens which are carried from plant to plant by insects such as bees. On the other hand, trees, grasses and weeds are wind-pollinated. The small, dry pollens can be dispersed widely by the wind currents.

What tests can be performed to check for pollen allergy as cause of sneezing and bronchitis-like complaints?
When pollen allergy is suspected, a medical specialist may perform skin tests to identify which pollens are responsible. Using his knowledge of pollens important in his geographical area at various times, the allergist injects a diluted amount of each individual pollen under the skin (intravenous skin test) or applies it to a scratch (scratch test) on the patient's arm or back.
A small raised area, known as "weal and flare reaction" will develop at the test site in an allergic person. The size of the weal will depend on the severity of the allergic reaction. If the medical history and physical examination strongly suggest pollen allergy, but skin tests are negative - a rare occurrence - the allergist may choose more direct testing, such as direct application of pollen examples to the mucosal membrane of the nose.
A modern test is the RAST test (which stands for radio-allergo-sorbent technique), in which samples of the patient's blood are used to determine the extent of immunological globulin production in response to a particular allergen.

What causes emphysema and what are the symptoms?
Physicians do not fully understand all the causes of emphysema. People with a history of bronchial irritation seem prone to it. Smoking is the most common cause. Air pollution and lung infections may contribute to its development. Heredity also may be involved.
The earliest symptoms are shortness of breath and cough, especially early in the morning, which usually develop slowly over a period of months or years. This is not rapid breathing after exercise, but laboured breathing which may occur after only mild exertion. Wheezing also may occur.

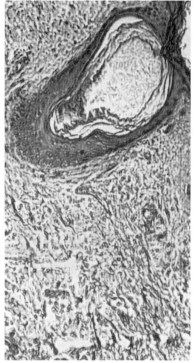

Unspecific allergic reaction characterized by the presence of small vesicles.

receive a penicillin jab. But your body may produce enough antibodies to stimulate a response the second or third time you are exposed to the antigen, or you may not have a reaction until years later.
Even with sufficient antibodies, however, you may remain symptom-free unless some secondary factors such as lowered resistance, stress, infection or hormonal changes occur at the time of exposure.
Allergy symptoms range in intensity from mildly annoying to severely debilitating. With some people, the symptoms come and go and may be scarcely noticeable; for others, they are a source of chronic misery and even total incapacitation. In extreme cases, some allergies can be fatal: each year in the United States, more than 5500 people die from asthma, and an unestimated number have fatal reactions to certain drugs and foods.
Some substances are more allergenic than others - that is, more likely to cause allergic reactions in a large number of individuals - but there is probably no substance that can't cause

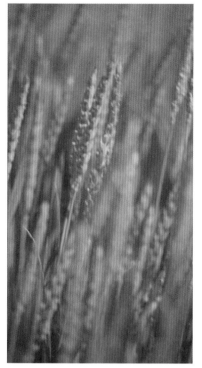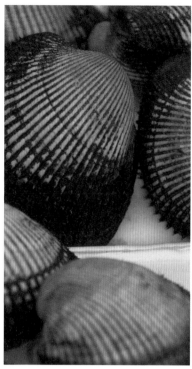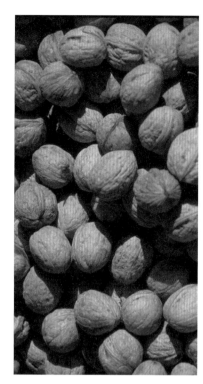

Many nutrients may cause allergic reactions (food allergy) such as grains, shellfishes, and nuts.

an allergic reaction in someone. Likewise, the same allergen might produce a different set and severity of symptoms in someone else.

Contact allergy

People with contact allergies break out in a rash when they touch certain objects or substances. The rash usually occurs after prolonged, recurrent contact and appears only at the site of contact (such as the hands).
This type of reaction may occur in all users of a particular substance such as a harsh chemical (primary irritation), or it may appear only in certain indi-

viduals who become sensitized to a substance that is harmless to others. Plants are common causes of contact allergies, particularly stinging nettle. Some people are so sensitive to these plants that they can break out simply by petting an animal that has brushed by the plants. A host of metals can also be allergens, including nickel, chrome

and mercury. A reaction may occur from a watchband, costume jewellery, zips or even silverware. Other common contact allergens are cosmetics, hair dyes, nail vanish, permanent waving and straightening solutions, deodorants, chemicals, cleaning products, plastic, rubber, resins, clothing dyes and more.

Simplified scheme to illustrate the relation between an antigen (A) and antibody (B). The top line shows the formation of an antigen-antibody reaction. In the second and third line, no reaction occurs.
Right: the grid shows a number of antigens (red) and antibodies (grey) combined in a kind of network. If the network is large enough, it will cause a physical allergic reaction.

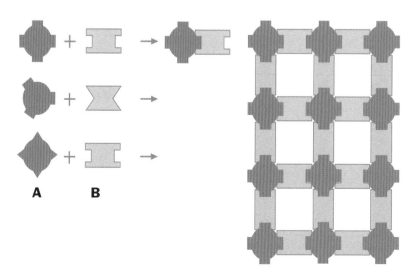

A

Allergy   Questions & Answers

I am sneezing all day; my doctor tells me I have an allergy to pollens. Which pollens are allergenic?

Pollens are the small, spherical or egg-shaped grains which, as the male germ cells of plants, are necessary for plant fertilization. While pollen allergy usually occurs first during childhood or young adulthood, it may develop at any age. At least two seasons of exposure to a pollen are generally necessary.

Not all pollens cause allergy. People often think that pollens of colourful, scented flowers such as roses are the source of their allergy. This is true for people like gardeners or florists, who spend a lot of time close to these flowers, but in general, tree, grass and weed pollens are the most frequent causes of pollen allergy. Pollens may be divided into two types: those carried by insects and those borne on the wind. Most flowers have large and waxy pollens which are carried from plant to plant by insects such as bees. On the other hand, trees, grasses and weeds are wind-pollinated. The small, dry pollens can be dispersed widely by the wind currents.

What tests can be performed to check for pollen allergy as cause of sneezing and bronchitis-like complaints?

When pollen allergy is suspected, a medical specialist may perform skin tests to identify which pollens are responsible. Using his knowledge of pollens important in his geographical area at various times, the allergist injects a diluted amount of each individual pollen under the skin (intravenous skin test) or applies it to a scratch (scratch test) on the patient's arm or back.

A small raised area, known as 'weal and flare reaction' will develop at the test site in an allergic person. The size of the weal will depend on the severity of the allergic reaction. If the medical history and physical examination strongly suggest pollen allergy, but skin tests are negative - a rare occurrence - the allergist may choose more direct testing, such as direct application of pollen examples to the mucosal membrane of the nose. A modern test is the RAST test (which stands for radio-allergo-sorbent technique), in which samples of the patient's blood are used to determine the extent of immunological globulin production in response to a particular allergen.

What is the best treatment for pollen allergy causing respiratory symptoms?

Three methods are available:
- avoidance of the allergen;
- medication (such as antihistamines);
- immunotherapy, sometimes called 'allergy shots' by the general public.

Such treatment will generally provide significant relief from the symptoms of allergy, although no actual cure has yet been found. Since it is not usually possible to eradicate allergenic pollen, complete avoidance of a particularly troublesome pollen involves moving to another location where the offending plant does not grow. However, this is not practical or even necessary for most sufferers and, for them, partial avoidance of troublesome pollens can be achieved without moving. Some people try to take their holidays at the height of their allergen's pollinating periods and choose a spot free of that pollen. The allergist might also suggest that air conditioning or an air filter should be used in the home.

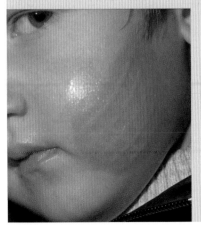

Drug allergies

With the proliferation of new drugs, the incidence of drug allergies has increased. Like contact allergies, drug reactions may occur in anyone, and some of these - although very few - are true drug allergies. Other drug reactions are side-effects, idiosyncrasies and toxic effects that a drug may have in any person who takes it.

Reactions can occur from both prescription and over-the-counter preparations taken by mouth, injected, used as suppositories, eye or nose drops, creams or ointments. Symptoms in drug reactions can run the gamut from immediate outbreaks of hives and dermatitis to flu-like symptoms appearing several days later.

In more serious incidences, drug reactions can cause anaphylactic shock (characterized by shortness of breath and a rapid fall in blood pressure), blood changes, disturbances in the digestive system and other organs, and inflammation of blood vessels and connective tissues.

Often a person is allergic to the source of the drug. For example, someone who is allergic to horses may be aller-

Microscopic view of the house dust mite (magnification x 250).

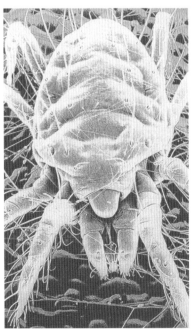

Advice for hayfever

- During pollen season, stay indoors as much as possible with windows closed. Use an air conditioning or air purification system if you can.
- Avoid mowing the lawn, raking leaves and other forms of yard work.
- Avoid activities in or near open fields where there are grasses.
- Avoid drives or hikes in the country where grasses could trigger your allergies.
- Take holidays in areas of the country where ragwort and other pollen producers are less prevalent: by coasts, in mountains, near large bodies of water.
- Use the allergy pills or antihistamines your doctor prescribes.
- Use nose drops occasionally for relief. They are only briefly effective and may damage nasal membranes if used too often.
- Use cotton handkerchiefs rather than paper tissues, which contain chemicals and fine paper dust.
- Avoid highly allergenic foods that may increase symptoms in susceptible individuals.
- Start a swimming program - you won't have to worry about pollen.

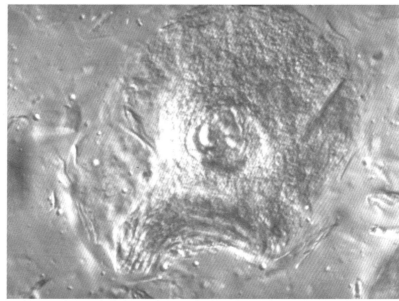

In this case of severe shell, damaged giant cells showed up in the urine.

Young baby suffering from lactose allergy.

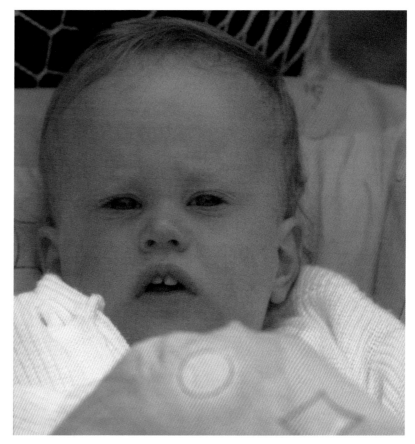

gic to an anti-tetanus serum derived from horses. Those who are allergic to eggs will probably react to virus vaccines (measles, mumps, influenza, rabies) that are grown on chicken or duck embryos.

Aspirin and any of the numerous drugs containing it, foods containing salicylates or salicylate additives, laxatives, sedatives, sleeping pills, tranquillizers, hormones, liver extract and insulin can also cause allergic reactions in some people.

New methods of treatment and cooperation between doctor and patient can make life much easier for the allergy sufferer. Besides adhering strictly to treatment, those with allergies can do a great deal to improve their condition by following a fit lifestyle that includes a well-balanced diet, exercise, plenty of rest and a minimum of stress and emotional upset.

ALZHEIMER'S DISEASE

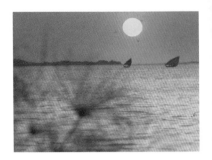

Introduction

Alzheimer's disease is a disorder that affects the brain's thinking and reasoning ability. It is the common cause of mental breakdown in older people, responsible for over half of all nursing home admissions. Although Alzheimer's usually begins in the elderly, it sometimes can start in the 40s and 50s. The cause and the essential nature of the disease process are not understood. It is not infectious or contagious, it tends to be inherited but not to the extent that every descendant of every Alzheimer's patient is afflicted. Alzheimer's disease appears to be related to a form of degeneration of certain brain cells. Specific alterations in brain cells can be found in a particular percentage of cases.

- *Dementia*
  A group of symptoms characterized by a decline in intellectual functioning severe enough to interfere with a persons's normal daily activities and social relationships.
- *Alzheimer's disease*
  The most common cause of dementia among older people. It is marked by progressive, irreversible declines in memory, performance of routine tasks, time and space orientation, language and communication skills, abstract thinking, and the ability to learn and carry out mathematical calculations. Other symptoms of Alzheimer's disease include personality changes and impairment of judgment.
- *Age-associated memory impairment*
  A decline in short-term memory that sometimes accompanies aging; also called benign senescent

forgetfulness. It does not progress to other cognitive impairments as Alzheimer's disease does.
- *Senile dementia*
  Am outdated term once used to refer to any form of dementia that occurred in older people.

Dementing disorders

Alzheimer's diseases belongs to the group of dementing disorders; a group of brain diseases that lead to the loss of mental functions, including memory and other intellectual and functional abilities, affecting today at least 500,000 inhabitants of the UK and 3-4 million Americans.
Dementia of the Alzheimer's type cannot now be prevented; its course cannot be slowed or reversed, though in many cases the severity of its impact on the individual or family may be reduced through early detection and appropriate treatment of associated problems.

Signs and symptoms

Alzheimer's patients suffer progressively increasing impairment of memory and other intellectual abilities. Although the problem may initially be manifested in such ways as forgetfulness, poor judgment, or difficulty making calculations and handling money, the cognitive losses ultimately leave the person confused, disoriented, and incapable of communicating normally.
Affected individuals undergo personality changes that may range from apathy and social withdrawal to quarrelsomeness and agitation, and frequently display various emotional reactions to their illness, such as anxi-

ety, depression, or suspiciousness. Other symptoms such as disturbed sleep, hallucinations, delusional ideas, or a tendency to wander aimlessly, are also common.
Over time, these individuals lose the ability for their own well-being. Eventually, they may lose elementary physical abilities, such as bladder and bowel control, and become totally dependent on others to provide for their personal needs and safety.
The peculiar tragedy of Alzheimer's disease and other related dementias is that they dissolve the mind and steal the humanity of the victim, leaving a body from which the person has largely been removed. In addition, abnormalities in the ability to communicate may occur that are not caused by disorientation but by brain abnormalities that can interfere with the ability to speak, understand speech, read or write.
There also may be a general physical showing - of movement, coordination, and reaction time - along with muscle rigidity. There may be loss of or change in appetite, such as disinterest in food or a demand for only one type of food, which can lead to malnutrition.
The individual leads an increasingly sedentary life, eventually taking to bed with its associated consequence of muscle contractures, pneumonia, and a propensity for infection, bed sores and other problems the patient may be unable to recognize or complain about in order for treatment to be undertaken in a timely way.
Caregivers face the agony of seeing their beloved ones' minds and personalities disappear from bodies that may frequently remain otherwise healthy, and shoulder heavy physical and social burdens for their loved ones' care, typically over prolonged periods

of incapacitation averaging 6-8 years and sometimes as long as 20 years.

Stages of the disorder

Until science comes up with good treatments, the best one can do is recognize its stages and give appropriate support and care. Not every patient exhibits the same symptoms, and the stages tend to overlap. But it helps to know the hallmarks of the disease and to have a plan for dealing with each stage before it arrives.

Stage 1: mild
This stage may last from two to four years.

Symptoms
- Increased forgetfulness that interferes with ability to hold job or complete household tasks.
- Forgets names for simnple things like bread or butter.
- Has trouble recognizing what numbers mean.
- Loses initiative and interest in favorite activities or hobbies.
- Decreased judgment that leads to, for example, wearing a bathrobe to the park.

What caregivers can do
- Make sure you have the right diagnosis. Many conditions can affect memory.
- Avoid correcting confused or faulty memories.
- Create a simnple 'orientation area' at home in which you keep essential items like keys, glasses, clock and calendar.
- Monitor driving habits.
- Plan for the future; decide when financial responsibilities should be turned over; set treatment options; designate a health-care proxy.
  Register with programs for reuniting lost or wandering Alzheimer's patients.

Stage 2: moderate
This stage may last from two to eight years.

Symptoms
- Unable to recognize close friends

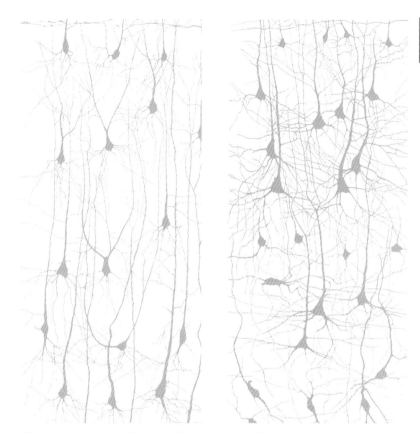

Cells in the cerebral cortex from an Alzheimer patient left) as compared to normal cells. The branches of the nerve cells are severely affected.

Macroscopic view of the brain of an Alzheimer patient.

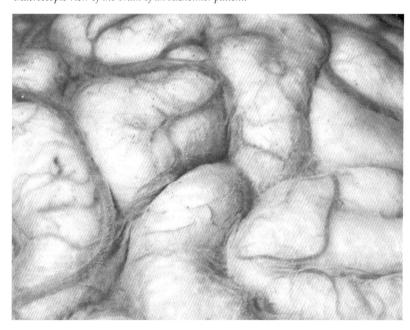

A

Summary of symptoms

Mild symptoms

- Confusion and memory loss
  Alzheimer's sufferers forget often, are unable to recall, and repeatedly ask the same question, forgetting the earlier answer. Patients may forget to pay household bills - forgetting what a bill is, why it needs to be paid - and even how to write a check or address an envelope.
- Disorientation; getting lost in familiar surroundings
  Anyone can temporarily misplace car keys or glasses. A person with Alzheimer's disease forgets often and may not be able to find belongings because they have put things in inappropriate places - an iron in the freezer, for example, or a loaf of bread in the washing machine.
  People with Alzheimer's disease may not know what year it is, where they live, who is the prime-minister or how to get to their neighbourhood grocery store. The disorientation is more than just momentary.
- Problems with routine tasks
  Occasionally, everyone gets distracted and forgets - for example, a step in a process. However, people with Alzheimer's disease may not only forget how to tie their shoes - they may not even remember to wear their shoes.
- Changes in personality and judgment
  People with Alzheimer's disease can have rapid mood swings for no apparent reason. Someone who was once calm, kind and loving may become mean, irritable and difficult. The patients may become passive and reluctant to get involved in business, social or family activities that they once enjoyed.
  Someone with Alzheimer's disease may forget to answer a ringing phone, turn off the faucet, care for a pet, or attend to any number of everyday activities that require conscientious thought. They may dress inappropriately, such as forgetting to wear a coat outdoors or wearing several shorts at a time.

Moderate symptoms

- Difficulty with activities of daily living, such as feeding and bathing
- Anxiety, suspiciousness, agitation
- Sleep disturbances
- Wandering, pacing
- Difficulty recognizing family and friends

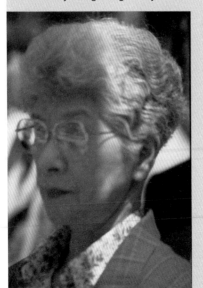

Severe symptoms

- Loss of speech
  A person with Alzheimer's disease may have trouble finding the right words, use inappropriate words or repeatedly say the same things - making speech virtually incomprehensible. Patients may also be completely unable to initiate conversation or they may misinterpret what others say.
- Loss of appetite; weight loss
- Loss of bladder and bowel control
- Total dependence on caregiver

and family.
- Wanders about, gets lost.
- Increased confusion, anxiety and personality changes.
- Forgets how to complete common daily tasks like getting dressed or brushing teeth.
- Delusions.
- Insomnia.

What caregivers can do
- Label drawers, closets, rooms and appliances as well as photos of family, friends and pets.
- Maintain familiar surroundings. Make sure hallways and bathrooms are well lighted at night. Install support rails and slip-proof surfaces in bath. Label hot-and-cold-water faucets.
- Take away car keys.
- Install door locks from the outside, or rig doors with alarms. Lay out articles of clothing one at a time.
- Brush your teeth at the same time to show how it is done.
- Start looking into residential care facilities, if that is what you want.

Stage 3: severe
This stage may last from one to three years.

Symptoms
- Unable to remember anything or process new information. Cannot recognize family.
- Cannot use or understand words but still responds to music, touch or eye contact.
- Difficulty eating, swallowing.
- Unable to dress, bathe or groom self; unable to control bladder and bowel function.
- Bedridden.

What caregivers can do
- Communicate often with patients who are institutionalized.
- Try to communicate in a different way, through exchange of old photos or through music.
- Minimize unneccessary blood tests and other painful procedures.
- You may not want to treat medical problems such as pneumonia and hip fractures as aggressively as you would for a healthy person.

Diagnostic tools

A definite diagnosis of Alzheimer's disease is still only possible during autopsy when the hallmark plaques and tangles can be detected. But with the tools now available, physicians and patients can count on 85 to 90 percent accuracy, according to studies in which clinical diagnosis was later confirmed by autopsy. The following diagnostic tools are available:

*   *Patient history*
    A detailed description of how and when symptoms developed; the patient's and family's medical history; and an assessment of the patient's emotional status and living environment.
*   *Physical examination and laboratory tests*
    Standard medical tests to help identify other possible causes of dementia.

Warning signs

*   Recent memory loss that affects job performance
*   Inability to learn new information
*   Difficulty with everyday tasks such as cooking or dressing oneself
*   Inability to remember simple words
*   Use of inappropriate words when communicating
*   Disorientation of time and place
*   Poor or decreased judgment
*   Problems with abstract thinking
*   Putting objects in appropriate places
*   Rapid changes in mood or behavior
*   Increased irritability, anxiety, depression, confusion, and restlessness
*   Prolonged loss of initiative

*   *Brain scans*
    Usually a computed tomography (CT) scan or magnetic resonance imaging (MRI) to detect strokes or tumors that could be causing symptoms of dementia.

*   *Neuropsychological testing*
    Usually several different tests in which patients answer questions or complete tasks that measure memory, language skills, ability to do arithmetic, and other abilities related to brain functioning.

Low-stress activities on a regular basis can help people feel independent (right). Such activities can also help relieve depression. Massage (left) can help relieve muscle tension.

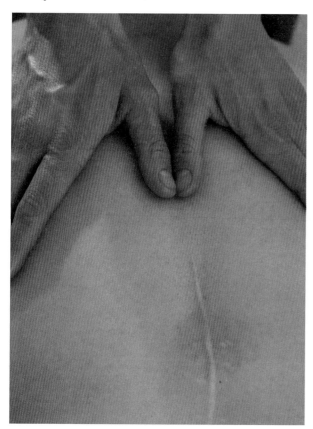
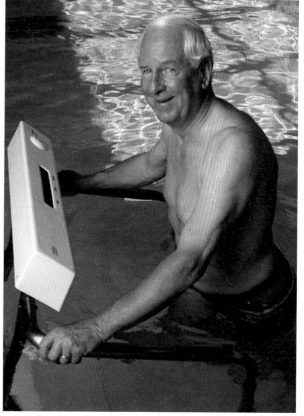

ANEMIA

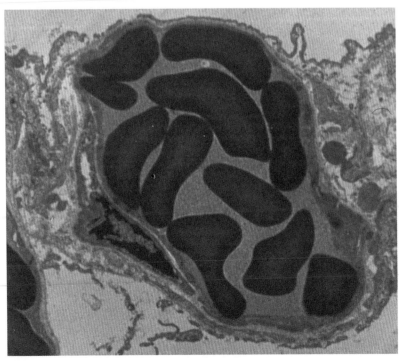

Blood

Blood is a thick red fluid filling the heart and blood vessels. It consists of plasma, a transparent fluid, that contains minute solid particles or corpuscles in it. These corpuscles or blood cells are of two types, the more numerous being the red corpuscles or cells (erythrocytes), which in normal human blood outnumber the white corpuscles or cells (leukocytes) by 500 to 1. Also present are minute circular bodies known as platelets, or thrombocytes.

Each of the enormous number of living cells which make up the body is supplied with materials to enable it to carry on its activities, and at the same time, materials resulting from its activities are removed.

Most cells are far from the source of supplies and the organs of elimination, hence the need for a medium to distribute supplies and collect materials not needed by cells. This need is met primarily by the blood and, to a lesser extent, by tissue fluid.

Blood is characterized by a number of specific physical properties. Its viscosity (pouring thickness) is about four to six times that of water - in other words, it flows four to six times more slowly than water under the same conditions. It is a little heavier than water; its specific gravity varies between 1.041 and 1.067, and in general, 1.058 is taken as a fair average. Blood has a characteristic odor, a salty taste, a pH value of approximately 7.35 to 7.45.

These ranges cover the values for both arterial and venous blood - that is, blood in the arteries and in the veins.

In the adult, blood volume is about one-thirteenth of body weight and plasma volume about one-twentieth of body weight.

Normally there is little variation in the quantity of blood. The ratio between blood quantity and tissue fluid quantity, however, is not constant, and many factors probably cause this ratio to change.

The quantity of blood varies with age, sex, the amount of muscle and fat in the body, activity, state of hydration, condition of the heart and blood vessels and many other factors. There are also wide and unpredictable individual variations. Studies reveal that prolonged bedrest results in a reduction in plasma volume.

The volume of cells and plasma is approximately equal. The percentage of the blood made up of red blood cells is called the hematocrit; the normal value is about 47 percent. The ratio varies in relation to hydration and other medical conditions.

Red blood cells

The red cells or erythrocytes are by far the most numerous of the blood cells; for every white cell there are about 500 red cells and about 300 platelets.

Under the microscope, red blood cells are seen to be homogeneous circular discs, without nuclei, and thicker on the circumference than in the middle. The average size is about 7.2 microns (1/3000 in). They have a yellowish-red tinge, and it is only when great num-

Red blood cells in a capillary.

bers of them are gathered together that a distinctly red color is produced. Red blood cells consist of a colorless, filmy, elastic framework, or stroma, in which hemoglobin, a red oxygen-carrying pigment, is deposited, surrounded by a delicate membrane.

The stroma is composed of protein and lipid substances including cholesterol. The blood group substances A and B and the Rhesus antigen are located in the stroma.

In the embryo, the first blood cells arise from certain types of cells in the yolk sac. The next phase of development is chiefly in the liver and to some extent in the spleen.

Development of red blood cells takes place in a fetus's bone marrow at about the fifth month and decreases in the liver as it increases in red bone marrow. Immature red blood cells, reticulocytes and normoblasts are sometimes found in the blood.

The life-span of red blood cells is thought to be about 120 days. When and how the red blood cells disintegrate are not known. One supposition is that as they age, they undergo hemolysis (breakdown) and fragmentation in the blood. Another is that they are destroyed in the spleen, lymph nodes and liver.

The average number of red blood cells in a cubic millimeter of normal blood is given as 5.5 million to 7 million for men and 4.5 million to 6 million for women.

Conditions of ill health may cause a marked diminution in number, and differences have also been observed when people are healthy.

The number varies because of several factors, such as:
- altitude;
- temperature;
- nutrition;
- lifestyle;
- age, being the greatest factor in the fetus and newborn child;
- the time of day, showing a reduction after meals.

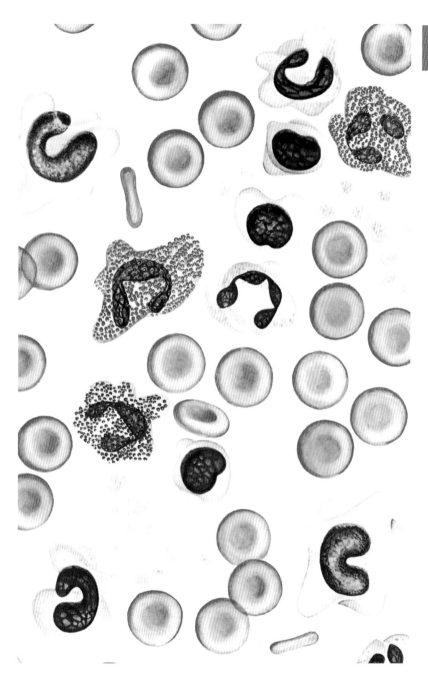

Drawing of the various cells in a normal blood preparation.
See for further explanation the legend of the illustration on page 151.

Hemoglobin
Hemoglobin comprises a complex protein molecule (globin) and a non-protein portion (hem), which contains iron. One red cell contains about 600 million molecules of hemoglobin. Under normal conditions, the adult body produces about 6-7 g of hemoglobin per day.

In the adult, 100 ml of normal blood contains, on average, between 12 and 19 g of hemoglobin - in males, the average is 14 to 18 g; in females, 11.5 to 16 g.

Hemolysis
This process, also called laking, is a serious condition in which disruption of the surrounding membrane of the red blood cell leads to the content of the cell passing into the plasma.

The red blood cell is then unable to

A

Anemia Questions & Answers

What are the causes of anemia?
Blood contains red cells that carry oxygen, white cells that deal with infection, and platelets that help in clotting. You cannot judge the health of your child's blood by the appearance of his skin; whether or not a child has pink cheeks depends on how close his small blood vessels are to the surface.
Anemia means that there is a lack of hemoglobin, the substance in the red cells that transports the oxygen from the air in the lungs to every part of the body.

What are the major symptoms of anemia?
To discover whether or not a child or adolescent is anemic the doctor looks at the lining of the eye (the conjunctiva) by pulling down the lower eyelid.
He also looks at the inside of the lips and at the palms of the hands. The color of the mucous membranes (the conjunctiva and the inside of the lips) gives a true picture, since they do not vary between individuals as the skin color does. If the doctor is in doubt he will have the child's blood tested for its level of hemoglobin.

Can lack of iron cause an anemia?
Iron deficiency anemia results from low or depleted stores of iron, which is needed to produce red blood cells. Iron deficiency anemia usually develops slowly, because it may take several months for the body's iron reserves to be used up. As the iron reserved are decreasing, the bone marrow gradually produces lower red blood cells. When the reserves are depleted, the red blood cells are not only fewer in number but also abnormally small.

How can disorders of bone marrow cells cause anemia?
When the bone marrow cells that develop into mature blood cells and platelets are damaged or suppressed, the bone marrow can shut down. This bone marrow failure is called aplastic anemia. The most common cause of aplastic anemia may be an autoimmune disorder, in which the immune system suppresses bone marrow stem cells. Other causes include:
- infection with parvovirus
- radiation exposure
- toxins (such as benzene)
- chemotherapy drugs.

Autoimmune disorders; what is the effect on red blood cells?
Autoimmune hemolytic anemia is a group of disorders characterized by a malfunction of the immune system that produces autoantibodies, which attack red blood cells as if they were substances foreign to the body.
Autoimmune hemolytic anemia is an uncommon group of disorders that can occur at any age. About half of the time, the cause of autoimmune hemolytic anemia cannot be determined. Autoimmune hemolytic anemia can also be caused by or occur with another disease, such as systemic lupus erythematosus, and rarely it follows the use of certain drugs, such as penicillin.
Destruction of red blood cells by autoantibodies may occur suddenly, or it may develop gradually. In some people, the destruction may stop after a period of time, whereas in other people, it persists and becomes chronic.

When is an anemia called a sickle cell disease?
Sickle cell disease is an inherited condition characterized by sickle (crescent)-shaped red blood cells and chronic anemia caused by excessive destruction of red blood cells.
In sickle cell disease, the red blood cells contain an abnormal form of hemoglobin that reduces the amount of oxygen in the cells. The reduced oxygen causes some of the red blood cells to become sickle-shaped.

exert its functions. The resulting colorless red blood cells are referred to as "ghosts."
Hemolysis may be brought about by the following factors or under the following circumstances:
- hypotonic solutions (solutions with a low salt concentration);
- foreign blood serums;
- agents such as snake venoms or other poisons;
- products of bacterial activity;
- immunizing agents;
- the addition of ether or chloroform;
- the addition of bile salts;
- alternate freezing and thawing;
- amyl alcohol or saponin;
- ammonia and other alkalis;
- incompatible transfusion of whole blood;
- certain types of allergic reactions.
Red blood cells that have lost their hemoglobin are incapable of serving as oxygen carriers.

Characteristics of anemia

The term *anemia* is applied to conditions associated with a deficiency of erythrocytes (red blood cells) or a deficiency of hemoglobin in those cells. A deficiency of erythrocytes can result from hemorrhage, hemolysis or inability to produce new erythrocytes due to lack of nutritious food, diseases of the bone marrow and various infections.
Except in cases of abnormal blood loss, anemia is the result of an imbalance between red blood cell production and destruction. The balance is normally maintained by proper functioning of the bone marrow (the spongelike tissue that fills the cavities of most bones).
Constant production and destruction of red blood cells is necessary because the cells naturally wear out after about four months. Old red blood cells must be destroyed, and young red blood cells must take their place.
In a number of different ways, this process can be disrupted, producing anemia. For each cause of anemia, treatment (and sometimes, signs and symptoms) is different.
The two major categories of causes are excessively rapid destruction of

A

Main functions of blood

The main functions of the blood are:
- To carry oxygen from the lungs to the tissues, and carbon dioxide from the tissues to the lungs.
- To carry nutrients absorbed from the intestine and transport them to the tissues for utilization.
- To carry products formed in one tissue to other tissues where they are used; in other words, to transport hormones to the tissues requiring them.
- To carry the waste products of metabolism to the organs of excretion - the lungs, the kidneys, intestine and skin.
- To aid in maintaining fluid balance between blood and tissues.
- To aid in maintaining the temperature of the body at a normal level.
- To aid in maintaining the normal acid-alkali balance of the tissues.
- To constitute a defence mechanism against the invasion of harmful organisms.
- To clot, preventing loss of blood after injury.

red blood cells or hemoglobin, and impairment of red blood cells or hemoglobin production.

Aplastic anemia

Aplastic anemia is a blood disorder resulting in the failure of the bone marrow to produce an sufficient amount of red blood cells. Aplastic anemia is generally categorized as severe or mild.

In the mild form of aplastic anemia, the blood cells are less drastically reduced in number. Sometimes, a deficiency of one type of blood cell precedes the full-blown development of aplastic anemia.

An individual case of aplastic anemia may initially be moderate and then become severe, or vice versa. Often, mild aplastic anemia develops into a severe form of the disease.

Mild aplastic anemia and, less frequently, severe aplastic anemia may resolve (blood cell levels return to normal). In moderate cases a patient may suffer frequent nosebleeds, occasional or mils infections, and mils anemia.

In severe cases, a patient may suffer from heavy or prolonged bleeding, frequently or severe infections, and severe anemia.

Aplastic anemia may be acquired or inherited. Acquired aplastic anemia occurs three times as often as the inherited variety. A child can acquire aplastic anemia at any age; inherited

aplastic anemia may be apparent at birth or become apparent later during childhood. It occurs most frequently before the age of 12.

Hemolytic anemia

Anemias caused by excessive destruction of red blood cells are called hemolytic anemias. Destruction of red blood cells may be short-term, long-term or intermittent.

The severity of any hemolytic anemia depends upon the difference between rates of red blood cell destruction and production. The outlook for a person with a hemolytic anemia depends upon the specific disorder involved.

Cause
Hemolytic anemia can be congenital (caused by abnormalities present at birth) or acquired. Each type of congenital anemia results from one of three types of defects.

■ *Hereditary spherocytosis and elliptocytosis*
In these cases defects occur in the structure of red blood cells. Examples of anemias caused by this type of

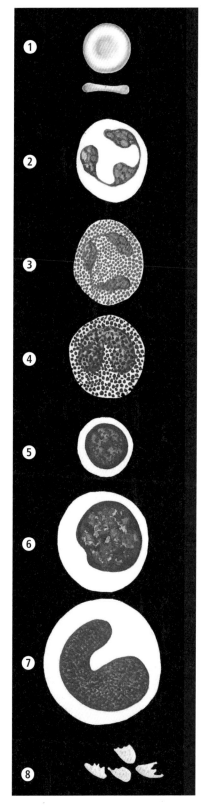

Schematic drawing of the main elements in e blood preparation.
1. Erythrocyte, 2. neutrophilic granulocyte, 3. basophilic granulocyte, 4. lymphocyte (old one), 6. lymphocyte (new one), 7. monocyte, 8. platelets.

defect are hereditary spherocytosis, in which red blood cells are shaped like spheres instead of disks, and ellepto-cytosis, in which red blood cells are shaped like ellipses (ovals)

■ Sickle cell anemia and thalassemia
The basic problem is a defect in the production of hemoglobin. In sickle cell anemia hemoglobin is abnormal and has a tendency to congeal (sickle), and in thalassemia the production of hemoglobin is reduced or never occurs.

■ G6PD deficiency
This disorder is characterized by a defect in an enzyme of red blood cells. G6PD deficiency is the most common disorder, in which the activity of the enzyme G6DP is greatly reduced. In the most common form of this deficiency, certain drugs or infections can induce episodes of hemolysis and subsequent anemia in affected persons.

Disorders
Each type of acquired hemolytic anemia results from one of two types of disorders: immunologic or nonim-munologic.

■ Immunologic disorders
These disorders are caused by anti-bodies, either passively acquired, as is the case of Rh incompatibility, or actively formed, as in some types of lupus erythematosus or lymphoma. These antibodies attack, reject, or crowd out red blood cells.

■ Nonimmunologic disorders
These disorders can be caused by poi-sons (toxins), such as certain drugs or chemicals, or infections, such as malaria. Exposure to these toxins of infections can cause excessive destruc-tion of red blood cells.

Treatment
Treatment varies for each type of hemolytic anemia and for each indi-vidual. For instance, some types of hemolytic anemia require replace-ment of lost iron, others require removal of the spleen. Inherited types of hemolytic anemia are not prevent-able. Anemia caused by nonimmulo-logic disorders can be prevented if the toxins or infections causing the disor-ders can be avoided.

Nutritional anemia

There are three types of nutritional anemias, which are distinguished by the size, shape, and color of the red blood cells: microcytic, macrocytic, and normocytic.

■ Microcytic anemias
The blood cells of a person with microcytic anemia are abnormally small and contain insufficient hemo-globin as a result of disorders that interfere with the production of heme (the iron-carrying component of hemoglobin) or of globin.
One example of a microcytic anemia is iron-deficiency anemia. Iron defi-ciency interferes with the production of heme and therefore of hemoglobin. Anemia occurs only after all the body's stored iron has been depleted and normal physical development begins to be affected.
Iron deficiency is the major cause of anemia during childhood. It is most common among preschool children and, in this age group, usually results from insufficient iron in the diet.
Although iron deficiency caused by an inadequate diet is preventable, the high incidence of subsequent anemia among preschool children remains a cause of concern to parents, physi-

Molecular structure of vitamin B_{12}, used for the treatment of certain types of anemias.

Causes of anemia due to decreased production of red blood cells

The major causes of anemia in this category are:
- Iron deficiency
- Vitamin B_{12} deficiency
- Folic acid deficiency
- Vitamin C deficiency
- Certain chronic diseases
- Multiple myelomas
- Leukemia
- Disorders of leukocytes
- Lymphoma
- Chronic infections
- Metastatic cancer

cians, and public health officials. The body's requirement for iron changes with age. Iron deficiency is most likely to occur at times when the need for iron is greater than normal: during pregnancy, during the first two years of life, and during pre-adolescence.

During adolescence, females lose iron when they menstruate and have a greater need for iron for the production of extra hemoglobin.

Mild cases of iron-deficiency anemia are treated by taking iron supplements at least an hour before meals so that the iron can pass into the intestines for absorption before food in the stomach interferes.

■ *Macrocytic anemias*

People with macrocytic anemia produce too few red blood cells; these red cells that are produced are abnormally large, but have normal concentrations of hemoglobin.

The most common macrocytic anemias are caused by folate deficiency and vitamin B_{12} deficiency. Both deficiencies cause anemia by stopping or slowing the development of red blood cells.

Folate deficiency can be caused by an inadequate diet, congenital or acquired intestinal malabsorption, or any condition - such as pregnancy, leukemia, or chronic hemolytic anemia - that stimulates increased production of red blood cells.

Vitamin B_{12} deficiency can be caused by an inadequate diet or insufficient intrinsic factor, both of which contribute to a decreased absorption of the vitamin by the intestines. Deficiency of intrinsic factor can be

present at birth or acquired; this condition is called pernicious anemia.

Folate deficiency is treated by the daily administration of oral folate and nutritional consultation. If vitamin B_{12}-deficiency is caused by inadequate dietary intake or other cause where intestinal absorption is normal, vitamin B_{12} supplements are given orally three times daily.

If intestinal absorption is the problem (as in pernicious anemia), injections of vitamin B_{12} are given, because taking pills would not help.

■ *Normocytic anemias*

The red blood cells of people with normocytic anemia are normal in size, shape, and concentrations of hemoglobin, but insufficient in number. Although normocytic anemias are caused by blood loss, in rare conditions vitamin E deficiency can bring on normocytic anemia.

The latter condition is treated by the administration of vitamin E supplements once a day. If this approach fails, vitamin E is given through injections.

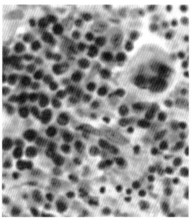
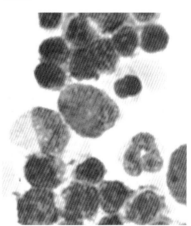

Blood preparation of a patient suffering from thalassemia, a special type of anemia. Thalassemia is an hereditary disease found in people of Mediterranean, Asian, and African ancestry. It is caused by impaired production of one of the polypeptide chains of the hemoglobin molecule. The patient shows severe hemolytic anemia. The peripheral blood smear shows microcytic, hypochromic red cells, probably due to the decreased synthesis of globin. The blood preparation shows basophilic stippling, increased polychromatophilia and numerous target cells.

Upper left: Bone marrow smear
Upper right: Bone marrow smear with normoblasts (young erythrocytes)
Lower left: Histiocytes with basophilic, polymorphic cells
Lower right: Normoblasts

Causes of anemia due to increased destruction of red blood cells

The major causes of anemia in this category are:
- Enlarged spleen
- Certain hereditary conditions
- Autoimmune reactions against red blood cells
- Sickle cell disease
- Thalassemia
- Hemoglobin disorders

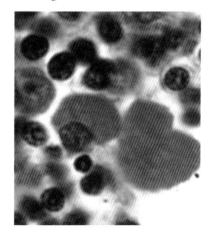
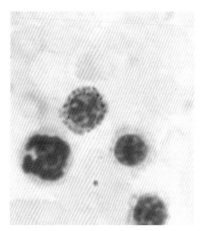

ANGINA PECTORIS

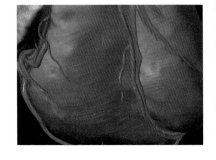

Introduction

Angina, or angina pectoris, is a recurring discomfort. It is usually located near the center of the chest. The pain or discomfort occurs when the blood supply to part of the heart muscle does not meet the heart's needs. As a result, the heart does not get enough oxygen and nutrients. The discomfort occurs most often during exercise or emotional stress. That is when the heart rate and blood pressure increase, and the heart muscle needs more oxygen.

Anginal pain or discomfort is usually brief, lasting just a few minutes. People describe it as a heaviness, tightness, oppressive pain, burning, pressure or squeezing. Usually it is located behind the breastbone. Sometimes it spreads to the arms, neck or jaws. It may also cause a numbness in the shoulders, arms or wrists.

Angina and heart attack

Angina is different from a heart attack. Both relate to the blood flow through the coronary arteries (which bring blood to the heart muscle), but there is a key difference. With angina, the blood flow is reduced, especially when the heart must do more work. This reduced blood flow to the heart muscle is temporary and leads to discomfort in the chest.

With a heart attack, the blood flow to

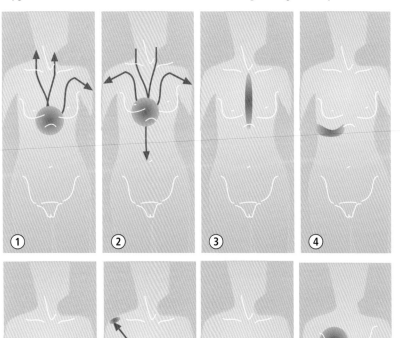

Angina pectoris is usually located behind the breastbone. Sometimes it spreads to the arms, neck or jaws. It may also cause a numbness in the shoulders, arms or wrists. Pain in the chest may also originate from other disorders or diseases.

Differential diagnosis of pain in the chest.

1. Characteristic distribution of pain of angina pectoris.

2. Thrombosis of a coronary artery; the pain may radiate toward the neck, arms and upper abdominal region.

3. Pain due to heartburn; a retrosternal sensation of warmth of burning occurring in waves and tending to rise upward toward the neck.

4. Herpes zoster of one of the thoracic segments of the spinal nerves.

5. Pleurisy, inflammation of the pleura.

6. Colicky pain of the gallbladder or one of the ducts of liver of gallbladder.

7. Pneumonia located in the lower lobe of the right lung.

8. Pneumothorax; air or gas in the pleural space, which may occur spontaneously, as a result of trauma or pathological process, or be introduced deliberately.

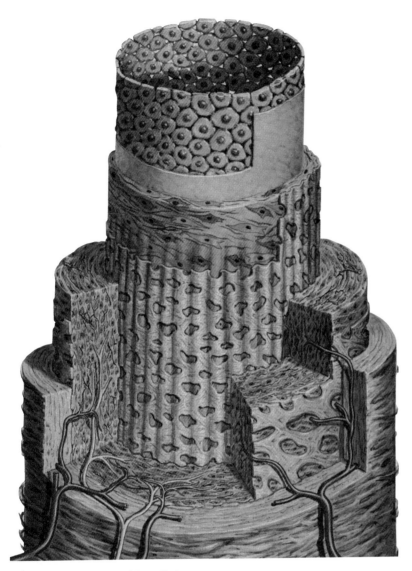

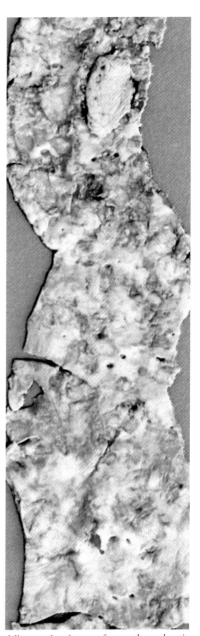

Schematic reconstruction of the wall of an artery.
1: Inner layer consisting of endothelial cells with a layer of loose connective tissue.
2: Middle layer consisting of smooth muscle cells and elastic fibers.
3: Outer layer consisting of a fibrous sheath mainly made up of collagen.
Atheromas will develop in the inner layer, eventually leading to the formation of emboli and blockage of the lumen resulting in angina or myocardial infarction.

Microscopic picture of an atherosclerotic arterial wall showing deposits of lipids, cholesterol and calcium. Atherosclerosis begins when the lining (intima or inner layer) of the artery is injured or deceased. Then certain white blood cells called monocytes are activated and move out of the bloodstream and through the lining of the artery into the artery's wall. Inside the lining, they are transformed into foam cells, which are cells that collect fatty materials, mainly cholesterol. Connective and elastic tissue materials also accumulate there, as may cell debris, cholesterol crystals, and calcium.

part of the heart muscle is suddenly cut off when a coronary artery os blocked. The chest pain that results is usually more severe and lasts longer. As a general rule, attacks of angina do not permanently damage the heart muscle; a heart attack does. many people who have angina have never had a heart attack, although angina can develop after one.

Causes of angina

Your body has a way to increase the amount of blood that flows to the heart muscle when a coronary artery is partly blocked. Other nearby arteries may expand and tiny branches may open up to carry more blood to the affected area. This is called collateral circulation.

Angina pectoris Questions & Answers

What is angina pectoris?
This heart disorder is defined as a severe but temporary attack of chest pain which may - among others - radiate to the left arm, resulting from lack of oxygen to the heart muscle. Angina pectoris (usually just called angina) occurs when the work and demand for oxygen by the heart muscle exceeds the ability of the coronary vessels to supply oxygen. The pain of angina pectoris is believed to be a direct manifestation of deficient blood supply to the heart muscle.

What are the signs and symptoms of angina pectoris?
The discomfort of angina pectoris, although highly variable, is most commonly felt beneath the breastbone. It may be a vague, barely troublesome ache, or it may rapidly become a severe, intense, crushing sensation. Pain may radiate to the left shoulder and down the inside of the left arm, even to the fingers. The pain may radiate straight through to the back, into the throat, the jaws, the teeth and occasionally even down the right arm. Anginal discomfort may be felt in the upper and lower abdomen.

How is angina pectoris triggered?
Angina pectoris is characteristically triggered by physical activity and usually persists for no more than a few minutes, subsiding with rest. The response to exertion is usually predictable, but in some, a given exercise may be tolerated one day but may precipitate again the next.Angina is worsened when the exertion follows a meal.
It is also exaggerated in cold weather, so that exertion without symptoms in the summer may induce angina in the winter. Walking into the wind or first contact with cold air on leaving a warm room may also precipitate an attack. Angina may occur at night or when the person is resting quietly and seemingly without stimulation. Nocturnal angina is frequently preceded by a dream that may be accompanied by striking changes in respiration, pulse rate, and blood pressure.

Are all attacks of angina pectoris equal in nature?
Attacks of angina pectoris may vary in frequency from several per day to occasional seizures separated by symptom-free intervals of weeks, months or years. They may increase in frequency to a fatal outcome or may gradually decrease or disappear if an adequate collateral coronary circulation develops - that is, if other arteries take over the work of the blocked one.
Since the characteristics of angina are usually constant for a given individual, any change in the pattern of angina-increased decreased threshold of stimulus (i.e., it takes less to bring on an attack), long duration - is viewed by the doctor as a serious increase of symptoms. Between attacks patients with angina pectoris may not have signs of heart disease. However, during attacks, the heart rate usually rises, blood pressure is frequently elevated and heart sounds become more distant.

How is angina pectoris diagnosed?
Angina pectoris is a clinical diagnosis which is based on a characteristic complaint of chest discomfort brought on by exertion and relieved by rest. Confirmation will often be obtained by the doctor in performing an electrocardiogram.

How is presently the outlook of angina pectoris?
The outlook of angina pectoris is better than has commonly been supposed and is improving with innovations in medical treatment. The major risk is sudden heart death. Three factors influence outcome:
- age;
- extent of coronary disease;
- function of the heart. Clinically, an annual mortality rate of 1.5 per cent has been reported in men with angina who also have a normal electrocardiogram in rest and normal blood pressure.
The rate rises to about 7½ per cent in those with high blood pressure.

What is the best treatment for angina pectoris?
The underlying disease, usually atherosclerosis, must be treated and risk factors reduced. For example, those who smoke should discontinue the habit, and a reduction of body weight enhances well-being and reduces the demand on the heart. High blood pressure should also be treated diligently. Specific medication, such as glyceryl trinitrate, is very important for the heart function.
The reasons for considering heart surgery to deal with angina pectoris are continually refined. The factors age, heart function and coronary disease must be evaluated when coronary artery surgery is being considered. It is generally agreed that a coronary bypass operation may be considered when the blood vessels are anatomically suitable in a patient whose angina pectoris is unresponsive to medical therapy and seriously interferes with normal activity.

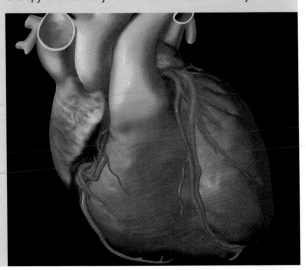

If the collateral circulation becomes well developed, anginal symptoms may decrease and even go away. This extra blood flow to the heart muscle can help prevent a heart attack. If a heart attack does occur, the permanent heart damage may be less severe. Angina and heart attack have the same root cause: atherosclerosis. This is the narrowing of the coronary arteries caused by deposits of fatty substances such as cholesterol. It usually starts early in life. Everyone has it to some degree by middle age.

Diagnosis

Usually your doctor can accurately diagnose angina from your description of symptoms. If you are suffering from it, it is possible for your physical examination and resting electrocardiogram to be entirely normal.
Consequently, your doctor may recommend an exercise test to increase your heart's demand for blood and oxygen. An electrocardiogram recorded during an exercise test can slow if your heart is not getting enough oxygen.
Sometimes it is hard to diagnose angina even after a medical history, a physical examination and an exercise test. If that is the case, your doctor may order a thallium stress test.
This is a special exercise test in which a radioisotope (thallium) is injected into a vein during exercise. It uses radioactivity detectors and computers to measure the blood flow to the heart muscle during exercise.
Your doctor may decide that a coronary arteriogram is necessary. This is an X-ray movie of your coronary arteries. It shows blood flow patterns as a radiopacque substance (a liquid that blocks X-rays) is injected into your arteries. If you have angina, an arteriogram will show if your coronary arteries are blocked or constricted, where the blockage is and how severe it is.

Medical treatment

Nitroglycerin usually works well to relieve chest discomfort from angina.

It can be sued to prevent discomfort, too. It is usually taken in tiny tablets, which are put under the tongue to dissolve. It may also be prescribed as an oral spray.
Nitroglycerin tablets are inexpensive and act quickly. Keep a fresh, sealed supply of them on hand at all times. As a general rule, avoid moving your tablets from their original, dark glass bottle, because they are sensitive to heat, light and air. Do not keep cotton in the bottle; it will absorb the nitroglycerin. And always use the medicine as directed by your physician.
Be sure to carry your nitroglycerin with you at all times. Take a tablet just before starting an activity you know is likely to cause anginal discomfort. Also, take a tablet if your discomfort

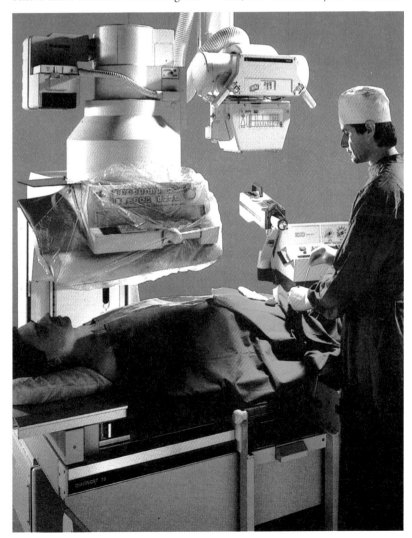

Coronary angioplasty in case of severe anginal symptoms. Generally angioplasty is preferred to bypass surgery because it is a less invasive procedure. A doctor inserts a balloon-tipped catheter into a large artery (usually the femoral artery), and threads the catheter through the connecting arteries and the aorta to the narrowed or blocked coronary artery. Then the cardiologist inflates the balloon to force the atheroma against the arterial wall and thus open the artery. Often, a collapsed tube made of wire mesh (a stent) is placed over the deflated balloon at the catheter's tip and inserted with the catheter. When the catheter reaches the atheroma, the balloon is inflated, opening up the stent. Then the balloon-tipped catheter is removed, and the stent is left in place to help keep the artery open.

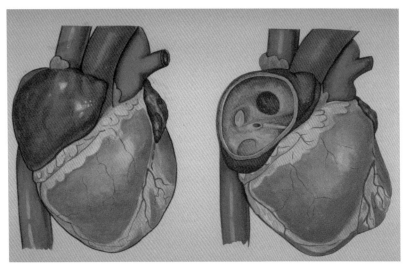

Deposit of fatty substances around the coronary arteries of the heart; this condition may cause narrowing of the arteries.

doesn't begin to go away within a minute or two after you have stopped the activity, or if discomfort occurs when you are not active. Tell your doctor what usually causes your angina so he or she can advise you about preventing attacks.

It may take several tablets a day to control your symptoms. Nitroglycerin is safe and not habit forming, so do not be afraid to take it. Ask your doctor what to do if nitroglycerin does not completely relieve your angina or if the pain starts to come more often and gets worse.

Some people who take nitroglycerin get a short headache or a felling of fullness in the head. Often these symptoms disappear after they have taken nitroglycerin several times. If you have this problem and it does not get better, your doctor may want to reduce the dosage in each tablet.

Microscopic picture of a narrowed artery.

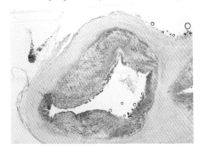

Surgery

If you keep having frequent or disabling angina despite using medications, or if your coronary arteries are badly blocked, you may need surgery. Your doctor may advise coronary artery bypass surgery on one or more of your arteries.

In this operation, a vein (taken from the leg or chest) is grafted onto the blocked artery, bypassing the blocked area. If more than one artery is blocked, each one may receive a bypass.

For a small percentage of people, another procedure, coronary angioplasty, may be advised. It is a technique in which the blockage in a coronary artery is dilated (stretched open) using an inflatable balloon on the top of a heart catheter.

Preventive measures

You can improve your condition by altering your way of life to reduce the chance of attacks of angina.

The suggestions that follow can help you live more comfortably with angina.

■ *Control your physical activity*
Learn what kinds of physical activities bring on your angina, and avoid doing them. Remember, it is how strenuous-

ly you exert yourself, not how long you do so, that causes angina. Some people can walk a mile or more without discomfort if they pace themselves. These same people may have an anginal attack if they walk rapidly for half a block.

Others can perform certain kinds of manual labour all day, but brief, intense physical effort will quickly bring chest discomfort. If sexual intercourse causes angina, discuss this with your doctor. Sometimes taking nitroglycerin can prevent angina during sex.

Many people find they are more prone to attacks of angina when they exert themselves in extremes of temperature (hot or cold) or after a heavy meal. You may find that what you can do easily in mild weather will cause chest discomfort if done in the cold and wind.

If this happens, cut back on your activities in winter weather and dress warmly whenever you are outdoors. Consult your doctor before you try to shovel snow or do other hard work in cold weather.

Moderate exercise may be good for you. many times symptoms of angina decrease when a person starts a program of progressive exercise. Ask your doctor about the best types and amounts of exercise for you. If your discomfort occurs during daily exercise, reduce your exercise and consult your doctor.

■ *Avoid emotional upsets*
Any kind of emotional upset, including outbursts of temper, can trigger angina. Excitement can also cause chest discomfort. Learning to control your emotions will help you control your angina.

Many people are surprised at how well they can control their emotions when they try.

Even so, it is impossible to avoid all emotional or anxiety-producing situations. Try to anticipate these situations and use your nitroglycerin in advance to help prevent chest discomfort. Some kinds of recurring emotional problems can be very hard to handle. If you are having difficulty, seek professional help.

If long-standing tensions seem to aggravate your angina, discuss them with your doctor, a clergyman or a family counsellor. Identify everyday situations in which you feel pressured and try to control them. Avoid time pressures like deadlines and over-crowded schedules. Also, do not insist on doing everything yourself.

Meditation and relaxation exercises are good ways to calm your emotions. Some doctors suggest that you totally relax all your muscles twice a day for 20 minutes. Others advise doing deep breathing exercises or concentrating on a pleasant thought or experience whenever you feel under stress.

If these practices do not seem to help, your doctor may recommend a mild tranquillizer. You may feel that taking tranquillizers is a sign of weakness or worry about becoming dependent upon them. If so, do not worry. Tranquillizers are safe and effective for controlling angina if you follow your doctor's advice.

■ *Adopt good eating habits*
Like exercise, digestion causes the heart to work harder. That means it needs more blood. Heavy meals can put a strain on your heart. You may find that you are especially pron to anginal discomfort after eating.

Try to avoid large meals and rich foods that leave you feeling stuffed. Relax for a while after eating. If you often get angina after meals, your doctor may advise you to use nitroglycerin before eating.

Extra weight can also aggravate angina. Many times a person's angina decreases or disappears after weight loss. Even if you are not overweight, your doctor may recommend that you control the amount of fat in your daily diet.

He or she may prescribe a diet or recommend one of the low-fat diet books available from your local American Heart Association.

■ *Check with your doctor about alcohol*
Drinking a moderate amount of alcohol helps some people relax and may not be harmful for you. But drinking too much alcohol can be potentially harmful, because it affects the heart. Some people with angina have other medical conditions that keep them from drinking alcohol. Ask your doctor's advice about drinking alcohol. And remember, if you are trying to lose weight, you should not drink too much. Alcoholic drinks are usually high in calories.

■ *Do not smoke cigarettes*
Cigarette smoking is bad fort general health. It is critical to avoid smoking if you have angina or any form of heart disease.

Cigarette smoking often makes angina worse, and it increases the risk of heart attack and other circulatory disorders.

■ *Control high blood pressure*
High blood pressure increases the risk of developing heart disease and other circulatory disorders. It also increases the heart's work and can aggravate angina. Controlling high blood pressure is essential, so follow your doctor's advice about treatment.

Healthy food is a prerequisite for the prevention of a myocardial infarction.

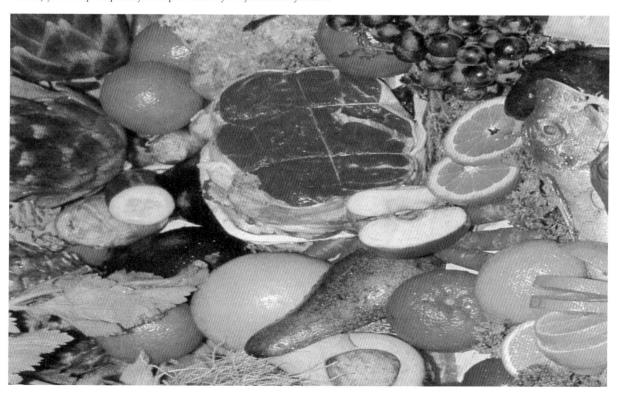

APPENDICITIS

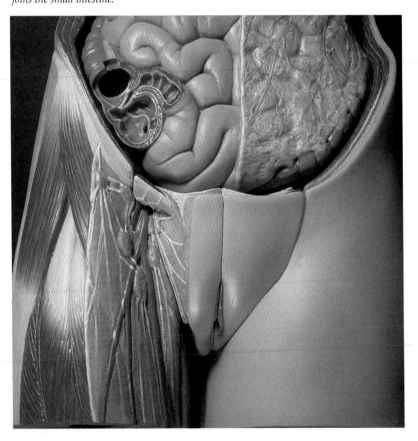

Description

Appendicitis is defined as an inflammation of the wormlike extension (appendix) of the caecum (large bowel), often caused by obstruction of its narrow opening, followed by swelling and bacterial infection. Acute appendicitis may lead to rupture of the organ, formation of an abscess or peritonitis (inflammation of the delicate membrane that lines the abdominal and pelvic cavities and also covers the organs contained in them).

Causes

Acute appendicitis is the most common inflammatory lesion within the abdominal cavity, and it can mimic almost any other lesion. It is the condition that should be thought of first when a patient presents his condition with abdominal pain to the doctor.

Despite its being so common, little is known about the etiology of acute appendicitis. It is believed that a mucosal lesion is the irritating factor, followed by a penetrating inflammatory process that by its own progression leads to inadequate blood supply of the appendiceal diverticulum and eventually to gangrene and perforation. The disease progresses much more rapidly in young children and in the elderly. The presence of a faecalith (stone composed of faeces) helps to explain the etiology as being on some sort of obstructive basis, and also increases the rapidity of the perforative process.

The appendix (here shown in a model of the abdomen in the left-hand part of the illustration) is a small finger-shaped tube projecting from the large intestine near the point where it joins the small intestine.

Symptoms

Less than half of the people with appendicitis have the combination of characteristic symptoms:
- nausea;
- vomiting;
- excruciating pain in the lower right abdomen.

Pain may begin suddenly in the upper abdomen or around the navel; then nausea and vomiting develop. After a few hours, the nausea passes, and the pain shifts to the right lower portion of the abdomen.

When a doctor presses on this area, it is tender, and when the pressure is released, the pain may increase sharply - a symptom called rebound tenderness. A fever is common.

Pain, particularly in infants and children, may be general rather than confined to the right lower portion of the abdomen. In older people and in pregnant women, the pain is usually less severe, and the area is less tender.

Diagnosis

The diagnosis is often difficult in young children because they are less likely to develop appendicitis and because vomiting may be the dominant symptom, overshadowing abdominal tenderness.

An elevated white blood cell count with a shift to the left (in the direction of immature cells) is a useful diagnostic aid although it may be absent or less evident in elderly patients. Nausea and vomiting are prominent in acute gastro-enteritis, and pain, when it occurs, is usually more generalized than in acute appendicitis.

Appendicitis may also mimic other abdominal disorders, such as:

▲ pancreatitis;
▲ regional enteritis;
▲ cholecystitis;
▲ pyelonephritis;
▲ spastic colon.

The patient with appendicitis may complain of periumbilical pain that, after several hours, becomes localized toward the flank, even down into the pelvis. The patient may have nausea, crampy pain in the abdomen, or constipation, although occasionally he or she may complain of some diarrhea.

Anorexia is frequently a reliable symptom and may be of great value in differentiating appendicitis from nay other abdominal complaints. Usually when patients who were first observed with abdominal pain in the lower abdomen begin to regain their appetite, the likelihood of them having appendicitis becomes more remote. Sometimes, acute appendicitis may be preceded by attacks of upper abdominal pain, diarrhea, nausea, and vomiting, which may be typical of acute gastro-enteritis, but as these subside the localized findings of appendicitis may begin. The persistence of pain in the right lower quadrant cannot be overlooked or disregarded. Radiation down into the testicles or labia, or down into the thighs tends more to make one think of

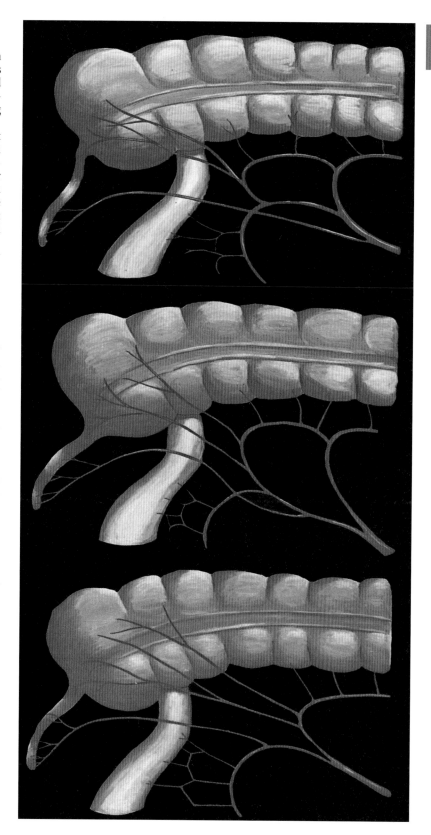

Variation in the blood supply of the appendix. If the bloodstream in one of the vessels is blocked, this may cause necrosis of the appendix. Appendicitis is the most common cause of sudden, severe abdominal pain.

A Appendicitis

Questions & Answers

What is appendicitis for kind of disease?

Appendicitis is an inflammation of the lining of the appendix which spreads to the other coats, thus involving the entire intestine structure. The appendix is a wormlike extension of the cecum (part of the large intestine), measuring 3-4 inches in length, located in the right lower portion of the abdomen at the very beginning of the large intestine. Normally, it is about the thickness of a pencil.

When involved in an acute inflammation, the appendix may become filled with pus. When the infection spreads through the wall of the appendix, it may become gangrenous and may rupture, causing an inflammatory process of the peritoneum, the lining of the abdominal cavity.

What is the function of the appendix?

It serves no function and is thought to be a remnant of our primitive past.

What causes appendicitis?

Appendicitis may be caused either by bacterial inflammation or by obstruction of the blood supply to the appendix by a hardened particle of faeces which blocks its passageway and presses upon the blood vessels in the region.

What are the signs of appendicitis in a child?

Children's symptoms often differ from those of adults. The pain stays around the navel instead of moving to the right side of the abdomen. In adults there is usually constipation, but in children there is often diarrhea. Vomiting is usual and there may or may not be a fever. The doctor confirms the diagnosis by examining the child's abdomen. This requires technical knowledge; don't try to diagnose appendicitis yourself. The more unwell your child, the more quickly you should get the doctor.

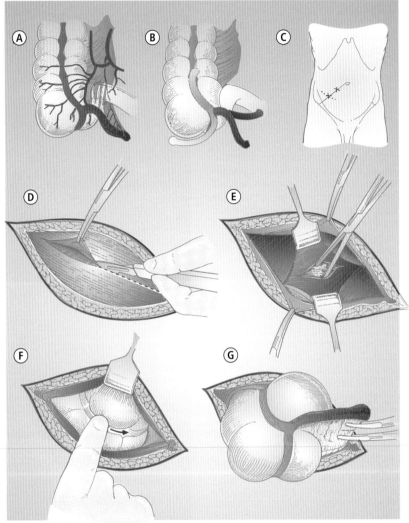

Anatomy in the region of the appendix (A); possible variations in the position of the appendix (B); centring the incision over McBurney's point (C); incision of the external oblique aponeurosis (D); separating the muscles along the lines of their fibers (E); using the taeniae coli to locate the appendix (F); removing the appendix, starting with he division of the mesoappendix (G-L); invaginating the stump (M); closing the wound.

ureteral colic. In a woman pain typical of either mittelschmerz or menstrual pain can be produced by the appendix lying on the Fallopian tube or the broad ligament. The pain of acute appendicitis may lack the usual referral phenomena if the appendix is lying behind the peritoneal cavity. In this case the onset of pain usually begins at this locus and remains there. Contact with the anterior abdominal wall produced much more severe pain on coughing or motion of ny sort, of course, exquisite tenderness on examination.

Treatment

With an early operation, the chances for success are great, the patient usually discharged within four to five days, and convalescence normally rapid and complete. With complications, the prognosis is more serious; if an abscess develops, final recovery may take several weeks. For a ruptured appendix, the prognosis is more serious. Fifty years ago, a rupture often was fatal. Antibiotics have lowered the death rate to nearly zero, but repeated

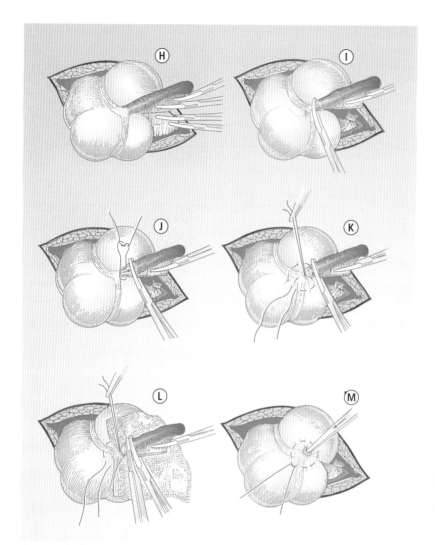

Anatomy in the region of the appendix (A); possible variations in the position of the appendix (B); centring the incision over McBurney's point (C); incision of the external oblique aponeurosis (D); separating the muscles along the lines of their fibers (E); using the taeniae coli to locate the appendix (F); removing the appendix, starting with he division of the mesoappendix (G-L); invaginating the stump (M); closing the wound.

How can I tell if I have an appendicitis?

Appendicitis is characterized by symptoms of generalized abdominal cramps, nausea or vomiting, and localization of pain to the right lower side of the abdomen. These symptoms persist over a period of several hours and tend to become more severe. There is also a slight temperature rise and an increase in pulse rate. Lack of appetite and constipation are also frequent findings in appendicitis. In a small number of cases, appendicitis can be successfully treated with large doses of antibiotic medicines. However, surgery is the best therapy. When performed for an early case of appendicitis, the procedure is not at all serious. When performed upon a patient whose appendix has ruptured and who has developed peritonitis, it is a serious operation.

What is the difference between acute appendicitis and recurrent appendicitis?

Acute appendicitis usually begins with abdominal cramps, nausea, vomiting and subsequent localization of pain to the lower side of the abdomen. This sequence of events takes place within a few hours' time. Recurrent appendicitis is characterized by repeated attacks of mild appendicitis which subside spontaneously, only to return at intervals of several months or years.

How common a condition is appendicitis?

Appendicitis is one of the most common of all surgical conditions within the abdomen. It is seen most often in young adults in their twenties, thirties or forties, although it can also occur in infants or in old people. It is also very common in children above three years of age.

operations and a long convalescence may be necessary.

Differential diagnosis

An acute appendicitis may be differentiated from any acute abdominal condition.
In very young and very old presentations may be atypical with misleading abdominal signs.
Specific differentiation may be made from the following conditions:

- gastro-enteritis
- urinary tract infection
- pelvic inflammatory disease
- ovarian cyst complication
- ruptured ectopic pregnancy
- perforated peptic ulcer
- cholecystitis
- testicular torsion
- Crohn's disease
- basal pneumonia
- pleurisy
- zoster
- trauma

ARTHRITIS

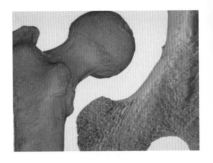

Description

The word arthritis is often loosely to describe any unexplained ache, but in true arthritis, joints are swollen, red, warm and tender.

Arthron means pertaining to the joint; *-itis* means inflammation. About 100 forms have been identified, including some that are not usually thought of as arthritis, such as gout and lupus erythematosus.

Many of us have an image of the arthritis sufferer: knees swollen, hands twisted and knobby. In fact, most arthritics lead full, productive lives with only moderate physical limitations.

Arthritic changes in a small bone. When a bone becomes infected, the soft, inner part (bone marrow) often swells.

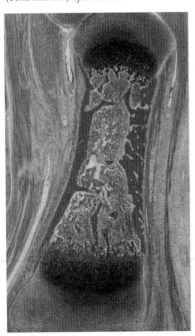

Arthritis is a major national problem, however, affecting thirteen million people in the United States, with 750,000 new cases every year. More than four million arthritics have some disability, and about 850,000 are seriously impaired (2004 data).

When you hear that someone has arthritis, it is most likely to be one of the two most widespread arthritic disorders - osteoarthritis or rheumatoid arthritis. These are usually chronic problems, conditions for which there is, to date, no cure, but which modern medicine can now do a good deal to control.

Two to three times more women than men are affected by osteoarthritis, and in the most serious form, rheumatoid arthritis, women have it three times as often.

Childhood arthritis also more common in girls than in boys. The reason for this is unknown, but researches are investigating the possibility that certain sex hormones may modify the body's defense system.

Osteoarthritis

This joint disease is a condition in which the cartilage that normally cushions a joint begins to deteriorate, causing pain and stiffness. Only rarely does inflammation become a problem in osteoarthritis.

The traditional wisdom was that this form of arthritis (once called rheumatism) was an inevitable "wear-and-tear" condition that would be visited upon us all if we lived long enough. However, many people live long lives without ever suffering stiff and creaky joints.

Osteoarthritis does take time to develop - usually dozens of years - so that most of the people who have it are at least middle-aged. And since women outlive men, more women are ultimately plagued with the condition.

Causes

Hundreds of researchers have spent years investigating the process of degeneration. Just about anything that subjects a joint to unnatural stress can lead to osteoarthritis:

▲ being overweight (that can cause strain on the knee and hip joints as well as the spine);
▲ congenital misalignment of bones (such as scoliosis);
▲ repeated occupational strain (the knees of auto mechanics who work in a squatting position, for example);
▲ poor posture that places continual strain on the joints;
▲ sports injuries that involve torn ligaments and cartilage.

Although more than one joint in the body can be affected, osteoarthritis rarely attacks several joints simultaneously, unlike some of the other forms of arthritis, nor does it roam from one joint to another.

Osteoarthritis attacks joints on an individual basis. Eventually, changes occur in and around the joint, and overgrowth of bone ends and thickening of surrounding tissues may change its size and appearance.

Sometimes, if a person avoids using the painful joint, nearby muscles may be affected - typically, weakening from disuse.

Treatment

The warning signs of a variety of arthritic conditions are often quite similar, so it's important to consult a doctor to determine if you have osteoarthritis and not some other kind of joint condition.

Treatment at an early stage is impor-

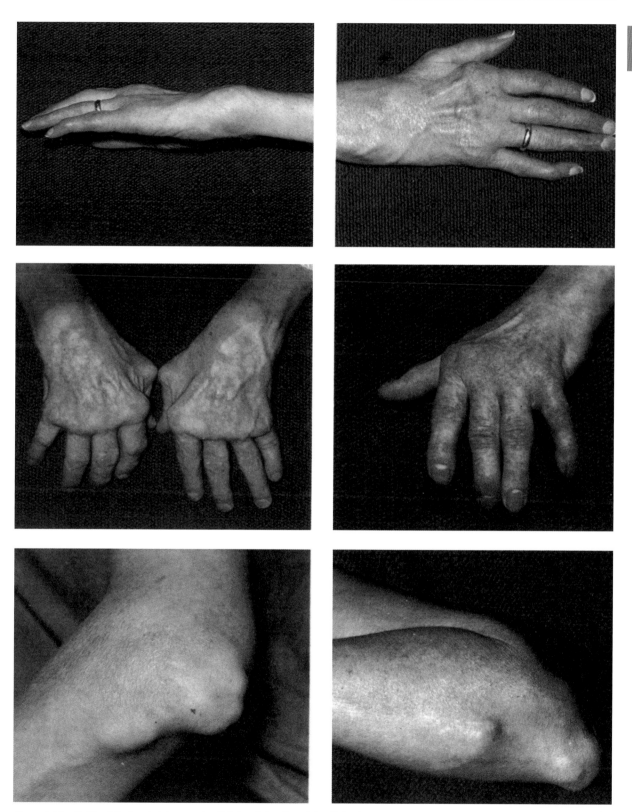

Reumatoid arthritis of the hands (above and middle) and the elbow joint (below).

A

Arthritis   Questions & Answers

What are the different types of arthritis?
Osteoarthritis, rheumatoid arthritis and gout are all very different conditions and it sometimes confuses people that they all be called arthritis.
▲ Osteoarthritis
The joints commonly involved are the small joints at the end of the fingers and base of the thumb, the joint at the base of the big toe, the spine, hips, knees and nek.
People suffering from osteoarthritis complain of a deep, aching pain in the affected joints. The pain is usually made worse by using the affected joint, and settles with rst. As the joints get more badly damaged the pain may be present most of the time, even when the joints are not being used, and can interfere with sleep.
▲ Rheumatoid arthritis
This medical condition is less common than osteoarthritis. It causes joint inflammation and damage and affects general health as well. Women are three times more likely to get it than men, but the cause is unknown. The joints of hands and feet become swollen, hot, stiff and painful.
▲ Gout
A type of arthritis where crystals of a substance called uric acid are deposited in a joint. The causes the joint to become red, swollen, hot, tender and agonizingly painful.

What causes the different types of arthritis?
▲ Osteoarthritis
The cause of this disease is unknown, but sometimes it runs in families. It is known that if a joint has been damaged in the past, then it is more prone to this type of arthritis in later life.
▲ Rheumatoid arthritis
This disease is due to the body's normal defence mechanisms attacking the lining of the joints. This causes inflammation and damage to all the structures affecting joints, and eventually damages the surfaces of the bones, making holes in them.

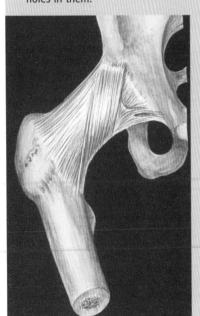

▲ Gout
This disease may be due to a metabolic disorder, but a common cause is also taking water tablets for some other medical problem such as high blood pressure. Gout is more common if you are overweight and if you drink a lot of alcohol.

What treatments are available?
A summary of available treatments for arthritis is given in the table. Many people with mild osteoarthritis do not need any treatment for their joints at all.
Simple painkillers such as aspirin and paracetamol can be very effective for the pain of arthritis if a lot of joints of large joints are involved.

tant, so don't ignore the signals your body may be sending. If any of the following symptoms persists for more than two weeks, consult your family physician:
▲ swelling in one or more joints;
▲ recurring pain or tenderness in any joint of your body;
▲ inability to move a joint properly or do normal activities;
▲ obvious redness and warmth in one or more joints;
▲ persistent early morning pain and stiffness in joints;
▲ unexplained weight loss, fever, weakness or fatigue combined with joint pain.
The aim of treatment is twofold: to relieve pain or discomfort, and to keep the affected joint operating as well as possible.
Once a diagnosis has been made, simple do-it-yourself measures often suffice, and continued professional care is not required.
Ordinary over-the-counter painkillers, such as paracetamol, ibuprofen or aspirin, are frequently enough to relieve discomfort.
Occasionally, stronger prescription painkillers may be needed, but doctors caution that these should not be used too often, since "masking" of discomfort can lead to overuse of the joint. Moist heat helps some people, but others find that cold packs are more effective.
While stress and strain are obviously not advisable, neither is prolonged immobilization. Research has shown that lack of use can encourage further breakdown of cartilage.
Apparently, some degree of movement is needed to sustain lubrication within the joint, allowing it to work smoothly.
If a weight-bearing joint is affected, losing excess weight is a good idea. Special exercises can help to strengthen muscles around the joint but these should be undertaken with professional guidance from a physiotherapist.
If cartilage has deteriorated to the point of causing constant pain, joint replacement surgery is another alternative. Known as arthroplasty, this procedure involves the complete replacement of joints by mechanical constructions using metals, plastics

and other materials. Since l990 this type of surgery has become increasingly common, especially for hip and knee joints.

Thus therapy may include regular exercises, particularly activities that involve smooth rather than jerky movement - swimming or walking in preference to tennis or jogging - and can be increased gradually. Aspirin and other drugs are used in moderation. Osteoarthritis can be helped, but the keys to controlling it are early diagnosis and prompt treatment.

Rheumatoid arthritis

Unlike osteoarthritis, rheumatoid arthritis often strikes young adults, and as many as 380,000 children have the disease worldwide. Fortunately, an estimated two-thirds of children with rheumatoid arthritis recover by the time they reach adulthood.

Women are more susceptible than men, comprising three out of every four victims. While the cause of rheumatoid arthritis is still unknown, recent research suggests a genetic predisposition to the disease, though it is not actually inherited.

Onset and development

The onset of rheumatoid arthritis is gradual, typically beginning with weakness, swelling and possibly pain in a few small joints, such as those of the hands or feet. Later, other joints may be affected.

The disease comes and goes unpredictably, in what is known as a "flare-and-remission" pattern. As it progresses, recurrent inflammation causes swelling and thickening of the membrane, called the synovia or synovium, that lines the joint.

Enzymes then attack and erode cartilage and other tissues, while spasms of surrounding muscles may pull the joint out of line. All this may be caused by the body's immune system being faulty and attacking the joints for no reason.

Rheumatoid arthritis can be severely crippling, as anyone knows who has seen the gnarled and twisted hands of a person who has the disease.

To date, there is no cure for rheumatoid arthritis, but the disease can be controlled. And with continued treatment, the possibility of severe crippling is minimal.

Treatment

Once rheumatoid arthritis has been diagnosed by a doctor, the aim of the therapy is threefold:
▲ to relieve pain;
▲ to reduce inflammation;
▲ to prevent joint damage that can lead to deformity.

Initial methods of treatment are usually the same ones used to relieve osteoarthritis.

All over the world, researchers are looking for new treatment methods. One promising avenue of investigation has been suggested by the discovery that the imbalance of the body's immune system characteristic of patients with rheumatoid arthritis is somehow corrected during pregnancy. About 75 per cent of pregnant rheumatoid arthritis patients have felt better, only to have the symptoms return after delivery.

■ Medicines
See survey in the table.

■ Physical therapy
Hot baths or showers, as well as hot packs or heat lamps, can relax and soothe an inflamed joint, and wax baths (coating hands or feet with melted wax so the heat transfers to the joints) can lessen pain. Paradoxically, as with osteoarthritis, if heat doesn't help, locally applied cold may.

Exercise can be vital in order to strengthen muscles and help prevent deformities that might otherwise be crippling. Passive exercise - gentle movement of a joint by another person - can also be helpful.

Many rheumatologists (doctors who specialize in arthritis disorders) work closely with physiotherapists and occupational therapists who show patients how to do appropriate exercises to help maximize mobility.

But when a joint is inflamed, exercising can increase pain and cause real damage, so during "flare-ups" doctors often suggest wearing plastic splints (especially on hands or fingers) to keep affected joints at rest and out of flexed, deformity-inducing positions.

When aspirin does not work or is irritating, prescription anti-inflammatory drugs may be required.

The success rate as well as the side-effects of these drugs is extremely variable from one patient to another, and trials of two, three or even half-a-dozen drugs may be needed until the ideal one is found. Even then, medication must be carefully monitored for efficacy.

Sometimes switching drugs may be called for if the patient develops a tolerance to one medication.

Other types of drugs are also used - with varying degrees of success - to treat the more advanced cases of rheumatoid arthritis. All of these potent drugs can cause a host of unpleasant and often dangerous side-effects, so doctors limit dosages, monitor side-effects carefully and rarely prescribe them for extended periods of time.

■ Surgical options
Remarkable progress in orthopedic surgery over the past few years has brought about a change in the kinds of surgery employed when, despite medication and other measures, a joint seems on its way to becoming permanently deformed.

Until a few years ago, one widely used technique was synovectomy - removal of the inflamed and thickened synovial membrane enveloping a joint. Unfortunately, the synovium grows back and the benefits usually disappear within three years after surgery.

A second choice is joint fusion, an extreme alternative used only when joints (mainly ankle and wrist joints) become completely dysfunctional. Fusion essentially "locks" the joint in position.

Obviously, this procedure is done only in cases when a person can no longer walk or when the wrist has already been rendered useless by the disease. After surgery, it is possible for patients to walk with the aid of crutches and to have limited use of their hands.

It is possible that fusion surgery will be phased out entirely as progress continues in joint-replacement surgery.

Replacement of the ball-and-socket joint of the hip is now considered almost routine. Only a decade ago, total knee replacement was strictly

A

Drugs used to treat rheumatoid artritis

Nonsteroidal anti-inflammatory drugs (NSAIDs)
All NSAIDs treat the symptoms and decrease inflammation but do not alter the course of the disease.

▲ Selected side effects
  - Upset stomach
  - Stomach ulcers
  - Increased blood pressure
  - Risk of adverse effects on the kidneys

▲ Examples
  • Aspirin
  • Ibuprofen
  • Naproxen
  • Celecoxib
  • Diclofenac
  • Salsalate
  • Indomethacin
  • Piroxicam
  • Sulindac
  • Tolmetin

Slow-acting drugs
All show-acting drugs can slow progression of joint damage as well as gradually decrease pain and swelling.

Gold compounds

▲ Selected side effects
  - Adverse effects on the kidneys
  - Rashes
  - Itchy skin
  - Decreased numbers of blood cells

▲ Examples
  • Auranofin
  • Ridaura
  • Mypocrisin

Penicillamine

▲ Selected side effects
  - Suppression of blood cell production
  - Muscle disease
  - Rash
  - Bad taste in the mouth

▲ Examples
  • Cuprimine
  • Depen

Hydroxychloroquine

▲ Selected side effects
  - Rashes
  - Muscle aches
  - Eye problems
▲ Example
  • Plaquenil

Sulfasalazine

▲ Selected side effects
  - Stomach upset
  - Liver problems
  - Blood cell disorders
  - Rashes

▲ Examples
  • Azaline
  • Salazopirin

Corticosteroids
Can reduce inflammation quickly, may not be useful long term because of side effects.

▲ Selected side effects
  - Numerous side effects throughout the body

▲ Examples
  • Prednisone
  • Orasone

Immunosuppressive drugs
Methotrexate or leflunomide can be used early for severe rheumatoid arthritis; can slow joint damage. Etanercept and infliximab show dramatic prompt response in most people; can slow joint damage.

▲ Selected side effects
  - Liver disease
  - Lung inflammation
  - Suppression of blood cell production
  - Risk of infection

▲ Examples
  • Methotrexate
  • Leflunomide
  • Cyclophosphamide
  • Etanercept
  • Infliximab

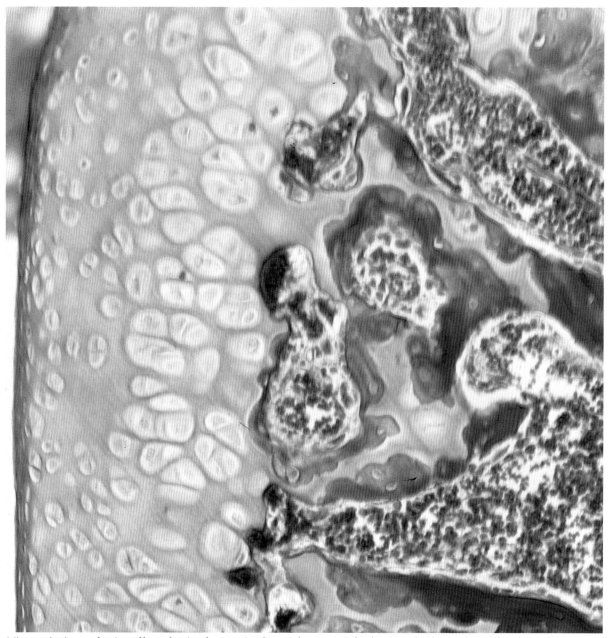

Microscopic picture of a piece of bone showing degenerative changes characteristic for rheumatoid arthritis. The cartilage, bone, and ligaments of the joint erode, causing deformity, instability, and scarring within the joint.

experimental; today, it is the second most common kind of arthroplasty. Silicone rubber implants have proven successful replacements for deformed finger joints, and both shoulder and elbow arthroplasty have now moved out of the experimental stage, although neither operation can yet be called common.

■ Diet

Research has shown that what you eat is unlikely to cause the disease, but in a 1996 study supported by the Arthritis Foundation, certain foods and chemicals were shown to produce symptoms in arthritis patients. Such evidence, backed up by the observations of family doctors, suggests that the link between diet and arthritis merits further investigation.

Common sense should tell you to avoid foods that seem to bother you, but totally eliminating any category of food can be dangerous. Most medical and nutritional experts agree that a well-balanced diet is essential for arthritis sufferers.

A

Protection of arthritic joints

Joints that have been affected by inflammation, swelling and arthritic changes can be damaged more easily than normal joints. Pressures - from outside and inside - can contribute to deformity.

And so you will be learning new ways of doing things that are part of your typical day - not only to avoid pain, but to protect your joints.

You will be changing some old habits - not yourself, just some habits. Each person with arthritis has different interests, desires and problems.

The principles of joint protection that follow are important to all, and you will see their value for you as you begin to apply them. If you do not understand any part as you read, or how it relates to you, you must ask your doctor or physiotherapist.

Be aware of body positioning

A position of flexion (bent knees, hips, elbows, fingers) can lead to deformity if held for long periods. The following tips should help:

▲ Lie face down, if possible, for 10, 15 or more minutes twice a day, with your feet over the end of the bed for total muscle relaxation. Your body weight helps to keep hips and knees straight. This is called "proning," and balances the time spent in a chair with hips and knees flexed.

▲ Sitting for long periods leaning on bent elbows is an easy habit to change. Relax your arms into your lap or rest them at a comfortable height on a table.

▲ Falling asleep with a pillow under your knees is forbidden.

▲ If propping your face on your hands is a comfortable habit, uncurl the fingers and straighten them against your cheek, chin in palm.

You can see that extension at all joints is being emphasized because it's important for movement. Changing position often is also important, to prevent stiffening.

Become an expert in body mechanics

You may have seen film of weightless astronauts bouncing as they walked on the moon, but those of us who are earthbound have to move our bodies against - or with - the forces of gravity.

▲ A tall ladder standing perfectly upright can be easily held in that position, but it takes a lot of strength to hold one that has begun to lean.

▲ So is it with your body: if you hold it erect, shoulders under your ears, and knees, hips and back straight, it balances. But begin to slouch and all of your muscles have to work harder to keep you `upright' against gravity. The result is greater fatigue and often pain.

▲ Good sitting posture also ensures that your arms are in the best functional position, and that your lungs have room to expand when you breathe. You'll tire less quickly, feel better and look better.

▲ Learn the most efficient way to get up from a chair: slide your buttocks forward, knees together, tuck your feet (flat on the floor) beneath you, lean forward so that your chin lines up with your knees.

▲ Now, with palms on the chair arms, push off as you push up with hips and knees. With your center of gravity brought forward this way, you're using good body mechanics, with all muscles working together.

▲ Remember, you have got to keep at it. When you are taking a bath, when you are brushing your teeth, when you're walking to work or around the house (glance in a shop window or a mirror), when you're sitting at the table, at your desk or in your car, think tall.

Avoid using muscles in one position for long periods

Sustained (static) grasp or position tires muscles quickly. Tired muscles cannot give your joints support, so:

▲ Stand if you can, for some of your work, but sit to work for a while before your legs get too tired. A high, sturdy stool makes getting up and down easier.

▲ Shift your weight from time to time when you do stand, so that different sets of muscles can share the work.

▲ Support your back against a wall or your arms on a shopping cart if you're talking to a friend at the shops. Lean against the sink if you're doing the dishes. It "underweights" the joints of hips and knees.

▲ To help, use a vegetable-holding cutting board, and non-skid material under mixing bowls or paint cans.

▲ Prop a book or newspaper on a flat pillow across your knees or on a bookstand or a table, just so that your fingers are not gripping. If you wear bifocals, consider separate reading glasses to avoid the chin-to-chest tilt that can give you a "pain in the neck."

▲ Activities such as vacuuming, ironing, cleaning windows or the family car, involving a repetitive, tiring motion as well as holding, are especially stressing and should be done for very short periods, if you can't get someone else to do them.

▲ Writing (with its static grasp) and knitting (with its close-to-the-body positioning) are activities that are very important to some people.

▲ If this is true of you, relax and stretch your hands and arms at least every ten minutes. But if you can, use an electric typewriter; and when you're knitting, consider a pillow in your lap to support your arms.

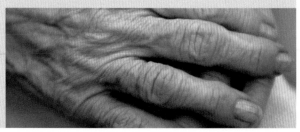

Protection of arthritic joints

Use the strongest joints available for any activity

Fingers are not for weight-bearing so push up on your palms, or use forearms on a firm table, or a trapeze to move about in bed.

▲ Use body weight to move objects: close a drawer with your "rear," move a chair with your hips.

▲ The thumb makes the hand an engineer's dream tool. Don't abuse yours. Use needle-nose pliers for tight pinch, use a small hammer for drawing pins, use a gadget to open your car door, an adaptation for your keys.

▲ You can substitute pinching movements by attaching tape loops where needed: a long loop inside each seam of your trousers and you can "hook" them on with your palms; a loop on each end of face flannels and towels, and you can bathe and dry your back or feet without tight pinching or squeezing.

Avoid activities involving a tight grip

There is reason to believe that, for the hand affected by arthritis, gripping objects tightly can cause harmful internal tensions around your joints by your own muscles, so:

▲ Choose kitchen and workshop tools for their fat handles and light weight.

▲ Wrap foam on the handles of tools you use often, to both enlarge and soften the gripping surface.

▲ Use an offset screwdriver and a longer spanner. Lever action uses power from large muscles of both arms and protects your hands from twisting forces.

▲ Hold objects palm-to-palm instead of gripping.

▲ Allow clothes you handwash to drip or wrap them in a towel rather than wringing them.

▲ Press moisture out of cleaning cloths or sponges instead of twisting.

▲ Stop and think when you are gripping objects - a golf club, a steam iron or the steering wheel of your car. It is usually possible to grip less tightly and still maintain good control.

Avoid ulnar (away from the thumb) pressures on the fingers

If you look at your fingers during your usual way of doing some familiar tasks, you'll see that they push against each other toward the small finger, rather than suppor-ting each other in good alignment, so:

▲ Hold your thick-handled knife like an icepick, and use a pulling action to cut. Your joints are more stable in this position and you get more power per pull, with less joint stress.

▲ Lift plates, bowls or pans by slipping the palms of both hands underneath. Don't grip the edges. Use oven gloves for hot stuff. Wear your wrist splints under rubber gloves for dishwashing.

▲ Open screw-top jars by leaning on the jar lid with the palm of your hand and using shoulder motion. Place the jar on a sponge-cloth in the sink bottom for good leverage and stability - and remind the family not to tighten them again.

▲ Hold a cup between both palms. Consider a thermal cup; it's safer and the heat feels good. And fill it only halfway.

Avoid lateral (sideways) pressures on individual finger joints

For dialling the telephone, slip a foam cylinder from a hair roller over a pencil and hold it, again, like an icepick.

▲ For opening tins, instead of a butterfly opener, use an electric opener on a surface low enough for leverage, or a wall-mounted rotary tin opener.

▲ Before you buy scissors, try out several electric types at the shop for weight and fit; there should be one that's right for you.

▲ For limited use, choose lightweight, freely moving scissors. Long handles with short blades are usually sufficient, and well-shaped grips are critical.

Respect pain

The body usually gives you the danger signal of pain if you place joints under harmful stress.

▲ Be alert for pain that lasts more than an hour after an activity, and is not just passing discomfort.

▲ Identify the cause so that the method can be changed or the time reduced. This applies to your exercise program as well; your therapist needs to be told.

Plan for a balance of rest and activity

You need eight to ten hours of sleep a night, and you should have at least one rest period during the day.

▲ Teach yourself to do part of a job, then stop for a short rest before you are tired. Have at least one chair that really fits you, comfortably supporting your arms, your back and your head.

▲ To remove the pressure of a chair edge on your thighs, make a simple footstool to park your feet on, for example, a slab of polystyrene.

▲ Consciously relax your body in a position of good alignment - neck to toes. And if you're sitting more than you're walking, do your footankle exercises hourly.

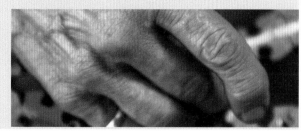

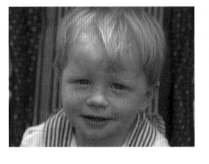

ASTHMA

Introduction

Bronchial asthma is a reversible obstruction of the airways not due to any other disease. Asthma is a common condition which affects up to 5 per cent of the population at some period of their lives.

In recent years there has been a more precise understanding of the underlying mechanisms of the body's immune defense systems, which have led to more rational guidelines for effective management of the condition. Changes in the immune defense system and in the control of the diameter of the airways are probably responsible for attacks of wheezing.

When individuals with sensitive bronchi (airway tubes) are subjected to stresses of different kinds, overt asthma attacks may occur.

Among the known stresses are:

▲ respiratory infections;
▲ certain types of exercise;
▲ emotional upset;
▲ changes in barometric pressure;
▲ changes in temperature;
▲ inhalation of cold air;
▲ inhalation of such irritants as petrol fumes, fresh paint and other noxious odours;
▲ inhalation of cigarette smoke;
▲ exposure to specific allergens.

Psychological factors may aggravate an asthmatic attack but are not a primary cause. Persons whose asthma is precipitated by exposure to something to which they are allergic - for instance airborne pollens, moulds, house dust, flakes of animal skin -are said to have allergic or extrinsic asthma, but they account for only about 10 to 20 per cent of adult asthma suf-

ferers. In perhaps 30 to 50 per cent of adult asthmatics, attacks appear not to be triggered by allergens, but by infection, irritants or emotional factors. These are said to have intrinsic asthma.

Symptoms and signs

Asthmatic attacks are characterized by the narrowing of the large and small airways due to spasm of the muscles of the bronchial tubes, edema (excess fluid in the tissues) and inflammation in the inner lining of the airways, and the production of mucus. Pathological findings in the airways of those who have died of severe asthmatic attacks have shown the presence of secretions, frequently in the form of extensive mucus plugs obstructing both large and small airways. The walls of the airways themselves show edema or swelling, thickening of the layer of smooth muscle cells and infiltration of certain types of white blood cells.

Individuals with asthma differ greatly in the frequency and degree of their symptoms. Some have only an occasional attack that is mild in degree and of brief duration, and otherwise are entirely free of symptoms.

Others have mild coughing and wheezing much of the time, punctuated by severe attacks following exposure to known allergens, infections, certain exercise or irritants. An asthma attack may begin acutely with bouts of wheezing, coughing and shortness of breath, or gradually with slowly increasing symptoms and signs of distress of the respiratory system.

In either case, the person usually first notices the onset of breathing that is difficult and becoming more rapid, coughing and tightness or pressure in the chest, and may even notice audible

Microscopic picture of the inside of the trachea. Part of the cartilage of the trachea is bent.

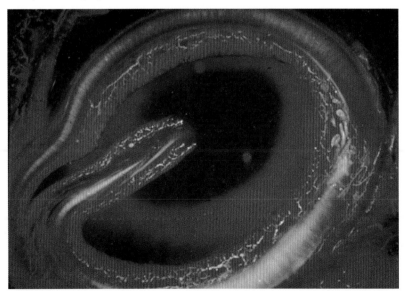

wheezes. All of this may subside quickly or may persist for hours or days, and abnormalities in the function of the airways and lungs may last for weeks or months after an acute attack.

The cough during an acute attack sounds tight and is generally free of mucus. Except in young children, who rarely expectorate, sputum with mucus is produced as the attack subsides.

In severe episodes, the person may not be able to speak more than a few words at a time without having to stop for breath. Fatigue and severe distress are evident in the rapid, shallow breathing.

The presence, absence or prominence of wheezes does not precisely match the severity of an asthma attack. The most reliable signs indicating a severe asthma attack include assessment of the degree of shortness of breath at rest, difficulty in talking and the use of accessory muscles of respiration.

Diagnosis

It is surprising that asthma often goes undiagnosed. There is, of course, little difficulty in identifying the child with a history of widespread eczema, and a family history of allergies, who suffers from recurrent wheezing.

Yet many children with persistent coughs, particularly at night, and wheezing episodes are regarded as suffering from bronchitis, triggered by infections of the airways. To distinguish between the two, many doctors have children blow deep breaths into a peak-flow meter; this measures the force of the breath.

After the first blow, the child breathes in a specific medicinal aerosol, and if, on blowing into the peak-flow meter a second time, there is more than a 15 per cent improvement, the doctor can safely diagnose asthma.

It is often difficult for the family doctor or specialist to estimate the severity of attacks in children and to tailor treatment accordingly. Because some parents persistently deny the severity of the condition, while others are overprotective to the point of preventing their child from taking part in any normal school activities because

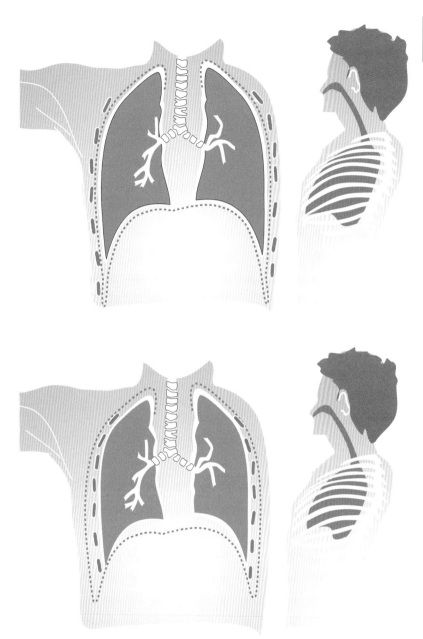

During breathing, the chest cavity is alternately compressed and expanded. The inflow of air during inhalation is made possible by the activity of the respiratory muscles. During inspiration, the volume of the chest is enlarged by tilting the ribs upward, and consequently the lungs are filled with air. The diaphragm, too, contracts during inspiration.
Left is a frontal view and right a side view of the chest.
To visualize the difference between inspiration and expiration, the position of the chest cavity and the diaphragm during expiration is drawn in broken lines.
Expiration: the ribs are tilted downward and the volume of the chest becomes smaller. The elasticity of the lungs pulls the diaphragm upward. The abdominal muscles push the contents of the abdomen against the diaphragm that yields the pressure. The revolving axis on the ribs is in the spinal column, hence the latitude of their displacement in the front part of the chest.

Asthma   Questions & Answers

What are the major characteristics of asthma?
Asthma is a disease characterized by an increased responsiveness of the windpipe (trachea) and bronchi to various stimuli and manifested by a widespread narrowing of the airways that changes in severity either spontaneously or as a result of therapy.

What is the incidence of asthma in Western countries?
About 3.5-4 per cent of the population suffer from asthma and as many as 6 per cent have had asthma during their lifetime (2005 data).
Symptomatic asthma is more prevalent in children than adults. Long-term follow-up studies of asthmatic children indicate that 50-70 per cent go into permanent or temporary symptom-free remission by adulthood.
And in many of these patients, symptoms significantly decrease in severity so that there is a good overall prognosis in the case of children that develop asthma. The prevalence rate for asthma is slightly higher in males than in females.

What are the characteristics of extrinsic asthma?
Patients are generally characterized as having either extrinsic (primarily caused by allergens) or intrinsic (not primarily caused by allergens) asthma.
Characteristics of extrinsic asthma are:

- a personal history or family history of allergy;

- seasonal variation in symptoms;

- positive skin tests;

- elevated levels of circulating immunoglobulin E (IgE) (one of the five classes of antibodies, produced in lymph tissue in response to the invasion of a foreign substance).

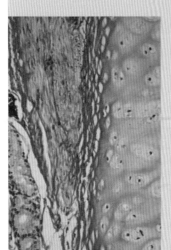

What are the characteristics of intrinsic asthma?
Patients with intrinsic asthma (not primarily caused by allergens) show the following characteristics:

- a negative family history of allergy;

- negative skin tests;

- development of polyps (benign growth from a mucous membrane) in the nose;

- sensitivity to aspirin and related chemical compounds.

About 2-10 per cent of asthmatic patients develop an acute asthma attack after taking as little as 300 mg of aspirin. Many patients, however, present characteristics of both extrinsic and intrinsic asthma.

What are the major characteristics of asthma in children?
Asthma is a disease characterized by an increased responsiveness of the windpipe (trachea) and bronchi to various stimuli and manifested by a widespread narrowing of the airways that changes in severity either spontaneously or as a result of therapy.

What is the incidence of asthma in developing countries?
About 5-7 per cent of the population of developing countries suffer from asthma and as many as 8 per cent have had asthma during their lifetime (1999 data).
Symptomatic asthma is more prevalent in children than adults. Long-term follow-up studies of asthmatic children indicate that 50-70 per cent go into permanent or temporary symptom-free remission by adulthood. And in many of these patients, symptoms significantly decrease in severity so that there is a good overall prognosis in the case of children that develop asthma. The prevalence rate for asthma is slightly higher in males than in females.

What are the characteristics of asthma caused by allergens?
Characteristics asthma caused by allergens are:

- a personal history or family history of allergy;

- seasonal variation in symptoms;

- positive skin tests;

- elevated levels of circulating immunoglobulin E (IgE) (one of the five classes of antibodies, produced in lymph tissue in response to the invasion of a foreign substance).

What are the characteristics of hereditary asthma?
Patients suffering from asthma due to hereditary factors show the following characteristics:

- a negative family history of allergy;

- negative skin tests;

- development of polyps (benign growth from a mucous membrane) in the nose;

- sensitivity to aspirin and related chemical compounds.

of mild wheezing. The extrinsic kind of asthma can best be shown by skin-prick testing, in which a number of allergens are pricked into the skin. This shows that the person has the capacity to respond in a particular way to an allergen.

It is possible, however, for people with extrinsic asthma to have negative skin tests to common allergens, and this often occurs in occupational asthma where high concentrations of particular industrial dusts and vapours can induce the development of extrinsic asthma. One type of allergic reaction is that in which the asthmatic reaction begins minutes after contact with the offending allergen, which is then cor-

respondingly easy to identify. However, asthma may be of later onset and begin one or two hours after contact with the offending allergen, and may last up to 24 hours.

There is, however, a combination of immediate and late asthma attacks, called dual asthma, the late component of which gives rise to symptoms occurring in the evening and during the night. If a person has this sort of reaction, they are likely to require urgent hospital admission.

Recurrent asthma, which may last over several days or even weeks, may follow a single exposure to an allergen over a short period of time with maximum falls in function of airways and lungs occurring during the night.

Diagnostic tests include:

▲ examination of the blood and the sputum;
▲ chest X-rays, CT-scans and MRI-scans;
▲ pulmonary (lung) function tests;
▲ allergy skin tests;
▲ exercise testing.

The diagnosis of asthma should be considered in any individual who wheezes. Asthma is the most likely diagnosis when the typical bouts of wheezing start in childhood or early adulthood and are interspersed with intervals without wheezing. In addition, more than 50 per cent of asthmatics have a family history of allergy or asthma.

Complications

A number of complications may occur during acute and severe attacks.

▲ *Pneumothorax*
Air or gas in the pleural cavity (the space between the lung and the membrane that covers it). This occurs when an over-dilated air sac in the lung ruptures, permitting communication between airways and the pleural cavity. It is first seen as a sudden worsening of the person's respiratory distress, accompanied by sharp chest pains.

▲ *Atelectasis*
The absence of air in air sacs, commonly called a collapsed lung. This condition usually involves the right middle lobe or an entire

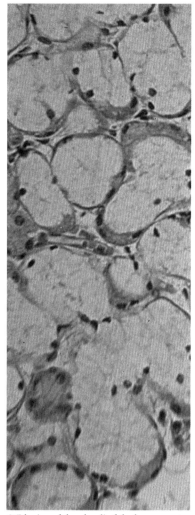

Widening of the alveoli of the lung, eventually leading to emphysema, a severe lung condition. This may lead to greatly limited breathing capacity.

lung. Unless the collapse involves a substantial amount of lung tissue, the atelectasis is usually only diagnosed as a result of X-ray examination.

▲ *Bronchiectasis*
Narrowing of the airways (bronchial tubes). This may lead to greatly limited breathing capacity and recurrent infections. Contrary to popular opinion, uncomplicated asthma rarely leads to chronic emphysema, especially in a nonsmoker. Emphysema is a gaseous distention of the air sacs.

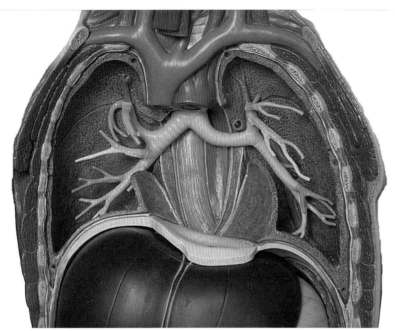

Model of the thoracic cavity showing the branching pattern of the main bronchi.

Bronchoscopic view of the inside of the main bronchi, showing dilatation of the bronchi due to severe asthma.

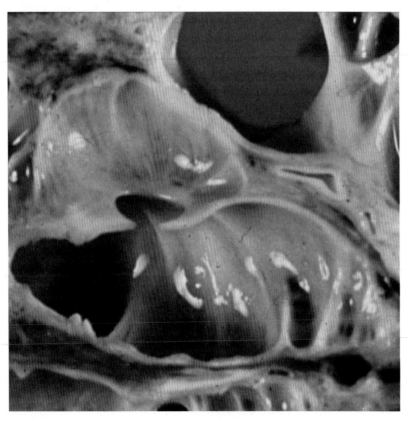

Asthma emergencies

The most important step is the recognition that the degree of severity is notoriously difficult. A good guide is the person's ability to speak, so that an attack may be considered severe if the person can only utter monosyllables or is completely unable to speak.

Examination of such sufferers may also show an irregular pulse or a heart rate over 130 beats per minute, cyanosis (bluish tinge of the lips, nails, face, etc.) and so on. Such signs suggest a medical emergency, and are indications that the person should immediately be admitted to hospital.

The initial treatment should be the administration of oxygen by face mask, together with an intravenous injection of a hydrocortisone preparation to reduce inflammation, followed by aminophylline that will relax the spasm of the bronchi.

Antibiotic treatment requires definite indications of a bacterial infection. In childhood, associated infections are very often caused by viruses, and are unresponsive to antibiotics, but in the older person, where the asthmatic attack may be superimposed on chronic airways obstruction, early use of an antibiotic may be valuable. The most frequently used bronchodilator (a drug that widens the airways) is aminophylline. A useful alternative is salbutamol, which is usually given by aerosol inhalation. However, since, in an asthma emergency, the person will almost certainly be unable to use a pressurized aerosol, the doctor will give the medication by other means.

Long-term management

Since there is a significant link between the presence of positive skin-prick tests to common allergens and a positive history of developing symptoms from them, in those with asthma and rhinitis (inflammation of the inner lining of the nose).

The doctor will carry out skin-prick tests to different allergens that are commonly involved, such as the house dust mite, grass and tree and shrub pollens. Those with allergic asthma usually develop asthma early in life in association with rhinitis and eczema.

Schematic reconstruction of the parts of the respiratory system.
1. Trachea (windpipe), 2. enlargement of the trachea, 3. diagram of the respiratory movements, 4. branches of bronchi, 5. microscopic enlargement of bronchi, 7. microscopic enlargement of lung vesicles.

They have a more favourable prognosis, and respond better to certain types of therapy. If, on the other hand, a child has only mild and occasional wheezing attacks, all that is usually required is a bronchodilator drug, such as salbutamol or ephedrine. Those children in whom attacks are infrequent but more severe should be offered inhalation therapy.

Where symptoms are more frequent, continuous therapy with salbutamol or theophylline compounds taken by mouth is required, with the additional use of inhaled salbutamol for acute attacks. Slow-release preparations may be prescribed by the doctor where nocturnal coughing is the problem. Those children who still remain uncontrolled should be referred to a specialist unit. A few years ago there was a vogue for attempting to reduce the house-mite population by beating mattresses and pillows out of doors, and enclosing them in plastic containers, washing linoleum, and cleaning and vacuuming carpets.

These are still worth trying, although only a small number of children appear to benefit by them. Similarly, desensitization injections are seldom of value except in the occasional individual who demonstrates an allergy to a single or predominant antigen.

Finally, it has been a common practice for doctors to present a reassuring attitude to parents that childhood asthma will improve and disappear before puberty. It is difficult, however, to predict which children are likely to get better beyond the fact that those most severely affected are least likely to improve.

Nor is there any evidence to show that prescribed therapy alters the natural history of the disease. There is undoubtedly, in about 25 per cent of cases, a tendency for relapse to occur in adult life, often after periods of more than 10 or 15 years.

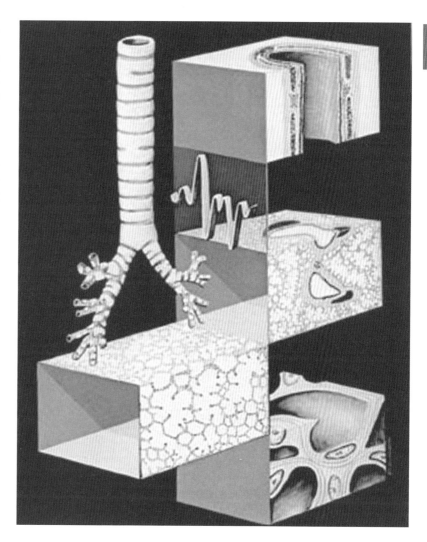

Model of a small; bronchus with arterial (red) and venous (blew blood supply).

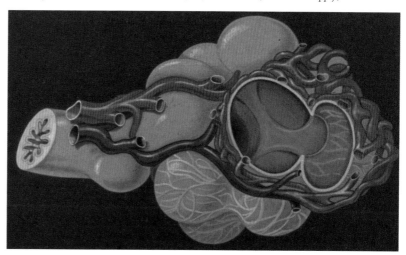

ATHEROSCLEROSIS

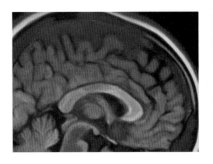

Description

Atherosclerosis is the formation of fatty deposits (containing cholesterol) in the inner lining of an artery, followed by scarring and deposits of calcium (calcification). It is commoner in older age groups, but in those with diabetes, disorders of fat metabolism and high blood pressure, its appearance may be earlier. Excess saturated fats in the blood may play a role in its formation. Narrowing or obstruction of brain arteries may lead to stroke, while that of coronary (heart) arteries causes angina pectoris (sharp chest pains) and coronary thrombosis (blockage of a heart artery by a clot). Reduced blood flow to the limbs may cause cramp on exertion, ulcers and gangrene. The complications of atherosclerosis are the major causes of death in the Western world, including the US and UK.

Deaths classified as due to 'degenerative and arteriosclerotic heart disease' represent 33-34 per cent of the total, and cerebral vascular disease (stroke) is the third most common cause of death after heart disease and cancer.

How the disease develops

The fatty deposit, or atheroma, is the major characteristic and represents the end of a process that begins with the depositing of lipids (fats) in the muscle cells of the wall of the blood vessel causing it to bulge inwards.

How atheroma develops remains unclear. It may be that the 'bulge' causes turbulence in the blood flowing past, high blood pressure and lack of oxygen, and following such injury, smooth muscle cells are damaged. Lipoproteins, especially low-density lipoproteins (LDL), become attached to the cells and stimulate their growth. This uptake of LDL can convert what ordinarily would be a limited tissue response to injury into atherosclerosis by introducing cholesterol, a major component of the LDL, into the vessel wall. In the end, an atheroma develops that may block the passage of blood.

Risk factors

If one or more of certain factors, known as 'risk factors,' are present in

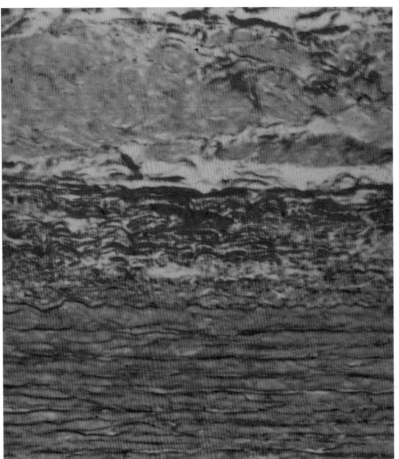

Microscopic picture of the wall of an atherosclerotic artery. The picture shows fatty deposits; beginning with the depositing of lipids in the muscle cells of the wall of the blood vessel causing it to bulge inward. The uptake of low-density lipoproteins can convert what ordinarily would be a limited response to injury into atherosclerosis by introducing cholesterol into the vessel wall.

individuals, the possibility of their suffering from atherosclerosis and its complications increases. Removal or modification of the risk factors in a population seems to diminish the incidence of the complications of atherosclerosis, such as coronary heart disease.

Major risk factors are:
· high blood pressure;
· elevated levels of lipids;
· cigarette smoking;
· diabetes;
· obesity.

Other presumed risk factors include:
· physical inactivity;
· certain types of behavioral patterns;
· certain types of personality;
· hardness of the drinking water;
· family history of premature atherosclerosis.

The risk of atherosclerosis also increases with age. The death rate from coronary heart disease among Caucasian men aged 25 to 34 is about ten in every 100,000; at age 55 to 64 it is nearly 1000 in every 100,000.

This relationship to age may be due to the time required for the atheromas to develop or to the duration of exposure to risk factors. Being male is an important risk factor; at ages 35 to 44 the death rate from coronary heart disease among men is 6.3 per cent.

Symptoms and signs

Atherosclerosis is characteristically silent until stenosis (narrowing of an artery), thrombosis (blood clot) or aneurysm (extreme bulging or rupture of an artery wall) develops. Symptoms and signs may develop gradually as the atheroma slowly narrows the inner cavity (the lumen) of an artery. Clinical findings occur in tissues (heart, brain, kidney, etc.) whose circulation depends on the affected artery.

Treatment

In many societies, the incidence of atherosclerosis is much lower than in ours, and attempts to prevent atherosclerosis by focusing on the risk factors seem useful. Diabetes and obesity

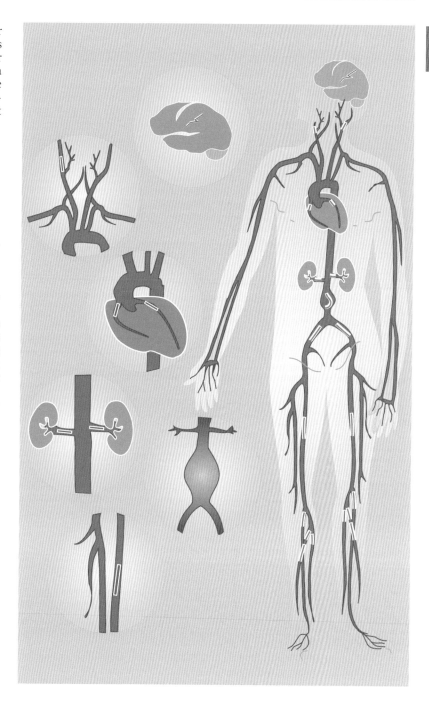

Predilection of the occurrence of atherosclerosis.
From top to bottom:
- brain arteries;
- branches of the aortic arch;
- coronary arteries of the heart;
- kidney arteries;
- abdominal aorta;
- leg arteries.

A

Atherosclerosis   Questions & Answers

What is atherosclerosis and what causes it?
The normal wall of an artery is strong, supple, and elastic so that it can expand and contract in adjustment to the changes in the blood pressure which take place with every heart contraction. When an artery becomes hardened or atherosclerotic, its walls are rigid and pipe-like instead of elastic. This is caused by abnormal deposits within the walls of the artery which cause gradual narrowing and may eventually seal the vessel completely so that no blood passes through it.
The exact cause of atherosclerosis is unknown but advancement have been made within recent years in investigations as to the cause. Current thinking tends to favour the theory that wear and tear upon the blood vessels and faulty metabolism of fatty substances (such as cholesterol) produce atherosclerosis.

Are some people more prone to atherosclerosis than others?
Atherosclerosis is more prone to develop in the following types of people:
• overweight people;
• people with diabetes;
• those who have a particularly high fat content within their blood;
• people with high blood pressure;
• people with lots of stress. Early atherosclerosis does exist in some families.
It is thought that there is an inborn factor which predisposes some people toward earlier hardening of their arteries.

What are the symptoms of atherosclerosis and how is the diagnosis made?
The symptoms will depend entirely upon the location and the degree of the condition. Basically, the symptoms are those caused by diminished blood flow through the artery. For example, if the coronary arteries of the heart are involved, the individual may experience angina pectoris upon exertion.
If the arteries of the legs are involved, the patient may experience intermittent claudication (severe cramps and pain in the muscles of the legs in walking). There are many ways in which the doctor can arrive at the diagnosis. For instance, an examination of the eye grounds through an ophthalmoscope will often reveal hardening of the arteries in the retina.
Hardening of the arteries of the arms and legs can often be determined simply upon feeling the vessels with the examining fingers. X-ray examination, arteriography and ultrasound research of various structures often will reveal the characteristic picture of hardened blood vessels.

What foods are high in cholesterol and saturated fats? How much cholesterol should I eat?
Fat and cholesterol circulating in the blood are deposited on the inner walls of the arteries. Most coronary disease is caused by blocked arteries. Cholesterol is found only in foods from animals, such as egg yolks, meat, fish, poultry and whole milk products. Saturated fat is usually hard at room temperature, like the fat in beef. It is also found in coconut and palm oils.
Vegetables, fruits, cereal grains and starches contain no cholesterol and little or no saturated fats. It is recommended that you eat no more than 100 milligrams of cholesterol a day for every 1,000 calories you take in, and no more than 300 mg total in a day, no matter how much you eat.

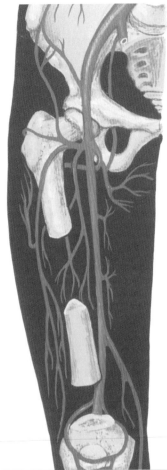

Course of the main artery (femoral artery) of the leg. In elderly people this artery can show atherosclerotic changes leading to diminished blood supply to the leg and foot.

should be treated early and adequately. Cigarette smoking should be limited or stopped. Regular exercise may help to prevent heart disease and may be a useful therapeutic measure.
Lowering blood pressure reduces the incidence of heart attacks, so individuals with high blood pressure should be identified and treated early. The intake of cholesterol and saturated and short-chain fatty acids, such as occur in meat and dairy products, should be reduced. Such a low-fat diet is consumed by many populations in the world and is well tolerated. Weight reduction to normal, or even slightly below current statistical norms, is recommended. Taking aspirin on a regular basis has a beneficial effect.

Eating to cut cholesterol

It is relatively easy to reduce your blood cholesterol. To do so, eat more low-fat, low-cholesterol foods and cut down on high-fat foods. Basically, it means eating more fruit, vegetables and whole grains in place of fatty meats and bakery goods; eating fresh poultry without skin and lean meats instead of fatty ones; and consuming low-fat or skim milk dairy products rather than whole milk dairy products.

Whole milk dairy products
Whole milk contains more saturated fat than low-fat or skim milk. In fact, about 45 per cent of the calories in whole milk comes from saturated fat. Whole milk also contains more cholesterol. Instead of whole milk, aim for low-fat (two per cent) milk, because only 30 per cent of its calories come from saturated fat. Skim milk has even less saturated fat. Using low-fat milk or skim milk works best, because they are rich in protein, calcium and other nutrients without being high in fat.

Butter, cream and ice cream
Save these dairy products for special occasions - they have even more fat than whole milk. And while you are at it, beware of butter and cream hidden in certain casserole and other dishes, bakery goods and desserts.

Cheese
Many people think they can eat cheese instead of meat because it is high in protein. Unfortunately, many cheeses are also high in saturated fatty acids. About 60 to 70 per cent of the calories in cheese comes from butterfat, about the same percentage as in ice cream. Instead of regular cheese, select low-fat cottage cheese, part-skim milk mozzarella, ricotta and other low-fat cheeses.

Eggs
One egg contains about 213 mg of cholesterol. It is recommended eating no more than four eggs per week, including those in cooking. Egg whites, however, do not contain cholesterol and are good protein sources, so they are fine. You can substitute two egg whites for each egg yolk in many recipes requiring eggs.

Meats
For most people, about six ounces of poultry, fish or lean meat daily is plenty.

▲ Beef, lamb, pork and veal
Look for lean cuts of these meats with a minimum of visible fat, and trim all outside fat before cooking. Most meats have about the same amount of cholesterol, roughly 77 mg in each three-ounce (cooked) serving. Red meat is okay to eat in moderation as long as it's lean.

▲ Processed meats
These include sausage, bologna, salami and hot dogs, which have about 70 to 80 per cent of their calories as fat.

Processed meats-even those with 'reduced fat' labels-are high in calories and saturated fat, so choose once in a while.

▲ Organ meats
These include liver, sweetbreads, kidney, brain and heart. Organ meats, except the heart, are extremely high in cholesterol. Eat them infrequently if you are on a cholesterol-lowering diet. Consider heart a red meat.

▲ Poultry
Eat chicken and turkey rather than duck and goose, which have a higher fat content. Chicken and turkey are also preferable to fatty red meat. Remember to remove the skin from poultry-that's where much of the fat is stored.

▲ Fish
Although fish can be either fatty or lean, it's among the best meats you can choose. That's because fatty fish usually comes from the deep sea and contains high amounts of omega-3 fatty acids.
Some scientists think this kind of fatty acid may be beneficial, but they are still studying this. Lean fish can come from either fresh or salt water and have little or no omega-3 fatty acids. Fish is not free of cholesterol, but it's very low in saturated fat. For a cholesterol-lowering diet, fish is better than lean red meat and much better than fatty red meat.
Many people are wondering whether to add fish oil to their diet, because they have heard about the benefits of omega-3 fatty acids. But because we do not really know what effect large doses of omega-3 oils would have, we recommend that you get your fish oil the natural way: by including fish in your diet regularly. Two or three times a week should be plenty.

▲ Shellfish
Shellfish is very low in fat, which is good, but shrimp and lobster contain a little more cholesterol than fish, meat or poultry. Choose these less often.

Bakery goods
Commercially baked goods are often made with egg yolk and saturated fats. Eating limited amounts is okay, but it is better to stick with home-made baked goods made with unsaturated oils and egg whites.

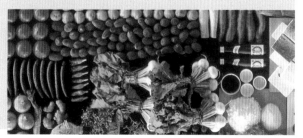

AUTISM

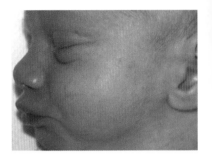

Description

Usually in the sense of infantile autism, a syndrome present from birth or beginning almost invariably in the first 30 months of life. Responses to auditory and visual stimuli are abnormal and there are usually severe difficulties in the understanding of spoken language. Autism is regarded as a social developmental disorder that may be an abnormality in the development of the brain due to damage during growth as a foetus, at birth or in the first year of life. Neuroimaging studies confirm what scientists long suspected: autistic brains don't react to facial cues the way normal brains do. One of the commonest descriptions of babies that might be autistic is that they are very good. They are very passive, very quiet. It is almost like not having a baby in the house. There is a minority who scream all the time without stopling and cannot be comforted, but that is a very much smaller group.

Test to investigate the intelligence level of young autistic children.

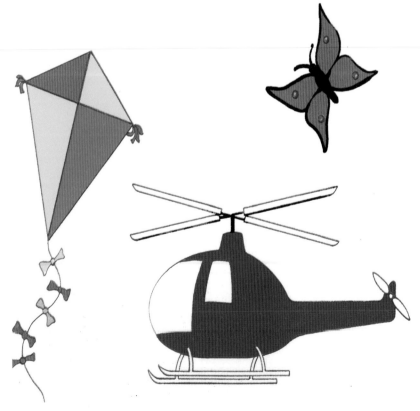

Cause

Despite considerable research, the cause of autism remains unknown. Experts do not know how the body malfunctions to produce the syndrome. Since autism severely restricts perception and communication, some experts have proposed that it is caused by problems with the brain centers that regulate sensory input and processing, especially of language.

Another question yet to be answered is why autism sometimes appears in conjunction with certain conditions present at birth (congenital). Such conditions include:

- encephalitis;
- mental retardation;
- PKU - phenylketonuria;
- retrolental fibroplasia;
- congenital rubella;
- congenital syphilis;
- tuberous sclerosis.

Experts speculate that the same factors that can cause these conditions may also lead to autism.

Medical researchers are investigating the possibility that autism may result in part from genetic factors. It is significant that the incidence of autism is 50 times greater among siblings of autistic children than in the general population. The incidence of other disorders, such as in language, also is higher than usual among families with autistic children.

One fact about the cause of autism has now become clear: the syndrome is not caused by improper parenting. It is certain that a child who is autistic is born with the disorder, that all different types of parents - regardless of their child-rearing practices - have autistic children, and that child-rearing practices have no bearing on the cause of the disorder.

The way parents respond to their

child's autism can, however, have some bearing on how far the child can go within the confines of his or her disabilities.

Diagnosis

Any child suspected by parents of having a developmental problem should be seen by a pediatrician, preferably one specializing in developmental disorders.

Although the signs and symptoms of autism are thought by experts to be evident in most cases from birth, parents may not notice them until the child is a toddler or even older. The majority of children are diagnosed at age 2 or 3, when their language deficits and social difficulties become obvious, especially compared with their peers' development.

Obtaining an accurate, detailed diagnosis for a child who seems to be autistic is absolutely essential. Because the behavioral problems associated with autism are so varied, the syndrome is easily mistaken for other disorders, especially when some problems are quite mild and others quite severe.

Parents should be especially wary of physicians who casually contend that their child is "slow" or is "mentally retarded with autistic tendencies (or features)". Although the degree of severity may vary, autism is diagnosed only when all its symptomatic behaviors are present.

The best place to obtain a thorough, precise diagnosis is a university-affiliated developmental evaluation clinic. These clinics are more likely than other facilities to have an interdisciplinary approach; they usually employ a team of specialists who are trained to rule out the wide variety of conditions that can easily be confused with autism.

Such conditions include:
- depression;
- hearing loss;
- developmental language disorders;
- mental retardation;
- abnormally slow development.

If parents have any doubts about a diagnosis - whether it is thorough or accurate, for example - they should

Categories of symptoms in autism

Social relationships

Autistic children have serious difficulty forming emotional attachments to parents and other people. This disability is sometimes apparent as early as infancy; a baby may, for example, be indifferent or even averse to being held.

In addition to having a continued lack of desire for affectionate physical contact, an autistic toddler characteristically does not make meaningful eye contact with other people, does not respond socially to others by smiling or using other facial expressions, and seems, in general, not to recognize people as individuals - or sometimes even as people. Typically, an autistic child seems to live in a world of his or her own.

Language

Language disorders are universal among autistic children. Although hearing difficulties are not a component of autism, young autistic children are often first thought to be deaf.

Experts believe that autistic children have great difficulty processing the meaning of speech, even though they hear clearly. Autistic children suffer from long delays in language development or, in severe cases, from a lifelong inability to speak.

If an autistic child does begin using language, it is usually not for communicative purposes, at least at the outset. Autistic children seem to enjoy language for its sound alone.

A characteristic feature of an autistic child's early use of language is echolalia, the tendency to repeat the sounds and words of others. While echoing may occur immediately after another person speaks, some autistic children have an unusual capacity for remembering whole passages from conversation or television programs for a surprisingly long period of time.

If an autistic child develops meaningful speech, it is often peppered with grammatical errors and other peculiarities. One common characteristic is a tendency to mix up pronouns: a child requesting an apple, for instance, may say "you want apple."

It is also common for autistic children to have difficulty remembering the names of objects, talking about abstract ideas, and using metaphors.

The speech of an autistic child tends to be flat, lacking tone, emotion, ant other subtleties. When tone does change, it is often inappropriate.

Appropriate nonverbal expressions of emotion, such as gestures and facial expressions, often do not accompany speech. All of these problems tend to persist through adulthood.

Behavior

Autistic children are very resistant to changes, such as new food, toys, furniture arrangement, and clothing. They often become excessively attached to particular inanimate objects.

They often repeat certain acts, such as rocking, hand flapping, or spinning objects in a repetitive manner. Some may injure themselves through repetitive behaviors such as head banging or biting themselves.

Intelligence

About 65 per cent of children with autism have some degree of mental retardation (an IQ less than 70). Their performance is uneven, they usually do better on tests of motor and spatial skills than on verbal tests, but specific tests such as the Childhood Autism Rating Scale, may help the evaluation.

In addition to giving standardized tests, a doctor should perform certain tests to look for underlying treatable or inherited medical disorders (such as hereditary disorders of metabolism and fragile X syndrome).

A

Autism   Questions & Answers

What is autism?
Autism is a disorder in which a young child cannot develop normal social relation-ships, uses language abnormally or not at all, behaves in compulsive and ritualis-tic ways, and may fail to develop normal intelligence. Autism, the most common of the pervasive developmental disorders, occurs in 5 of 10,000 children. The disorder is 2 to 4 times more common in boys than in girls. Autism is different from mental retardation, although many children with autism have both.

What is a pervasive mental disorder?
Pervasive mental disorders comprise a group of related conditions (for instance autism, Asperger's disorder) that all involve some combination of impaired social relationships, stereotyped or ritualistic behavior, abnormal, language development, and intellectual impairment.

What causes autism in children?
Medical scientists just do not know yet. Since it rarely occurs in more than one fam-ily member, it does not appear to be inherited. The specific cause of autism is not fully known, although it is clearly a biologically determined disorder.
While theories have been advanced about parental involvement, none have been proved. So far, we do know why autistic children seem to suffer from impairment of their cognitive and/or perceptual functioning.
As a result, they appear to have a limited ability to understand, communicate, learn and participate in social relations-hips.

What are the symptoms of autism?
The symptoms vary from child to child. Generally, the youngsters may have severe-ly impaired speech or not talk at all. They may not relate at all to family members or others around them. They may get very upset about minor changes in their envi-ronment.
Their intellectual development may seem to be normal in some areas, but abnor-mal in others. Some are known for repetitive and peculiar body motions, such as constant rocking.
Some appear insensitive to pain. Most do not relate normally to such stimuli as noise or light.
The great variance in the behavior of autistic children can further be indicated by the fact that some are hyperactive, while others are very passive.

What can be done for autistic children?
It depends on the severity and range of handicaps with which the child is dealing. Certainly, a complete physical, neurological and psychological examination of such children is warranted at an early age - as soon as the abnormal symptoms appear. Sometimes the problem is not autism but some other disorder.
If autism is the problem, the child will need special educational and psychological attention. Once upon a time, these youngsters were simply sent to state insti-tutions and nothing was done to help them. This should not be the case today.
In small classes, autistic children get one-to-one attention from their teachers. They are slowly taught to communicate, and to manage simple chores.
With this kind of care, many are able to transfer to normal public schools. Others will need sheltered environment all their lives. Yet all deserve and can benefit from special education.

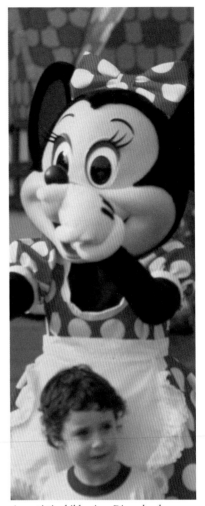

An autistic child enjoys Disneyland.

seek a second opinion. In addition, children diagnosed as autistic should be reevaluated at least once a year so that their treatment can be adapted to their current needs.

Signs

The major signs of autism are usually apparent in toddlers:
- No pointing by one year.
- No babbling by one year; no single words by 16 months; no two-word phrases by 24 months.
- Any loss of language skills at any time.
- No pretend playing and little interest in making friends.
- Extremely short attention span

and no response when called by name.
- Indifference to others; little or no eye contact.
- Repetitive body movements, such as hand flapping, rocking.
- Fixations on a single object, such as spinning fan.
- Usually strong resistance to changes in routines; intense tantrums.
- Oversensitivity to certain textures or smelts.

Treatment

There is no cure for autism, but there are many treatments that can make a difference.
▲ *Speech therapy*
   Can help overcome communication and language barriers.
▲ *Occupational therapy*
   Helps with sensory integration and motor skills.
▲ *Behavioral therapy*
   Improves cognitive skills and reduces inappropriate behavior.
▲ *Educational therapy*
   A highly structured approach works best.
▲ Medication
   Can reduce some symptoms.
▲ *Special diets*
   Eliminating certain food groups, such as dairy, helps some children..

Autism   Questions & Answers

What are pervasive deviopmental disorders?
Pervasive developmental disorders comprise a group of related conditions that all involve some combination of impaired social relationships, stereotypes or ritualistic behaviors, abnormal language development and use, and in some cases, intellectual impairment.

What is Asperger's disorder?
Asperger's disorder is a pervasive developmental disorder closely to autism but less severe.

What are the major symptoms of Asperger's disorder?
Children with Asperger's disorder have impaired social interactions similar to those of children with autism, as well as stereotypes or repetitive behaviors and mannerisms and non-functional rituals. However, language skills are normal and sometimes superior to those of an average child, and IQ is normal.

Are children with Asperger's disorder function normally?
Children with Asperger's disorder tend to function at a higher level than children with autism and may be able to function independently. Children with Asperger's disorder respond well to psychotherapy.

Brain mechanisms inovlved in autism

▲ The autistic brain differs in several ways from a typical brain. Scientists are trying to determine whether the differences are the cause of the result of autism.
▲ The frontal lobes, home to higher reasoning, are greatly enlarged, due mainly to excess white matter, the brain's connector cables. The brains of kids who develop autism are growing at an unusual rate by age 2 and have puzzling signs of inflammation.
▲ The corpus callosum is undersize. This band of tissue links the left and right hemispheres of the brain. Activity across diverse regions of the brain is poorly coordinated in autistic people, more like a jam session than a symphony.
▲ The amygdala is also enlarged. This area plays a role in sizing up threats in the environment and in emotional and social behavior. Its size may be related to the high level of anxiety in autistic people.
▲ The hippocampus is about 10% larger than normal. This area is vital to memory. One possibility is that this structure become enlarged because autistic children rely on memory to interpret situations that most people process elsewhere.

Test to investigate the intelligence level of young autistic children.

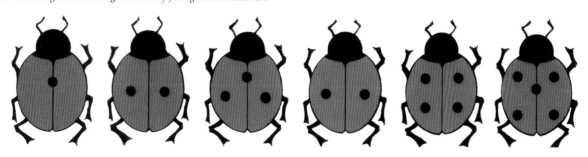

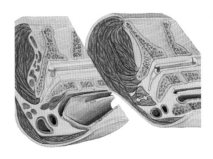

BACK PAIN

Definition

Back pain or low back pain is commonly called lumbago: pain in the lumbar and/or sacral region of the back. Although low back pain (with or without pain also radiating down the leg) is an extremely common symptom, there is no general agreement as to its cause.

In consequence, many doctors' first response to patients with such a complaint is one of despair, and this may be a reasonable response when one

Back view of the lower part of the trunk to show the relationship between the spinal nerves and lumbar vertebral column. The back is vulnerable to most forms of arthritis, but the commonest is the kind caused over the years by wear and tear - osteoarthritis.

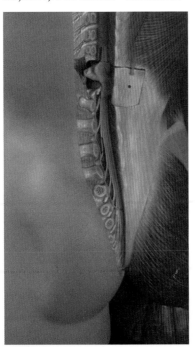

considers the list of possible causes. Anyone can have back pain. In fact, 10 percent of all people in western Europe and the United States have back pain in a given year. Back pain can occur at any age in both men and women. However, it may occur slightly more in women beginning at middle age, probably due to osteoporosis.

Causes

The following are important (but non common) causes of low back pain.
- *Congenital*: for instance, the fusing together of lumbar vertebrae.
- *Traumatic*: i.e. injury, not only of bone but also of soft tissue.
- *Inflammatory*: acute and chronic with a recent reoccurrence of bone and joint tuberculosis in the forefront of the mind.
- *Tumors*: primary in bone and nervous tissues; secondary mainly from breast, thyroid and prostate glands and kidney.
- *Metabolic*: for instance, osteoporosis.
- *Rheumatic*: ankylosing spondylitis, osteochondritis, gout, rheumatoid arthritis.
- *Bone disease*: for example, Paget's disease.
- *Pelvic disease*: for instance, endometriosis, impacted ovarian cysts and so on.

In addition to these important but less common causes, there are the more common causes that must be considered in every case. These include:
- disk prolapse;
- strained ligaments as a result of postural and occupational faults
- disturbances of function in joints (apophyses) that have bony projections (e.g. the vertebrae of the spine);
- sacro-iliac joint disturbance, spondylosis and osteoarthritis of the spine.

Ruptured intervertebral disk
This may be the most painful, yet easiest condition to identify. A ruptured or herniated disk is one that bulges and extends into the spinal canal, pressing on the nerve roots. This condition causes the nerve roots to become irritated. On occasion, a ruptured disk can occur after bending and lifting over. However, it usually occurs for no apparent reason.

A ruptured disk may cause back pain and muscle spasms, but a more common symptom is sciatic. This is severe pain spreading down one leg and often into the foot. Sometimes it is the only symptom of a ruptured disk.

A ruptured disk can generally be detected by a physical examination alone. Occasionally, a myelogram. CT-scans, or MRI-scans are necessary to confirm the diagnosis and determine if surgery is necessary. Treatment includes bed rest, traction, heat, muscle relaxants, and/or weight reduction. Surgery is rarely used, but may be required if pain is prolonged and severe.

Injuries and accidents
Have you ever moved a piece of furniture that did not seem too heavy, only to feel pain in your back next day? Have you ever stretched for something that was just a little out of your reach, and felt a twinge in your back? Many back injuries are caused by an unexpected twist or sudden motion. This usually results in muscle strain.

Fortunately, most of us have not experienced back injury from a blow or fall. These injuries could cause fractures (broken bones) in the spinal column, accompanied by tenderness over the fractured vertebrae.

There may also be muscle spasms at the fracture. Back movement will be limited. Pain is usually immediate, although it may not occur for days. Spinal fractures are more common in older women with osteoporosis.

Injuries can also damage the spinal cord and nerves. Be especially concerned about any pain that travels down one or both legs. This could be a sign of nerve damage. However, paralysis as a result of low back pain is extremely rare.

With neither an injury or accident, severe muscle spasm usually last 48-72 hours. They are generally followed by days or weeks of less severe pain. It usually takes 2-4 weeks to heal; completely from a mild back injury. It could take up to 6-12 weeks if there are strained ligaments or if the strain is more severe. Severe back injury from a fall or accident may require hospitalization and a longer recovery period.

Arthritis

Arthritis means joint inflammation. Joint inflammation can cause the area surrounding the joints to become warm, red, painful, and swollen. There are over 100 kinds of arthritis. Some forms of arthritis cause aches and pains near and around joints, but not in the joints themselves.

Sometimes arthritis affects the muscles, tendons, ligaments, and other parts of the body. Certain forms of arthritis, such as those listed below, can cause back pain.

Ankylosing spondylitis

This form of arthritis causes the joints in the spine to become stiff and swollen. With time, stiff joints can grow together (fuse). The most common symptoms are pain and stiffness in the hip and low back, which continue for more than three months. Ankylosing spondylitis is most common in men ages 20-40.

Osteoarthritis

This form of arthritis breaks down the soft, elastic material (cartilage) that cushions the spinal joints and other joints in the body. Low back pain can be aggravated when osteoarthritis affects the hips of the knees.

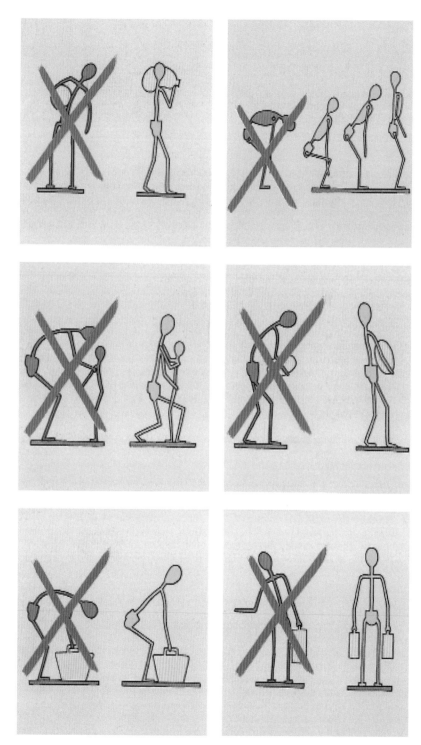

Many back injuries are caused by an unexpected twist or sudden motion, by lifting heavy boxes, or carrying parcels in the wrong way. The left part of each figure illustrates the wrong way of carrying weights or lifting children, the right part of the illustration shows the right way to lift or carry objects. During posture training, an occupational or physical; therapist will teach you healthier ways to sit, stand, sleep, and lift objects.

B

Back pain   Questions & Answers

What is meant by back pain or low back pain?

Low back pain or back pain is a common disorder caused by symptoms affecting the spine, its surrounding muscles or spinal nerves. It is the leading cause of disability for those aged 19 to 45 and is the second most common cause of missed work days (after the common cold) for adults younger than 45.

What is the source of most back pains?

Back pains aches are among the most common human ailments. Most chronic low back pain is not due to any disease or hidden abnormality. They are usually the result of the way we live - getting overweight, not exercising enough, having poor posture, and not carrying things properly.

Because humans walk in an upright position, all of our upper body weight rests on our lower back. Sudden low back pain usually result from exercise, aging, injury, a fall, lifting a heavy object improperly, or shovelling snow. The pain comes from a sprain (injury to the ligaments) or a strain (injury to the muscles).

What is meant by the term slipped disk?

The term slipped disk is not really an accurate one. The disk doesn't slip; rather is ruptured. The spine consists of rounded, cube-like bones called vertebrae, separated from each other by spongy cushions of tissue called intervertebral disks. Nerves from the spinal cord pass between the vertebrae going to different parts of the body. The disks cushion the vertebrae as they move, when the back bends or turns. In essence, the disks are shock absorbers for whatever jarring, pressure, or sudden movement changes your body undergoes. The entire weight of your upper body rests on the lower portion of the spine. That is why ruptured disks most commonly occur in the lower back.

The disk is composed of a strong, fibrous ring of tissue - like a small inner-tube - and is filled with a softer, spongy material. When excessive pressure is placed on the disk, the "inner-tube" portion tears, and the softer, spongy material bulges out into the spinal canal. As it bulges out, it presses on nerves in your spine leading to sensations of severe pain. Sometimes the pain extends from the back down into one or both legs.

Who may get a ruptured disk?

Although it sometimes happens to young adults, ruptured disks occur most often in people 25 years or older because disks begin to lose some of their fluid as we age. As this drying out or degeneration of the disk continues, it stands a greater chance of rupturing. In some people, even a minor slip of lifting a heavy object can cause a rupture.

A variety of different conditions, some of them serious illnesses, can cause low back pain. This is why you should see your doctor if any severe back pain occurs, or even lesser back pain that does not respond to rest within 10 days. However, even before then, see your doctor if you develop any leg pain or tingling sensations or weakness in your feet or legs.

How is a ruptured disk being treated?

Treatment usually requires bed rest (sometimes for several weeks), use of a heating pad and/or hot baths to relax the muscles and promote healing, anti-inflammatory medication which also relieves pain, and muscle relaxants. Most people respond to such treatment. If it is not effective, or if there is severe weakness, surgery may be indicated. A ruptured disk is not always diagnosed in an easy way. A variety of tests, including special X-rays, CT-scans, and/or magnetic resonance imaging (MRI), may be necessary.

Osteoarthritis can also directly affect the spine, which may cause back pain. However, back pain is more commonly associated with osteoarthritis of the hips and knees.

Osteoporosis

This is a type of bone disorder which causes bones to become thin and weak.

Fragile bones such as these can break more easily, especially bones in the spinal column.

Rheumatoid arthritis

This form of arthritis causes any joints to become stiff, painful, and swollen. It can affect the neck and, more rarely, the joints in the lower back.

Polymyalgia rheumatica

This form of arthritis causes muscle pain, aching, and stiffness in the neck and shoulders, low back, thighs, and hips. It can last a few months or many years. Most people experience severe stiffness in the morning.

Paget's disease

This is a type of bone disorder. The bones most commonly affected are in the low back, pelvis, tailbone, skull, and long bones of the legs. It is slightly more common in men than in women. If often begins between 50-70 years of age.

Back pain may be a symptom, but most often there are no obvious symptoms. Paget's disease is usually discovered on an X-ray or bone scan done for reasons other than pain.

Fibrositis

Most people with fibrositis experience pain and stiffness around joints, muscles, tendons and ligaments. The pain can last for weeks, months, or years. It can vary from day to day.

Often times, the symptoms go away by themselves. This condition is usually related to stress, sleep problems, or depression. It occurs most often in women aged 20-50.

Spinal stenosis

In spinal stenosis the spinal canal narrows. This squeezes the back nerves, putting pressure on them. It is the pressure that causes back pain.

Numbness, pain, and weakness in the legs can also occur.

The most common symptom of spinal stenosis is pain that gets worse while walking and is relieved by sitting down. Spinal stenosis more commonly occurs in older adults who already have osteoarthritis and advanced disk disease.

Symptoms and signs

Acute back pain is characterized by the following signs and symptoms:
▲ pain usually lasting a few days or 6-12 days;
▲ pain may be mild or severe;
▲ pain may occasionally be caused by an accident or injury;
▲ about 80 per cent of all back pain is acute.

Major characteristics of chronic back pain are:
▲ pain usually lasts more than 3 months;
▲ pain may be mild or severe;
▲ pain may be related to other illnesses;
▲ about 10 per cent of all back pain is chronic.

Diagnosis

It is essential that the doctor takes an adequate medical history in every case. Too often back pain sufferers are given short shrift and treated as though they were all alike. This is as unwarranted as treating all persons with
abdominal pain in the same way.

It is important to elicit details of the onset and unfolding of the pattern of pain -the story of trauma or incident at the onset, the nature, site and radiation of pain, alleviating or exacerbating factors (e.g. posture), variation with time during the day. The presence of morning stiffness for longer than one hour must be investigated as must neurological symptoms such as paraesthesia (tingling, numbness, etc.) or muscular weakness.

Aggravation by coughing, sneezing or laughing are signs that the dura mater (the outer membrane covering the spinal cord and the brain) may be

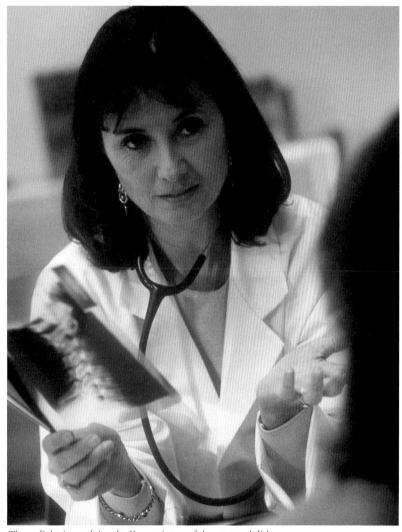

The radiologist explains the X-ray picture of the ruptured disk.

involved. Every patient must also be asked about alteration in bowel and bladder function since the onset of pain.

Incontinence or retention of urine constitute a surgical emergency for which a neurosurgeon must be consulted as a matter of urgency since delay may result in irreversible loss of bladder control. In addition, the doctor will pay attention to the patient's physical activities at work, in the home and during recreation. The person's previous medical history is important, too. Recurrence and increasing frequency and severity of attacks of back pain commonly occur, while the history of, say, a mastectomy

(removal of a breast) or other major surgery may be of great diagnostic significance.

Any physical examination must start with a conscious appraisal of the person's state of well-being. Recent weight loss is particularly significant, and the person's gait is important as an indicator of severe pain.

With the patient standing, the range of forward, lateral and backward bending can be measured and compared with the norm for his/her age and physique. The level of the iliac crests (the tops of the hipbones) should be observed, for this may indicate a difference in leg length and may sometimes explain a scoliosis (side-

B

ways curvature of the spine).
Leg length difference is more common in those with low back pain than in others. It is important to ask patients who are in bed when seen for the first time to stand on the floor if it is at all possible, otherwise an acute scoliosis may be missed that would not be obvious if he/she is only examined lying down.
The person is then asked to sit, and if the iliac crests level up, then the difference when standing is probably due to leg length inequality. The usual difference is between 0.5 cm and 3 cm. With the patient supine a neurological examination is carried out.
Muscle power against resistance is tested for hip flexors, knee extensors, foot dorsiflexors, plantar flexors and great toe extensors. Straight leg raising is also done. Hip movement is tested, especially in those at and beyond middle age, and the pulses that can be felt in the legs (e.g. in the groin) are examined. Knee and ankle reflexes and plantar responses are elicited.
With the person lying on his/her stomach, resisted knee flexion is tested as is palpation of the contracted buttock muscle - weakness of one gluteus maximus muscle of vertebral muscles at each level should be assessed by light pressure about 2 cm on either side of the spine. A line joining the iliac crests crosses the fourth lumbar vertebra.
Mobility between the lumbar vertebrae can be assessed with the person lying on his/her side, the hips and knees bent and the legs supported by the examiner with one hand while the other hand feels the intervals between the vertebrae in the lumbar region during gentle passive bending and straightening of that part of the spine by the hand supporting the legs.

X-rays
Straight spinal X-rays are of limited usefulness. There is no correlation between radiological findings and symptoms and signs in the majority of cases. Degenerative changes in the lumbar spine are extremely common. Narrowing of disk spaces, osteophytes (bony outgrowths) on the vertebrae and osteoarthritic changes in apophyseal joints can be seen in a high pro-

portion of persons over the age of 55. These changes never regress, and since the attacks of low back pain tend to be recurrent, it is impossible to know whether they relate to the current attack or to a previous one.
Straight X-rays are useful for:
▲ diagnosis of bone disease and bone erosion;.
▲ diagnosis of spondylosis and spondylolisthesis, and here X-rays taken at any angle are necessary;
▲ diagnosis of leg-length difference. Standing views including the heads of the femurs (thighbones) enable direct measurements to be made.

CT-scan and MRI-scan
CT-scans are made with a special machine. The information from the scan is then sent into a computer. The computer can display images of the area on a TV-like screen, or store them for permanent record. A CT-scan gives the factor a three-dimensional view of the back. It is particularly useful in determining if there is a ruptured disk.
NMR produces very clear pictures of the skeletal system. Unlike many other tests, the NMR does not use X-rays or radioactive dyes. It is very useful in getting clearer images of soft tissues such as muscles, cartilage, ligaments, tendons, and blood vessels, in addition to bone structure.

Myelography
A myelogram may be ordered to detect problems such as spinal stenosis or spinal cord tumors. If back surgery is being considered, many neurosurgeons will require a myelogram beforehand.
During a myelogram, an injection is given into the spinal canal. It contains a special material (called contrast medium). X-rays will then be taken of the area. The contrast medium can make problem areas more visible on the X-ray.

Bone scan
Occasionally bone scans are done to look for damage or tumors in the bones themselves. However, back pain is rarely due to diseases of the bones. During a bone scan, the patient will be asked to take a very small amount

of radioactive material. A special radioactive detecting machine will then be used to scan the area of concern.

Blood tests
If your doctor orders blood tests for you, a laboratory technician will carefully draw a small amount of blood from your arm, which will be tested in the laboratory. Any one of the following blood tests may be ordered:
- erythrocyte sedimentation rate;
- hematocrit;
- hemoglobin;
- white blood cell count;
- HLA B-27 test;
- rheumatic factor tests;
- chemical profile.

Treatment

Many back problems go away in a matter of days or weeks and do not come back. However, the longer back problems last, the more likely they are to come back again.
Doctors generally prescribe one or more treatments. For some back conditions, the doctor may refer you to another specialist such as an orthopaedist, rheumatologist, physiatrist, physical or occupational therapist, psychologist, psychiatrist, or surgeon.

■ *Rest*
The first treatment doctors usually recommend for acute back pain is bed rest. Different people require different amounts of rest. Usually 2 days staying in bed, except to go to the bathroom, will be enough to ease your back pain.
You may want to ask the doctor if special pillows or devices are necessary. Sometimes, these aids give additional support to your neck, back, or feet.

■ *Heat and cold*
Many people have found that hot and cold treatments help relieve back pain. You might try both to find out which works best for you.
Heat relaxes muscles and soothes painful areas. There are many ways to apply heat: some people like hot showers or baths, while others prefer using heat lamps, heating pads, or

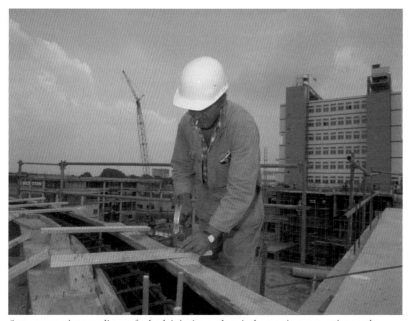
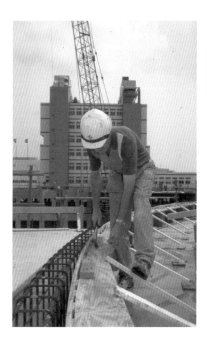

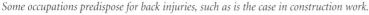
Some occupations predispose for back injuries, such as is the case in construction work.

warm compresses.

Cold has a numbing effect. This often helps relieve pain. You might try one of these methods for applying cold.
- an ice bag;
- a slush pack;
- a large ice cube used to massage the area;
- frozen package of vegetables (peas work best).

Exercises

For many people, the key to a healthy back is proper exercise. Some exercises are designed to strengthen your back and stomach muscles, while other exercises will keep you totally fit. There are even exercises to improve your posture.

The right kind of exercise program may help keep your back problem under control. It can make it easier for you to continue doing your daily exercises. You may need to temporarily refrain from strenuous exercise if it aggravates your back pain.

Posture training

If poor posture is a factor, then posture training may help relieve your back pain. During posture training, an occupational or physical therapist will teach you healthier ways to sit, stand, sleep, and lift objects.

Weight control

Do not be surprised if your doctor recommends weight loss as one way of reducing your back pain and improving your general health. The best way to lose weight is with a balanced diet along with regular exercise. Be sure to avoid fad diets or fast weight loss programs. These can be harmful and cause new problems for you, instead of solving old ones.

Stress management

Every day of our line is filled with some kind of stress. It is a part of daily living. In fact, any situation can cause stress such as work, personal relationships, raising children, paying bills, the death of a loved one, or a new experience.

TENS devices

TENS (Transcutaneous Electrical Nerve Stimulation) is a small battery-operated device used to stimulate nerves and block pain. If you use a TENS device, it should not hurt. When the unit is turned on, electrical signals are sent to the nerves in that area. These signals tend to block the pain.

Check with your doctor to find out if a TENS unit would work for you. A physical therapist can show you the proper way to use it. You might con-

sider trying it out a few times before buying your own unit.

Medications

Many times medication is not necessary. However, if your back pain is not relieved using other forms of treatment, your doctor can prescribe the proper medications. The medication chosen depends on the back pain. For example, there are medications called analgesics which can relieve pain. Other medications, called muscle relaxants, are prescribed to relax tight muscles. If your back pain is due to arthritis, your doctor can give you medication that will reduce inflammation, as well as relieve your back pain. The most common medications prescribed are called nonsteroidal anti-inflammatory drugs (NSAID). This means they are not cortisone-like drugs and they can reduce inflammation. Aspirin is one NSAID. More often, NSAID medications which cause less stomach distress are prescribed.

Surgery

Very few people with back pain need surgery. Most people can be treated successfully with rest, exercise, and medication. An orthopaedist or neurosurgeon will help you decide if a back operation is necessary.

BIRD FLU

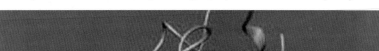

Introduction

Avian influenza, or "bird flu", is a contagious disease of animals caused by viruses that normally infect only birds and, less commonly, pigs. Avian influenza viruses are highly species-specific, but have, on rare occasions, crossed the species barrier to infect humans.

In domestic poultry, infection with avian influenza viruses causes two main forms of disease, distinguished by low and high extremes of virulence. The so-called "low pathogenic" form commonly causes only mild symptoms (ruffled feathers, a drop in egg production) and may easily go undetected. The highly pathogenic form is far more dramatic. It spreads very rapidly through poultry flocks, causes disease affecting multiple internal organs, and has a mortality that can approach 100 percent, often within 48 hours.

Causative agents

Avian influenza is caused by influenza A viruses. Influenza viruses are grouped into three types, designated A, B, and C. Influenza A and B viruses are of concern for human health. Only influenza A viruses can cause pandemics.

Influenza A viruses have 16 H subtypes and 9 N subtypes.

Only viruses of the H5 and H7 subtypes are known to cause the highly pathogenic form of the disease. However, not all viruses of the H5 and H7 subtypes are highly pathogenic and not all will cause severe disease in poultry. On present understanding, H5 and H7 viruses are introduced to poultry flocks in their low pathogenic form. When allowed to circulate in poultry populations, the viruses can mutate, usually within a few months, into the highly pathogenic form.

This is why the presence of an H5 or H7 virus in poultry is always cause for concern, even when the initial signs of infection are mild.

The H subtypes are epidemiologically most important, as they govern the ability of the virus to bind to and enter cells, where multiplication of the virus then occurs. The N subtypes govern the release of newly formed virus from the cells.

The causative agent of avian influenza, the H5N1 virus, has proved to be especially tenacious. Despite the death or destruction of an estimated 150 million birds, the virus is now considered endemic in many parts of Indonesia and Viet Nam and in some parts of Cambodia, China, Thailand, and possibly also the Lao People's Democratic Republic. Control of the disease in poultry is expected to take several years. The H5N1 virus is also of particular concern for human health, as explained below.

Spread by migratory birds

The role of migratory birds in the spread of highly pathogenic avian

Model of the H5N1 virus detected by various groups of scientists in the latter part of 2005.

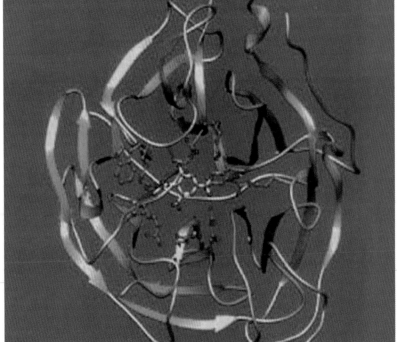

influenza is not fully understood. Wild waterfowl are considered the natural reservoir of all influenza A viruses.

They have probably carried influenza viruses, with no apparent harm, for centuries. They are known to carry viruses of the H5 and H7 subtypes, but usually in the low pathogenic form.

Considerable circumstantial evidence suggests that migratory birds can introduce low pathogenic H5 and H7 viruses to poultry flocks, which then mutate to the highly pathogenic form. In the past, highly pathogenic viruses have been isolated from migratory birds on very rare occasions involving a few birds, usually found dead within the flight range of a poultry outbreak. This finding long suggested that wild waterfowl are not agents for the onward transmission of these viruses. Recent events make it likely that some migratory birds are now directly spreading the H5N1 virus in its highly pathogenic form. Further spread to new areas is expected.

The current outbreaks of highly pathogenic avian influenza, which began in South-east Asia in mid-2003, are the largest and most severe on record. Never before in the history of this disease have so many countries been simultaneously affected, resulting in the loss of so many birds.

From mid-December 2003 through early February 2004, poultry outbreaks caused by the H5N1 virus were reported in eight Asian nations, listed in order of reporting:

- Republic of Korea
- Viet Nam
- Japan
- Thailand
- Cambodia
- Lao People's Democratic Republic
- Indonesia
- China.

Most of these countries had never before experienced an outbreak of highly pathogenic avian influenza in their histories.

In early August 2004, Malaysia reported its first outbreak of H5N1 in poultry, becoming the ninth Asian nation affected.

Russia reported its first H5N1 outbreak in poultry in late July 2005, followed by reports of disease in adjacent

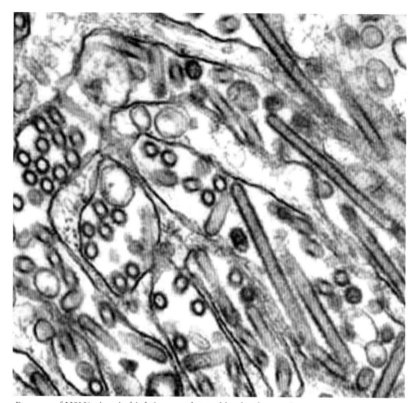

Presence of H5N1 virus in bird tissue as detected by the elctronmicroccope.

parts of Kazakhstan in early August. Deaths of wild birds from highly pathogenic H5N1 were reported in both countries.

Almost simultaneously, Mongolia reported the detection of H5N1 in dead migratory birds. In October 2005, H5N1 was confirmed in poultry in Turkey and Romania. Outbreaks in wild and domestic birds are under investigation elsewhere.

Japan, the Republic of Korea, and Malaysia have announced control of their poultry outbreaks and are now considered free of the disease. In the other affected areas, outbreaks are continuing with varying degrees of severity.

Danger of H5N1 virus

▲ The H5N1 subtype of the virus that causes avian flu is the most deadly to humans, killing almost 50 per cent of those infected.

▲ Symptoms include:
  • Fever
  • Cough
  • Sore throat
  • Muscle aches
  • Pneumonia
  • Acute respiratory distress

▲ The only way to catch bird flu is by coming into contact with an infected chicken or bird, or a contaminated surface.

Bird flu   Questions & Answers

What is avian influenza?

Avian influenza, or "bird flu", is a contagious disease of animals caused by viruses that normally infect only birds and, less commonly, pigs. Avian influenza viruses are highly species-specific, but have, on rare occasions, crossed the species barrier to infect humans.

What kind of disease may occur in poultry?

In domestic poultry, infection with avian influenza viruses causes two main forms of disease, distinguished by low and high extremes of virulence.
- The so-called "low pathogenic" form commonly causes only mild symptoms (ruffled feathers, a drop in egg production) and may easily go undetected.
- The highly pathogenic form is far more dramatic. It spreads very rapidly through poultry flocks, causes disease affecting multiple internal organs, and has a mortality that can approach 100 percent, often within 48 hours.

Which viruses cause highly pathogenic disease?

Influenza A viruses have 16 H subtypes and 9 N subtypes. Only viruses of the H5 and H7 subtypes are known to cause the highly pathogenic form of the disease. However, not all viruses of the H5 and H7 subtypes are highly pathogenic and not all will cause severe disease in poultry.

Do migratory birds spread highly pathogenic avian influenza viruses?

The role of migratory birds in the spread of highly pathogenic avian influenza is not fully understood. Wild waterfowl are considered the natural reservoir of all influenza A viruses. They have probably carried influenza viruses, with no apparent harm, for centuries. They are known to carry viruses of the H5 and H7 subtypes, but usually in the low pathogenic form.

Recent events make it likely that some migratory birds are directly spreading the H5N1 virus in its highly pathogenic form. Further spread to new areas is expected.

What is special about the current outbreaks in poultry?

The current outbreaks of highly pathogenic avian influenza, which began in Southeast Asia in mid-2003, are the largest and most severe on record. Never before in the history of this disease have so many countries been simultaneously affected, resulting in the loss of so many birds.

The causative agent, the H5N1 virus, has proved to be especially tenacious. Despite the death or destruction of an estimated 150 million birds, the virus is now considered endemic in many parts of Indonesia and Vietnam and in some parts of Cambodia, China, Thailand, and possibly also the Lao People's Democratic Republic. Control of the disease in poultry is expected to take several years.

Which countries have been affected by outbreaks in poultry?

From mid-December 2003 through early February 2004, poultry outbreaks caused by the H5N1 virus were reported in eight Asian nations (listed in order of reporting): the Republic of Korea, Viet Nam, Japan, Thailand, Cambodia, Lao People's Democratic Republic, Indonesia, and China. Most of these countries had never before experienced an outbreak of highly pathogenic avian influenza in their histories.In early August 2004, Malaysia reported its first outbreak of H5N1 in poultry, becoming the ninth Asian nation affected. Russia reported its first H5N1 outbreak in poultry in late July 2005, followed by reports of disease in adjacent parts of Kazakhstan in early August.

In October through December 2005, H5N1 was confirmed in poultry in China, Indonesia, Turkey, Russia and Romania. Outbreaks in wild and domestic birds are under investigation elsewhere.

Implications for human health

The widespread persistence of H5N1 in poultry populations poses two main risks for human health.

- The first is the risk of direct infection when the virus passes from poultry to humans, resulting in very severe disease. Of the few avian influenza viruses that have crossed the species barrier to infect humans, H5N1 has caused the largest number of cases of severe disease and death in humans.
  Unlike normal seasonal influenza, where infection causes only mild respiratory symptoms in most people, the disease caused by H5N1 follows an unusually aggressive clinical course, with rapid deterioration and high fatality.
  Primary viral pneumonia and multi-organ failure are common. In the present outbreak, more than half of those infected with the virus have died. Most cases have occurred in previously healthy children and young adults.

- A second risk, of even greater concern, is that the virus - if given enough opportunities - will change into a form that is highly infectious for humans and spreads easily from person to person. Such a change could mark the start of a global outbreak (a pandemic).

In the current outbreak, laboratory-confirmed human cases have been reported in four countries:
- Cambodia
- Indonesia
- Thailand
- Viet Nam

Hong Kong has experienced two outbreaks in the past. In 1997, in the first recorded instance of human infection with H5N1, the virus infected 18 people and killed 6 of them. In early 2003, the virus caused two infections, with one death, in a Hong Kong family with a recent travel history to southern China.

System of human infection

Direct contact with infected poultry, or surfaces and objects contaminated by their faeces, is presently considered the main route of human infection. To date, most human cases have occurred in rural or periurban areas where many households keep small poultry flocks, which often roam freely, sometimes entering homes or sharing outdoor areas where children play. As infected birds shed large quantities of virus in their faeces, opportunities for exposure to infected droppings or to environments contaminated by the virus are abundant under such conditions. Moreover, because many households in Asia depend on poultry for income and food, many families sell or slaughter and consume birds when signs of illness appear in a flock, and this practice has proved difficult to change. Exposure is considered most likely during slaughter, defeathering, butchering, and preparation of poultry for cooking.

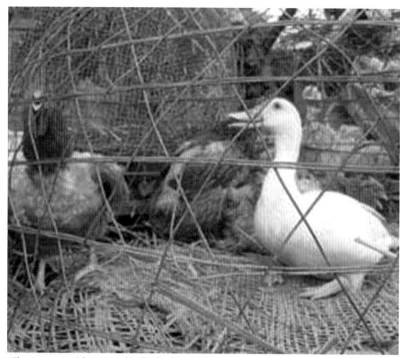

Close contact with various kinds of infected birds may cause transmission to humans.

■ *Poultry and poultry products*

Poultry and poultry products can safely be eaten, though certain precautions should be followed in countries currently experiencing outbreaks. In areas free of the disease, poultry and poultry products can be prepared and consumed as usual (following good hygienic practices and proper cooking), with no fear of acquiring infection with the H5N1 virus.

In areas experiencing outbreaks, poultry and poultry products can also be safely consumed provided these items are properly cooked and properly handled during food preparation. The H5N1 virus is sensitive to heat. Normal temperatures used for cooking (70 °C in all parts of the food) will kill the virus. Consumers need to be sure that all parts of the poultry are fully cooked (no "pink" parts) and that eggs, too, are properly cooked (no "runny" yolks).

Consumers should also be aware of the risk of cross-contamination. Juices from raw poultry and poultry products should never be allowed, during food preparation, to touch or mix with items eaten raw. When handling raw poultry or raw poultry products,

persons involved in food preparation should wash their hands thoroughly and clean and disinfect surfaces in contact with the poultry products Soap and hot water are sufficient for this purpose.

In areas experiencing outbreaks in poultry, raw eggs should not be used in foods that will not be further heat-treated as, for example by cooking or baking.

Avian influenza is not transmitted through cooked food. To date, no evidence indicates that anyone has become infected following the consumption of properly cooked poultry or poultry products, even when these foods were contaminated with the H5N1 virus.

Spread from birds to humans

The virus does not spread easily from birds to humans. Though more than 100 human cases have occurred in the current outbreak, this is a small number compared with the huge number of birds affected and the numerous associated opportunities for human exposure, especially in areas where

backyard flocks are common. It is not presently understood why some people, and not others, become infected following similar exposures.

Pandemic risk

- ▲ pandemic can start when three conditions have been met:
- ▲ a new influenza virus subtype emerges;
- ▲ it infects humans, causing serious illness;
- ▲ it spreads easily and sustainably among humans.

The H5N1 virus amply meets the first two conditions: it is a new virus for humans (H5N1 viruses have never circulated widely among people), and it has infected more than 100 humans, killing over half of them. No one will have immunity should an H5N1-like pandemic virus emerge.

All prerequisites for the start of a pandemic have therefore been met save one: the establishment of efficient and sustained human-to-human transmission of the virus.

The risk that the H5N1 virus will

B

Bird flu   Questions & Answers

What are the implications for human health?

The widespread persistence of H5N1 in poultry populations poses two main risks for human health.

▲ The first is the risk of direct infection when the virus passes from poultry to humans, resulting in very severe disease. Of the few avian influenza viruses that have crossed the species barrier to infect humans, H5N1 has caused the largest number of cases of severe disease and death in humans. Unlike normal seasonal influenza, where infection causes only mild respiratory symptoms in most people, the disease caused by H5N1 follows an unusually aggressive clinical course, with rapid deterioration and high fatality. Primary viral pneumonia and multi-organ failure are common. In the present outbreak, more than half of those infected with the virus have died. Most cases have occurred in previously healthy children and young adults.

▲ A second risk, of even greater concern, is that the virus – if given enough opportunities – will change into a form that is highly infectious for humans and spreads easily from person to person. Such a change could mark the start of a global outbreak (a pandemic).

Where have human cases occurred?

In the current outbreak, laboratory-confirmed human cases have been reported in six countries: Cambodia, Indonesia, Thailand, Turkey, China and Vietnam.

Hong Kong has experienced two outbreaks in the past. In 1997, in the first recorded instance of human infection with H5N1, the virus infected 18 people and killed 6 of them. In early 2003, the virus caused two infections, with one death, in a Hong Kong family with a recent travel history to southern China.

From the outbeaks in 2005 and 2005, the World Health Organization has reported 150 human cases, of which 82 people so far have died.

How do people become infected?

Direct contact with infected poultry, or surfaces and objects contaminated by their faeces, is presently considered the main route of human infection. To date, most human cases have occurred in rural or periurban areas where many households keep small poultry flocks, which often roam freely, sometimes entering homes or sharing outdoor areas where children play. As infected birds shed large quantities of virus in their faeces, opportunities for exposure to infected droppings or to environments contaminated by the virus are abundant under such conditions.

Is it safe to eat poultry and poultry products?

Yes, though certain precautions should be followed in countries currently experiencing outbreaks. In areas free of the disease, poultry and poultry products can be prepared and consumed as usual (following good hygienic practices and proper cooking), with no fear of acquiring infection with the H5N1 virus.

In areas experiencing outbreaks, poultry and poultry products can also be safely consumed provided these items are properly cooked and properly handled during food preparation. The H5N1 virus is sensitive to heat. Normal temperatures used for cooking (70°C in all parts of the food) will kill the virus. Consumers need to be sure that all parts of the poultry are fully cooked (no "pink" parts) and that eggs, too, are properly cooked (no "runny" yolks).

In areas experiencing outbreaks in poultry, raw eggs should not be used in foods that will not be further heat-treated as, for example by cooking or baking.

Avian influenza is not transmitted through cooked food. To date, no evidence indicates that anyone has become infected following the consumption of properly cooked poultry or poultry products, even when these foods were contaminated with the H5N1 virus.

acquire this ability will persist as long as opportunities for human infections occur. These opportunities, in turn, will persist as long as the virus continues to circulate in birds, and this situation could endure for some years to come.

■ *Reassortment and adaptive mutation*

The virus can improve its transmissibility among humans via two principal mechanisms.

▲ The first is a "reassortment" event, in which genetic material is exchanged between human and avian viruses during co-infection of a human or pig. Reassortment could result in a fully transmissible pandemic virus, announced by a sudden surge of cases with explosive spread.

▲ The second mechanism is a more gradual process of adaptive mutation, whereby the capability of the virus to bind to human cells increases during subsequent infections of humans.

Adaptive mutation, expressed initially as small clusters of human cases with some evidence of human-to-human transmission, would probably give the world some time to take defensive action.

Human-to-human transmission

The significance of limited human-to-human transmission is rare, but instances of limited human-to-human transmission of H5N1 and other avian influenza viruses have occurred in association with outbreaks in poultry and should not be a cause for alarm. In no instance has the virus spread beyond a first generation of close contacts or caused illness in the general community. Data from these incidents suggest that transmission requires very close contact with an ill person. Such incidents must be thoroughly investigated but - provided the investigation indicates that transmission from person to person is very limited - such incidents will not change the WHO overall assessment of the pandemic risk. There have been a number of instances of avian influenza infection occurring among close family members. It is often impossible to determine if human-to-human transmission has occurred since the family members are exposed to the same animal and environmental sources as well as to one another.

Pandemic influenza

The risk of pandemic influenza is serious. With the H5N1 virus now firmly entrenched in large parts of Asia, the risk that more human cases will occur will persist. Each additional human case gives the virus an opportunity to improve its transmissibility in humans, and thus develop into a pandemic strain.

The recent spread of the virus to poultry and wild birds in new areas further broadens opportunities for human cases to occur. While neither the timing nor the severity of the next pandemic can be predicted, the probability that a pandemic will occur has increased.

Treatment with medicines

Two drugs (in the neuraminidase inhibitors class), oseltamivir (commercially known as Tamiflu) and zanamivir (commercially known as Relenza) can reduce the severity and duration of illness caused by seasonal influenza. The efficacy of the neuraminidase inhibitors depends on their administration within 48 hours after symptom onset. For cases of human infection with H5N1, the drugs may improve prospects of survival, if administered early, but clinical data are limited. The H5N1 virus is expected to be susceptible to the neuraminidase inhibitors.

An older class of antiviral drugs, the M2 inhibitors amantadine and rimantadine, could potentially be used against pandemic influenza, but resistance to these drugs can develop rapidly and this could significantly limit their effectiveness against pandemic influenza. Some currently circulating H5N1 strains are fully resistant to these the M2 inhibitors. However, should a new virus emerge

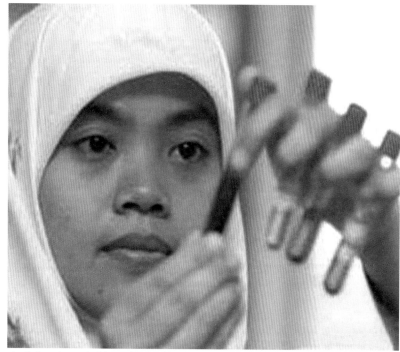

An Indonesian technician collecting blood samples from infected birds.

through reassortment, the M2 inhibitors might be effective.

For the neuraminidase inhibitors, the main constraints - which are substantial - involve limited production capacity and a price that is prohibitively high for many countries. At present manufacturing capacity, which has recently quadrupled, it will take a decade to produce enough oseltamivir to treat 20 percent of the world's population. The manufacturing process for oseltamivir is complex and time-consuming, and is not easily transferred to other facilities.

So far, most fatal pneumonia seen in cases of H5N1 infection has resulted from the effects of the virus, and cannot be treated with antibiotics.

Vaccination against bird flu in Indonesia. For animals a vaccine is available. Vaccines for humans against a pandemic virus are not yet available. Although a vaccine against H5NI virus for humans is under development in several countries, no vaccine is ready for commercial production and no vaccines are expected to be widely available until several months after the start of a pandemic.

Nonetheless, since influenza is often complicated by secondary bacterial infection of the lungs, antibiotics could be life-saving in the case of late-onset pneumonia. WHO regards it as prudent for countries to ensure adequate supplies of antibiotics in advance.

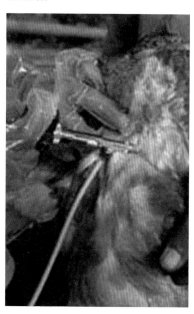

BLADDER ILLNESSES

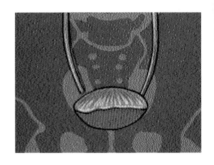

Introduction

The bladder is an expandable, muscular sac. Urine accumulates in the bladder as it is arriving from the kidneys via de ureters. The bladder gradually increases in size to accommodate an increasing volume of urine. When the bladder is full, nerve signals are sent to the brain to convey the need to urinate. A sphincter located at the bladder's outlet, where the bladder and urethra meet, opens to allow urine to flow out. Simultaneously, the bladder wall contracts automatically, creating pressure that forces the urine down the urethra. Voluntarily tightening the muscles of the abdominal wall assists by adding extra pressure. The sphincters through which the ureters enter the bladder remain tightly shut to prevent urine from flowing back up the ureters toward the kidneys.

Major disorders of the bladder are:
- urinary incontinence;
- infection of the bladder (*cystitis*);
- bladder cancer.

Urinary incontinence

Definition
Incontinence is the involuntary loss of urine. It is a symptom that may be manifested regardless of age. It should not be considered a natural consequence of ageing. Classification includes:
- stress incontinence;
- urge or reflex incontinence;
- overflow incontinence;
- continuous or total incontinence;
- mixed incontinence;
- functional incontinence.

Physiology of continence
In a normal woman continence is maintained by five mechanisms.

- The bladder detrusor muscle comprises most of the bladder musculature and is that portion of the bladder which contracts to effect micturition. It is stimulated by cholinergic receptors that are under the control of sacral parasympathetic nerves.
- The bladder neck (internal sphincter) is closed when the bladder is fully distended. It is rich in adrenergic receptors. The upper one-third of the urethra lies above the pelvic diaphragm. Therefore, in normal circumstances, any abdominal pressure is transmitted equally to the bladder and the proximal urethra, effectively preventing leakage of urine.
- The muscles of the urethra consist of longitudinal and circular fibers, primarily of smooth muscle, surrounded by modified striated muscle. In its resting state, the urethra is held closed by these muscles, which are also rich in alpha-adrenergic receptors.
- The external sphincter is a ring of striated muscle surrounding the distal urethra. This sphincter is under voluntary control. Although it may be used to interrupt the urinary stream, it does not have sufficient tone in the resting state to preserve continence in the absence of proper bladder neck function.
- The inner lining (mucosa) of the urethra is under estrogenic influence, and undergoes atrophic changes at the time of menopause. This can be severe enough to cause incontinence or contribute to stress incontinence.

Stress incontinence
Stress incontinence is the inability to hold urine when intra-abdominal pressure is increased. Activities that commonly precipitate episodes of stress urinary incontinence include:
- coughing;
- laughing;
- straining;
- dancing;
- sneezing;
- lifting;
- bending;
- jogging.

Stress urinary incontinence must be distinguished from "giggle" incontinence, a cerebrospinal reflex phenomenon seen in some adolescent girls who experience leakage of urine when they giggle but not during other activities related to stress urinary incontinence.

Stress urinary incontinence is most often associated with a history of vaginal delivery, ageing (estrogen deficiency), obesity, chronic cough (asthma, smoking), or chronic obstipation.

The etiological factors enumerated above can cause the bladder neck and upper one-third of the urethra to prolapse through the pelvic diaphragm. When this happens, coughing, straining, and other manoeuvres that increase intra-abdominal pressure will transmit this pressure to the bladder detrusor muscle but not to the bladder neck or the urethra, in which case abdominal pressure in the bladder will be greater than pressure in the outflow tract, resulting in loss of urine.

Pelvic (Kegel) exercises are designed to improve the strength of the pelvic floor musculature, which in turn will suspend the proximal urethra. They often are helpful for women with mild to moderate stress urinary incontinence not associated with a large cystocele or rectocele.

Estrogen therapy counteracts atrophy of the inner lining of the urethra, which is a contributing factor to stress urinary incontinence in post-menopausal women. A vaginal estro-gen creme such as conjugated equine estrogens, 2,5 g three times a week for 12 weeks, inserted using a vaginal applicator, may be prescribed for postmenopausal women with stress urinary incontinence.

A wide variety of operations continue to be used to stress urinary inconti-nence. Most surgical procedures are aimed at elevating the bladder neck and bringing the proximal urethra back into the abdominal cavity. Most women with moderate to severe symptoms fail to improve with con-servative management and require an operation.

Urge incontinence

Urge or reflex incontinence is sudden voiding caused by involuntary bladder contraction. Besides sudden loss of urine, which is perceived by the patient, symptoms include frequency and urgency. In contrast to stress uri-nary incontinence, in which loss of urine is associated only with activities that increase intra-abdominal pres-sure, urine loss can occur at any time. Most commonly, involuntary bladder contractions occur without a known neurologic lesions. Such idiopathic urge incontinence is termed detrusor instability. Approximately 20 per cent of adult women suffer from it, and the incidence rises with age.

Involuntary bladder contraction may result from a known underlying neu-rological condition (for example, cerebrovascular accident, Parkinson's disease, prolapsed intervertebral disk, spinal cord injury, or multiple sclero-sis). This is then termed hyperreflexic bladder.

The drugs used to control detrusor instability or hyperreflexia are prima-rily anticholinergic agents. The dosage needed to control bladder contrac-tions may lead to side effects such as dryness of the mouth or constipation.

Patients with severe symptoms who do not respond to pharmacologic treatment may benefit from disten-tion of the bladder with 1-2 litre of water. The procedure is performed under epidural block. If successful, it may be repeated as needed for recur-rence of symptoms.

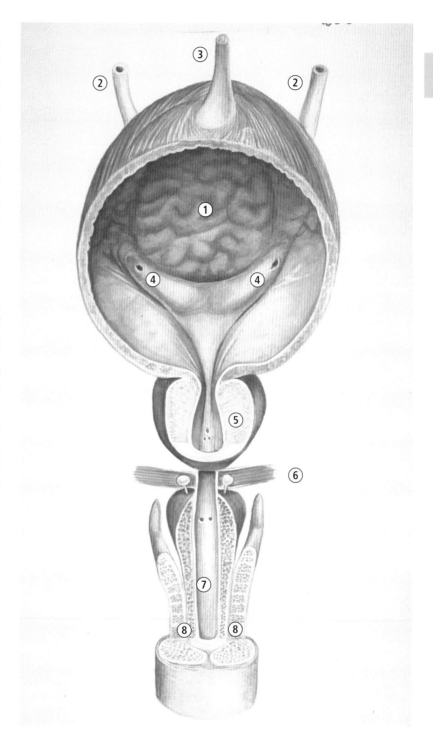

Schematic drawing of the male urinary sys-tem.
1. Inner part of the bladder
2. urethra
3. ureter
4. opening of the urethra
5. prostate gland
6. muscle of the pelvic floor
7. urethra
8. corpora cavernosa

Incontinence Questions & Answers

What is urinary incontinence?

Urinary incontinence is involuntary loss of urine during the day or night. Urge incontinence is characterized principally by an urgent desire to void followed by involuntary loss of urine.

It may occur alone or with varying degrees of stress incontinence. In the absence of urinary tract infection the most common causes are:

▲ neurological bladder disorder;

▲ multiple sclerosis;

▲ bladder stones;

▲ tumor.

The therapy is directed towards the underlying cause.

What is stress incontinence?

Stress incontinence is the involuntary loss of urine on coughing, straining, sneezing, lifting, or any manoeuvre that suddenly increases the pressure in the abdominal cavity. In men, stress incontinence is seen occasionally following an operation on the prostate gland or trauma to the bladder neck.

In women, stress incontinence is the most common cause of involuntary loss of urine. It is usually due caused by multiple pregnancy or aging. Mild cases may respond to a series of specific exercises of the muscles of the pelvic floor (Kegel's exercises). More severe cases require surgical correction.

How occurs overflow incontinence?

Overflow incontinence occurs when the bladder becomes acutely or chronically overdistended and the pressure in the urinary bladder increases overcoming the resistance of the bladder sphincter.

Urine than dribbles from the urethra, and the patient may be unable to initiate or maintain a good urinary stream. The condition is usually associated with a disorder of the urethra or spinal cord.

What are the characteristic symptoms of total incontinence of the urinary bladder?

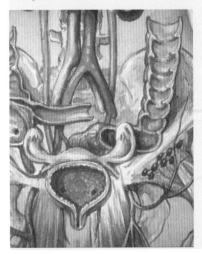

Total incontinence of the urinary bladder sphincter is characterized by a constant involuntary dripping of urine from the urethra day and night without bladder distention. The condition is usually due to trauma or damage to the bladder neck. Surgical procedures are the only treatment.

Psychogenic incontinence is occasionally seen in children and even in adults who have underlying emotional disturbances. Diagnosis can be established only after all other causes of incontinence are ruled out. Treatment consists of medicines and psychotherapy.

Overflow incontinence

In this condition, the patient has chronic urinary retention. Eventually, there is sufficient urine in the bladder to result in involuntary overflow, resulting in incontinence.

The most common cause of overflow incontinence is diabetes, which greatly reduces detrusor activity. Other neurologic deficits that may cause detrusor atony include lumbosacral nerve disease (for instance, compression from prolapsed intervertebral disc, spinal tumors, myelomeningocele, multiple sclerosis) and high spinal cord injury.

The role of surgery in treating outflow obstruction is limited to the correction of urethral obstruction. Appropriate operations include urethral dilation for stricture and correction of urethral angulation. Sphincterectomy may be performed in spinal cord injury patients who are unable to relax the sphincter.

Continuous incontinence

In sharp contrast to the preceding types of incontinence, in which the patient can always tell when urine loss occurs, leakage of urine is imperceptible to the patient with continuous or total incontinence. She is generally unaware of her incontinence as it occurs.

Multiple operations on the urethra may cause severe periurethral fibrosis, precluding proper closure of the urethra and resulting in urethral incompetence.

The failure to perceive urination is critical. Predisposing conditions, such as prior irradiation, will be sought by the doctor. Physical examination of the vestibule in incontinent children may reveal congenital abnormalities. Treatment is determined by the primary cause. Continuous incontinence resulting from urethral fibrosis may be managed by the pubovaginal sling procedure, periurethral injection, or an artificial urinary sphincter.

Mixed and functional incontinence

In many patients, a history of severe urgency and less of urine may be concomitant with a history of loss of urine during coughing, sneezing, or walking. Such a combination of symptoms may result from an overactive detrusor muscle in combination with an incompetent urethra.

Some women with incontinence may have normal bladder and urethral function with no detectable abnormality on urodynamic testing. Patients with Alzheimer's disease, Parkinson's disease, or severe arthritis may find it difficult to reach the bathroom and undress themselves in time to urinate in the appropriate place.

Easy accessibility and availability of toilet facilities as well as possible clothing modifications are important factors in maintaining continence, and thereby dignity, in this group.

Bladder infections

Cystitis is an infection of the inner lining of the urinary bladder. The urinary bladder is a membranous sac serving as receptacle for the collection and secretion of urine. The organ is connected to the outside of the body by the urethra.

The urinary bladder, which is generally referred to simply as the bladder, is a hollow organ lying behind the junction of the pubic bones (symphysis) and in front of the rectum, and is surrounded by peritoneum. The empty bladder is the size of an orange, with a very thick wall and practically no central cavity.

Both kidneys secrete a steady stream of urine droplets and these are stored in the reservoir of the bladder. The capacity of the bladder is so great that, under normal conditions, it needs only be emptied once or twice every 24 hours.

Depending upon age, its maximum capacity ranges from 200 to 900 mL, but when the bladder contains about 400 mL in adults, all the sensory nerves in the area are stimulated, and this brings about contraction of the bladder muscles so that urination can take place.

The inner lining of the bladder consists of a layer of mucous membrane which, when the bladder is empty, falls into many folds. Next there are three layers of smooth muscle fibers that enable the bladder to adapt itself to the varying content.

At the outlet of the bladder, this muscular tissue forms a ring or sphincter,

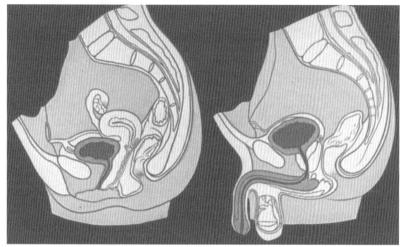

Side view of the lower part of the trunk. Topography of the urinary bladder. Left: the female bladder is located between the symphysis and vagina/uterus. Right: the male bladder is located between the symphysis and rectum.

which is regulated by the voluntary nervous system. The sphincter, which consists partly of smooth and partly of striated muscle tissue, serves to regulate the discharge of urine from the bladder.

The tension (tone) of the muscles of the bladder wall and that of the sphincter muscles are mutually adjusted. Thus, when the bladder is extremely full, tension is high in the wall muscles, and in the striated muscle of the sphincter, up until the moment when a signal from the brain opens it to allow urine to pass.

The emptying of the bladder is brought about by an intricate system of nerve signals. In infants there is only one reflex: when the bladder wall is stretched to a certain point, urination occurs. During the second year of life, conscious control of the bladder function generally takes over, and as a result, children become capable of controlling their urination voluntarily.

Causes

Bladder infections are common in women, particularly during the reproductive years. Some women develop bladder infections repeatedly. Bacteria in the vagina may travel to the urethra and into the bladder.

Women often develop bladder infections after engaging in sexual intercourse, probably because the urethra

was bruised during sex. The most common cause of recurring bladder infection of the prostate.

The majority of women experience at least one such infection in the course of a lifetime and 20 per cent of women have had more than one episode.

Escherichia coli is responsible for the majority of urinary tract infections acquired outside the hospital. Enterobacter aerogenes frequently

Cystitis

Factors contributing to bacterial urinary tract infections

Ascending infections

- Blockage (for example, by stones) anywhere in the urinary tract.
- Abnormal bladder function that prevents proper emptying, such as occurs in neurological diseases.
- Leaking of the valve between the ureter and the bladder.
- Insertion of a urinary catheter or an instrument by a doctor.

Blood-borne infections

- Infection in the bloodstream.
- Infection of the heart valves.

B

Cystitis   Questions & Answers

How are bladder diseases examined?

A special method for examination of the bladder is cystoscopy. This endoscopic technique is useful for the direct examination of the inside of the bladder.

The thin cystoscope uses a system of lenses to illuminate the bladder and is inserted through the urethra. Cystoscopy may show stones, infections and tumors, but also abnormalities in the transport of urine through one of the ureters.

What is a cystitis?

Cystitis is bacterial infection. It is a common bladder disorder, especially in women. Normal urine is usually almost free of bacteria, but there are many bacteria around the anus, and on the skin surrounding the exit of the urethra.

When the bladder is not working properly and, at the same time, the lower part of the body is chilled in cold weather, bacteria may invade the urethra and cause inflammation of the bladder.

What are the symptoms of the acute form of cystitis?

The acute form of cystitis is characterized by a frequent urge to urinate; such urination is painful and only small amounts of urine are passed. There is pain just before and after urination, and blood often appears at the end as well. Depending on the type of bacteria present, a specific type medicine will be administered.

What are the causes of a chronic cystitis?

A chronic, long-lasting infection may be due, among other conditions, to a stone in the bladder, to a tumor or to obstruction of the urethra. A urologist is usually called upon for advice and treatment.

How are stones formed in the urinary bladder?

Stones in the bladder are either formed on the spot or descend into the bladder from the kidneys. They almost invariably give rise to painful and copious urination and sometimes cause blood in the urine.

Occasionally the sufferer notices that the stream of his or her urine is suddenly broken off. This can happen when the stone in the bladder blocks off the urethral entrance. The doctor will always seek to confirm the presence of a bladder stone by means of a cystoscope or X-rays. When using a cystoscope the doctor can sometimes dispose of the stone immediately by crushing it up and washing the fragments away.

How can I prevent bladder infection?

▲ Drink lots of fluid every day. Try to drink a glass of water every two or three hours. For active infection, drink enough to pour out a good stream of urine every hour.

▲ Urinate frequently and try to empty your bladder completely each time. Never try to hold your urine once your bladder feels full.

▲ Keep the bacteria in your bowels and anus away from your urethra by wiping yourself front to back after urinating or having a bowel movement. Wash your genitals from front to back with plain water or very mild soap at least once a day.

▲ Any sexual activity that irritates the urethra, puts pressure on the bladder or spreads bacteria from the anus to the vagina or urethra can contribute to cystitis (bladder infection). If you tend to get cystitis after sex despite a number of precautions, you may want to ask your doctor for preventive tablets (i.e. sulfa, ampicillin, nitrofurantoin); a single dose of a tablet after sex has been shown effective in preventing infections and is usually not associated with the same negative effects as prolonged courses of antibiotics.

▲ Some birth control methods can contribute to or aggravate a urinary tract infection. Women who take oral contraceptives have a higher rate of cystitis than those not on the pill. Some diaphragm users find that the rim pressing against the urethra and contribute to infection.

▲ If you use sanitary napkins during your period, the blood on the pad provides a convenient bridge for bacteria from your anus to travel to your urethra. Change pads frequently and wash your genitals twice a day when you are menstruating.

▲ Tight jeans, bicycling or horseback riding may cause trauma to the urethra. When you engage in sports that can provoke cystitis in you, wear loose clothing and try to drink extra water.

▲ Caffeine and alcohol irritate the bladder. If you don't want to stop using them, try to drink less of them and drink enough water to dilute them.

▲ Diets high in refined sugars and starches may predispose some women to urinary tract infections.

▲ Keep up your resistance by eating and resting well and finding ways to reduce stress in your life as much as possible.

causes such infections as well. Postmenopausal women are especially susceptible to bacterial colonisation of the urinary tract because of atrophic vaginal and urethral mucosal lining. Any condition that causes incomplete emptying of the bladder (for instance, meatal stenosis, urethral stricture, infrequent voiding) is associated with an increased incidence of urinary tract infections.

Symptoms

Bladder infections usually produce a frequent, urgent desire to urinate and a burning or painful sensation during urination. Frequency, urgency and dysuria are characteristic. The dysuria (pain during urination) is experienced at the end of urination in contrast to the dysuria of vulvitis, which occurs at the beginning of voiding. Pain of a sensation of heaviness may be present in the suprapubic region. Gross hematuria (blood in the urine may be present. Fever is rarely present in patients with cystitis.

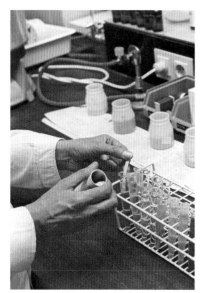

Laboratory analysis of urine to investigate the cause of bladder infections.

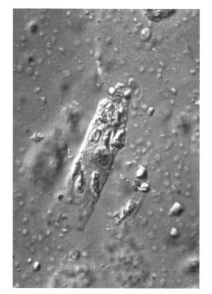

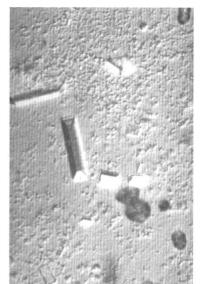

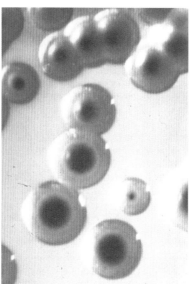

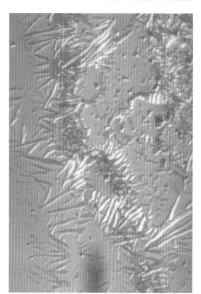

Diagnosis

The diagnosis of a urinary tract infection is made by appropriate examination of a midstream clean-catch urine specimen. A presumptive diagnosis may be established immediately on the basis of dipstick or microscopic examination of a urine specimen.

Microscopic examination of a spun sediment reveals numerous white blood cells and bacteria. A definite diagnosis is established with urine culture, which identifies both the pathogen and its spectrum of antibiotic sensitivity.

Treatment

Pending culture results, empiric antibiotic therapy may be instituted in patients with symptoms suggestive of urinary tract infection. Asymptomatic bacteriuria and community-acquired cystitis are usually caused by Escherichia coli, which is sensitive to a wide variety of antimicrobial agents. The treatment regimen should begin with an antimicrobial drug to which the organism Escherichia coli is sensitive. Therapy may be revised later if the patient does not respond and if the culture and sensitivity report demonstrates that the pathogen is resistant to the chosen antimicrobial agent. One should drink at least 2 litres of fluid daily. Often, symptoms

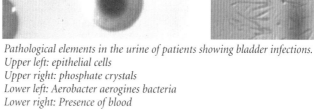

Pathological elements in the urine of patients showing bladder infections.
Upper left: epithelial cells
Upper right: phosphate crystals
Lower left: Aerobacter aerogines bacteria
Lower right: Presence of blood

can be relieved by making the urine alkaline, which involves drinking baking soda dissolved in water.

Bladder cancer

The urinary bladder may be the site of benign and malignant tumors. Most bladder cancers develop in the inside

lining of the bladder. The cancer often looks like a small mushroom attached to the bladder wall. It may also be called a papillary tumor. Often, more than one tumor is present. Research shows clearly that environmental agents are a leading cause of bladder cancer, and evidence points to aniline dye, used in rubber and cable industries, as a specific causative agent. It was demonstrated that the compound betanaphthylamine, used in the dye manufacturing process, was carcinogenic. This substance belongs to a group of chemicals called aromatic hydrocarbons.

An association between smoking and cancer of the bladder has been reported in several studies and some scientists believe that the role of smoking as a causative factor is well-established. Schistosomiasis, a parasitic infection that irritates the bladder, common in some parts of the world, is another environmental cause.

Symptoms

The most common warning sign of bladder cancer is blood in the urine. Depending on the amount of blood present, the colour of the urine can turn faintly rusty to deep red. Pain during urination can also be a sign of bladder cancer. A need to urinate often or urgently may be another warning sign. Often, bladder tumors cause no symptoms.

When symptoms do occur, they are not sure signs of cancer. They may also be caused by infections, benign tumors, bladder stones, or other problems. It is important to see a physician to find out the cause of the symptoms. Any illness should be diagnosed and treated as early as possible.

Diagnosis

To diagnose bladder cancer, the physician will take the patient's medical history and do a complete physical examination. Sometimes, the physician can feel a large tumor during a rectal or vaginal examination. In addition, urine samples are checked under the microscope to see whether any cancer cells are present.

Often, the physician wants to have an X-ray called an intravenous pyelogram (IVP). This test lets the physician see the kidneys, ureters, and bladder on an X-ray.

An IVP normally causes little discomfort, although a few patients have nausea, dizziness, or pain from the procedure.

The physician may also look directly into the bladder with an instrument called a cystoscope. In this test, a thin, lighted tube is inserted into the bladder through the urethra. If the physi-

cian sees any abnormal areas, samples of tissue can be removed through the cystoscope. This is called a biopsy. A pathologist examines the tissue under the microscope to see whether cancer cells are present. A biopsy is needed to make a definite diagnosis of bladder cancer.

Treatment

Treatment for bladder cancer depends on a number of factors. Among these are how quickly the cancer is growing; the number, size, and location of the tumors; whether the cancer has spread to other organs, and the patient's age and general health. The physician will develop a treatment plan to fit each patient's need.

■ Staging

Before treatment begins, it is important for the physician to know exactly where the cancer is located and whether it has spread from its original location. Staging procedures include a complete physical examination and additional blood tests and scans.

The physician may want the patient to have a CT-scan. A CT-scan is a series of X-rays put together by a computer to form a three-dimensional picture. Ultrasound is a procedure that creates pictures of the inside of the body using high-frequency sound waves. The echoes make an image on a video screen that is much like a television.

Sometimes the physician asks for magnetic resonance imaging (MRI). In this scan, a cross-sectional image (like a CT-scan) is produced on a screen with the use of a powerful magnet instead of X-rays.

■ Planning treatment

Before starting treatment, the patient might want a doctor to review the diagnosis and the suggested treatment plan. A short delay will not reduce the chances that treatment will be successful.

There are a number of ways to get a second opinion. The patient's physician can discuss the case with other physicians who treat bladder cancer. Patients may also get the name of another physician from the local medical society, nearby hospitals or medical universities, and asks for detailed information.

■ Methods of treatment

Early (superficial) bladder cancer (in which the tumors are found on the inside surface of the bladder wall) generally can be treated using the cystoscope in a procedure called transurethral resection. The cystoscope can remove all or part of the tumor or destroy it with an electric current.

When several tumors are present in the bladder or when there is a risk that the cancer will recur, transurethral resection may be followed by treatment with drugs. Anticancer drugs (chemotherapy) may be put directly into the bladder.

Radiation therapy (also called radiotherapy) may be needed when the cancer cannot be removed with transurethral resection because it involves a larger area of the bladder. X-rays destroy the ability of cancer cells to grow and multiply. Internal radiation therapy, with the radioactive material placed in the bladder, which comes from a machine located outside the body. For internal radiation therapy, radioactive material is inserted into the bladder through the cystoscope. This puts cancer-killing rays as close as possible to the side of the cancer while sparing most of the healthy tissues around it. The patient stays in the hospital for this treatment for between 4 and 7 days. For external radiation treatments, the patient goes to the hospital or clinic each day. Usually, treatments are given 5 days a week for 5 to 6 weeks. This schedule helps to protect normal tissue by spreading out the total dose radiation.

When the cancer involves much of the surface of the bladder or has grown into the bladder wall, standard treatment is to remove the entire bladder. In this operation, the surgeon removes the bladder as well as nearby organs. In women, this operation includes removing the uterus, fallopian tubes, ovaries, and part of the vagina. In men, the prostate gland and seminal vesicles are removed. Research is under way to find treatments that spare the bladder.

When cancer involves the pelvis or has spread to other parts of the body, the physician may suggest chemotherapy, the use of anticancer drugs that travel through the bloodstream to reach cancer cells in all parts of the body. Drugs used to treat cancer may be given in different ways: some are given by mouth; others are injected into a muscle or a blood vessel. Chemotherapy is usually given in cycles - a treatment period, followed by a rest period, than another treatment period, and so on. The patient usually receives chemotherapy as an outpatient at the hospital, at the doctor's office, or a home. Sometimes the patient may need to stay in the hospital for a short while.

Side effects of treatment

The methods used to treat bladder cancer are very powerful. It is hard to limit the effects of treatment so that only cancer cells are destroyed; healthy tissue may also be damaged. That is why treatment may cause unpleasant side effects. Side effects depend on the type of treatment used and on the part of the body being treated.

When the bladder is removed, the patient needs a new way to store and pass urine. Various methods are used. In one, the surgeon uses a piece of the person's small intestine to form a new pipeline. The ureters are attached to one end, and the other end is brought out through an opening in the wall of the abdomen. This new opening is called a stoma. It is also called an ostomy or a urostomy. A flat bag fits over the stoma to collect urine and it is held in place with a special adhesive. A specially trained nurse or enterostomal therapist will show the patient how to care for the ostomy.

A new method uses part of the small intestine to make a new storage pouch (called a continent reservoir) inside the body. The urine collects there and does not empty into a bag. Instead, the patient learns to use a tube (catheter) to drain the urine through the stoma. Other methods are being developed that connect a pouch made

from the small intestine to a remaining part of the urethra. When this procedure is possible, a stoma and a bag are not necessary because urine leaves the body through the urethra.

Radical cystectomy causes infertility in both men and women. This operation can also lead to sexual problems. In the past, nearly all men were impotent after this procedure, but improvements in surgery have made it possible to prevent this in many men. In women, the vagina may be narrower or shallower, and intercourse may be difficult. During radiation therapy, patients may become very tired as the treatment continues. Rasing as much as possible is important. radiation therapy to the lower abdomen may cause nausea, vomiting, or diarrhea. Usually, the physician can suggest certain foods or medications to ease these problems. Radiation therapy can also cause problems with fertility and can make sexual intercourse uncomfortable.

Chemotherapy causes side effects because it damages not only cancer cells but other rapidly growing cells as well. The side effects of chemotherapy depend on the specific drugs that are given. In addition, each patient reacts differently. Chemotherapy commonly

affects blood-forming cells and cells that line the digestive tract.

As a result, patients may have side effects such as lowered resistance and vomiting, less energy, and mouth sores. They may also lose their hair. These are short-term side effects that usually end after treatment stops. When drugs are put directly into the bladder, these side effects may be limited. However, it is common for the bladder to be irritated. Loss of appetite can be a serious problem for patients during therapy. Patients who eat well may be better able to withstand the side effects of their treatment, so good nutrition is an important part of the treatment plan. Eating well means getting enough calories to prevent weight loss and having enough protein to build and repair muscles, organs, skin, and hair.

Many patients find that eating several small meals and snacks during the day is easier than trying to eat three large meals. The side effects that patients have during cancer treatment vary for each person. They may even be different from one treatment to the next. Physicians try to plan treatment to keep problems to a minimum. Fortunately, most side effects are temporary.

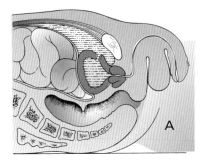
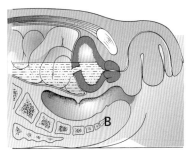
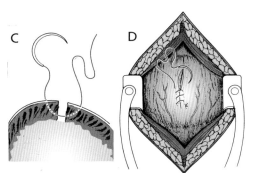

Management of ruptured bladder. Extraperitoneal rupture (A); intraperitoneal rupture (B); repairing an intraperitoneal tear with seromuscular stitches, taking care not to include the mucosa (C, D); burying the first layer of seromuscular stitches with a second (E).

BRAIN CANCER

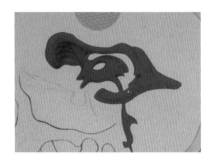

Description

Cancers of the brain, like other cancers, are diseases of the body's cells. Although cells of various organs differ in shape and function, all cells reproduce themselves by dividing. Normal growth and repair of tissue take place in this orderly manner. When cell division is not orderly and controlled, abnormal growth occurs. Cancers that begin in the brain or spinal cord seldom spread (metastasize) to other locations. But metastasis to the brain from cancers of other body sites is common.

Lateral view of the brain (MRI-scan).

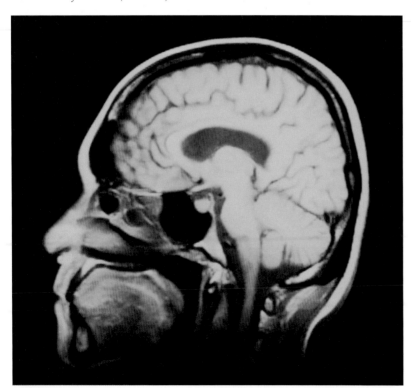

Symptoms

Brain cancer symptoms are varied and depend upon what part of the brain is involved. Any of the symptoms may be caused by a condition other than cancer. Brain tumors show a number of general symptoms such as headaches, a dull feeling in the head, vomiting, dilation of the pupil in the eye, epilepsy, bradypsychism and bradycardia, all dependent on the location of the tumor. However, one should realize that these symptoms are not specific; headache is, in 99 per cent of cases, not a sign of a brain tumor.

■ *Headache*
Headaches are the most common symptom. They may indicate a growing tumor's increasing pressure on normal tissue in and around the brain. Any new or persistent severe headache should be reported to a physician. Headache often occurs in form of attacks, which may be severe, and sometimes unbearable, for the patient. Often the patient reports that the headaches are most violent in the early hours of the morning and subsequently decrease gradually.
A more specific location of headache, however severe, rarely yields any information as to the site of the tumor. For instance, a tumor in the back part of the skull may cause pain at the back of the head, but it may also give rise to pain exclusively in the forehead. With other tumors in other regions, the headache may also be felt some distance away from the site of the tumor. In the case of some tumors located near the surface of the skull, a constant, strictly localized headache may give an indication as to the site, but these are exceptions.
Finally, it should be noted that headache may also be completely absent in some cases of brain tumor. Furthermore, it is often noted that a headache that is present at first may disappear completely, for some inexplicable reason, during the subsequent course of the disease.

■ *Dull feeling in the head*
This constitutes a second group of vague but very frequent symptoms of a brain tumor. There may be a dull feeling in the head, dizziness and other vague complaints. If the dizziness is accompanied by attacks in which there is also a sensation of rotation and a tendency to fall, it is probably that the brain tumor will be locat-

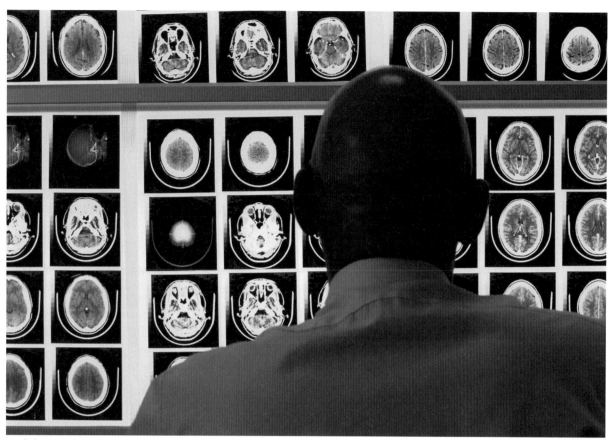

Radiologist studying brain scans.

ed in the back part of the brain. However, tumors in other regions may also bring about such a dizziness, because the increased pressure in the brain may be transmitted to one or both labyrinths, the organ of balance (equilibrium) in the inner ears. If the complaints of the patient about a decreased mental capacity can be recorded objectively, this symptom, too, may help, in a limited way, to locate the site of the tumor.

■ Vomiting
Vomiting due to a disorder of the function of the brain may often be recognized because of its sudden explosive character and the almost complete absence of either preceding or subsequent nausea. The attacks of vomiting and headache may often coincide. The frequency of the vomiting is highly variable. If vomiting is the initial symptom and is a frequent daily occurrence, it constitutes an argument

in favour of the tumor being located in the back part of the brain.

■ Dilation of the pupil of the eye
This is in principle an objective sign. It may be present for a long time before any disorder of vision occurs. In more than 95 per cent of the cases of dilation of the pupil of the eye, there exists a space-occupying tumor in the brain. If the dilation of the pupil is much more pronounced in one eye than in the other, it generally constitutes an argument in favour of the location of the tumor in the cerebral hemisphere on the same side as the eye with the greater amount of congestion.

■ Epilepsy
The occurrence of epileptic attacks is very frequent, and usually an early symptom of a brain tumor. It is very useful for physicians of they can supplement the date of the person's medical history by personal observation of

an attack. Brain tumors give rise to epilepsy in the majority of cases. If the epileptic attacks repeatedly exhibit certain constant focal phenomena, and this applies particularly to Jacksonian attacks, it is possible to determine the site of the tumor with a greater or lesser degree of certainty on the basis of these findings.

■ Bradypsychism
A general slowing-down of the psychological process - bradypsychism - is a symptom that is frequently encountered, particularly in the case of large tumors in the cerebral hemispheres. Occasionally, the patient exhibits more extensive psychological disorders, sometimes even genuine psychoses, and these will cause major problems in daily living.

■ Bradycardia
Sometimes a slowing down of heart activity (bradycardia) is noticed.

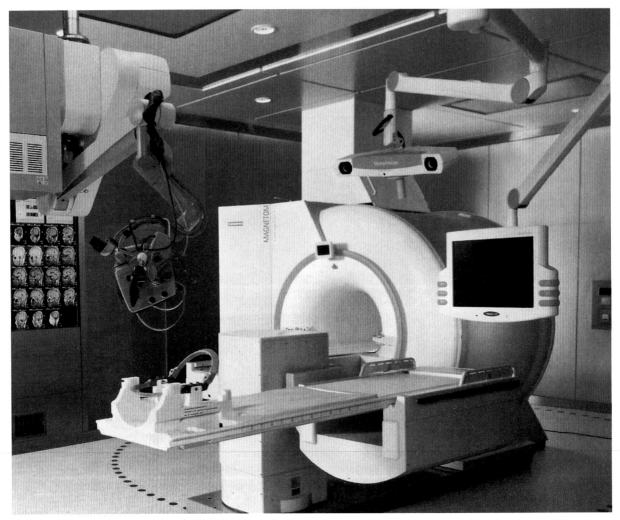

Apparatus for magnetic resonance imaging (MRI).
Medical images can be produced by the interaction of biological tissue (for example the brain or spinal cord) with a number of different types of electromagnetic radiation. Biological tissue is generally opaque to intermediate wavelength radiation, such as the ultraviolet, infrared, or microwave bands. However, the body is relatively transparent to short wavelength radiation (e.g. X-rays) which interact with atomic electrons, and to long wavelength, low frequency radio waves which interact with atomic nuclei.
Radiographic techniques (conventional X-ray, or X-ray computerized tomography) produce a shadow image resulting from the attenuation of X-ray photons by the body. Contrast differences are based on variations in tissue density, which are often very small. Overlapping structures are indistinguishable unless an alternate imaging angle is available. Furthermore, the use of ionizing radiation may entail unacceptably large doses when the need for serial monitoring is indicated.
Images can also be produced using ultrasound, where the signal brightness is the result of the relative amount of reflected signal. Ultrasound techniques avoid the use of ionizing radiation, but offer relatively poor spatial resolution. Further, ultrasound is limited by the availability of a clear acoustic window between the external surface and the region of interest. This is especially restrictive in thoracic imaging where bone and lung tissue overlap.
Magnetic resonance images, however, are noninvasive, do not employ ionizing radiation, and rely on a different principle for image production. A magnetic resonance image represents the relative response of specific nuclei to absorb radio frequency energy.
Like radiography or ultrasound, this image is a function of density - in this case, the distribution of nuclei being observed. However, image contrast is influenced by other physical factors, including differences in the ability to re-emit the absorbed radio frequency signal, and flow phenomena.
MRI offers the unique ability to acquire images in virtually any orientation, without repositioning the patient. This translates into greater convenience for medical staff and minimized patient discomfort. Plus, magnetic resonance provides chemical information not measurable with conventional radiography or ultrasonography. It is the combination of versatility, sensitivity and specificity as a diagnostic modality that has accelerated the acceptance of MRI.

Local symptom of brain tumors

The local symptoms are listed in the order in which they usually occur.

- Left frontal area
  - Epileptic attacks
  - Psychological disorders
  - Motor aphasia (difficulty in speaking)
  - Hemiparesis (slight paralysis of one side of the body)

- Right frontal area
  - Epileptic attacks
  - Psychological disorders
  - Hemiparesis

- Left temporal area
  - Epileptic attacks
  - Sensory aphasia (difficulty in understanding speech)
  - Hemiparesis
  - Hemianopia (loss of half the usual area of vision)
  - Psychological disorders

- Right temporal area
  - Epileptic attacks
  - Hemiparesis
  - Hemianopia
  - Psychological disorders

- Cerebellum
  - Ataxia (uncoordinated movement) with decreased tendon reflexes
  - Corneal areflexia (inability of the cornea of the eye to react to light)
  - Nystagmus (fine, jerky movements of the eyeballs)

- Midbrain
  - Diminished reactions of the pupils of the eyes
  - Vertical disorder of gaze
  - Ataxia
  - Increased tendon reflexes

- Brain stem
  - Horizontal disorders of gaze
  - Alternating hemiplegia (severe paralysis of one side of the body)
  - Absence of dilation of pupil of the eye

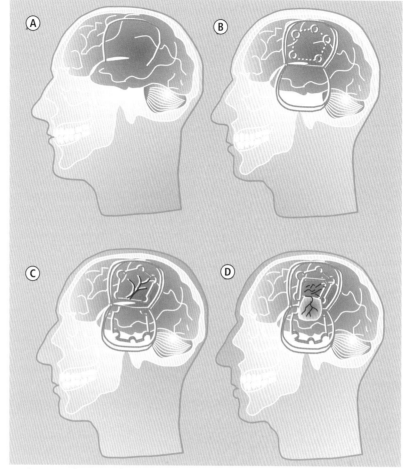

Brain surgery for a superficially located brain tumor.
A-D various phases od the operation.

Diagnosis

Diagnosis by a physician starts with questions about symptoms, followed by an examination for physical signs that may point to a tumor.

Examination of the eye with an instrument called an ophthalmoscope lets the physician see the retina (the sensory membrane on the inside of the eye) and the optic nerve, which connects the retina with the brain.

A tumor pressing anywhere along the route of this nerve swells it, causing a visible condition called papilloedema. The physician may also check your muscle function, reflexes and ability to feel pin pricks.

A number of specific examinations to detect brain tumors are now available.

Treatment

Your physician will consider a number of factors in determining the best treatment for you. Among these are your medical history, your general health, and the type and location of the tumor you have. Cancerous brain tumors may be treated by surgery, radiation or anticancer drugs. These methods are often used in combination. Your treatment must be tailored to your individual needs.

Surgery is the oldest method of treating brain tumors. Steady advances have been made since the first operations, beginning this century. A brain surgeon (neurosurgeon) may be able to completely remove a benign tumor or cancer that is encapsulated (enclosed in a membrane or sac).

BREAST CANCER

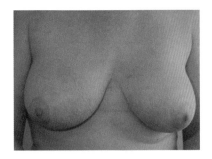

Description

Women's breast come in sizes and shapes. Each woman's breasts change during her life because of age, the monthly menstrual cycle, pregnancy, menopause, or taking birth control pills or other hormones. Besides normal changes in sizes and shapes also pathological growth can occur in the breasts, both benign and malignant (cancer). It is important to find breast cancer as early as possible. If cancer is found early, there are choices for treatment. With prompt treatment, the outlook is good. Physicians encourage women to take an active role in the early detection of breast cancer by:
- practising monthly breast self-examination;

Model of the female breast. East breast is located anterior to the pectoral muscles and extend in a convex structure from the lateral margin of the breast bone to the anterior border of the axilla.
There are from 15 to 20 lobes of glandular tissue arranged radially within the breast. Each is embedded in fat and connective tissue.

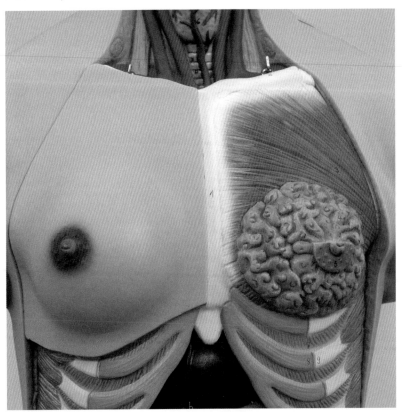

- having a yearly breast examination;
- getting a routine mammography after the age 40.

Women are often confused about what their breasts are supposed to feel like. It is normal for the breasts to feel lumpy and uneven. Sometimes the breasts are swollen and tender, especially right before a menstrual period. By doing monthly breast self-examination, women learn what is normal for their own breasts, and they are more likely to find anything unusual that might be a warning sign of cancer. Any changes should be reported to the doctor.

The second step of early detection is for a woman to have her breasts checked regularly by her physician. Mammograms (X-rays of the breast) can find many breasts cancers before they can be felt. Mammography, together with a breast examination by a health professional, can reduce the number of deaths cancer. Starting at age 40, a woman should have a mammogram every 1 to 2 years. When she reached 50 she should have a mammogram every year.

Symptoms

Breast cancer can cause many symptoms. Some warning signs to watch for include:
- a lump or thickening in the breast or in the axilla (armpit);
- a change in the size or shape of the breast;
- discharge from the nipple;
- a change in the colour or feel of the skin of the breast or areola (such as dimpling, puckering, or scaliness).

Pain is usually not an early warning sign of breast cancer. However, a

B

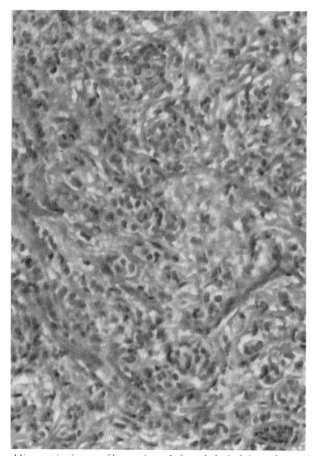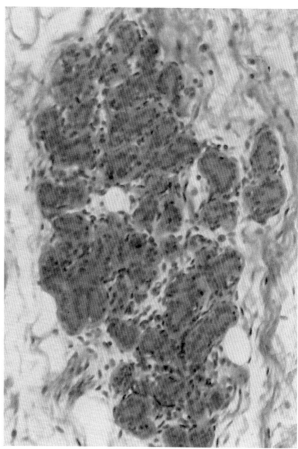

Microscopic pictures of breast tissue. Left: pathological tissue changes indicative for cancer; right: normal tissue.

woman should see her physician if she notices changes in her breasts. Changes may be caused by cancer or by other less serious problems. Only a physician can tell for sure. Early diagnosis is very important because breast cancer can be treated best before it has spread. The earlier breast cancer is found and treated, the better a woman's chances for complete recovery.

Diagnosis

To diagnose breast cancer, a woman's physician does a careful physical examination and asks her personal and family medical history. In addition to checking general signs of health (temperature, pulse, blood pressure, and so on), the doctor may do one or more of these examinations.

Palpation

By carefully feeling the breast, the physician can tell a lot about a breast lump - its size, its texture, and whether it is movable.

Aspiration

The physician may use a thin needle to remove fluid or a small amount of tissue from a breast lump. This may show whether the lump is a fluid-filled cyst (not cancer) or a solid mass (which may or may not be cancer).

Mammography

X-rays of the breast can give the physician important information about a breast lump. Also, a mammogram can show tumors too small to be felt.

Biopsy

A biopsy is surgery to take out part or all of a lump or suspicious area. This tissue is examined under a microscope by a pathologist. A biopsy is the only sure way to know whether cancer is present. Four out of five breasts lumps are not cancer. If a woman has a fluid-filled cyst, it most likely can be drained by fine needle aspiration.
If the lump is a benign tumor, it often can be removed by surgery with no further problems. Some lumps may not need any treatment, but the physician may want to check the woman regularly. If the biopsy shows that the lump is cancer, other special laboratory tests may be done on the tissue to learn more about the cancer. Also, the woman will have other tests to find out whether the cancer has spread from the breast to other parts of her body.

B

Breast cancer Questions & Answers

What is breast cancer?
Mammary carcinoma is the technical name for this all too common cancer; growth and multiplication of malignant cells affecting the female breast.

What is the incidence of breast cancer?
One out nine women in the UK will develop breast cancer during their lifetime. Early detection can save life, and mortality rates are falling due to effective treatment and raised awareness of the disease.

Who is most at risk from breast cancer?
The risk of developing breast cancer increases with age and 80% of cases occur in women over the age of 50. It is relatively rare in teenagers and women in their 20s.

How important is my family history?
Only about 5%-10% of breast cancers are hereditary and just because a close family member has had breast cancer it doesn't necessarily mean that there is hereditary breast cancer in your family. If you are concerned that breast cancer may run in your family your physician will be able to give you further advice.

How can I protect myself?
• Be aware of the condition of your breasts throughout your life. While being breast aware cannot prevent cancer developing, being aware of how your breasts look and feel normally will help to ensure that you spot problems as early as possible and get proper treatment before serious illness arises.

• Most breast changes, including lumps, will prove to be benign (harmless), but you should always report them to your physician to be certain.

• A healthy lifestyle can help to reduce the risk of any type of cancer. Try to cut down the amount of fat and increase the amount of fiber in your diet, making sure you eat at least five portions of fruit or vegetables a day. Exercise regularly, drink a sensible amount of alcohol (two to three units per day or less) and stop smoking.

What is the most common form of treatment?
The most common form of treatment is a lumpectomy in which only the cancer itself is removed, but if it is too large for this procedure a simple mastectomy, in which only the breast is removed, may be performed, leaving a cosmetically acceptable scar and scope for later plastic reconstruction of the breast. Only the lymph nodes under the arm will be removed at the same time. A course of radiotherapy and/or chemotherapy (drugs) may also be given.

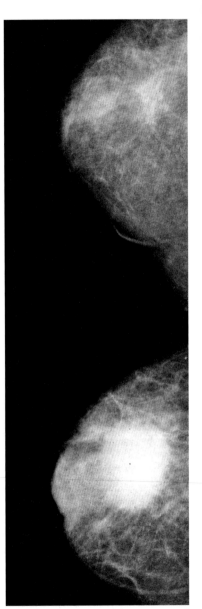

Mammograms. Upper picture: normal appearance of mammary tissue; bottom picture: presence of a tumor.

Treatment

Treatment depends on the type of breast cancer and how far it is spread, as well as on a woman's age, menopausal status, and general health. T
he physician will develop a treatment plan to fit a woman's individual needs. Before treatment a woman might want a second physician to review her diagnosis and treatment plan. A short delay will not reduce her chances that her treatment will be successful.

Methods of treatment
Breast cancer is treated with surgery, radiation therapy, chemotherapy, and hormone therapy. The physician may use just one method or combine them, depending on the patient's need. In some cases, the patient may be referred to other physicians who specialize in the different kinds of cancer treatment. Surgery is the most common treatment. The surgeon removes the tumor in the breast and, usually, the lymph nodes under the arm. The lymph nodes are removed because they filter the lymph that flows through the breast and other parts of the body, and they are one of the first places where breast cancer spreads. Cancer cells in the lymph nodes mean that there may be cancer elsewhere in the body.

Radiation therapy

Radiation therapy uses high-powered rays to damage cancer cells and stop them from growing. Like surgery, radiation therapy is a local treatment and affects only the cells in the treated area. Radiation may come from an X-ray machine outside the body (external radiation). It can also come from radioactive materials placed directly in the breast through thin plastic tubes (implant radiation). Sometimes both are used.

The patient goes to the hospital or clinic each day for external radiation treatments. Usually treatments are given 5 days a week for 5 to 6 weeks. At the end of that time, an extra "boost" of radiation is usually given to the tumor site. The boost may be either external or internal (using an implant). Patients usually stay in the hospital for a short time for implant radiation.

Chemotherapy

Chemotherapy uses drugs to kill cancer cells. The physician may use one drug or a combination. Chemotherapy may be given by mouth or by injection into a muscle or vein. The drugs enter the bloodstream and travel through the body. Chemotherapy is given in cycles: a treatment period followed by a rest period, then another treatment, and so on. This type of treatment is called systemic therapy. Depending on which drugs are given, most patients have chemotherapy as an outpatient at the hospital, at the doctor's office, or at home. Sometimes the patient may need to stay in the hospital for a short while.

Hormone therapy

Hormone therapy is used to keep cancer cells from getting the hormones they need to grow. This treatment may include the use of drugs that change the way hormones work, or surgery that removes organs such as the ovaries that make hormones. Like chemotherapy, hormone therapy can act on cells all over the body.

Treatment choices

Breast cancer is very treatable. The choice of treatment depends on the stage of the cancer (whether it is just in the breast or has spread to other

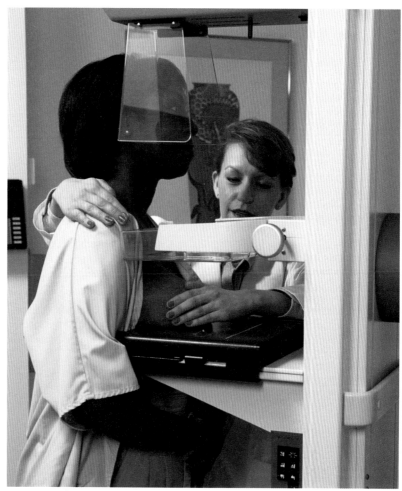

Mammography. X-rays of the breast are taken to detect abnormal areas. A technician positions the woman's breast on top of an X-ray plate.

Staging system for breast cancer

▲ Carcinoma in situ is very early breast cancer. Cancer is found in a local area and in only a few layers of cells.

▲ Stage I means the tumor is no larger than 2 centimeters and has not spread beyond the breast.

▲ Stage II means the tumor is from 2 to 5 cm and/or has spread to the lymph nodes in the arm (axilla).

▲ Stage III means the cancer is larger than 5 cm. It involves more of the underarm lymph nodes, and/or it has spread to other lymph nodes or to other tissues near the breast.

▲ Stage IV means the cancer has spread to other organs of the body, most often to the bones, liver, lungs, or brain.

B

Breast self-examination   Questions & Answers

How will I know what is normal?

- It is less a question of what is normal, than what is normal for you, and you will get to know that by being breast aware. Your breasts will change and develop during your life, and will be affected by hormonal changes during your menstrual cycle, pregnancy, breast-feeding and the menopause as well as by weight loss or gain.

- You will notice that just before your period your breasts may become enlarged, tender and lumpy. This is because your body is preparing for pregnancy. Usually, after your period, your breasts will return to normal because you are not pregnant. However some women experience tender, lumpy breasts throughout their menstrual cycle.

- Your breast tissue will change after the menopause, becoming softer and, in some cases, smaller. However, if you are taking estrogens (hormone replacement therapy) your breasts will feel firmer and sometimes tender.

How should I be breast aware?

Get into the habit of looking at and feeling your breasts from time to time. One way of looking is using a mirror, so that you can see your breasts from different angles.

You may find feeling your breasts is easier to do with a soapy hand in the bath or shower and you may prefer to do it lying down. You can decide what is convenient for you and what you are comfortable with.

What changes should I look for?

- A change in size, in one or both of your breasts.
- A nipple that has become inverted (pulled in) or changed its position or shape.
- A rash around the nipple.
- Any discharge coming from your nipples.
- Puckering or dimpling of the skin.
- A swelling in your armpit or under your collarbone (where your lymph nodes or glands are).
- A lump or thickening in your breast that feels different from the rest of your breast tissue.
- Constant pain in one part of your breast or armpit.

What is the breast awareness five point code?

- Know   Know what is normal for you and what to look and feel for.
- Look   Look at your breasts for any changes.
- Feel   Feel your breasts for any changes.
- Talk   Talk to your physician if you find any changes.
- Act   Act by attending routine breast screening if you are 50+.

If you notice any changes, it is really important to see your general physician.

places), the type of breast cancer, and certain characteristics of the cancer cells (such as how fast they are growing). The patient's age, menopausal status, and general health are also important. Decisions about treatment are also based on the experience of the physician and the desires of the patient.

Recovering from treatment

Recovery from treatment is important for every breast cancer patient. Recovery will be different for each woman, depending on the extent of the disease and the treatment she receives. Exercising after surgery can help a woman regain motion and strength in her arm and shoulder. It can also reduce pain and stiffness in her neck and back.

Carefully planned exercises should be started as soon as the physician says the woman is ready, often within a day or so after surgery. At first, exercises are gentle and can even be done in bed. Gradually, the exercises are more active, and regular exercise should become part of a woman's normal activities. Women who have a mastectomy and immediate breast reconstruction have different exercise needs that the physician or physical therapist will explain.

Lymphedema after surgery can be reduced or prevented with exercises and by resting with the arm propped up on a pillow. If lymphedema becomes a problem later on, the woman should tell her physician, who may suggest other exercises.

Some women with lymphedema wear an elastic sleeve or use an elastic cuff to improve lymph circulation. Other approaches - including medication, a low-salt diet, or a machine that compresses the arm - may be suggested by the physician.

After a mastectomy, some women choose to wear a breast form (*prosthesis*). Other have breast reconstruction. Each choice has its pros and cons, and what is right for one woman may not be right for another. What is important is that nearly all breast cancer patients have a choice. It may be helpful to talk with a plastic surgeon before mastectomy is done, but reconstruction is still possible years later.

Follow-up care

Regular follow-up examinations are very important after breast cancer. The physician will continue to check the patient closely to be sure that the cancer has not returned. Checkups usually include examinations of the chest, axilla, and neck.

From time to time, the patient will have a complete physical examination, blood and urine tests, a mammogram, and other X-rays. The physician sometimes orders scans (special X-rays) and other tests, too. A woman who has had breast cancer should check both the treated area and her

B

Self-examination of the breasts. Use your right hand to examine your left breast and vice versa. With one arm at your side (A, B):

▲ *Keep your fingers together and use the flat of the fingers, not the tips. Start from the collar bone above your breast.*

▲ *Investigate the four quadrants of the breast or trace a continuous spiral round your breast moving your fingers in small circles. Feel gently but firmly for any unusual hump.*

▲ *Now repeat this examination, but this time bend your arm at the elbow and raise it above your head (C, D).*

▲ *Finally examine your armpit (E, F). Use the flat of your fingers and small circular movements to feel for any lumps. Start right up in the hollow of your armpit and gradually work your way down towards your breast.*

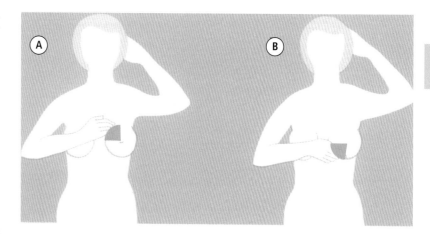

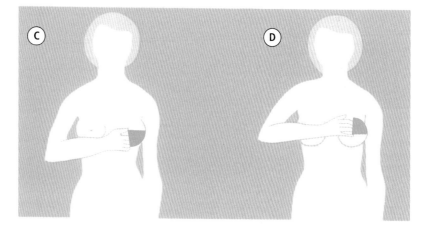

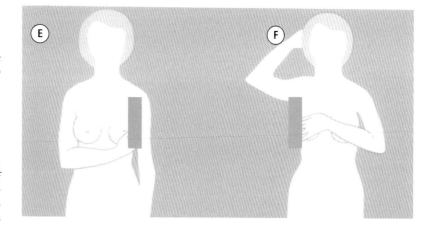

other breast each month. She should report any changes to her physician right away.

Also, she should tell her doctor about other physical problems if they come up, such as:

- pain;
- loss of appetite;
- loss of weight;
- changes in menstrual periods;
- unusual or lasting digestive problems;
- coughing or hoarseness;
- headaches;
- dizziness;
- blurred vision.

These problems may be a sign that the cancer has returned, but they can also be signs of many other problems. Only the physician can tell for sure.

Adjusting to the disease

The diagnosis of breast cancer can change a woman's life and the lives of those close to her. It is natural for the patient and her family and friends to have many different and sometimes confusing emotions. Women and their loved ones may feel frightened, angry, or depressed. These are normal reactions that people have when faced with a serious health problem.

Others in the same situation have found that they cope with their emotions better if they can talk openly about their illness and their feelings with those who love them. Concerns about what the future holds - as well as worries about tests, treatments, a hospital stay, etc. - are common. Talking with doctors, nurses, or other members of the health care team may help to calm fears and ease confusion. A woman can take an active part in decisions about her medical care by asking questions about breast cancer and her treatment choices. Patients, family members, and friends often find it helpful to write down ques-

B

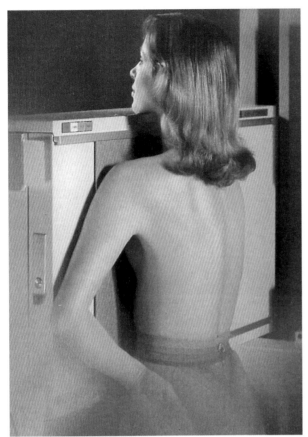
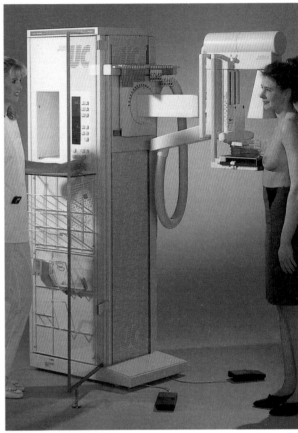

X-ray investigation of the thoracic cavity. X-rays of the thoracic cavity are taken to detect abnormal areas in the mammary glands and thoracic structures.

Different types of surgery for breast cancer

▲ Modified radical mastectomy removes the breast, the lymph nodes in the axilla, and the lining over the chest muscles (but leaves the muscles). This is the most common surgery for breast cancer.

▲ Lumpectomy removes just the breast lump and is followed by radiation therapy. Most surgeons also remove the lymph nodes- in the axilla.

▲ Total or simple mastectomy removes just the breast. Sometimes the arm lymph nodes closest to the breasts also are removed.

▲ Partial or segmental mastectomy removes the tumor, some of the normal breast tissue around it, and the lining over the chest muscle below the tumor. Usually some of the arm lymph nodes are removed. In most cases, radiation therapy follows surgery.

▲ Radical mastectomy removes the breast, chest muscles, all of the lymph nodes in the axilla, and some additional fat and skin. This operation was the standard for many years. It is still used on occasion but for most patients, less extensive surgery is just as effective.

tions to ask the doctor as they think of them. Taking notes during visits to the doctor helps them remember what was said.

Breast reconstruction
As cancer specialists have developed better ways to treat breast disease, plastic surgeons are increasingly at their sides and have made dramatic strides in breast reconstruction. There has been a revolution in their ability to create soft, natural-looking and feeling breasts. Often they can now perform such reconstructions during the same operation as the mastectomy, so women do not have to face the trauma of breast loss. Some twenty years ago, breast reconstruction was rare. The prevailing opinion was that the desire for reconstruction was a vain impulse.

Although some physicians continue to be hesitant about reconstruction,

Questions to ask the physician about breast cancer

- What is the extent of my breast cancer?
- How can it be treated?
- How successful is the treatment likely to be?
- What are my treatment choices?
- What are the benefits of treatment?
- What are the risks and side effects of treatment?
- How will I look after treatment?
- Will I need to change my normal activities?
- For how long?
- Can I keep working during treatment?
- How often will I need to have checkups?

the attitudes of many have dramatically changed as research has documented that the integrity of the woman's self-image - her sense of wholeness as well as her outlook on life, rather than attractiveness - is what is really at stake.
There are no data to support the fear that reconstruction might promote or hide recurrent cancer or impair the ability of physicians to treat such a recurrence.
In fact, some physicians suggest that because the immune system in general does a better job when the patient has a positive attitude, women who have reconstruction and suffer less depression may do better in terms of fighting cancer. Another factor responsible for the increasing number of reconstructions is that the surgical options available now are far more sophisticated than even a few years ago.

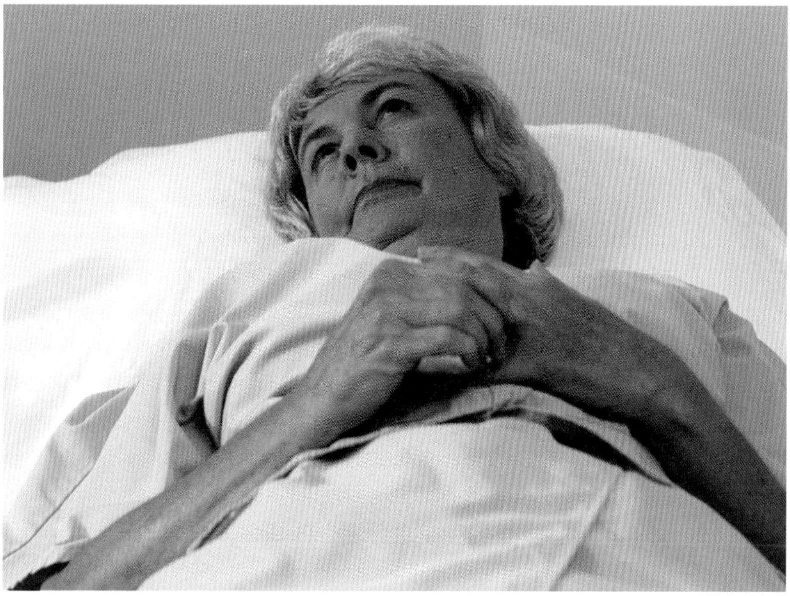

A patient waiting for breast reconstruction.

Silicone implant. Reconstruction of the breast may be performed at the same time as the mastectomy or later.

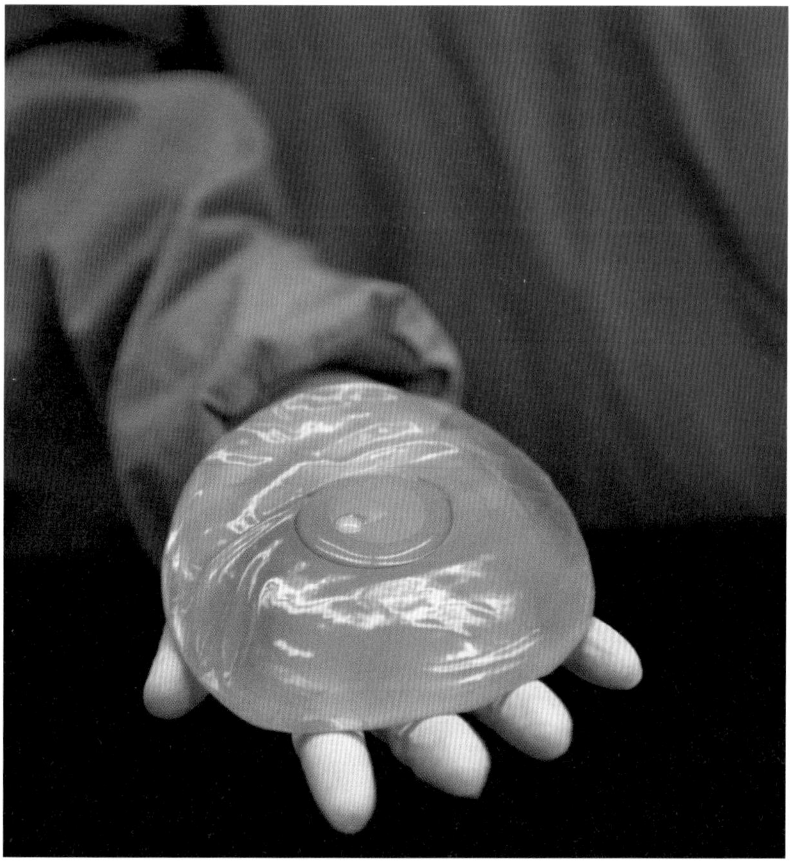

BRONCHITIS AND BRONCHIOLITIS

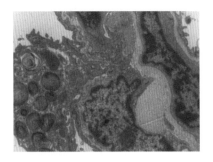

Bronchitis

Bronchitis is a very common infection of the major tubes (bronchi), that carry air within the lungs, but it occurs in two very different forms, acute and chronic.

Acute bronchitis

The acute form is commonly caused by viruses, occasionally by bacteria, and rarely by fungi. It spreads easily from one person to another on the breath. The symptoms include:
- fever
- chest aches
- pains
- headache
- tiredness
- productive cough

The diagnosis is confirmed but listening to the chest through a stethoscope. In early stages, X-rays may be normal, but later show characteristic changes. Sputum may be cultured to identify any bacteria present, and the correct antibiotic to treat it.

Viral infections settle with time, rest, inhalations, bronchodilators and physiotherapy.

Chronic bronchitis

This form of bronchitis is a long term inflammation of the larger airways in the lungs. The cause may be repeated attacks of acute bronchitis, long-standing allergies, or constant irritation of the bronchi by noxious gases, particularly those found in tobacco smoke, Physiotherapy, bronchodilators, and antibiotics if a bacterial infection is present, are the main treatments. It is a semi-permanent condition for which there is no effective cure, but treatment can keep the condition under control for many years. Sometimes it may progress to emphysema.

Bronchiolitis

Description

Bronchiolitis is an infection of the small breathing tubes (*bronchioles*) of the lungs. It occurs most often in infants. Bronchiolitis is sometimes confused with bronchitis, which is an infection of the larger, more central airways. Bronchiolitis is almost always caused by a virus. The infection causes the small airways in the lungs to swell. This blocks the flow of air through the lungs and makes it hard for the baby to breathe.

The virus is spread by contact with an infected person's mucus or saliva. If often spreads through families, child-care centers, and hospital wards. Careful hand washing can help prevent the spread of this infection.

Patient recovering from a severe bronchitis resulting in a pneumonia.

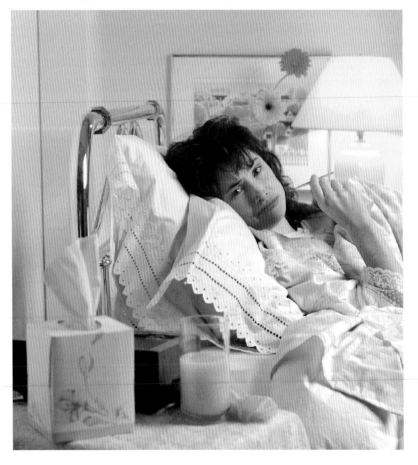

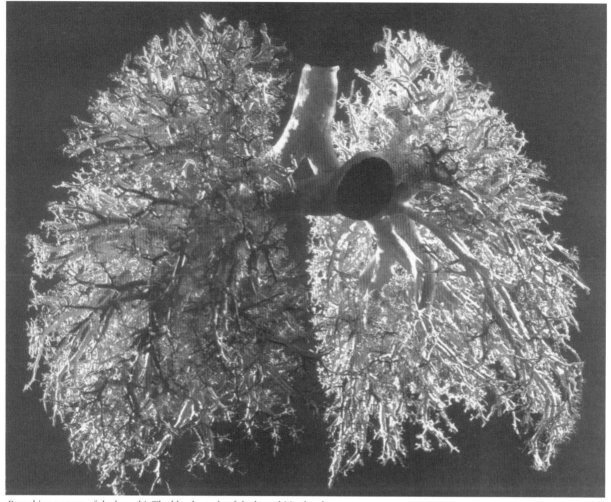

Branching pattern of the bronchi. The blood supply of the bronchi is also shown.

Signs and symptoms

A baby who develops bronchiolitis often starts off with signs of a cold, such as a runny nose, a mild cough, and a fever. After a day or two his cough may get worse. The following signs may mean he is having trouble breathing:

- He may widen his nostrils and squeeze the muscles under his rib cage to try to get more air in and out of his lungs.
- When he breathes he may grunt and tighten his stomach muscles.
- He will make a high-pitched whistling sound, called a wheeze, each time he breathes out.
- He may not take fluids well because he is working so hard to breathe that he has trouble sucking and swallowing.

Contact your doctor

- ▲ If your baby shows signs of trouble breathing, or if his fever lasts more than 24 hours (or is present at all in an infant under 3 months of age), call your pediatrician.

- ▲ If your baby is taking less that her normal amount of fluids.

- ▲ If your baby has a dry mouth and is crying without tears.

- ▲ If you think your child has bronchiolitis and your child has any of the following conditions, call your pediatrician:
  - Cystic fibrosis
  - Congenital heart disease
  - Bronchopulmonary dysplasia
  - Immune deficiency disease
  - Organ transplant
  - A cancer for which she is receiving chemotherapy

B

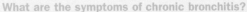

What is the cause of an acute bronchitis?

An acute bronchitis is an acute inflammatory disorder of the windpipe and bronchi, generally self-limited and with eventual complete healing and return of function. Though commonly mild, bronchitis may be serious in debilitated patients and in those with chronic lung or heart disease. Pneumonia is a critical complication.

When does acute bronchitis occur?

Acute infectious bronchitis is most prevalent in winter. It may develop after a common cold or other viral infection of the nose and pharynx, throat, or tracheobronchial tree, often with secondary infections by bacteria.Exposure to air pollutants and, possibly, chilling, fatigue, and malnutrition are predisposing or contributory factors.

When do recurrent attacks of bronchitis occur?

Recurrent attacks of bronchitis often complicate diseases, which impair bronchial clearance mechanisms. Repeated infections may be associated with:
- chronic sinusitis;
- bronchiectasis;
- bronchopulmonary allergy;
- enlarged tonsils;
- adenoids.

What are the major symptoms of bronchitis?

Onset of cough usually signals onset of bronchitis. The cough is initially dry and nonproductive, but small amounts of viscous sputum are raised after a few hours or days; it later becomes more abundant. Frankly purulent sputum suggests a superimposed bacterial infection.In a severe uncomplicated case, fever to 38.3°C to 38.9°C may be present for up to 3 to 5 days, after which acute symptoms subside; though cough may continue for several weeks. Persistent fever suggests complicating pneumonia. Pulmonary signs are few in uncomplicated acute bronchitis. Scattered high- or lowpitched rhonchi may be heard by the doctor, as well as occasional crackling or moist rales at the bases of the lungs. Wheezing, especially after cough, is commonly noted.

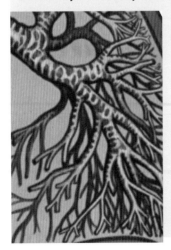

When do complications of acute bronchitis occur?

Serious complications are usually seen only in patients with an underlying chronic respiratory disorder. In such patients, acute bronchitis may lead to severe blood gas abnormalities (acute respiratory failure).

What are the symptoms of chronic bronchitis?

Chronic bronchitis is a condition associated with prolonged exposure to nonspecific bronchial irritants and accompanied by increased secretion of mucus and certain structural changes in the bronchi. The disorder is usually associated with cigarette smoking and is characterized by chronic productive coughing.

When does chronic obstructive bronchitis occur?

The term chronic obstructive bronchitis is used when chronic bronchitis is associated with extensive abnormalities of the small airways leading to clinically significant airways obstruction. The disease is thought to begin early in life, though significant symptoms and disability usually do not occur until middle age. Mild ventilatory abnormalities may be discernible long before the onset of significant clinical symptoms. A mild 'smoker's cough' is often present many years before onset of exertional dyspnoea.

Cough and sputum production are extremely variable. One patient may admit only to 'clearing my chest' on awakening in the morning or after smoking the first cigarette of the day. Another may describe a severe disabling cough. Wheezing also varies in character and intensity. Asthma-like episodes may occur with acute infections. A mild chronic wheeze that is most obvious on reclining may be noted. Many patients deny having any wheeze.

What is the best treatment for a severe bronchitis?

Therapy does not cure, but relieves symptoms and controls potentially fatal exacerbations. It may also slow progression of the disorder. Treatment is directed at alleviating conditions that cause symptoms and excessive disability (for instance, infection, spasm of the bronchi, increased secretion of mucus, decrease of oxygen in the blood, and unnecessary limitation of physical activity). Avoidance of bronchial irritants (especially cessation of smoking) is of primary importance.

What is a chronic bronchitis?

A chronic bronchitis is a condition associated with prolonged exposure to nonspecific bronchial irritants and accompanied by increased secretion of mucus and certain structural changes in the bronchi. The disorder is usually associated with cigarette smoking and characterized by chronic productive cough.

What is a chronic obstructive bronchitis?

A chronic obstructive bronchitis is a chronic bronchitis associated with extensive abnormalities of the small airways leading to clinically significant airways obstruction.

What is a chronic obstructive emphysema?

A chronic obstructive emphysema is pulmonary emphysema accompanied by obstruction of the airways; the major features of the disease can be explained by emphysematous changes in the lungs.

▲ If it gets very hard for him to breathe, you may notice a bluish tint around his lips and fingertips. This tells you that his airways are so blocked that there is not enough oxygen getting into the blood.

Home treatment

There are no medications you can use to treat bronchiolitis at home. Antibiotics, which treat bacteria, are not helpful for bronchiolitis because it is almost always caused by a virus.

However, you can ease your child's cold symptoms. Try the following suggestions:

▲ Thin the mucus using mild salt-solution nose drops recommended by your pediatrician. Never use nonprescription nose drops that contain any medication. Only use salt-solution nose drops.

▲ Clear your baby's nose with a suction bulb.

▲ Place a cool-mist humidifier (vaporizer) in your baby's room. Set it close to her. Be sure to clean and dry the humidifier each day to keep bacteria or mold from growing. Do not use hot water vaporizers.

▲ If your baby has a fever, give her acetaminophen. Be sure to follow the recommended dosage for your child's ge. Do not give aspirin

▲ Be sure your baby drinks lots of fluid so he does not become dehydrated. Her may prefer clear fluids rather than milk or formula.

Professional treatment

If your baby is having mild to moderate trouble breathing, your pediatrician may try using a drug that opens up the breathing tubes, which seems to help some infants. Some children with bronchiolitis need to be hospitalized, either for breathing problems or dehydration. Your pediatrician will treat your baby's breathing problems with oxygen and medication. The dehydration will be treated with a special liquid diet or with fluids given intravenously. Very rarely an infant will not respond to any of these treatments. She might have to be put on a breathing machine. This usually is only a temporary measure to help her until her body is able to overcome the infection.

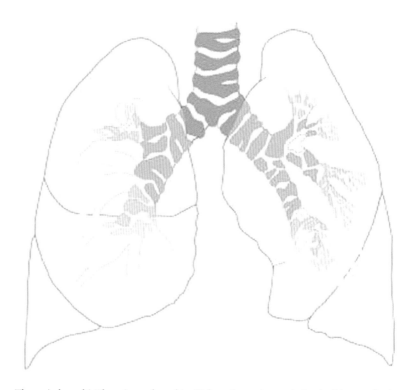

The main bronchi. The primary bronchi split from the trachea at the level, of the superior border of the fifth thoracic vertebra. The right bronchus differs from the left that it is shorter and wider and takes a more vertical course. Foreign bodies from the trachea usually enter the right bronchus because of these characteristics.

Pathological lung condition due to chronic bronchitis lasting more than 10 months.

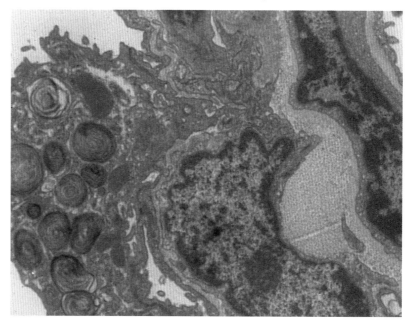

CANCER

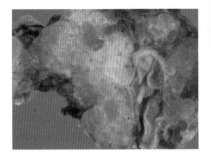

Description

The word cancer is derived from the Greek word for "crab," karkinos. Among its many synonyms are "malignant tumor", "carcinoma" and "malignant neoplasm." This last word also comes from the Greek and means "new growth."

Cancer is a term that stands for a large group of diseases that afflict both humans and animals. Cancer can arise in any organ or tissue of the body. Its main characteristic is an abnormal, seemingly unrestricted growth of cells. The resultant mass, or tumor, compresses, invades and destroys normal adjacent tissues.

Cancer cells can break off and leave the original mass and be carried by the blood or lymph systems to distant sites in the body. There they set up secondary growths, or metastases, further attacking and destroying the organs involved. At the present time, at least 100 different types of cancer have been classified by their appearance under the microscope, and by the site in the body from which they arise. The 30 trillion cells of the normal, healthy body live in a complex, interdependent condominium, regulating one another's proliferation. Indeed, normal cells reproduce only when instructed to do so by other cells in their vicinity. Such unceasing collaboration ensures that each tissue maintains a size and architecture appropriate to the body's needs.

Cancer cells, in stark contrast, violate this scheme; they become deaf to the usual controls on proliferation and follow their own internal agenda for reproduction. They also possess an even more insidious property - the ability to migrate from the site where they began, invading nearby tissues and forming masses at distant sites in the body. Tumors composed of such malignant cells become more and more aggressive over time, and they become lethal when they disrupt the tissues and organs needed for the survival of the organism as a whole.

Some cancers grow very slowly, and destroy neighbouring tissue by only a limited spread. Others spread rapidly to distant sites. Most cancers occur in older people, but a few forms are found most often in children. We know a great deal about some cancers and can prevent their occurrence, but our knowledge regarding the causes of many others is still entirely lacking.

Cancer cells do not necessarily appear to be strikingly different from normal cells. The body's normal repair (regeneration) of damaged tissue may, for a limited time, look quite "wild" in appearance under the microscope.

On the other hand, a tumor that could be fatal if located in a vital area such as the brain can seem benign, or innocent, in microscopic appearance. In addition, although cancer tissues are generally characterized by a rapid growth rate, cell division and tissue growth in normal pregnancy may proceed at an even greater pace. The most important difference is that the normal process stops when it has reached its end point, as in the healing of a cut or the completion of a pregnancy, whereas the cancerous process is uncontrolled.

The diseases grouped under the name cancer are second only to heart disease as killers of the people of the Western countries, including the UK and the United States. This is true in other

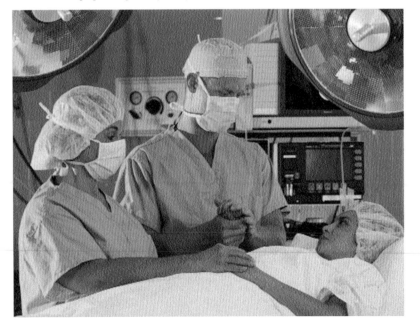

The anesthetist prepares a patient for major surgery

countries where infectious diseases and malnutrition play only a relatively unimportant role in causing deaths. A cure for cancer is not going to show up anytime soon - almost certainly not in the next decade. In fact, there may never be a single cure, one drug that will bring every cancer patient back to glowing good health, in part because every type of cancer, from brain to breast to bowel, is different. Now for the good news: during the next 10 years, doctors will be given tools for detecting the earliest stages of many cancers - in some cases when they are only a few cells strong - and suppressing them before they have a chance to progress to malignancy. Beyond that, nobody can make predictions with any accuracy, but there is reason to hope that within the next 25 years new drugs will be available to ameliorate most if not all cancers and maybe even cure some of them.

Risks of specific types of cancer

However, this static growth is by no means true of certain specific types of cancers. For example, lung cancer among men, relatively rare only 40 years ago, is now their top cancer killer. As important as the rise in lung cancer deaths has been the impressive drop in Western countries of deaths from cancer of the stomach.

During the past 30 years, in both women and men, this type of cancer has dropped in occurrence and in the number of deaths by about 50 per cent. The reasons for this are not understood, but laboratory studies and studies of population groups have focused on the dietary factors that may be involved. These may provide us with leads for the further reduction of this important form of cancer.

During the last 30 years these has also been a steady increase in reported deaths from leukaemia and related cancers of the blood and lymphatic systems. There has been a decrease in deaths from cancer of the uterine cervix (neck of the womb) in women. Part of this decrease is due to the detection of a greater proportion of uterine cancer cases at earlier, more

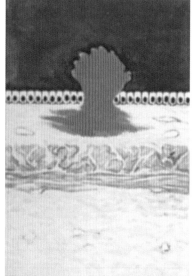

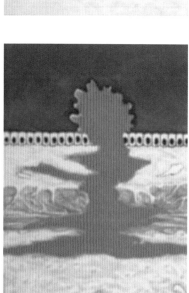

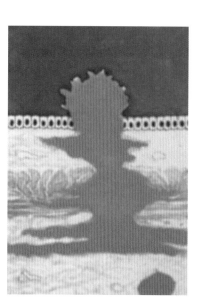

Various stages in the development of bladder cancer.
Upper left: Infiltration of the mucosal layer.
Upper right: Infiltration of the muscle layer.
Bottom left: Invasion of the perivesicular layer.
Bottom right: Spread to the lymph glands.

curable stages by the use of a cell examination technique known as the cervical smear, "scrape" or Pap test ("Pap" after Dr George N. Papanicolaou who developed the technique). Death from cancer in women is caused most frequently by cancers of the breast, the large intestine and the uterus.

Among men, death comes most often from cancers of the lung, prostate and large intestine. The skin is the most common site of cancer for both men and women, but most patients with this type of cancer are successfully treated and do not die of the disease. Careful studies going back to the last century show that human beings of all

C

Major cancers

Bladder cancer

Risk factors
- whites get bladder cancer twice as often as black people do
- men get bladder cancer two to three times as often as women do
- this cancer develops two to three times more often in cigarette smokers than in nonsmokers
- workers in the rubber, chemical and leather industries are at higher risk, as are hairdressers, metal workers, printers, painters, textile workers, truck drivers

Warning signs
- blood in urine
- pain during urination
- urgent need to urinate
- frequent need to urinate

Detection and diagnosis
- a tumor can sometimes be felt during rectal examination
- a tumor can sometimes be felt during vaginal examination
- cancer cells are sometimes seen in urine samples under a microscope
- cystoscopy (examination of the bladder with an instrument inserted in the urethra) can reveal abnormal areas
- biopsy is needed to confirm diagnosis

Treatment
- early-stage cancer confined to the bladder wall can often be removed with a cystoscope
- if several tumors are present, doctors may remove them and then infuse the bladder with a solution containing bacteria able to stimulate the immune system
- chemotherapeutic drugs may also be out directly into the bladder to lower risk of recurrence
- if the cancer cannot be easily removed, radiation may be needed
- if the cancer has spread through the bladder wall, the bladder may be removed
- chemotherapy may be needed after metastasis

Five-year survival rates
- all stages: about 80 per cent
- localized: about 93 per cent
- distant spread: about 5 per cent

Under study
- mutations in the p 53 gene that might signal tumor aggressiveness
- changes in certain proteins found in cell nuclei
- bladder-sparing surgery with chemotherapy
- interferon or interleukin-2 therapy for early-stage disease
- photodynamic therapy (using laser light and a photosensitizer to kill tumor cells)
- the analysis of DNA alterations and proteins from cell nuclei to detect recurrences

Breast cancer

Risk factors
- inherited mutations in the BRCA1 or BRCA2 genes
- increasing age
- early onset of menstruation
- late menopause
- never having had children
- having a first child after age 30
- personal or family history of breast cancer
- possibly a high-fat diet

Warning signs
- a painless lump in the breast is typical;
- there may occasionally be pain
- any change in the shape, colour or texture of the breast
- any change in the shape, colour or texture of the nipple
- discharge from or tenderness in the nipple

Detection and diagnosis
- self-examination
- clinical breast examination
- mammograms

Treatment
- for localized tumors, mastectomy (removal of the whole breast) may be appropriate
- breast-conserving surgery (removal of a tumor and some surrounding tissue, sometimes called lumpectomy) followed by local radiation is often preferable
- either procedure may be followed by additional chemotherapy or hormone-blocking therapy
- if tumor cells have high levels of receptors for the hormones estrogen and progesterone, it is a good sign because hormone-blocking therapy may stop their growth

Five-year survival rates
- all stages: about 83 per cent
- localized: about 95 per cent
- regional spread: about 75 per cent
- distant spread: about 20 per cent

Controversies
- tests for detecting inherited mutations in the BRCA1 and BRCA2 genes have become available, but doctors have not reached a consensus on their use
- value of chemotherapy for elderly patients
- value of routine mammography in women younger than 50 years of age

Under study
- biochemical and genetic markers
- density of blood vessels in a tumor may help indicate its aggressiveness
- high-dose chemotherapy followed by reconstruction of damaged bone marrow
- chemotherapy before surgery
- immunotherapy, including immunotoxins (molecules that combine a toxic agent with an antibody that binds to tumor cells)
- new chemotherapies and drug combination
- Tamoxifen, a drug that suppresses the effects of estrogen, may help prevent breast cancer in some women at high risk

Major cancers

Colorectal cancer

Risk factors
- family history of colorectal cancer
- polyps
- inflammatory bowel disease
- specific genetic mutations have been linked to familial adenomatous polyposis, which can develop into colon cancer
- rise in risk for people living in industrial or urban area
- physical inactivity
- exposure to certain chemicals
- high-fat or low-fiber diet

Warning signs
- blood in the stool
- any change in bowel habits
- general stomach discomfort
- unaccountable weight loss

Detection and diagnosis
- annual digital rectal examination recommended for people older than 40
- stool blood tests recommended for people older than 40
- sigmoidoscopy every three to five years after age 50
- if possible problems are found, colonoscopy may be used
- a patient's prognosis is poorer if the bowel is obstructed or perforated or if the pretreatment levels of certain marker substances (carcinoembryonic antigen and carbohydrate antigen 19-9) in the blood serum are high

Treatment
- surgery to remove the tumor
- sometimes combined with radiation or chemotherapy, or both
- if the disease has spread to the lymph nodes, chemotherapy with fluoroucil appears to be worthwhile
- chemotherapy combined with radiotherapy is used against intermediate and advanced rectal cancer
- surgical removal of metastases in the liver may prolong survival in some patients

Five-year survival rates
- all stages: about 60 per cent
- localised: about 90 per cent

Controversies
- the benefit of chemotherapy without evidence of lymph node involvement is uncertain
- the value of radiation in advanced cases is under study
- to treat liver metastases, implantable drug pumps and infusion ports are sometimes used, but their worth is unproved

Under study
- various genetic tests looking for the ras oncogene, characteristic changes in colorectal cell DNA and mutation affecting DNA repair
- combinations of chemotherapy and immunotherapy are under investigation for postoperative patients with cancerous lymph nodes
- biological therapy and surgery that spares a patient's sphincter are being evaluated

Kidney cancer

Risk factors
- males have twice the risk of females
- cigarette smokers have twice the risk of nonsmokers
- excess weight increases risk for some types of disease
- coke-oven workers and asbestos workers have higher rates of kidney cancer

Warning signs
- blood in urine
- lump in area of the kidney
- occasionally, signs include high blood pressure or an abnormal number of red blood cells

Detection and diagnosis
- X-ray of kidneys, involving injected dyes
- CT scans
- magnetic resonance imaging (MRI) scans
- arteriograms
- ultrasound examinations
- biopsy needed to confirm diagnosis

Treatment
- removal of all of part of the effected kidney, usually with the adjoining adrenal gland
- radiotherapy
- embolization, a procedure to block blood vessels
- interleukin-2, a system that plays a role in the immune system, is approved for use but can produce severe toxic side effects

Five-year survival rates
- all stages: about 56 per cent
- localized: about 88 per cent
- distant spread: about 10 per cent

Under study
- mutations of the von Hippel-Lindau gene in biopsy samples may indicate cancer
- well-documented cases of spontaneous remission without therapy
- biological therapeutic drugs, including interleukin-2 and interferon
- biological therapy after surgery for early-stage kidney cancer
- new anticancer drugs

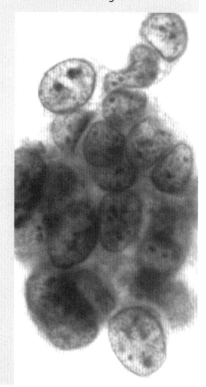

Major cancers

C

Leukemia

Characteristics
- contrary to common belief, leukemia strikes many more adults than children
- acute lymphocytic leukemia is the most common form among children
- in adults the common types are acute myelogenous leukemia and chronic lymphocytic leukemia

Risk factors
- certain genetic abnormalities, including Down's syndrome, Bloom syndrome and ataxia-telangiectasia
- excessive exposure to ionizing radiation
- some chemicals such as benzene, found in lead-free gasoline
- exposure to virus HLTV-I

Warning signs
- fatigue
- paleness
- weight loss
- repeated infections
- ready bruising
- nosebleeds

Detection and diagnosis
- blood tests that look for abnormal white blood cells
- bone marrow biopsy

Treatment
- chemotherapy is the first-line treatment
- various combinations of anticancer drugs are employed in sequence
- transfusions of blood components and antibiotics are used to minimize the danger from infections

- radiotherapy of the central nervous system is used against acute lymphocytic leukaemia and may also be used against other types
- bone marrow transplants in combination with chemotherapy can treat chronic myelogenous leukaemia
- interferon therapy has also shown value

Five-year survival rates
- chronic lymphocytic leukaemia: about 68 per cent
- acute lymphocytic leukaemia: about 55 per cent
- chronic myelogenous leukaemia: about 27 per cent
- acute myelogenous leukaemia: about 12 per cent

Lung cancer

Characteristic
- incidence has been declining in men since the 1980s but is still rising in women
- small cell lung cancer spreads rapidly

Risk factors
- cigarette smoking (linked to 85 to 90 per cent of all cases)
- exposure in the workplace to certain substances, including asbestos and some organic chemicals
- radiation exposure
- radon exposure (especially in smokers)
- environmental tobacco smoke

Warning signs
- persistent cough
- sputum streaked with blood
- wheezy breathing
- chest or shoulder pain
- swelling in face or neck
- recurring pneumonia or bronchitis

Detection and diagnosis
- chest X-ray
- analysis of cells in sputum
- fiber-optic examination of the bronchial passages

Treatment
- small cell cancer: chemotherapy alone or with radiation
- radiation may be given to the chest or, in some cases, to the brain, to kill metastases
- localized nonsmall cell cancers: surgery of the affected part
- advanced cases: radiation, chemotherapy, laser therapy or some combinations

Five-year survival rates
- all stages: about 13 per cent
- localized: about 48 per cent
- regional spread: about 17 per cent

Controversies
- ventilation equipment can prevent radon from accumulating in basements

Under study
- several new chemical agents (including taxol, taxotere, topotecan, irinotecan, vinorelbine)
- biological agents
- gene therapy using "antisense" approaches to reestablish activity of the tumor suppressor protein p53
- gene therapy to turn off oncogenes

Major cancers

Non-Hodgkin lymphoma

Non-Hodgkin's lymphoma includes about 10 different types of disease. Lymphoblastic and small noncleaved types are the most aggressive.

Risk factors
- because lowered immune system function raises susceptibility to this group of diseases, infectious agents such as HIV, which causes AIDS, increase risk
- recipients of organ transplants are at higher risk because of immunosuppressive drug they must take
- further possible dangers include occupational exposure to herbicides and other environmental chemicals

Warning signs
- enlarged lymph nodes
- generalized itching
- night sweats
- anaemia
- weight loss

Detection and diagnosis
- biopsy of affected lymph nodes
- X-rays of the lymphatic system
- computed tomographic scans
- ultrasonography

Treatment
- chromosome rearrangements associated with different forms of the disease offer clues how well or badly the cancer cells may respond to therapy
- asymptomatic low-grade lymphomas may be treated with radiation or left untreated
- chemotherapy is commonly used, because results with this approach have improved
- patients with higher-grade lymphomas are given chemotherapy and radiation
- relapses are common and may be treated with high-dosage chemotherapy in combination with bone marrow transplants
Five-year survival rates
- overall: about 50 per cent
- grade is more important than tumor stage
- people with low-grade tumors have a good chance of surviving longer than 10 years

Controversies
- researchers disagree about the classification and proper treatment of some uncommon types of non-Hodgkin's lymphomas

Under study
- various ways of improving the efficacy and safety of bone marrow transplantation
- monoclonal antibodies directed as lymphoma cells

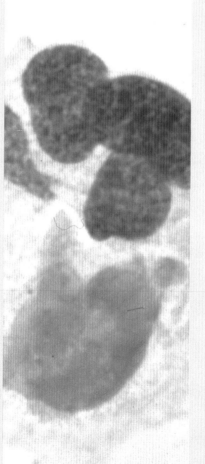

Ovarian cancer

Risk factors
- increasing age
- never been pregnant
- family history of breast cancer
- family history of ovarian cancer
- living in an industrial country
- inherited mutated BRCA1 or possibly BRCA2 gene

Warning signs
- enlargement of the abdomen
- rarely, abnormal vaginal bleeding
- in women older than 40 years, vague digestive discomfort
- often, few symptoms appear

Detection and diagnosis
- periodic, thorough pelvic examinations
- transvaginal ultrasound
- test for tumor marker substance (CA 125 antigen) in women suspected of having ovarian cancer
- biopsy is the definitive test
- women older than 40 should have cancer-related physical checkup each year

Treatment
- surgical removal of one or both ovaries, the uterus and the fallopian tubes
- in very young women, only the involved ovary may be removed
- radiation is commonly employed
- chemotherapy is sometimes used
- doctors measure levels of CA 125 and other substances to monitor responses to therapy

Five-year survival rates
- all stages: about 45 per cent
- localized: about 90 per cent
- regional spread: about 50 per cent

Controversies
- testing of mutated BRCA1 gene as an indicator of high risk
- doctors disagree over whether chemotherapy is valuable as an adjunct to surgery for early-stage disease

C

C

Major cancers

Pancreatic cancer

Risk factors
- increasing age
- cigarette smoking
- chronic pancreatitis
- diabetes
- cirrhosis
- incidence is high in countries with high-fat diets

Warning signs
- usually none until disease is advanced

Detection and diagnosis
- biopsy

Treatment
- tumors that are not small and confined to the pancreas are hard to treat
- surgery, radiation and standard anticancer drugs can be used if the cancer has not metastasized
- to alleviate the pain of the disease, radiotherapy, surgical procedures to clear the bile ducts, and nerve blocks can be effective

Five-year survival rates
- all stages: about 4 per cent
- localized about 12 per cent

Controversies
- increasing age

Under study
- the use of ultrasound imaging and CT scans for detecting cancers sooner
- octreotide, a biological agent that has stabilized disease in a few patients
- new surgical techniques that may improve quality of life
- drugs that improve tumor sensitivity to radiation
- various biological therapies
- new anticancer agents

Prostate cancer

Risk factors
- increasing age
- possibly a high-fat diet
- the cancer may tend to run in families

Warning signs
- urine flow is weak
- urine flow is interrupted or difficult to control
- frequent need to urinate
- back or pelvic pain

Detection and diagnosis
- every man older than 50 years should have a digital rectal examination annually
- a prostate-specific antigen (PSA) blood test can signal the presence of prostate abnormalities at an early stage
- transrectal ultrasound evaluation can confirm suspicious results form other tests
- examination of the amount of DNA in abnormal cells can indicate how aggressive a cancer may be

Treatment
- removal of prostate is routine
- radiotherapy is also widely used as an alternative or supplement to prostatectomy
- against metastatic disease, drugs can block cancer cells from receiving the male hormones they need to grow

Five-year survival rates
- all stages: 85 per cent
- localized: about 98 per cent
- regional spread: about 92 per cent

Controversies
- the merits of PSA testing for detecting asymptomatic disease and the best approach for handling localized tumors are intensely debated

Under study
- detailed genetic analysis of tumor cells may help predict their aggressiveness
- radiation therapy with beams that are controlled so as to maximize radiation dose to the tumor with the smallest amount of collateral exposure
- finasteride, a drug used to relieve symptoms caused by benign enlargement of the prostate, may prevent cancer

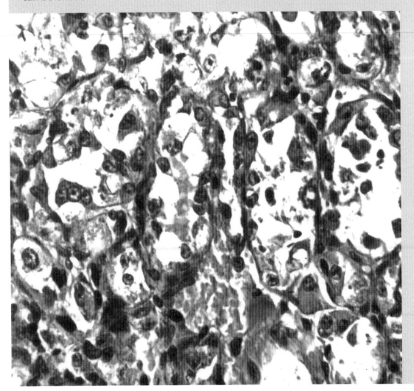

Major cancers

Skin melanoma

Melanoma of the skin accounts for three quarters of all deaths from skin cancer. The incidence has increased by 4 per cent each year since 1975 in developed countries.

Risk factors
- exposure to the sun, especially during childhood
- the cancer occurs more frequently in people who have fair skin that burns or freckles easily
- white people are 40 times more likely than black people to develop melanoma

Warning signs
- a change in size, colour, texture or shape of a mole
- a change in size, colour, texture or shape of a darkly pigmented skin area
- the appearance of a new, abnormal mole
- spontaneous bleeding from a mole
- changes in other bumps or nodules in the skin are also suspect

Detection and diagnosis
- early detection is crucial
- adults should practice self-examination of the skin once a month
- report to a physician any bleeding or sudden change in size or colour involving a mole-like growth
- biopsy may be needed to confirm diagnosis

Treatment
- surgical removal of the melanoma

Five-year survival rates
- all stages: about 85 per cent
- localized: about 93 per cent
- regional spread: about 60 per cent

Under study
- biological therapies, including interleukin-2 and interferon
- therapeutic vaccines containing melanoma antigens, which are showing considerable promise

Uterine cancer

Risk factors
Cervical cancer
- sexual intercourse before age 18
- many sexual partners
- cigarette smoking
- low socioeconomic status
Endometrial cancer
- exposure to estrogen, including estrogen replacement therapy not accompanied by progestin
- tamoxifen treatment
- early onset of menstruation
- late menopause
- never having been pregnant
- other medical conditions:
  diabetes
  gallbladder disease
  hypertension
  obesity

Warning signs
- abnormal uterine bleeding
- pain occurs later in the course of disease

Detection and diagnosis
- pap smear tests can find abnormal cells prefiguring cervical cancer
- pelvic examinations are more effective at detecting endometrial cancer
- women at high risk should have an endometrial tissue sample evaluated at menopause

Results of a Pap test for cervical cancer
■ Class 1
The Pap test is completely normal; no abnormal cells are present.

■ Class 2
Some cells are abnormal, but none suggests cancer. The abnormal cells may be due to an inflammation and/or infection. The Pap test should be repeated in 3 to 6 months.

■ Class 3
Dysplasia is present. A follow-up Pap test and a biopsy may be needed.

■ Class 4
Carcinoma in situ is found. A follow-up Pap test and biopsy are needed.

■ Class 5
The Pap test reveals invasive cancer of the cervix. A biopsy is necessary.

Treatment
Cervical cancer
- surgery or radiation, or both
- precancerous cells in the cervix may be eliminated by cryotherapy, electrocoagulation or local surgery
Endometrial cancer
- surgery, possibly with radiation and either hormone treatments or chemotherapy

Five-year survival rates
Cervical cancer
- all stages: about 68 per cent
- localized: about 90 per cent
- regional spread: about 50 per cent
Endometrial cancer
- all stages: about 83 per cent
- localized: about 95 per cent
- regional spread: about 65 per cent

Controversies
- experts disagree over whether it may be reasonable to delay treatment of early-stage cervical cancer detected during pregnancy to improve the chances of cervical of the foetus

Under study
- tests for mutations in genes regulating DNA repair may help warn of endometrial cancer

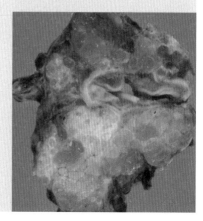

C

Modifiable determinants of cancer risks

Smoking
Lung cancer mortality rates are about 22 times higher for current male smokers, and 12 times higher for current female smokers, than for those who have never smoked. Smoking accounts for about 30 per cent of all cancer deaths in the United States. Tobacco use is responsible for nearly 1 in 5 deaths in the United States. Smoking is associated with cancer of the lung, mouth, nasal cavities, pharynx, larynx, esophagus, stomach, pancreas, liver, uterine cervix, kidney, bladder, and myeloid leukemia.

Nutrition and Diet
Risk for colon, rectum, breast (among postmenopausal women), kidney, prostate, and endometrial cancers increases in obese patients. While a diet high in fat may be a factor in the development of certain cancers, particularly cancer of the colon and rectum, prostate, and endometrium, the link between obesity and cancer is more the result of imbalance between caloric intake and energy expenditure than fat per se. Eating 5 or more servings of fruits and vegetables each day, and eating other foods from plant sources (especially grains and beans), may reduce risk for many cancers. Physical activity can help protect against some cancers.

Sunlight
Many of the 1 million skin cancers that are diagnosed annually in the United States could have been prevented by protection from the sun's rays. Epidemiological evidence shows that sun exposure is a major factor in the development of melanoma and that the incidence rates are increasing around the world.

Alcohol
Heavy drinking, especially when accompanied by cigarette smoking or smokeless tobacco use, increases risk of cancers of the mouth, larynx, pharynx, esophagus, and liver. Studies have also noted an association between regular alcohol consumption and an increased risk of breast cancer.

Smokeless tobacco
Use of chewing tobacco or snuff increases risk of cancers of the mouth and pharynx. The excess risk of cancer of the cheek and gum may reach nearly 50-fold among long-term snuff users.

Estrogen
Estrogen replacement therapy to control menopausal symptoms can increase the risk of endometrial cancer. However, adding progesterone to estrogen helps to minimize this risk. Most studies suggest that long-term use (5 years or more) of hormone replacement therapy after menopause increases the risk of breast cancer, and recent studies suggest that risk from taking hormones exceed benefits. The benefits and risks of the use of hormones by menopausal women should be discussed carefully by the woman and her doctor.

Radiation
Excessive exposure to ionizing radiation can increase cancer risk. Medical and dental X-rays are adjusted to deliver the lowest dose possible without sacrificing image quality. Excessive radon exposure in the home may increase lung cancer risk, especially in cigarette smokers.

Environmental hazards
Exposure to various chemicals (including benzene, asbestos, vinyl chloride, arsenic and aflatoxin) increases risk of various cancers. Risk of lung cancer from asbestos is greatly increased when combined with smoking.

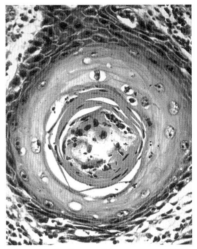

Macroscopic picture of larynx cancer. This epithelial type of cancer occurs more often in men.

races, living in all parts of the world, develop cancer of one type or another. Reports of primitive people that are "immune" to cancer have all proved to be wrong. These groups, whether they be Eskimos or South American tribes, for example, usually consist of small numbers of people who, due to lack of adequate medical care and other advantages, do not live to middle or older age when diagnosed cancer is most frequent.

Immunity

Some of the greatest triumphs of medicine are closely associated with research on immunity, which has enabled physicians to protect people against a wide variety of bacterial and viral diseases. It was long known that individuals recovering from diseases such as smallpox were nearly always safe from catching the disease again: in other words, they were immune.
Partial immunity to a specific agent is manifested by the development of mild disease, or, in fact, by infections that produce no recognizable symptoms. Such immunity, induced by deliberate exposure to many attenuated (weak) strains of agents, provides future protection against more virulent strains. Early experiences with transplanted tumors, before the development of inbred strains of laboratory animals, gave rise to hopes that immunity to

cancerous tumors could also be induced. It is now established that many cancers in humans as well as in animals do have antigens (reaction-causing proteins) that evoke immune reactions in body fluids or cells. Tumor antigens include proteins that resemble those found in embryonic tissues but not in adult tissues; and proteins that are formed from interactions between viruses and cell components in the cell membrane or in the cell nucleus. Tumors produced by chemicals or tumors that arise spontaneously have weaker and more diversified antigens. Interesting attempts, too, have been made to immunize patients against cancer by the use of antisera produced in animals injected with a patient's tumor, or by "vaccination" with products of the tumor. Since cancer varies so much in its effect on different individuals, this may indicate that some persons are more resistant than others to the disease. For example, in some patients, cancer of the breast will grow very rapidly and kill the individual within a few months after diagnosis, while in others, this type of tumor will progress slowly. Moreover, in some patients, the disease will spread widely while the primary tumor is still small, whereas in others, large tumors will remain localized for many years. Some untreated tumors, including the neuroblastomas of childhood and melanomas of the eye, even undergo seemingly permanent regressions. The possibility exists that these tumors stimulate a form of immune response in the patient.

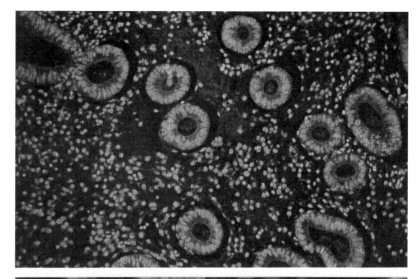

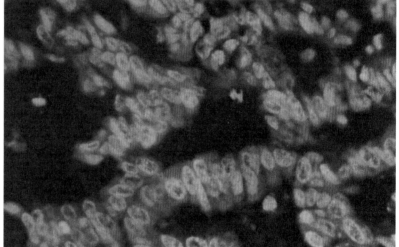

Microscopic picture of uterine cells seen through a fluorescence microscope. Upper illustration: normal tissue: bottom illustration: malignant cells showing polymorphia.

Sarcoma; microscopic picture of malignant spindle-shaped cells

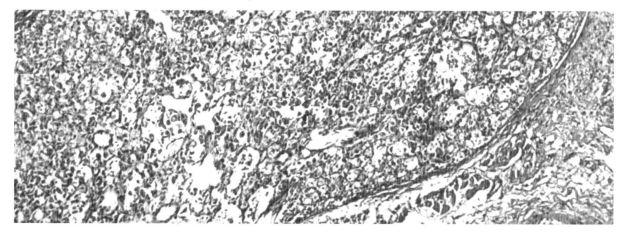

CATARACT

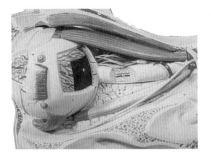

Description

A cataract is a cloudiness (opacity) in the eye's lens that impairs vision. Approximately 20 per cent of the individuals in our country who are considered legally blind have cataracts as an underlying cause. A cataract is an opacity of the crystalline lens. At present, drug therapy is not a treatment for cataracts but only an aid for certain symptoms. The treatment of cataracts involves surgical removal of the opacity.

Symptoms and diagnosis

Juvenile or adult cataract is characterized by progressive, painless loss of vision. The cause may be: senile degeneration, X-rays, heat from infrared exposure, systemic diseases (for instance, diabetes). systemic medications (e.g., corticosteroids). The cardinal symptom is a progressive, painless loss of vision. The degree of loss depends on the location and extent of the opacity. When the opacity is in the central lens nucleus (nuclear cataract), myopia develops in the early stages, so that a presbyopic patient may discover that he can read without his glasses ("second sight"). Pain occurs if the cataract swells and produces secondary glaucoma.

Opacity beneath the posterior lens capsule affects vision out of proportion to the degree of cloudiness because the opacity is located at the crossing point of the rays of light from the viewed object. Such cataracts are particularly troublesome in bright light. Well-developed cataracts appear as grey opacities in the lens. Ophthalmoscopic examination of the dilated pupil with the instrument held at about 30 cm away will usually disclose subtle opacities. Small cataracts stand out as dark defects in the red reflex. A large cataract may obliterate the red reflex.

Red refractions and eyeglass prescriptions changes help maintain useful vision during cataract development. Occasionally, chronic pupillary dilation is helpful for small lens opacities. When useful vision is lost, lens extraction is necessary; it can be accomplished by removal of the lens intact, or by emulsification followed by irrigation and aspiration. Age is no contraindication to surgery.

Prevention

There are several things people can do to try to prevent cataracts. Consistent

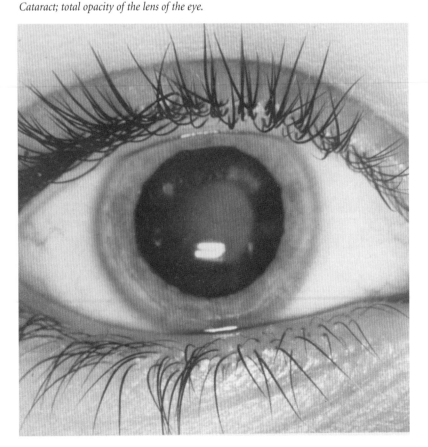

Cataract; total opacity of the lens of the eye.

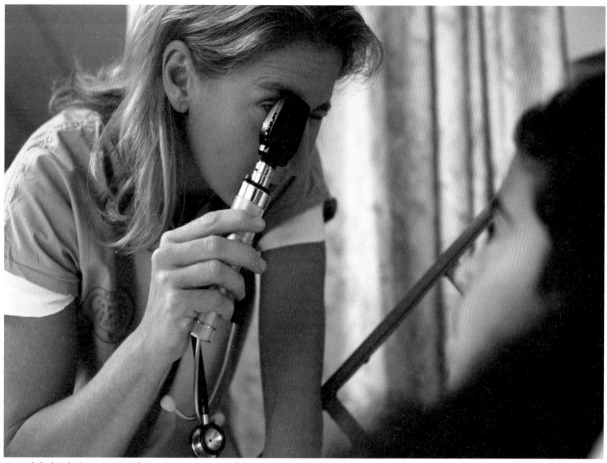

An ophthalmologist examines the various structures of the eye.

use of sunglasses with a coating to filter ultraviolet light will protect the eyes form bright sunlight and may help.

Not smoking is useful and has other health advantages. people with diabetes should work with their doctor to be sure the level of sugar in their blood is well controlled.

A diet high in vitamin C, vitamin A, and substances known as carotenoids (contained in vegetables such as spinach and kale) may protect against cataracts.

Estrogen use by women after menopause may also be protective, but estrogen should not be used solely for this purpose.

Finally, people who are taking corticosteroids for extended periods might discuss with their doctor the possibility of using a different drug.

Cataract: partial opacity of the eye.

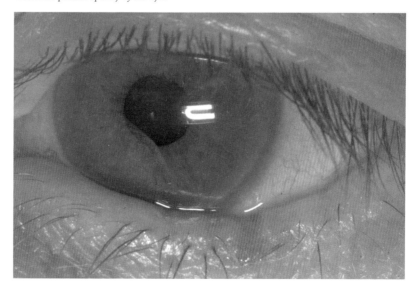

C

Cataract Questions & Answers

How do cataracts develop?

A cataract is not a growth or tumor of the eye. It is simply a loss of clearness of the eye; if not treated, this loss can lead to blindness. In the normal eye, the lens is so clear that you do not know it is there. With age, it yellows somewhat and vision becomes slightly hazy in almost all aged people.

In some people, the yellowing becomes so severe that the lens gets cloudy. As it becomes difficult for light rays to pass through the cloudy lens, vision begins to fall, starting with dimmed or blurred vision. Eventually, the lens may become completely opaque.

The most common cause of cataract is the normal, gradual change in lenses as we age. However, cataracts can occur at any age in life, even in babies. Physical injuries and certain illnesses can promote their development. Cataracts also seem to run in some families more than in others.

How are cataracts diagnosed?

Cataracts can be detected by an ophthalmologist during a regular eye examination with an instrument that lights the inside of your eye. Cataracts usually develop slowly. It may take years for surgery to be necessary. Some may never become that severe. The size, location, and density of the cataract determine the extent of the vision loss.

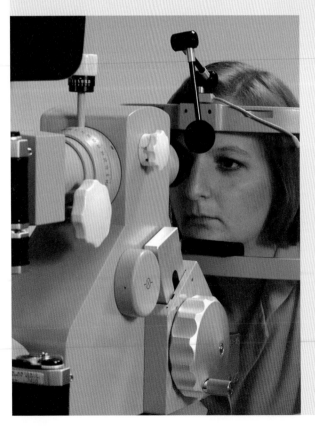

Can cataract be treated effectively?

No eye drops, salves, or medicines can treat cataracts. The only satisfactory treatment is surgical removal of the cloudy lens. Without a lens, the eye cannot focus normally. To assure vision after surgery, you have three options. Cataract eyeglasses are the oldest and least expensive choice but have rather thick lenses; however, they limit side vision and make objects look larger than normal.

Next come special contact lenses, which may be standard dailywear lenses or extended wear lenses that may be worn for a month or more without changing. However, some people with certain health conditions cannot wear contact lenses. The most recent choice is the intraocular lens which is implanted in the eye during surgery and which results in normal postoperative visions.

What are the most common eye injuries?

he most common injury is getting a foreign object in the eye. Other frequent injuries are:
- contusions;
- open wounds;
- burns.

Almost half of all vision impairment due to injury results from accidents in the home. Others occur at work, at school - particularly in laboratory or shop classes - or during sports participation or other recreational activities. Baseball, basketball, racquet sports - such as tennis, badminton, racquetball, and squash - account for the greatest number of sports injuries.

How can I prevent injuries to the eye?

When any risk of eye injury is possible - such as when participating in sports, shop classes or home construction - eyes should be shielded from potential hazards. A wide variety of such equipment is available.
They include:
- ▲ a sturdy eyeglass frame with industrial strength, impact-resistant lenses;
- ▲ special sports frames with such features as padded bridges, deep-grooved eyewires, etc.

What are the most common eye infections?

Eyes have excellent defenses to protect us against infections: tears which wash germs away, eye lids which blink to push away invading particles, and tear drainage which washes debris out to the nose, to be swallowed into the digestive system for disposal. When one of the systems breaks down, eye infections occur - ranging from simple problems you can self-treat to vision-threatening disorders that warrant immediate medical care.

Simple viral conjunctivitis, also called pink eye, is the most common eye infection. It is caused by germs similar to those that cause colds. Symptoms are redness with a thin watery discharge. Running a close second are styes, an infection of an oil gland at the base of an eyelash outside the eye.

Cataract operation; intracapsular removal of cataract.

A. Position of the patient as seen by the eye surgeon.
B. Incision in the cornea.
C-E. Removal of the pieces of the cataract.
F-G. Placement of the new, artificial, lens.
H. Extra fluid is injected.
I. If necessary, closing of the incision.

Cataract surgery can be performed on a person of any age. The eye surgeon makes a small incision in the eye and removes the cataract by breaking it up with ultrasound and taking out the pieces. When all the cataract pieces have been removed, the surgeon replaces the cataract with an artificial lens.

Surgery to remove cataracts is almost always performed under local anesthesia, in which the eye surface is numbed with an injection or eye drops.

The procedure normally takes about 30 minutes, and the person can go home the same day. No sutures are usually needed, because the incision into the eye is small and can seal itself.

Treatment

Until vision is significantly impaired, eyeglasses and contact lenses may improve a person's vision. Wearing sunglasses in bright light and using lamps that provide over-the-shoulder lightning may decrease glare and aid vision.

Rarely, drugs that keep the pupil dilates may be used to help vision if the cataract is located in the center of the lens.

The only treatment that provides a cure for cataracts is surgery; there are no eye drops or drugs that will make cataracts go away.

Occasionally, cataracts will cause changes (such as swelling of the cataract or glaucoma) that lead doctors to recommend the cataract be removed quickly.

However, most times people should have surgery only when their vision is so impaired by cataracts that they feel unsafe, uncomfortable, or unable to perform daily tasks.

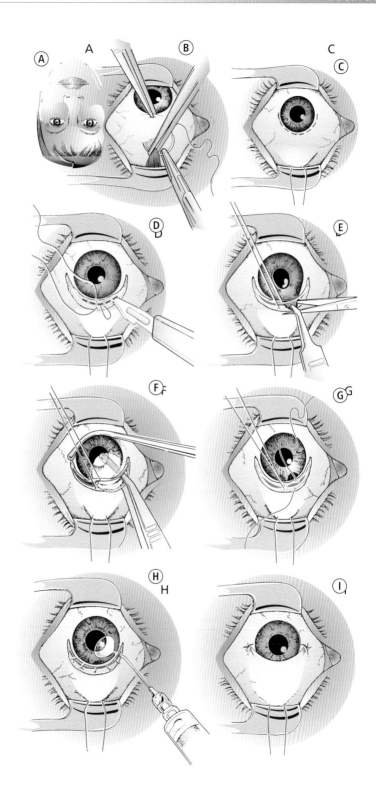

CERVIX DISORDERS

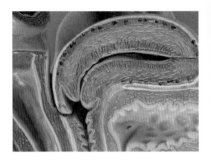

Introduction

Disorders of the cervix - the lower, narrow end of the uterus - are very common. Most of these disorders are not serious and can be treated easily. Others can be very serious and may require more involved treatment.

Do not take chances if you think you may have a problem - do not let fear keep you from seeing a doctor. In this case, what you do not know can hurt you. Here are two guidelines to help you stay healthy:

▲ Have a complete pelvic exam, including a Pap smear, once a year. A Pap test may detect a problem before you are aware that something is wrong.

▲ Report problems promptly. If you have unexpected vaginal bleeding or discharge, or if you notice any other sign that something could be wrong, do not wait. See your doctor right away.

As is true of many other problems, the best results occur when cervical disorders are treated early.

Cervicitis

Cervicitis is an inflammation of the cervix that may or may not produce symptoms. It is common in women during their childbearing years. It may occur as a result of these factors:

▲ Acute (short, severe) infection, especially those that can be sexually transmitted:
  • bacteria such as gonorrhea or chlamydia
  • viruses, such as the one that cause herpes or genital warts
  • Trichomonas, an organism that can cause vaginal infection

▲ Irritation from a foreign body, such as an intrauterine device (IUD) or contraceptive sponge, a forgotten tampon, or a pessary (a device placed in the vagina to hold sagging pelvic organs in place).

Symptoms

Cervicitis may produce some or none of the following symptoms:

▲ leukorrhea, a thick vaginal discharge that may have a bad odor;

▲ tenderness or pain in the pelvic region;

▲ slight vaginal bleeding between periods or after intercourse.

Diagnosis and treatment

There are several factors that may lead to the diagnosis of cervicitis. These include:

▲ Culture or other diagnostic test.

▲ Results of a Pap test (in which a sample of cells is taken from the cervix and looked at under a microscope).

▲ Results of colposcopy (viewing of the cervix under magnification with a special instrument).

The type of treatment for cervicitis depends on the cause. If the cervicitis is caused by an infection of the cervix, it is usually treated with oral medication. In very rare cases, minor surgery may be required. With surgery, infected tissue is removed to allow healing and permit a new layer of normal cells to grow over the affected area. Several methods of surgical treatment are available.

▲ *Cryotherapy* ("cold cautery"): freezing agents, such as liquid nitrogen, are applied to the affected area.

▲ *Electrocoagulation* ("hot cautery"): destroys the affected cervical tissue with heat.

▲ *Laser treatment*: a high-intensity beam of light is used to remove abnormal tissue or growths.

Benign growths

Other types of cervical disorders include growths or problems caused by viruses. Polyps are benign (noncancerous) growths or tumors that commonly appear on the cervix. They vary in size and may cause irregular vaginal bleeding. Condyloma, also called genital warts, are spreading growths that are caused by a virus. Although they are usually few in number, they may join together to form large masses.

Another cervical disorder occurs when there is a change in the cells on the surface of the cervix. At one time, these changes were called dysplasia, or carcinoma *in situ* (CIS). More recently, the term cervical intra-epithelial neoplasia, or CIN, is most often used to describe this disorder.

Cervical intra-epithelial neoplasia (CIN)

In CIN, normal, noncancerous cells are it is particularly common in young women and teenagers. It is often linked to a viral infection passed on during intercourse. It is more likely to occur in women who have had multiple sexual partners, or whose male partners have had multiple partners.

Although milder forms of these "precancerous" changes may go away on their own, they as well as other more severe forms can develop into cancer if they are not treated.

■ *Diagnosis*

A screening test called a Pap test is useful to detect these problems at an early stage. For most women, a Pap test done annually, starting at age 18 or when a woman becomes sexually active, is the best screening method for detecting abnormal changes in the cervix.

A Pap test can be done in the doctor's office during a regular pelvic exam. Your doctor will explain to you what the results mean. If abnormal cells are detected through the Pap test, colposcopy and biopsy may be recommended to diagnose the problem specifically.

■ *Colposcopy*
This is a direct viewing of the cervix through a special magnifying instrument called a colposcope. It allows the doctor to detect abnormalities of the cervix that cannot be seen directly with the eye. A speculum like the one used during a Pap test is placed in the vagina. The colposcope is than positioned so that the cervix can be seen. The cervix will be cleansed with a

Results of a Pap test for cervical cancer

■ **Class 1**
The Pap test is completely normal; no abnormal cells are present.

■ **Class 2**
Some cells are abnormal, but none suggests cancer. The abnormal cells may be due to an inflammation and/or infection. The Pap test should be repeated in 3 to 6 months.

■ **Class 3**
Dysplasia is present. A follow-up Pap test and a biopsy may be needed.

■ **Class 4**
Carcinoma in situ is found. A follow-up Pap test and biopsy are needed.

■ **Class 5**
The Pap test reveals invasive cancer of the cervix. A biopsy is necessary.

Spectroscopic picture of Herpes virus, responsible for many cervical infections.

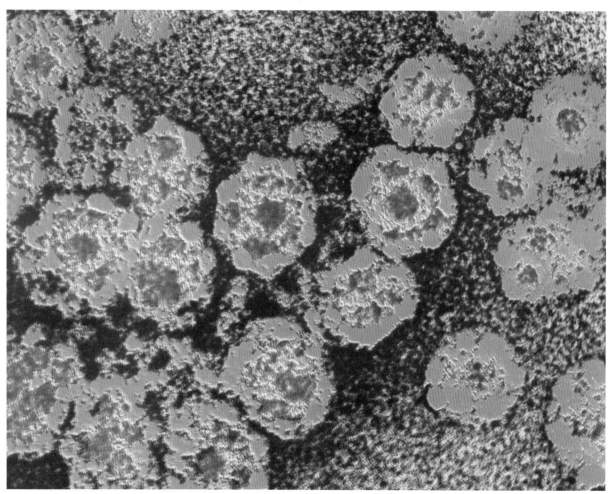

C

Cervical cancer   Questions & Answers

What is cervical cancer?
Cancer of the cervix of the uterus involves the part of the womb which opens into the top of the vagina. It is one of the more common form of female cancers.

What is the incidence of cervical cancer?
Although much less common than breast cancer, there are still 3,000 new cases of cervical cancer diagnosed each year in the UK. But with the introduction of screening, cervical smear tests have helped prevent many cases of the disease.
Regular smear tests can detect precancerous changes in the cells of the cervix and treatment can stop the cancer before it starts.

Who is most at risk from cervical cancer?
• Women who begin having unprotected sex at an early age.
• Women who have had unprotected sex with many partners.
• Women who smoke.
• Women who are taking immunosuppressant drugs.
• Women who have a family history of cervical cancer.

What are the symptoms?
The symptoms are not always visible, but some women will notice abnormal vaginal bleeding after sex. In later stages, symptoms can include:
• A watery, bloodstained vaginal discharge with an offensive odour.
• Pelvic pain.
• Pain during intercourse.
If you notice any of these symptoms, it is important to see your physician as soon as possible.

How will my general physician know I have cervical cancer?
Your physician will probably perform a ceder lining can become thinner, increasing your risk of cystitis and other infections.
Estrogen loss can also aggravate pelvic floor muscles already weakened by childbirth, and lead to problems in controlling the urge to pass urine. The medical term for this condition is stress incontinence, and it can cause small amounts of urine to leak out of your body when you sneeze, cough or run.
Pelvic floor exercises can help to relieve this embarrassing problem, so there is no need to suffer, simply ask your doctor for advice.

dilute vinegar solution that in some cases causes a slight burning. The exam usually takes less that half an hour. Because some doctors do not have the special equipment needed to perform this test in their offices, you may be referred to another doctor or go to a special clinic for this test.

■ *Biopsy*
When abnormalities of the cervix are seen by colposcopy, it is necessary to remove small pieces of cervical tissue for study to accurately diagnose the problem. This is usually done in the doctor's office or clinic. You may have some mild cramping or pinching sensation.

Because CIN may precede cancer by some years, early detection is important. CIN can be readily detected by a Pap test and can be diagnosed by colposcopy and cervical biopsy. Occasionally, a procedure called conization may be needed. In this surgical procedure, a cone-shaped wedge of the cervix is removed and examined under a microscope by a pathologist, someone who is specially trained in the study of disease. It may take about a week to 10 days to get these results.

Treatment
The type of treatment used for CIN depends on how extensive it is. CIN can be treated with cryotherapy, electrocoagulation, laser therapy, or conization.

Cervical cancer

Description
The various parts of the uterus or womb may be the site of benign of malignant tumors or growths. Cancer that develops in the cervix of the uterus is called cervical cancer and is one of the common cancers. About six per cent of all cancers in women are malignant tumors in the cervix of the uterus. When cervical cancer spreads, it usually travels through the lymphatic system. Cancer cells are carried along by lymph, an almost colourless fluid discharged by tissue into the lymphatic system. Lymph nodes scattered along this system filter bacteria and abnormal substances such as cancer cells. For this reason, surgeons often remove lymph nodes near the uterus to learn whether they contain cancer cells. Cancer of the cervix also can spread through the bloodstream.
Because cancer can spread, it is important for the physician to find ours as early as possible if the tumor is present and whether it is benign or malignant. As soon as a diagnosis is made, the doctor can begin treatment to control the disease. In some women, the cells in the cervix may go through a series of changes. Normal, healthy cells may become irregular in size and shape, and lose their normal orientation (a condition known as dysplasia).
Dysplasia is not cancer, although it may develop into very clear cancer of the cervix. Dysplastic cells undergoing mitosis have the same general appearance under the microscope as cancer cells; however, dysplastic cells do not invade nearby healthy tissues.
Dysplasia is classified as mild, moderate, or severe, depending on how abnormal the cells appear under the microscope. The condition develops most often in women between the ages of 25 and 35, but it can appear in other age groups as well.

Early detection
Very early cancer of the cervix (also called carcinoma in situ) involves only

the top layer of cervical cells and does not invade deeper layers of cervical tissue for many months, perhaps years. It is the earliest form of cervical cancer that can be detected. Although very early cervical cancer develops most often in women between the ages of 30 and 40, it can occur in younger and older women.

Invasive cervical cancer is cancer that has spread deeper into the cervix and/or nearby tissues or organs. It occurs most often in women between the ages of 40 and 60. Most cases of invasive cervical cancer could be prevented if all women had pelvic examinations and Pap tests regularly. A pelvic examination of the uterus, ovaries, fallopian tubes, urinary bladder, and rectum.

The physician feels these organs for any abnormality in their shape or size. During a pelvic examination, a speculum is used to widen the opening of the vagina so that the physician can see the upper portion of the vagina and the cervix.

■ *Pap test*

The Pap test (named after dr. G. Papanicolaou) is a simple, painless test to detect abnormal cells in and around the cervix. A Pap test can be done in a doctor's office, clinic or hospital. The physician collects a sample of cells from the cervix and upper vagina with a wooden scraper or cotton swab and places the sample on a glass slide.

The slide is sent to a medical laboratory for evaluation. The results of the Pap test usually are given by class (see the data below). All women who are 18 or older or who have had sexual intercourse should have regular annual check-ups.

These checkups should include a pelvic examination and a Pap test. After a woman has had three or more normal annual Pap tests, the examination may be done less often, as her physician advises. Women who are at increased risk of developing cancer of the cervix may need to be examined more often.

The need for a Pap test following a hysterectomy (surgical removal of the uterus) depends on the reason for the surgery and the type of procedure done.

▲ If the hysterectomy was a treatment for cancer, regular Pap tests should continue.
▲ If the cervix was not removed (partial hysterectomy), Pap tests are still needed.
▲ For most women who have had the uterus and cervix removed (total hysterectomy), regular pelvic examinations are important, but Pap tests are not needed.
▲ Women who were exposed to the drug diethylstilbestrol (DES) before birth should have a pelvic examination and a Pap test at least once a year starting at age 14 or when they begin menstruating, whichever is earlier.

Symptoms

Dysplasia and early cervical cancer seldom cause symptoms. They can only be detected by a pelvic examination and a Pap test. Symptoms generally do not appear until cervical cancer becomes invasive.

The most common symptom of cervical cancer is abnormal bleeding. Bleeding may start and stop between regular menstrual periods, or it may occur after sexual intercourse, douching, or a pelvic examination.

Menstrual bleeding may last longer and be heavier than usual. Increased vaginal discharge is another symptom of cervical cancer.

Pain is not an early warning sign of the disease. These symptoms are not sure signs of cervical cancer; however, it is important for a woman to see her physician if any symptoms lasts longer than 2 weeks. Any illness should be diagnosed and treated as early as possible. Early diagnosis is especially important for cervical cancer.

Diagnosis

If the pelvic examination or the Pap test shows any abnormality, the physician will do more tests to find out what the problem is. When a vaginal infection is the suspected cause of an abnormal Pap test, the physician will treat the infection and then repeat the Pap test. If an infection is not the reason for the abnormal Pap test, the physician may remove a small amount of tissue for further evaluation (biopsy).

Biopsy is mandatory if a suspicious lesion (a viable mass or an ulcer) is

Malignant growth in the epithelial tissue of the cervix. The cancer is characterized by chaotic growth, different sizes of cells and irregular mitosis (cell division). This malignant growth has been photographed by a special technique using a fluorescent microscope. The nuclei of the cells show up as yellow-green; RNA (nuclei acid) appears red. The presence of nucleic acid points to cell division.

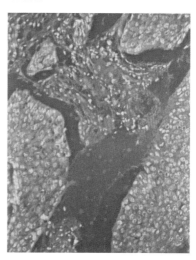

C

seen. The physician may use a number of procedures to pinpoint areas that should be biopsied. These tests usually are done in the physician's office. In the Schiller test, an iodine solution is applied to the cervix. Healthy cells turn brown; abnormal cells turn white or yellow.

In another procedure, the physician may use an instrument much like a microscope (called a colposcope) to look at the cervix. Small samples of abnormal tissue are taken for further examination.

In some cases the doctor must remove larger samples of tissue to make a diagnosis.

These samples are obtained most often by conization (cone biopsy) or dilatation and curettage (D&C).

In a conization, the physician removes a cone-shaped piece of tissue from the cervix and cervical canal. In a D&C, the physician dilates (widens) the cervix and inserts a curette (a small spoon-shaped instrument) to scrape tissue from the cervical canal and the inner lining of the uterus. A brief hospital stay may be needed for these procedures.

If a woman has cervical cancer, it is important to find out whether the disease has spread from the cervix to other parts of the body. Staging procedures include a thorough physical examination that is done under anesthesia, as well as blood and urine tests and a chest X-ray.

Physicians may also use ultrasound to view the inside of the body. In this procedure, high-frequency sound waves that cannot be heard, echo off tissues and organs, and the echoes produced can be seen on a screen.

Healthy tissues and tumors produce different echoes. Because cancer of the cervix can spread to the bladder, colon, and rectum, the physician may ask for special examination of these areas too.

Treatment

The physician considers a number of factors to determine the best treatment for dysplasia (abnormal cells) and cervical cancer. Among these factors are the extent of the disease, as well as the age and general health of the woman. How dysplasia is treated depends on its severity.

▲ *Mild dysplasia* may not require any treatment, but it should be checked regularly for any changes.

▲ *Moderate dysplasia* usually is treated by cryosurgery (freezing) or cauterization (burning). These methods destroy abnormal areas of the cervix without harming surrounding healthy tissues. Conization is the usual treatment for severe dysplasia.

Recently, lasers have been used to treat dysplasia. The laser uses a powerful beam of light to destroy abnormal cells, leaving the normal cells underneath unharmed.

Treatment of cervical cancer may involve surgery, radiation therapy, or chemotherapy. Surgery may remove only a small area of abnormal tissue, or it may remove the cervix, uterus, and other nearby tissues.

Radiation therapy uses high-energy rays to kill cancer cells. Radiation may be given from a machine located outside the body (external radiation therapy) or from radioactive material placed inside the body (internal radiation therapy). Chemotherapy is the use of anticancer drugs to treat cancer. Sometimes, a combination of these methods is used.

Treating very early cervical cancer

Treatment for very early cervical cancer depends on the age of the woman and on the preferences of the patient and her physician. Treatment may involve cryosurgery, cauterization, conization, laser treatment, or hysterectomy.

Conization is the usual treatment for young women who wish to have children. Most women who do not want to have additional children are treated with total hysterectomy (removal of the cervix and body of the uterus).

Treating invasive cervical cancer

Treatment of invasive cancer of the cervix depends on the extent of the disease. Patients whose cancer has invaded only the cervix and those whose disease has extended into the tissues next to the cervix or the upper vagina can be treated effectively with either surgery or radiation therapy.

Surgery may be a total hysterectomy (removal of the cervix and uterus) or a radical hysterectomy (removal of the cervix, uterus, upper vagina, and the lymph nodes in the area). Both external and internal radiation therapy can be used to treat invasive cervical cancer. Patients with cancer that has spread to the pelvis, to the lower part of the vagina, or to the ureters are treated with radiation therapy alone. Again, both external and internal radiation therapy can be used. Patients with cervical cancer that has spread to the bladder, rectum, or distant parts of the body may receive chemotherapy, in addition to surgery or radiation therapy.

Chemotherapy is also used to treat patients whose disease recurs following treatment with surgery or radiation therapy.

Experts disagree over whether it may be reasonable to delay treatment of early-stage cervical cancer detected during pregnancy to improve the chances of survival of the foetus.

Side effects of treatment

The treatment used against cancer must be very powerful. It is rarely possible to limit the effects of treatment so that only cancer cells are destroyed. Normal, healthy cells may be damaged at the same time. This is why treatment often causes side effects.

Hysterectomy is major surgery. After the operation, the hospital stay usually lasts about one week. For several days after surgery, patients may have

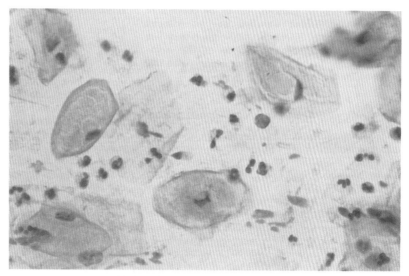
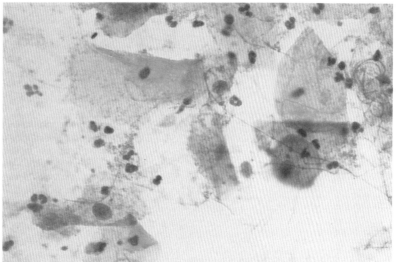
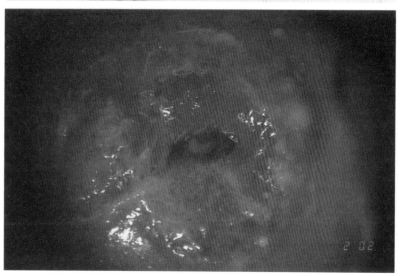

Microscopic pictures of the cervix based on Pap smears and macroscopic photographs.
Upper: Cervical smear from a pregnant woman showing several navicular cells. They contain yellow-stained glycogen. The cell borders are thick and sharp.
Middle: Cervical smear showing superficial and intermediate squamous cells, leukocytes and some bacteria.
Lower: Macroscopic picture of a normal cervix showing columnar epithelium.

C

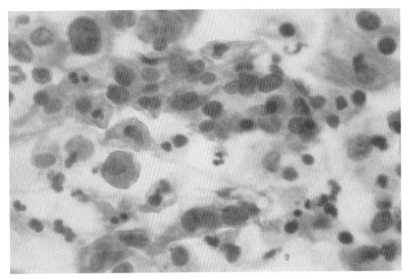

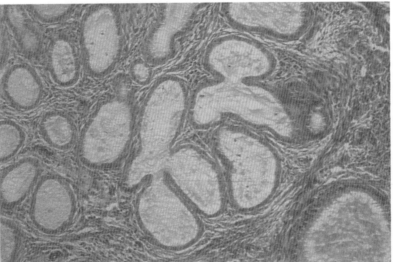

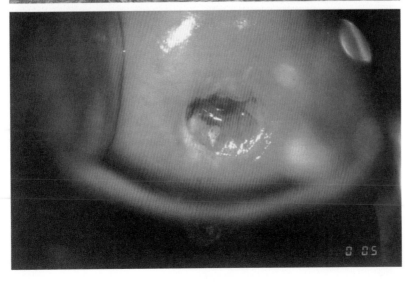

problems emptying their bladder and having normal bowel movements. The lower abdomen will be sore. Normal activities, including sexual intercourse, usually can be resumed in 4 to 8 weeks.

Women who have had their uterus removed no longer have menstrual periods. When the ovaries are not removed, women do not go through menopause (change of life) because their ovaries still produce hormones. If the ovaries are removed or damaged by radiation therapy, menopause will occur. Hot flashes or other symptoms of menopause caused by treatment may be more severe than those from a natural menopause.

Sexual desire and the ability to have intercourse usually are not affected by hysterectomy. However, many women have an emotionally difficult time after a hysterectomy. They may have feelings of deep loss because they are no longer able to become pregnant.

Radiation therapy destroys the ability of cells to grow and divide. Both normal and diseased cells are affected, but most normal cells are able to recover quickly. Patients usually receive external radiation therapy as an outpatient. Treatment are given 5 days a week for several weeks. This schedule helps to protect healthy tissues by spreading out the total dose of radiation. Weekend rest breaks allow the normal cells to repair themselves.

Internal radiation therapy puts cancer-killing rays as close as possible to the side of the cancer while sparing most of the healthy tissue around it. This type of radiation therapy requires a short hospital stay. A radiation implant, a capsule containing

Microscopic pictures of the cervix based on Pap smears and macroscopic photographs.
Upper: Cervical smear with numerous squamous cells, many of which have enlarged and hyperchromatic nuclei. The smear is characteristic for a reactive process, indicating a cervicitis.
Middle: Cervical smear showing gland proliferation. Secretions are seen in the gland's lumen. The picture is indicative for a benign proliferation of the cervix.
Lower: Macroscopic picture of the cervix showing a lesion with coarse punctuation; a preinvasive lesion of the cervix.

radioactive material, is inserted through the vagina into the cervix and uterus. The implant usually is left in place for 2 or 3 days.

During radiation therapy, patients may notice a number of side effects, which usually disappear when treatment is completed. Patients may be unusually tired, and they may have skin reactions (redness or dryness) in the area being treated.

It is important to rest as much as possible and to treat the skin gently. Patients also may have diarrhea and frequent and uncomfortable urination. Patients can expect to stop menstruating and may have other symptoms of menopause.

Treatment can cause dryness, itching, or burning in the vagina. Intercourse may be painful, and some women are advised not to have intercourse at this time. Most women can resume sexual activity within a few weeks after treatment ends.

The anticancer drugs used in chemotherapy travel through the bloodstream to almost every part of the body. Drugs used to treat cancer maybe given to patients in different ways: some are given by mouth; others are injected into a muscle, a vein, or an artery.

Chemotherapy is most often given in cycles - a treatment period, followed by a rest period, than another treatment period, and so on.

Depending on the drugs that are used, the patient may need to stay in the hospital for a few days so that the effects of the drugs can be watched. Sometimes, the patient may receive treatment at the hospital clinic, at the physician's office, or at home.

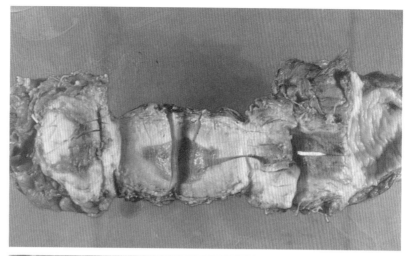

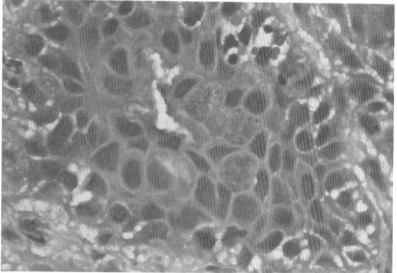

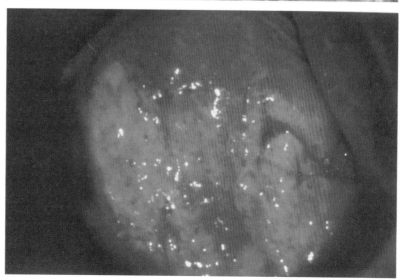

Microscopic pictures of the cervix based on Pap smears and macroscopic photographs.
Upper: Macroscopic picture of a specimen from a woman with squamous cell cancer of the cervix. The uterus (center) is flanked by the bladder (left) and the rectum (right).
Middle: High-power view of an endosquamous cancer of the cervix with squamous cells surrounding a slitlike lumen.
Lower: Colpophotograph of the cervix of a 15-year-old girl. The cervix was replaced by a 5 to 6 cm tumor characteristic for a malignant lymphoma.

CHILD BIRTH

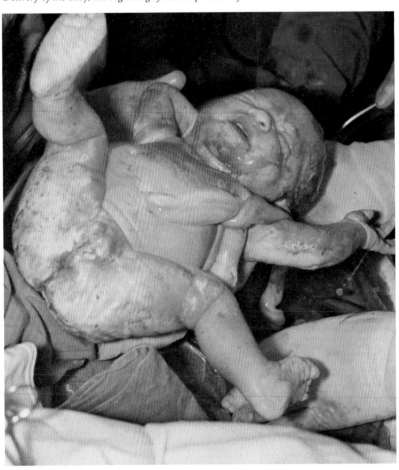

Introduction

Birth is the act of expelling the young from the mother's body; the emergence from the mother's womb (uterus) marking the beginning of an independent life. The birth process is triggered by hormonal changes in the woman's bloodstream.

Mild labor pains (contractions of the muscles of the uterus) are usually the first sign that a woman is about to give birth. This is the first stage of labor, usually lasting about 14 hours. The contractions push the baby downwards, usually head first, which breaks the membranes surrounding the baby, and the amniotic fluid escapes. (Sometimes, however, the waters break before there are any contrac-

tions.) In the second stage of labor, stronger contractions push the baby through the cervix and vagina (the birth canal). This is the most painful part and usually lasts less than two hours. Anesthetics or analgesics are often given, and delivery aided by hand or obstetric forceps.

A cesarean section (surgical removal of the baby) may be performed if great difficulty occurs. Some women choose natural childbirth in which no painkillers are used, but pain is minimized by the distraction of relaxation exercises. As soon as the baby is born, its nose and mouth are cleared of fluid and breathing starts, whereupon the umbilical cord is cut and tied.

In the third stage of labor, the placenta is expelled from the uterus and bleeding is stopped by further contractions.

Labor

Labor is the process by which the products of conception including the fetus and placenta are expelled from the pregnant uterus to the outside environment. This process can occur at any time during the period of gestation when the foetus is at varying stages of development.

Normal labor in the human is said to occur when it results in a mature living baby, i.e. of more than 2500 g (5 lb 8 oz), usually within two or three weeks of the expected date of delivery. In spite of much research, the mechanism that initiates labor is unknown. An old suggestion that labor starts when the fetus outgrows its oxygen supply must be incorrect because the fetus may die of asphyxia and yet be retained in the uterus for several weeks. Recent research indicates that both hormones from the placenta and

Delivery of the baby, the beginning of an independent life.

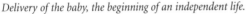

C

the woman's pituitary gland play an important role in the initiation of delivery.

The possibility that the fetus might control its own time of expulsion from the uterus has always been attractive, as it would explain why birth occurs in various species when the fetus has reached an adequate state of development to cope with existence in the outside world and yet is not too large to cause difficulties at delivery.

It appears that no single factor is responsible for the onset of labor. Both fetal and maternal hormones, as well as local mechanical factors and concentrations of various substances in the blood, influence uterine activity through the final common pathway of increasing the contractibility of the muscle layer of the uterus.

The mechanisms involved in a normal birth are fourfold:

▲ The expulsive forces, i.e., the uterine contractions, augmented at a later stage by voluntary efforts.
▲ Cervical effacement (thinning) and dilation.
▲ The shape and size of the fetus, especially the fetal skull since it is usually the part to come out first.
▲ The shape and size of the birth canal, especially the bony pelvis, although the soft tissues are important in the later stages of expulsion.

For convenience, labor may be considered as three stages, which follow in a continuous sequence.

▲ The first stage of labor extends from the onset of labor until full dilation of the cervix.
▲ The second stage of labor extends from full dilation of the cervix until the completion of delivery of the baby.
▲ The third stage of labor extends from delivery of the baby until completion of expulsion of the placenta.

First stage

It is usually difficult to determine with any accuracy when labor begins. Established labor is characterized by regular coordinated uterine contrac-

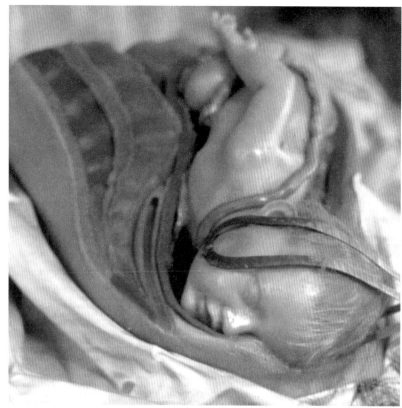

Model of forceps delivery. Forceps or a vacuum extractor may be used to help with delivery. Forceps are placed around the baby's head. A vacuum extractor uses suction to adhere to the baby's head. With either device, the baby is gently pulled out as the woman pushes.

In the United States, almost all babies are born in hospitals, but some women want to have their babies at home. However, because unexpected complications can occur during or shortly after labor, most experts do not advise delivery at home.

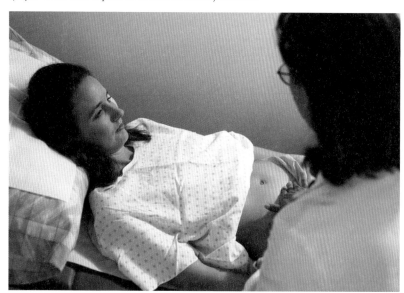

C

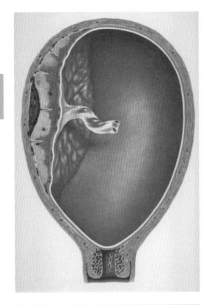

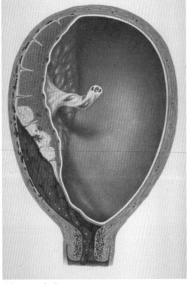

Abnormal placentas.
Upper figure: The placenta detaches from the uterine wall, causing the uterus to bleed.
Lower figure: The placenta is located over or near the cervix (placenta previa), causing painless bleeding that suddenly begins late in pregnancy.

tions which become progressively more painful.

However, some women may have apparently strong uterine contractions that do not develop into established labor, and it is impossible to distinguish these false labor pains from true labor other than by obser-

vation over a period of hours to see if they are progressive. In addition, a small minority have no first-stage-of-labor pains at all.

Initially, though, contractions are often felt as a dull ache low in the back but later they become more severe and are felt most in the lower abdomen.

The onset of painful uterine contractions may be preceded by a vaginal discharge of blood and mucus, often referred to as a "show." This may vary from a slight pink discharge to obvious bleeding and is due to the cervix beginning to shorten, so allowing the cervical plug of mucus to escape into the vagina.

It may be difficult to distinguish between a heavy show and a hemorrhage due to separation of the placenta from the uterus wall. In a minority of woman the onset of uterine contractions may coincide with, or be preceded by, rupture of the fetal membranes and the escape of amniotic fluid via the vagina - the "breaking of the waters."

It is not known why the membranes should rupture early in labor in some women while in the majority they remain intact until the second stage. Rupture of the membranes at term is usually followed by the onset of uterine contractions within 24 hours.

As the first stage of labor progresses, the uterine contractions increase in strength and frequency. In well-established labor, contractions should occur every two to four minutes and last 40-60 seconds. Less frequent or shorter contractions may be relatively ineffective and more frequent or more prolonged contractions may be harmful to the fetus.

The attending midwife or doctor has three responsibilities during the conduct of the first stage of delivery:

▲ To detect early signs of impending danger to the fetus by regularly listening to the fetal heart and the inspection of amniotic fluid.
▲ To ensure that the mother is as comfortable as possible and is not at unnecessary risk.
▲ To observe that steady progress in terms of dilation of the cervix and descent of the head is being made. Descent of the head is usually recognized by abdominal palpation

but it may be necessary to repeat the vaginal examination.

The average duration of the first stage of normal labor for a first child is about 14 hours, and is usually 7-8 hours for the second and following children. However, there is a wide variation in its length and pattern. The rate of dilation of the cervix is not even.

Second stage

Towards the end of the first stage the character of the contractions alters. As the head reaches the pelvic floor it stimulates a reflex, a sensation to bear down during each uterine contraction.

Most women welcome this change because they feel that they can actively help to expel the baby. However, if this sensation occurs before the cervix is fully dilated, the impulse should be resisted because any attempt to expel the baby before full dilation may result in the cervix being pushed down the birth canal in front of the head, where it becomes trapped.

This desire to bear down is often accompanied by a desire to defecate. As the cervix reaches full dilation small tears may occur and cause slight bleeding. Furthermore, the membranes commonly rupture spontaneously.

Consequently, the signs which herald the onset of the second stage are:

▲ The desire to bear down and possibly defecate.
▲ Vaginal bleeding.
▲ Spontaneous rupture of the membranes.

If these features are missed, the next sign may be bulging and gaping of the vagina and appearance of the fetal head. The importance in recognizing the onset of the second stage is to allow time to prepare for delivery and to assess the rate of progress.

The position the woman adopts for delivery is largely one of custom and convenience. In many primitive cultures, women deliver in the crouched, squatting position that adds gravity to the force of uterine contractions. This position is becoming more and more popular among American and European woman.

In most Western countries, woman deliver lying on their backs with their legs open and held up in stirrups. This position is relatively comfortable for the woman and, perhaps more significant, convenient for the attendants.

During each uterine contraction, the woman is encouraged to bear down for as long as possible at each contraction. When the head shows at the entrance of the vagina, the perineum (the skin area between the vagina and anus) is swabbed with an antiseptic solution, and the legs and thighs are draped with sterile towels.

After the head first appears, it usually advances with each contraction and retreats less each time until the skin of the perineum stretches thinly; this stage is often called the "crowning" of the head. If the perineum becomes very stretched and looks as if it may tear, a small relieving incision or episiotomy is made.

An episiotomy may minimize damage to the perineum, reduce the length of the second stage and possibly prevent damage to the fetal head by prolonged arrest on the pelvic floor. However, an episiotomy may also cause substantial

Stages of labor
Labor occurs in three main stages. The first stage (which has two phases: initial and active) is labor proper. In it, contractions cause the cervix to open gradually and to thin and pull back until it merges with the rest of the uterus (upper figures).

The second and third stages constitute delivery of the baby (second and third row of figures) and the placenta (fourth row of figures).

First stage: From the beginning of labor to the fill opening (dilatation) of the cervix - to about 4 inches.

Second stage: from the complete opening of the cervix to delivery of the baby. This stage averages about 45 to 60 minutes in the first pregnancy and 15 to 309 minutes in subsequent pregnancies.

Third stage: From delivery of the baby to delivery of the placenta. This stage usually lasts only a few minutes but may last up to 30 minutes.

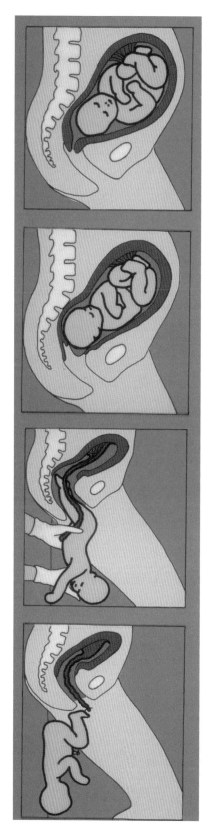
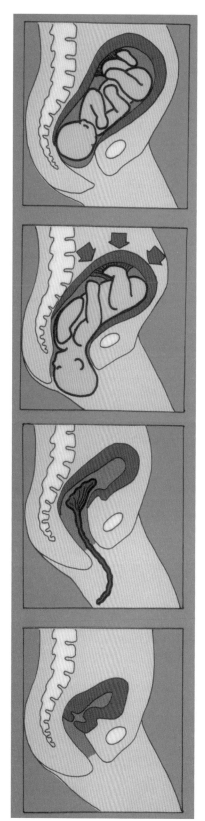

C

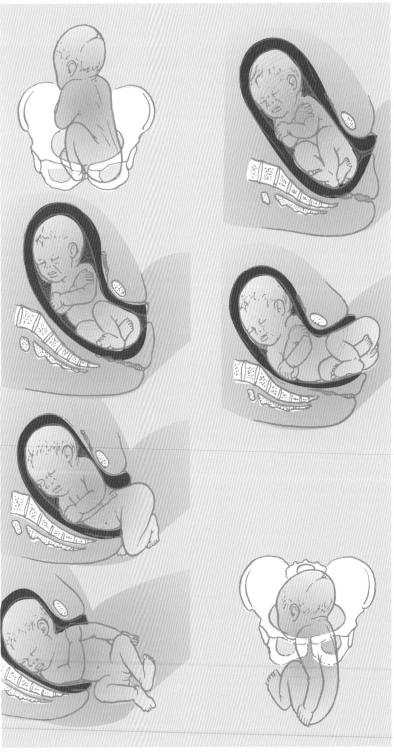

Breech delivery.
Breech presentation, in which the buttocks present first, occurs in 2 to 3% of full-term deliveries. When delivered vaginally, babies that present buttocks first are more likely to be injured than those that present head first.

bleeding and its repair can cause extreme discomfort in the puerperium (the six-week period following delivery).

As the head is delivered, the perineum is supported by a pad held in the right hand of the attendant while the fingers of the left grasp the top of the head of the baby to control its delivery.

Every effort is being made by the midwife or doctor to ensure slow delivery of the head by obtaining the woman's cooperation, because a rapid, uncontrolled delivery of the head may cause brain damage and tear the perineum severely.

It is often possible to deliver the head gently between contractions.

Once the head is delivered, the midwife or doctor uses a finger to feel if there is a loop of umbilical cord around the neck of the baby. After the head has rotated externally it is grasped between the palms of the hands without exerting pressure on any one area.

By exerting pressure from the back during the next uterine contraction, the shoulder in front can be induced to slip out. The head is then lifted so that the shoulder at the back and the rest of the baby follows.

When the baby has been delivered, it usually cries spontaneously, taking several deep breaths that expand its lungs. The umbilical cord is clamped in two places and then cut, and the umbilical stump is safely secured either by a rubber band or by a small disposable plastic clamp.

There is considerable argument over the optimal time at which the cord should be clamped. At the time of delivery the blood volume of the infant is about 300 ml, and another volume of 100 ml (about 3.5 fl. oz) of blood is trapped within the placenta. If clamping of the cord is delayed for a few minutes and the infant is held at a level below the uterus, a major part of the placental blood volume is transferred to the infant; conversely, immediate clamping withholds this volume of blood from the infant.

The average duration of the second stage is about 50 minutes (maximum about two hours) in women who deliver for the first time and about 20-25 minutes in other women.

Third stage

Immediately following delivery of the baby, the upper part of the uterus may be felt just below the navel. Contractions of the uterus continue intermittently and the placenta separates and descends into the lower part of the uterus and vagina. Placental separation usually occurs within three to four minutes of delivery but its expulsion from the uterus may be delayed longer either by weakness of the uterus muscles or by being held in place by uterine spasm.

After delivery of the infant, there is usually a steady trickle of blood from the vagina and, when the placenta separates, an additional gush of blood. Descent of the placenta is indicated by the lengthening of the umbilical cord.

When the placenta is expelled from the uterus, a length of about 75 mm (3 in) of cord descends with it. At the same time the uterus assumes a globular shape and rises to a slightly higher level in the abdomen, at or just below the navel.

The classical signs of placental separation and descent are:

▲ Fresh vaginal bleeding.
▲ Lengthening of the umbilical cord.
▲ Change in the shape and height of the uterus.

Relief of pain in labor

Labor is almost invariably painful but the enthusiasm with which midwives and doctors attempt to relieve this pain varies widely throughout the world. Many women demand and are given painless labor by the regular use of regional and inhalation anesthesia. Others labor without anesthesia or with only small doses of the narcotic pain reliever, pethidine.

All the analgesic and anesthetic agents in routine use (except spinal anesthetics) freely cross the placenta and may affect the fetus. Unfortunately most of them cause a slowing of breathing. Although this is usually insignificant in the woman, it may be critical for the fetus at the time of delivery when there must be a rapid and efficient

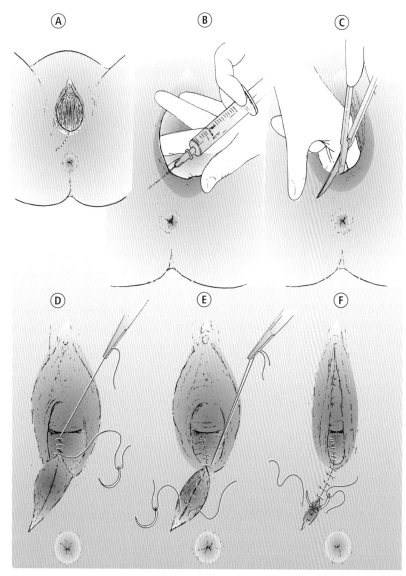

Episiotomy. Line of incision (A); infiltrating tissues with local anesthetic (B); making the incision, while inserting two fingers to protect the baby's head (C); repairing the wound in three layers by first suturing the vaginal mucosa and submucosa in one layer (D), then suturing the muscle layer (E), and finally suturing the skin (F).

transition from breathing via the placenta to breathing via the lungs.

The fetus may also be influenced by the actions of anesthetics on the woman. Thus use of some inhalation analgesics such as a mixture of nitrous oxide and air ("gas and air") may reduce the oxygen content of air breathed in, while methods that induce maternal hypotension (lowering of blood pressure) may reduce the amount of blood going to the placenta.

These fetal hazards are aggravated if the foetus is already at risk, either because of some prolonged complication such as high blood pressure, or by an episode of hypoxia (decrease of oxygen in the blood).

Regional anesthesia (numbing of only a specific part of the body) can be achieved in various ways. The pain of labor is transmitted by sensory fibers from the uterus and cervix that enter

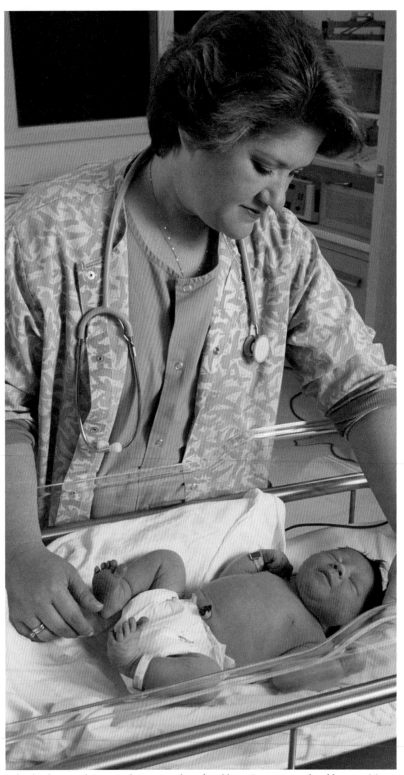

After birth, a newborn may have a number of problems. Doctors may be able to anticipate many problems by monitoring fetal growth and development, particularly using ultrasound. Many newborns with problems are cared for in a neonatal intensive care unit (NICU).

the spinal cord at the lower thoracic and upper lumbar levels.

The pain experienced at the time of delivery is transmitted mainly by the nerves of the vulva and perineum (those in the area between the legs). Consequently a nerve block can be effective if made in the epidural space of the spine up to the level of the tenth thoracic segment. Low spinal anesthesia involves the injection of a local anesthetic into the cerebrospinal fluid (that which surrounds the spinal cord), but this method often causes headache.

Epidural anesthesia (where an injection is made near the spinal canal but not into it) has less risk of causing headache and is easier to control. Most local anesthetics are effective for only one or two hours.

Psychoprophylaxis was first made popular by the British obstetrician, Dr Grantly Dick-Read, in 1933 under the name of "natural childbirth."

Apart from extensive preparation involving the teaching of the mechanism of childbirth, it depends to a large extent on achieving good muscular relaxation by controlled breathing. Generally, muscular tension is reduced, pain is lessened, labor is shortened and blood loss reduced. It is likely that the relief of pain is achieved by reducing anxiety through better instruction and some autohypnosis and distraction, rather than by controlled breathing.

Cesarean section

Surgical incision through the abdomen and uterus for removal of a foetus, performed when conditions (e.g. maternal hemorrhage, a placenta that is over the birth canal, foetal distress, baby too large for passage through mother's pelvis) for normal vaginal delivery are deemed hazardous for mother or baby.

Julius Caesar was purportedly delivered from his dead mother, alive and well, after her belly was cut open immediately upon her demise, giving rise to the common name for the operative delivery of a baby.

In the last 2000 years the operation has been considerably refined to the point where about a quarter of all

Vaginal Delivery or Cesarean Section

▲ For a Cesarean section, an incision is made in the upper part or lower part of the uterus. A lower incision is more common.

▲ The lower part of the uterus has fewer blood vessels, so that less blood is usually lost. Also, the healed scar is less likely to open in subsequent deliveries. A lower incision may be horizontal or vertical.

▲ Usually, an upper incision is used when the placenta covering the cervix, when the fetus lies horizontally, or when the fetus is very premature.

▲ The choice of having a vaginal delivery or a repeat Cesarian section is usually offered to women who have had a lower incision. Vaginal delivery is successful in about three forth of these women.

babies are now delivered in this manner.

The operation is extremely safe for both mother and child. A spinal or epidural anesthetic is given to the mother, and the baby is usually delivered within five minutes.

A general anesthetic is these days only given in some specific circumstances. After delivery the longer and more complex task of repairing the womb and abdominal muscles is undertaken. In most cases, the scar of a cesarean is low and horizontal, below the bikini line, to avoid any disfigurement.

Recovery from a cesarean is slower than for normal childbirth, but most women leave hospital within seven days. It does not affect breast feeding or the chances of future pregnancies, and does not increase the risk of miscarriage. Attitudes towards Cesarean section largely determine the frequency with which this operation is used.

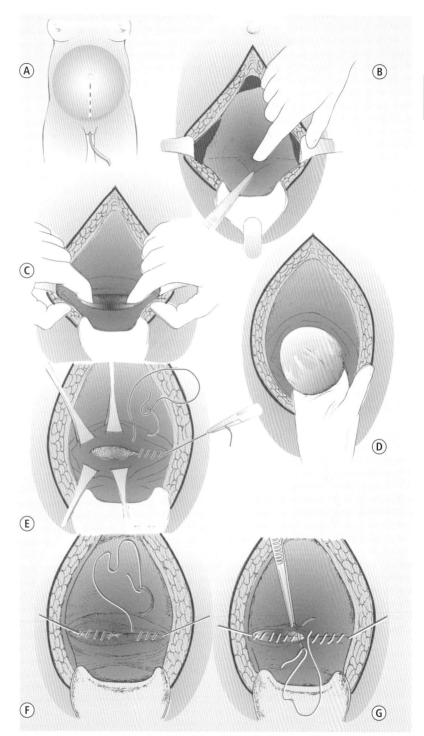

Lower-segment caesarean section. Site of the midline (A); incision of the loose peritoneum covering the anterior surface of the lower uterine segment (B); blunt incision on either side of the uterus (C); insinuation of the fingers between the lower uterine flap and the head of the baby (D); delivery of the baby. Suturing of the uterine wall (E); inserting the second layer of suture, taking the muscles and burying the first layer (F); inserting the peritoneal layer of suture (G).

CHILD HEALTH CARE

Health supervision

The objectives of baby and child care are:

▲ prevention of disease through routine immunizations and through educational means (parental instruction on nutrition, accident prevention, sanitation, etc.);

▲ early detection of disease through interview, physical examination, and screening procedures;

▲ early treatment of disease;

▲ provision of guidance in child rearing to afford optimal conditions for normal emotional and intellectual development.

To meet these objectives, child and parent are seen by the doctor at regular intervals throughout the early years of life. The frequency of these visits and their content are determined by the child's age, the population served, and the physician's opinion of their value.

Inquiries as to the infant's intellectual and psychosocial development will be considered an aspect of preventive health care.

Personal adaptive development (social, language, gross motor, fine motor) can be estimated by using the Denver Developmental Screening Test (DDST). Routine testing will be started at age 4 to 6 months, and can be repeated into early childhood.

Assessing the parents' perception of their child and the interactions between parents and infant cannot be accomplished easily by any convenient, standardized method.

Nonetheless, the physician will attempt to determine the parents' feelings and attitudes toward their child. This should begin with the first contact in the hospital, when the parents and the physician can discuss the vicissitudes of raising children.

In subsequent discussions, parental attitudes may be identified tactfully by determining how parents feel they are being affected by caring for a new baby, how they cope with difficult situations, or how easily they can obtain help when feeling tired or short-tempered.

Assessing the parents' perception of their child and the interactions between parents and infants can not be accomplished easily by any conventional, standardized method.

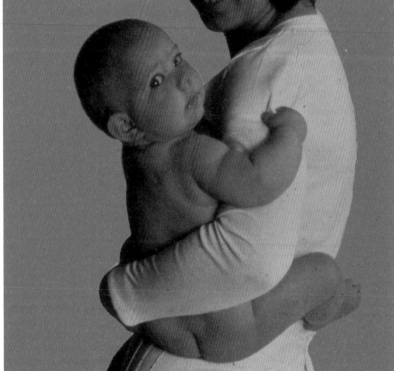

Failure to thrive

One of the most serious problems in child care concerns the failure to thrive. This problem is defined as the failure of growth and development to meet realistic expectations because of genetic, physical, or psychosocial factors. Growth and development in children are sensitive indicators of their state of health.

Failure to thrive most often presents in an infant as insufficient weight gain, in a child as shortness, and in the early teenager as a combination of shortness and lack of sexual development.

Presented with a patient who is failing to thrive, the physician will first determine if indeed the child is not reaching his or her potential. The expectations of the parents or other concerned individuals may be realistic and pathologic causes are involved, or they may be unrealistic, which can lead to psychologic problems.

Causes

Any pathological process that is severe enough to interfere with normal metabolism will inhibit body growth. When the deranged metabolism is related to acute illness, as is unusually the case, it is of brief duration and has little or no long-range effects on growth or development.

With prolonged or frequent abnormalities, however, growth will almost certainly be impeded and possibly permanently affected.

The causes can be physical, psychosocial, or both. Malnutrition is often a mediating influence, particularly in the younger child. Failure to thrive may be only one of many manifestations of a complex disease process and may even go unnoticed, overshadowed by the severity of other symptoms.

■ Genetic defects

Tall parents as a rule have tall children; short parents, short children. However, children inherit not only this potential for ultimate development but also the pattern for obtaining it.

Parents who were small as children, with a late onset of puberty and a late cessation of growth (eventually falling within the normal range), may have offspring who follow the same pattern, which is a form of constitutional delay.

These parents may seek help in hurrying along their children's growth so that the youngsters will not suffer the indignities the parents did.

■ Organ defects

Deficiency of thyroid hormone, or of specific pituitary hormones, leads to profound growth retardation and, in the case of thyroid deficiency, also to developmental delay.

Lack of sex hormones or their pituitary trophic hormones causes failure

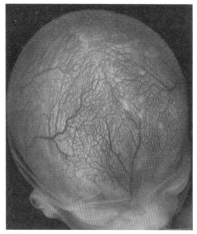
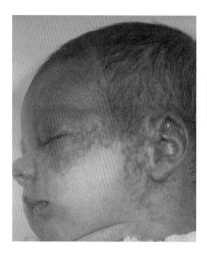

Failure to thrive.
The two photographs show children who suffered from failure to thrive, due to a disturbance of the thyroid gland. Deficiency of thyroid hormones or of specific pituitary hormones, leads to profound growth retardation, and, in the case of thyroid deficiency, also to developmental delay.

of secondary sexual development and its accompanying growth spurt. Excesses of adrenocortical hormones interfere with growth.

Damage to the brain may lead to feeding difficulties or to changes in endocrine function that affect growth and development.

Because the kidneys eliminate the toxic waste products of metabolism and help to maintain a normal electrolyte concentration, chronic kidney failure with uremia leads to growth failure.

■ Malnutrition

The problem of malnutrition is intrinsically interwoven with the complex etiology of failure to thrive and may be caused by inadequate food intake, malabsorption, or faulty metabolism.

Specific deficiencies of essential nutrients, as well as general malnutrition, may cause profound growth retardation, as in marasmus, kwashiorkor, or rickets.

■ Psychosocial and environmental influences

A supportive, loving parent-child interaction is important for satisfactory nutrition, growth, and development. If physically or emotionally deprived, infants and young children may stop growing.

Parental withdrawal, rejection, or hos-

tility, all of which can cause emotional deprivation, can result from a number of causes, including an unwanted pregnancy, the death of another child, parental jealousy or insecurity, or disappointment over the sex, appearance, or growth of the child.

The socioeconomic status of the family may be an important factor in the child's growth, since it can affect nutrition, living conditions, and parental attitudes.

Environmental factors that may interfere with growth include exposure to infections, parasitic infestations and intoxication by a variety of foreign substances.

■ Unknown causes

A form of constitutional delay is seen in some children whose growth inexplicably appears to stand still for a period of time.

Occasionally, this can be related to some stressful event such as a family move, a hospitalization, or some intercurrent illness. As inexplicably as it stopped, growth starts once again.

The lost growth may not be regained, but an approximate normal rate of development is maintained from that point on.

As in the hereditary form of constitutional delay, pubescence and final cessation of growth are delayed, so that these children ultimately achieve a reasonably normal adult stature.

Medicines - Important rules for treatment of children

C

Rule number one
- Let your doctor - and only your doctor - prescribe medication and dosage.
- When your child is sick, it sometimes seems as if everybody is an expert on how to cure him. Your mother, your mother-in-law, your next-door neighbor, all your friends and relatives - they certainly mean well. But their home remedies could be ineffective, or outdated, or actually harmful. Your doctor is highly trained, experienced. He has access to the latest medical information. He is the only person qualified to diagnose your child's health problems.

Rule number two
- If you have any doubt about your doctor's instructions, ask for additional information.
- For example: Instructions on a bottle of medicine read: "One teaspoon every four hours." Does "every four hours" mean day and night? Should you wake your child during the night to give it to him? Or is it better to let him sleep through?
- Do not be afraid to ask questions. It is important that you understand the instructions clearly. It can often prevent mistakes in dosage and treatment.

Rule number three
- Be sure to follow your doctor's instructions. Apply the right medication in the right place.
- Many problems have to be treated in a way that may seem to be indirect. For example: middle ear infections are usually treated with oral medication or sometimes with nose drops.
- Sometimes drops in the ear (externally) are prescribed, but these are to relieve pain, not to cure the middle ear infection. Follow the instructions exactly.
- If your doctor prescribes a suppositorium for vomiting, the body absorbs the medicine in suppositories just as efficiently as it does the medicine in pills - sometimes more so. Besides, when the stomach's contents are involuntarily coming out of one end, it is much easier to get the medication into the other end.

Rule number four
- Read and follow the directions on the medicine container. Read the label carefully.
- Not all medications should be kept in a medicine chest. For example, suppositories need to be stored in a refrigerator.
- Some medicines become outdated. They lose their effectiveness and should be thrown out.

Rule number five
- Let your doctor know if you think you should stop the medication.
- There are times when a child does not or cannot accept the medicine. You are the one who is with your sick child constantly. You are the first to notice if your child is having a bad reaction to his medication. This does happen.

- He may vomit before the medicine does him any good. he may have an allergic reaction, such as a rash.
- Your doctor may want to suspend the medication. He may suggest a different one - or a different method of giving the same one.

Rule number six
- Do not give medication to any child other than the one for whom it was prescribed.
- Two children with the same symptoms may have entirely different illnesses. Even if they have the same illness, the dosage for your baby may not be enough for his brother or sister.
- Giving too small a dose to an older child can be just as dangerous as giving an overdose to an infant.
- Just because your child seems to be getting better, you should not stop giving certain medications. For example: a medicine such as an antibiotic may be prescribed for ten days. Your child's problem seems to clear up in three days.
- Your doctor will have sound reasons for wanting you to give the entire prescription. Often the symptoms will clear up, but the illness itself is not completely cured.

Rule number seven
- Do not give old medicine to your child without first consulting your doctor.
- Many different illnesses have symptoms that appear the same. Many medications are no longer effective after sitting six months on the shelf.

Rule number eight
- Do not hide from your child the fact that you are giving him medicine.
- It is not a good idea to hide medicine from your child by mixing it in food or drink. Worst of all, he will probably discover the medicine anyway and learn to distrust you. This will make it more difficult next time.
- He may develop a dislike for the particular food or drink in which he discovers the hidden medicine.
- If he does not finish all of the bottle or food, he ends up by not taking all his medicine.

Rule number nine
- Suppose your child has trouble swallowing pills - you have to give him a bitter-tasting medicine (which does not happen too often these days). Then you can mix it with something more palpable. A little bit of apple-sauce, for example - or a teaspoon of honey.
- But let him know what you are doing. Let him help you with it, if he is old enough. He should understand that this medicine is necessary so he can get well.

Rule number ten
- Some medicines, like penicillin G, do not absorb well if mixed with food. As you get new medication, it is a good idea to check with your doctor.

Primordial dwarfism is a type of growth failure frequently associated with a variety of congenital abnormalities, many of which appear as minor structural defects.

These children are frequently small at birth despite normal gestational age, and manifest no obvious cause for their lack of growth. It has been assumed that their cells do not respond to environmental and controlling mechanisms as do normal cells.

Diagnosis

The family history, including prenatal, birth, neonatal, psychosocial, and family information, is of particular importance, because often the physical examination is not unusual except for the smaller-than-normal height and weight measurement.

Information from the antepartal and neonatal periods provides important diagnostic clues:

▲ Was the pregnancy complicated by such factors as inadequate prenatal care, toxemia, maternal diseases (e.g., diabetes or thyroid disease).
▲ Was the infant premature or small for gestational age?
▲ Was there birth trauma?
▲ Did the expectant mother use drugs or alcohol in excessive

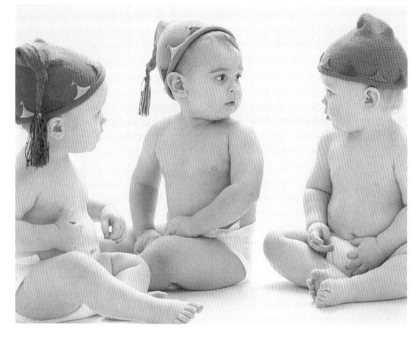

amounts?

The family history should include:

• age-related heights of relatives in order to give an indication of genetic potential;
• developmental patterns such as the time of the mother's menarche and the age when the father stopped growing;
• any stressful events affecting atti-

tudes toward the child, such as a sibling's death;
• the kind of relationship that exists between the mother and child;
• the emotional climate in the home.

All obtainable previously recorded heights, weights, and head circumferences are plotted on any of the standard growth charts (keeping in mind

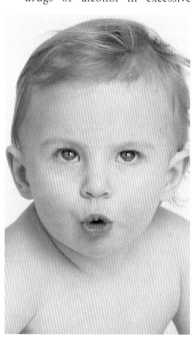

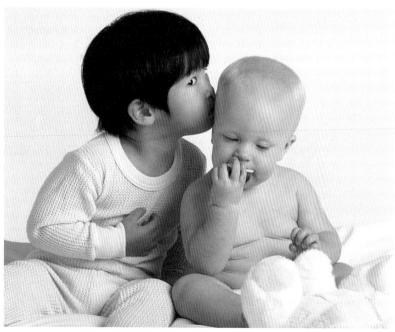

Developmental milestones from 3 months to 15 years

Watching a young child is a wonderful and unique experience for a parent. Learning to sit up, and talk are some of the more major developmental milestones your child will achieve. But your child's growth is a complex and ongoing process. Your children are constantly going through a number of physical and mental stages.

Although no two children develop at the same rate, they should be able to do certain things at certain ages. As a parent, you are in the best position to note your child's development, and you can use the milestones described below as guidelines.

For the first year use the milestones listed for each age to see how your child is developing. Try to answer the questions fore this period with Yes or No. Remember, a No answer to any of these questions does not necessarily mean that there is a problem. Every child develops at his own pace and may sometimes develop more slowly in certain areas than other children the same age. Keep in mind that milestones should be used only as guidelines.

For the second period (2 years to 15 years) the milestones are differently described to make it easy for you to check the various developmental capabilities and abilities of your child.

Plan to talk about these guidelines with your pediatrician during your next office visit if you note the following:
▲ Major differences between your child's development and the milestones.
▲ Your child does not yet do many of the things usually done at her age.

3 months

When your baby is lying on his back, does he move each of his arms equally well?
- Does your baby make sounds such as gurgling, cooing, babbling, or other noises besides crying?
- Does your baby respond to your voice?
- Are your baby's hands frequently open?
- When you hold your baby in the upright position, can she support her head for more than a moment?

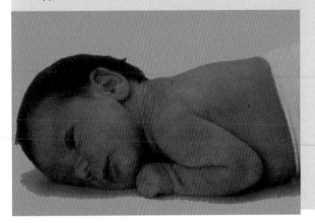

6 months
- Have you seen your baby play with his hands by touching them together?
- Does your baby turn her head to sounds that originate out of the immediate area?
- Has your baby rolled over from his stomach to his back and from back to stomach?
- When your baby is on his stomach, can be support his weight on outstretched hands?
- Does your baby see small objects such as crumbs?
- Does your baby produce a string of sounds?
- Does your baby begin to relax when you read him a bedtime story?
- Does your baby notice herself and her actions in a mirror?
- Does your baby reach out for you to pick him up?

9 months
When your baby is playing and you come up quietly behind her, does she sometimes turn her head as though she hears you? It is important that you see her respond to quiet sounds or whispers.
- Can your baby sit without support and without holding up his body with his hands?
- Does your baby crawl or creep on her hands and knees?
- Does your baby hold his bottle?
- Does your baby deliberately drop or throw toys?
- Does your baby bang, strike, and shake her toys?
- When you show your baby a book, does he get excited, then try to grab and taste it?
- Is your baby wary of unfamiliar people?
- Does your baby make sounds that use vowels and consonants?

12 months
When you hide something or around a corner, and then reappear, does your baby look for you and eagerly plan for you to reappear?
- Does your baby pull up to stand?
- Does your baby walk holding on to furniture?
- Does your baby make "ma-ma" or "da-da" sounds?
- Is your baby to locate sounds by turning his head?
- Does your baby imitate familiar adult behavior, such as using a cup or telephone?
- Does your baby turn her book face up, but turn several pages at once?
- Does your baby look for and find toys?
- Does your baby eagerly explore objects and spaces?

15-16 months
- Walks; has given up crawling
- Is able to build a tower of two cubes
- Uses characteristic jargon or individualized vocalizations
- Indicates his/her wants
- Puts wooden beads into box

Developmental milestones from 3 months to 15 years

1½ years
- Walks up stairs with one hand held
- Climbs up on chairs
- Builds a tower of three or four cubes
- Makes vertical strokes with a crayon
- Partially feeds self

2 years
- Runs without falling
- Goes up and down stairs alone
- Says a two- or three-word sentence
- Can point out eyes, ears, nose, mouth, hair, hands

3 years
- Rides a tricycle
- Roughly copies a circle
- Gives his or her full name
- Tells his or her sex
- Repeats three digits
- Is able to play by him/herself
- Feeds self

4 years
- Finishes an incomplete drawing of a person
- Goes up and down stairs without help, one foot at a time
- Is able to dress self partially
- Performs simple tasks
- Washes and dries hands and face
- Takes part in simple group activities

5 years
- Draws recognizable objects
- Copies a square
- Defines common objects in terms of their use
- s able to dress self almost entirely
- Plays in groups

6 years
- Locates glaring omissions in pictures of familiar objects
- Differentiates between morning and afternoon
- Knows right from left
- Can be trusted in familiar surroundings outside his own immediate neighborhood
- Can print his/her name

7 years
- Copies a diamond
- Repeats five digits
- Uses pencil for writing
- Can bath self with assistance
- Goes to bed unassisted

8 years
- Can name days of week
- Uses a table knife

- Reads time to nearest quarter hour
- Remembers major features of short children's story
- Specifies essential similarities and differences of pairs of objects

9 years
- Performs simple subtraction
- Reads comics, film titles and television items
- Baths self without help

10 years
- Repeats six digits forward
- Gives sensible reasons for common choices in everyday situations
- Goes freely about the whole community
- Uses judgement in making purchases

11 years
- Classifies objects according to type or use
- Uses telephone, including use of directory
- Mails coupons in response to advertisements
- Writes letter on own initiative

12 years
- Makes useful articles or repairs things
- Can be left alone at home and can care for younger children

13-15 years
- Unscrambles words in jumbled sentence to produce sense
- Able to grasp and apply general rules
- Takes complete care of dress
- Buys appropriate articles

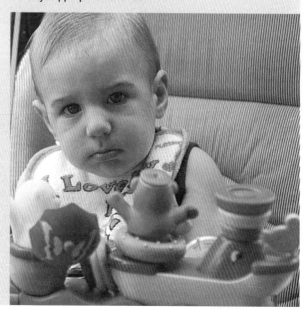

C

Guidelines for child health supervision

Age
If a child comes under care for the first time at any point on the schedule, or if any items are not accomplished at the suggested age, the schedule should be brought up to date at the earliest possible time.

History
At these points, history may suffice; if problem suggested, a standard testing method will be used by the physician.

Developmental/behavioral assessment
By history, and appropriate physical examination; if suspicious, by specific objective developmental testing.

Physical examination
At each visit, a complete physical examination will be performed, with infant totally unclothed, older child undressed and suitably draped.

Procedures
These may be modified, depending on entry point into schedule and individual need.

Hereditary/metabolic screening
PKU (phenylketonuria) and thyroid testing will be done at about 2 weeks. Infants initially screened before 24 hours of age should be rescreened.

Immunization
Vaccination or immunization may vary from country to country.

Tuberculin test
In some regions or countries testing is performed at 12 months of age and every 1 to 2 years later. In many countries tuberculosis is of exceedingly low occurrence and the physician may elect not to retest routinely or to use longer intervals.

Blood analysis - hematocrit and hemoglobin
Present medical evidence suggests the need for re-evaluation of the frequency and timing of hemoglobin or hematocrit tests. One determination is therefore suggested during each period. performance of additional tests is left to the individual practice experience.

Urinalysis
Present medical evidence suggest the need for evaluation of the frequency and timing of urine analysis. One determination is therefore suggested during each time period. performance of additional tests is left to the individual practice experience.

Anticipatory guidance
Appropriate discussion and counseling should be an integral part of each visit for care.

Initial dental referral
Subsequent examinations as prescribed by the dentist.

---

the potential validity if the figures are obtained from different sources).

This set of data, along with the parents' height, will show how far below his expected growth the child is. The child's growth, although within the normal range on the standard chart, may be abnormal based on his own growth potential.

The data may also indicate when growth stopped, and it will give values for annual growth increments. If a standstill period is found, the physical and psychosocial events of that time are investigated. If the child is small but his or her annual height and weight increments are appropriate for age, constitutional delay is likely.

In general, children who fail to thrive because of some pathologic process grow at less that the normal rate and tend to fall progressively behind their peers.

In addition to evaluating data on physical growth and development, psychomotor development will be assessed, searching for possible lesions in the central nervous system.

Physical examination
Height, weight, and body proportion measurements are obtained (e.g., upper to lower body segment ratios, arm span versus height).

From the height and weight, a height age and weight age (the age at which each measurement matches the median on standard growth charts) can be determined.

A weight age considerably below height is suggestive for a nutritional disorder. The maintenance of infantile body proportions suggests developmental delay as well as growth failure, as seen in a decreased function of the thyroid gland.

Minor structural abnormalities, such as high-arched palate, low-set ears, hypoplastic nails, shortened metacarpals, or inability to fully extent joints, will be sought by the examining physician. Their presence suggests Turner's syndrome in a female or primordial dwarfism in the male or female. In the older child, pubertal development is assessed. The earliest manifestation in a girl will usually be budding of the breasts; in the male, testicular enlargement. In general, a testis longer that 2.5 cm (1 inch) is a stimulated testis.

■ *Neglect or abuse*

The physician will be alert for signs of neglect or abuse. These can include:

▲ signs of poor hygiene;
▲ skin lesions such as ecchymoses or burns;
▲ fractures (old or new);
▲ bruises about the mouth or eye;
▲ evidence of injury to the brain;
▲ evidence of injury to internal abdominal organs.

If there are serious questions about the child's growth rate, a period of simple observation mat be indicated prior to an extensive laboratory investigation.

Special studies

Special laboratory or other studies may be indicated to evaluate more completely the function of other organ systems or to detect other causes.

In a girl who is short, and especially if she is sexually underdeveloped and beyond the normal age for puberty, Turner's syndrome is possible. Either a buccal smear for sex chromatin or chromosomal analysis of peripheral blood would be diagnostic.

If emotional deprivation or any other disturbed parent-child relationship is suspected, removing the child from the environment, generally to a hospital for observation, may be helpful for both diagnosis and treatment.

Hypothalamic-pituitary function will be evaluated in children whose growth rate is less than optimal, who do not have multiple abnormalities, and in whom no abnormality is identified by the above procedures.

Treatment

Treatment depends on the cause - it may be as simple as providing a proper diet or as complex as the transplant of a kidney. When malnutrition is a factor, nutritional rehabilitation is of primary importance and must often be implemented while diagnostic studies are being made. When psychosocial factors are involved, treatment must include management of the family and living conditions.

If the period of failure to thrive has been relatively short, and its cause corrected, one can generally anticipate a period of catch-up growth followed

Scheme health supervision 1

	a	b	c	d	e	f
Infancy						
By 1 mo	*	*	*	-	s	s
2 mo	*	*	*	-	s	s
4 mo	*	*	*	-	s	s
6 mo	*	*	*	-	s	s
9 mo	*	*	*	-	s	s
12 mo	*	*	*	-	s	s
Early childhood						
15 mo	*	*	-	-	s	s
18 mo	*	*	-	-	s	s
24 mo	*	*	-	-	s	s
3 yr	*	*	-	*	o	s
4 yr	*	*	-	*	o	o
Late childhood						
5 yr	*	*	-	*	o	o
6 yr	*	*	-	*	o	s
8 yr	*	*	-	*	o	s
10 yr	*	*	-	*	s	s
12 yr	*	*	-	*	o	o
Adolescence						
14 yr	*	*	-	*	o	s
16 yr	*	*	-	*	s	s
18 yr	*	*	-	*	o	o
20+ yr	*	*	-	*	o	s

a : History (initial/internal)
b : Measurements: height and weight
c : Head circumference
d : Blood pressure
e : Sensory screening: vision
f : Sensory screening: hearing
    s = subjective, by history
    o = objective, by standard method

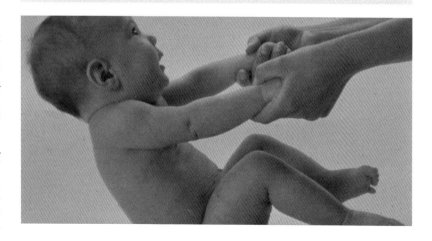

C

Scheme health supervision 2

	g	h	j	k	l	m
Infancy						
By 1 mo	*	*	*	-	-	-
2 mo	*	*	-	*	-	-
4 mo	*	*	-	*	-	-
6 mo	*	*	-	*	-	*
9 mo	*	*	-	-	*	-
12 mo	*	*	-	-	-	-
Early childhood						
15 mo	*	*	-	*	-	-
18 mo	*	*	-	*	-	-
24 mo	*	*	-	-	*	*
3 yr	*	*	-	-	-	-
4 yr	*	*	-	-	-	-
Late childhood						
5 yr	*	*	-	*	-	-
6 yr	*	*	-	-	-	-
8 yr	*	*	-	-	*	*
10 yr	*	*	-	-	-	-
12 yr	*	*	-	-	-	-
Adolescence						
14 yr	*	*	-	*	-	-
16 yr	*	*	-	-	-	-
18 yr	*	*	-	-	*	*
20+ yr	*	*	-	-	-	-

g : Developmental/behavioral assessment
h : Physical examination
j : Hereditary/metabolic screening
k : Immunization
l : Blood analysis; hematocrit, hemoglobin
m : Urinalysis

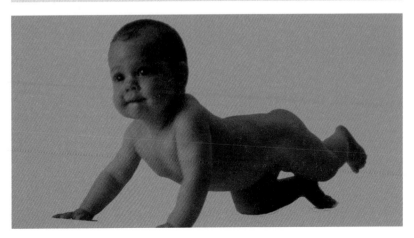

by return to a normal pattern.

If the period of failure to thrive has been prolonged, its effect may be long-lasting and return to normal height and weight for age may never be achieved.

Those children with constitutional delay are, in general, best reassured that they will reach a normal height without treatment. Anabolic steroids or sex hormones have been used on occasion, with controversial results. They increase bone development relatively faster than height, in effect potentially reducing the growing period and thus the ultimate height. Their use should therefore be restricted to those children who are having severe psychologic problems because of their small size and who thoroughly understand and accept the possible risks.

Child handicap

Description

A child handicap is defined as any disadvantage possessed by one child as compared with others, especially physical or emotional disability.

Probably the most helpless creatures in the world are newborn babies. From the moment they are born, they are dependent on other people for their everyday needs.

If their parents or other adults around them do not give them food, they starve. If they do not dress them in warm clothing and wrap them snugly in blankets, they catch cold and die.

If they do not keep them clean, they lie in their own body wastes, unable to move themselves to a dry place. About the only thing newborn babies can do is cry when they need attention. If they do not get it, they do not survive. In their helpless state at birth, infants are extremely vulnerable - that is, they are easily hurt or upset if they are not handled with extreme care. They have no way to defend themselves from any sort of danger that might threaten.

Tiny babies have suffocated under their blankets because they did not have the strength to throw the covers off. There are even reports of babies killed by rats, which would never attack a stronger person.

Because they are so vulnerable, infants need the utmost protection by their parents and the other adults around them. As babies grow older, they grow stronger and become less vulnerable. With a bit more flesh on their bones, they are able to withstand greater temperature changes and do not catch cold so easily.

They can move themselves about and delight in kicking off their covers despite the cold. Their stomach grows bigger and can hold more food so that they do not need to eat so often.

Though still vulnerable in the sense that any small creature is more or less at the mercy of the bigger creatures around it, young children who develop normally begin to feel at home in their surroundings and learn to take the ups and downs of everyday living in their stride.

Deficiencies

In the course of growing up, some children still have deficiencies which make it difficult for them to adjust to the people and things around them, and which make them vulnerable in some ways.

They might not be able to see or to hear well. A bone deformity or mild nervous system damage may keep a child from crawling and walking like other children. Some babies, for one reason or another get off to a bad start in life and, as they grow older, continue to be easily upset.

Illness or constant disturbing experiences during the first six months of life may influence their behavior for the rest of their lives. All babies need peace and quietness, to be comfortable during the early months when their bodies are learning to do their work and their minds are beginning to take shape.

Those who experience constant pain, anger or anxiety in the very early months may develop emotional disturbances or even mental illness later on. Children with handicaps are vulnerable in ways that require special handling. They need more help from their parents or supporting adults than do other children.

Teachers and parents must be aware of why certain children are sensitive and must help them learn to do things for themselves. Adults must provide support when it is needed, but they must not be overprotective. These children

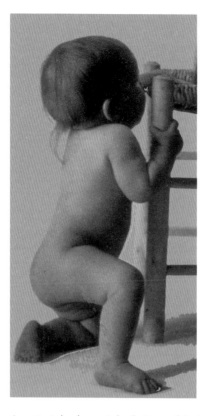
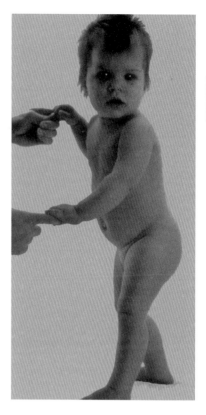

Important developmental milestones of the infant's first year. At nine mine months the child crawls and creeps on hands and knees (lower figure), and stands holding on to someone or something (upper right photographs). The child also works to get a toy out of reach (upper left photograph), standing holding on to a chair.
A few months later the infant walks by holding furniture and may walk one or two stapes without support.

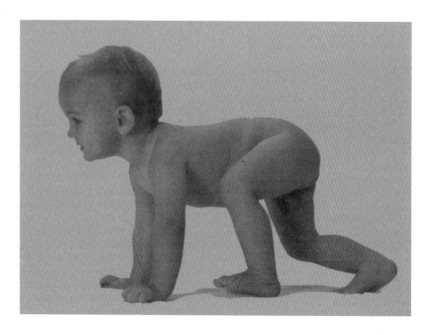

have to compete in a world of normal, healthy people, and they must learn to overcome or live with their handicaps.

Adapting to a handicap

Overcoming a handicap may be as simple as providing glasses to correct poor vision, or it may be as difficult as laboriously exercising underdeveloped muscles until they are strong enough to hold up the body and allow the child to walk without braces.

When children are vulnerable emotionally, they may need to talk about and act out the feelings that worry them. When children suffer from several handicaps at once, the effects can build up until they can no longer cope with the difficulties they are faced with. Thus they need a helping hand to show them how to keep from becoming overwhelmed.

As children become more successful in adapting to their handicaps and in overcoming their disabilities, they become less vulnerable.

They do not need so much special attention, are better able to deal with other children and can begin to make their way in a competitive world.

Physical handicaps

One of the most heart-rending sights in the world is a crippled child. Everyone who sees him or her instinctively wants to hold out a helping hand. For example, a girl must wear a brace on her left leg because of a weakness from polio. Everyone recognizes that she has difficulties and no one expects her to keep up with other children in activities requiring two strong legs.

This girl may be called a "vulnerable." The fact that she is vulnerable in a way that is obvious to everyone may make it easier for her to live with her handicap.

In fact, her parents and teacher feel so sorry for her that they often do things for her that she can do for herself, and sometimes she gets more attention that is good for her. If she can be encouraged to exercise, the leg will grow stronger, and she will be able to join in more activities.

Poor vision

If you have ever looked at a television set when the antenna connection has come loose, you know how annoying it is to see four or five fuzzy figures instead of one clear picture on the screen.

You may watch for a while if the program is really interesting, but before long, your eyes will probably begin to ache and you will turn off the set in disgust.

There are children who see fuzzy images of everything they look at because they have a defect in their eyes. Until the defect is corrected, these children never get a clear picture of the world around them.

Children with faulty vision may have an incorrect idea about the world because their reasoning is also based on incomplete information. Unless their vision is corrected with glasses, they will continue to go through life with "fuzzy" thoughts.

Children with poor vision have been mistakenly thought to be stupid because they couldn't learn to read. Actually, they could not learn to read because they couldn't see the letters clearly. They may also have only a dim idea of the layout of their nursery or junior school and feel too unsure of themselves to play about freely.

Paintings would be merely blurs of color to them, and they might be afraid to walk alone in a play area for fear of falling over things or bumping into people that they could not see.

A person with good vision cannot imagine what sorts of shadowy monsters may lurk in the corners for the child who cannot see that far. Obviously, the first step in helping these vulnerable children is to see that their eyes are examined and that corrective glasses are prescribed.

Once their world comes into focus, their vulnerability may disappear without any further help from parents and teachers. It may be a holdover from the days when they could not play as the other children did, and they may need some extra help from the adults in their lives to join in activities.

Loss of hearing

Television again may help us to understand the plight of children who are hard of hearing. Turn off the sound for a minute and try to follow the action of a story just by looking.

Unless you have had special training in lip reading, you will probably soon lose track of what is happening. Children whose hearing is defective go through life seeing lips move and not knowing what they are saying. Children with a hearing loss really have two handicaps to overcome: deafness and difficulty in speech.

Babies learn to talk by hearing other people say words and eventually by imitating them. If their ears never hear other words, or if the sounds that come to their ears are fuzzy and indistinct, they do not have a clear idea what sounds they are expected to imitate, and may voice meaningless syllables thinking they are talking.

Realizing that nobody understands them, they may begin to withdraw and lapse into a hopeless silence. There are many different kinds of hearing problems. Children may be able to hear if someone looks directly at them and speaks very distinctly, but when directions are given from distance, the children's ears may not be able to separate the words from the normal background noises. In addition, they may be able to understand a man's deeper voice better than a woman's higher-pitched voice.

Children who cannot hear directions are very likely to break rules without meaning to. If someone speaks to them and they do not hear, they will not answer and it may mistakenly be considered that they are sullen and unresponsive, given to sudden outbursts of anger. Once a hearing loss is identified, it frequently can be helped or corrected with a hearing aid. Now it is up to parents and teachers to help the children catch up with their hearing classmates.

They probably will need more individual conversation with adults to expand their speaking ability. They may not be able to pronounce words correctly at first and may even need some special exercises to help them speak so that they are understood. Nothing can be more frustrating than to say something and discover that nobody understands you.

Hard-of-hearing children may also need some help in paying attention to directions. Children who cannot hear what it being said, soon learn not to listen. Parents and teachers may have to remind them to listen when they speak, and they must also remember to look directly at these children and speak clearly.

At storytime if teachers reserve a nearby place, but not always in the favored spot on their laps, they will make it easier for these children to hear the story.

Children with a loss of hearing may also have to be reminded to speak softly and not to tap their feet during stories, for people who do not hear well themselves cannot know how annoying noises may be to people with normal hearing.

A severe cold may leave the ear passages clogged and a child may suffer a temporary loss of hearing. If a child suddenly begins to ignore directions and does not answer when spoken to, the teacher might check his or her hearing before disciplining the child for his or her behavior.

Psychological vulnerabilities

All new parents experience the same nagging fears right after their babies are born.

▲ Are they normal?

▲ Do they have ten fingers and ten toes?

▲ Two arms and legs?

▲ Are all parts in their proper place?

Not until they hold their babies for the first time and determine for themselves that they are indeed normal, do their worries leave them. If only we could be sure that a baby is healthy just by counting fingers and toes. Unfortunately most defects are hidden within the body. Physical defects, such as poor eyesight or a faulty heart valve, eventually show up in a medical examination, but there are children who have no obvious problems, yet have trouble adjusting to life itself.

Somehow they do not seem to be well put together. Their impulses tend to run away with them and they quickly develop reputations as "behavior problems." A new situation or a sudden change is likely to disturb them, they find it hard to concentrate and their attention span is short.

Some of these are the children who become the "slow learners," the "juvenile delinquents" and the "dropouts" that society is so concerned about today.

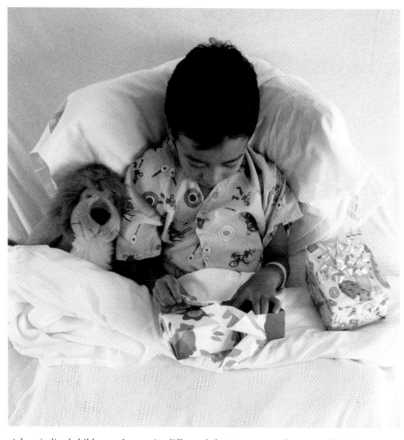

A hospitalized child may show quite different behavior patterns that normally is the case.

Studies have shown that many of these so-called "problem" children got off to a poor start in life. Unborn babies may not develop properly if their mothers do not have adequate medical attention during pregnancy, particularly if it is a difficult pregnancy. Very slow, long labors or some other difficulties at birth can get babies off to a poor start, particularly if there is no qualified medical person in attendance. An unusually slow birth may result in a shortage of oxygen to the baby, a condition that may cause some brain damage. There is no question that premature babies often get off to a bad start. If they happen to be born without medical attention, their first weeks are extremely risky, and babies who survive such conditions are often affected in some way.

Even if the pregnancy and birth are normal, experiences in the first six months can upset babies so that they have difficulty adjusting to life.

After birth, a baby's body and brain continue to develop and to become better organized. During these first few months he needs to be quiet and comfortable so that nothing interferes with his important growth and maturation.

It is thought by some that disturbing experiences in infancy may also have some later effect on the way children think and on their attitudes towards life.

They may not be able to accept the everyday changes and pressures that come to everyone. They may find that normal relationships with other people overtax their patience. Life may become too much to cope with.

When children like this become adults, they may be nervous or even suffer from mental illness. The way children are handled in early childhood may help overcame some of the emotional difficulties they carry with them from infancy.

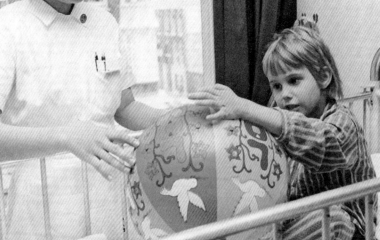

CHILDHOOD INFECTIONS

Introduction

Throughout human history infectious diseases have been responsible for more death and morbidity in childhood than any other single cause. Causative pathogens interact with deprivation, malnutrition, overcrowding, and poor sanitation to give rise to human disease; consequently economic improvement, planned hous-

ing, clear water, and sewage disposal are as critical to controlling these diseases as immunization and antibiotics.

The eradication of smallpox in the 1970s remains the only complete victory of humans over a specific infectious agent. Against this solitary triumph have to be placed the rise in antibiotic-resistant organisms, the emergence of new infections (most

notably the human immunodeficiency virus, HIV, and also bird flu that may infect humans and cause a pandemic), as well as the reappearance of conditions such as polio and diphtheria when immunization rates have fallen.

In addition, infections such as gastroenteritis, measles, pneumonia, and tuberculosis, which rarely kill in North America or Europe, still have high mortality rates in parts of the developing world. Measles has a mortality rate of 30 per cent or more in some areas of Africa.

The need for continuous vigilance means that most countries have systems for the notification of infectious diseases to public health authorities.

In the US, infectious diseases are the commonest reason for a child consulting a primary care physician or being admitted as an emergency to hospital. Many such cases are relatively minor viral infections, but they may cause both misery to the child and great anxiety in some families.

Serious infections such as bacterial meningitis, herpetic encephalitic, or staphylococcal pneumonia occur rarely but can kill or lead to significant disability. Recognition and early aggressive treatment of the child with a serious infection is essential to prevent the rapid deterioration which may occur in such cases.

Chickenpox

Chickenpox is an acute viral disease of children. The time between exposure to someone with chicken pox and the beginning of the illness (incubation period) is 14 to 21 days. Children are infectious from one day before the rash appears until the blisters dry and crust over (seven days). It spreads very

Infant recovering from severe intestinal infection.

easily.

Chickenpox is usually ushered in by mild symptoms that are followed shortly by a skin eruption appearing in crops and characterized by red pimples that become fluid-filled vesicles, which then burst and crust over.

n *Treatment*

Mild cases require only treatment of symptoms, e.g. calamine lotion to relieve the itching. Local or systemic antihistamines may be used in severe cases. Affected children should be kept at home until the vesicles have crusted over, as they are contagious until then. Chicken pox is usually a relatively mild disease in childhood.

Croup

Croup is a contagious viral infection of the upper airways that causes cough and sometimes difficulty breathing, especially breathing in. The illness causes swelling of the lining of the airways, particularly the area just below the voice box. Parainfluenza virus is the most common cause, but croup can be caused by other viruses, such as the respiratory syncytial virus or an influenza virus.

Different types of croup.
Generally two types of croup are being distinguished.

■ *Viral croup*
This is the most common type and is the result of a viral infection in the voice box and windpipe. This kind of croup often starts with a cold that slowly turns into a barking cough. Your child's voice will become hoarse and her breathing will get noisier. She may make a coarse musical sound each time she breathes in, called stridor. Most children with viral croup have a low fever.

■ *Spasmodic croup*
This type of croup is usually caused by a mild upper respiratory infection or allergy. It can be scary because it comes on suddenly in the middle of the night. You child may go to bed with a mild cold and wake up in a few hours, gasping for breath.
He will be hoarse and have stridor when he breathes in. He also may have

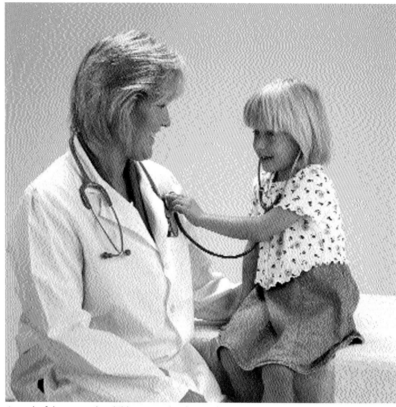

In a playful manner the child gets used to hospital routine.

a cough that sounds like a seal barking. Most children with spasmodic croup do not have a fever. It is probably similar to asthma and often responds to asthma medicines.

Diphtheria

Diphtheria is an acute, contagious infection caused by the bacterium *Corynebacterium diphtheriae*, which produces a toxin affecting the whole body and characterized by severe inflammation of the throat and larynx with production of a membrane lining the throat, along with fever, chills, malaise, brassy cough, and, in some cases by impaired function of the heart muscle and peripheral nerves. It is now a rare childhood disease, because of routine immunization (DTP) against the disease.
Rapid, early treatment is critical and involves diphtheria antitoxin injection, antibiotics (to kill the bacteria but do not remove the toxin), and

medications to control or prevent complications.
In severe cases a tracheotomy (cut into the front of the throat) is performed to allow air into the lungs. It can be totally prevented by vaccination in infancy.
Severe cases may affect the heart, nose, skin and nerves. Survivors may be affected for life by damage to the heart and lungs. The death rate varies from 10 per cent to 30 per cent, and most deaths occur within the first day or two. Survivors improve in a few days, but must be kept at rest for at least three weeks to prevent complications, as it will take this time for all the toxin to be removed from the body.

Erythema infectiosum (Fifth disease)

Erythema infectiosum is a contagious viral infection that causes a blotchy or raised red rash with mild illness. The

Childhoofd infections Questions & Answers

C

What is croup?
Croup is an infection that causes a swelling of the voice box (larynx) and windpipe (trachea), making the airway just below the vocal cords become narrow. This makes breathing noisy and difficult.

Who gets croup?
Most children get infectious croup once or twice, and some children get croup whenever they have a respiratory illness. Children are more likely to get croup between 6 months and 3 years of age. After age 3, it is not as common because the windpipe is larger and swelling is less likely to get in the way of breathing. Croup can occur at any time of the year, but is more common in the winter months.

What is the best initial treatment for croup?
If your child wakes up in the middle of the night with croup, take her into the bathroom. Close the door and turn the shower on the hottest setting to let the bathroom steam up. Sit in the steamy bathroom with your child. Within 15 to 20 minutes, the warm, moist air should help her breathing.

How about the following days?
The following 2 to 3 days, try to use a cold-water vaporizer or humidifier in your child's room. Sometimes another attack of croup will occur the same night or the next. If it does, repeat the steam treatment in the bathroom. Steam almost always works. If it does not, take your child outdoors for a few minutes. Inhaling moist, cool night air may also help open the air passages so that she can breathe more freely.
If that does not help, call your pediatrician. If your child's breathing becomes a serious struggle or if your child looks blue, call for emergency medical services.

What shouldn't I do?
Never try to open your child's airway with your finger. Breathing is being blocked by swollen tissue out of your reach, so you cannot clear it away. Besides, putting your finger in your child's throat will only upset her. This makes her breathing even more difficult.
For the same reason, do not force your child to throw up. If she does vomit, hold her head down and then quickly sit her back up once she is finished.

Are medicines helpful?
If your child has viral croup and is not breathing better after the steam treatment, your pediatrician may prescribe a steroid medication to reduce swelling. Steroids can be inhaled, taken by mouth, or given by injection. Treatment with a few doses of steroids should do no harm.
For spasmodic croup, your pediatrician may recommend a bronchodilator to help your child's breathing.
Antibiotics, which treat bacteria, are not helpful because croup is almost always caused by a virus or allergy.
Cough syrups are of little use too, because they do not affect the larynx or trachea, where the infection is located. These also may get in the way of your child coughing up the mucus form the infection.

fifth disease occurs most often during the spring months, often in geographically limited outbreaks among children and adolescents. Infection is spread mainly by breathing in small droplets that have been breathed out by an infected person. Symptoms begin about 4 tot 14 days after infection. Symptoms can vary and some children have none. However, a child with erythema infectiosum typically has a low fever, feels mildly ill, and develops red cheeks that often look like they have been slapped. Within a day or two, a rash appears, especially on the palms or soles. The rash can be itchy and consists of raised, blotchy red areas and lacy patterns, particularly on areas of the arms not covered by clothing.
The illness generally lasts 5 to 10 days. Over the next several weeks the rash may temporarily reappear in response to sunlight, exercise, heat, fever, or emotional stress.

■ *Diagnosis and treatment*
A doctor makes the diagnosis based on the characteristic appearance of the rash. Blood tests can help identify the virus, although these are rarely performed. Treatment is aimed at relieving the fever and pain.

German measles

Rubella is the medical term for German measles. Acquired rubella is a mild, preventable disease, which before a vaccination was developed, was common among childhood. Today adults and adolescents (who are 15 years old or older) who have not been immunized are most susceptible to contracting the disease.
German measles is a viral disease and is usually accompanied by a characteristic rash. However, the disease is often confused with other viral disease and often goes misdiagnosed.
The disease may occur with only very mild symptoms and the child may not be very sick. The first indication of the disease among children is usually a rash of tiny, flat or slightly raised, pink-red spots that may appear behind the ears, on the forehead, around the mouth, or elsewhere on the face.

Within a day the rash spreads to the trunk, then to the arms and possibly legs. By the time the rash appears on the arms and legs, it may have started to fade on the face and may linger on the trunk only in the form of flushed-looking patches. In some rubella cases no rash appears at all.

■ *Treatment*
After a physician has diagnosed childhood rubella, home treatment is fairly simple. A fever-reducing medication may be helpful. Calamine lotion may relieve itching. Generally the child can get a usual diet.

Measles

Measles is a serious infectious disease that each year used to affect tens of thousands of American children between 5 and 10 years old. Today, as a result of a highly successful immunization program, the incidence of measles has been reduced dramatically.
The disease still afflicts a small number of children, adolescents, and young adults who have not been vaccinated, who may have received defective vaccine, or who were vaccinated before their first birthday.
The disease makes children quite uncomfortable. Measles is characterized by
- rising fever
- cough
- runny nose
- sore throat
- red, watery eyes
- characteristic rash

The rash usually first appears on the forehead end behind the ears and then spreads to cover the entire body. Initial symptoms commonly appear 9 to 12 days after exposure to the disease. Symptoms occasionally develop as early as 6 days after exposure. Measles usually lasts from 7 to 9 days or until fever has subsides and the rash has faded. This disease is rarely life-threatening, although younger children can develop several serious complications.

■ *Treatment*
Home treatment of measles focuses on relieving symptoms. Bed rest and

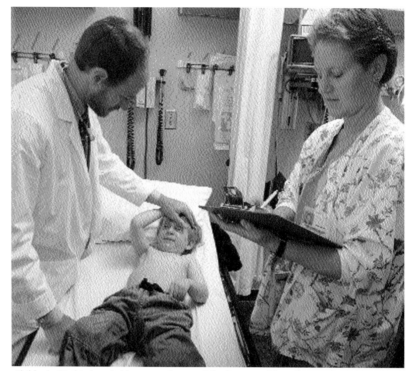
Child admitted to hospital because of severe infection caused by unknown virus.

plenty of fluids are helpful during the fever. A mild fever-reducing medication may be helpful.

Mumps

Mumps is a viral infection of the salivary glands. The period between exposure and illness (incubation period) is about 14 to 21 days. Children are infectious until de parotid gland swelling disappears.
Children have swelling of the salivary glands, most commonly the parotid gland located just in front of and below the ears. Chewing lemons or pickles makes the pain worse. A low-grade fever and headache may accompany swelling.
There is no rash. Problems may include swelling and pain of the testicles as well as inflammation of the brain or pancreas.
The best way to help a child is to reduce discomfort with acetaminophen. Encourage fluids and avoid sour substances and citrus fruits. If testicular pain develops, rest, support and pain medicines are usually adequate.

After identifying the illness as mumps (as opposed to swollen lymph nodes), your doctor will examine your child for complications and will suggest specific measures, if necessary.

Poliomyelitis

Polio or infantile paralysis is a viral disease that in its very severe form affects the central nervous system (brain, spinal cord). Polio is characterized primarily by high fever, headache, and an overall achy feeling. Additional signs include stiffness of the neck and back, vomiting, and irritability. These signs and symptoms may last for 3 to 4 days and then disappear. In most cases the disease progresses no further.
In paralytic poliomyelitis, a second phase of illness occurs in which symptoms recur, the brain and spinal cord are generally involved, and paralysis appears, involving any or all of the voluntary muscles. In the majority of diagnosed polio cases, paralysis appears by the third or fourth day of the illness if it occurs at all.

C

■ *Treatment*

Although there is no cure for the disease, a child with nonparalytic polio can be treated at home. Treatment is aimed at relieving fever and headache. If examination reveals or symptoms suggest any form of paralysis, a child should be hospitalized.

Immunization is the only protection against the poliovirus. The law requires that children be immunized against polio before entering public school.

Rashes in children

Rashes in children come in many sizes, colors and shapes. It is hard to distinguish different type of skin problems; the following list may help to sort out some of the more common ones.

Rashes that are red without bumps
- Measles
- Rubella
- Roseola
- Scarlet fever
- Erythema infectiosum (Fifth disease)

Rashes that are red with bumps
- Acne
- Candidiasis
- Contact dermatitis
- Diaper rash
- Eczema
- Hives
- Impetigo
- Insect bite
- Ringworm

Rashes with blisters
- Chicken pox
- Herpes zoster
- Impetigo (bullous)
- Insect bite
- Scabies

Call your pediatrician if
- The rash is purple, red or blood-like
- Burn-like
- Red, blue or tender to the touch
- Red-streaking
- Pustular

Scarlet fever

Scarlet fever is a bacterial infection characterized by fever, rash, and usually a sore throat. The disease and its complications were severe among children in industrialized countries until the 1940s, when penicillin became widely available. Scarlet fever now occurs less often end has become considerably milder.

Scarlet fever is generally the same disease as strep throat with a rash added. The rash in scarlet fever is sometimes confused with that of measles, German measles, toxic syndrome, heat rash, or sunburn

■ *Complications*

Scarlet fever results when streptococci infecting a person - usually in the throat - release a toxin. This toxin leads to a widespread, pink-red rash that is most obvious on the abdomen, on the sides of the chest, and in the skinfolds. The rash does not itch or hurt. Other symptoms include a pale area around the mouth, a flushed face, and dark red lines in the skinfolds.

■ *Treatment*

People with strep throat and scarlet fever usually get better in 2 weeks, even without treatment. Nevertheless, antibiotics can shorten the duration of symptoms and help prevent serious complications (such as rheumatic fever). Antibiotics also help prevent the spread of the infection to the middle ear, sinuses, and mastoid bone as well as to other people.

Whooping cough

Whooping cough is a severe infection of the respiratory tract (nose, throat, windpipe, and lungs) that causes serious, prolonged breathing problems. Whooping cough gets its name from the loud whooping sound heard after a series of uncontrollable coughs. The person who is ill tries to make a full breath quickly after a coughing spasm, and the whooping sound results.

Whooping cough is caused by infection with a particular bacterium. The bacteria are carried in mucus droplets produced when en infected person coughs or sneezes. Because of its persistence, whooping cough weakens those children who contract the disease. Whooping cough, which an unimmunized child can develop within 5 to 10 days after exposure, may result in illness for as long as 2 months, especially among the very young.

Children under years old generally become more severely ill with whooping cough than do older ones. Moderate cases of the disease produce less severe symptoms, and the child may recover in less than 2 weeks.

■ *Treatment*

Severely ill infants and older children often require hospitalization for diagnosis and care. Infants in the inflammation stage may suddenly require emergency care if a thick mucus discharge blocks normal breathing. Older children with mild to moderate symptoms may be able to receive adequate care at home throughout the course of the disease.

At home a child should be kept comfortable and as relaxed as possible in order to try to avoid coughing up. Keeping an older child occupied may be a challenge, because someone who does not have a high fever may try to do too much.

Attention to adequate nutrition is important, especially when vomiting is a problem. During the long course of the illness, children need continual encouragement and reassurance.

An antibiotic given very early in the illness to shorten the period of contagiousness may block further progress of whooping cough. Infants suffering from whooping cough may require suctioning to clear the nose and airways in the lungs in addition to oxygen and, rarely, ventilation to assist their breathing.

Immunizations

Vaccines are available today to prevent the most severe communicable disease of childhood. The most common vaccines for children are those for:
- diphtheria
- German measles
- measles
- mumps

Protecting against infectious disease

In the United States and most European countries, vaccines are available for the following diseases

Adenovirus
- Selected people
- All children and adults

Anthrax
- Selected people

Cholera
- Selected people

Diphtheria
- All children and adults

Hemophilus influenzae B
- Selected adults
- All children

Hepatitis A
- Selected adults
- All children

Hepatitis B
- Selected adults
- All children

Influenza
- Selected people

Japanese encephalitis
- Selected people

Measles
- All children and adults

Meningococcal meningitis
- Selected people

Mumps
- All children and adults

Pertussis (whooping cough)
- All children and adults

Plague
- Selected people

Pneumococcal infection
- Selected adults
- All children

Polio
- All children and adults

Rabies
- Selected people

Rubella (German measles)
- All children and adults

Smallpox
- Not currently recommended

Tetanus
- All children and adults

Tuberculosis
- Selected people

Typhoid
- All children and adults

Varicella (chickenpox)
- Selected adults
- All children

Yellow fever
- Selected people

- polio
- tetanus
- whooping cough

Even though it may seem that vaccines have virtually eliminated these diseases, they continue to occur in the United States, Canada and most other countries of the world. It is very important, therefore, that parents see that their children receive all needed immunizations.

Public health authorities estimate that one in three preschoolers has not had all the recommended immunizations and that as many as half of all children under 11 years old are not completely protected. Because of the possibilities of epidemics, health officials periodically initiate local campaigns to reach all unimmunized children. Currently, health departments in all 50 US states require parents to present proof of certain immunizations before their children begin school and, in some cases, at the beginning of each school year.

Immunization is based on a remarkably simple principle. Many infectious diseases can be contracted only once during a lifetime because in the process of recovery the body produces a permanent defense response against the organism causing the particular illness. Immunization artificially triggers this defense response so that a person can become immune without actually contracting the disease.

All vaccines are delivered by injection except the one against polio, which is usually given orally. Vaccinations are often delayed if a child is running a fever, redness, and mild to moderate muscle soreness at the site of injection for a day or two. A mild rash, 5 top 10 days in duration, may develop after a child receives the measles vaccine.

If a child has ever experienced a convulsion (seizure), parents should so advise the physician before the DTP vaccine is given. The physician may decide to omit the pertussis vaccine because of the possibility of a severe reaction for a child who has had a convulsion, previous vaccine reactions, or who suffers from suppressed immunity.

Vaccines are best administered at specified times in early childhood, when "peak immunity" can be obtained. During the first few months of life, the vaccines create only transient immunity, so dosages must be scheduled at designated intervals throughout childhood to ensure maximum protection.

Although every health team administers vaccines and maintains records of a child's immunizations, parents should keep their own up-to-date record at home. Parents should also think about preparing their children psychologically for immunizations. For children, the diseases against which they are being protected are unknown and abstract, but the brief pain of a needle is immediate and vivid.

A child may miss an immunization inoculation or a whole series of regular infant and toddler examinations have not been performed. If an initial DTP shot or OPV dose has been given, the usual schedule can be resumed where it left off (the whole series need not be started over). If an entire series is missed, a physician usually will begin a catch-up schedule for the child's age and need for immediate protection.

CHRONIC FATIGUE SYNDROME

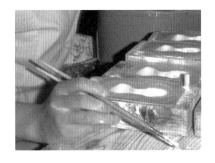

Description

This syndrome is characterised by a persistent tiredness and easy fatigue that persists for many months for no obvious reason. No specific single cause has been determined. It is possible that it is actually several diseases that overlap with their symptoms, and may be due to a combination of infection, immune deficiencies, autoimmune type condition (where the body rejects its own tissue), chronic inflammation, stress and psychiatric disturbances. The diagnosis can only be confirmed if in the list in the table, both major criteria are met, plus six symptoms and two signs from the minor criteria. There are no specific diagnostic tests, but numerous blood tests may show minor abnormalities. Tests are also performed to exclude any other possible cause.

There is no specific treatment available, but patients can benefit by having an understanding doctor who may suggest exercise programmes, and prescribe antidepressants, anti-inflammatory medication, steroids and other drugs that may be helpful.

Diagnosis

According to the Centers for Disease Control and Prevention, a diagnosis of chronic fatigue syndrome requires the following:

▲ Medically unexplained persistent or recurring fatigue of at least 6 months' duration that is new or had a definite beginning, is not due to exercise, is not substantially relieved by rest, and substantially interferes with work-related, educational , social, or personal activities. At least four of the following symptoms:
  • Pour memory for recent events
  • Reduced concentration severe enough to interfere with work-related, educational, social or personal activities

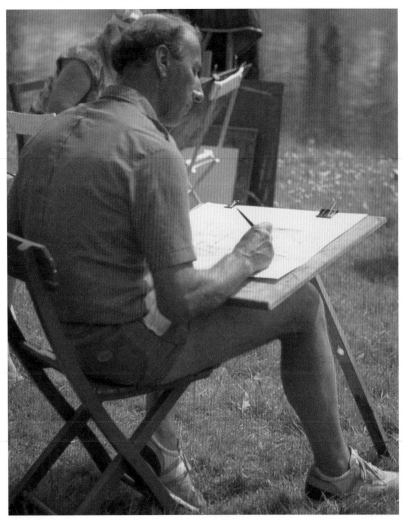

Adequate rest balanced by some activity is an essential part of the recovery program. Some doctors believe that chronic fatigue syndrome is due to psychological factors; therefor individual psychotherapy may be helpful. Others believe that the disorder is caused by physical agents, such as viruses and chemicals, or by abnormalities in the immune system. In the latter case, the strengthening of the immune system may be helpful.

Chronic fatigue syndrome   Questions & Answers

Why am I tired all the time?
You may be the victim of chronic fatigue.

- Have you been tired (fatigued) for along time - more than six months - even though you are getting enough rest and are not working too hard?

- Has your doctor been unable to find illnesses that could explain your symptoms?

- Are you able to do less that half of what you used to do, because you feel tired?

- Have you a number of general symptoms such as sore throat, mild fever or chills?

In that case you may be suffering from the Chronic Fatigue Immune Dysfunction Syndrome (CFIDS).

What are the major symptoms of the Chronic Fatigue Immune Dysfunction Syndrome (CFIDS)?
The major characteristics of this syndrome are the following:
- mild fever or chills;
- sore throat;
- unexplained muscle aches or weakness;
- headaches that are different from the kind you usually get, or headaches that make your whole head hurt;
- confusion
- trouble thinking and concentrating;
- feeling very tired for more than 24 hours after exercise that did not bother you before;
- trouble sleeping.

What causes Chronic Fatigue Immune Dysfunction Syndrome (CFIDS)
No one is certain about what causes CFIDS. The symptoms of Chronic Fatigue Immune Dysfunction Syndrome (CFIDS) may be caused by an immune system that is not working well. Or CFIDS may be caused by some kind of virus. Researchers are still looking for the cause of CFIDS.

How is Chronic Fatigue Immune Dysfunction Syndrome (CFIDS) treated?
The first step is to see if there is a medical cause for your fatigue. Your doctor will probably want to review your symptoms and medical history, and give you a physical examination. Your doctor also want to do some blood tests, but laboratory testing is not often helpful.
Some of the symptoms, such as muscle aches, sleep problems, anxiety and depression, can be treated with medicine. The medicine is intended only to reduce your symptoms and allow you to be more active, not to cure the fatigue. So far, there is no medicine that "cures" the entire syndrome. Most patients improve with time.

How can I improve my outlook and my ability to function in case of Chronic Fatigue Immune Dysfunction Syndrome (CFIDS)
- Keep a daily dairy to identify times when you have the most energy. Plan your activities for the times you ave the most energy.

- Keep up some level of activity and exercise, within your abilities. Your doctor can help you plan an appropriate exercise program to maintain your strength at whatever level is possible. Exercise can help your body and your mind.

- Give yourself "permission" to recognize and express your feelings, such as sadness, anger and frustration. You need to grieve for the energy you have lost.

- Emotional support is important in coping with a chronic health problem. Ask for support from family and friends. Look for support groups or counselling in your community. Your doctor is another important source of help.

I am suffering from Chronic Fatigue Immune Dysfunction Syndrome; what should I do about not being able to think clearly or remember things the way I used to?
Memory and concentration are often affected by chronic fatigue. You can cope by keeping lists and making notes to remind yourself of important things. Also, give yourself more time to do things that take concentration.
If possible, do these things at the time of day when your energy level is highest. Medicine may also help you sleep better, which might improve your memory and concentration.

What can I expect from my doctor in case of Chronic Fatigue Immune Dysfunction Syndrome (CFIDS)?
Your doctor can work with you to provide symptom relief and to help you find ways of coping with the changes Chronic Fatigue Immune Dysfunction Syndrome (CFIDS) makes in your life. Chronic fatigue affects you physically, emotionally and socially.
When you address all of these factors, you have the best chance of adjusting to your illness and feeling more satisfied with your life.If you have CFIDS, a good long-term relationship with your doctor helps. This relationship is the key that helps you feel less frustrated.

C

Chronic fatigue syndrome   Major and minor criteria

Major criteria
- New, persistent or intermittent, debilitating fatigue severe enough to reduce or impair average daily activity below 50 per cent of normal activity for a period of more than six months.
- Exclusion of all other causes by thorough clinical evaluation, and blood tests.

Minor criteria - Symptoms
- Generalised fatigue lasting more than 24 hours following levels of exertion that would have been easily tolerated previously.
- Vague headache, without specific symptoms of migraine.
- Unexplained general muscle weakness.
- Muscle pains.
- Arthritis that moves from joint to joint without any apparent damage to the joint.

- One or more of the following problems:
  - avoidance of bright lights
  - forgetfulness
  - irritability
  - confusion
  - poor concentration
  - depression
  - intermittent visual disturbances
  - difficulty thinking
- Inability to sleep, or excessive sleepiness.
- Rapid onset over hours or days of major criteria.

Minor criteria - Signs
Documented by a physician on at least two occasions at least a month apart.
- Mild fever greater than 38.6°C)
- Sore throat with no pus present.
- Tender enlarged lymph nodes in neck or arm pit.

Chronic fatigue syndrome   Questions & Answers

What is chronic fatigue syndrome (CFS)?
It is a term that explains a specific pattern of symptoms, chiefly severe fatigue. Muscle and joint pain, headache, flu-like symptoms and sleep disturbance are also common. Some people also suffer irritable bowel problems, dizziness, difficulty concentrating and complain of a poor short-term memory. Depression and anxiety can be an added problem, although they may be a reactioneto feeling ill all the time.
Many people still call this condition ME, or myalgic ncephalomyelitis, which means muscle pain and inflammation of the brain. However, since the brain is not inflamed, this is not medically correct.

What causes it?
Scientists and doctors don't know for sure, but the condition often starts after an infection. Physical of psychological stress can also be triggers. It is likely that infections and stress cause ripples in the immune system that makes it malfunction.

How is it diagnosed?
There are no definitive tests, but an experienced doctor can make a diagnosis from the history alone. These may be done to exclude other disorders, for instance blood tests to check thyroid, liver and kidney function and a full blood count.

What distinguishes the illness?
The fatigue often follows a specific pattern. Many sufferers find that when they exert themselves, either mentally of physically, they feel fine at the time but are exhausted a day or so later. This delayed response is very common.

How is it treated?
Adequate rest balanced by some activity is an essential part of the recovery programm. However, people often find it hard to accept this and try to struggle on. This can lead to a relapse.
The next part of the programm is graded exercise or pacing. Tuis is not regarded an exercise regime, but a way of keeping as fit as possible without making the condition worse.

Are there medications?
There is no treatment to cure CFS but drugs can relieve some symptoms. Low-dose antidepressants can help restore disturbed sleep patterns and reduce sensitivity to pain, while antispasmodic drugs can relieve bowel problems.
Special diets are popular with alternative therapists, although there is no particular diet that has been proven to be effective for everyone.

- Sore throat
- Muscle pain
- Tender lymph nodes in the neck or armpits
- Pain in more than one joint without joint swelling or tenderness
- Headaches that differ from previous headaches in terms of type, pattern, or severity
▲ Unrefreshing sleep
▲ Persistent feeling of illness for at least 24 hours after exercise

These symptoms must have been present persistently or recurrently during but not before, the period of fatigue.

Treatment

In most cases, symptoms of chronic fatigue syndrome lessen over time. Regular aerobic exercise, such as walking, swimming, cycling, or jogging, under close medical supervision may reduce fatigue and improve physical function. Psychotherapy, including individual and group behavioral therapy, may be helpful as well.

Drug therapy has had mixed results. Antidepressants and corticosteroids have been useful in some cases, although their safety and effectiveness in the treatment of chronic fatigue syndrome have not been established.

A number of other treatments, including use of interferons and antiviral drugs, have been mostly disappointing. Excessive periods of prolonged rest may worsen symptoms of chronic fatigue syndrome.

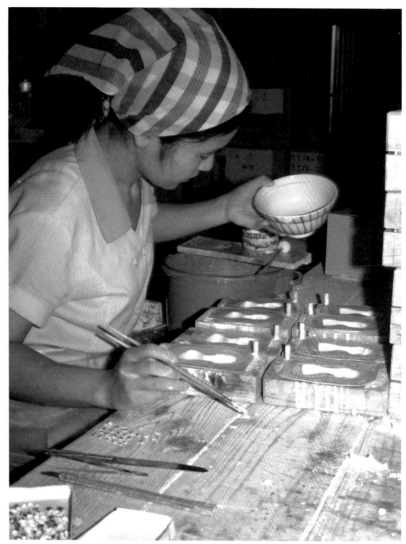

Painting, as integral part of psychotherapy, may be helpful in the treatment of chronic fatigue syndrome.

COLORECTAL CANCER

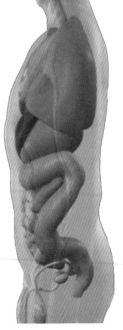

Description

The lowest portion of the digestive system is the colon. It is also called the large bowel or large intestine. The colon is at least 1.5-2 metres of the intestine. The last 20-25 cm of the colon is the rectum.

Every year, more than 400,000 people die of cancer of the colon and rectum. About half of all cases of cancer of the colon can be cured by surgery, and early detection can greatly improve this percentage. Over the next 12 months, an estimated 437,000 people worldwide will die of the disease. But the good news is, it does not have to be this way. Provided it is caught in its earliest, most treatable stages, colorectal cancer is curable more than 90 per cent of the time.

A simple test for occult blood (not visible to the naked eye) can indicate whether further tests should be made for the presence of this type of cancer. Everyone who is over 40 or who has chronic digestive problems should have this test regularly. Cure is twice as likely if the disease is discovered before symptoms occur.

About 25 per cent of colorectal cancers are triggered by a genetic predisposition that has been present since birth. The rest of the time, normal genes become damaged with age or exposure to the toxic brew of wastes that collect in the colon.

Researchers have identified the genes responsible for at least two types of hereditary colon cancer - dubbed FAP and HNPCC that trigger malignant growths in people in their 30s and 40s. But it can be tough to tell who has these genes, since they are often camouflaged by normal ones.

Symptoms

When an illness affects the colon or rectum, a number of symptoms appear. The ones listed below are warning signs of a possible problem:
- ▲ diarrhea or constipation;
- ▲ blood in or on the stool (either bright red or very dark in colour);
- ▲ stools that are narrower than usual;
- ▲ general stomach discomfort (bloating, fullness, cramps);
- ▲ frequent gas pains;
- ▲ a feeling that the bowel does not empty completely;
- ▲ loss of weight with no known reason;
- s constant tiredness.

These symptoms can be caused by a number of problems - such as flu, ulcers, an inflamed colon, or cancer. It is important to see a physician if any of these symptoms lasts as long as two weeks. Any disease should be diagnosed and treated as soon as possible, and this is especially true for cancer of the colon and rectum.

Diagnosis

When a person's symptoms suggest that there might be cancer in the colon or rectum, the physician will ask about the patient's medical history and will conduct a complete examina-

Frontal view (left) and lateral view (right) of the thoracic and abdomina, cavities. The large intestine or colon occupied a sizable part of the abdominal cavity.

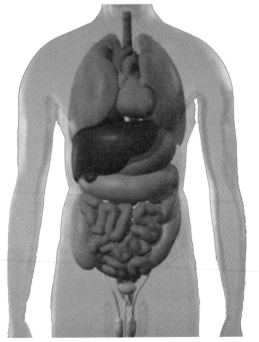

C

Major parts of the abdominal organs:
1. stomach, 2. duodenum, 3. small intestine,
4. large intestine (ascending colon), 5.
appendix, 6. sigmoid.

tion. In addition to checking the general signs of health (temperature, pulse, blood pressure, and so on), the physician usually does several other examinations.

▲ To check the rectal area, the physician inserts a lubricated, gloved finger into the rectum and gently feels for any lumps.

▲ The physician may also do a "procto" to look at the rectum and the lower end of the colon.

For this examination, a thin, lighted instrument called a sigmoidoscope is inserted into the rectum. Some of these scopes are rigid, others are flexible, allowing the doctor to see higher up in the colon. About 50 per cent of colon and rectum cancers can be found with the procto examination.

After these first steps, the physician may order some laboratory tests and other examinations.

The physician may ask the patient for a stool sample to find out if there is blood in the stool. For this test, the patient places a small amount of stool (called a "smear") on a plastic slide or piece of special paper. The sample is then sent to a laboratory to be examined.

Sometimes the physician wants to see the entire length of the colon. For this examination, the physician uses a colonoscope, which is a thin, flexible tube with a light at the end. If an abnormal growth is found, the physician will remove a small sample for examination in the laboratory. The procedure is called a biopsy.

In many cases, the physician can use a colonoscope to remove the whole growth. A biopsy is the only sure way to know if the tumor is cancer. The physician may also ask for a "lower GI - gastrointestinal - series" or "barium enema".

This is an X-ray of the colon that is taken after a thick solution of barium is pumped into the bowel through an enema tube. The barium shows an outline of the colon on the X-ray. It helps the doctor to see tumors or other suspicious areas that were not

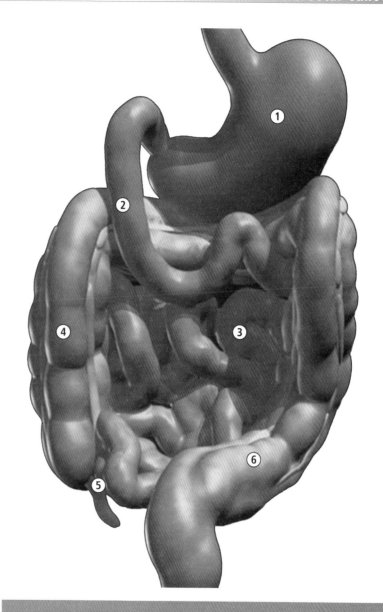

Staging of colorectal cancer

■ Stage 0
Cancer is limited to the inner layer of the colon covering the polyp.

■ Stage 1
Cancer spreads to the space between the inner layer and muscle layer of the large intestine.

■ Stage 2
Cancer invades the muscle layer and outer layer of the colon or rectum.

■ Stage 3
Cancer extends through the outer layer of the colon or rectum into nearby lymph nodes.

■ Stage 4
Cancer spreads to other organs, such as the liver or lungs.

Colorectal cancer Questions & Answers

What types of tumors occur in the colon?

Tumors of the colon are usually polyps or cancers. The tendency of some persons to form polyps is nowhere more strikingly exemplified than in the rare disorder known as congenital polyposis, in which the colon may be studded with hundreds or thousands of small polyps.

The kind of colon that can produce so many polyps eventually produces cancers as well; therefore, these patients should have their colons removed surgically as soon as the diagnosis is made. Another peculiar form of polyp is the villous adenoma, a slowly growing, fern-like structure that spreads along the surface for some distance. It possesses the potential for local recurrence after locally being resected, or it may develop into a full-blown cancer.

What are the characteristics of a colorectal cancer?

Cancer of the colon is in the Western world a more common tumor than is cancer of the stomach, and it occurs in both sexes about equally. Symptoms are highly variable, the main unifying feature being blood in the stools, but this may be only detectable by chemical testing.

Cancers compress the lumen of the colon to produce obstruction, they attach to neighbouring structures to produce pain, and they perforate to give rise to peritonitis. They may also metastasize to distant organs before causing local symptoms.

What are the symptoms of a colorectal cancer?

When an illness affects the colon or rectum, a number of symptoms may appear. The ones listed below are warning signs of a possible problem:
- diarrhea or constipation;
- blood in or on the stool (either bright red or very dark in colour);
- stools that are narrower than usual;
- general stomach discomfort (bloating, fullness, cramps);
- frequent gas pains;
- a feeling that the bowel does not empty completely;
- loss of weight with no known reason;
- constant tiredness.

How is the diagnosis of a colorectal disease made?

When a person's symptoms suggest that there might be cancer in the colon or rectum, the doctor will ask about the patient's medical history and will conduct a complete examination. In addition to checking the general signs of health (temperature, pulse, blood pressure, and so on), the doctor usually does several other examinations.
- To check the rectal area, the doctor inserts a lubricated, gloved finger into the rectum and gently feels for any bumps.
- The doctor may also do a "procto" to look for suspected tissue and to be if the tumor is cancer. The doctor may also ask for a "lower GI gastrointestinal - series" or "barium enema".

What are the main ways to treat cancer of the colon?

There are three main ways to treat cancer of the colon: surgery, radiation therapy, and chemotherapy. Another method, called immunotherapy, is now being studied in clinical trials. The doctor may use just one method or combine them. The decision is based on the patient's individual needs. In some cases, the patient may be referred to specialists in the different kinds of cancer treatment.

found in other tests.

If a tumor is benign, it most likely can be removed with no further problems. However, if the tumor is cancer, the physician may want to start planning further diagnostic tests or treatment.

Treatment

The first step in treatment usually is finding out the stage of the cancer. Staging tests show whether the disease has spread from its starting point in the colon or rectum to other parts of the body. Staging is very important because it helps the physician plan the best treatment. During staging, the physician will often order X-rays or other scans of the lungs, liver, kidneys, and bladder. Sometimes a special blood test - the carcino-embryonic

Presence of multiple polyps in the large intestine. Polyps may show malignant degeneration.

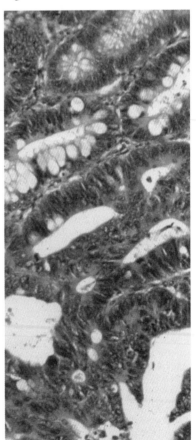

antigen (CEA) assay - is done to detect substances that may increase in the blood of a person with colon or rectal cancer.

The same test may be used later to find out how the patient is responding to treatment. The physician will develop a treatment plan to fit the patient's medical history, age and general health, and the extent and location of the cancer. Before starting treatment, the patient may want a second physician to review the diagnosis and treatment plan. There are three main ways to treat cancer of the colon:

▲ surgery;
▲ radiation
▲ chemotherapy.

Another method, called immunotherapy, is now being studied in clinical trials. The physician may use just one method or combine them. Biological therapy and surgery that spares a patient's sphincter are also being evaluated. The decision is based on the patient's individual needs. In some cases, the patient may be referred to specialists in the different kinds of cancer treatment.

Survival rates of colorectal cancer

■ Stage 0
More than 95% of people with cancer at this stage survive at least 5 years.

■ Stage 1
More than 90% of people with cancer at this stage survive at least 5 years.

■ Stage 2
About 55 to 85% of people with cancer at this stage survive at least 5 years.

■ Stage 3
About 20 to 55% of people with cancer at this stage survive at least 5 years.

■ Stage 4
Fewer than 1% of people with cancer at this stage survive at least 5 years.

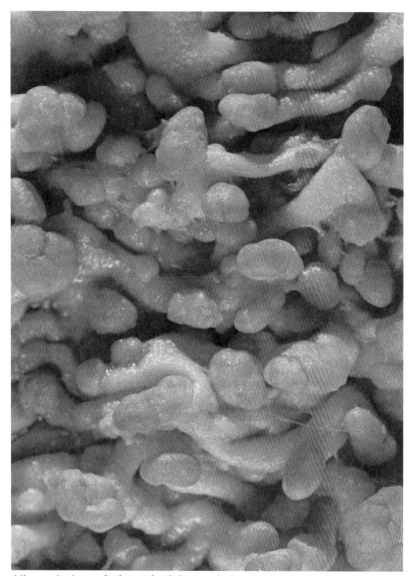

Microscopic picture of polyps. A family history of polyps increases the risk of colorectal cancer.

Detection guideline for colorectal cancer

Beginning at age 50, both men and women should follow one of these testing schedules:
▲ Yearly fecal occult blood test, or flexible sigmoidoscopy every 5 years.
▲ Yearly fecal occult blood test plus flexible sigmoidoscopy every 5 years.
▲ Colonoscopy every 10 years.
▲ Double-contrast barium enema every 5-10 years.

Persons known to be at increased risk for colorectal cancer (due to inflammatory bowel disease, personal or family history, etc.) need to begin screening at an early age and may need more frequent screening.

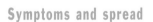

COMMON COLD

Description

Adults average about two to four colds a year, although the range varies widely. Women, especially those aged 20-30 years, have more colds than men, possibly because of their closer contact with children.

On average, individuals older than 60 have fewer than one cold a year. Colds are most prevalent among children, and seem to be related to the youngsters' relative lack of resistance to infection and to contacts with other children in day-care centers and schools. Children have about 6-10 colds a year.

Causes

More than 200 different viruses are known to cause the symptoms of the common cold. Rhinoviruses (from the Greek rhin, meaning nose) caused an estimated 30 to 35 percent of all adult colds, and are most active in early fall, spring, and summer.

Coronaviruses are believed to cause a large percentage of all adult colds. They induce colds primarily in the winter and early spring. Of the more than 30 isolated strains, three or four infect humans,

Although many people are convinced that a cold results from exposure to cold weather, or from getting chilled or overheated, these conditions in fact have little or no effect on the development or severity of a cold. Nor is susceptibility apparently related to factors such as exercise, diet, or enlarged tonsils or adenoids.

Viruses cause infection by overcoming the body's complex defence system. The body's first line of defence is mucus, produced by the membranes in the nose and throat. Mucus traps the material we inhale: pollen, dust, bacteria, and viruses.

When a virus penetrates the mucus and enters a cell, it commandeers the protein-making machinery to manufacture new viruses which, in turn, attack surrounding cells.

Symptoms and spread

Cold symptoms are probably the result of the body's immune response to the viral invasions. Virus-infected cells in the nose send out signals that recruit specialized white blood cells to the site of the infection.

In turn, these cells emit a range of immune system chemicals such as kinins. These chemicals probably lead to the symptoms of the common cold by causing swelling and inflammation of the nasal membranes, leakage of proteins and fluid from capillaries and lymph vessels, and the increased production of mucus.

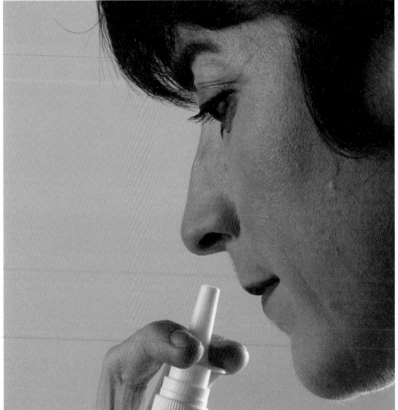

Antihistamines and other decongestants may relieve the symptoms of a common cold.

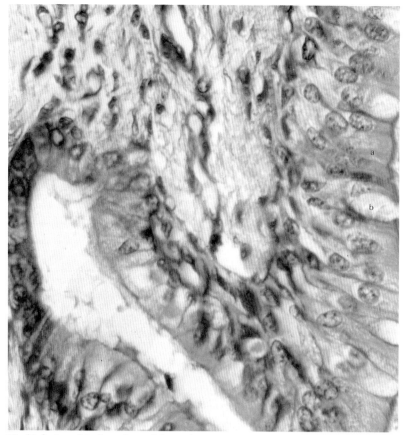

Viral infection of the inner layer of the trachea.

Depending on the virus type, any or all of the following routes of transmission may be common:

▲ Touching infectious respiratory secretions on skin and on environmental surfaces and then touching the eyes or nose.

▲ Inhaling relatively large particles of respiratory secretions transported briefly in the air.

▲ Inhaling droplets nuclei, smaller infectious particles suspended in the air for long periods of time.

Prevention

Handwashing is the simplest and most effective way to keep from getting rhinovirus colds. Not touching the nose or eyes is another. Individuals with colds should always sneeze and cough into a facial tissue, and promptly throw it away. If possible, one should avoid close, prolonged exposure to persons who have colds. Because rhinoviruses can survive up to three hours outside the nasal passages on inanimate objects and skin, cleaning environmental surfaces with a virus-killing disinfectant might help prevent spread of infection.

Treatment

Only symptomatic treatment is available for uncomplicated cases of the common cold:

- bed rest;
- plenty of fluids;
- gargling with warm salt water;
- petroleum jelly for a raw nose;
- aspirin or acetaminophen to relieve headache or fever.

Nonprescription cold remedies, including decongestants and cough suppressants, may relieve some cold symptoms but will not prevent, cure, or even shorten the duration of illness. Nonprescription antihistamines may have some effect in relieving inflammatory responses such as runny nose and watery eyes.

Antibiotics do not kill viruses. These prescription drugs should be used only for rare bacterial complications, such as sinusitis or ear infections, that can develop as secondary infections. The use of antibiotic "just in case" will not prevent secondary bacterial infections.

Many people are convinced that taking large quantities of vitamin C will prevent colds or relieve symptoms. To test this theory, several large-scale, controlled studies involving children and adults have been conducted. To date, no conclusive data has shown that large doses of vitamin C prevent colds. The vitamin may reduce the severity or duration of symptoms, but there is no definitive evidence.

CONSTIPATION

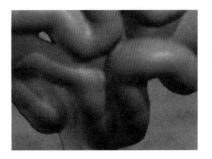

Description

Constipation is defined as difficulty in having bowel movements because of loss of muscle tone in the intestine, very hard stools, or other causes (for instance, intestinal obstruction).

Patients who complain of constipation may refer to the number, consistency, or size of stools, difficulty in passing stool, or a feeling of incomplete evacuation.

Normally, adults have at least three bowel movements a week, and normal stool weight is 35-225 g/day. Faecal impaction is a complication of severe constipation and is most common in nonambulatory nursing home patients.

Causes

Constipation is defined as difficulty in having bowel movements because of loss of muscle tone in the intestine, very hard stools, or other causes (for instance, intestinal obstruction).

Causes of constipation are numerous. Idiopathic constipation often begins in childhood or adolescence. Constipation of recent origin in adults suggests an organic or medicine-induced cause.

Constipation of organic origin may be due to:

▲ decreased function of the thyroid gland;
▲ too large colon (megacolon);
▲ stricture;
▲ lesions (benign of malignant).

Symptoms

If constipation does occur, complex symptoms of varying degrees may develop. Typical symptoms include the following:

▲ anorexia;
▲ dull headache;
▲ lassitude;
▲ low back pain;
▲ abdominal distention;
▲ lower abdominal distress.

Abdominal discomfort and inadequate response to increasing varieties and doses of laxatives are frequent. Although only limited quantitative data are available, some studies indicate that the range of bowel movement frequency in humans is from 3 times/day to 3 times/week.

These latter individuals are usually symptom-free and do not have any specific abnormality related to their individual pattern of defecation. Therefore, constipation cannot be defined solely in terms of the number of bowel movements in any given period.

Treatment

Constipation that does not have an organic cause can often be alleviated without the use of a laxative product. The following factors are very important in returning to a relatively normal state:

▲ adequate fiber in the diet;
▲ retraining to respond to the urge to defecate;
▲ physical exercise;
▲ adequate fluid intake;
▲ relaxation to reduce emotional stress and its effects on defecation.

A diet consisting of high-fiber foods and plenty of fluid (4-6 glasses of water/day) will help relieve chronic constipation.

Dietary fiber is that part of whole grain, vegetables, fruits, and nuts that resist digestion in the gastrointestinal tract. It is composed of carbohydrates (cellulose, hemicellulose, polysaccharides, pectin) and a nonocarbohydrate, lignin.

Food fiber content, which is expressed in terms of crude fiber residue after treatment will dilute acid and alkali, has a significant effect on bowel habits.

Because fiber holds water, in persons with a higher fiber intake, stools tend to be softer, bulkier, and heavier and probably pass the colon more rapidly.

The patient should learn not to ignore the urge to defecate and should allow adequate time for elimination. A relaxed, unhurried atmosphere can be very important in aiding elimination.

The patient will be encouraged to set a regular pattern for bathroom visits. Mornings, particularly after breakfast, seem to be a very good time.

Having a specific time period set aside for elimination may help the body adjust itself to producing a regular stool.

The ideal laxative would be non-irritating and non-toxic, would act only on the descending and sigmoid colon, and would produce a normally formed stool within a few hours. Its action would then cease, and normal bowel activity would resume. Since a laxative that meets these criteria is not presently available, proper selection of such an agent depends upon the etiology of the constipation.

Laxative drugs have been classified according to site of action, intensity of action, chemical structure, or mechanism of action.

The most meaningful classification is the mechanism of action, whereby laxatives are classified as bulk forming, emollients, lubricants, saline and stimulants.

Constipation   Questions & Answers

What is constipation?

Constipation is defined as difficulty in having bowel movements because of loss of muscle tone in the intestine, very hard stools, or other causes (for instance, intestinal obstruction).

What are the major causes of constipation?

Causes of constipation are numerous. Idiopathic constipation often begins in childhood or adolescence. Constipation of recent origin in adults suggests an organic or medicine-induced cause.

Constipation of organic origin may be due to:
- decreased function of the thyroid gland;
- too large colon (megacolon);
- stricture;
- lesions (benign of malignant).

What are the major symptoms of constipation?

If constipation does occur, complex symptoms of varying degrees may develop. Typical symptoms include the following:
- anorexia;
- dull headache;
- lassitude;
- low back pain;
- abdominal distention;
- ower abdominal distress.

Abdominal discomfort and inadequate response to increasing varieties and doses of laxatives are frequent.

What is the best treatment of constipation?

Constipation that does not have an organic cause can often be alleviated without the use of a laxative product. The following factors are very important in returning to a relatively normal state:
- adequate fiber in the diet;
- etraining to respond to the urge to defecate;
- physical exercise;
- adequate fluid intake;
- relaxation to reduce emotional stress and its effects on defecation.

What is the best diet for constipation?

A diet consisting of high-fiber foods and plenty of fluid (4-6 glasses of water/day) will help relieve chronic constipation. Dietary fiber is that part of whole grain, vegetables, fruits, and nuts that resist digestion in the gastrointestinal tract.

It is composed of carbohydrates (cellulose, hemicellulose, polysaccharides, pectin) and a nonocarbohydrate, lignin. Food fiber content, which is expressed in terms of crude fiber residue after treatment will dilute acid and alkali, has a significant effect on bowel habits.

Because fiber holds water, in persons with a higher fiber intake, stools tend to be softer, bulkier, and heavier and probably pass the colon more rapidly.

What are bulk-forming laxatives?

To this group belong products such as methylcellulose, carboxymethyl cellulose and plantago seeds. Because they approximate most closely the physiologic mechanism in promoting evacuation, bulk-forming products are the recommended choice as initial therapy for constipation.

These laxatives are natural and semi-synthetic polysaccharides and cellulose derivatives that dissolve or swell in the intestinal fluid, forming emollient gels that facilitate the passage of the intestinal contents and stimulate peristalsis. They are usually effective in 12-24 hours but may require as long as 3 days in some individuals.

What are emollient laxatives?

Dioctylsulfosuccinate is a surfactant which, when taken orally, increases the wetting efficiency of intestinal fluid and facilitates admixture of aqueous and fatty substances to soften the faecal mass. The medicine does not retard absorption of nutrients from the intestinal tract. In many cases of faecal impaction, a solution of this medicine is added to the enema fluid. Emollient laxatives should be used only for short-term therapy (less than 1 week without physician consultation) where hard faecal masses are present. Either in acute perianal disease in which elimination of painful stools is desired or in which the avoidance of straining at the stool is desirable (for instance, following myocardial infarction).

What are lubricant laxatives?

Liquid petrolatum and certain digestible plant oils, such as olive oil, soften faecal contents by coating them and thus preventing colonic absorption of faecal water. Liquid petrolatum is useful when it is used judiciously in cases that require the maintenance of a soft stool to avoid straining (for instance, after abdominal surgery, or in cases of hernia, high blood pressure, or myocardial infarction). However, routine use in these cases is probably not indicated.

What are stimulant laxatives?

Stimulant laxatives (such as aloe, castor oil, rhubarb) increase the propulsive peristaltic activity of the intestine by local irritation of the mucosa or by a more selective action on the nerve plexus of the intestinal smooth muscle. Depending on the laxative, the site of action may be the small intestine, the large intestine, or both. Intensity of action is proportional to dosage, but individually effective doses vary.

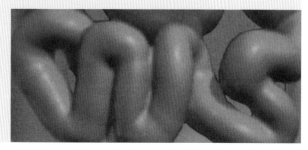

CONTRACEPTION

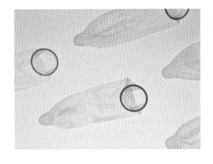

Introduction

The prevention of conception or pregnancy. In order to prevent the birth of unwanted children, one or both parents can use contraception to avoid pregnancy temporarily, or sterilisation to prevent pregnancy permanently. Contraceptive methods include:
- oral contraceptives (birth control pills)
- male condoms
- female condoms
- preparations that stop or kill sperm on contact (spermicides - in vaginal foams, creams, gels and suppositories)
- withdrawal before ejaculation
- diaphragms
- male sterilisation

- female sterilisation
- cervical caps
- rhythm methods
- contraceptive implants
- injectable contraceptives
- intrauterine devices (IUDs)

Contraceptives may be used by a person who is physically able to conceive a baby and has sexual relations with someone of the opposite sex but does not want to have a baby right away. After learning about the advantages and disadvantages of various contraceptive methods, a person can choose the most suitable method.

Contraceptives must be used correctly to be effective. They are more likely to fail when used by people who are younger, have less education, or are less motivated to prevent pregnancy.

From 5 to 15 per cent of women using contraceptive methods designed for use at the time of sexual intercourse (diaphragm, condom, foam, withdrawal) become pregnant during the first year of use.

Generally, these methods are less effective in preventing pregnancy that are oral contraceptives, implants, injectable contraceptives and intrauterine devices, which provide longer-term protection and do not require last-minute decisions.

From 0,1 to 3 per cent of women using these longer-term contraceptive methods become pregnant during the first year of use.

Contraceptive methods

Male condom
Male condoms are the most used form of contraception. They work by creating a barrier that physically traps the sperm released during ejaculation. Not only are condoms one of the easiest ways to enjoy safer sex, but, if used correctly, they are up to 90 per cent effective in preventing pregnancy and they are one of the best forms of protection against sexually transmitted infections including HIV.

Female condom
The female condom is a soft, fine sheath that is inserted into the vagina (like a tampon) to create a barrier against sperm. Up to 95 per cent effective in preventing pregnancy, female condoms also help to protect both partners against sexually transmitted infections including HIV. Female condoms are made from polyurethane.

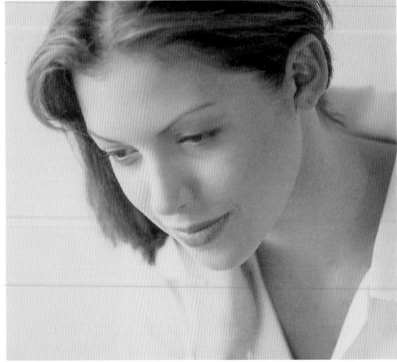

Selection of a good contraceptive method is an important decision in life.

Designed to gently line the vagina, so you don't have to worry about using the right size, female condoms can also be inserted before sex begins.

Spermicides and lubricants

Spermnicides are chemical substances which kill sperm. Available in many different forms, including jellies, foams and pessaries, they can be inserted into the vagina before sex but, on their own, they are not a reliable form of contraception. They should be used along with condoms, diaphragms and caps to provide extra protection. Lubricants are very useful if you or your partner are experiencing vaginal dryness, This can occur for a number of reasons: feeling tired and stressed, hormonal changes during the menstiual cycle, pregnancy and the menopause.

Lubricants are available in different forms so choose the one that best suits your needs. Pessaries can be inserted discreetly into the vagina, whilst creams and gels can be gently rubbed onto the erect penis before it is gently inserted into the vagina.

Condoms not only prevent conception or pregnancy but are also very effective against sexually transmitted diseases such as AIDS.

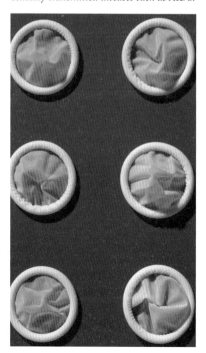

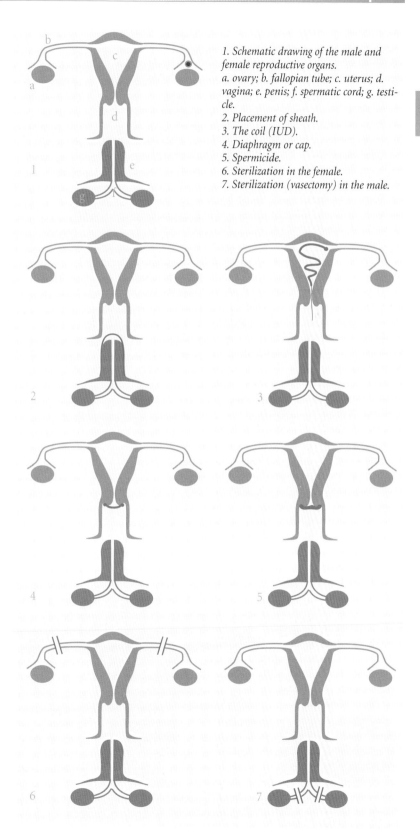

1. Schematic drawing of the male and female reproductive organs.
a. ovary; b. fallopian tube; c. uterus; d. vagina; e. penis; f. spermatic cord; g. testicle.
2. Placement of sheath.
3. The coil (IUD).
4. Diaphragm or cap.
5. Spermicide.
6. Sterilization in the female.
7. Sterilization (vasectomy) in the male.

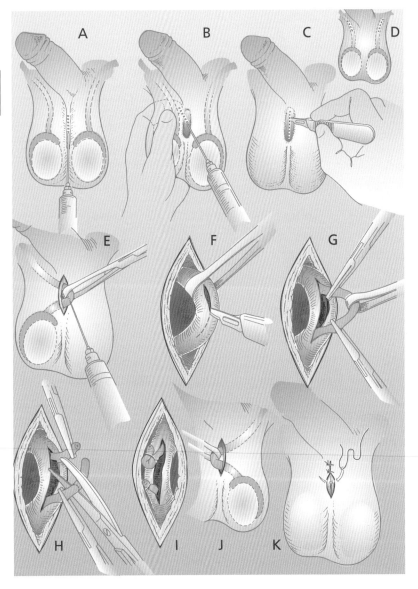

Various steps in vasectomy, the sterilization procedure in men (A-K). It involves cutting (E-H) and sealing (I) the vasa deferentia (the tubes that carry sperm from the testes). A vasectomy, which is performed by a urologist in the office, takes about 20 minutes and requires only local anesthesia (B). Through a small incision on each side of the scrotum (C), a section of each vas deferens is removed and the open ends of the tubes are sealed off (E).

Diaphragms and caps

Diaphragms and caps are barrier methods of contraception. This means that, like condoms, they prevent the sperm reaching an egg.

▲ Diaphragms are soft, rubber domes which you wear inside your vagina to cover your cervix.

▲ Caps can be rubber or silicone and are smaller than diaphragms and they cover the cervix directly.

Used correctly a rubber/latex diaphragm or cap is up to 96 per cent effective in preventing pregnancy. It will also help to protect you from cervical cancer and some sexually transmitted infections, but this does not include HIV.

Hormone-based contraception

There are two main types of contraceptive pill, the combined pill (containing estrogen and progestogen) and the progestogen-only pill. Within these types there are also a number of brands of pill, which may contain different doses of these hormones and have different effects on your body.

Natural methods of contraception
There are several methods of monitoring a woman's fertility naturally. These are based on recognising the bodily changes which occur throughout the menstrual cycle. Monitoring these changes helps to pinpoint the time of the months when you are most likely to become pregnant (ovulation). The most common method of natural family planning involves observing and recording changes in your cervical secretions, waking body temperature and menstrual cycle length. Persona is a special method to tell you on which days eou are most likely to become pregnant. If you wish

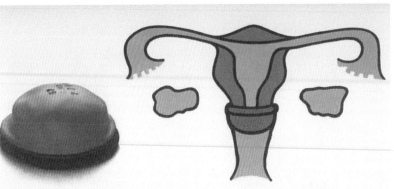

A cap is a barrier method of contraception. Caps can be rubber or silicone and are smaller than diaphragms and they cover the cervix directly.

to have sex on these days, you can then use a barrier contraceptive.

Long-acting contraception

The contraceptive methods free you from having to remember to take regular precautions against pregnancy, but will not protect you from sexually transmitted diseases. Long-acting contraceptives last between 3 months and 10 years.

- Injections - 2 to 3 months (depending on type)
- intrauterine system - 5 years
- mplants - 3 years
- intrauterine devise - 3 tot 10 years

Permanent contraception

Both sterilisation (for women) and vasectomy (for men) involve a simple and relatively minor operation. In women, this operation involves tying, cutting or blocking the Fallopian tubes to prevent the egg from meeting the sperm.

In man, the same procedure is applied to the tubes (vas deferens) that carry sperm from the testicles to the penis. In both cases, egg and sperm are absorbed naturally by the body.

Emergency contraception

The emergency hormonal contraceptive pill is the most common type of emergency contraception and works by:

- stopping ovaries from releasing an egg;
- preventing sperm from fertilising any egg you may have already released;
- stopping a fertilised egg from attaching itself to the womb lining.

Intrauterine devices (IUDs) are inserted by a doctor into a woman's uterus through the vagina (upper figures). IUD's are made of molded plastic. One type releases copper from a copper wire wrapped around the base; the other type releases a progestin. A plastic string is attached , so that a woman can check to make sure the device is still in place. Rarely, the uterus is perforated during insertion. Usually, perforation does not cause symptoms.

Removal by a doctor (lower figures) is also quick and usually causes minimal discomfort. IUD's kill or immobilize sperm and prevent fertilization of the egg.

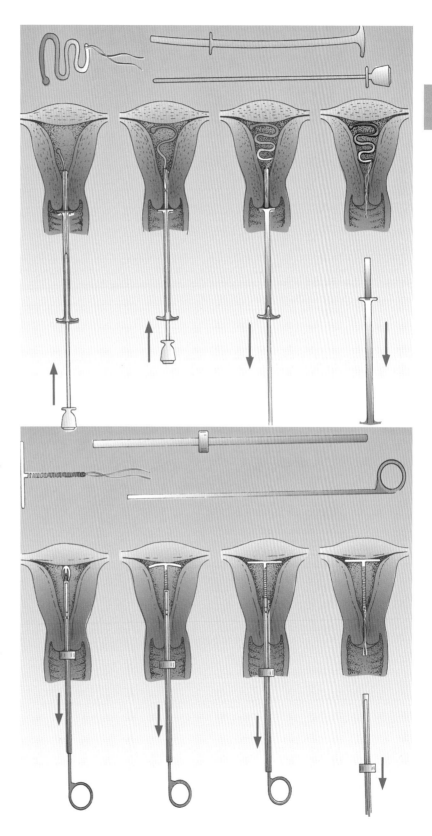

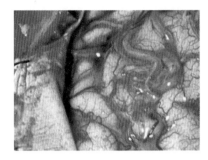

CVA

Description

This condition or disorder affects the blood vessels of the brain. Cerebrovascular accident is the commonest cause of neurological disability in our country.

Although vascular injury to the brain can occur as part of a number of relatively rare diseases, most cerebrovascular illnesses are the result of degeneration of the vessel wall (atherosclerosis), high blood pressure (hypertension) or a combination of both.

The major specific types of cerebrovascular disease are:

▲ insufficient blood to the brain due to transient disturbance of the blood flow;

▲ cerebral infarction (blockage of a blood vessel in the brain and the death of tissue) due either to embolism or to thrombosis;

▲ cerebral hemorrhage.

The terms "stroke" and "cerebrovascular accident" are commonly applied to the clinical syndromes that accompany either ischemic (lack of blood and the oxygen it carries) or hemorrhagic (bleeding) lesions.

Ischemic syndromes

These are defined as cerebrovascular disorders caused by insufficient circulation of blood in the brain. Normally, an adequate blood flow to the brain is ensured by an efficient collateral system: blood gets round any blockage by flowing from one carotid artery to the other, from one vertebral artery to the other and to the carotids via the circle of Willis.

Congenital defects and the changes that atherosclerosis makes in the blood vessels impair these compensatory mechanisms, so that brain ischemia and consequent neurological symptoms can result from interruption in the blood flow to the brain.

If the blood supply to the ischemic region is promptly restored, the brain tissue recovers and symptoms disappear, but if ischemia lasts for more than a few minutes, infarction results and neurological damage is permanent. Atheroma (deposition of hard yellow plaques of fatty material in the inner lining of arteries) that underlies most thromboses (blood clots formed on damaged artery walls), may affect any of the major brain arteries.

Large atheromas are more commonly found outside the skull, affecting the common carotid artery and vertebral artery at their origins. An obstruction can occur either in these large arteries outside the brain or in any of the smaller arteries inside the brain. Whether ischemia and infarction occur depends upon the efficiency of collateral circulation.

Thrombosis inside the skull may occur in one of the large arteries at the base of the brain, in deep perforating arteries, or in small branches in the cortex, but the main trunk of the middle cerebral artery and its branches are the most common sites.

Localization of a hemorrhage in the brain stem, causing a severe cerebrovascular accident.

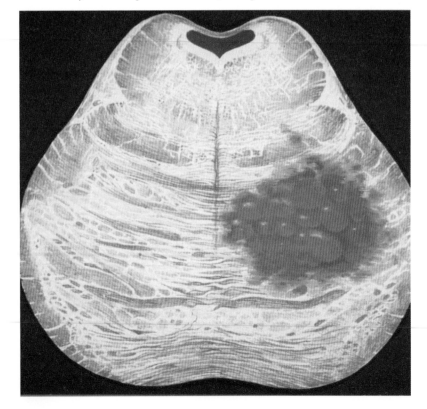

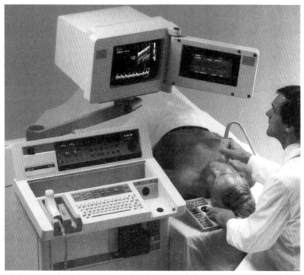

Color Doppler ultrasonography showing different rates of blood flow in different colors. This method is used mainly to measure blood flow through the arteries in the neck (carotid arteries) or through the arteries at the base of the brain. This method can help access the risk of CVA.

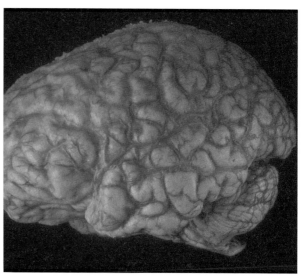

Outer surface of the brain showing dilated vessels as a result of a CVA in another part of the brain.

Cerebral emboli (fragments of clot, air bubbles, etc. that block an artery) originate in vessels outside the brain and skull and usually derive from atheromas in the large arteries in the neck or chest or - in children as well as adults - from thrombi in damaged hearts. The fragments, which lodge temporarily or permanently in major or minor branches of the cerebral arterial tree, may come from an accumulation of blood platelets, fibrin and cholesterol on the surface of plaques in atherosclerosis or from abnormal growths on the heart valves.

Transient ischemic attacks (TIA) are of sudden onset and brief duration (less than 24 hours), and reflect the improper functioning in the distribution of the arterial system of the brain. The attacks are usually recurrent and at times come before a stroke. They are most common in the middle-aged and elderly. A transient ischemic attack can occasionally occur in children in whom severe cardiovascular disease produces emboli.

High blood pressure, atherosclerosis, heart disease and diabetes can predispose a person to these attacks, but the immediate cause can seldom be ascertained. Transient ischemic attacks occur suddenly, last from two or three minutes to half an hour (seldom more than one or two hours), and then disappear, leaving behind neurological symptoms. Consciousness remains intact throughout the episode. Symptoms depend on the arterial system affected. If the carotid artery is affected, blindness or hemiparesis (slight paralysis of half of the body) may occur; aphasia (difficulty in speaking) indicates involvement of the dominant hemisphere.

When the vertebral or basilar artery is involved, symptoms reflect a disorder of the brainstem, characterized by confusion, dizziness and sometimes weakness of one of the legs or arms. The patient may have several attacks daily, or only two or three over several years. As far as the treatment is concerned, in addition to treating the atherosclerosis, hypertension, or other underlying disorder, the specialist may suggest vascular surgery. Anticoagulant drugs (which suppress clotting) may be indicated.

Stroke

A stroke is another type of cerebrovascular disease. There are differences between a "stroke in evolution" and a "completed stroke."

A stroke in evolution is the clinical condition manifested by neurological defects that increase over a 24- to 48-hour period, reflecting an enlarging infarction (blockage of an artery) or progressive edema (swelling), usually in the territory of the middle cerebral artery.

A completed stroke is the clinical condition manifested by defects in the brain of varying severity, usually abrupt in onset and either fatal or showing variable improvement, resulting from infarction of brain tissue due to atherosclerosis, high blood pressure, thrombosis or embolism. In a stroke in evolution, paralysis in one side of the body (often beginning in one arm) increases painlessly and without headache or fever over several hours or a day or two.

There may be periods of stability, but the paralysis may be continuous. Acute completed stroke is by far the more common condition: symptoms develop rapidly and typically are at their worst within a few minutes.

In either stroke in evolution or acute completed stroke, defects may worsen and consciousness may become clouded during the next few days because of edema in the brain, or, less

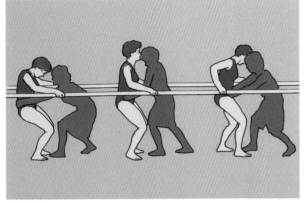
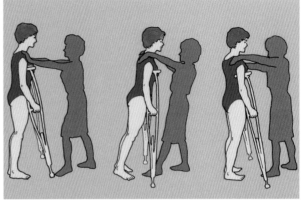
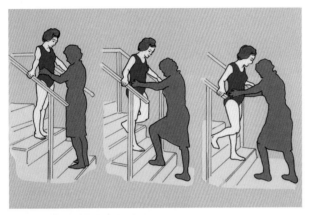
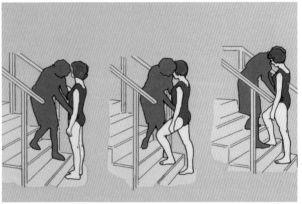

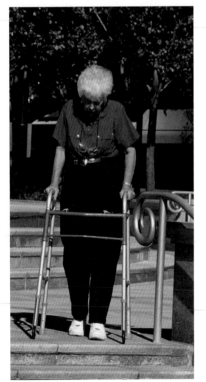

Intensive rehabilitation can help many people help overcome disabilities after a stroke. The exercises and training (upper illustrations) help develop the plasticity of the brain and teach the person new ways to use muscles unaffected by the stroke to compensate for losses in function.

often, from extension of the infarct (blockage).

The treatment of a stroke should be in the hands of a specialist. The eventual extent of recovery depends on the patient's age and general state of health as well as on the site and size of infarction or edema.

Hypertensive encephalopathy

This is an acute or subacute condition in patients with severe high blood pressure, and is marked by headache, confusion or stupor, and convulsions. Often the doctor finds rapidly changing neurological abnormalities, including blindness, hemiparesis and sensory defects.

Although both ischemic and hemorrhagic stroke are common in patients with high blood pressure, hypertensive encephalopathy is an additional, specific brain disorder confined to patients with a severe condition of high blood pressure.

The diagnosis depends on the characteristic clinical picture and the exclusion of other possible illnesses. The treatment consists of deliberate but progressive reduction of the blood pressure to nearly normal ranges by the use of specific drugs.

Hemorrhagic syndromes

These are disorders of the brain caused by bleeding into brain tissue or spaces surrounded by membranes within the skull. A hemorrhage usually results from rupture of an atherosclerotic vessel exposed to high blood pressure. Such a hemorrhage usually begins abruptly with headache, followed by steadily increasing neurological defects.

Large hemorrhages produce hemiparesis very often, difficult breathing, pinpoint pupils and coma, and may occur at onset or develop gradually. Nausea, vomiting, delirium and seizures are also common.

Large hemorrhages are fatal within a few days in more than 50 per cent of patients. In those who survive, consciousness returns and neurological symptoms gradually recede as blood is reabsorbed.

Some degree of impairment usually remains, including a speech disorder if the dominant hemisphere was affected, but a reasonable degree of functional recovery most often occurs. Therapy following hemorrhage is similar to that for ischemic stroke except that anticoagulants are contra-indicated.

Subarachnoid hemorrhage is usually a secondary bleeding into the subarachnoid space due to head injury. Spontaneous hemorrhage is usually from a ruptured aneurysm (swelling of an artery wall). Even with surgical treatment, subarachnoid hemorrhage leaves many patients with residual neurological damage.

Rehabilitation

Intensive rehabilitation can help many people to overcome disability despite the impairment of some brain tissue. Other parts of the brain can assume tasks previously performed by the damaged part.

If activities of daily living are started as soon as possible, the patient will maintain strength in his unaffected extremity and trunk muscles, will be more alert, and will have a more hopeful attitude. In addition, it may aid him in regaining some strength on his weak side.

Depending on the condition of the patient, it may be necessary to increase activities gradually. However, some patients can progress at a rapid rate. In either case, frequent rest periods should be provided between activities so that the work is not too strenuous.

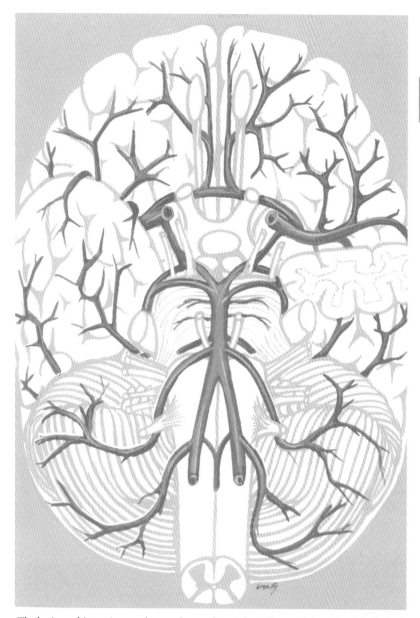

The brain and its main vascular supply seen from below. The arterial supply of the brain is derived from two sources. The carotis arteries (middle) supply the front part of the brain (top), and the two vertebral arteries (below) that fuse beneath the medulla to form the basilar artery supply the hind part of the brain. Cerebrovasvcular accidents are due to insufficient circulation of blood in either of the two arterial systems.

As soon as it is indicated by the doctor, the patient should begin activities such as rolling over in bed (using a side rail if necessary), changing his position in bed, lifting his hips on the bedpan, partially bathing himself, and feeding himself with his strong hand. If this is his left hand and he is left-handed, he should not encounter many difficulties except for not having his other hand to help. If his left hand is strong, and he is right-handed, he will be very awkward at first but with encouragement, he should learn to feed himself with his left hand.

DEAFNESS

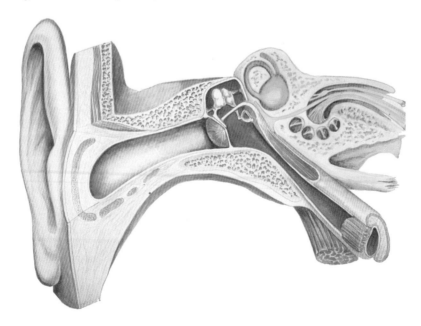

Description

Hearing loss may be due to a number of different causes. In order for a sound to be heard, it must first be conducted through the ear canal to the membrane (eardrum) inside. If this canal is blocked by wax or a foreign body, this will impair hearing. Beyond the eardrum are three little bones that are connected to each other. The sound wave that makes the eardrum vibrate moves these bones. As a result, tiny hair-like structures, the nerve endings in the inner ear, are stimulated, sending a signal to the hearing center in the brain, which interprets the sound.

When deafness is of the conductive type, the eardrum cannot make these bones vibrate, the nerve endings deep inside the ear are not stimulated, and no message is sent to the brain.

This form of deafness can usually be corrected by surgery. Other causes of conductive deafness are an infection with pus or fluid in the ear, or a perforated eardrum.

By contrast, nerve or perceptive deafness stems from damage not to the bones or the eardrum, but to the hearing nerve itself, which is then unable to transmit to the brain the message it receives from the vibrating eardrum and bones. Although a brain tumor is sometimes responsible, the usual cause of nerve injury is atherosclerosis of the blood vessels supplying the nerve or injury due to excessive noise. Nerve or perceptive deafness is the type one usually finds in older people. It progresses very slowly and does not often cause severe deafness. More commonly, the ability to discriminate high-pitched sounds is lost. Telephones may go unanswered, and the conversation of some women, especially in a noisy room, may be poorly understood.

Unlike the conductive form of deafness, surgery cannot help such sufferers, and even hearing aids are of limited use. Incidentally, noise not only causes deafness but also raises blood pressure and heart rate.

Tests

In reaching diagnoses, medical histories as given by patients and especially by their relatives are often most valuable. The Rinne test (tuning fork test) is useful as a simple and practical means of comparing air and bone conduction responses to a vibrating fork and thus differentiating between conductive and perceptive deafness prior to full evaluation by a specialist.

■ *Rinne test*
When the conduction mechanism of the middle ear is normal, not surprisingly the usual route of sound transmission is the more efficient, hence air-conducted sound appears louder than it does by bone conduction (Rinne positive).

This is the case in all normal ears and in ears with hearing loss due to disease of the perceptive apparatus (nerves and brain centers).

On the other hand, when defects of the conduction mechanisms impair the passage of sound through the middle ear, hearing is better by bone conduction than by air conduction (Rinne negative).

From left to right: outer ear, middle ear, inner ear. The inner ear is the essential part of hearing, located in the hard portion of the temporal bone of the skull.

Weber test

In the Weber test, a vibrating fork placed on the vertex (crown of the head) will sound louder in the better-hearing ear in perceptive deafness and louder in the worse-hearing ear in conductive deafness.

Understanding the Weber test depends on remembering that a sound stimulus from the vertex reaches both temporal bones (i.e. those next to the ear) at the same time and with equal intensity.

Although most of the sound stimulates the cochlea in the inner ear, some of it is normally passed to the external ear canal via the conduction mechanism working in the reverse direction to that which is physically normal.

Audiometry

To investigate the extent of deafness, specific audiometric apparatus will be employed. The audiometer is used to ascertain the quantity of hearing loss. With this electronic device, acoustic stimuli of specific frequencies are delivered at specific intensities in order to determine the person's hearing threshold for each frequency.

The hearing for each ear is measured from 125 or 250 to 8000 Hz by air conduction (using earphones) and by bone conduction (using an oscillator in contact with the head). Hearing loss is measured in decibels (Db), which equal ten times the logarithm of the ratio of acoustic power of a stimulus required to achieve hearing threshold in someone with possible deafness to the acoustic power required to achieve threshold in a normal individual. Test results are plotted on a graph called an audiogram.

Hearing aids

All hearing aids comprise a microphone, an amplifier and a receiver. They are often most useful for conduction hearing loss but they can also be helpful in certain forms of perceptive deafness.

Although the amount of assistance that any hard-of-hearing individual can expect from an aid can be predicted with fair accuracy by special hear-

Deafness   Questions & Answers

How does hearing loss occur?
There are two main types: conductive and sensory-neural. Conductive problems involve damage or disease to the outer or middle ear, which blocks sound from reaching the inner ear. Sensory-neural problems involve damage to the inner ear or auditory nerve, which sends electrical signals to the brain. People with this type of problem can hear sound but may not be able to understand what they hear.

What are the causes of hearing loss?
Many factors may cause hearing loss. Inheritance either of poor hearing or of a trait making hearing structures susceptible to disease can be involved. Birth defects can be a cause, if an infant's hearing has been damaged by maternal disease or by medication taken by the mother during pregnancy. A major cause of hearing loss in children is disease, such as the complications of chickenpox, mumps and measles.
Excessive noise in your environment, as well as accidents, can damage hearing and produce permanent hearing loss. Hearing loss also occurs in many people as they age, but the degree of difficulty resulting from aging varies greatly from person to person and affects men more than women.

What is presbycusis?
Presbycusis is defined as age-associated hearing loss; a type of sensory-neural hearing loss. The condition occurs in the elderly due to deterioration of the ear's tiny inner ear hair cells which send electrical sound impulses to the brain where sounds are received and processed.

What can be done about hearing loss?
That depends on the cause of the problem. Hearing problems, like all physical illness, are best treated as soon as symptoms develop. If left untreated, particularly in children, it can be compounded by speech, language, reading, behavioral and learning problems. To communicate well, you must be able to hear. Sometimes medical treatment or surgical procedures can completely restore normal hearing. In other instances, a hearing aid and/or audiologic rehabilitation (including auditory training and lip-reading) may be needed. If a hearing aid is necessary, be sure yours is recommended by a health professional, not a salesperson. he best way, if possible, is to prevent hearing loss. One of the best ways of prevention is to avoid exposure to excessive noise.

ing tests, the most certain way of reaching a decision is by trying one or several aids in the environment where help is most needed.

Although behind-the-ear or glasses-frame aids are often preferred (because they are less conspicuous and "hear" at ear level), their performance is less satisfactory than the body aid (placed directly in the ear) in cases of extreme deafness. Unfortunately, none gives the high fidelity required for musical appreciation.

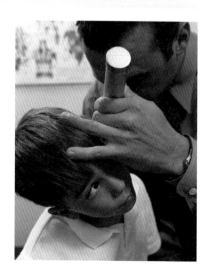

A young child complained about hearing problems. The doctor uses an otoscope to examine the eardrum.

DEATH

D

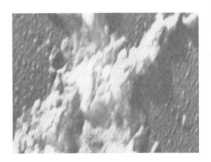

Introduction

Death is the complete and irreversible cessation of life in an organism or part of an organism. The moment of death is conventionally accepted as the time when the heart ceases to beat, there is no breathing and the brain shows no evidence of function. Ophthalmoscopic examination of the eye shows that columns of blood in small vessels are interrupted and static.

Since it is now possible to resuscitate and maintain heart function and to take over breathing mechanically, it is not uncommon for the brain to have suffered irreversible death but for "life" to be maintained artificially.

Brain death

The concept of "brain death" has been introduced. In this, reversible causes have been eliminated, and there is no spontaneous breathing, no movement and no specific reflexes seen on two occasions. When this state is reached, artificial life support systems can be reasonably discontinued as brain death already occurred. The electroencephalograph (EEG) has been used to diagnose brain death but is now considered unreliable on its own. After death, enzymes are released that begin the process of autolysis (decomposition), which later involves bacteria. In the hours following death, changes occur in muscle that cause rigidity (rigor mortis).

Following death, anatomical examination of the body (autopsy) may be performed. Embalming and burial or cremation are the usual practices for disposal of bodies in Western society. Death of part of an organism (necrosis), such as occurs following lack of blood supply, consists of loss of cell organization, autolysis and gangrene. The part may separate or be absorbed but if it becomes infected, this is liable to spread to living tissue.

Cells may also die as part of the normal turnover of a structure (for example, skin or blood cells), because of compression (for example, by a tumor), or as part of a degenerative disease. They then undergo characteristic changes.

Criteria of death

The entire body does not die at the same rate; breathing and heart action may stop, but other functions may continue. In humans, for example, the kidneys, skin, bone, liver, pancreas, cornea and heart have been transplanted into needy recipients and may continue to function for quite a long period of time.

From ancient times to the present, it has been evident that, when respiration and heart action stopped, the brain would die in a few minutes. Cessation of the heartbeat was therefore synonymous with death. Now, however, technology permits the heart and lungs to be bypassed through the use of a heart-lung machine.

Patients' hearts may even be removed while they are thus artificially maintained, as during a heart transplant. It is more common, however, to use such a machine on a patient who, because of some medical condition, is totally unable to sustain respiration on his or her own and who is completely unreceptive and unresponsive to outside stimuli.

When on the artificial respirator, such an individual may maintain a heartbeat. Yet is that person truly alive? If the respirator is turned off, how long will he or she remain alive? What happens to the brain of a person who is maintained on a respirator for some time? These troublesome questions have serious ethical, religious and

Electron microscopic view of typhoid bacilli, causing the death of hundreds of people in a recent epidemic in Indonesia.

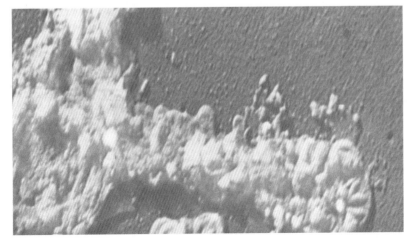

legal implications and make apparent the need to redefine and update the criteria for determining death.

The sequence of events towards the cessation of life suggests four stages:
- a time of impending death;
- a period of reversibility, with or without residual change;
- a period of irreversibility;
- absolute death, as set forth in the current legal definition.

The state of the brain has become a significant issue in the determination of death. The obligation of the doctor is to determine when the brain is no longer functioning and has no possibility of being restored; such a brain, for all practical purposes, may then be declared dead.

The condition has been variously designated as
- irreversible coma
- cerebral death
- brain death
- artificial survival

The vital organs - those essential in maintaining life - are the lungs, heart and brain. A failing respiration can be maintained by a machine. A stopped heart can sometimes be restarted and stimulated to go on unaided, but if it stops permanently, death automatically occurs. What happens, however, if the brain dies before the heart, and the breathing mechanism controlled by the now-dead lower brain centers stops? This can occur after head injury, stroke, brain tumor and a number of other illnesses.

As the disease process affects more and more of the brain, the lower part - the brain stem - which regulates such vital functions as breathing and heartbeat, finally fails. Breathing stops, and - after hours or days and even if a respirator is used - the heart ultimately stops.

Two conditions may then exist. When breathing and the heartbeat stop completely for more than seven to eight minutes, the brain dies, and total death ensues. When the brain is totally dead, breathing stops first and then the heartbeat, before death occurs. It is easy to detect when respiratory or heart function has ceased, but the determination of brain death is more difficult and must be made by a doctor. A person should be considered dead if, in the announced opinion of a

Brain-death criteria

(1) Total unresponsiveness to any type of stimulation, sound, noise or even pain.

(2) Inability to breathe on one's own.

(3) Absence of cephalic reflexes (certain reflex responses in and around the head, including coughing, swallowing, selected eye movements, pupils dilated wider than 4 mm).

(4) Electrocerebral silence (a flat brain wave on an electroen-cephalogram that shows no evidence of biological activity from the brain) for at least 30 continuous minutes.

(5) A confirmatory test indicating absence of blood flow through the brain for 30 consecutive minutes.

These criteria should guard against a premature dia-gnosis of brain death in instances of drug overdose and certain diseases in which pathological processes simulate brain death. In such instances, the condition may be alleviated by treatment. Thus sedative drug intake - determined by history, evidence about the patient or blood test - must be ruled out before a diagnosis of death.

doctor based on ordinary standards of medical practice, he or she has experienced an irreversible cessation of spontaneous respiratory and circulatory function.

In the event that adequate means of support preclude a determination that these functions have ceased - that is, the person is kept "alive" by mechanical means - he or she will be considered dead if, in the announced opinion of a doctor based on ordinary standards of medical practice, he or she has experienced an irreversible cessation of spontaneous brain function. Death will have occurred at the time when relevant functions ceased.

Causes of death

Death may be natural or unnatural, and while the circumstances often allow a reasonable diagnosis to be made as to the cause of death, only autopsy can provide accurate information.

Natural death
Natural death is often assumed to be due to coronary thrombosis ("heart attack"), and it is indeed true that the commonest cause is ischemic (blood-starved) heart disease, though not necessarily the result of thrombosis (a clotting up of an artery, particularly in the heart). Sometimes in cases where an apparently healthy person has died almost instantly, autopsy discloses a well-established heart condition that might have been present for several days or longer.

Other common causes of death are acute hypertensive heart failure (that is, one due to very high blood pressure), pulmonary embolism (a clot that has travelled to the lung) and subarachnoid or cerebral hemorrhage ("stroke").

Unnatural death
The principal causes of unnatural death are:
- Mechanical violence including the rising toll of road traffic accidents, industrial mishaps or disasters, sexual and other forms of assault and homicide.
- Physical agencies such as heat, cold, electricity or radiation.
- Deprivation involving the complete or partial lack of basic essentials such as water, food or warmth.
- Poisoning, which includes chemicals and drugs, anesthetics, intravenous infusions and blood transfusions.

DEMENTIA

D

Description

Dementia is an acquired, overall disorder of the intellect. The psychiatric aspects include not only a deficiency of memory, judgement and thought, but also a loss of emotional depth and the power of independent thought and action.

Not every case of dementia - broadly defined as a progressive or permanent - decline in intellectual function - is caused by Alzheimer's disease. In fact, there are dozens of conditions that can cause or mimic dementia, including:
- depression;
- drug overdose;
- dehydration;
- anemia;

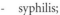

- syphilis;
- viral infections;
- vitamin deficiencies.

Many of these are reversible if they are treated promptly, so it is important to get the proper diagnosis when you or someone you love starts experiencing serious mental deterioration. In the majority of cases, this condition is due to a diffuse disease of or injury to the cortex of the cerebral hemispheres of the brain.

The principal indications of the presence of developing dementia are:
- general slowing-down of thought processes;
- rapid intellectual fatigue;
- difficulties of immediate memory;
- mental impoverishment with a tendency to repeat thoughts and actions;
- loss of physical spontaneity.

Clinical picture

The most common clinical picture is of slow disintegration of personality and intellect due to impaired judgement and insight and the loss of emotions. However, the progression of the disease is usually more painful to the beholder than to the sufferer, whose interests become restricted, outlook becomes rigid, conceptual thinking becomes more difficult, and some poverty of thought becomes apparent. Familiar tasks may be performed well, but acquiring new skills is difficult. Initiative is diminished, and the person may be easily distracted. In addition, a larger defect eventually develops, involving all aspects of higher brain functions.

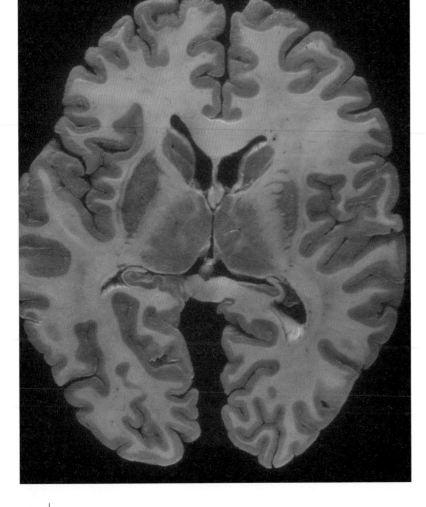

Section of the brain showing microscopic signs of dementia.

Dementia

Diseases and conditions that may result in symptoms of dementia		

DEGENERATIVE DISEASES
- Alzheimer's disease
- Pick's disease
- Huntington's chorea
- Senility

MECHANICAL CONDITIONS
- Injury
- Occult hydrocephalus
- Subdural hematoma (bruising and swelling in the skull)

METABOLIC CONDITIONS
- Hypothyroidism (reduced function of the thyroid)

- Hypercalcaemia (too much calcium in the blood)
- Hypoxia (too little oxygen)
- Wilson's disease (too much copper in the tissues)
- Uremia (excess urea in the blood, as found in kidney failure)
- Hepatic coma (coma due to liver failure)
- Carbon dioxide poisoning

VASCULAR DISEASES
- Atherosclerosis
- Collagen disease

INFECTIOUS DISEASES
- AIDS
- Chronic meningitis
- Creutzfeldt-Jakob disease

POISONING
- Metals
- Bromides
- Alcohol
- Barbiturates
- Belladonna alkaloids
- Organic phosphates
- Hallucinogens

VITAMIN DEFICIENCY
- Vitamin B1
- Vitamin B6
- Vitamin B12
- Niacin
- Folic acid

Along with the disorders in the functions of thinking, specific disturbances of speech (aphasia), movement (apraxia) and recognition of perceptions (agnosia) may be discernible. In some, dysfunction in thinking ability is preceded by modifications in their usual behavior and emotional responses.

Typically, emotions are blunted, but in early stages they may be excessive. Normal personality traits may become exaggerated or caricatured, and depression is common. If mood changes (depression, anxiety or elation) are sustained, the disorder may be misdiagnosed.

Diagnosis

In making an objective diagnosis of developing or more advanced dementia, doctors are confronted with considerable difficulties, because the usual methods of elementary psychological examination only make it possible to assess certain mental functions that are only partially correlated with the intelligence as such, irrespective of how the latter is defined.

Diagnosis can be tricky. Psychological tests go only so far because patients showing signs of dementia are often uncommunicative; failure to remember or fully answer questions can be as easily caused by severe depression as by full-fledged dementia.

Doctors typically conduct a battery of tests, which can include blood counts, chest X-rays and tests of thyroid function. Important are also CAT-scans or magnetic resonance images (MRI-scans) of the brain. These are particularly good at revealing structural problems caused by ministrokes, blood clots, tumors and fluid buildup.

Device to train memory and concentration of patients with dementia.

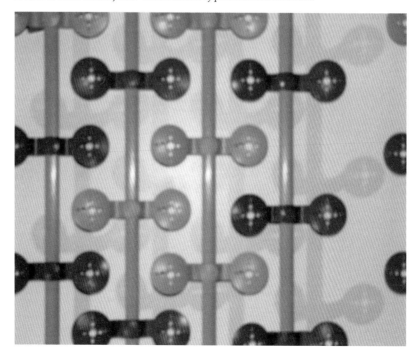

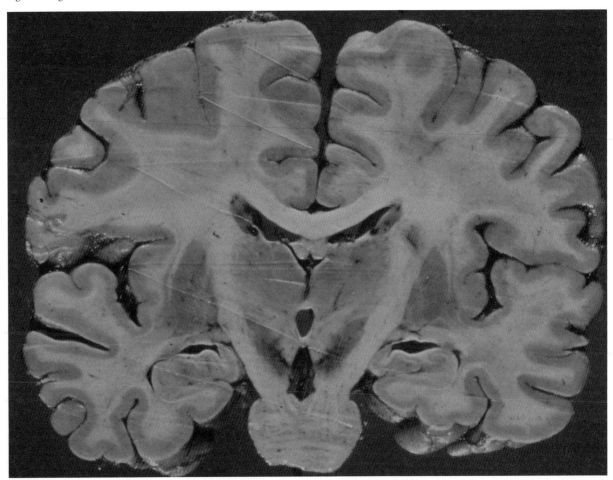

DEPRESSION

Description

Feeling depressed is a normal and natural response to the experiences of loss, failure and undeserved bad luck that anyone might suffer. It has been pointed out that without depression we would lack much of the world's great tragic literature, music and art and we would be less than, or at any rate other than, human. In some cases, however, depression becomes something more than just normal feelings of the blues or a letdown.

A large number of people suffer from what psychiatrists and psychologists call "depressive illness," which is more intense and lasts longer than common down-in-the-dumps feelings.

Sometimes a serious bout can begin ordinarily enough with an event such as the loss of a loved one or a change to a worse or more difficult job, but the depression often persists and becomes

Frontal section of the brain of a patient who committed suicide at the age of 40 years. Examination of the brain did not show specific pathological changes.

Physical disorders than can cause depression

Depression may occur with, or be caused by, a number of physical disorders directly (such as when thyroid disease affects hormone levels, which can induce depression) or indirectly (such as when rheumatoid arthritis causes pain and disability, which can lead to depression). Often, depression that results from a physical disorder has both direct and indirect causes.

Infections
• AIDS
• Influenza
• Syphilis
• Tuberculosis
• Viral hepatitis
• Viral pneumonia

Hormonal disorders
• Addison's disease
• Cushing's syndrome
• Parathyroid disorder
• Hypopituitarism
• Estrogen deficit

Neurological disorders
• Brain tumors
• Dementia
• Head injury
• Parkinson's disease
• Stroke
• Temporal lobe epilepsy

Cancers
• Ovary cancer
• Colorectal cancer
• Lung cancer
• Metastatic cancer
• Pancreas cancer

Side effects of drugs
• Withdrawal from amphetamines
• Certain antipsychotic drugs
• Certain beta-blockers
• Methyldopa
• Reserpine
• Vinblastine and vincristine

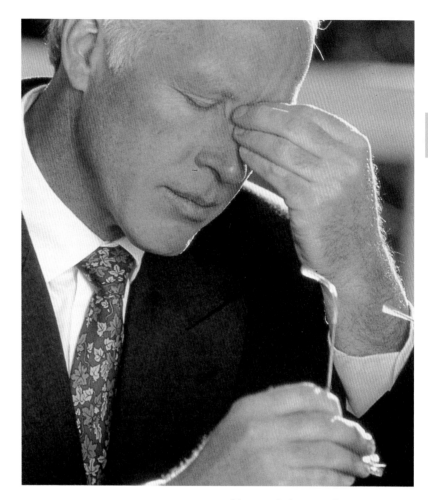

worse. At times, in very severe cases there does not seem to have been any circumstance serious enough to have caused the depression.

Researchers are not sure, even today, whether depressive illness is an aggravated form of normal depression or whether it is something entirely different. Some sufferers have described their feelings during a depressive illness as being quite distinct from any blue feelings they had ever experienced.

Depression can show itself in many ways and with different degrees of intensity. There is a variety of possible symptoms, particularly in the milder forms of the illness, called "depressive neuroses."

Often those who go to their doctors with general complaints or feelings of "not being myself" do not know that depression may be behind these feelings.

Signs of depression

Some psychiatrists suggest that the key feature in depression is change. The sufferers become different from the way they were before the onset of their depression, and may even become the opposite of their usual selves. There are many examples: the businessman who becomes a vagrant, the mother who wants to harm her children and herself, the gourmet who develops an aversion to food, the sexually active woman who develops an aversion to sex.

Instead of seeking gratification and pleasure, depressed people avoid it; instead of taking care of themselves, they neglect themselves and their appearance. Their drive to survive gives way to suicidal wishes; their drive to succeed and achieve turns into passive withdrawal. In general, the most obvious and typical sign of

Depression   Questions & Answers

What is a depression?

A depression is a feeling of intense sadness; it may follow a recent loss or other sad event but is out of proportion to that event and persists beyond an appropriate length of time.

Who gets depressed and what causes severe depression?

Everyone has blue moods now and then. Sometimes there is a good reason for feeling down. But depression is different. It may start without reason and continue for months or years. Even if there seems to be a good cause, the degree of depression may be completely out of proportion to the problem.

People in every age group, from children through the elderly, can develop severe depression. At any given time, between 4 and 5 per cent of the population suffers from major depression. Unfortunately, less than half of them get properly diagnosed and treated.

The cause of severe depression is unclear. A tendency toward depression may be inherited. It may be caused by physiologic dysfunction of the brain, rather than just psychological problems.

Medicines may be a vital part of the therapy, but they will not cure depression. So never take someone's else tranquilizers or pep pills. Medication can help ease your distress and clear your thinking.

How do severely depressed people feel?

Severely depressed people have a feeling of great sadness and a sense of misery all over. They may have a look of sadness and hopelessness that other people notice. They tend to lose interest in people and activities around them. They often express pessimism, guilt and self-depreciation.

Such depression can distort your outlook on life. You may not be able to see the good side of anything, including yourself. If these feelings are allowed to persist, you may think about suicide - which you would never consider if you were feeling better. Suicidal feelings are a sure sign that you need hell to cope with depression.

What are the major symptoms of a depression?

Many depressed people experience one or more of the following physical symptoms:

- weight loss or gain
- leeplessness
- loss of appetite
- fatigue
- loss of sexual desire
- dizziness

Sometimes they attribute their problems to these symptoms and do not recognize that they are depressed. If you are depressed for more than two weeks, or if your depression interferes with your work, or social life, then you probably have a serious depression and should see your physician.

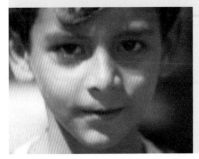

What is meant by a transient depression?

A transient depression occurs when someone becomes temporarily depressed in reaction to certain holidays (holiday blues) or meaningful anniversaries, such as the anniversary of a loved one's death; during the premenstrual phase, or during the first 2 weeks after giving birth.

depressive illness is a gloomy mood of sadness, loneliness and apathy. However, if periods of deep depression seem to alternate with periods of extreme elation, this too points to serious depressive illness. Seriously depressed people see themselves in a very negative way. They are convinced that they are "alone" and hopeless and often reproach or blame themselves for ordinary faults and shortcomings that they exaggerate.

They are very pessimistic about themselves, about the world and their future. They become less interested in what is going on around them and do not get satisfaction out of the things they used to enjoy.

Fatigue, disturbed sleep and especially waking much earlier than usual are quite common; or, feeling constantly tired, they may want to sleep more than usual. They may lose their appetite and lose weight, or eat more than normally and gain weight.

Another characteristic, particularly evident in women, is crying spells, whether or not there is something to cry about. Many of these spells are short-lasting and fairly common, but if the symptom persists, professional assistance should be sought.

Some depressive illness may not even show the usual telltale signs of moody sadness and dejection. In these cases, the underlying depression may mask itself in physical discomfort or it may contribute to alcoholism or addiction to a drug.

Chronic fatigue and boredom, as well as habitual underachievement, may be unrecognized forms of depression. There is even evidence that the hyperkinetic (overly active) child may be compensating for an underlying depression, because the same drugs that relieve depression in adults seem to help hyperactive children as well.

Depressives share the common feeling that they have lost something very important to them, though often this is not really the case. From a feeling of loss, these depressed people progress to unrealistic convictions that they are losers and will always be losers, that they must be worthless and "bad" and perhaps not fit to live. They may even attempt suicide.

So many seriously depressed people do attempt suicide, in fact, that

Warning signs

Depression is not simply "the blues" or a problem that can be wished away. It is a collection of symptoms that lasts two weeks or more and interferes with the ability to enjoy activities that used to bring pleasure.

These symptoms or warning signs include:
- Feeling of emptiness, guilt, hopelessness, or despair
- Lack of energy
- Feeling irritable or overwhelmed - as if everything is too much
- Difficulty thinking or concentrating
- Loss is interest in sex
- Changes in eating or sleeping patterns

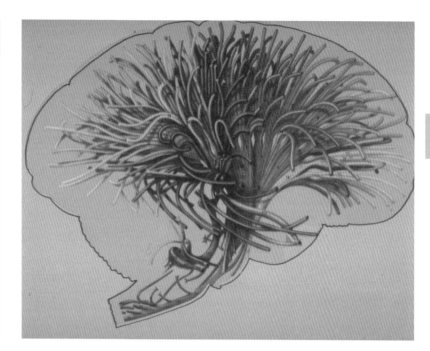

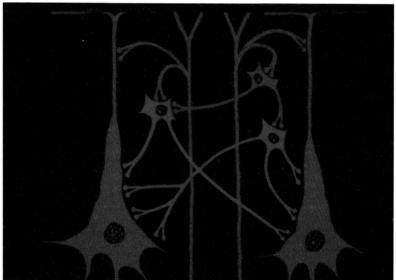

According to some scientists depression is primarily caused by a lack of connectivity of nerve cells in the cerebral cortex.

depressive illness may be considered the only "fatal" mental illness. Not all those suffering from depressive illness will attempt suicide, nor are all those who attempt suicide necessarily suffering from depressive illness, but the relationship is striking.

It is estimated that as many as 75 per cent of those who attempt suicide are seriously depressed, and other studies indicate that people hospitalized for depression at some time in their lives are about 36 times more likely to commit suicide than are non-depressed people, with the greatest risk being during or immediately following hospitalization.

After the age of 40, the possibility of suicide increases in severely depressed persons. Almost twice as many women as men suffer from depressive illness and almost twice as many women attempt suicide, but three times more men than women succeed. Aside from the danger of suicide, depression is a tragic condition that often leads to broken homes, ruined friendships and careers and disrupted lives.

The course of the illness

Generally, the beginning of any depressive episode is clear-cut and well-defined. The depression progresses until it has reached its most severe point, then the person begins to improve spontaneously and steadily until the episode is over. There is a tendency for all types of depressive illness to recur, but the intervals between episodes are free of symptoms. Attacks before the age of 30 tend to be shorter than those after this age. They may last for a few days, a few months or for several years.

The average duration of the attacks among hospitalized patients is a little more than six months, and among those not needing hospitalization, about three months.

It is wise to get professional help as soon as a depressive illness is suspected.

Drugs used to treat depression

Tricyclics and related drugs

Once the mainstay of treatment, now used infrequently. They often cause sedation and lead to weight gain. Side effects are usually more pronounced in older people. There is also the danger of serious, potentially life-threatening toxicity in overdose.

■ *Selected side effects*
- Sedation
- Weight gain
- Increased heart rate
- Decreased blood pressure
- Dry mouth
- Confusion
- lurred vision
- Constipation
- Difficulty urinating
- Delayed orgasm
- Seizures

■ *Examples*
- Amitriptyline
- Amoxapine
- Clomipramine
- Doxepin
- mipramine
- Maprotiline
- Nortriptyline
- Imipranine
- Trimipramine

Selective serotonin reuptake inhibitors

Most commonly used class of antidepressants. Also effective for dysthymia, generalized anxiety disorder, obsessive-compulsive disorder, panic disorder, phobic disorder, posttraumatic stress disorder and premenstrual dysphoric disorder. There exists a less serious risk of toxicity on overdosage.

■ *Selected side effects*
- Sexual dysfunction
- Nausea
- Diarrhea
- Headache
- Weight loss
- Withdrawal syndrome
- Forgetfulness
- Blunting of emotions

■ *Examples*
- Citalopram
- Fluoxetine
- Fluvoxamine
- Paroxetine
- Sertraline

Monoamine oxidase inhibitors

These drugs, also called MAOIs may be effective when other antidepressants have failed but are rarely the first choice in treatment. People who use MAOIs must adhere to a number of dietary restrictions and follow special precautions.

■ *Selected side effects*
- Insomnia
- Weight gain
- Sexual dysfunction
- Pin-and-needles sensation
- Lowered blood pressure
- Severe high blood pressure

■ *Examples*
- Phenelzinee
- Tranylcypromine

Psychostimulants

These drugs are generally not effective when used alone. Often used in combination with antidepressants.

■ *Selected side effects*
- Nervousness
- Tremor
- Insomnia
- Dry mouth

■ *Examples*
- Dextroamphetamine
- Methylphenidate

Newer drugs

New drugs have become available that are as effective as selective serotonin reuptake inhibitors but may have fewer and less severe side effects for some people. Most of the side effects can be prevented or minimized when low doses are used and when changes in dosages are made slowly.

■ *Selected side effects*
- Headache
- Dry mouth
- Weight gain
- Mild sedation

■ *Examples*
- Bupropion
- Mirtazapine
- Nefazodone
- Trazodone
- Venlafaxine

Susceptibilities

Anyone can become depressively ill, but some people are more susceptible than others. As mentioned above, twice as many women as men suffer from depressive illness, though the reasons are unclear.

Some researchers speculate that a woman's hormonal cycle may have some effect on her vulnerability, and also that our culture makes it easier for women to show signs of depression - such as tearfulness and hypersensitivity. Also, married persons seem more prone to depression than unmarried individuals.

There is wide agreement that both hereditary and environmental factors play an important part in depressive illness. Studies have shown rather conclusively that depression is more likely to occur in a person with a family history of depressive illness.

Some investigators have found that nearly 25 per cent of patients had mentally ill mothers and more than 15 per cent had depressed fathers. More specifically, present studies provide some convincing evidence that a dominant gene or genes on the X-chromosome may be a necessary condition for the development of at least one form of manic-depressive illness. This means that a mother (who possesses two X-chromosomes) can pass on the tendency to a son (xy) or a daughter (xx), but a father (who has X and Y chromosomes) can only pass it to a daughter.

Further studies have indicated that a manic-depressive can pass on a tendency towards either unipolar depression or manic-depression, suggesting that at least two genes are involved. There is also much evidence to support the importance of a stressful situation or event in the actual onset of a depressive episode.

A National Institute of Mental Health (US) study found that each of 40 depressed persons had suffered from several personal problems in the year preceding his or her breakdown - the most common being a threat to the individual's sexual identity. Other personal traumas included divorce, moving to another community, physical illness and the death of a loved one.

The interaction of heredity and stress, which can result in serious depression in some people and not in others, is a matter for continuing research. Another major area of research on depression involves chemical changes in the body that take place during depressed states.

Whether these chemical changes cause depression or are caused by the illness is not yet clearly understood, but significant abnormalities can be demonstrated in the functioning of many body systems during the peak of a depressive illness - even malfunctioning within the brain itself. A relatively new research approach - inducing depression in animals - may provide some insight into the dynamics and causes of the illness.

Until about ten years ago, depression was thought to be unique to humans, but researchers now believe it afflicts all higher forms of life, including monkeys, geese, dogs, parrots and other animals. If depression can be induced in animal models, scientists have reasoned, they may obtain valuable insights that apply to human situations.

One group of studies has already demonstrated that monkeys appear to take on many of the outer behavioral characteristics of human depression if they are separated from their mothers at an early age and kept isolated.

This kind of separation seems to affect humans in much the same way. Using monkeys and other animals,

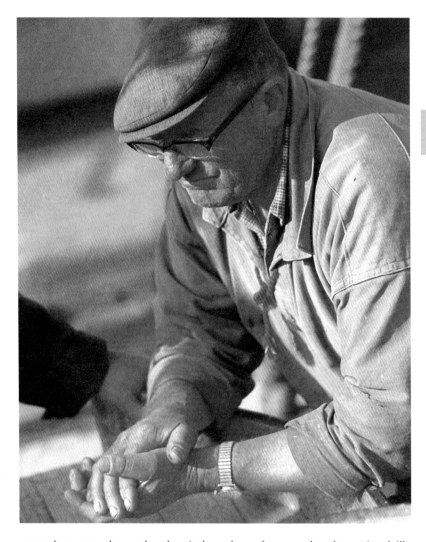

researchers can also make chemical tests and try drug treatments that would not be possible with humans.

Treatment

Although depressive illness is the leading cause of psychiatric hospital admissions, it is also among the psychiatric disorders that are most responsive to treatment.

Behavioral scientists do not fully understand how depression works or what causes it, but with current treatment even a severe, incapacitating depressive illness

will usually respond within a matter of two to six months. Much of the credit for this optimistic outlook is due to advances in the use of various

drugs for mental and emotional illnesses, coupled with psychotherapy.

To date, no single drug has been found effective for all kinds of depression. Unipolar and bipolar depression respond to different drugs entirely, giving added support to genetic evidence that the two forms of serious depression may be entirely separate.

Unipolar depression is treated mainly with two groups of drugs - those of the tricyclic chemical family and those that inhibit the monoamine oxidase (MAO) enzyme that, in health, destroys substances in the brain that act on nerve transmission. Recently, a third type of antidepressant drug has been developed, of which Prozac is a well-known representative.

Bipolar (manic-depressive) illness seems most responsive to lithium car-

Depression Symptoms			
The 15 most frequently occurring symptoms in endogenous depression (ranked in order of frequency)		**The 15 most frequently occurring symptoms in psychogenic (reactive) depression (ranged in order of frequency)**	
Males	Females	Males	Females
1. Lack of energy	Sadness	1. Sadness	Sadness
2. Sadness	Joylessness	2. Joylessness	Joylessness
3. Joylessness	Lack of energy	3. Anxiety	Anxiety
4. Anxiety	Anxiety	4. Lack of energy	Lack of energy
5. Loss of interest	Loss of interest	5. Loss of interest	Tension
6. Loss of ability to concentrate	Lack of appetite	6. Ideas of inadequacy, etc.	Aggression, irritability
7. Tension	Loss of ability to concentrate	7. Tension	Inability to fall asleep
8. Ideas of inadequacy, etc.	Tension	8. Disruption of social functioning	Lack of appetite
9. Disruption of social functioning	Disruption of social functioning	9. Hopelessness	Suicidal ideas
10. Slowness and retardation of thought etc.	Ideas of inadequacy	10. Loss of ability to concentrate	Loss of interest
11. Hopelessness	Hopelessness	11. Aggression, irritability	Ideas of inadequacy
12. Indecisiveness	Fitful, restless sleep	12. Indecisiveness	Hopelessness
13. Decrease of sex drive	Indecisiveness	13. Suicidal ideas	Loss of ability to
14. Slowing down of body and mind	Inability to fall asleep	14. Inability to fall asleep	Disruption of social functioning
15. Inability to fall asleep	Early awakening	15. Lack of appetite	Fitful, restless sleep

bonate, a drug that has been used for many years.

Research has indicated that lithium is highly effective in the treatment of acute manic attack. In one study, 80 per cent of the manic patients treated with lithium responded favourably, and other results suggest that lithium may also help relieve the depressed phase of manic-depressive illness. Some researchers believe that daily doses of lithium can protect susceptible individuals from depressive relapses.

In Scandinavia, lithium is an established treatment for prevention of recurring mood disorders, but in the US and Britain, most scientists are withholding judgement on the broad claims for lithium until further studies, now in progress, provide more information.

Drugs are not as effective in providing relief from the less severe forms of depression.

These are the depressive neuroses, which account for the greatest proportion of hospitalized patients. Except for bedtime sedation, drugs do not seem particularly helpful, and electroconvulsive therapy (ECT) is now believed to be inappropriate.

The main treatment is psychotherapy, either on an individual or group basis. Other treatments include milieu therapy (a carefully structured environment), occupational therapy and psychodrama.

Until biological and drug research claimed the limelight during the past decade, there was much interest in attacking depression through studies of the psychological, social and cultural aspects of these illnesses.

There are many theories about the psychological nature of depression. Freud considered depression to be an expression of hostile feelings directed towards one's self, and today, the most widely accepted theory suggests that depression results from a feeling of helplessness following a loss of self-esteem.

Results of a recent five-year research project, supported by the US National Institutes of Health, propose yet another approach. The main cause of depression, the researchers suggest, may be that some people perceive or see situations incorrectly, which affects how they feel.

In other words, rather than thinking they are inadequate and alone because they feel sad and lonely, depressed persons may feel sad and lonely because they think they are inadequate and alone.

Psychotherapists who hold this view deal primarily with the faulty thought processes of sufferers, rather than being concerned mainly with elevating their low moods.

New approaches to treatment have been suggested by mental health authorities who are studying depression from this point of view. They have found that, regardless of this low opinion of themselves held by psy-

D

chotically depressed persons, they perform just as well as "normal" subjects in a series of complex intellectual and motor tasks.

One group of researchers gave depressed patients a series of verbal tasks, guaranteeing that the patients would meet with success. As they began to experience success in performing the tasks, the depressed patients began to show increased optimism, improvement in their mood and self-image and a surprising improvement in performance of later tasks.

How families and friends can help

Friends and family members can do a great deal to relieve sufferers of the more moderate forms of depression. Keeping the depressed person busy and active often helps, as depression tends to feed on itself.

A moderately depressed person becomes apathetic and inactive and, as a result of the inactivity becomes more depressed, more withdrawn, even more inactive, and the vicious circle grows.

Sometimes such a person finds it hard to get organized to do even routine chores, and a schedule of constructive and pleasurable activities to fill the day can help. And a sympathetic ear can sometimes work wonders.

Another aid, often prescribed by doctors, is a change of scene - a week off from work or a holiday away from home may help depressed people to get away from situations that may be getting them down.

If friendly interest and efforts to take their minds off their troubles do not seem to comfort these depressed persons, it is wise for them to see a doctor. Just talking with the doctor may help, or the doctor may prescribe a mild anti-depressant or recommend further counselling or psychotherapy. The haunting possibility of suicide must always be taken into consideration in cases of depression. Although the depression may appear relatively mild, this does not by any means exclude the possibility of suicide, because seemingly mild depression sometimes has much deeper roots.

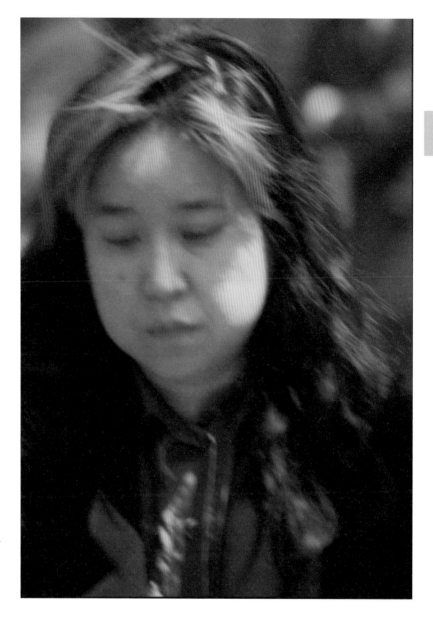

If depressed feelings linger beyond what seems reasonable and normal, if there seems no apparent reason for a persistent feeling of unhappiness and gloom, professional help should be sought. It is not true, as many people believe, that a person who talks about suicide will not attempt it. Those who attempt suicide often appeal first for help by threatening to do so.

Even when there is little or no danger of suicide, a doctor should be consulted when depressive illness is suspected. Everyone has suffered an unpleasant bout of the blues, but this is a very minor indication of the kind of mental pain that serious depression can inflict.

Much can be done to restore the happiness and well-being of depressed people, to relieve their families, friends and co-workers of the terrible burden imposed by depressive illness. But it is important to diagnose depressive illness as early in its onset as possible.

Modern medicine can help, but early identification plays a large part in the effectiveness of treatment and the speed of recovery.

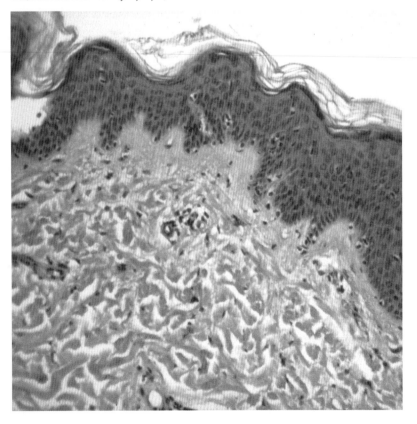

DERMATITIS

D

Introduction

Disorders and diseases of the skin are so varied and so common that dermatology is a specialty in the practice of medicine. The most remarkable fact about this field of medicine is how much there remains to be learned about it.

Although most microorganisms are parasites and thus pathogenic to man, there are numerous species that live on the skin at peace with us. Under certain conditions these microorganisms may become pathogenic and cause serious skin diseases.

Skin infection or dermatitis is not a specific illness but a general term for any inflammation of the skin. In the last decades it has been found that a great many such inflammations are allergic reactions.

Skin (cutaneous) infections (dermatitis) may be caused by bacteria, fungi, viruses, or parasites. Many, but not all, bacterial and fungal infections are amenable to topical therapy. Careful assessment of the conditions must be made before appropriate treatment can be recommended.

Bacterial infections

Bacterial skin infections are classified as pyodermas since pus is usually present. They are principally caused by Streptococci and Staphylococci. The lesions result from external infection or reinfection and may be superficial or involve deeper dermal tissue.

These pyodermic infections may be either primary (in which no previous dermatoses exist) or secondary (in which a predisposing dermal problem preceded the infection).

Other organisms may be present in secondary pyodermas, including gram-negative bacteria (Pseudomonas aeruginosa), which are especially prevalent on warm moist skin such as axillae, ear canals, and interdigital spaces.

Infections by pathogenic organisms are related to the breakdown of the skin's disinfecting protective mechanisms or to the development of an abundance of colonies of pathogenic organisms.

A breakdown of the normal ecological balance may be enhanced by alterations in the skin's other defense mechanisms. Normally, the stratum corneum has only about 10 per cent water content, which ensures elasticity but is generally below that needed to support luxuriant microbial growth.

An increase in moisture content may allow microbial growth, leading to infection. A break in the intact surface has a deleterious effect on the skin's defensive properties, allowing large numbers of pathogenic organisms to be introduced into the inner layers.

Skin disorders may occur in all three layers of the skin: Form top to bottom: epidermis, dermis, subcutaneous tissue (fatty layer).

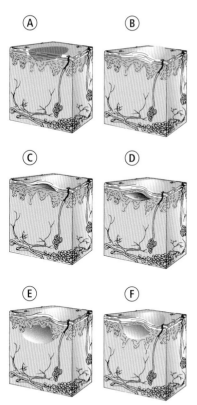

Schematic drawing showing major marks and growth of the skin.
A. Macula (flat, discolored spot).
B. Urticaria.
C. Superficial vesicles.
D. Subcutaneous vesicle-formation.
E. Pustule (blister containing pus).

In addition, infection may be predisposed by a number of external factors such as:
- excessive scrubbing of the skin (especially with strong detergents);
- excessive exposure to water;
- occlusion;
- increasing the skin temperature;
- excessive sweating or bathing;
- injury.

Thus the presence and severity of microbial skin infection generally is dependent on the condition of the skin's defense mechanism, the number of pathogenic organisms present, and the supportive nutrient environment for those organisms.
The main pyodermic infections are:
- impetigo;
- ecthyma;
- folliculitis;
- furuncles (boils);
- carbuncles;
- erysipelas;
- sweat gland infections;
- ecthyma;
- pyonychia.

Fungal infections

Infections caused by fungi, often called dermatomycoses, are among the most common cutaneous disorders. Characteristically, they exhibit single or multiple lesions that may have mild scaling or deep granulomas (inflamed nodules).
Superficial infections affect the air, nails, and skin and are generally caused by three types of fungi:
- Trichophyton;
- Microsporum;
- Epidermophyton.

Candida species may also be involved. Fungal infections of hairless skin are generally superficial, and the organisms are found in or on the uppermost skin layers. In fungal infections of areas covered with heavy hair, the infections are much deeper because of hair follicle penetration.

Viral infections

Infections by viruses may occur directly in or on the skin and present as:
- warts;
- molluscum contagiosum;
- herpes simplex;
- HIV.

Chicken pox and measles are systemic viral diseases that also have important diagnostic dermatologic manifestations.
Herpes zoster infections also present with skin manifestations and affect a nerve or group of nerves of the same area.

Treatment

The use of non-prescription topical antimicrobial products should be limited to superficial conditions that involve minimal areas, when no predisposing illnesses exist.
Self-administered topical products

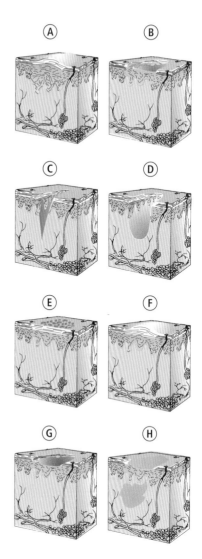

Schematic drawing showing major marks and growth of the skin.
A. Papule (solid bump).
B. Erosion (Loss of part or all of the top surface of the skin).
C. Excoriation.
D. Ulcer.
E. Lichenification.
F. Keratosis.
G. Crust (scab).
H. Scar.

should be viewed as extensions of supportive treatment (proper cleaning, proper hygiene, and clean bandaging), and not as "miracle" treatments.
Medical attention should be sought in all but the most superficial, uncompli-

Dermatitis   Questions & Answers

D

How are bacterial infections of the skin classified?

Bacterial skin infections are classified as pyodermas since pus is usually present. They are principally caused by Streptococci and Staphylococci. The lesions result from external infection or reinfection and may be superficial or involve deeper dermal tissue.

What are pyodermic infections of the skin?

The pyodermic infections may be either primary (in which no previous dermatoses exist) or secondary (in which a predisposing dermal problem preceded the infection). Other organisms may be present in secondary pyodermas, including gram-negative bacteria (Pseudomonas aeruginosa), which are especially prevalent on warm moist skin such as axillae, ear canals, and interdigital spaces.

How develops a pyodermic infection?

Infections by pathogenic organisms are related to the breakdown of the skin's disinfecting protective mechanisms or to the development of an abundance of colonies of pathogenic organisms. A breakdown of the normal ecological balance may be enhanced by alterations in the skin's other defense mechanisms.

Normally, the stratum corneum has only about 10 per cent water content, which ensures elasticity but is generally below that needed to support luxuriant microbial growth. An increase in moisture content may allow microbial growth, leading to infection.

A break in the intact surface has a deleterious effect on the skin's defensive properties, allowing large numbers of pathogenic organisms to be introduced into the inner layers.

What are the main pyodermic infections?

The main pyodermic infections are:
- impetigo;
- ecthyma;
- folliculitis;
- furuncles (boils);
- carbuncles;
- erysipelas;
- sweat gland infections;
- ecthyma;
- pyonychia.

What is impetigo?

Impetigo vulgaris (Latin impetigo = attack), caused by Streptococci and/or Staphylococci, probably is the most superficial of the pyodermas, mainly involving the surface areas. Direct contact with the lesions or infected exudate generally is required for its transmission.

How does impetigo of the skin develop?

The lesions start with small red spots that rapidly evolve into characteristic vesicles (tiny sacs or blisters) filled with amber fluid. Exudate collects and forms yellow or brown crusts on the skin's surface, surrounded by a zone of redness (erythema).

The eruptions may be circular with clear central areas and may occur in groups. The exposed parts of the body are most easily affected, but no area of skin is immune to reinfection from within.

What causes impetigo?

Impetigo is most common in children and is highly contagious. Failure to treat impetigo adequately will greatly increase the risk of secondary kidney ailment (acute glomerulonephritis), with resultant increase in morbidity/mortality.

Generally, in primary impetigo the responsible bacteria cause the infection directly. Some forms, however, occur secondarily to the presence of other infections, injury, or the general breakdown of skin defences.

What is erysipelas?

Erysipelas (meaning red skin), caused by beta-hemolytic Streptococci, is a cellulitis characterized by a rapidly spreading, red and edematous plaque. This superficial infection has sharply established borders and a glistening surface. It occurs most often on the scalp and face, and the organisms enter through a break in the skin. The disorder is usually accompanied by fever, chills, and malaise.

What is a furuncle or boil?

Furuncles are pus-producing skin diseases generally caused by Staphylococci located in or around hair follicles. The lesion may start as a superficial folliculitis but develops into a deep nodule.

The fully established furuncle or boil has elevated swelling, is erythematous, and is very painful. Furuncles are most common in males. Hairy areas and areas subject to maceration and friction (collar, waist, buttocks, and thighs) seem most vulnerable.

How does a furuncle develop?

The initial redness and swelling stage is followed by thinning of the skin around the primary follicle, centralized pustulation, destruction of the pilosebaceous structure, discharge of the cord (plug), and central ulceration. Scarring often occurs. Chronic furunculosis is common, with new lesions appearing intermittently for months or years.

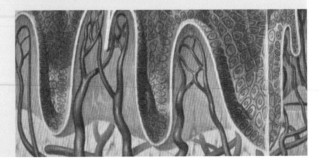

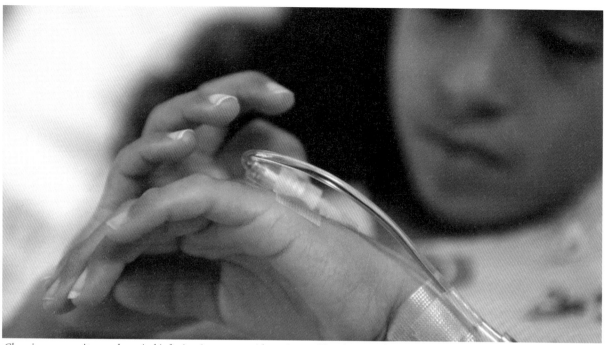

Chronic eczema mit secondary viral infection (treatment with corticosteroid and antiviral medicines).

cated skin infections, especially if it appears that systemic medication is needed.

Deep-seated and complicated secondary infections require medical attention. Improper lancing as self-treatment may cause scarring and spreading of the infected exudate.

Only the most superficial, minor cutaneous infections are amenable to topical anti-infective therapy. In more severe cases of bacterial infection, systemic therapy is required.

In athlete's feet it is essential that the feet and the spaces between the toes are kept as dry as possible. Wash the feet with water as soap tends to soften the skin and offers a favourable culture medium for the fungi.

Medical treatment will be directed to the patient's clinical presentation and, when necessary, cultures of the lesion to determine the infecting organism.

Minor surgical procedures such as debridement, curettage, and liquid nitrogen are indicated in the treatment of some dermatoses. Such procedures must be performed by a dermatologist.

Erythema due to a bacterial infection.

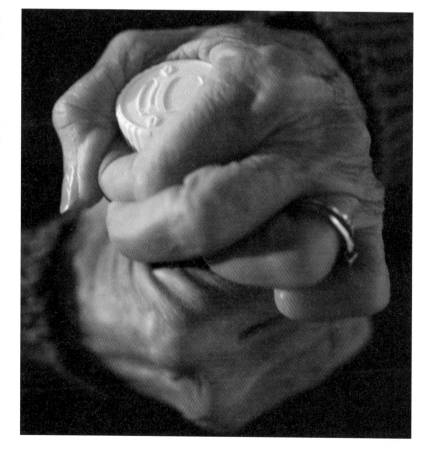

DIABETES

D

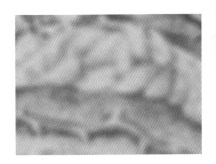

Description

Diabetes is a common disease, characterized by the absence or inadequate secretion of insulin. In diabetes, the body is unable to convert certain foods into the heat and energy necessary for normal activity. Doctors often use the full name diabetes mellitus, rather than diabetes alone, to distinguish this disorder from diabetes insipidus, a relatively rare disorder.

Normally, the sugars and starches (carbohydrates) in the food we eat are processed by our digestive juices into a form of sugar called glucose or blood sugar, and this is the fuel which enables our bodies to function. It is burned as needed for energy or stored for later use. Insulin, a hormone produced by the pancreas, is one of the major regulators of the use of our fuel supply.

When the right amount of insulin is present at the right time, the right amount of glucose is taken into the cells, burned or released for use by the body. In the diabetic individual, there is an impairment of insulin activity. Either the body does not produce enough insulin, or the available insulin is somehow blocked or inactivated by other substances within the body and it is prevented from performing its primary function.

Because of this impairment, glucose is not properly utilized by the body and excessive amounts accumulate in the blood and tissues and overflow into the urine. Too much glucose in the blood and glucose in the urine are signs of diabetes.

Forms of diabetes

There are two main forms of diabetes, which differ from each other in several ways. The more serious of the two is type 1 diabetes ,mellitus (insulin-dependent diabetes), formerly called juvenile diabetes, in which there is a total or substantial lack of insulin, and daily injections of the hormone are necessary for survival.

Before the discovery of insulin over 60 years ago and its subsequent production from the pancreas of animals, juvenile diabetics did not live more than a year or two after the onset of the disease.

■ Type 1 diabetes mellitus

People with type 1 diabetes mellitus (insulin-dependent diabetes) provide little or no insulin at all. Although 6 per cent of the western population has some form of diabetes, only about 10 percent of all diabetics have type 1. Most people who have type 1 diabetes developed the disease before age 30.

Scientists believe that an environmental factor - possibly a viral infection or a nutritional factor in childhood or early adulthood - causes the immune system to destroy the insulin-producing cells in the pancreas. Some genetic predisposition most likely needed for this to happen.

Whatever the cause, in type 1 diabetes more than 90 per cent of the insulin-producing cells (beta cells) of the pancreas are permanently destroyed. The resulting insulin deficiency is severe, and to survive, a person with type 1 diabetes must regularly inject insulin.

■ Type 2 diabetes mellitus

In type 2 diabetes mellitus (non-insulin dependent diabetes), the pancreas continues to manufacture insulin, sometimes even at higher than normal levels. However, the body develops resistance to its effects, resulting in a relative insulin deficiency.

Type 2 diabetes may occur in children and adolescents but usually begins after age 30 and becomes progressively more common with age, About 15 per cent of the people over age 70 have type 2 diabetes.

Obesity is a risk factor for type 2 diabetes; 80 to 90 per cent of the people with this disease are obese. Other less common causes of diabetes are abnormally high levels of corticosteroids, pregnancy, drugs, and poisons that interfere with the production of effects on insulin, resulting in high blood sugar levels.

In general, women are more susceptible to type 2 diabetes mellitus than men, and the disease tends to occur most frequently in certain "high-risk" groups - close relatives of individuals who have diabetes, people who are overweight or over forty, women who have given birth to large infants (weighing over 4.5 kg (10 lb.)).

Causes, symptoms and diagnosis

The basic cause of the loss of insulin production or activity in diabetes is not known. While there appears to be a strong hereditary factor in diabetes, leading to the belief that it has a tendency to "run in families," not all cases fall into this category.

Consequently, other possible causes are continually being explored - previous severe virus infections, environmental factors, some forms of auto-immunity such as a lack of a diabetes-preventing gene.

Thus far there is no conclusive evidence linking diabetes to these possible causes. A fact that does seem clear, however, is that obesity worsens and may even precipitate diabetes.

The early symptoms of diabetes stem from the increased amount of sugar in the blood and urine. Since the kidneys excrete excessive amounts of water along with the excess sugar, uncontrolled diabetics are likely to urinate frequently and to be constantly thirsty.

Because the sugar in their blood is not being converted to energy, they will be weak, tired and hungry. Because of the calories lost in the urine, they will lose weight, no matter how much they eat. Common symptoms that can be easily recognized and that should be brought to the prompt attention of a doctor include:

- excessive urination
- increased thirst
- rapid loss of weight with increased appetite and food intake
- general weakness, drowsiness and fatigue
- visual disturbances, such as blurring;
- slow healing of cuts and bruises;
- skin disorders, such as boils, infections and intense itching, especially around the genital areas.

Some diabetics, especially those with the milder maturity-onset form, may experience none of these symptoms, or the symptoms may be so vague - just a "run down" feeling - that they go unrecognized.

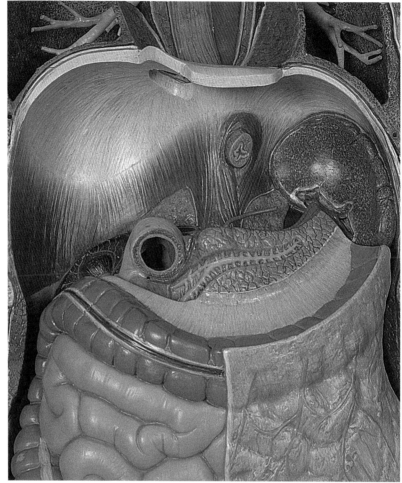

The pancreas is a large, lobulated gland located in the upper part of the abdomen. It has both exocrine and endocrine functions, secreting externally through a duct and internally into the blood or lymph, respectively. The pancreatic islands of Langerhans, constituting about 2 per cent of the glandular tissue, are scattered throughout the pancreas. The islets produce two polypeptide hormones, insulin and glucagon.
The overall effect of insulin on intermediary metabolism is:
• to increase the utilization and decrease the production of glucose;
• to increase the storage and decrease the mobilization and oxidation of fatty acids;
• to increase the formation of protein (increasing cellular uptake of amino acids and the synthesis of proteins from amino acids).

Sometimes the only way that this so-called "hidden" type of diabetes is detected is when the sufferer goes to the doctor for a completely different reason - say, for an examination for life assurance.

Even when there are no symptoms, a doctor can detect the possibility of diabetes by testing small samples of the urine and blood for sugar. In such cases, a more complicated diagnostic procedure, the glucose tolerance test, is administered. In this, the level of glucose in the blood is measured before and at timed intervals after drinking a prepared glucose drink.

Treatment

Since no two cases of diabetes are exactly alike, treatment must be prescribed on an individual basis. The doctor and patient are mainly con-

D

Diabetes   Questions & Answers

What is the difference between type 1 and type 2 diabetes?

People with type 1 diabetes produce little or no insulin at all. In type 2I diabetes, the pancreas continues to manufacture insulin, sometimes even at higher than normal levels. However, the body develops resistance to its effects, resulting in a relative insulin deficiency

Can anyone suffer a so-called hypo-attack?

Hypo stands for hypoglycemia: too little sugar in the blood. This condition may result when the balance of insulin, diet and exercise is disrupted, for instance by not eating enough, engaging in too much strenuous exercise or by taking too much insulin.

Hypoglycemia is the most common complication of insulin therapy and occurs when the diabetic fails to eat, engages in too much exercise, or is prescribed more insulin than is needed.

What are the major symptoms of a hypo-attack and what can be done about it?

important symptoms of a hypo-attack are the following

- tremor
- hunger
- irritability
- headache
- ocalized numbness
- nausea
- blurred vision
- loss of consciousness

Prompt relief can usually be attained by taking a couple of teaspoons of sugar in water and then, when the diabetic is more alert, a biscuit or some other sugary food. In all cases, symptoms should be reported to a doctor, and nothing should be given to someone who has become unconscious - emergency treatment is then needed.

How can hyperglycemia (too much sugar in the blood) occur?

This condition can occur when a diabetic fails to take sufficient insulin or follow a meal plan, and other contributory causes can be infection and illness.

In this condition, which is the opposite of a hypo-attack, fat is burned to supply energy and this produces an increasingly acid condition of the blood and other body fluids (acidosis) due to the accumulation of s-called ketone substances, including acetone.

What are the major symptoms of too much sugar in the blood (hyperglycemia)?

The major symptoms of hyperglycemia are the following:

- drowsiness
- headache
- blurred vision
- apid breathing

Acetone and high blood sugar levels can be detected in the routine urine tests and should be immediately reported to a doctor, for if it progresses, it too can lead to loss of consciousness and coma.

As diabetics are more susceptible to infections than other individuals, even minor wounds should receive careful attention. Serious infections should be promptly reported to the doctor, and they are frequently a precipitating factor in acidosis and diabetic coma.

cerned with diet, exercise and insulin when needed.

Some form of exercise and dietary regulation are necessary in every case of diabetes. In juvenile diabetes, insulin must be taken regularly to replenish the subject's own supply.

■ Diet

Years ago, diabetics' diets were rigid and unappealing, but today they may be varied and are much more satisfying. For the most part, diabetics can eat the same foods as the rest of the family (lean meat, fish, eggs, bread, cereal products, vegetables, fruits within reason), cutting down only on sugar, and sugar-rich foods such as cakes, soft drinks and other sweets, and fats found in fatty meats, most cheeses, butter, margarine, nuts, etc.

Only, recently have diabetics been urged to eat more foods containing dietary fiber - also a type of carbohydrate but one that is not involved in sugar metabolism. Thus, eating plenty of wholemeal bread and pasta, jacket potatoes, brown rice, bran cereals, etc., as long as this is evenly distributed throughout the day, can be an advantage.

Doctors, however, must decide on the appropriate diets to meet their patients' special needs. Diets are sometimes written in precise terms - 30 g (1 oz) meat, a slice of bread, 230 mL (8 fl. oz) milk - but with the help of "exchange lists," menus can be endlessly varied. For the overweight patient, some form of weight-reducing diet is essential, for it will greatly improve the abnormality of sugar metabolism.

■ Physical activity

Exercise in the form of work and play is also important if a person has diabetes. A normal amount of regular exercise increases the ability of the body to use food. Here again, doctors must decide what is best for each patient, balancing diet and medication with the level of activity.

Some of our star athletes have insulin-dependent diabetes. With proper care, young diabetics can engage in sports and other vigorous activities and should be encouraged to do so, for this is important to their emotional as well as physical development.

D

■ Insulin

Insulin, a hormone that is prepared from pancreas extracts from cattle and pigs, must be taken by injection as the digestive juices in the stomach would destroy it if it were taken by mouth. In recent years, new and improved forms of insulin have been developed that are of a higher purity than the earlier ones.

Substances that caused allergies in some diabetics have been removed and the incidence of hypersensitive reactions, such as skin rashes and pitting of the skin, has been diminished. In addition, measurement of prescribed doses is now simpler, reducing the changes of error.

All diabetics (type 1 and type 2) must take insulin in order to use blood sugar in a comparatively normal manner. In order to gain their freedom and independence, type I diabetics must, as soon as possible, assume full responsibility for their own care.

For the rest of their lives they will have to take insulin injections daily, give themselves the jabs at precise times in precise doses, and balance the dosage with their food intake and physical activity.

Three times a week to several times a day, as an indirect check on their blood sugar level, they will have to perform urine and blood tests. The responsible performance of these activities will permit juvenile diabetics to participate in a productive life. Infants, young children and the disabled who cannot perform these tasks need the assistance of individuals who are trained in the procedure.

■ Taking tablets

Since 1970, chemical compounds, taken by mouth, have been available for the treatment of maturity-onset diabetes. While these drugs have been widely used, a recent ten-year study of their effects in controlling diabetes, conducted at 12 leading medical centers, has raised some doubt as to their value in controlling the disease and its complications and, in fact, doubts about their safety.

New developments in oral antidiabetics have superseded most of the disadvantages and side effects of the medicines developed in the 1970s and 1980s.

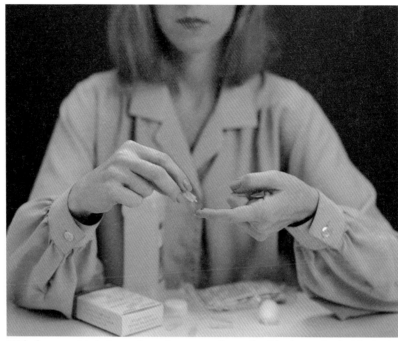

With the present techniques, the patient can easily monitor blood sugar levels. Monitoring blood sugar levels is an essential part of diabetic care. People with diabetes must adjust their diet, exercise and drugs to control blood sugar levels.

Blood sugar levels can be measured easily at home or anywhere. Most sugar monitoring devices use a drop of blood obtained by pricking the tip of the finger with a small lancet. The lancet holds a tiny needle that can be jabbed into the finger or placed in a syringe-loaded device that easily and quickly pierces the skin.

Then, a drop of blood is placed on a reagent strip. In response to sugar, the reagent strip undergoes some chemical changes. The amount of sugar in the blood is then indicated by specific color changes of the strip.

"Hypo" attacks and high blood sugar reactions

"Hypo" attacks are due to hypoglycemia (too little sugar in the blood) and may result when the diet-exercise-insulin balance is disrupted - by not eating enough, engaging in too much strenuous exercise or by taking too much insulin.

Symptoms include:
- tremor
- hunger
- sweating
- headache
- nausea
- blurred vision and
- eventually, if not promptly treated, loss of consciousness (diabetic coma).

Prompt relief can usually be attained by taking a couple of teaspoons of sugar in water and then, when the diabetic is more alert, a biscuit or some other sugary food.

In all cases, symptoms should be reported to a doctor, and nothing should be given to someone who has become unconscious - emergency treatment is then needed.

■ Hyperglycemia

Hyperglycemia (too much sugar in the blood) can occur when a diabetic fails to take sufficient insulin or follow a meal plan, and other contributory causes can be infection and illness. In this condition, which is the opposite of a "hypo" attack, fat is burned to supply energy and this produces an increasingly acid condition of the blood and other body fluids (acidosis) due to the accumulation of so-called ketone substances, including acetone. Usual symptoms are:

Diabetes - What you can do

D

Left untreated, type 2 diabetes can damage the heart, kidneys, nervous system and eyes. You can minimise your risk by taking a few simple steps to keep your blood sugar within bounds.

Diet and exercise

Start by planning your meals and increasing your physical activity; 30 minutes daily is the goal. You can help stabilise blood-sugar levels by eating several small meals (breakfast, lunch and dinner plus two snacks) each day at the same time, and choosing high-fiber and low-fat-foods, such as raw fruits and vegetables, beans and unrefined whole grains.

Drugs

If changing your diet and getting more active are not enough to keep glucose un der control, there are several medications that can help:

■ *Sulphonylureas*

These drugs activate the pancreas to release more insulin. For instance:
- Amaryl
- Daonil
- Diabenese
- Diamicron
- Euglucon
- Glibenclamide
- Minidiab
- Rastinon

■ *Meglitinides*

Like sulphonylureas, these trigger the pancreas to chum out insulin.

■ *Buguanides*

This class of drugs signals the liver to produce less glucose and sensitizes muscle tissue to absorb more glucose from the blood. For instance:
- Diabex
- Diaformin
- Glucophage
- Metformin

■ *Thiazolidinediones*

The most recent additions to the diabetic medicine chest, these pills improve insulin's ability to push glucose into muscle and fat tissue. For instance:
- Avandia
- Rezulin
- Rosiglitazone
- Troflitazone

■ *Alpha-glucosidases*

Acting in the intestine, these drugs block conversion of starches in bread and pastas into glucose.

Insulin

Depending on how long blood-sugar levels remain high, and other health factors, some type 2 diabetics may need insulin. While there are different types of insulin that can be delivered in various ways, for type 2 diabetics, injections (either with a needle and a syringe or an insulin pen, which contains a needle and a cartridge of variable doses of insulin) are the most convenient. Many benefit from a combination of oral drugs and insulin to control glucose levels.

Tests

Once you have been diagnosed with diabetes, it is important to keep track of your blood-glucose levels. This can be done in several ways:

■ *HBA1C*

Also known as the glycated hemoglobin test, HBA1C is a blood test that provides a record of glucose levels over two to three months. Glucose in the blood attaches to hemoglobin, a protein in red blood cells that ferries oxygen, forming glycated hemoglobin. Because the red blood cells circulate in the body for several months, levels of glycated hemoglobin are a good marker for average blood-glucose levels over time.

■ *Urine*

When the body cannot make enough insulin, and blood-sugar levels get too high, it begins to break down fat, forming ketones. These compounds spill out into the urine, signalling too little insulin at work.

■ *Finger prick*

The most common way to keep track of blood-sugar levels - pricking the finger for blood before meals and bed - has become more convenient and less painful than it used to be. Automatic lances make the drawing of blood easier, and computerized devices can record readings automatically.

■ *Glucowatch*

Only one device approved by the European Union provides glucose measurements without puncturing the skin. Worn on the wrist, it uses tiny electric current to gently draw body fluid from the skin up to six times an hour for as long as 13 hours.

- nausea
- drowsiness
- extreme thirst
- headache
- blurred vision
- abdominal pains
- rapid breathing

Acetone and high blood sugar levels can be detected in the routine urine tests and should be immediately reported to a doctor, for if it progresses, it too can lead to loss of consciousness and coma.

As diabetics are more susceptible to infections than other individuals, even minor wounds should receive careful attention. Serious infections should be promptly reported to the doctor, as they are frequently a precipitating factor in acidosis and diabetic coma.

Complications

Diabetes is a complex, multi-faceted disorder that affects the entire body and involves more than an impaired production or activity of insulin. Despite satisfactory control of blood sugar levels through diet and the administration of insulin, in many cases the long-term complications of diabetes develop, primarily those affecting blood vessels, nerves, the kidneys and the eyes.

While both type 1 and type 2 diabetics are susceptible to these complications, in general it is the juvenile diabetics who are more severely affected. Although present-day methods of treatment have improved, complications usually occur at some time in the course of the disease. While treatment of the these has improved in recent years,

More than one-third of all individuals with diabetes do not know that they have the disease until one of its life-threatening complications occurs. Potential complications include:

▲ *Blindness*
Diabetes is the leading cause of blindness in people aged 20 to 70.
▲ *Kidney disease*
Ten per cent to twenty per cent of all people with diabetes develop kidney disease.
▲ *Amputations*
Diabetes is the most frequent

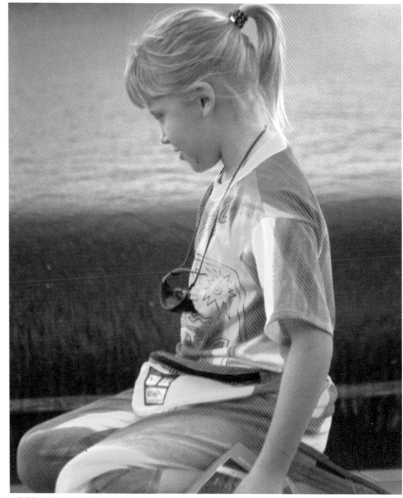

Child with type 1 diabetes. The pancreas produces little or no insulin. Most people who have type 1 diabetes develop the disease before age 30. Scientists believe that an environmental factor - possibly a viral infection or a nutritional factor in childhood or early adulthood - causes the immune system to destroy the insulin-producing cells of the pancreas. A genetic predisposition may make some people more susceptible to the environmental factor.

cause of non-traumatic lower limb amputations. The risk of a leg amputation is 15 to 40 times greater for a person with diabetes than for the population.
▲ *Heart disease and stroke*
People with diabetes are 2 to 4 times more likely to have heart disease, and they are 2 to 4 times more likely to suffer a stroke.

Treatment through diet

Whether you are overweight or not, the cornerstone of treatment will be a diet. In many cases, diabetes can be controlled by diet alone. If you are "diet controlled," that does not mean that you are cured. Rather, it means you are fortunate to be able to control your disease simply by watching what you eat.

To most people, the word "diet" means a restriction only in the number of calories consumed; the kind of diet that is designed for weight loss.

A "diet" can also mean a daily plan in which the kinds and amounts of foods chosen and the timing of the meals are important. Both types of diets can play a part in treating diabetes.

D

Diabetes emergencies

High blood sugar reaction

Signs and symptoms
- Skin: red and dry
- Temperature: lowered
- Breath: sickly sweet odour or acetone

First aid treatment
- Treat as you would for shock
- Place in semi-inclining position
- In case of vomiting turn head to one side
- Do not give anything, e.g. sugar or alcoholic beverages, unless you are not sure that it is a high blood sugar reaction; in that case, give sugar.

Hypo attack

Signs and symptoms
- Skin: pale, clammy and covered with cold sweat
- Breathing: normal or shallow
- Breath: no odour of acetone

First aid treatment
- If the victim is conscious, give him/her sugar (sugar, bar of chocolate or sweet drink)
- If unconscious, call emergency services

Because it is often difficult to determine the difference between the two types diabetic emergencies, sugar should be given to any semi-conscious diabetic even though he or she may be suffering from a high blood sugar reaction.

The reason for this is that a "hypo" attack (too little sugar) that goes on to diabetic coma can quickly cause brain damage or death, while a high blood sugar reaction takes relatively longer to cause damage, and the amount of sugar given will make little difference to the outcome.

For some type 2 diabetics, avoiding simple sugars may be all that is required. Many others will need to restrict calories as well. For those whose diabetes is harder to control, special attention has to be paid to the distribution of food throughout the day.

General principles
There is no specific "diabetic diet." Rather, the best diet for controlling diabetes depends a great deal on the individual. For those who are overweight - the large majority of all type II diabetics - the first emphasis will be on weight loss. Often, weight loss may be the only treatment needed. Many diabetics will also need to follow a set of principles or guidelines for planning a wide variety of well-balanced and nutritious meals. The aim of this kind of diet is to help your body make better use of carbohydrates. This is done with ordinary foods, with an emphasis on choosing the right amounts from all the major food categories. In fact, a good diet for diabetics is an excellent one for everybody. Besides making good use of carbohydrates, the diet should be low in fats, especially saturated fats, and should eliminate random eating. The diabetic diet is a good base for a weight loss diet, since it is made up of well-balanced everyday foods. What particular diet plan is right for you will depend on a number of things. Especially important factors are how high your blood sugar is, whether you need to lose weight (and how much), how much insulin of your own is available, and what other kinds of treatments you require. Your age, normal activities, and overall health will be taken into account.

Most likely, your diet will include many of your favourite foods and will be planned to fit in with your eating and lifestyle preferences. It has been estimated that if all type II diabetics followed the right meal plan, only a small percentage would need additional kinds of treatment. Studies have shown that the number of insulin receptor sites increases with the right diet. This increase makes the body's insulin supply work better.

Planning a diet
Your doctor will probably discuss with you and give you some guidelines. If you need to lose just a few pounds or make simple changes, you may be able to carry on by yourself. However, if you need to cut way down on your calories or make a big change from your former eating habits, you may need help from a dietitian or diet counsellor. Your doctor may advise you or refer you to one.
Diet counselling can be especially helpful for diabetes because:
- The wrong diet could be harmful
- What to eat and what to avoid should fit your individual needs
- You need to change your eating habits
- With proper planning, a diet can still be pleasurable
- You can be advised to set realistic goals
- You can learn why fad diets, crash diets, and some reducing aids seldom work
- You must understand how your diet interacts with the rest of your treatment program
- You must balance your meals and snacks with your usual physical activities and with en exercise program, if one is recommended.

Spacing meals
Among the things that is important is the timing of your meals. If your diabetes is controllable by diet alone, the

guidelines will be relatively simple. You should spread your meals fairly evenly throughout the day, including snacks if recommended.

Spacing your meals like this will help keep your blood sugar more stable. And you should eat about the same amount each day. On days when you are more active than usual, you may need extra food.

Your doctor or diet counsellor will help you plan for this. In general, if your diabetes is controlled by diet alone, you do not need to worry if you occasionally skip a meal or eat later than usual. However, try not to let that become a habit, and do not overeat at the next meal because you skipped one.

If you are injecting insulin or taking medicine for your diabetes, you may need to pay much closer attention to when and what you eat because you risk developing low blood sugar if meals are missed.

Excess weight

Most adults gain weight over the years unless they consciously try not to. And it is easy to see how this happens. On the average, the body needs 10 fewer calories a day for each year of age over 25.

One hundred extra calories a day (about 10 potato chips) adds up to about 10 pounds a year. Unfortunately, it also gets harder to lose weight as you get older.

For some people with type 2 diabetes, excess weight and the disease may be connected in a way that makes weight loss even more difficult. Excess weight increases the body's demand for insulin, and insulin actually stimulates the appetite.

Insulin also promotes the storage of excess food as fat.

By breaking this vicious cycle - that is, by losing weight - your insulin needs drop, your own available insulin works better, and your appetite is not overstimulated.

If your diet is based on a daily allowance of calories, your doctor or dietitian will figure out how many you should have each day.

The number will depend on your ideal weight (not your current weight) and your normal work and daily activities.

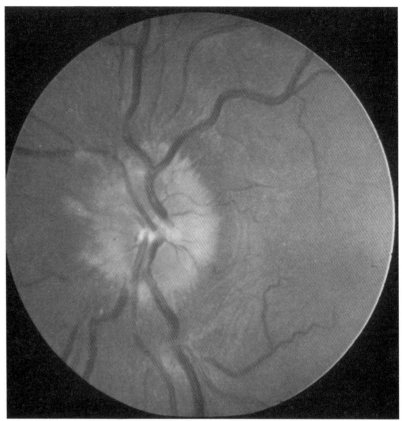

Damage to the small blood vessels in the retina of a diabetic patient. The result is decreased vision and, ultimately, blindness.

Foot care

Poor circulation means that the blood vessels in your feet and legs may be obstructed, therefore not allowing enough blood to flow through them. Perhaps you have bad veins, which can cause blood to pool in your feet and legs, making them feel cold or look blue.

This can lead to aching and cramping, and your legs may become easily injured. In addition, if you have diabetes-related neuropathy you will not feel pain or sense heat, and are more prone to injury.

Infections and complications are more likely to occur in legs and feet that are injured, which means that you need to take special precautions. Always keep your legs and feet warm, clean, and protected from any possible injuries.

One of the best ways to prevent injury to your feet is to wear the right type of shoes and socks. Going barefoot, even while in the house, may cause injury.

Good foot care also means that you should wash yout feet every day with warm water and mild soap. Try to avoid hot water.

Dry your feet thoroughly, especially between the toes. As you dry them, inspect them carefully to see if there is redness or dryness, or if there are any cracks on the feet or between the toes.

Never wear socks that have holes at the toe or heel area.

Do not use commercially prepared foot soaks, which may irritate the skin. Instead, medicated powder can reduce the possibility of developing fungus, and can help make your feet feel more comfortable.

See your physician promptly if your feet or toes are injured in any way. He or she may be able to give you more tips on proper foot care.

DIARRHEA

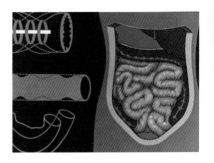

Description

Diarrhea is the abnormally frequent passage of watery stools. The frequency of bowel movements varies with the individual. Some healthy adults may have as many as three stools per day, others may defecate once in 2 or more days.

The mean daily faecal weight is 100-150 g. In Diarrhea there can be an increase of from 150-300 g. The major factor contributing to Diarrhea is exertion of excess water that normally is reabsorbed from the intestine. Disruption in the water absorption process resulting in accumulation in the intestine of even a few hundred millilitres of water may cause Diarrhea.

Diarrhea usually is viewed and treated as a symptom of undiagnosed and presumed minor and transient gastrointestinal disorder. More than 50 conditions, including major diseases involving the kidneys, heart, liver, thyroid, and lungs, are associated with Diarrhea. Often, Diarrhea is only one of many symptoms associated with a major illness.

Acute Diarrhea is characterized by a sudden onset of frequent, liquid stools accompanied by the following symptoms:

▲ weakness;
▲ flatulence;
▲ pain;
▲ often fever and vomiting.

Chronic Diarrhea is the persistent or recurrent passage of unformed stools and usually is the result of multiple factors.

The variability in the origins of Diarrhea make identification of the pathophysiologic mechanism difficult and may make a complete physical examination necessary, including supportive clinical laboratory tests.

Acute Diarrhea

Acute Diarrhea may be infectious, toxic, medicine-induced, or dietary in origin. It may also be the result of acute or chronic illness. Infectious Diarrhea in adults is usually bacterial while viral Diarrhea is more commonly seen in children.

Two general mechanisms may be involved in the development of Diarrhea: decreased absorption and increased secretion. The alimentary canal maintains a balance between absorption and secretion of gastrointestinal fluids.

Infectious Diarrhea

Although the causative agent is not readily identified in most cases of acute Diarrhea, the bacterial pathogens most commonly responsible for Diarrhea in our country are:

- Escherichia coli;
- Shigella;
- Salmonella;
- Campylobacter (Helicobacter pylori);
- Staphylococcus.

Patients with Diarrhea caused by toxin-producing agents (for instance, Escherichia coli, Staphylococcus aureus) clinically present with a "cholera-like" syndrome, which primarily involves the small bowel. The patient experiences an abrupt onset of large volumes of watery stools, variable nausea, vomiting, and cramps, possibly with a low-grade fever. Invasive organisms (for instance, Shigella, Salmonella) produce a "dysentery-like" syndrome if the large bowel is the site of attack. This type of diarrhea is characterized by:

- fever;
- abdominal crampy pain;
- tenesmus (straining);
- frequent small-volume stools that may contain blood and pus.

When the patient is first seen by the doctor, a careful medical history is essential for him to identifying a cause. For example, staphylococci grow rapidly in food (ham and milk) producing a toxin. Upon ingestion, the toxin quickly (within 1-2 hours) provokes the Diarrhea attack. In contrast, the incubation period for Salmonella is 12-24 hours.

An infectious, inflammatory disease of the bowel is characterized by:

▲ fever;
▲ malaise;
▲ muscle aching;
▲ profound abdominal discomfort;
▲ severe anorexia.

The treatment of infectious Diarrhea is based upon treating the spread of the pathogenic bacteria, generally with a prescribed antibiotic or other anti-infective agent and fluid support. In many instances the illness is self-limiting, a normal function of the alimentary tract is restored with or without treatment in 24-48 hours.

Infantile diarrhea

Diarrhea in infants and young children is a common paediatric problem, and the cause is difficult to identify, although it is frequent caused by a viral infection of the intestinal tract. Diet and systemic and local infections, such as otitis media, are other known causes or acute diarrheal episodes in children.

Rotaviruses have been implicated as the cause of about 50 per cent of all infantile diarrhea. Clinical features include a 12-48 hour incubation period, vomiting, watery diarrhea, and a low-grade fever. The illness usually is self-limiting, lasting 5-8 days. Generally, it requires only symptomatic therapy.

Evidence has demonstrated that breast feeding is effective in preventing viral diarrhea. In children, particularly infants, acute diarrhea may cause severe, and possibly dangerous, dehydration and electrolyte imbalance.

In the newborn, water may comprise 75 per cent of the total body weight; water loss in severe diarrhea may be 10 per cent or more of body weight. After 8-10 bowel movements in 24 hours, a 2-month-old infant could lose enough fluid to cause circulatory collapse and kidney failure. For this reason, moderate to severe diarrhea in infants should receive an immediate doctor's evaluation.

Traveller's diarrhea (turista)

The acute diarrhea that frequently develops among tourists visiting foreign countries. With warm climates and relatively poor sanitation usually cannot be traced to known pathogens. Usually Escherichia coli is the most common cause of traveller's diarrhea in tropical and subtropical countries. It probably results from an extensive alteration in the bacterial flora of the gut caused by exposure, through food and drill to a markedly different microbial population. Traveller's diarrhea is characterized by the following symptoms:
- sudden onset of loose stools
- nausea
- occasional vomiting
- abdominal cramping

Children seem particularly susceptible, and most cases develop during the first week of exposure to the new location.

Medicine-induced diarrhea

Diarrhea is frequently a side effect of medicine administration. All antibiotics can produce adverse gastrointestinal symptoms including diarrhea, but severity depends largely on the specific antibiotic.

Antibiotics that have a broad spectrum of activity against aerobic and anaerobic (anaerobe is a microorganism that thrives without oxygen) micro-organisms frequently

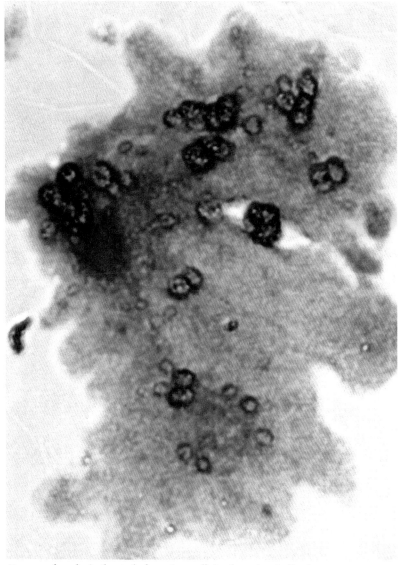

Presence of ameba in the stool of a patient suffering from chronic diarrhea.

cause diarrhea. The processes may account for antibiotic induced diarrhea:
- Diarrhea associated with the first few doses is attributed to mild irritant properties of the drug itself.
- Diarrhea beginning within a few days of the initial antibiotic therapy is due most likely to a disruption in the normal intestinal flora.

In general, orally administered antibiotics are not completely absorbed. The unabsorbed fraction of the dose may be irritating to the intestinal mucosa, cause alterations in intestinal motility, and induce diarrhea. Even the soluble antibiotics may cause irritation if they form strong acidic solutions, such as tetracycline hydrochloride. Some antibiotics affect intestinal absorption of nutrients, even at usual dosage levels.

The following antibiotics are reported to cause colitis, a severe and persistent diarrhea:
- Chloramphenicol
- Neomycin
- Cephalosporins
- Tetracycline

Diarrhea   Questions & Answers

What is diarrhea?

Diarrhea is the abnormally frequent passage of watery stools. The frequency of bowel movements varies with the individual. Some healthy adults may have as many as three stools per day, others may defecate once in 2 or more days. The mean daily faecal weight is 100-150 g. In diarrhea there can be an increase of from 150-300 g.

What is the major factor contributing to diarrhea?

The major factor contributing to diarrhea is exertion of excess water that normally is reabsorbed from the intestine. Disruption in the water absorption process resulting in accumulation in the intestine of even a few hundred millilitres of water may cause diarrhea.

Diarrhea usually is viewed and treated as a symptom of undiagnosed and presumed minor and transient gastrointestinal disorder. More than 50 conditions, including major diseases involving the kidneys, heart, liver, thyroid, and lungs, are associated with diarrhea. Often, diarrhea is only one of many symptoms associated with a major illness.

What are the major characteristics of acute diarrhea?

Acute diarrhea is characterized by a sudden onset of frequent, liquid stools accompanied by the following symptoms:
- weakness;
- latulence;
- pain;
- often fever and vomiting.

What is chronic diarrhea?

Chronic diarrhea is the persistent or recurrent passage of unformed stools and usually is the result of multiple factors. The variability in the origins of diarrhea make identification of the pathophysiologic mechanism difficult and may make a complete physical examination necessary, including supportive clinical laboratory tests.

What are the major causes of acute diarrhea?

Acute diarrhea may be infectious, toxic, medicine-induced, or dietary in origin. It may also be the result of acute or chronic illness. Infectious diarrhea in adults is usually bacterial while viral diarrhea is more commonly seen in children. Two general mechanisms may be involved in the development of diarrhea: decreased absorption and increased secretion. The alimentary canal maintains a balance between absorption and secretion of gastrointestinal fluids.

What are the causes of a dysentery-like syndrome?

Invasive organisms (for instance, Shigella, Salmonella) produce a 'dysentery-like' syndrome if the large bowel is the site of attack. This type is characterized by:
- fever;
- abdominal crampy pain;
- tenesmus (straining);
- frequent small-volume stools that may contain blood and pus.

How is infectious diarrhea treated?

The treatment of infectious diarrhea is based upon treating the spread of the pathogenic bacteria, generally with a prescribed antibiotic or other anti-infective agent and fluid support.

- Sulfonamides
- Ampicillin
- Lincomycin
- Clindamycin
- Metronidazole

Other medicines, such as cathartics, which are irritating to the intestinal mucosa, may precipitate diarrhea, as may drugs that cause the retention of salts and water in the intestinal lumen.

Certain antacid preparations contain magnesium to prevent the constipating effects of aluminum and calcium. Depending on the dose taken and the individual, these types of antacid preparations may induce diarrhea. Medicines that alter autonomic control of intestinal motility also may cause diarrhea.

Food-induced diarrhea

Food tolerance, caused by allergy, or the ingestion of foods that are excessively fatty, spicy, or contain a high degree of roughage or a large number of seeds, can also provoke diarrhea. If diarrhea occurs in more than one person within 24 hours of ingestion of the same food, it is likely that a preformed toxin (food poison) has been ingested.

Food tolerance and diarrhea may be associated with disaccharidase deficiency (lactase deficiency). Carbohydrates in the diet commonly include lactose and sucrose, which are hydrolysed to monosaccharides. These enzymatic activities are reduced in intestinal disorders such as infectious diarrhea, congenital disaccharide deficiency, and gastrointestinal allergy.

Chronic diarrhea

Chronic diarrhea is usually the result of multiple factors and therefore can be difficult to diagnose. The condition may be defined as los of watery stools lasting more than 2 weeks.

It may be caused by a disease of the bowel or may be a secondary manifestation of a systemic disease. Determining chronic diarrhea can be very difficult because it does not always involve frequent daily passage of watery stools.

Three categories of chronic diarrhea can be described:

- ▲ frequent, small, formed stools with tenesmus (straining);
- ▲ large, oily, malodorous, formed stools;
- ▲ frequent, voluminous, loosely formed stools.

The patient may complain of weight loss, fever, anxiety/depression, nausea, vomiting, abdominal tenderness. Psychogenic factors are frequent causes of chronic diarrhea. Psychogenic diarrhea is usually characterized by small, frequent stools and abdominal pain.

The stools may be watery and may follow a normal bowel movement or may appear shortly after eating. Psychogenic diarrhea is related to emotional stress that may periodically increase the parasympathetic nervous system impulses to the gastrointestinal tract.

The diarrhea may alternate with constipation. Patients complaining of chronic diarrhea that appears to be psychogenically related should consult a physician.

In chronic diarrhea, the most significant finding is usually a medical history of previous bouts of diarrhea and complaints of anorexia, weight loss, and chronic weakness. These patients generally have histories of poor health. The following symptoms needs the consultation of a doctor:

- bloody stools
- abdominal tenderness
- high fever
- dehydration
- weight loss of greater than 5 per cent of body weight;
- diarrhea that has lasted 5-7 days.

Stool character gives valuable information about diarrhea. For example, undigested food particles in the stool indicate small bowel irritation; black, tarry stools can indicate upper gastrointestinal bleeding (for instance, from the stomach), and red stools suggest possible lower bowel bleeding, or simply the recent ingestion of red-coloured food such as beets or drug products.

Diarrhea from the small bowel probably is manifested as a marked outpouring of fluid high in potassium and bicarbonate. A paste-like or semi-

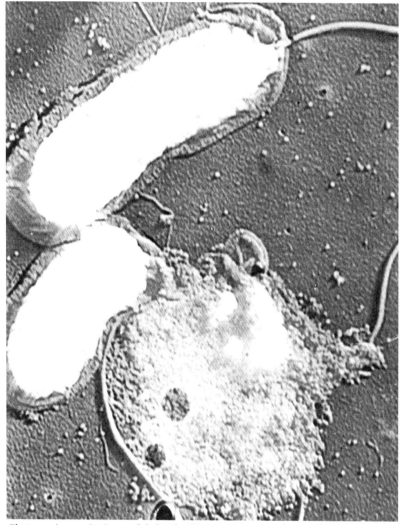

Electron microscopic picture of cholera bacilli, causative agents of severe diarrhea.

solid loose stool is indicative of colon-type diarrhea.

Treatment

Diarrhea is a symptom, and symptomatic relief must not be interpreted as being a cure for the underlying cause. Symptomatic relief generally suffices in simple functional diarrhea that is only temporary and relatively uncomplicated. Quite a few non-prescription products are available; however, the pharmacist will exercise caution in recommending their use in self-medication. Certain diseases that cause diarrhea might be serious or treated

more effectively with agents specific for the underlying cause.

Many remedies have been tried for curing traveller's diarrhea. Antibiotics have not been effective in the treatment of this form of diarrhea; however, doxycycline has been effective in the prevention of diarrhea.

It has been suggested that travellers to areas where hygiene and sanitation are poor may prevent diarrhea by eating only recently peeled and thoroughly cooked foods and by drinking only boiled or bottled water, bottled carbonated soft drinks, beer, or wine. Tap water used for brushing teeth or for ice in drinks may be a source of infection.

DISABILITY

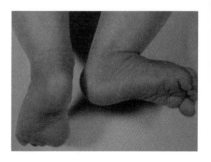

Description

A disability is any restriction or lack (resulting from an impairment) of ability to perform an activity within the range considered normal for a human being. Disability is characterized by excesses or deficiencies in the customarily expected performance of activities and in behavior, and these may be temporary or permanent, reversible or irreversible, and progressive or regressive. Disabilities may arise as a direct consequence of impairment or as a response by the individual, particularly psychologically, to a physical, sensory or other impairment, and as such it reflects disturbances at the level of the person. Disability is concerned with abilities, in the form of composite activities and behaviors, that are generally accepted as essential components of everyday life.

Examples include disturbances in behaving in an appropriate manner, in personal care (such as control of the bowels and the ability to wash and feed oneself), in the performance of other activities of daily living, and in locomotor activities (such as the ability to walk).

Behavior disabilities

Awareness disabilities

A behavior disability refers to a lack of awareness and the inability of individuals to conduct themselves "normally," both in everyday activities and towards others, and includes a decreased ability to learn. Self-awareness disability includes the disturbance in the ability of an individual to develop or maintain a mental representation of the identity of his or her own self or body ("body image") and

its continuity over time.

It also concerns the disturbance of behavior produced by confusion with consciousness or a sense of identity, resulting in inappropriate interpretation of and response to external events, which expresses itself in agitation, restlessness and noisiness.

A disability in body-image orientation includes a disturbance in the mental representation of the individual's body, such as an inability in differentiating right from left, phantom-limb experiences and other related phenomena.

Disturbance of appearance includes careless dress or make-up and an appearance that is considered bizarre (such as special clothes or ornaments with idiosyncratic meanings, which may be related to delusions), of very inappropriate taste or conspicuously out of fashion. Other disturbance of self-presentation refers to that of the ability to present a favorable image in social situations, such as by inattention to such social routines as greetings, partings, thanking, apologizing, excusing and reciprocation of these, and lack of presence (e.g. total absence of originality or excessive conformity in demeanour). Disabilities relating to location in time and space result from the inability of individuals to correctly locate external objects, events and themselves in relation to the dimensions of time and space.

A special kind of behavior disability is "conduct out of context." It refers to conduct that is generally appropriate but which is inappropriate to the place, the time or the person's age.

In this category are "cultural shock" (such as that found among immigrants), living under different identities (e.g. transvestites, and blacks "passing" for white), pseudo- feeble-mindedness and breaking taboos.

A personal-safety disability is a disturbance in the ability to avoid hazards to the integrity of the individual's body, such as being in danger of self-injury or because of an inability to safeguard the self from danger. Situational behavior has to do with the capacity to register and understand relationships between objects and persons in situations of daily living.

Disabilities in the course of life

A number of various disabilities may develop in the course of life:

- ▲ *Situation comprehension disability*: disturbance of the capacity to perceive, register or understand relationships between things and people.
- ▲ *Situation interpretation disability*: false interpretation of the relationships between and meaning of things and people.
- ▲ *Situation coping disability*: disturbance of the ability to perform everyday activities in specific situations, such as outside the home or in the presence of particular animals or other things.
- ▲ *Disabilities in relationships.*

Family-role disabilities

Among the family-role disabilities, four special types can be distinguished:

- ▲ *Disability in participation in household activities.* This includes customary common activities - having meals together, doing domestic chores, going out or visiting together, playing games and watching television, etc. - and conduct during these activities, as well as household decision-making, e.g. decisions about children and money.
- ▲ *Disability in the emotional role of marriage.* This involves the emo-

tional relationship with a steady partner or spouse, as well as communication (such as talking about children, news and ordinary events), ability to show affection and warmth (but excluding acceptable customary outbursts of anger or irritability), and engendering a feeling in the partner of being a source of support.
▲ *Sexual marital role disability*. This includes disturbance in sexual relations with a steady partner, including the frequency of sexual intercourse and whether both partners find sexual relations satisfactory.
▲ *Parental role disability*. This involves the undertaking and performance of child care tasks appropriate to the individual's position in the household (such as, for small children, feeding, putting to bed or taking to school, and, for older children, looking after their needs) and taking an interest in the child(ren) (such as playing with and reading to them and taking an interest in their problems or schoolwork).

■ *Disabilities in occupational roles*
Occupational-role disability refers to disturbance of the ability to organize and participate in routine activities connected with the occupation of time, and is not just confined to the performance of work. In this field, various disabilities may occur:
▲ *Motivation*: interference with the ability to work because of a severe impairment of drive.
▲ *Cooperation*: inability to cooperate with others and in the give-and-take of social interaction.
▲ *Work routine*: problems in other aspects of conformity to work routine, such as going to work regularly and on time, and observing rules.
▲ *Organizing daily routine*: disturbance in the ability to give enough time to certain activities and difficulty in making decisions about day-to-day matters.
▲ *Work performance*: other inadequacies in performance and output.
▲ *Recreation*: lack of interest in leisure activities such as watching television, listening to the radio,

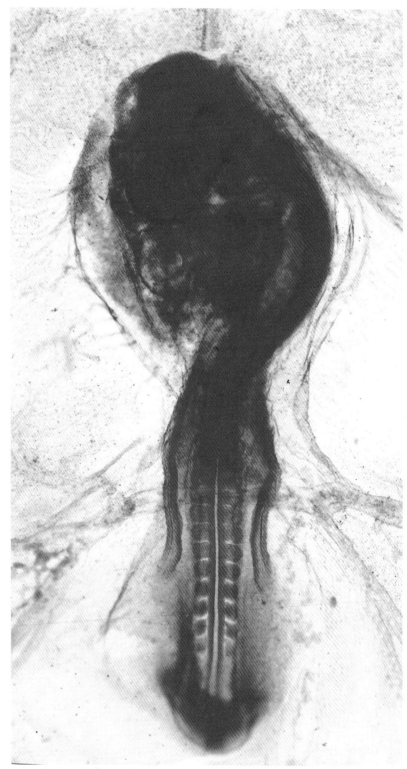

Microphotograph of an early embryo (about four weeks old) to show the development of the spinal cord. At this stage the embryo is very susceptible for environmental factors that can damage the spinal cord. Such a damage may cause locomotor disabilities.

Categories of disability

1. Behavior disabilities

◼ Awareness disability
- Self-awareness disability
- Disability relating to location in time and space
- Other identification disability
- Personal safety disability
- Disability relating to situational behavior
- Knowledge acquisition disability
- Other educational disability

◼ Disabilities in relationships
- Family role disability
- Occupational role disability
- Other behavior disability

2. Communication disabilities

◼ Speaking disabilities
- Disability in understanding speech
- Disability in talking
- Other speaking disability

◼ Listening disabilities
- Disability in listening to speech
- Other listening disability

◼ Seeing disabilities
- Disability in gross visual tasks
- Disability in detailed visual tasks
- Other disability in seeing and related activities

◼ Other communication disabilities
- Disability in writing
- Other communication disability

3. Personal care disabilities

◼ Excretion disabilities
- Controlled excretory difficulty
- Uncontrolled excretory difficulty
- Other excretion disability

◼ Personal hygiene disabilities
- Bathing disability
- Other personal hygiene disability

◼ Dressing disabilities
- Clothing disability
- Other dressing disability

◼ Feeding and other personal care disabilities
- Disability in preliminaries to feeding
- Other feeding disability

4. Locomotor disabilities

◼ Ambulation disabilities
- Walking disability
- Traversing disability
- Climbing disability
- Running disability
- Other ambulation disability

◼ Confining disability
- Transfer disability
- Transport disability

◼ Other locomotor disabilities
- Lifting disability
- Other locomotor disability

5. Body disposition disabilities

◼ Domestic disability
- Subsistence disability
- Household disability

◼ Body movement disabilities
- Retrieval disability
- Reaching disability
- Other disability in arm function
- Kneeling disability
- Crouching disability
- Other body movement disability

◼ Other body disposition disabilities
- Postural disability
- Other body disposition disability

6. Dexterity disabilities

◼ Daily activity disability
- Environmental modulation disability
- Other daily activity disability

◼ Manual activity disabilities
- Fingering disability
- Gripping disability
- Holding disability
- Handedness disability
- Other manual activity disability

◼ Other dexterity disabilities
- Food control disability
- Other body control disability
- Other dexterity disability

7. Situational disabilities

◼ Dependence and endurance disabilities
- Circumstantial dependence
- Disability in endurance

◼ Environmental disabilities
- Disability related to temperature tolerance
- Disability related to tolerance to other climatic features
- Disability relating to tolerance to noise
- Disability relating to tolerance to light
- Disability relating to tolerance to work stresses
- Disability relating to tolerance to other environmental factors

◼ Other situational disabilities

---

reading newspapers or books, participating in games and hobbies and in local and world events.

▲ *Crisis conduct:* unsatisfactory or inappropriate responses to incidents such as sickness, accidents or other incidents affecting family members or involving other people, or emergencies and other experiences customarily requiring quick decisions and action.

◼ *Social-role disabilities*
There may also exist an indifference to accepted social standards - for example, embarrassing conduct such as making sexual suggestions or advances, lacking restraint in scratch-ing genitals, passing "wind" loudly or irreverence (e.g. singing, making facetious silly jokes or flippant remarks). Other social-role disabilities include such unacceptable conduct as picking arguments, arrogance, irrational anger, marked irritability or other friction arising in social situations outside the home, say:

D

Outlook reflects the likely course of the individual's disability status.

0. Not disabled
No disability present.

1. Recovery potential
There is a disability present but diminishing, and recovery without ultimate restriction in functional performance is expected.

2. Improvement potential
There is a disability present but diminishing, though the individual is likely to be left with residual restriction in functional performance.

3. Assistance potential
The disability exists in a stable or static state, but functional performance could be improved by provision of aids, assistance or other support.

4. Stable disability
The disability exists in a stable or static state with no outlook for improvement in functional performance.

5. Amelioration potential
The disability is increasing, but functional performance could be improved by provision of aids, assistance or other support.

6. Deterioration disability
The disability is increasing with no outlook for amelioration.

▲ with supervisors, co-workers or customers, if the individual engages in outside work;
▲ with neighbours and other people in the community, if the individual has a domestic role;
▲ with teachers, administrators and fellow students, if the individual is a student;
▲ with fellow residents, if the individual lives in communal accommodation.

Communication disabilities

This group of disabilities refers to an individual's ability to generate and emit messages and to receive and understand messages - that is, speaking, listening, seeing and other communication disabilities. A disability in understanding speech includes the loss or restriction of the ability to understand the meaning of verbal messages.
If the disability has to do with talking, there is loss or restriction of the ability to produce audible verbal messages and to convey meaning through speech. A disability of vision includes the loss of or reduction in the ability to execute tasks requiring adequate distant or peripheral vision, or adequate visual acuity (that required for reading, recognition of faces, writing and visual manipulation). Sometimes there exists a writing disability, when there is a loss of or reduction in the ability to encode language into written words and to execute written messages or to make marks. Other communication disabilities may occur with symbolic communication, nonverbal expression and nonverbal communication:

▲ *Symbolic communication*: loss or restriction of the ability to understand signs and symbols associated with conventional codes, e.g. traffic lights and signs, and pictograms, and to read maps, simple diagrams and other schematic representations of objects.
▲ *Nonverbal expression*: loss of restriction of the ability to convey information by gesture, expression and related means.
▲ *Nonverbal communication*: loss or restriction of the ability to receive information by gesture, expression and related means.

Personal-care disabilities

This group of disabilities refers to the ability of individuals to look after themselves in regard to basic physiological activities, such as excretion and feeding, and to care for themselves, e.g. hygiene and dressing.
An excretion disability usually is concerned with difficulty in the control of

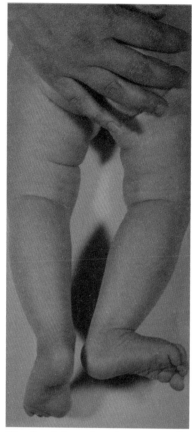

Disorder of the embryonic neuromuscular apparatus resulting in malformation of the skeleton of the legs.

the bowels and of urination. Normal control can sometimes be achieved, or other means can be devised to achieve acceptable behavior, through the use of adaptive devices, electrical stimulators, special protective clothing or by some other means.

Locomotor disabilities

This group of disabilities refers to the ability of individuals to execute distinctive activities associated with moving, both themselves and objects, from place to place, such as walking, traversing, climbing stairs, lying down, sitting and standing and moving between these positions, and reaching for bed or chair. Other disabilities in this area include those involving personal transport and lifting.

DISEASE

D

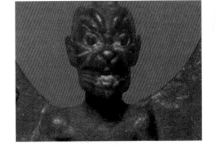

Introduction

A disease is a disturbance of normal body function in an organism. Medicine and surgery are concerned with the recognition or diagnosis of disease and with treatment aimed at its cure. Disease is usually brought to a person's attention by symptoms through which he or she becomes aware of some abnormality of, or change in, body function.

Common examples of symptoms are:
- pain
- headache
- fever
- cough
- shortness of breath
- dyspepsia
- constipation
- diarrhea
- loss of blood
- lumps
- paralysis
- numbness
- loss of consciousness

Diagnosis is made on the basis of such symptoms as well as from signs discovered on physical examination and from laboratory and X-ray or scan investigations; the functional disorder is analyzed and possible causes are examined.

Causes of physical disease are legion, but certain categories are recognized:
- trauma (injury);
- congenital (inborn);
- infectious, inflammatory;
- vascular (to do with the heart and/or blood vessels);
- tumor;
- degenerative;
- deficiency;
- metabolic;
- poison;
- occupational;
- iatrogenic (induced by a doctor).

▲ Trauma to the body may cause skin lacerations and bone fractures as well as disorders specific to the organ involved (for example, contusion).

▲ Congenital diseases include hereditary conditions (i.e., those passed on genetically) and diseases beginning in the fetus, such as those due to drugs or maternal infection during pregnancy.

▲ Infectious diseases include those caused by viruses, bacteria and parasites, and such illnesses may be acute or chronic and are usually communicable; insects, animals and human carriers may be important in their spread and epidemics may occur. Inflammation is often the result of infection, but inflammatory disease can also result from disordered immunity and other causes.

▲ In vascular diseases, organs become diseased as a result of disease in their blood supply; examples are

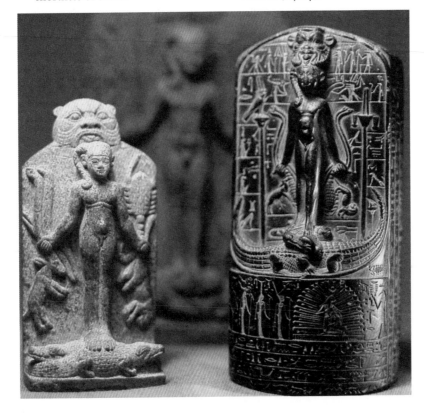

Small statues depicting the Egyptian gods Horus and Isis, employed for the treatment of snake bites. Example of magic medicine. The cause of medicine, as the centuries passed, made little appreciable progress in the Nile Valley. It was initiate medicine, practiced for the purpose of ridding patients of demonic powers. All cures were revealed by the gods.

D

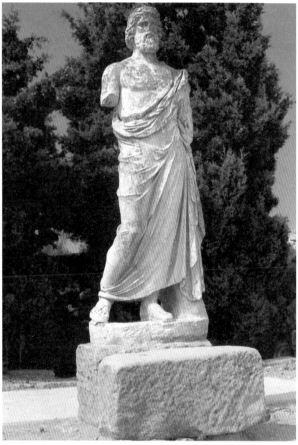
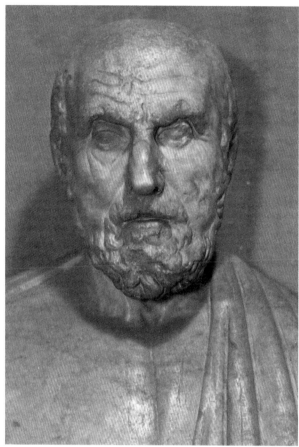

Statues of Hippocrates, the founder of scientific medicine. In the 5th century BC he wrote at treatise on symptoms and syndromes. The Hippocratic Oath is renowned through the centuries for setting a high standard of professional conduct. In the fifth century BC it symbolized the spirit informing the famous school of Cos under the inspired leadership of Hippocrates.

atherosclerosis, aneurysms, thrombosis and embolism.

▲ Tumors, including benign growths, cancer and lymphoma, are diseases in which abnormal growth of a structure occurs and leads to a lump, pressure on or spread to other organs, as well as distant effects such as emaciation, hormone production and neuritis (inflamed nerves).

▲ In degenerative disease, death or premature ageing of parts of an organ or system lead to a gradual impairment of function.

▲ Deficiency diseases result from inadequate intake of nutrients, such as vitamins, minerals, calcium, iron and trace substances; disorders of their fine control and that of hormones leads to metabolic disease.

▲ Poisoning is the toxic action of chemicals on body systems, some of which may be particularly sensitive to a given poison. An increasingly recognized side-effect of industrialization is the occurrence of occupational diseases, in which chemicals, dusts or moulds encountered at work cause disease - especially pneumoconiosis (a result of coal dust) and other lung disease, and certain cancers.

▲ An iatrogenic disease is one produced by the intervention of doctors, in an attempt to treat or prevent some other disease. The altered anatomy of diseased structures is described as "pathological."

▲ Psychiatric disease, including psychoses (schizophrenia and severe depression) and neuroses, are

functional disturbances of the brain, in which structural abnormalities are not recognizable; they may represent subtle disturbances of brain metabolism.

Treatment of disease by surgery or drugs is usual, but success is variable; a number of conditions are so mild that symptoms may be suppressed until the illnesses have run their natural course.

Acute and chronic disease

In colloquial speech, "acute" tends to indicate something sharp or intense, whereas "chronic" implies severity in terms of being objectionable or very bad. For this reason, a person can become alarmed when he or she learns that the official name for

Health and disease: present status

■ Arthritis

Some 17 million people worldwide suffer enduring pain caused by rheumatoid arthritis, a condition in which the body's immune system erodes the cartilage and bone near joints. While doctors do not know why the body turns against itself, they are exploring some promising prospects for relief. One involves mimicking the activity that dampens the immune system in pregnant women, allowing their bodies to adjust to the presence of the foreign foetus. Some doctors believe repeated vaccination of properly prepared foreign cells will curb the immune reaction enough to hinder the inflammation of arthritis. Other researchers are genetically engineering cells into knuckles, where they can teach the immune system to stop attacking the body's own cartilage.

■ Asthma

The death rate from asthma, which attacks over 175 million people worldwide annually, has grown some 5 per cent each year since the late 1980s. Much of that rise has occurred in urban areas, where dust mites, cigarette smoke and cockroach droppings are among many factors that can help trigger an attack.

A quick squirt from a steroid inhaler usually relaxes constricted breathing passages and helps an asthmatic breathe normally, but other drugs are under review that may reduce the need for inhalers.

■ Baldness

Microsurgery and gene guns are the newest weapons doctors are using to coax stubborn hair follicles to bloom again. Microsurgically implanted grafts with one or two hairs each result in less puckering and bleeding than do larger implants with more hairs.

Recently, researchers studying a genetic disorder that causes hair and tooth loss identified the first gene that may be associated with baldness. They speculate that the gene codes for substances that create the necessary environment for continued hair growth.

Perhaps the least invasive treatment for hair loss, however, remains minoxidil, now available without prescription. When used continuously for at least four months, it prompts thinning hair to grow in some people.

■ Bone fractures

Many people know ultrasound as the device that gives them the first grainy, in-utero glimpse of their baby. Now doctors are using it to speed up bone healing. Even a sonogram's low-intensity waves are enough to stimulate bone-cell formation. When treated within seven days, stress fractures heal as much as 40 per cent faster than they would without treatment. Patients take home a portable device and zap the fracture for about 20 minutes a day until their doctor deems the fracture healed.

■ Burns

For severe burn patients, the first priority is to restore the damaged skin that is the body's first line of defence against microbes. To lessen the need for taking extensive skin grafts from other areas of a burn patient's already weakened body, several biotechnology companies have developed grafts made from collagen, a fibrous protein that is a natural component of skin and other tissues.

The laboratory-grown collagen serves as a permanent scaffolding, in areas in which both the upper epidermis and deeper dermal layers of skin have been burned. Once grafted, new skin cells and blood vessels grow around the template within a few weeks, regenerating the skin.

■ Cholera

120,000 deaths a year. Crowded living conditions and lack of clean drinking water allow Vibrio cholerae to thrive. Regions of India and South America, as well as refugee camps in Somalia and Zaïre, have become breeding grounds for new, aggressive strains. Researchers hope to have an effective vaccine by the year 2001.

■ Common cold

Rhinovirus, with its more than 100 identified strains, has been around for many thousands of years. With age comes wisdom, which in the case of this virus means the ability to resist every concoction - from chicken soup to zinc lozenges. So far, modern medicine has its merits match. Still the best treatment: aspirin, rest and lots of fluids.

■ Diabetes

For most of the more than 200 million people who have Type 1 or Type 2 diabetes, insulin injections timed up to one hour before each meal are a routine part of dining. The diabetic either does not make enough insulin to digest sugars or does not use the insulin efficiently.

New classes of drugs may make keeping track of sugar levels easier. Some of these work in the small intestine to inhibit the absorption of carbohydrates (which raise blood-sugar levels) after a meal, while others stop the liver from producing excess amounts of sugar.

■ Diphtheria

8,000 deaths a year. An effective vaccine against diphtheria exists, but the numerous outbreaks in Eastern Europe and Russia beginning 1990 demonstrate the importance of maintaining immunization programmes. Last year 54,000 cases were reported worldwide, and as many as 25 per cent of these infected died.

Top causes of death and disability

2000
1 Respiratory infections
2 Diarrheal diseases
3 Complications of birth
4 Severe depression
5 Heart disease
6 Stroke
7 Tuberculosis
8 Measles
9 Traffic accidents
10 Congenital anomalies

2020
(Projections by the Harvard School of Public Health)
1 Heart diseases
2 Severe depression
3 Traffic accidents
4 Stroke
5 Chronic pulmonary disease
6 Respiratory infections
7 Tuberculosis
8 War injuries
9 Diarrheal diseases
10 HIV/AIDS

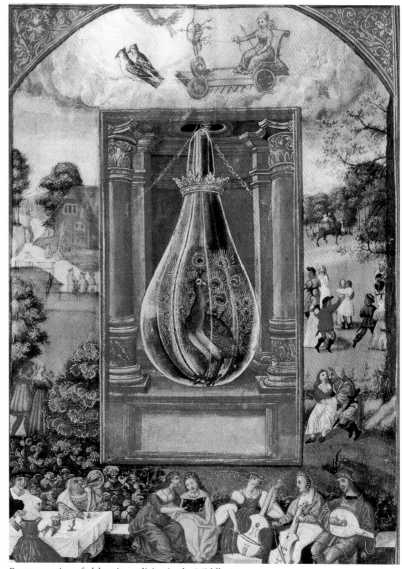

Representation of alchemic medicine in the Middle Ages.

his/her condition includes the latter term - e.g. chronic bronchitis.

However, professional usage of these two words remains closer to their etymology. Thus "acute" means "ending in a sharp point," implying a finite duration that, classically, culminates in a crisis. On the other hand, "chronic," which is derived from a word meaning "time" indicates "long-continued."

The characteristics of acute disease may be exemplified by acute infections. The onset of the condition is frequently sudden, when there may be almost total prostration, not least because rest is commonly regarded as facilitating recovery. Furthermore, there is the prospect of a limited period in this state.

Most acute diseases are self-limiting, some may be life-threatening, but the remainder, because of their finite duration, pose a minimal threat to the subject.

Chronic disease presents different challenges. The onset is usually slow; there may be a gradual progression of symptoms, or more permanent problems may develop as the sequel to a number of acute episodes. The confidence and hopes of sufferers are undermined; the experience is usually difficult to account for, no end is in sight, and self-perception - the sense of identity - is assaulted by changes in the body and its functional performance.

The restriction of activity, though at times severe, nevertheless usually falls short of total incapacity until very late in the course of the disease.

Acceptance of the existence of the disease by others can be more difficult when a degree of independence is possible, not least because obligations cannot be suspended indefinitely; some way of coming to terms with the altered situation therefore becomes necessary.

Finally, the persistence of the problems implicitly reveals limitations in medical treatment, so that professional advice is often accepted with less assurance. The impact of the condition on the individual, though important, does not dominate the scene to

Health and disease: present status

Emphysema
Whether because of smoking, a genetic condition or simple age, parts of the lung tissue of more than 25 million emphysema patients worldwide become too thin and often shred. The newest surgical treatments for the condition focus on preserving as much healthy tissue as possible by rolling up the torn portion of the lung like a window shade. Surgeons then secure the roll by lining it with cow muscle and stapling the tissue together.

Flue (influenza)
Each year health officials race to stay ahead of the wily flu virus, which is constantly changing, by concocting new mixes of vaccines to head off novel strains. One the horizon are more sophisticated vaccines that incorporate a snippet of viral genome that is common to many strains. Once inoculated, a person would be protected against a number of different flu viruses for more than a year. From bird flu 23 people died in 2005.

Heart disease
More people in the western world die from this disease each year than from any other condition, prompting physicians to explore a host of ways to keep hearts healthy. For patients whose only resource is a heart transplant, one bold method, pioneered by a Brazilian surgeon, involves increasing the efficiency of the heart by cutting away a portion of the muscle of the left ventricle, the chamber from which blood is pumped to the rest of the body. Surgeons at several facilities in the US, Japan and UK have begun using the technique in trials and hope to improve on its current 40 per cent death rate.

Hepatitis C
Some 100 million people infected. Identified in 1989, hepatitis C is a major cause of cirrhosis of the liver and liver cancer. Transmission occurs commonly through transfusion of tainted blood. Interferon sometimes halts the infection but is too expensive for most of the developing world. To date, there is no vaccine.

Hernia
Hernia surgery is synonymous with painful and slow recovery, which is one reason that only 20 per cent sufferers seek surgical treatment. In repairing a serious groin hernia, surgeons generally stitch in a synthetic screen to cover a tear in the abdominal wall from which a portion of the intestine may protrude. Now, however, they can simply plug the opening with a cone-shaped mesh device. Plugging rather than patching the hole causes less strain on the surrounding tissue and reduces the extent of both surgery and recovery time.

Hearing loss
The most common cause of hearing loss in developed countries is nerve deafness, affecting more than 200 million people worldwide. Unlike their predecessors generations ago, however, today's hearing-impaired have at their disposal hearing aids with the power of microcomputers. Once fitted for the individual ear, these sophisticated devices automatically filter out background noise and deliver amplified, focused sound equally efficiently whether in a quiet office or a noisy restaurant.

HIV infection
HIV infection and AIDS have reached epidemic proportions. Through december 2005, more than 37 million cases were reported worldwide. In the United States more than 805,000 cases of AIDS and 457,000 deaths were reported up to december 2005. In parts of Africa, more than 30 per cent of the adult population (between the ages of 15 and 45) is infected, threatening to nearly eliminate a whole generation.

Hypertension
One in four people in the western world has high blood pressure, but fully a third of them are not aware of their condition, in which the heart pumps blood through the body with excessive force. Untreated, the constant pounding on the vessels can result in hardened arteries and an enlarged heart, both risk factors for a heart attack.
Traditionally, doctors could do little for their hypertensive patients other than advice them to adhere to a low-salt and low-fat diet. Today a flood of medications, including diuretics, calcium channel blockers, angiotensin-converting enzyme, or ACE, inhibitors and betablockers give physicians and patients alike many options.

Impotence
Continued failure to become aroused may signal a medical problem. The immediate cause of impotence is a lack of blood flow to the penis, and a wide range of treatments is available, Men can take pills that dilate the blood vessels and help facilitate an erection, or they can use vacuum instruments that draw blood into the penis. On the more invasive side, they can inject drugs into the base of the penis that dilate blood vessels, or patients can undergo surgery for penile implants.

Lyme disease
Often packed into the bodies of ticks, no bigger than the head of a pin are bacteria that cause flu-like symptoms in more than a million people each year. The best-known illness is Lyme disease, which, left untreated, can lead to arthritis, paralysis of facial nerves and meningitis. Antibiotics are the standard treatment.

Malaria
2.7 million deaths a year. Malaria is spread to humans by mosquitoes, and 90 per cent of all cases occur in Africa. Strains of the parasite that are increasingly resistant to available drugs keep outbreaks alive. As a result, researchers have begun field-testing some of the 15 to 20 malaria vaccines currently in development.

the exclusion of all else.

The person's health, or lack of it, has to be set against his or her background and responsibilities.

Symptoms reflecting impairments and disabilities call for attempts at amelioration in their own right. The sensitivity of others can also be taxed: virtually everyone experiences an acute disease at some time, so that it is not too difficult to project oneself into the situation of the patient, but personal knowledge of chronic suffering is much less wide-spread.

Development of disease

The principal events in the development of disease are:

- Something abnormal occurs within the individual. This may be present at birth or acquired later. A chain of circumstances (the etiology) gives rise to changes in the structure or functioning of the body (the pathology). Pathological changes may or may not make themselves evident; when they do, they are described as "manifestations," which in medical parlance are usually distinguished as symptoms and signs. These features are the components of the medical model of disease.
- Someone becomes aware of such an occurrence. Most often the individual him/herself becomes aware of disease symptoms, usually referred to as "clinical disease." However, it is also necessary to encompass two other types of experience:
- Not infrequently, symptoms may develop that cannot currently be linked to any underlying disease process. Most health professionals would attribute such symptoms to a disturbance - as yet unidentified - of some essential structure or process within the body.
- In contrast, some deviation may be identified of which the patient him/herself is unaware. Such pathology without symptoms sometimes constitutes "subclinical disease," which is encountered with increasing frequency as screening programs have been extended. In behavioral terms,

such individuals have become or been made aware that they are unhealthy. Their disease heralds the recognition of impairments - abnormalities of body structure and appearance and/or of organ or system function, resulting from any cause.

- The performance or behavior of the individual may be altered as a result of this awareness, i.e. there may be disability. Common activities may become restricted, and in this way, others come to recognize the experience. Also relevant are psychological responses to the presence of disease, part of so-called "illness behavior" and "sickness phenomena" - behavior by individuals in response to the expectations others have of them when they are ill.
- Either the awareness itself, or the altered behavior or performance to which this gives rise, may place the individual at a disadvantage relative to others, i.e. that person may become handicapped.

This reflects the response of society to the individual's experience, be this expressed in attitudes, such as attaching a stigma to a certain illness or disability, or in behavior, which may include legislation.

The explicit concern with the value attached to an individual's performance or status obviously makes this the most problematical result of disease. The major consequences of disease are: impairment, disability and handicap, which will be discussed in detail.

Impairment

In the context of health experience, an impairment is any loss or abnormality of psychological, physical or anatomical structure or function. The term "impairment" is more inclusive than "disorder" in that it also covers losses; e.g. the loss of a leg is an impairment, but not a disorder.

Impairment is characterized by losses or abnormalities that may be temporary or permanent, and it includes the existence or occurrence of an anomaly, defect or loss in a limb, organ, tis-

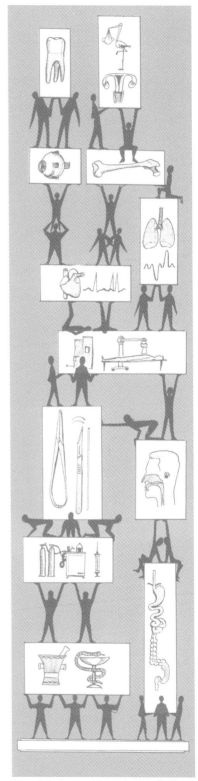

Pictorial schema of the various medical specialists.

Common illnesses

Health and disease: present status

Menopause
Postmenopausal women are at higher risk for heart disease and osteoporosis (among other things, estrogen prevents the build-up of plaque in blood vessels and protects bone from thinning). On the plus side, the drop in estrogen reduces the risk of developing breast cancer. Estrogen-replacement therapy - whether by pill, skin patch, or injection - provides just enough estrogen to prevent the unpleasant symptoms of menopause while offering protection against heart disease and osteoporosis.

Before starting hormone-replacement therapy, those with a family history of breast cancer should, in consultation with a physician, weigh their risk of breast cancer against that of heart disease and osteoporosis.

Migraine
No ordinary headache, a migraine results when tightened blood vessels in the brain repeatedly expand, squeeze surrounding nerves and then constrict again, resulting in excruciating pain that often leaves sufferers unable to function for days at a time.

Migraines are triggered by a variety of sources, from caffeine to changes in weather to menstrual periods - catalysts, doctors believe, that result in a flood of serotonin that causes blood vessels in the brain to contract. New drugs, which block serotonin and prevent vessels from swelling initially, give relief.

Pain
From headache sufferers to cancer patients, millions of people live with pain, sometimes mild, sometimes crippling. Researchers are currently testing, in animals, a more convenient and safer way to deliver relief. Researchers have packed a button-size insert with a powerful narcotic. Implanted under the skin, the device releases analgesic into the bloodstream continuously for three months.

Sleep disorders
▲ *Snoring*: muscles at the back of the mouth relax during sleep, obstructing the airway and vibrating with each breath.
   More than 300 devices, from nose tapers to surgery, aim to open air passages.
▲ *Sleep apnoea*: also caused by relaxed muscles at the back of the mouth, apnoea reduces oxygen flow to the brain as breathing stops for about 10 seconds at a time.

Surgery that removes soft tissue at the back of the mouth can help and drugs can stimulate normal breathing
▲ *Narcolepsy*: sudden irresistible daytime episodes of sleepiness affect millions of people each year. There is no cure, but drugs are being tested. Meanwhile, short voluntary naps and avoidance of alcohol are
Insomnia: a continued inability to fall asleep that affects about 10 per cent of people in the western world, insomnia can last for days, even weeks.
For most, adopting a schedule of limited time in bed and regular wake-up times can help. Some people also rely on melatonin, but researchers say there is still no proof that it works.

Spinal cord injuries
Currently no therapy exists to restore torn or damaged spinal-cord nerves, but certain drugs developed in the past decade can tip the scales in the patient's favour. One, administered in the first eight hours after injury, protects nerve cells from damage caused by the body's immune system, which immediately floods the affected site with powerful toxins. Other drugs helps surviving nerve cells transmit their electrical signals from spinal cord to muscle.

Tuberculosis
22 million infected. Tuberculosis has made a comeback by forming a deadly partnership with AIDS. About one-third of AIDS-related deaths each year may be due to tuberculosis. Even in developed nations, the number of cases jumped 17 per cent from 1990 to 2005. Of greatest concern is the shrinking number of antibiotics that can battle the disease.

Ulcers
More than a decade ago, the prevailing wisdom held that ulcers resulted from too much acid in the stomach. Milk, antacids and other drugs that slowed the stomach's acid secretion topped physicians' treatment options. Today doctors know that almost all cases of ulcers that occur in the first part of the intestine and 80 per cent of those in the stomach are caused by a bacterium Helicobacter pylori. So if an ulcer cannot be traced to triggers such as aspirin, caffeine or stress, doctors now prescribe antibiotics.

sue or other structure of the body, including mental function.
Impairment is not contingent upon how the state arose or developed; both ascribed and achieved states, such as genetic abnormality or the consequences of a road traffic accident, are included.

Disability

In the context of health experience, a disability is any restriction or lack (resulting from an impairment) of ability to perform an activity in the manner or within the range considered normal for a human being.

Disability represents a departure from the norm in terms of performances of the individual, as opposed to that of an organ or mechanism.
The concept is characterized by excesses or deficiencies of customarily expected behavior or activity, and these may be temporary or perma-

nent, reversible or irreversible and progressive or regressive.

Disability takes form as the individual becomes aware of a change in his or her identity. Customary expectations embrace integrated functioning in physical, psychological and social terms and it is unrealistic to expect a neat separation between medical and social aspects of activity. For instance, physical incapacities and socially deviant behaviors equally transgress what is expected of the individual.

Handicap

In the context of health experience, a handicap is a disadvantage for a given individual, resulting from an impairment or a disability, that limits or prevents the fulfilment of a role that is normal (depending on age, sex and social and cultural factors) for that individual.

The state of being handicapped is relative to other people. Handicap is characterized by the difference between the individual's performance or status and the expectations of the particular group of which he or she is a member.

Disadvantage accrues as a result of his/her being unable to conform to the norms of this group. Handicap is thus a social phenomenon, representing the social and environmental consequence for the individual stemming from the presence of impairments and disabilities, and it results in discrimination by other people.

Thus the individual's own intention is of no immediate concern; disadvantage can arise when the individual deviates in spite of his/her own wishes, but it can also develop when the deviation is inadvertent or the product of his/her own choice.

The three consequences of disease could be linked in the following manner: disease > impairment > disability > handicap. Although this graphic representation suggests a simple linear progression along the full sequence, the situation is, in fact, more complex.

In the first place, handicap may result from impairment without there being a disability. For example, disfigurement may give rise to problems in

dealing with the rest of society, and it may thus constitute a very real disadvantage, to say nothing of the embarrassment that the disfigured individual may feel.

Similarly, a child with coeliac disease (an intestinal sensitivity to the protein gluten in certain grains), who is functionally limited, may be able to live a fairly normal life and not suffer any restriction in activity, but could nevertheless suffer disadvantage by virtue of his or her inability to partake of a normal diet.

Other examples of the above mentioned consequences of disease are:

▲ A child born with a fingernail missing has a malformation - a structural impairment, but this does not in any way interfere with the function of the hand and so there is no disability; the impairment is not particularly evident, and so disadvantage or handicap would be unlikely.

▲ A very short-sighted or diabetic individual suffers a functional impairment but, because this can be corrected or abolished by aids, appliances or drugs, he or she would not necessarily be disabled. However, the non-disabled juvenile diabetic could still be handicapped if the disadvantage is considerable, e.g. by not being allowed to eat sweets like other children or by having to give him/herself regular injections.

▲ Individuals with red-green colour blindness have an impairment, but it would be unlikely to lead to restriction of activity; whether the impairment constitutes a handicap would depend on circumstances. If their occupations were agricultural, they might well be unaware of their impairment, but they would be at a disadvantage if they aspired to become railway engineers, because they would be prevented from following this occupation.

▲ A subnormal intelligence is an impairment, but it may not lead to appreciable activity restriction. Factors other than the impairment may determine the handicap because the disadvantage may be minimal if the individual lives in a remote rural community. Whereas

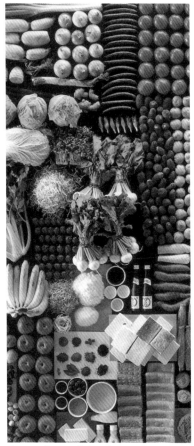

Present-day medicine plays more attention to healthy food than in the past.

it could be severe in the child of university graduates living in a large city, of whom more might be expected.

▲ Perhaps the most graphic example of someone who is handicapped without being disabled is the individual who has recovered from an acute psychotic episode but who bears the stigma of having been a "mental patient."

▲ Finally, the same handicap can arise in different situations, and therefore as a result of different disabilities. Thus, personal hygiene might be difficult to maintain, but the reasons for this could be very different, as when someone accustomed to washing in a washbasin is compared to some whose ablutions are performed in a lake, or in a fast-moving river.

EAR DISORDERS

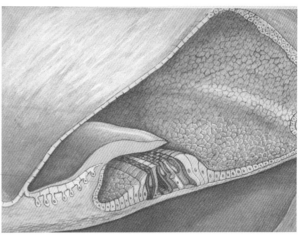

General aspects

Predisposing factors often lead to the breakdown of natural barriers of the normal ear canal; hairs in the outer half of the meatus, the size of the ear canal and its isthmus, and cerum collectively prevent the introduction of foreign material that may cause injury or infection.

The integrity of the skin layers and the acid pH of the canal provide protection against infection. Infection usually is preceded by an alteration of the protective acid Ph of the canal.

Certain conditions and activities contribute to the breakdown of natural barriers of the normal ear canal. Warm humid climates, inside environments with intense heat and humidity, accompanied by sweating, and exposure to water (swimming and diving) during the summer months have been implicated. The increased exposure to moisture may result in tissue maceration that breaks down the protective barrier of the skin, alters the pH of the skin, and predisposes the ear canal to infection. There is a positive correlation between the amount of water exposure in the ear canal and the incidence of external otitis.

Disorders of the auricle

The disorders associated with the auricle, the part of the ear not within the head, are generally minor and involve lacerations, boils, and dermatitis. These conditions are generally self-limiting.

Trauma
Lacerations, including scrapes and cuts, involving only the auricle skin usually heal spontaneously. A wound that does not heal normally should be checked by a physician. Deep wounds that may involve injury to the cartilage also require examination by a physician. Injury to the auricle that does not perforate the cartilage may cause subcutaneous bleeding and produce a hematoma.

A hematoma requires aspiration or incision by a physician, since the red-blue swelling may obliterate normal auricular contours and frequently results in inflammation and a cartilage disorder or "cauliflower ear." The swelling can also cause local pruritus and pain upon touch.

Boils
Furuncles or boils are usually localized infections of the hair follicles. The cause is uncertain. Fatigue and emotional stress appear to predispose to furuncles. Anaemia and diabetes as well as malnutrition have been found to be predisposing factors in some populations. In a high percentage of cases in young adults, no specific

Microscopic drawings of part of the sensory systems of the inner ear.
Left Bony labyrinth; series of interconnecting canals and cavities in the hard portion of the temporal bone.
Right: Enlargement of the tectorial membrane, organ of Corti and basilar membrane.

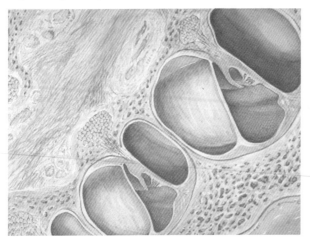

causative or predisposing factor has been established. Poor body hygiene is generally contributory to boils. Boils often involve the external auditory meatus. They usually begin as a red papule and may progress into a round or conical superficial pustule with a core of pus and erythema around the base.

The lesion gradually enlarges, becomes firm, then softens and opens spontaneously (after few days to as long as 2 weeks), discharging the purulent contents. Because the skin is very taut, minimal swelling may cause severe pain.

Boils are usually self-limiting, they may be severe, and multiple. Deeper lesions may lead to perichondritis (inflammation of the connective tissue). The pus-producing organism found in boils is usually Staphylococcus aureus.

Small boils may be treated by good hygiene combined with topical compresses. Hot compresses of saline solution may be applied to the auricle and the side of the face. Cases in which boils do not respond rapidly to topical dressings should consult a doctor.

Perichondritis

This is an inflammation involving the perichondrium (the fibrous connective tissue surrounding the ear cartilage), usually following a poorly treated or untreated burn, injury, or local infection. The onset of perichondritis is characterized by a sensation of heat and stiffness of the auricle with pronounced pain.

As the condition progresses, an exudate forms and the auricle becomes dark, diffuse, and swollen. The entire auricle becomes shiny red with uniform thickening caused by edema and inflammation. The lesions usually are confined to the cartilaginous tissue of the auricle and external canal. Constitutional disturbances may include generalized fever and malaise. Perichondritis frequently results in severe auricular deformity, and atresia (a pathologic closure) of the external auditory canal may occur.

Dermatitis of the ear

An inflammatory condition of the skin may result from an abrasion of

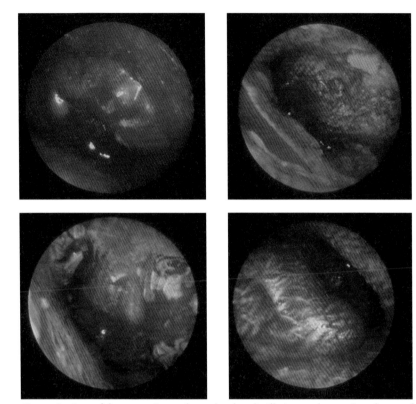

Otoscopic views of the tympanic membrane (eardrum). All pictures show various degrees of infectious processes of the eardrum, usually in connection with middle ear infections.

the auricle and, if untreated, may develop into an infection of these skin layers. Inflammatory conditions such as seborrhoea, psoriasis, and contact dermatitis also may affect the skin of the auricle and the external ear canal. Contact dermatitis also may be caused by an allergic response to jewelry, cosmetics, detergents, or topical drug applications. The lesions may spread to the auditory canal, neck, and facial areas. The symptoms of dermatitis of the ear usually include itching and local redness followed by vesication, weeping, and erythema. The lesions form scales and yellow crusts on the skin. They may spread to adjacent unaffected areas, and excessive scratching may cause them to become infected. Topical drugs should be used cautiously with dermatitis because of their potential allergic reactions, which could exacerbate the condition. Seborrhoeic dermatitis of the ear is usually associated with dandruff. Treatment with dandruff-control shampoos is recommended.

Itching of the ear

An itchy ear canal is a common symptom and may mask the pre-inflammatory stages of acute external otitis. Itching can also occur without visible lesions of the ear. Patients with chronic external otitis experience itching due to dry ears because of the absence of cerumen.

Itching is a very common complaint with chronic external otitis and may be due to eczema of the skin around the ears, infections, seborrhoeic dermatitis, psoriasis, contact dermatitis, or neurodermatitis.

Itching commonly begins as an annoying itch-scratch cycle that results in trauma, infection, epidermal barrier destruction, and inflammation of the affected areas. Ear scratching has been shown to be a nervous habit that may be addictive. Careful observation to determine the cause of itching often is helpful prior to any attempt to afford symptomatic relief and to correct the problem.

Ear disorders   Questions & Answers

How common are ear infections in childhood?

Next to the common cold, an ear infection is the most common childhood illness. In fact, most children has had one ear infection by the time they are 3 years old. Most of the time, ear infections clear up without causing any lasting problems. But, if they occur often or are not treated, they can lead to hearing loss and other damage.

How do ear infections in children develop?

When a child has a cold, nose or throat infection, or allergy, the eustachian tube can become blocked, causing a buildup of fluid in the middle ear. If this fluid becomes infected by bacteria or a virus, it can cause swelling of the eardrum and pain in the ear. This type of ear infection is called acute otitis media.

What is otitis media with effusion?

Often after the symptoms of acute otitis media clear up, fluid remains in the ear. Acute otitis media then develops into another kind of ear problem called otitis media with effusion.

This condition is harder to detect than acute otitis media because, except for the fluid and some hearing loss that is usually mild, there are often no other noticeable symptoms. This fluid often lasts for up to 3 months and, in most cases, disappears on its own. The child's hearing then returns to normal.

What are risk factors for developing childhood ear infection?

The are several risk factors for developing childhood ear infection, including:

■ *Age*

Infants and young children are more likely to get ear infections. The size and shape of their eustachian tubes make it easier for fluid to build up. Ear infections occur most often in children between 3 months and 3 years of age.

■ *Sex*

Boys have more ear infections than girls.

n Heredity

Ear infections can run in families. Children are more likely to have repeated middle-ear infections if a parent or sibling also had repeated ear infections.

■ *Colds/Allergies*

Colds often lead to ear infections. Children in group child care settings have a higher chance of passing their colds to each other because they are exposed to more germs and viruses from other children. Allergies that cause stuffy noses can also lead to ear infections.

■ *Tobacco smoke*

Children who breathe in someone else's tobacco smoke have a higher risk of developing health problems, including ear infections.

■ *Bottle feeding*

Babies who are bottle-fed get more ear infections than breastfed babies.

How can parents help reduce some of the risks of ear infections?

Parents can help reduce some of the risks of ear infections. For instance:

▲ Breastfed instead of bottle-feed
▲ Keep your chlld away from tobacco smoke, especially in your home or car
▲ Try to keep your child's hands clean

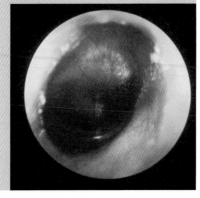

Aural drainage

The drainage or discharge may be blood, watery fluid (serum), or purulent or mucoid material. Head trauma may cause leakage of cerebrospinal fluid. The origin of the fluid may be due to an infection of the external ear canal. A ruptured tympanic membrane usually produces serum-like fluid.

Any trauma to the ear canal may cause bleeding and, if infected, the ear may exude a purulent fluid from which the causative organisms may be cultured and appropriate antibiotics prescribed.

Disorders of the external auditory canal

Common disorders of the auditory canal are:

- boils
- otomycosis
- presence of foreign objects
- impacted cerumen
- external otitis

Boils

Boils of the external auditory canal are pathologically similar to those found on the auricle and external auditory meatus. Symptoms include pain of the infected site, which is usually exacerbated by mastication.

The auditory meatal opening may be partly occluded by swelling; however, hearing is impaired only if the opening is completely occluded. Edema and pain over the mastoid bone directly behind the auricle may occur. Traction of the auricle or tragus is very painful.

Patients with boils in the external auditory canal should consult a doctor because unresolved conditions may lead to a generalized infection of the entire external auditory canal.

Otomycosis

External fungal infection of the ear - otomycosis - is more common in warmer, tropical climates than in mild, temperate zones.

Aspergillus species and Candida species are the most common causative agents. Antibiotic treatment of a bacterial ear infection, with resultant suppression of normal bacterial flora, may predispose an individual to a mycotic external ear infection.

A superficial mycotic infection of the external auditory meatus is characterized by pruritus with a feeling of fullness and pressure in the ear. Pain may be present, increasing with mastication and traction on the pinna and the tragus.

The fungus forms a mass of epithelial debris, exudate, and cerumen and, in the acute stage, may clog the external auditory meatus. Hearing may be impaired.

Depending on the nature of the fungus, the colour of the mass may vary. The skin lining the external auditory canal and the tympanic membrane becomes beefy-red and scaly and may be eroded or ulcerated.

A scant, colourless mucoid discharge is common. Otomycosis is particularly serious in diabetic patients. Mycotic ear infections must be treated by a physician.

Foreign objects in the ear

Young children often use the ear canal for inserting small items such as beans, peas, marbles, pebbles, or beads. If the objects become lodged in the ear canal, they may cause significant hearing loss.

Vegetable seeds, such as dried beans or dried peas, lodged in the external auditory meatus swell when moistened during bathing or swimming and become wedged in the bony portion of the canal, causing severe pain. Furthermore, if an obstruction of the external auditory meatus is not removed promptly, acute bacterial otitis may result. Insects may enter the meatus and cause distress by beating their wings and crawling.

Foreign objects lodged in the ear canal may not cause symptoms and may be found only during a routine physical examination. usually, a hearing deficiency or pain is observed with pressure in the ear during mastication. An exudate may form because of secondary bacterial infection.

Mechanical removal should be reserved for a physician because unskilled attempts at removal often result in damage to the skin surrounding the external auditory meatus.

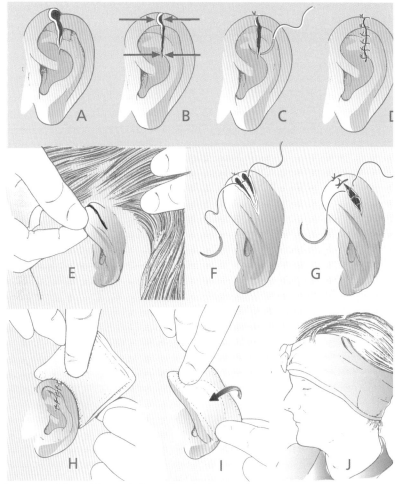

Severe cut of the auricle, surgical procedure (A-J).
For lacerations of the external ear that penetrate the cartilage and the skin on both sides, the edges of the torn skin are sewn together, the cartilage is splinted together externally with cotton wool and a protective dressing is applied.

Earache - When to contact your doctor

▲ If, despite a painkiller, the child still has a bad earache after twelve hours.

▲ If the child still has a slight earache after three days.

▲ If the child gets a runny ear.

▲ Have the child examined by a doctor if you suspect an ear infection, especially if the child is still too young to say so itself.

▲ When the area surrounding the ear is painful.

▲ If a child has a runny ear and ther pain and/or fever does not lessen contact your doctor immediately.

Ear disorders   Questions & Answers

What are the major symptoms of an ear infection in childhood?
Your child may have a number of symptoms during an ear infection. Knowing what thoese symptoms are may help you treat some of them more quickly and get medical care, if needed.

■ *Pain*
The most common symptom of an ear infection is pain. While older children are able to tell you when their ears hurt, younger children may only appear irritable and cry. This may be more noticable during feeding because sucking and swallowing may cause painful pressure changes in the middle ear.

■ *Fever*
Another sign of an ear infection is a temperature ranging from 100 °F to 104 °F.

■ *Ear drainage*
You might also notice yellow or white fluid, possible blood-tinged, draining from your child's ear. The fluid may have a foul odor and will look different from normal earwax (which is orange-yellow or reddish-brown).

■ *Difficulty hearing*
Druing and after an ear infection, your child may have trouble hearing for several weeks. This occurs because the fluid behind the eardrum gets in the way of sound transmission. This is usually temporary and clears up after the fluid from the midle ear drains away.

Are there any other reasons besides an ear infection why my child's ears may hurt?
There are other reasons besides an ear infection why your child's ears may hurt. In these cases, your child probably has en earache, not an ear infection. Ear pain can be caused by:
▲ an infection of the skin of the ear canal
▲ blocked or plugged eustachian tubes from colds or allergies
▲ a sore throat or sore gums

Do children show behavioral problems due to diffisulty in hearing?
Because your child can have trouble hearing without other symptoms of an ear infection, watch for the following changes in behavior (especially during or after a cold) that may mean he or she cannot hear well:
▲ talking softly or in a muffled way
▲ saying "huh?" or "what?" more than usual
▲ not responding to sounds
▲ having more trouble understanding language in noisy rooms
▲ listening with TV oi radio turned up louder than usual
If you think your child may have difficulty hearing, contact your pediatrician. Being able to hear and listen to others talk helps a child learn speech and language. This is especially important during the first few years of life.

Can complications develop from a simple ear infection?
While your child is young and at higher risk for ear infections, it is important for you to know the symptoms and to get child treatment if an infection develops. Although it is very rare, complications from untreated ear infections can develop, including:
- infection of the iner ear
- infection of the skull behind the ear
- infection of the membranes around the brain
- scarring or thickening of the eardrum
- facial paralysis
- permanent hearing loss

Impacted cerumen
The accumulation of cerumen in the external auditory meatus may be caused by any of these factors:
• overactive ceruminous glands
• abnormally shaped external auditory meatus
• abnormal cerumen secreted by the ceruminous glands
Overactive ceruminous glands cause cerumen to accumulate in the external auditory canal. A tortuous or small canal or abnormal narrowing of the canal may not permit normal migration of the cerumen to the outside, allowing cerumen to accumulate. Abnormal cerumen may be dried or softer than normal cerumen and may interfere with the normal epithelial migration. It is often packed deeper into the external auditory meatus by repeated attempts to remove it, which is the most common cause of impacted cerumen.
In general, there usually is no cerumen in the inner half of the external auditory canal unless it has been pushed there. In elderly persons, cerumen is frequently admixed with long hairs in the external auditory canal, preventing normal expulsion and forming a matted obstruction in the ear.

External otitis
Inflammation of the skin lining the external auditory canal often due to infection is one of the most common diseases of the ear. It is very painful and annoying. The external auditory canal is considered a blind canal lined with skin. It is a dark, warm cul-de-sac that is well suited for collecting moisture.
Prolonged exposure to moisture tends to disrupt the continuity of the epithelial cells, causing skin maceration and fissures, which provide a fertile area for bacterial growth.
Factors contributing to susceptibility to external otitis include:
• race
• heredity
• age
• sex
• climate
• diet
• occupational background
The most common causative organisms of external otitis include

Pseudomonas species, also Staphylococcus species, Bacillus species, and Proteus species. Fungi may be the causative organism in some cases.

Often the patient first complains of an itching feeling. Then within a few hours or up to 24 hours later, the complaints are followed by feeling of wetness of the ear canal and discomfort leading to pain.

The amount of wetness may vary from minimal to frank otorrhea (discharge). Any secondary hearing loss may be caused by epithelial debris mixed with purulent discharge causing blockage.

A bacterial infection of the external auditory canal leads to inflammation and epidermal destruction of the tympanic membrane. The infection may progress through the fibrous layer of the tympanic membrane and cause perforation and spreading of the infection into the middle ear, resulting in intense pain and discomfort.

Symptoms of acute external otitis are related to the severity of the pathologic conditions. There usually is mild to moderate pain that becomes pronounced by pulling upward on the auricle or by pressing on the tragus. There may be a discharge. Hearing loss may occur if the ear canal is obstructed by swelling and edema or by debris.

Chronic external otitis usually is caused by the persistence of predisposing factors.

The most common symptom is itching, which prompts patients to attempt to scratch the ear canal to reduce or relieve the itch. This scratching can cause the skin to become broken.

Disorders of the middle ear

Disorders involving the middle ear should not be treated with nonprescription products. Although some symptoms of middle ear disorders are the same as those of external ear disorders, others are not.

All bacterial infections of the middle ear should be promptly evaluated and treated by a physician. The usual treatment is systemic antibiotics.

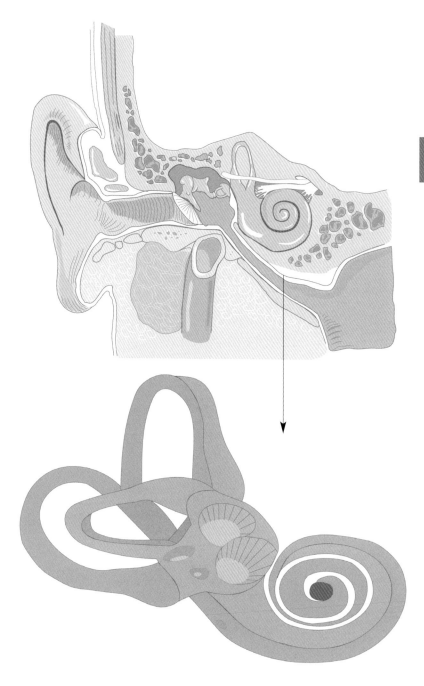

Above: cross section of the right ear. From left to right: outer ear with auricle and external acoustic meatus; middle ear with ossicles and inner ear with semicircular canals and cochlea. Below: magnification of part of the inner ear. The cochlea looks like a small shell. The modiolus forming the core of the cochlea contains small openings in its base for the nerves that extend up the center of the modiolus, giving off filaments which extend into the lamina to innervate the membranous labyrinth.

The membraneous labyrinth is a series of intercommunicating membranous canals and chambers contained within the bony labyrinth.

Ear disorders   Questions & Answers

What is tinnitus?

Tinnitus is defined as noise originating in the ear rather than in the environment. It is very common - 10 to 15% of people experience some degree of tinnitus.

Is tinnitus a deases?

No. Tinnitus is not a disease in itself. It is a symptom of a problem in your hearing mechanisms.

What causes tinnitus?

The exact cause of tinnitus is unknown. However, there are sources that may trigger or worsen tinnitus such as:
- degenerative inner ear changes due to aging
- ear infections
- excessive sound exposure

These changes may also lead to hearing loss or balance disorders. More severe problems that can contribute to the development of tinnitus are:
- Menière disease
- autoimmune disorders
- cardiovascular disease
- tumor in the hearing nerve

What kind of noise is being heard?

The noise heard by people with tinnitus may be a buzzing, ringing, roaring, whistling, or hissing sound. Some people hear more complex sounds that vary over time. These sounds are more noticeable in a quiet environment and when the person is not concentrating on something else. Thus, tinnitus tends to be most disturbing to people when they are trying to sleep.

However, the experience of tinnitus is highly individual, some people are very disturbed by their symptoms, and others find them quite bearable.

How is tinnitus diagnosed?

An otologist or otorhinolaryngologist, also known as an ENT (ear, nose, throat) doctor, can diagnose tinnitus. The physician will do a physical examination and special testing. Tests may include an audiogram to check your hearing, an auditory brain stem response test that detects brain waves in response to sound, and an MRI to check for a tumor in the hearing nerve.

How is tinnitus treated?

If an underlying disease such as diabetes, hypertension, or lupus is detected, stabilizing that particular disease or illness may ease your tinnitus.

If a tumor is found, treatment for tinnitus depends on the size of the tumor as well as your age and health status.

For most types of tinnitus, therapy may include medication, masking - a form of psychoacoustical training - or a combination of both.

Masking devices, such as white sound machines or devices worn like hearing aids, can reduce your awareness of the tinnitus.

Finally, biofeedback, behavioral or tinnitus retraining therapy (TRT) can teach you to reduce your perception of - or sensitivity to - the sound that tinnitus produces.

What kind of medication is prescribed?

Several categories of drugs - none of which were originally developed for tinnitus - may help. These include tranquilizers such as Xanax, antidepressants such as Elavil, and anti-seizure drugs such as Neurontin. Beyond oral prescription drugs, doctors can use medications such as steroids, and put them directly into the inner ear with a micro-catheter or wick that stays in place for 2 to 4 weeks.

■ Otitis media

Middle ear infection is an inflammatory condition that occurs most often during childhood. Conditions that interfere with eustachian tube function predispose individuals to otitis media.

Such conditions are:
- ▲ upper respiratory tract infection;
- ▲ allergy;
- ▲ adenoid disorders;
- ▲ cleft palate.

Blockage of the eustachian tube allows oxygen in the middle ear cleft to be absorbed. This leaves a relative negative pressure or vacuum that results in transudation (movement) of fluid into the middle ear cleft.

Nose blowing and sneezing against occluded nostrils may worsen the condition and therefore should be avoided. If the fluid in the middle ear cavity remains sterile, the condition is referred to as serous otitis media and is most often of viral origin; if it becomes infected, it is called purulent otitis media and is most often of bacterial origin.

Children often experience repeated episodes of eustachian tube obstruction caused by masses of adenoids that become edematous and block the eustachian tube openings, resulting in otitis media.

The most common symptoms in the acute phase of purulent otitis media are:
- pain;
- hearing loss;
- constitutional disturbances such as fever.

Severity of symptoms increases as the condition worsens. Pain arises from the pressure of the fluids in the middle ear. This causes an outward tension on the tympanic membrane, which is innervated by sensory nerves. The rapid production of fluid and tension in a short period is responsible for the acute pain described as sharp, knife-like, and steady.

The pain usually does not increase with mastication or when traction is applied to the auricle or tragus. If patients are not treated promptly, the pressure inside the middle ear may increase, leading to distention and bulging of the tympanic membrane. As bulging increases, so does necrosis, leading to perforation and escape of purulent material from the middle ear. The condition worsens as the fluid accumulates and fills the middle ear cleft. The sensation of fullness is associated with voice resonance, a congested feeling in the ears, a hollow sound, or a popping or cracking noise in the ears especially during swallowing or yawning. The condition should promptly be treated by a physician.

■ Chronic otitis media
In chronic serous otitis media, the fluid in the middle ear may be thin and serous or thick and viscous ("glue ear").
Chronic serous otitis media occurs most often in small children.
It may be caused by inadequate treatment of previous episodes of otitis media or by recurrent upper respiratory tract infections associated with a dysfunction of the eustachian tube.
The most common symptom is impaired hearing, but the onset is often insidious, and the child may have no symptoms. Frequently, parents accuse the child of being inattentive and disobedient. Pain is usually absent. The diagnosis is performed by visual inspection of the tympanic membrane.
The tympanic membrane appears yellow to orange and lustreless, and its flexibility is lost. It is not perforated but often appears to be retracted. Often long-standing fluid becomes more and more viscous, thus the term "glue ear."
Treatment may involve evacuation of the fluid by aspiration through an incision in the tympanic membrane and implantation of a temporary, pressure-equalizing tube.
This procedure usually is performed in both ears. The pressure-equalizing tubes permit the atmospheric pressure to equalize with the middle ear, assisting in the return of normal hearing. It is not uncommon for children during the first 10 years of life to wear the tubes for 6-12 months.

■ Tympanic membrane perforation
The most common cause of traumatic perforation of the tympanic membrane are water sports, such as diving or water-skiing. Any corrosive agent introduced into the ear canal may produce tympanic membrane perfo-

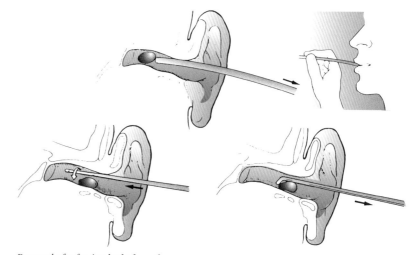
Removal of a foreign body from the ear.
Above: removal by suction. Below: removal using a hook.

ration.
Other causes of the perforation include:
▲ blows to the head with a clubbed hand;
▲ foreign objects entering the ear canal with excessive force;
▲ forceful irrigation of the ear canal.
At the moment of injury, the pain is severe, but it decreases rapidly. Hearing acuity usually diminishes. An untreated injury may lead to otitis media. Other complications may include tinnitus, nausea, and vertigo, and may progress to mastoiditis. Any patient suspected of having an acute perforated tympanic membrane should be examined thoroughly by a physician.

■ Barotrauma
Barotrauma occurs during quick descent from high altitude. The middle ear fails to ventilate, resulting in a negative pressure in the middle ear.
This negative pressure causes a suction and forces the tympanic membrane to retract, causing pain. In addition, oedema is formed, with transudation and hemorrhage into the middle ear space.
Barotrauma may also occur in individuals who fly during an upper respiratory tract infection or any condition associated with impaired eustachian tube ventilation. Upon examination, the tympanic membrane appears inflamed and retracted and is similar

to that seen with acute otitis media.
Pretreatment with antihistamines and/or decongestants may help to avoid serious symptoms during air travel for patients susceptible to barotrauma. Treatment of acute episodes consists of oral decongestants, antihistamines and autoinflation of the eustachian tube.

Class with a small group of children with hearing problems.

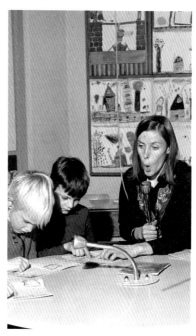

EATING DISORDERS

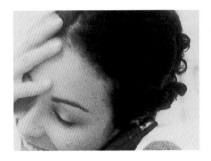

Introduction

Each year millions of people in the United States develop serious and sometimes life-threatening eating disorders. The vast majority - more than 90 percent - of those afflicted with eating disorders are adolescent and young adult women.

One reason that women in this age group are particularly vulnerable to eating disorders is their tendency to go on strict diets to achieve an "ideal" figure. Researchers have found that such stringent dieting can play a key role in triggering eating disorders.

Eating disorders are grouped into three main categories:

▲ refusing to maintain a minimally normal body weight - anorexia nervosa;
▲ bingeing and purging - bulimia nervosa;
▲ binging without purging - binge eating disorder.

Binging is the rapid consumption of large amounts of food in a short period ot time accompanied by a feeling of loss of control. Purging is selfinduced vomiting or misuse of laxatives or enemas.

Anorexia nervosa

Anorexia nervosa is a disorder of self-starvation which manifests itself in an extreme aversion to food and can cause psychological, endocrine and gynaecological problems.

It almost exclusively affects adolescent white girls, with symptoms involving a refusal to eat, large weight loss, a bizarre preoccupation with food, hyperactivity, a distorted body image and cessation of menstruation.

Although the symptoms can be corrected if the patient is diagnosed and treated in time, about 10-15 percent of anorexia patients die, usually after losing at least half their normal body weight.

Anorexia patients typically come from white, middle to upper-middle class families that place heavy emphasis on high achievement, perfection, eating patterns and physical appearance. There never has been a documented case of anorexia nervosa in a black male or female. A newly diagnosed patient often is described by her parents as a "model child," usually because she is obedient, compliant, and a good student.

Although most teenagers experience some feelings of youthful rebellion, persons with anorexia usually do not outwardly exhibit these feelings, tending instead to be childish in their thinking, in their need for parental approval, and in their lack of independence.

Psychologists theorize that the patient's desire to control her own life manifests itself in the realm of eating - the only area, in the patient's mind, where she has the ability to direct her own life.

In striving for perfection and approval, a person with anorexia may begin to diet in order to lose just a few pounds. Dieting does not stop there, however, and an abnormal concern with dieting is established. Nobody knows what triggers the disease process, but suddenly, losing five or ten pounds is not enough.

The anorexia patient becomes intent on losing weight. It is not uncommon for someone who develops this disorder to starve herself until she weighs just 60 or 70 pounds.

Throughout the starvation process she either denies being hungry or claims to feel full after eating just a few bites.

Characteristics

Most researchers agree that the number of patients with anorexia nervosa is increasing. Recent estimates suggest that out of every 200 girls in Western countries between the ages of 12 and 18, one will develop anorexia to some degree.

Therapists find that persons with anorexia usually lack self-esteem and feel they can gain admiration by losing weight and becoming thin. While most anorexia nervosa patients are female, about 6 percent are adolescent boys. Occasionally the disorder is found in older women and in children as young as eight years old.

Some researchers believe that certain characteristics are common to the families of persons who develop the disorder. Although this "typical" family model may not apply to all patients, it is common in many.

Researchers describe these families as warm and loving on the surface. Evidently, this loving atmosphere masks a series of underlying problems in which family members are excessively involved in each other's lives, and overly dependent on one another. Apparently, they often are unable to deal with conflicts within the family. Either they deny that conflicts exist, or they become so overwhelmed by numerous petty conflicts that they are unable to recognize real problems.

Symptoms

Psychological symptoms such as social withdrawal, obsessive-compulsiveness and depression often precede or accompany anorexia nervosa. The patient's distorted view of herself and the world around her are the cause of these psychological disturbances.

Distortion of body image is another prevalent symptom. While most normal females can give an accurate esti-

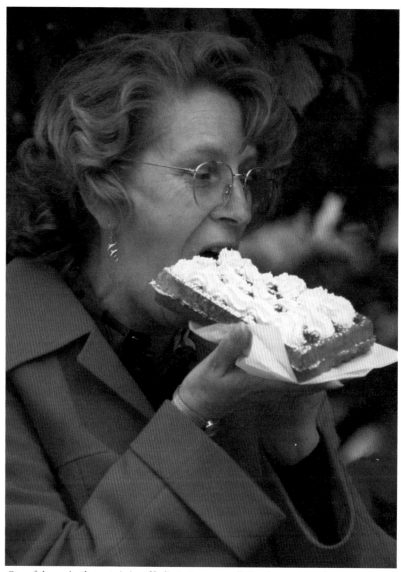

mate of their body weight, anorectic patients tend to perceive themselves as markedly larger than they really are. When questioned, most feel that their emaciated state (70-80 lbs.) is either "just right" or "too fat."

Profound physical symptoms also occur in cases of extreme starvation. These include:

- loss of head hair
- growth of fine body hair
- constipation
- intolerance of cold temperatures
- low pulse rate
- shallow breathing

Certain endocrine functions a;so become impaired. In females these result in a cessation of menstruation (amenorrhoea) and the absence of ovulation. Menstruation usually will not resume until endocrine balance is restored. Ovulation is suppressed because production of certain necessary hormones decreases.

Anorexia in boys has effects similar to those in girls; severe weight loss, psycho-social problems and interruption of normal reproductive system processes.

Causes of anorexia

While the cause of anorexia is still unknown, a combination of psychological, environmental and physiological factors are associated with development of the disorder. Researchers have discovered that a part of the brain called the hypothalamus begins to work improperly after the onset of anorexia.

The hypothalamus controls such activities as maintenance of water balance, regulation of boy temperature, secretion of the endocrine glands and sugar and fat metabolism.

In anorexia patients, this improper functioning may result in lower blood pressure and body temperature, a lack of sexual interest and hormonal changes resulting in amenorrhea and reduced production of thyroid hormone.

Some scientists are studying the possibility that abnormalities in certain endocrine functions may actually precede the onset of anorexia. Further studies are needed, however, to determine of anorexia patients have a biological predisposition to develop the illness.

One of the main characteristics of bulimia is uncontrolled and excessive eating.

Treatment

Treatment for anorexia nervosa is usually threefold, consisting of:

- nutritional therapy
- individual psychotherapy
- family counselling.

A team made up of pediatricians, psychiatrists, social workers and nurses often administers treatment. Some physicians hospitalize patients until they are nutritionally stable. Others prefer to work with patients in the family setting.

But no matter where therapy is started, the most urgent concern of the physician is getting the patient to eat and gain weight. This is accomplished by gradually adding calories to the patient's daily intake.

If she is hospitalized, privileges are sometimes granted in return for weight gain. This is known as a behavioral contract, and privileges may include such desirable activities as leaving the hospital for an afternoon's outing.

Physicians and hospital staff make every effort to ensure that the patient does not feel overwhelmed and powerless. Instead, weight gain is encour-

Goals of Treatment

▲ Eating disorder sufferers may not admit they are ill and may resist treatment. Early diagnosis and a comprehensive treatment program are essential to recovery. Some patients may need immediate hospitalization.

▲ For anorexia, treatment usually follows 3 established steps:
  • weight restoration
  • treatment of accompanying psychological disturbances
  • achieving long-term remission or recovery

▲ Medications may be helpful in treating undelying depression or anxiety.

▲ Families are sometimes involved in the therapeutic process.

▲ Normal body weight
▲ Consequences of potassium depletion
  • Weakness
  • Cardiac arrythmia
  • Kidney impairment
▲ Other consequences
  • Swollen parotid glands
  • Pitted teeth

Bingeing (rapidly and quickly consuming relatively large amounts of food while feeling a loss of control (is followed by intense distress as well as by purging, rigorous dieting, and excessive exercising.

Many differences in symptoms are apparent between anorectics and bulimics. Anorexia nervosa patients are not obese before onset of their illness. Typically, they are good student who become socially withdrawn before becoming ill and often come from families who fit the anorexia prototype described above.

Bulimics, on the other hand, usually are extroverted before their illness, are inclined to be overweight, have voracious appetites and have episodes of binge eating. Anorexia patients often have a better chance of returning to normal weight because their eating patterns, unlike the of bulimics, have been altered for a relatively short time.

aged in an atmosphere in which the patient feels in control of her situation, and in which she wants to gain weight.

Individual psychotherapy is necessary in the treatment of anorexia to help the patient understand the disease process and its effects. Therapy focuses on the patient's relationship with her family and friends, and the reasons she may have fallen into a pattern of self-starvation. As a patient begins to learn more about her condition, she is often more willing to try to help herself recover.

In cases of severe depression, drugs such as antidepressants are part of the therapy. Behavior improvement generally occurs rapidly in these cases and the patient is able to respond more quickly to treatment. The third aspect of treatment, family therapy, is supportive in nature. It examines how the patient and her parents relate to each other.

Persons with anorexia often become a source of family tension because refusals to eat cause frustration in the parents. The goal of family therapy is to help family members relate more effectively to one another, to encourage more mature thinking in the anorectic patient and to help all family members work together for the well-being of the patient and the family unit.

In treating anorexia, it is extremely important to remember that immediate success does not guarantee a permanent cure. Sometimes, even after successful hospital treatment and return to a normal weight, patients suffer relapses. Follow-up therapy lasting three to five years is recommended if the patient is to be completely cured.

Bulimia nervosa

The term bulimia refers to episodes of uncontrolled and excessive eating, sometimes called binge eating. The symptoms of bulimia sometimes occur in anorexia nervosa.

Bulimia nervosa is a disorder characterized by repeated episodes of binge eating followed by purging (well-induced vomiting or taking laxatives, diuretics, or both) rigorous dieting, or excessive exercising to counteract the effects of bingeing.

Patient with bulimnia indulge in "food binges," and then purge themselves through vomiting immediately after eating or through the use of laxatives or diuretics. While on the surface these patients may appear to be well adjusted socially, this serious disease is particularly hard to overcome because it usually has been a pattern of behavior for a long time.

Characteristics

The major clinical features of bulimia are
▲ Excessive concern with shape and weight
▲ Binge eating
▲ Behavior to prevent weight gain
  • Dietary restraint
  • Self-induced vomiting
  • Excessive exercise
  • Purging

Treatment

A doctor suspects bulimia nervosa if a person is overly concerned about weight gain and has wide fluctuations in weight, especially with evidence of excessive laxative use. Other clues include swollen salivary glands in the cheeks, scars on the knuckles from using the fingers to induce vomiting, erosion of tooth enamel from stomach acid, and a low level of potassium detected in a blood test. The diagnosis is not confirmed until the person describes bingepurge behavior.

The two approaches to treatment are psychotherapy and drugs. Psychotherapy, generally best conducted by a therapist with experience in eating disorders, may be very effective. An antidepressive drug often can help control bulimia nervosa, even when a person is not obviously depressed, but the disorder may return after the drug is discontinued. Most of the treatment aspects of anorexia also apply to bulimia. The usual treatment is a form of cognitive behavior therapy designed to reduce dietary restraint and to increase control over eating and vomiting.

Patients are encouraged to keep records of their food intake and episodes of vomiting, and to identify and avoid any emotional changes that regularly provoke episodes of bulimia. It has been reported that antidepressant medication benefits non-depressed patients with bulimia nervosa, but until the evidence is stronger such medication is better for patients with an associated depressive disorder.

Binge eating disorder

In this disorder, bingeing contributes to excessive caloric intake and consequent weight gain. Unlike bulimia nervosa, binge eating disorder occurs most commonly in people who are obese and becomes more prevalent with increasing body weight. People who have binge eating disorder tend to be older than those having anorexia nervosa or bulimia nervosa, and more (nearly half) are men.

The foods that binge eaters typically choose (binge foods) are high in calories (for example, cake and ice cream), and binges usually occur in secrecy. They eat large quantities of food and do not stop until they are uncomfortably full. People who have binge eating disorder are distressed by it, and about 50 percent of obese binge eaters are depressed.

Although this disorder does not cause the physical problems that can occur with bulimia nervosa, it may lead to complications of obesity. Usually, they have more difficulty losing weight and keeping it off than do people with other serious weight problems.

Treatment

Behavior therapy, as it is used to treat obesity, may be the best treatment for binge eating disorder. Behavior therapy has been shown to reduce body weight and the frequency of bingeing, even when no special attention is given to binge eating. Cognitive-behavior therapy markedly reduces the frequency of bingeing as well, but without reducing body weight.

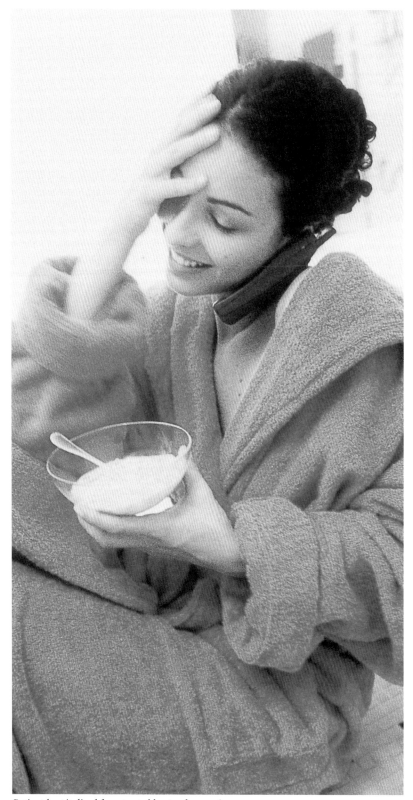

Patient hospitalized for repeated bouts of anorexia nervosa.

ECZEMA

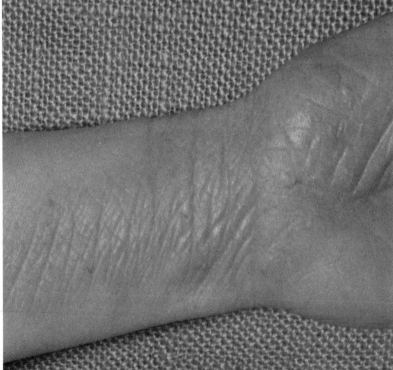

Introduction

Disorders and diseases of the skin are so varied and so common that dermatology is a specialty in the practice of medicine.

The most remarkable fact about this field of medicine is how much there remains to be learned about it.

More than 95 per cent of all skin diseases and disorders are among the following ailments: acne, eczema, infections, psoriasi, tumors.

Eczema is a collective term for many inflammatory conditions of the skin. The term *dermatitis* is often used as a synonym for eczema, although in fact "dermatitis" means any inflammation of the skin. All eczemas are forms of dermatitis, but dermatitis is not always eczema; for example, common sunburn is dermatitis but not eczema. An eczema causes one or more of the following physical changes to the skin:

▲ erythema (blood congestion);
▲ infiltration of plasma into the tissues;
▲ vesicles (blisters);

▲ papules (pimples).

Secondary changes include:

▲ erosion of tissue;
▲ exudation of fluid on the skin;
▲ crusts;
▲ lichenification (thickened areas of itchy skin);
▲ scaling.

The eczemas commonly show rapid changes in the clinical features and striking differences between different sites.

Causes

Contact dermatitis, due to contact with chemical agents, constitutes a group for which the cause is known. Scratching and stasis (sluggish blood in the veins) are other causes, but in many cases the reasons for eczema are obscure.

In all types of eczematous dermatitis, including contact dermatitis, many factors may exist that predispose, trigger or aggravate the condition. Microorganisms (bacteria and fungi) may play an important role in the genesis of many of the eczemas.

Fungal infections often produce a reaction that is probably due to an allergic response to metabolites of the fungi. Remote allergic reactions also occur.

Dermatitis can become secondarily infected with disease-causing bacteria, and the risk is greatest when the skin is scratched or when blisters have burst, the protective barrier then being completely broken down.

Atopic eczema

Atopic eczema, which tends to run in families together with hay fever and asthma, is usually seen on the elbows

Chronic eczema disorder followed by lichenification.

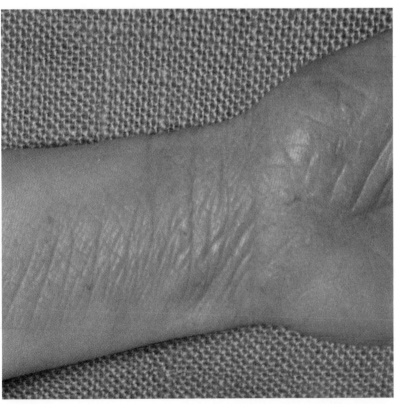

and knees as well as on areas such as the fronts of the ankles, the backs of the forearms just below the elbows and the upper eyelids.

It often begins on the face in infants only a few months old. It is a common form of eczema in childhood and may persist into adult life, although every year that passes increases its chances of disappearing.

More rarely, the condition can develop for the first time in older children or adults; the hands may become involved in young adults. Older children who still have atopic eczema should think carefully about which jobs they take up, so that they can try to avoid any substances that might aggravate the condition.

Seborrheic eczema

This condition is common in mild form in adults of every age and sometimes also occurs in children.

It affects a few individuals more severely. In its mild form, it leads to liberal scaling in the eyebrows, in the ears, in the folds of the skin around the nose and in the groin and on the chest and back.

In severe cases the facial rash may become more extensive, or the armpits and all of the groin may become involved. It tends to run a chronic, mild, fluctuating course. Its cause is essentially unknown.

Stasis eczema

Stasis or varicose eczema - due to an impaired flow of blood in the veins - has become less common in recent years as improved medical care has decreased the number of people with untreated varicose vein problems.

Its pattern is perhaps the easiest of all to recognize, primarily involving the lower third of the leg. It is important to realize that all eczema has a tendency to spread beyond its original site, however, and widespread unclassified eczema may sometimes be mainly due to stasis.

Another important point about stasis eczema is that people who suffer from it tend to take large numbers of prescribed and nonprescribed drugs,

Causes of contact eczema

Cosmetics
- hair-removing chemicals
- nail polish
- nail polish remover
- deodorants
- moisturizer
- after shave lotions
- perfumes
- sunscreens

also: nickel in jewelry

Plants
- poison ivy
- poison oak
- poison sumach

- ragweed
- primrose

Drugs in skin creams
- penicillin
- sulphonamide
- neomycin
- antihistamines
- antiseptics
- stabilizers

Chemicals used in clothing manufacture
- tanning agents in shoes
- rubber accelerators
- antioxidants in gloves

some of which can induce allergic reactions.

Discoid eczema

Discoid or mummular eczema is probably the most poorly understood eczema of all. It is recognized by the presence of multiple coin-shaped patches of eczema that tend to favour the surfaces of the limbs, including the hands and feet, but can become widespread.

It is commoner in the over-40s than the younger age groups. It sometimes lasts for a matter of weeks but frequently becomes chronic. Usually no discernable cause can be found for it.

Contact eczema

This type of eczema is due to substances in contact with the surface of the skin. Contact factors capable of inducing eczema enter the skin from the outside and produce damage within it. They can be divided into contact irritants and contact sensitizers.

Contact irritants damage the skin by a direct chemical effect: acids, alkalis and organic solvents are familiar examples. They are frequently encountered at work, but in many cases the cause is unknown.

Contact sensitization form a signifi-

cant minority of occupational eczemas. Common occupational contact sensitizers are:
- chromate in cement;
- epoxy resins in additives;
- chemical additives in rubber.

Other domestic contact sensitizers are plants such as primula and chrysanthemum, dyes in clothing materials, resin in nail varnish and nickel found in zips, coins and much "gold" jewellery.

Contact eczema is often hard to distinguish from the various forms of endogenous eczema (i.e., eczema resulting from some process within the body), particularly when it affects the hands.

Treatment

Eczema can usually be controlled by a judicious combination of emollients and steroids applied to the skin, with the occasional use of antibiotics either taken by mouth or on the skin. Emollients are particularly useful for those with atopic eczema.

In the acute stage of eczema, all that may be useful to apply are soothing and cooling creams, ointments or liquids.

A fluorinated steroid cream or ointment becomes effective as soon as the acute stage has settled but should be substituted, after a few days, by a more diluted preparation.

ENDOCRINE GLAND DISORDERS

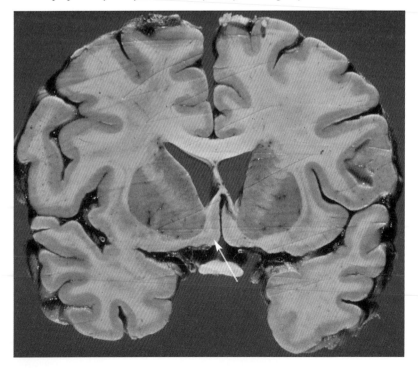

E

Introduction

The endocrine system consists of glands or parts of glands whose secretions (called hormones) are distributed in the human body by means of the bloodstream rather than being discharged through ducts. The glandular tissues of the endocrine system have in common that they secrete into the bloodstream "chemical messengers" that regulate and integrate body functions.

One of the characteristics of the endocrine glands is their wanderlust, their tendency to leave their source and look for work elsewhere. The human embryo develops gills like those of primitive fishes, but parts of these turn into endocrine glands and leave their birthplace at the sides of the throat in the course of their embryonic development.

The pituitary gland, the thyroid, the parathyroids and the thymus develop in part from these primitive gills. The two adrenal glands do not migrate far. They form in the peritoneum of the abdomen and then settle on top of the kidneys. A group of cells from the neighboring sympathetic nervous system migrates into the adrenal glands and forms a core there. Thus the adrenal glands become double organs, with a nervous core or marrow and a glandular cortex or bark.

The cortex produces a series of steroids, the corticosteroids, which have wide-ranging effects. The core functions in conjunction with the sympathetic nervous system, regulating the blood pressure, the heart action and other activities of the body, through the secretion of adrenalin and noradrenaline.

Another double organ is the pancreas. Its ordinary glandular tissue produces the various digestive enzymes that serve to open the molecular chains of proteins, carbohydrates, and fats. In this digestive gland there settled an endocrine gland in the form of little islands of tissue that fabricate the hormones insulin and glucagon.

Similar double organs are the sex glands. These produce the germinating cells, the sperm cells in the man and the egg cells (ova) in a woman; they also produce sex hormones that flow through the blood and give rise to such secondary traits as the beard of the male and the breasts of the female.

One gland, the pituitary or hypophysis, hangs under the brain like a fire bell, serving to regulate all the endocrine glands. An outstanding example of the transformation of an old organ is the pineal body or epiphysis. Among the ancestors of man there must have been a reptile that spent its days lying lazy in the mud of primordial swamps, looking toward the sky through a third eye that developed out of the midbrain.

Only some reptiles of an almost vanished prehistoric past around Australia still possess faint remnants of such an eye. In man this remnant has been transformed into a small cone-shaped body on the roof of the brain, the pineal body.

Its function in man is unknown; some

Microscopic picture of cells of the endocrine system synthesizing enzymes.

believe it is merely investigial while others believe that it is an endocrine gland whose secretions affect the gonads either directly or via the anterior part of the pituitary gland.

Hormones

A hormone is a complex chemical product produced and secreted by endocrine (ductless) glands that ravels through the bloodstream and controls and regulates the
activity of another organs or groups of cells - its target organ.
For instance, growth hormone released by the pituitary body controls the growth of long bones in the body. Hormones are produced and released by the endocrine system.
This is a network of endocrine glands of the following organs: pituitary gland or body, hypothalamus, thyroid, thymus, parathyroids, adrenal medulla, adrenal cortex, islets of Langerhans in the pancreas, gonads, thymus, pineal gland or epiphysis and groups of cells in the stomach and intestines.
Along with the nervous system, the endocrine system coordinates and regulates many of the activities in the body, including growth, metabolism, sexual development,
and reproduction.
The hormones perform three basic functions:
▲ hormones enable and promote physical, sexual and mental development;
▲ hormones enable and promote the adjustment of performance level; the ability of organs and organ systems to modify their activity to meet the demands made upon hem is lost in the absence of certain hormones;
▲ hormones are necessary to keep certain physiological parameters constant (e.g., osmotic pressure and the blood glucose level). These hormones have a homeostatic function.
Hormones are effective in very low concentrations. They do not serve as a substrate for the biochemical processes they "control". In some cases (e.g., ADH, adrenalin) the response of the target organ has a more or less strict

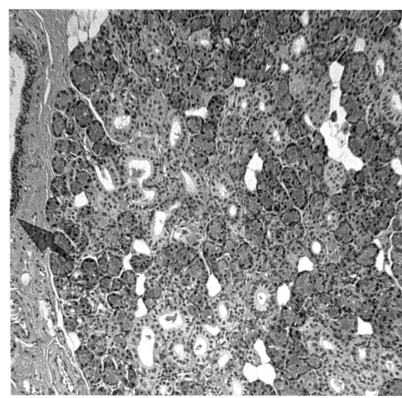

Frontal section of the brain showing the location of the hypothalamus (arrow), regulator of the endocrine system in the body.

quantitative relation to the concentration of the hormone in the blood. In cybernetic terminology these hormones can be called "information carriers" - a situation than emphasizes the above-mentioned analogy to the nervous system.

The pituitary gland

The hypophysis or pituitary gland is the master gland of the body. Compared with other endocrine glands, it produces the largest number of hormones, including some that control the other endocrine glands of the body.
If the pituitary gland is the master, the hypothalamus may be regarded as the supermaster gland. This explains that many changes in the function of the brain lead to alterations in function of the endocrine glands, showing a close relationship between endocrine and neural regulation of many organs and tissues.

It appears that virtually all substances produced by the hypothalamus and the pituitary gland are secreted in a pulse-like or burst-like fashion, some of the hormones have definite circadian or diurnal rhythmicity with increased secretion during specific hours of the day; other hormones have still longer ultradian rhythms. The pituitary consists of three parts: the anterior, middle and posterior pituitary.

Anterior pituitary
Under the microscope the anterior pituitary is seen to be made up of nests of cells separated by blood vessels and connective tissue. The cells are of three sorts: acidophil (taking up, and thus stained by acid dyes); basophil (stained by basic days) and chromophobe (without special affinity for dyes). Usually these stain red, blue and grey respectively.
The acidophil cells produce growth hormone and also a hormone which stimulates milk production in preg-

Endocrine gland disorders   Questions & Answers

What is the endocrine system?
The endocrine system consists of glands or parts of glands whose secretions (called hormones) are distributed in the human body by means of the bloodstream rather than being discharged through ducts. The glandular tissues of the endocrine system have in common that they secrete into the bloodstream "chemical messengers" that regulate and integrate body functions.

What is a hormone?
A hormone is a complex chemical product produced and secreted by endocrine (ductess) glands that ravels through the bloodstream and controls and regulates the activity of another organs or groups of cells - its target organ. For instance, growth hormone released by the pituitary body controls the growth of long bones in the body.

What types of organs produce hormones?
Hormones are produced and released by the endocrine system. This is a network of endocrine glands of the following organs:
• pituitary gland
• hypothalamus
• thyroid
• thymus
• parathyroids
• adrenal medulla
• adrenal cortex
• islets of Langerhans in the pancreas
• gonads
• thymus
• pineal gland or epiphysis
• groups of cells in the stomach and intestines.

What is the major function of the endocrine system?
Along with the nervous system, the endocrine system coordinates and regulates many of the activities in the body, including growth, metabolism, sexual development, and reproduction.

What is the relationship of the endocrine system to the human life cycle?
Unlike the heart or skin or stomach, the hormonal glands do not work in the same way from the birth of the body to its death. The life of man has three divisions.
▲ The first part is childhood, during which he grows; in this period the growth hormone from the pituitary is particularly active, while the gonads or sex glands are at rest.
▲ Then comes puberty, so called from the pubes, the hair around the genitals. This hair appears only after the gonads begin to work, and they start only after the growth hormone is slowing down and the body has grown to a certain size.
▲ In the third division of life, some thirty to forty years after the onset of the function of the gonads, these latter glands usually begin to wither. A woman's menstruation ends and with it her fertility; the man may loose part of his potency.

How important are the endocrine glands for human life?
The endocrine glands and their hormones determine part of the fate of man. A child with an underactive thyroid gland remains stunted physiologically, a cretin is mentally and sluggish in temperament. The endocrine glands may well be called the glands of our destiny.

What is the specific definition of a hormone?
The difficulty in formulating a precise definition of the term "hormone" is particularly well illustrated by the catecholamines noradrenalin and adrenalin. When their production in and release from the adrenal medulla is being considered adrenalin and noradrenaline are usually called hormones, but in their role as signal mediators at the sympathetic nerve endings they are called "transmitter substances." The hormone concept has become even more vague since it has been realized that the so-called regulatory hypothalamic hormones act not only as hormones in the strict sense but also have what appears to be a transmitter function or a modulating influence on the function of other transmitter systems.

What are the basic functions of hormones?
The hormones perform three basic functions:
▲ hormones enable and promote physical, sexual and mental development;
▲ hormones enable and promote the adjustment of performance level; the ability of organs and organ systems to modify their activity to meet the demands made upon them is lost in the absence of certain hormones;
▲ hormones are necessary to keep certain physiological parameters constant (e.g., osmotic pressure and the blood glucose level). These hormones have a homeostatic function.

What is the significance of hormones as information carriers?
Hormones are effective in very low concentrations. They do not serve as a substrate for the biochemical processes they "control". In some cases (e.g., ADH, adrenalin) the response of the target organ has a more or less strict quantitative relation to the concentration of the hormone in the blood. In cybernetic terminology these hormones can be called "information carriers" - a situation than emphasizes the above-mentioned analogy to the nervous system.

How do hormones regulate bodily functions?
When considering hormones as elements in regulating systems, it is useful to divide them into two classes. In one group, which includes adrenaline, noradrenaline, ADH and others, the rate of secretion and the blood concentration undergo wide fluctuations; the rate of secretion is adjusted to the changing situation. The most typical example of the second group is thyroxin; the blood concentration of this hormone is normally kept constant.

Anterior pituitary

Location
Base of the brain
Hormone
Growth hormone (STH)
Normal function
Affects skeletal growth, protein synthesis, blood glucose concentration
Excess secretion
Gigantism, acromegaly
Diminished secretion
Dwarfism
Hormone
Trophic hormones such as
- TSH: stimulates thyroid
- ACTH: stimulates adrenal cortex
- FSH: stimulates ovarian follicles, testes
- LH: stimulates gonads
Normal function
Stimulates target endocrine gland and is regulated by feedback mechanisms
Excess secretion
Oversecretion of hormones by the target glands
Diminished secretion
Undersecretion of hormones by target glands

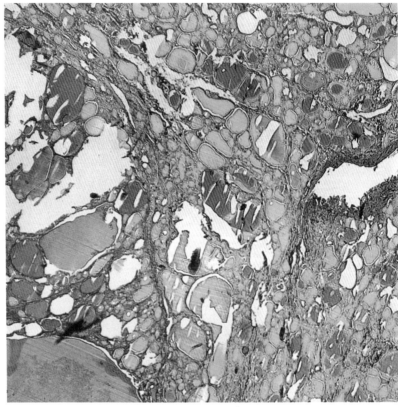

Microscopic picture of endocrine cells of the pituitary body.

nancy. The basophils secrete hormones which stimulate the thyroid, adrenal cortex, ovaries and testes. Some chromophobes secrete hormones while some are probably inactive forms of other cell types. The hormones are usually known by their abbreviated names: there is ACTH (adrenocorticotroop hormone), which stimulates the functioning of the adrenal cortex.

The anterior pituitary also secretes a hormone known as TSH (thyroid stimulating hormone). All these hormones are secreted upon the release of hormonelike substances from the hypothalamus, an important part of the brain involved in the regulation of autonomic and vital functions of the body. The activating substances of the hypothalamus reach the anterior pituitary via an intricate network of blood vessels.

One of the most important hormones manufactured by the anterior pituitary is a growth hormone. If too much of this is produced by the pitu-

itary, a growing child becomes a giant. If not enough growth hormone is produced, the child will become a midget.

In rare cases the pituitary begins oversecreting growth hormone after the end of childhood; when this happens the bones of the hands, feet and chin continue to grow until they become abnormally large and produce a condition known as acromegaly. Disorders of the anterior pituitary may be associated either with under- or oversecretion of its trophic (also called tropic) hormones. Underactivity of the gland diminishes the activity of the target organs and may lead to underactivity of the thyroid gland (hypothyroidism), failure of the gonadal glands and, in children, dwarfism.

The onset of the symptoms and signs of underactivity of the anterior pituitary (hypopituitarism) is most often insidious and may not be recognized as abnormal by the patient but occasionally may be sudden or dramatic.

Posterior pituitary

Location
Base of the brain
Hormone
Vasopressin
Normal function
Control of blood pressure; reabsorption of water by kidney tubules
Excess secretion
Increased blood pressure; glycogen converted to glucose
Diminished secretion
Decreased blood pressure; excess sugar changed to fat; kidney tubules not reabsorbing water
Hormone
Oxytocin
Normal function
Contractions of the uterus
Excess secretion
-
Diminished secretion
Disturbance of tone of uterine muscles

Thyroid

Location
Two lobes on either side of the larynx (voice box)
Hormone
- Thyroxin
- Triiodothyronine
Normal function
Controls rate of oxidation in cells
Excess secretion
Increased oxidation; increased irritability; nervousness; exophthalmus; goitre
Diminished secretion
- In a child: cretinism
- In an adult: myxoedemic goitre

Treatment is directed toward replacing the hormones of the hypofunctioning target organs. When the condition is due to a tumor, specific treatment will be directed to the tumor as well. Many cases of pituitary disorder are caused by tumors, some of which erode part of the base of the skull and press on neighbouring parts, especially the optic tract system, hypothalamus and other brain structures. In this way visual disturbances and other brain disorders arise.

A curious condition may occur when the production of prolactin is disturbed. In such cases galactorrhoea may develop, which means lactation in men, or in women who are not breast-feeding a infant. In both sexes, a tumor secreting prolactin is the cause. The treatment will be in the

Parathyroids

Hormone
Parahormone
Normal function
Regulates amount of calcium and phosp-hate in blood; some influence on irritability of nerve cells and muscle fibers
Excess secretion
Trembling due to lack of muscular control
Diminished secretion
Contractions of muscles (tetany)

hands of a team of specialists in an university hospital.

Posterior pituitary

The posterior part of the pituitary is really an extension of the brain, unlike the anterior part which is derived from the palate of the embryo. It contains nerve fibers, connective tissue and blood vessels. The hormones are produced in the adjoining hypothalamus and are passed along nerve fibers in the stalk of the gland to be stored in the posterior pituitary.

Disorders of the posterior pituitary may lead to diabetes insipidus, a disturbance of the antidiuretic hormone (ADH). Diabetes insipidus is an uncommon metabolic disorder (a rare condition accounting for about 1 per 10,000 known as acromegaly).

Thyroid gland

The first organ recognized as an endocrine gland was the thyroid. It consists of two bodies like small walnuts; they are connected by an isthmus beside the larynx (voice box). It is the most conspicuous of the endocrine glands because it is directly under the skin and can be felt by touch when it becomes enlarged. See Thyroid disorders.

Parathyroid glands

The parathyroids are four small glands attached to the thyroid gland, which act to maintain normal levels of calcium and phosphate in the blood and thus normal function of muscles and nerves.

The parathyroid hormones parahormone (consisting of 84 amino acids), calcitonin, and vitamin D (by some also considered as a hormone) are considered the principal regulators of calcium and phosphorus homeostasis. The most important actions of parahormone are:

▲ rapid mobilization of calcium and phosphate from bone and the long-term acceleration of bone resorption;
▲ increase in reabsorption of calcium in the tubules of the kidney;
▲ increase in absorption of calcium

in the intestines;
▲ decrease in reabsorption of phosphate in the tubules of the kidney.

Hyperparathyroidism

Overactivity of the parathyroids may be caused by hormone-producing tumors of the glands (primary hyperparathyroidism) or for some unknown reason (secondary parathyroidism).

Lesser degrees of increase in calcium in the blood are without symptoms, moderate elevations lead to chronic illness associated with the following symptoms:
· weakness
· lassitude
· depressed mood
· nausea and vomiting
· symptoms of a peptic ulcer
· constipation
· occasionally thirst

Mobilization of calcium from the bones may lead to the formation of cysts in the bowel and "spontaneous" fractures. Deposition of calcium in the tissues may affect the cornea and joints and may also lead to the formation of kidney stones. The treatment of primary hyperparathyroidism is surgical removal of the tumor which is usually responsible for the disease.

Hypoparathyroidism

A decrease in the function of the parathyroid glands (hypoparathyroidism) most commonly results from injury or disturbance in blood supply during operations for removal of the thyroid gland.

The symptoms of tetany are the best known manifestations of the illness. The sensory symptoms are usually the first to appear, consisting of abnormal sensations such as tingling or pins and needles, but also numbness.

The motor symptoms may vary from muscle cramps with occasional twitching, problems with swallowing and speech disorders. Epilepsy may also occur. Recovery of function usually occurs and the symptoms of the illness disappear spontaneously within a few months after operation but may occur later.

Other cases, those occurring in children, have no known cause. Some may be defective due to development of the glands. Others are probably due to an autoimmune disorder. The object of treatment is to restore the concentration of calcium in the blood to normal.

Thymus

The thymus has been long a mystery; it has not yet been shown to secrete a hormone but it nevertheless exerts a powerful influence on the whole body, especially in the early part of life.

It is a fatty bilobate gland at the root of the neck and in the front part of the chest. Its outer part contains millions of dividing lymphocytes (a kind of white blood cell) while the inner zone contains primitive cells.

It is known to be large in infancy and then to diminish steadily until a remnant remains in adults. It has now been demonstrated that the thymus is necessary in the late stages of embryonic development and in early infancy to develop the immunity mechanisms.

The thymus is of utmost importance in the body's defences against infection, for in the first few weeks of life the lymphocytes produced in it migrate into the bloodstream and colonize lymph nodes all over the body. Lymphocytes manufacture antibodies and are vital for immunity.

If the thymus of newborn animals is damaged, there is a marked stunting of growth, development is retarded and there is a great susceptibility to infections - due to the reduction of the number of lymphocytes and impairment of antibody formation.

The reduced resistance to infection which is brought about by corticosteroid treatment is paralleled by a shrinkage of the thymus and lymphoid tissue generally. This will lead ultimately to a lowered capacity for antibody formation.

Pancreas

The islets of the pancreas are marked by the wanderlust of the endocrine glands. Early in evolution, hormonal tissues immigrated in small groups into the big digestive gland behind the stomach.

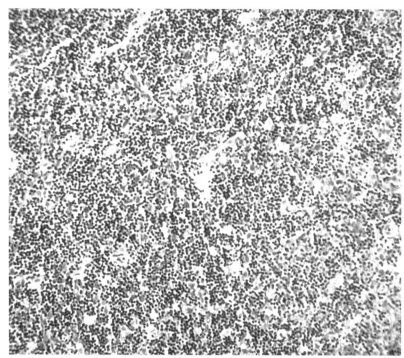
Microscopic picture of cells in the thymus.

There they became islets of hormonal tissue producing insulin and glucagon. The alpha cells of the islets secrete glucagon, which raises the blood glucose level by stimulating the breakdown of liver glycogen.

The function of glucagon in the body is uncertain, but it is of minor importance compared with insulin, that is produced and released by the beta cells.

Insulin controls the burning of sugar in the cells for the production of energy. How it does this is not completely known but it is believed that it permits sugar to pass through the walls of the cells so that it can undergo metabolism inside the cell.

Adrenal glands

The suprarenal or adrenal glands, each perched over one of the kidneys, are double glands. The yellow-brown triangular glands lie close to the upper end of the kidneys alongside the vertebral column (spine). Like all endocrine glands they have a rich blood supply. See Adrenal gland disorders

The four parathyroid glands (3) are attached to the thyroid gland (2) lying in the neck region close to the trachea (4) and esophagus (1).

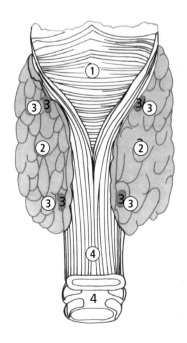

EPILEPSY

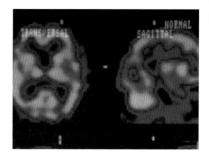

Description

Epilepsy is not a kind of insanity; only a small percentage of affected people suffer brain damage and deterioration. Epileptics are not, contrary to common belief in the past, inferior people, nor are epileptics particularly superior, even though a number of exceptional people have had epilepsy, including Socrates, Julius Caesar, Napoleon, Paganini, Peter the Great, Lord Byron, Dostojevsky, Flaubert, and many others.

Neurologist examining the scans of a patient with severe epileptic attacks.

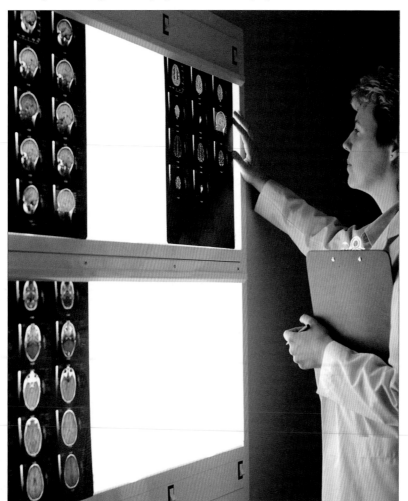

Epilepsy is defined as a recurrent paroxysmal disorder of brain function characterized by sudden, brief attacks of altered consciousness, motor activity, sensory phenomena, or inappropriate behavior.

Convulsive seizures, the most common form of an attack, begin with loss of consciousness and motor control, and tonic and clonic jerking of all extremities, but any recurrent seizure pattern may be termed epilepsy.

Causes

Epilepsy may be classified as idiopathic or symptomatic. Idiopathic means of unknown origin. No obvious cause can be found in about 70 per cent of adults and a smaller percentage of children under age 3 years. Some authorities believe that idiopathic epilepsy is due to a microscopic scar in the brain resulting from birth trauma or other injury, and, indeed, many patients classed during life as idiopathic show evidence of a causative lesion at autopsy. However, it is more likely that unexplained, predominantly inherited metabolic abnormalities underlie most idiopathic cases. Idiopathic epilepsy generally begins between ages 2 and 14. Seizures before age 2 are usually related to developmental defects, birth injuries, or a metabolic disease affecting the brain; those beginning after age 25 are usually secondary to brain trauma, tumors, or other organic brain diseases.

Convulsive seizures may be associated with a variety of brain or systemic disorders, as a result of focal or generalized disturbance of cortical function. The major causes of seizures are listed in the table. The seizures are only transient in many of these conditions and do not recur once the illness ends.

Symptoms and signs

Epilepsy affects about 1.5 per cent of the population; chronically recurring seizures are perhaps 25 per cent that frequent.

Most patients have only one type of seizure; about 30 per cent have two or more types. About 90 per cent experience grand mal seizures, either alone (60 per cent) or in combination with other seizures (30 per cent). Absence (petit mal) attacks occur in about 25 per cent. Psychomotor attacks occur in about 18 per cent.

Partial seizures begin focally with a specific sensory, motor, or psychic aberration that reflects the affected part of the brain hemispheres where the seizure originates. Aura are focal manifestations that immediately precede generalized convulsions and that also reflect where the seizure begins. Sometimes a focal lesion of the hemispheres activates deeper parts of the brain so rapidly that it produces a generalized grand mal seizure before any focal sign appears.

Generalized seizures usually affect both consciousness and motor function from the onset. The seizure itself is initiated in the deeper part of the brain and frequently has a genetic or metabolic cause.

■ Partial seizures

Common manifestations of partial or focal lesions are dependent on the site of dysfunction; they include:
- localized twitching of muscles;
- localized numbness or tingling;
- chewing movements or smacking of lips;
- olfactory hallucinations;
- visual hallucinations (formed images);
- visual disorders (flashes of light);
- complex autonomic behaviorism.

Most partial lesions are characterized by a variety of patterns of onset. In most instances, the patient has a 1- to 2-minute loss of contact with the surroundings. The patient at first may stagger, perform autonomic purposeless movements, and utter unintelligible sounds.

He does not understand what is said and may resist aid. mental confusion continues for another 1 or 2 minutes after the attack is apparently over.

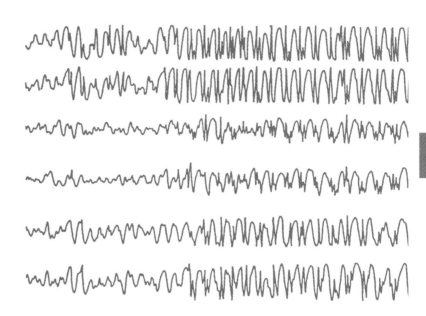

Characteristic electrical activity of the brain during an epileptic seizure of the petit mal type.

An eight-channel recording of a person with marked epileptic seizures.

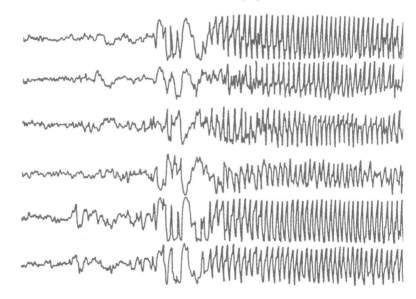

■ Generalized seizures

These can be minor or major in their manifestations. Absence (petit mal) attacks are brief generalized seizures manifested by a 10- to 30-second loss of consciousness, with eye or muscle flutterings at a rate of 3 per second, and with or without loss of muscle tone. The patient suddenly stops any activity in which he is engaged and resumes it after the attack. Petit mal seizures are genetically determined and occur predominantly in children; they never begin after age 20.

The attacks are likely to occur several or many times a day, often when the

E

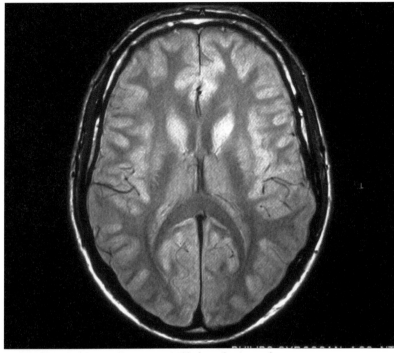

Brain section showing small scars responsible for epileptic attacks.

Causes of seizures

Increase in body temperature
- acute infection
- heat stroke

Central nervous system infections
- meningitis
- encephalitis
- brain abscess
- syphilis
- rabies
- tetanus
- some forms of malaria
- toxoplasmosis

Metabolic disturbances
- low glucose blood content
- phenylketonuria

Toxic agents
- camphor
- pentylenetetrazol
- strychnine
- picrotoxin
- lead
- alcohol

Lack of brain oxygen
- anesthesia
- carbon monoxide poisoning
- breath-holding

Brain defects
- congenital
- developmental

Cerebral swelling
- hypertension
- eclampsia

Brain trauma
- skull fracture
- birth injury

Withdrawal syndromes
- alcohol
- hypnotic drugs
- tranquillizers

patient is sitting quietly. They are infrequent during exercise. petit mal attacks rarely indicate gross brain damage, and many patients are highly intelligent.

Infantile spasms are characterized by sudden flexion of the arms, forward flexion of the trunk, and extension of the legs.

The attacks last only a few seconds but may be repeated many times a day. They are restricted to the first three years of life, often to be replaced by other forms of attack. Brain damage is usually evident.

Grand-mal seizures occasionally begin with a sinking or rising sensation in the upper part of the abdomen (the aura) followed by an outcry.

The seizure continues with loss of consciousness; falling, and tonic, then clonic, contractions of the muscles of the extremities, trunk, and head. Urinary and faecal incontinence may occur. The attacks usually last two to five minutes.

It may be preceded by a prodromal mood change, and may be followed by a state with deep sleep, headache, muscle soreness or, at times, focal motor or sensory phenomena. The attacks may appear at any age.

Prognosis

Drug therapy can completely control grand mal seizures in more than 60 per cent of cases and greatly reduce the frequency in seizures in another 30 per cent; can control petit mal seizures in 50 per cent and reduce the frequency in 40 per cent, and can control psychomotor attacks in 35 per cent and reduce its frequency in 55 per cent. Newer anticonvulsant agents promise to improve these results even more.

Most patients with epilepsy are normal between attacks, although overuse of anticonvulsants can dull alertness.

Progressive mental deterioration is usually related to an accompanying neurologic disease that itself caused the seizures.

The outlook is better when no brain lesion is demonstrable. About 75 per cent of non-institutionalized patients with epilepsy are mentally normal. 15

per cent show a slight reduction in intellect, and 10 per cent have a moderate to pronounced impairment.

Management and treatment

In idiopathic epilepsy, treatment is prima-rily control of seizures. In symptomatic epilepsy, the associated disease musty be treated as well. Continued anticonvulsant treatment is usually needed in those cases that a brain lesion had to be removed surgically.

A normal life will be encouraged. Moderate exercise is recommended; such sports as swimming and horseback riding are permitted with proper safeguards.

Members of the family will be taught a common sense attitude toward the patient's illness.

Instead of overprotection and oversolicitude, sympathetic support will be directed against feelings of inferiority, self-consciousness, and other emotional handicaps, and emphasis placed on preventing invalidism.

Institutional care is advisable only for patients with severe mental retardation or with attacks that are frequent, violent, and not controlled by medication.

New drugs are available for previously intractable seizure types, and the widespre-ad availability of accurate estimations of drug levels has made clinical management more secure and effective. No single drug controls all types of seizures, and diffe-rent drugs are required for different pa-tients. Furthermore, some patients may require several drugs.

For the newly diagnosed patient with a seizure disorder, the single first drug of choice for the particular type of epilepsy is selected, starting with relatively low doses and increasing over a week or so to the standard therapeutic dose.

After about a week at such dosage, blood levels are obtai-ned to determine the individual's response to the medicine and, if appropriate, whether the effective therapeutic level has been reached. If seizures continue, the daily drug dosage is increased by small increments as doses rise above the usual.

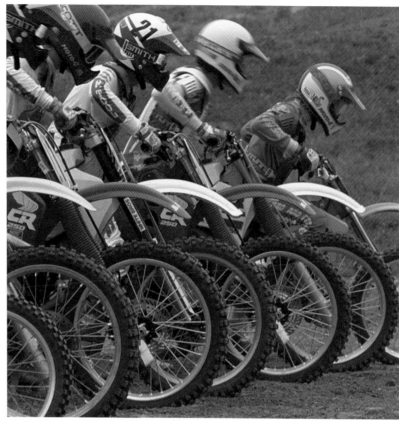

Sports like motorbiking is only allowed for persons free of seizures.

Classification of seizures

1. Partial seizures

A. Partial seizures with elementary symptoms (generally without impairment of con-scious-ness)
- with motor symptoms
- with special sensory or somatic symptoms
- compound forms

B. Partial seizures with complex symptoms (generally with impair-ment of consciousness)
- with impairment of conscious-ness only
- with cognitive symptoms
- with affective symptoms
- with psychosensory symptoms
- with psychomotor symptoms (automatism)
- compound forms

C. Partial seizures, secondarily generalized

2. Symmetrical seizures
- symmetrical and without local onset
- absences (petit mal)
- massive epileptic clonus
- infantile spasms
- clonic seizures
- tonic seizures
- atonic seizures
- akinetic seizures

3. Unilateral seizures

4. Unclassified epileptic seizures

ESOPHAGEAL DISORDERS

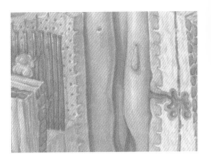

Description

Dysphagia is one of the most common signs of a disturbance of the function of the esophagus. It is defined as a subjective awareness of difficulty in swallowing due to impaired progression of matter from the pharynx to the stomach. The usual complaint is that the food "gets stuck" on the way down. The feeing may be accompanied by pain.

Dysphagia is the major symptom of esophageal transport disorders. The transport of liquids and solids may be impeded by organic lesions of the pharynx, esophagus and adjacent organs or by functional derangements of the nervous system and musculature.

Motor disorders causing dysfunction of the esophagus involve the smooth muscle of the esophagus. They produce dysphagia for both solids and fluids by impairing the peristalsis of the esophagus, thus interrupting the smooth transport of a bolus in the esophagus.

From the onset of symptoms, the presence of dysphagia for both liquids and solids accurately distinguishes motor from obstructive causes. The condition of dysphagia should not be confused with globus hystericus (globus sensation), a feeling of having a lump in the throat that is unrelated to swallowing and occurs without impaired transport. This condition is often noted in association with feelings of grief, and is generally emotional in etiology.

■ Pain

The second important common symptom of disturbance of the esophagus is pain. Chest or back pain is classified as heartburn, pain during swallowing or spontaneous esophageal motor disorder pain.

Heartburn, caused by reflux of contents of the stomach into the esophagus, is a burning pain behind the breast bone that rises in the chest or even face.

It usually occurs after meals or when the patient is lying down, and is frequently accompanied by regurgitation of contents of the stomach into the mouth.

Pain during swallowing (also called adynophagia) may occur with or without dysphagia and may be due to destruction of the mucosal layer of the esophagus induced by the following conditions:

- reflux from the stomach;
- bacterial infections;
- fungal infections;
- tumors;
- chemical agents.

The patient may describe the pain as a burning sensation or a tightness below the breast bone typically elicited by very hot or very cold food or liquid.

Onset is prompt on swallowing. Severe squeezing chest pain, brought on by swallowing cold beverages and invariably associated with dysphagia, is characteristic of esophageal motor disorders.

Obstructive disorders

The esophagus may be compressed by adjacent organs or extrinsic (from outside) benign or malignant tumors (cancer). The symptom is dysphagia for solids, similar to intrinsic (from within) obstruction of the esophagus. Obstruction from outside may occur in the following situations:

- an enlarged left atrium of the heart;
- aneurysm of the aorta;
- enlarged thyroid gland;
- bony exostoses;
- extrinsic tumor; most common from the lung.

The most serious cause of dysphagia - cancer - usually presents with progressive dysphagia for solids over several weeks, associated with marked weight loss. Cancer may occur in any portion of the esophagus and may appear as a structure, mass or plaque.

The tumor is best diagnosed by X-ray or scan, followed by endoscopy with biopsy. Tumors are most frequently squamous cell carcinoma with about 5 per cent of esophageal cancer being adenocarcinoma.

Conditions associated with an increased frequency of esophageal cancer are:

- achalasia;
- lye stricture;
- esophageal webs.

The treatment of squamous cell cancer is either surgical resection or radiation therapy; adenocarcinoma is treated by surgery alone. The overall prognosis is rather poor.

Esophageal webs are defined as thin, membranous mucosal structures that grow across the lumen, usually in the upper part of the esophagus. Esophageal webs may develop rarely in patients with untreated severe iron deficiency anemia, even more rarely, without an overt anemia.

Motor disorders

The major motor disorder is called achalasia or cardiospasm. This condition is defined as a neurogenic esophageal disorder of unknown cause resulting in impairment of peristalsis and relaxation of the lower part of the esophagus.

The condition may be due to a disturbance in function of the myenteric nervous network of the esophagus that results in denervation of the muscles of the esophagus. Achalasia may occur at any age, but usually begins between ages 20 ad 40.

Dysphagia for both solids and liquids is the major symptom: onset is insidious and progression is gradual over many months or years. Increased pressure of the lower sphincter of the esophagus produced obstruction with secondary dilatation of the esophagus and a tendency towards regurgitation and aspiration when the patient lies down.

Regurgitation of undigested food during the night occurs in about one-third of the patients and may cause aspiration with lung abscess, bronchiectasis or pneumonia.

Chest pain is less common, but may occur upon swallowing or spontaneously. Weight loss is usually mild to moderate but may become marked in untreated cases. X-ray studies and scans of the esophagus demonstrate the absence of progressive peristaltic contractions during swallowing.

The esophagus is dilated and frequently reaches enormous proportions, but is narrowed and beaklike at the lower esophageal sphincter. Regurgitation during night with coughing suggests possible aspiration. Lung complications secondary to aspiration are difficult to manage. The incidence of esophageal cancer in patients with achalasia is about 5 per cent.

The aim of the treatment is to reduce the pressure and this the obstruction at the lower esophageal sphincter. Forceful or pneumatic dilation of the sphincter is indicated initially, since results are satisfactory in about 80 per cent of the patients; repeated dilations may be needed.

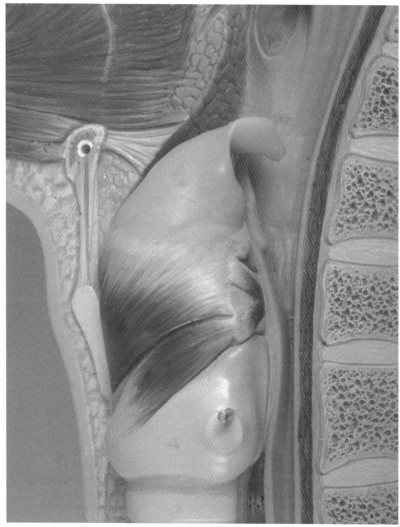

In the neck region and thoracic cavity the esophagus is located just in front of the spine.

Diverticula

A diverticulum is a sac or pouch of a canal or organ. There are several types of diverticula in the esophagus, each with a different cause. A pharyngeal diverticulum is an outpouching of the mucosa and submucosa. It probably results from incoordination between propulsion of the pharynx and relax-

ation of the cricopharyngeal muscle. The diverticula occurring in the middle part of the esophagus are either due to traction from inflammatory lesions in the mediastinum or secondary to motor disorders. Specific treatment is usually not required, though surgical resection of the diverticulum is occasionally necessary.

Hiatus hernia

This condition is defined as the protrusion of the stomach above the diaphragm. The cause is unknown, but a hiatus hernia may be a congenital abnormality or secondary to trau-

ma.

In a sliding hiatus hernia, the junction between esophagus and cardia of the stomach and a portion of the stomach are above the diaphragm. One side of the herniated stomach is covered with peritoneum.

A sliding hiatus hernia is common and may be seen by X-ray in more than 40 per cent of the population. Most patients do not show any signs or symptoms.

Although reflux occurs in a few patients, it is doubtful whether the hernia is the cause since reflux may also be found in patients with no demonstrable hernia on X-ray. Chest pain without reflux can also occur. A

Esophageal disorders   Questions & Answers

What conditions cause inflammation of the esophagus?

Inflammation of the esophagus (esophagitis) is found in association either with a hernia of the diaphragm (hiatus hernia) or with an ulcer in the stomach.

In hiatus hernia, a portion of the stomach protrudes into the chest cavity through a widening of the opening in the diaphragm. This permits stomach contents and juices to go up into the esophagus, where this often causes irritation and sets up a secondary inflammatory reaction.

Patients with ulcers in the duodenum are also prone to regurgitate highly acid contents from the stomach into the lower portion of the esophagus. They may create an esophagitis. It is a serious condition because it can result in a rupture of the esophagus, bleeding, or stricture formation, with consequent interference with swallowing.

Is achalasia (esophageal spasm) a common disorder of the esophagus?

Achalasia is a condition in which certain nerves of the esophagus are absent, probably since birth. As a result of this deficiency, there is inability of the lower part of the esophagus to dilate and relax.

As a consequence of this continued spasm, the esophagus above the area of spasm becomes tremendously widened and dilated. This condition is thought to be associated with a birth deformity in which there is absence of certain nerve elements within the wall of the esophagus.

The most common complaint is swallowing. This symptom becomes progressive and severe. In addition, there is often a foul odour to the breath because of retained food particles within the esophagus.

What is a globus sensation?

A globus sensation (lump in the throat, globus hystericus) is the subjective sensation of a lump or mass in the throat. No specific cause has been established. The sensation may result from esophageal reflux or from frequent swallowing and drying of the throat associated with anxiety or other emotional states.

Globus is probably a physiologic manifestation of certain mood states. It is not associated with a specific psychiatric disorder or set of stress factors. Certain individuals may have an inherent or learned predisposition to respond in this manner. The sensation resembles the normal reaction of being "choked up" during events that elicit grief, pride, or even happiness from mastery or hardship; suppression of sadness is most often implicated.

What causes varicose veins of the esophagus?

Varicose veins of the esophagus are caused by obstruction of the portal circulation, that is, the circulation of blood through the liver. This is seen in cirrhosis of the liver. Since blood cannot get from the intestinal tract through the liver, it bypasses that organ and travels along the veins of the esophagus.

This vastly increased blood volume causes the esophageal veins to dilate and become varicosed. Eventually, when the veins become too distended and dilated, they may rupture and cause a tremendous hemorrhage.

Conditions associated with an increased frequency of esophageal cancer are:
- achalasia;
- lye stricture;
- esophageal webs.

The treatment of squamous cell cancer is either surgical resection or radiation therapy; adenocarcinoma is treated by surgery alone. The overall prognosis is rather poor.

Gastroesophageal reflux

Description

Gastroesophageal reflux is the flow of gastric or duodenal contents across the gastroesophageal junction back into the esophagus. The effects depend on the mixture of stomach acid, pepsin, bile salts, and pancreatic enzymes refluxing into the esophageal mucosa.

Although gastroesophageal reflux may be without symptoms, the most common patient complaint is discomfort behind the breast bone, which radiates upward and is aggravated in the recumbent position. Reflux esophagitis is also aggravated by the following conditions:
- obesity
- tight garments about the abdomen
- pregnancy

The patient may refer to these symptoms as "heartburn", "indigestion", or "sour stomach". The regurgitation of fluid while sleeping or bending over is conclusive evidence of gastroesophageal reflux.

Other less common symptoms include:
- painful swallowing
- difficult swallowing
- hemorrhage
- lung complaints by choking on stomach contents

Although gastroesophageal reflux may exist simultaneously with a hiatus hernia (protrusion of part of the stomach through the diaphragm), the terms are not synonymous.

Gastroesophageal reflux and hiatus hernia are two separate clinical entities, and one has no effect on the other. In fact only about 5 per cent of patients with hiatal hernia complain of reflux symptoms. Hiatus hernia is a

sliding hiatus hernia usually requires no specific therapy, but any accompanying reflux must be treated.

Tumors

Tumors of the esophagus may be either benign or malignant growths.

Cancer may occur in any portion of the esophagus and may appear as a structure, mass or plaque.

The tumor is best diagnosed by X-ray or scan, followed by endoscopy with biopsy. Tumors are most frequently squamous cell carcinoma with about 5 per cent of esophageal cancer being adenocarcinoma.

rather common disorder and in many cases produces no symptoms.

Cause and diagnosis

There is general agreement that dysfunction of the lower esophageal sphincter is the cause of reflux. Symptoms have been associated with unexplained, inappropriate, and transient relaxation of the lower esophageal sphincter. However, there is no explanation for the dysfunction of this sphincter. Other factors that may be associated with reflux are disordered peristalsis and delayed stomach emptying.

Gastroesophageal reflux is related to stomach volume. Overeating which increases stomach volume enhances reflux, and this is especially true at bedtime. A cycle of events occurs in which reflux causes inflammation and damage leading to esophagitis (inflammation of the lining of the esophagus).

Esophagitis could result in defective peristalsis and incompetent lower esophageal sphincter. An appropriate medical history as taken by the family doctor and prompt relief by acid neutralization usually indicate gastroesophageal reflux.

The doctor may feel that further diagnostic testing should be performed if disorders or diseases of the heart, gallbladder, stomach or duodenum are suspected. The techniques used to diagnose gastroesophageal reflux include the following:

- radiography (X-rays) of the esophagus
- endoscopy of the esophagus
- biopsy of the mucosa of the esophagus;
- manometry (measuring of pressure) of the esophagus
- computer scanning methods (CT-scan, MRI-scan).

Treatment

The treatment of gastroesophageal reflux is divided into three phases:

▲ phase I involves dietary and life style changes, measures to improve acid clearance and antacids;
▲ phase II utilizes specific medicines;
▲ phase III is antireflux surgery. Although most therapy with med-

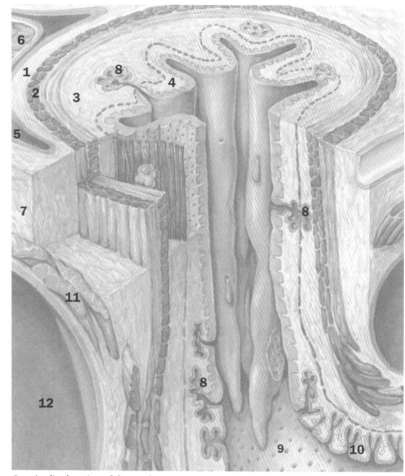

Longitudinal section of the esophagus.
1. Serous layer; 2. muscular layer; 3. submucosal layer; 4. mucosal layer; 5. pleural cavity; 6. lung tissue; 7. connective tissue; 8. glands in the wall of the esophagus; 9. gastric mucosa; 10. cardia glands; 11. diaphragm; 12. abdominal cavity.

icines is aimed at improving the tone of the lower esophageal sphincter and/or neutralizing stomach acid, some very effective results can be obtained if the patient changes his or her life style.

Smoking, and the ingestion of fatty foods, coffee, and chocolate, which can decrease lower esophageal sphincter tone, will be discouraged by the doctor. The patient will be asked if he is taking any medicines known to decrease lower esophageal sphincter tone. These medicines include theophylline, diazepam, verapamil and anticholinergics.

Individuals should eat slowly and not recline after meals. Carbonated beverages will also increase pressure in the stomach and should be avoided. Perhaps the most effective treatment is to utilize gravity to diminish the gastroesophageal pressure gradient by elevating the head of the bed with 15 cm blocks.

Weight loss is also successful in decreasing symptoms.

Bethanechol and antacids have been used to increase competence of the lower esophageal sphincter.

Alginic acid has been used to provide a physical barrier that will be neutral if refluxed, although there is controversy regarding the efficacy. Antireflux surgery is indicated only if other therapies fail.

EYE DISORDERS

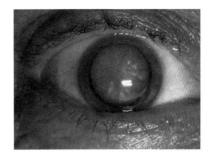

Introduction

Many of the skin receptors provide us with general information about our closest surroundings. But we also need to perceive the dangerous and desirable at a distance.

It is not enough to know in what direction something lies; we must also decide how far away it is and what it looks like. For this purpose man has a pair of special sense organs - the eyes. Very simply, the eye consists of a transparent part at the front that focuses images on to a light-sensitive layer at the back. Several comparisons can be made with the camera to make the eye easier to understand; for instance, the transparent part corresponds to the lens and the light-sensitive part, or retina, corresponds to the film.

Causes of common eye disorders

Some eye complaints are nonspecific, so that the physician will perform a complete history and examination of all parts of the eye and its accessory organs to identify the source of the complaint. The patient will be asked about the location and duration of the symptoms; the presence and nature of any pain, discharge, or redness; and any change in visual acuity.

Unless chemicals requiring immediate irrigation have splashed into the eye, the first step in eye evaluation is to record the visual acuity. The physician will test the vision by having the patient wear his lenses or glasses and look at an eye chart some 6 meters away. Covering each eye indicates that the patient sees at 6 meters what the average person sees at 12 meters. Gross inspection of the glasses will provide an approximation of the degree of nearsightedness, far-sightedness, astigmatism. Visual fields and eye motility may also be determined at this time.

Under a focal light and magnification, systemic examination of the eye will then be performed. The eyelids are examined for lesions of the margins and subcutaneous tissues.

The cornea will be inspected closely. The size and shape of the pupil and their reaction to light and accommodation will be noted. Ocular tension

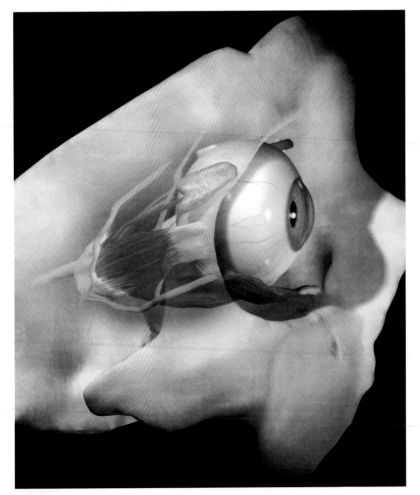

The eye from front and side in the eye socket showing the extra-ocular eye muscles and the surrounding tissues. The eyeball, or globe, occupies the front half of the cavity of the socket (orbit), where it is embedded in fat and connective tissue and projects slightly beyond the socket's opening.

360

and depth of the anterior chamber will also be investigated.

An ophthalmoscope and ultrasonography (use of high frequency sound waves) are being employed to investigate the various structures of the eye. Eye inflammation and/or discomfort may be due to several conditions, including:

▲ anatomical anomalies (such as incomplete closure of the eyelids);
▲ abnormal physiologic conditions (such as dry eye syndrome - keratoconjunctivitis sicca;
▲ allergic response;
▲ infection;
▲ irritants (including excessive ultraviolet radiation, drying winds, volatile chemical components of smog, and chemicals in fertilizers, pesticides, cleaning agents, and cosmetics).

Conditions due to physical causes (such as burns, lacerations, and concussions) or conditions associated with specific disease states should be referred immediately to a physician.

Conditions of the eyelids

Black eye

The skin layer covering the eye is very thin and, consequently, very delicate. Patients with injured or inflamed eyelids should consult a physician.

For immediate treatment of so-called "black eye," cold compresses in the initial 24 hours after injury followed by warm applications are helpful. These patients should consult their physician to rule out any other eye injury.

Irritation

Irritation may range from slight inflammation to severe chemical burns. Chemical burns of the eyelids or external ocular tissues must be treated immediately by copious irrigation with sterile water or saline. If these are not available, tap water should be used.

The offending agent must be diluted and removed quickly before extensive tissue damage occurs. Flushing should be continuous until the patient sees the physician or is in the emergency room. Patients should consult a physician as soon as possible after injury

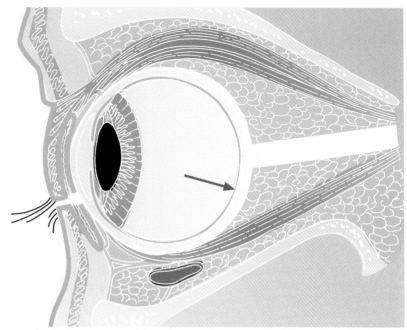

Longitudinal cross-section of the right eye and surrounding tissues. The arrow indicates the retina.

The eyeball may be considered as a hollow sphere, whose wall consists of three concentric coats and whose cavity is filled with three types of refracting fluid: the vitreous humor, filling the rear three-quarters of the cavity; the crystalline lens, in front of this; and the aqueous humor, between the lens and the cornea.

Electron microscopic picture of the rods and cones of the retina.

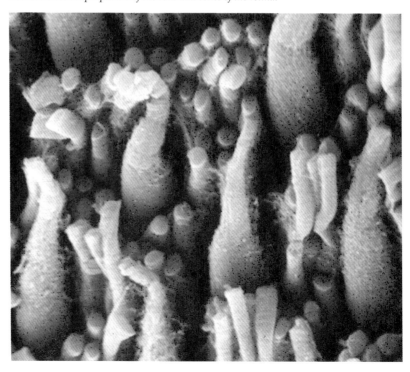

Eye disorders Questions & Answers

What is in general the best treatment for a common eye infection?
Warm, wet compresses applied a few times a day for 5 to 15 minutes usually bring improvement within a day or so. They usually will bring external styes to a "head" to allow them to rupture and clear up. If the infection fills your eye with "goop," you can irrigate it away with a sterile eye wash. Such infections with thick discharge, however, may be bacterial and not viral, and may require treatment with antibiotic eye drops if they are of more than mild severity.

How are more serious eye infections treated?
Usually with prescription eye drops or ointments, rather than systemic drugs given as pills or injections. Eyes respond best to topical medication. If your problems seems like more than a simple stye or pink eye, or lasts more than a few days, see your physician. Also head for professional care right away if redness and discharge are accompanied by pain, sensitivity to light, or any change in vision or the size of your pupils. Over-the-counter drugs, such as boric acid and yellow mercuric oxide, have generally fallen into disfavor for treating even minor eye infections. They may mask symptoms, but not affect underlying causes, thus delaying you from getting prompt professional care when needed.

What can be done about prevention of eye infections?
Some eye infections can be prevented. Avoid rubbing your eyes because your fingers transmit a large dose of germs. If you wear contact lenses, be sure to clean and disinfect them daily. Never put a lens in your mouth to moisten it and then put it in your eye.

What are the major causes of blindness?
The leading causes of blindness in our country are the following:
- accidents, which injure the eyes;
- cataracts, which are due to a clouding of the lens in front of the eye;
- diabetes, which is the leading cause of blindness;
- glaucoma, which has been called "the sneak thief of sight" because it has few warning signs;
- infections, for which the risk is increased if you uses extended wear contact lenses;
- macular degeneration, a leading cause of blindness in our older population.

How can blindness be prevented in our population?
Regular medical eye examinations are essential to detect treatable causes of vision loss. Adults over 35 should have eye checks every two years, or more often if prescribed due to a particular risk.

How can macular degeneration of the eye occur?
The macula is the tissue in the central portion of the retina, which is located at the back of the eye. The middle of the macula is responsible for our central vision. When it is damaged or diseased, central vision begins to blur. As a result, you develop difficulty in reading small print and seeing distant objects such as street signs. However, macular degeneration does not affect side vision, so that the patient is still able to get around independently. Senile macular degeneration is one of the most common causes of blindness. When the disease begins, small blood vessels may grow in the macular region between the retina and its supporting layer of tissue.

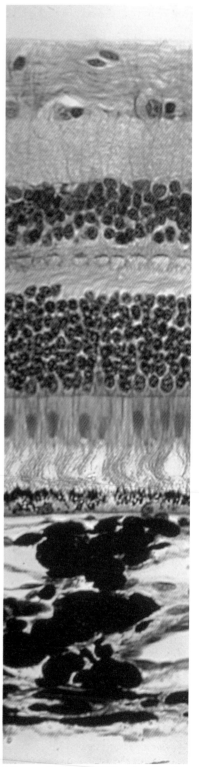

Microscopic picture of the retina showing the various types of nerve cells and the rods and cones (sensory cells).

for follow-up evaluation and treatment.

Inflammation of only the lid margins (blepharitis) may result from:

- associated seborrhoeic dermatitis of the scalp
- infection with Staphylococcus aureus
- contact dermatitis due to chemical fumes
- drugs used to treat ocular inflammation
- irritation from eye strain caused by improper refraction or rubbing of the eyes

Symptoms are hyperemia of the lid margins and associated skin scaling. The main complaint is redness of the lids, burning and itching of the eyes, and photophobia, concomitant with conjunctivitis. Vision usually remains normal.

Symptomatic treatment with nonprescription decongestants is not satisfactory. Symptoms will recur unless the underlying problem is effectively treated.

Infections

Hordeolum (stye) is an acute suppurative inflammation of the eyelash follicle or sebaceous or sweat gland. As with pustules anywhere in the body, the most common cause is Staphylococcus aureus.

The principal symptoms are:

- pain
- acute tenderness in the area around the hordeolum
- localized redness
- swelling

Touching and squeezing the stye may cause the infection to spread and should be avoided. Hordeola usually are self-limiting and respond well to warm moist compresses of tap water applied 3 to 4 times/day for 10-15 minutes.

This helps bring stye to a "head," leading to drainage. Antibiotic ointment

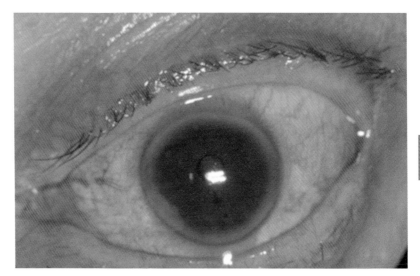

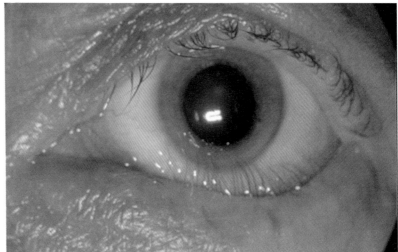

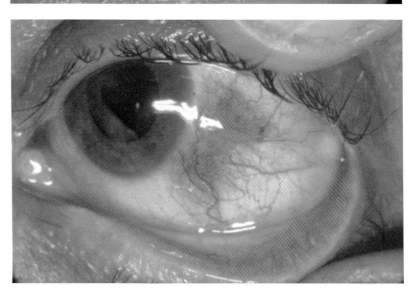

Various eye conditions as shown by macroscopic examination.
From top to bottom:
- aging disorder of the eye;
- entropion (the eyelid is turned in against the eyeball);
- infection of the cornea with characteristic hyperemic blood vessels.

Eye disorders   Questions & Answers

What is in general the best treatment for a common eye infection?
Warm, wet compresses applied a few times a day for 5 to 15 minutes usually bring improvement within a day or so. They usually will bring external styes to a "head" to allow them to rupture and clear up. If the infection fills your eye with "goop," you can irrigate it away with a sterile eye wash. Such infections with thick discharge, however, may be bacterial and not viral, and may require treatment with antibiotic eye drops if they are of more than mild severity.

How are more serious eye infections treated?
Usually with prescription eye drops or ointments, rather than systemic drugs given as pills or injections. Eyes respond best to topical medication. If your problems seems like more than a simple stye or pink eye, or lasts more than a few days, see your physician. Also head for professional care right away if redness and discharge are accompanied by pain, sensitivity to light, or any change in vision or the size of your pupils.

What about over-the-counter drugs?
Over-the-counter drugs, such as boric acid and yellow mercuric oxide, have generally fallen into disfavor for treating even minor eye infections. They may mask symptoms, but not affect underlying causes, thus delaying you from getting prompt professional care when needed.

What can be done about prevention of eye infections?
Some eye infections can be prevented. Avoid rubbing your eyes because your fingers transmit a large dose of germs. If you wear contact lenses, be sure to clean and disinfect them daily. Never put a lens in your mouth to moisten it and then put it in your eye.

What is astigmatism?
Astigmatism is an irregularity in the curvature (curved differently in different directions) of the cornea or lens that causes light traveling in different planes to be focused differently. For example, vertical lines may be in focus when horizontal lines are not (or vice versa). The irregularity can be in any plane, however, and is often different in each eye.
A person with astigmatism (each eye should be tested separately) tends to see certain lines more boldly (that is, in better focus) than the others.
Astigmatism is correctable with prescription eyeglasses or contact lenses. It often occurs together with nearsightedness or farsightedness.

What causes color blindness?
Color blindness affects how people perceive certain colors. It is usually present from birth and is nearly always due to an X-linked recessive gene, which means that it nearly always occurs in men who have the gene. Women, who are not usually affected themselves, can pass the gene for color blindness on to their children. Although color blindness is sometimes due to a problem with how the brain interprets color (rather than a problem with the eyes), usually people with color blindness lack certain photoreceptors at the back of the eye.

What is the most common type of color blindness?
Most cases of color blindness are due to a relative deficiency or abnormality of one of the photoreceptor types. Red-green color blindness is the most common form. Blue-yellow color blindness is usually due to acquired rather than inherited disease and may be caused by optic nerve disease.

may be applied under a physician's care or supervision.

Cosmetic agents frequently become contaminated with microorganisms. Contamination is associated with length and frequency of use, personal habits, product formulations, and presence or absence of preservatives. Because cosmetics are a source of ocular infections, patients should be advised to avoid wearing eye make-up for at least a week before ocular surgery. Mascara should not be used to hide blepharitis because it may aggravate and prolong the condition.

Foreign bodies
Foreign bodies are the most frequent cause of eye injury. Lint, dust, and similar objects can be removed from the eye by flushing with normal saline, an eye wash or water.

However, metallic or nonmetallic foreign bodies that are blown into the eye may cause serious problems if not removed. If the foreign body is small and not readily seen with the naked eye, fluorescein will be used to outline the particle.

If the foreign body is lodged in the conjunctival area, it should be removed by a physician. If the foreign body is deeply placed, it may require removal in the operating room.

External ocular disorders

Disorders affecting the external eye are chemical burn, conjunctivitis, and conditions of the lacrimal system. Conjunctivitis may be due to causes ranging from a foreign body to an allergic reaction; careful and accurate patient assessment is essential.

Conjunctivitis
Inflammation of the conjunctiva (conjunctivitis) is a common external eye problem. Its symptoms are a diffusely reddened eye with a purulent or serous discharge accompanied by itching, stinging, or a scratching, "foreign body" sensation. If the patient has not experienced pain or blurred vision, conjunctivitis is a likely diagnosis.

Conjunctivitis may be caused by foreign bodies, contusions or lacerations, or parasitic infestations. Most foreign bodies may be removed easily with irrigation or a cotton-tipped applicator provided no damage has occurred to deeper structures. If removal is difficult, the patient should consult a physician; the eye may have been irritated by rubbing, causing corneal epithelial abrasions which may lead to infection.

Patients with contusions or lacerations of the conjunctiva should consult an ophthalmologist for assessment of possible trauma to the globe or conjunctiva. Conjunctival irritation due to foreign bodies, chemical irritants, or allergies generally is treated by removing the cause and administering nonprescription decongestants.

A clue to chemical conjunctivitis, caused by airborne irritants such as smoke, smog, or garden sprays, is that both eyes are involved. Allergic conjunctivitis usually occurs on warm, windy days in the spring and during hay fever season. Typical symptoms, such as wheeling, congestion, stinging, watering, and itching, affect both eyes.

Bacterial conjunctivitis usually is self-limiting and does not impair vision. If the patient awakens with the eyelids stuck together by dried exudate or if there is discharge or signs of swelling of the local lymph nodes, the cause is probably bacterial.

Consultation of a physician is needed, since recovery may be hastened with appropriate prescription drugs, such as sulphonamide or another antibiotic-containing ophthalmic product.

Without treatment, most bacterial conjunctivitis lasts 10-14 days, although Staphylococcus and Moraxella species infections may become chronic.

Corneal infections may exhibit symptoms similar to those of bacterial conjunctivitis. These infections are more serious and may obliterate vision rapidly. An accurate diagnosis is important.

Viral conjunctivitis may resemble chemically induced conjunctivitis; symptoms may include red, perhaps swollen, watery, itching eyes and swollen lymph nodes. Unlike chemical irritations, however, viral conjunctivitis often is accompanied by systemic symptoms.

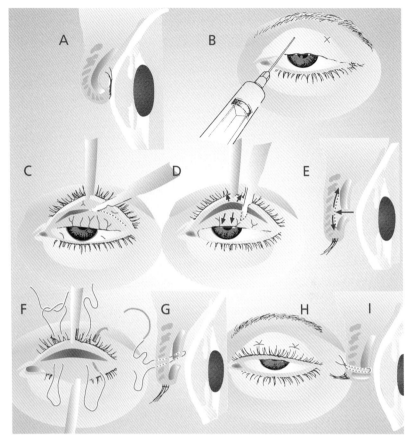

Surgical correction of an entropion. Both entropion and ectropion can irritate the eyes, causing watering and redness. Eye drops and ointments can be used to keep the eye moist and sooth irritation. Occasionally, entropion can lead to corneal ulcer. In that case entropion can be treated by surgery - for instance, to preserve sight if damage to the eyes (such as by corneal ulcer) has occurred. The various steps (A-I) of the surgery for entropion are shown.

Opacity due to deposits of lipids and calcium.

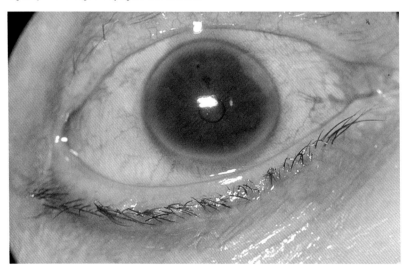

Eye disorders Questions & Answers

What are the major causes of blindness?
The leading causes of blindness in our country are the following:
▲ accidents, which injure the eyes;
▲ cataracts, which are due to a clouding of the lens in front of the eye;
▲ diabetes, which is the leading cause of blindness in the working population;
▲ glaucoma, which has been called "the sneak thief of sight" because it has few warning signs;
▲ infections, for which the risk is increased if you uses extended wear contact lenses;
▲ macular degeneration, a leading cause of blindness in our older population.

How can blindness be prevented in our popu-lation?
Regular medical eye examinations are essential to detect treatable causes of vision loss. Adults over 35 should have eye checks every two years, or more often if prescribed due to a particular risk.

How can macular degeneration of the eye occur?
The macula is the tissue in the central portion of the retina, which is located at the back of the eye. The middle of the macula is responsible for our central vision. When it is damaged or diseased, central vision begins to blur. As a result, you develop difficulty in reading small print and seeing distant objects such as street signs. However, macular degeneration does not affect side vision, so that the patient is still able to get around independently. Senile macular degeneration is one of the most common causes of blindness. When the disease begins, small blood vessels may grow in the macular region between the retina and its supporting layer of tissue.

How can macula degeneration be treated?
If the blood vessels of the retina leak blood, the retinal cells which are responsible for central vision can be damaged. Macular degeneration is painless and usually develops gradually. Until recently, doctors could to little to help these patients. However, they have now developed a new treatment, using krypton laser light to seal off the newly formed abnormal blood vessels. This can reduce or slow down vision loss. However, to be successful, laser treatment must begin early - preferably even before symptoms appear. Macular degeneration can be detected by your eye doctor as part of a regular eye check-up.

I have often problems with eye strain; what are the causes?
Eye strain has nothing to do with overuse, although its symptoms may appear when you change the demands you make on your eyes. The classic signs of eye strain are:
• achiness
• tension around the eye
• blurred vision
• headache
• fatigue
• nausea
This can lead to lower performance levels and greater irritability. Many people suffering with eye strain think they are neurotic and waste years in psychotherapy before they find out they have a vision problem. Others just avoid close work as much as posslble and even change careers to avoid the strain.
Eye strain is caused by eye coordination problems involving eye muscle balance - bringing your eyes together to join the separate images they see into a single clear picture. While eye coordination problems can occur at any age, they often do not cause symptoms until the late teens or 20s or 30s.

Lacrimal disorders
The therapy of inflammation of the lacrimal gland (dacryoadenitis) is determined by the cause. Assessment should be made by a physician. Decreased tear production may be associated with aging, physical trauma, and infection (trachoma). Symptoms are burning and constant "foreign body" sensation and reddened and dry eyes. Treatment is tear replacement with artificial tear products. Continued self-medication of a dry eye syndrome without professional diagnosis may cause an exacerbation of the underlying condition due to the delay in medical treatment.
Some allergic reactions may cause excessive tearing and watery eyes. Cold water compresses and cool, clean eye washes are beneficial for symptomatic relief, as are nonprescription vasoconstrictors. If, as in hay fever, the causative agent cannot be removed, oral antihistamines may be useful.

Internal eye conditions

Internal eye conditions may have far greater consequences than conditions of the external eye. Early diagnosis may help prevent partial or total loss of vision.

Glaucoma
Glaucoma is characterized by increased pressure in the eyeball, causing degeneration of the optic disk and defects in the visual field. It may be classified as either primary (including open-angle, narrow angle, or hypersecretion glaucoma), congenital, or secondary.
The most common form is primary open-angle glaucoma. Initial treatment of open-angle and secondary glaucoma may be medical; narrow-angle and congenital glaucoma treatment is generally surgical. Most chronic open-angle glaucoma will eventually require surgical intervention.
▲ Primary open-angle glaucoma occurs as a result of decreased outflow (drainage) of aqueous humor from the anterior chamber of the eye. In patients with this disorder, the chamber angles appear normal. The decreased

outflow is most likely caused by degenerative changes in the trabecular meshwork of Schlemm.

Open-angle glaucoma causes no early symptoms, and some loss of vision usually occurs late in the progress of the disease. Both eyes are nearly always involved, although one eye may be more severely affected.

▲ Secondary glaucoma also occurs due to increased outflow. Foreign bodies or tumors obstructing the trabecular meshwork, ocular inflammation, ocular trauma, hemorrhage, and topical corticosteroid therapy are causes of secondary glaucoma.

▲ Narrow-angle glaucoma (angle-closure or acute glaucoma) is characterized by a sudden onset of blurred vision followed by excruciating pain that may be accompanied by nausea and vomiting.

It occurs with sudden increase in intra-ocular tension due to a block of the anterior chamber angle by the root of the iris, which cut off all aqueous outflow. The chamber angle is anatomically closed. Any abnormal dilation of the pupil or swelling of the iris or lens may produce this obstruction.

There is no pain with open-angle glaucoma. Narrow-angle glaucoma can be very dangerous and requires immediate consultation of a physician.

Cataracts

Approximately 20 per cent of the individuals in our country who are considered legally blind have cataracts as an underlying cause. A cataract is an opacity of the crystalline lens. At present, drug therapy is not a treatment for cataracts but only an aid for certain symptoms. The treatment of cataracts involves surgical removal of the opacity.

Juvenile or adult cataract is characterized by progressive, painless loss of vision. The cause may be:

· senile degeneration
· X-rays
· heat from infrared exposure
· systemic diseases (for instance, diabetes)
· systemic medications (e.g., corticosteroids).

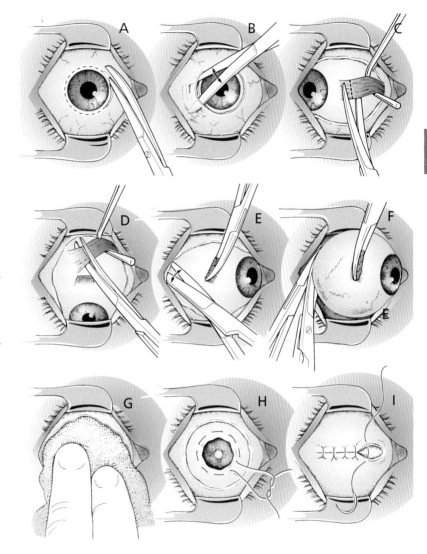

Enucleation of the eye because of the presence of a malignant tumor. Incising the conjunctiva all around the limbus (A); dissecting the conjunctiva and the fascial sheath from the sclera (B); identifying and cutting the rectus muscles, leaving a small fringe on the globe (C); identifying and cutting the tendons of the oblique muscles (D); freeing the globe from the fascial sheath (E); identifying, clamping and dividing the optic nerve (F); applying pressure over gauze after removing the globe (G); closing the fascial sheath with a purse-string suture (H); suturing the conjunctiva (I).

The cardinal symptom is a progressive, painless loss of vision. The degree of loss depends on the location and extent of the opacity. When the opacity is in the central lens nucleus (nuclear cataract), myopia develops in the early stages, so that a presbyopic patient may discover that he can read without his glasses ("second sight"). Pain occurs if the cataract swells and produces secondary glaucoma. Opacity beneath the posterior lens capsule affects vision out of proportion to the degree of cloudiness because the opacity is located at the crossing point of the rays of light from the viewed object. Such cataracts are particularly troublesome in bright light. Well-developed cataracts appear as grey opacities in the lens.

Eye irritation - Self-care

▲ Always be sure to wear protective goggles when using power tools or when under a sunray lamp. If a substance gets into your eye and it is not an acid or other caustic substance then try repeated rinsing with lukewarm water.

▲ If a caustic substance, such as an acid, gets in the eyes go straight to your local accident & emergency department.

▲ For any eye soreness: Cleanse the eyes with cool boiled water or cold tea. Often the eyelashes become stuck together. Soak crusts away using wet cotton wool. It is quite safe to cleanse the inside of the lower eyelid using moist cotton wool.

▲ Never use cotton wool in the eyes. It leaves small pieces of cotton behind. Always use wet cotton wool, a piece of gauze or tissue.

▲ *Contact your doctor*
  • If the eyes are discharging pus
  • If they are not better after 5-7 days
  • If vision remains disturbed
  • If the eyes are painful, even if there is no pus

▲ *Contact your doctor immediately*
  • If you think that there is something in the eye and you cannot rinse it out yourself
  • If the eye is painful or if you have arc eye
  • If you have been drilling metal
  • If there is a change in your vision that you haven't experienced before
  • If the eye of your child is so red that the eye white is no longer visible

Ophthalmoscopic examination of the dilated pupil with the instrument held at about 30 cm away will usually disclose subtle opacities. Small cataracts stand out as dark defects in the red reflex. A large cataract may obliterate the red reflex. Red refractions and eyeglass prescriptions changes help maintain useful vision during cataract development. Occasionally, chronic pupillary dilation is helpful for small lens opacities.

When useful vision is lost, lens extraction is necessary; it can be accomplished by removal of the lens intact, or by emulsification followed by irrigation and aspiration. Age is no contraindication to surgery.

Visual disorders

One of the commonest visual symptoms is the sensation of small, black objects floating in front of the eye. These move with the eye but lag slightly at the beginning of an eye movement and overshoot when the movement stops. They are due to cells and fragments of debris in the vitreous cavity of the eye.

Blind area in the field of vision occasionally force people to seek medical advice. Any condition that causes failure of function of part of the retina, the optic nerve, or the optic pathway to the brain, can cause such a blind spot, and the symptom requires careful investigation.

There is a naturally occurring "blind spot" in each visual field that corresponds with the lack of retinal elements where the optic nerve enters the eye. The brain is so skilful in filling in the visual pattern that the normal blind spot can be detected only by special methods.

Flashing lights in the field of vision are caused by stimulation of the retina by mechanical means. Most commonly this occurs when the vitreous body becomes degenerate. Similar symptoms also arise when the retina becomes detached, causing flashing lights to be seen.

Night blindness and defects of color perception

Defective vision under reduced illumination may be a rare congenital condition or may be acquired as a result of severe deficiency of vitamin A.

Defective color vision affects about four per cent of men and 0.5 per cent of women. Total color blindness is

Common choices of blindness

Cataract
- Most common cause
- Can be cured with surgery

Infection
- Most common preventable cause

Diabetes
- One of the most common cause
- Often preventable
- Laser treatment shows vision loss

Macular degeneration
- Affect central vision
- Preventable and treatable in fewer than 10 % of people

Glaucoma
- Highly treatable
- If treated early should not lead to blindness

extremely rare and is nearly always associated with poor vision in ordinary light.

The color-defective person is rarely aware of his disability until special matching tests are used, when it is discovered that he is unable to distinguish between hues in one or other part of the visual spectrum. Other visual functions are perfectly normal, and the only disadvantage is the restriction of certain types of occupation.

Eyestrain

Asthenopia, or eyestrain, is the term used to describe symptoms of fatigue and discomfort following the use of the eyes.

Although such symptoms may result from intensive close work, particularly if this is unaccustomed, in people with perfectly normal eyes, they may indicate abnormalities of muscle balance or refractive errors.

Eyestrain is more likely to be manifest during periods of fatigue or stress and is common among students working for examinations. Refractive errors require correction and muscle imbalance treatment. Psychological factors are often more important than physical factors.

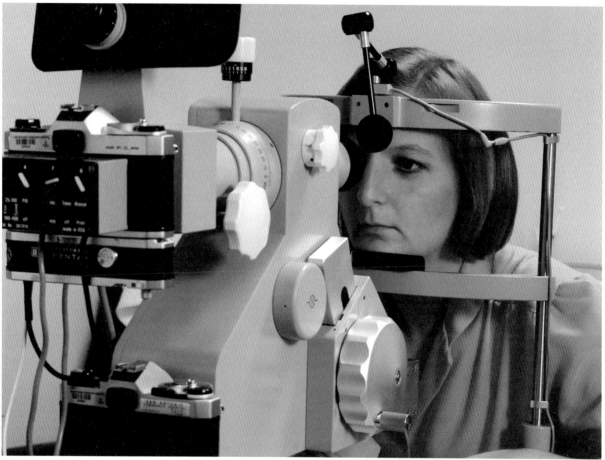

Examination of the eye after penetration of a small foreign body.

Refractive errors

In a normal eye rays of light from distant objects come to a focus on the retina. In near vision (nearsightedness), the refractive power of the eye is increased by altering the shape of the lens to focus the image on the retina. A twelve-year old can focus on an object 10 cm away from the eye but, with age, the ability of the lens to alter its shape decreases so that at the age of 40 the shortest distance at which an object can be kept in focus is about 25 cm.

■ *Presbyopia and hypermetropia*

The near point continues to recede with age until fine print, for example, cannot be read at a normal reading distance. This condition is known as presbyopia; it is corrected by the use of convex lenses for reading.

In some eyes rays of light from distant objects are not brought to a focus on the retina but are focused on a plane in front of the retina, as in myopia (short sight; nearsightedness), or behind the retina, as in hypermetropia (long sight; farsightedness).

■ *Myopia*

In myopia, near objects are brought into focus on the retina but distant objects can only be seen clearly with the aid of concave lenses.

In hypermetropia, distant objects can usually be brought into focus by using the accommodative power of the lens, and in young people there is usually sufficient accommodation to enable them to see reasonably near to them. The constant accommodative effort required, however, may produce symptoms, and the necessity for accommodating for distance can be overcome by wearing convex glasses or lenses.

■ *Astigmatism*

Another type of refractive error is astigmatism. In this condition the refractive power of the eye varies in different axes because of variation in curvature so that vision at all distances is distorted and can only be corrected by the use of cylindrical lenses or contact lenses.

Minor degrees of refractive error are extremely common.

The refractive state is genetically determined and there are marked racial differences.

Although most refractive errors are rarely accompanied by any serious disease of the eyes, hypermetropia is a factor in the development of some kinds of squint and high degrees of myopia are often associated with serious degenerative changes within the eye.

FEVER

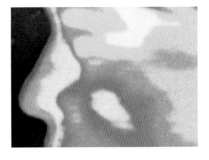

Description

In case of fever body temperature raises as a protective response to infection and injury. The elevated body temperature enhances the body's defense mechanisms, although it can cause discomfort for the person. Temperature is considered elevated when it is higher than 100° F as measured by an oral thermometer.

Although 98,6° F is considered "normal" temperature, body temperature varies throughout the day, being lowest in the early morning and highest in the late afternoon - sometimes reaching 99,9° F.

Causes of fever

Substances that cause fever are called pyrogens. Pyrogens can come from inside or outside the body. Microorganisms and the substances they produce (such as toxins) are examples of pyrogens formed outside the body. Pyrogens formed inside the body are usually produced by monocytes.

Pyrogens from outside the body cause fever by stimulating the body to release its own pyrogens. However, infection is not the sole cause of fever;

fever may also result from inflammation, cancer, or allergic reactions.

In summary, the causes of fever may be distinguished in general causes, acute causes, and chronic or recurrent causes. Some examples of those best known general causes are:

- *General causes*
- Infection
- Cancer
- Allergic reaction
- Hormone disorders such as hyperthyroidism
- Autoimmune diseases

Fever of unknown origin in a child showing also an eating disorder.

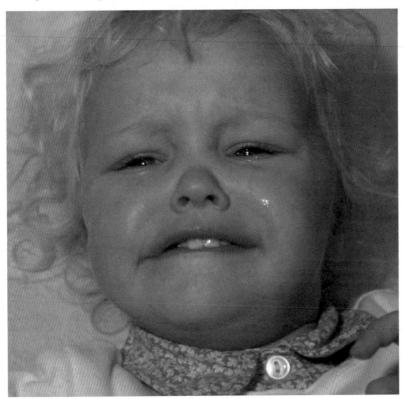

Febrile convulsion

▲ A fever that rises quickly may bring about a febrile convulsion. This is more often known as a fit or seizure.

▲ Keep calm with your child. The convulsion will usually only last for a few minutes.

▲ Your child will not be able to talk and will have muscle spasms. Your child's eyes will be rolling.

▲ After the convulsion your child will naturally go to sleep. Your child's breathing will be normal. If your child is unconscious, breathing will be loud and very heavy.

▲ Gently place your child on its side or stomach, with the head down and to one side.

▲ Following a fit it may be appropriate for your child to be admitted to hospital for observation and further treatment if necessary.

- Excessive exercise
- Excessive exposure to the sun
- Certain drugs, including anesthetics
- Damage to the hypothalamus

Acute fever
- Bacterial infections, such as earaches
- Viral infections, such as colds, influenza
- Allergic or toxic reactions to certain drugs or poisons
- Heat stroke
- Dehydration, often occurring in children as a result of diarrhea

Chronic or recurrent fever
This type of fever occurs repeatedly over time. Major examples are:
- Chronic inflammatory diseases of connective tissue such as arthritis
- Chronic inflammatory disease os the gastrointestinal tract, such as Crohn's disease
- Infections commonly associated with cystic fibrosis
- Tumors and cancers such as leukemia and lymphoma
- Disorders of the central nervous system, such as brain tumors
- Endocrine gland disorders, such as hyperthyroidism

Fever of unknown origin (FUO)

A fever of unknown origin is a prolonged elevation of temperature the cause of which is very difficult to diagnose. It is a sign of disease itself, and may affect a child at any age.
A fever designated FUO usually has three general characteristics:

▲ An elevation of more than 100.5° F (38.1° C) as measured several times over several days. To confirm the existence of a prolonged fever, it is necessary to obtain repeated temperature readings that clearly lie above the normal range. For a young child, rectal temperature readings are preferred.

▲ A duration of one week or more.

▲ A cause that remains unidentified even after investigation in a hospital for at least 1 week. If examina-

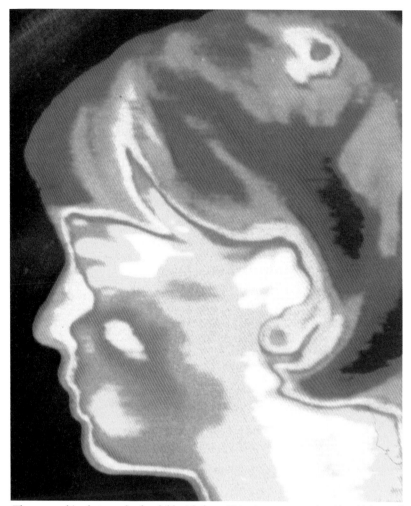

Thermographic photograph of a child with fever. This picture was made with a high-speed infraredcamera and shows differences of temperature in the various tissues of the face.

Emergency action
Contact your doctor immediately

▲ If your child shows any signs of neck cramp or pain when bending the head, or vomits all the time.

▲ If you have a temperature of over 104° F (40° C).

▲ If you have a stiff neck or vomiting. You may have a headache that does not go away as well and you may feel listless.

▲ If your child feels or appears listless, even if there is no fever or a low fever, your child could be very ill.

▲ If you have a rash.

Fever in children Questions & Answers

When has my child a fever?

Most pediatricians consider any thermometer reading above 38°C a sign of a fever. This number may vary depending on the method used for taking your child's temperature.

What are signs and symptoms of a fever in a child?

If your child has a fever, her heart and breathing rates naturally will speed up. You may notice that your child feels warm. She may appear flushed or perspire more than usual. Her body also will require more fluids. Some children feel fine when they have a fever. However, most will have symptoms of the illness that is causing a fever. Your child may have an ear ache, a sore throat, a rash, or a stomach ache. These signs can provide important clues as to the cause of your child's fever.

How do I manage a mild fever?

A child older than 6 months of age who has a temperature below 101°F (38.3°C) probably does not need to be treated for fever, unless the child is uncomfortable. Observe her behavior. If she is easting and sleeping well and is able to play, you may wait to see if the fever improves by itself. In the meantime:

- Keep her room comfortably cool.
- Make sure that she is dressed in light clothing.
- Encourage her to drink fluids such as water, diluted fruit juices, or a commercially prepared oral electrolyte solution.
- Be sure she does not overexert herself.

When should I call our paediatrician?

Call your paediatrician immediately if your child has a fever and

- looks very ill, is unusually drowsy, or is very fussy.
- Has been in an extremely hot place, such as an overheated car.
- Has additional symptoms such as a stiff neck, severe headache, severe sore throat, severe ear pain, an unexplained rash, or repeated vomiting or diarrhea.
- Has a condition that suppresses immune responses, such as sickle-cell disease or cancer, or is taking corticosteroids.
- Is younger than 2 months of age and has a rectal temperature of 102°F (39°C) or higher.

What if my child has a febrile seizure?

In some young children, fever can trigger seizures. These are usually harmless. However, they can be frightening. When this happens your child may look strange for a few minutes. Turn her head to the side; do not put anything into his mouth; call your pediatrician. Your pediatrician should always examine your child after a febrile seizure.

What is the cause of a fever of unknown origin (FUO)?

The causes of FUO usually fall into four broad categories:

- viral and bacterial infections
- inflammations of connective tissue (ligaments and tendons)
- malignancies
- miscellaneous illnesses

Other signs and symptoms of these diseases can be subtle or nonexistent in early stages of development, and fever can be the predominant or only indication of illness. Causes of FUO tend to vary, depending on whether a child is older or younger than 6 years. Younger children more often have viral and bacterial infections underlying prolonged fever. For older children an inflammation of connective tissue more often underlies a prolonged fever.

tion and testing of a child with a prolonged fever over a week or more at home fails to identify a cause, a physician may recommend hospitalization for further evaluation.

Extended observation in a hospital of a child with a fever allows a variety of experts to study the child in a controlled environment, evaluate various test findings, and consult about possible causes. If a cause cannot be identified after an entire week of such procedures and observation, then the puzzling is designated FUO and investigation continues, usually until a cause is found or the fever subsides spontaneously.

FUO may be accompanied by signs and symptoms typical of those appearing with any fever. Fever may remain nearly constant or may fluctuate by several degrees during the day or night.

In some children FUO resists diagnosis. Estimates vary, but perhaps 10 percent of all FUOs go undiagnosed. Fever reduction methods may be successful in some cases, while other children may recover spontaneously before diagnosis can be made.

Causes of FUO tend to vary, depending on whether a child is older or younger than 6 years. Younger children more often have viral and bacterial infections underlying prolonged fever. For older children an inflammation of connective tissue more often underlies a prolonged fever.

Treatment

Whether and when to call a medical professional for assistance for a child with fever depends upon several factors, including a child's age, overall health before beginning of fever, associated symptoms of illness, a parent's experience in caring for ill children, and the individual's physician's own policy about reporting fever.

If a child 3 years of age or older has a fever of less than 102° F (38.8° C) unaccompanied by any other signs or symptoms (except indications of mild illness, such as a decrease in appetite and activity), a parent can wait a day or two before consulting a physician. Such a wait-and-see attitude applies especially with older children who can reliably report symptoms. If any fever persists beyond several days, a physician should be informed regardless of the child's overall condition. If a parent has any doubt about what to do for a feverish child, a physician should be consulted.

As soon as a child begins to run a fever, one impulse is to treat and so eliminate it. Yielding to such an impulse immediately, however, may not be wise.

Fever reduction usually provides some immediate comfort, whatever the underlying cause of fever may be. If the fever is below 102°F (38.8° C), parents may want to reduce a fever to alleviate a child's discomfort. If any question exists about the advisability of trying to reduce a child's fever, regardless of degree, parents should consult the physician.

Three methods of fever reduction are available:

- radiational cooling to allow excess heat to leave a child's body;
- sponge baths to increase circulation to the skin and to allow heat to be absorbed by the lukewarm water touching the child's body;
- medication to reduce or eliminate fever.

Fever · Self-care

What you can do yourself

- You must drink a lot. If you have a fever you will lose a lot of fluid. Always replace lost fluid. Make sure the ill person has enough to drink.
- Keep the room at a comfortable temperature. Open the windows to let enough fresh are in occasionally.
- Sponge your body with lukewarm water. This will make you feel more comfortable.
- If you have a thermometer then take your temperature.
- If your child has a fever then watch carefully for any further symptoms.
- If your child is not at all its normal self then give paracetamol. Read the instructions on the pack carefully.

Adults and children over 13 years

Aspirin is more effective in reducing a temperature than paracetamol. Read the instructions on the packet carefully for the correct dosage. Do not give aspirin to children under 13 years of age. Do not take aspirin if you are allergic to it.

Contact your doctor
- If you feel feverish and have a long-standing or serious medical problem.
- If your fever comes back after a few days of feeling normal.
- If your child's fever returns after 2 days, and your child becomes unwell again.

- If your fever does not go away within 3 days, and you do not know when you have the fever.
- If you feel listless.
- If you have been to the tropics or a very hot country recently.

Children over 1 year

Contact your doctor
- If your child is confused or drowsy, whatever its temperature.
- If your child is vomiting (being sick) all the time.
- If you think your child is in pain.
- If your child is short of breath.
- If your child has a fever and diarrhea or vomiting or does not want to drink, after 24 hours.

Babies

Contact your doctor
- If the soft spot on top of your baby's head (fontanelle) is tight or bulging.
- If your baby moans when you lift its legs to change a dirty nappy.
- If the baby is being very sick (not just posseting).
- If your baby is not drinking much.
- If your baby gets diarrhea.
- If your baby has a fit, seizure or convulsion.
- If your baby has a fever which does not go away after 2 days. Speak to your doctor about this, even if the baby seems to be normal and is drinking enough.

FOOT CONDITIONS

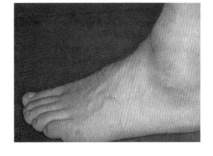

Description

There are 26 small bones in the foot, held together by a variety of ligaments, muscles and tendons. The normal foot should have two arches, one running lengthways along the foot from toe to heel, and another across the middle of the foot, higher on the inside and touching the ground at the outer border of the foot.

The feet are constantly exposed to shock and injury with every step, and when jumping or running are added, it is amazing that the feet do not suffer more injuries, as it is often only a small area on the ball of the foot that is taking the entire weight. Overweight people are more susceptible to foot injury because of the pressure on their feet is so much greater.

Any condition that can affect muscles, bone, tendons, ligaments, skin or even fat tissue can cause pain in the foot. Examples include heel spures, bone cancer, erythema nodosum. vasculitis, pernicious anemia, Morton's neuroma, Dupuytren contractures, Marfan syndrome, blood clots in veins, and impingement syndromes.

Foot conditions are common, with over one person in three suffering problems at some time. Corns, calluses, bunions, ingrown toenails and sweaty feet are the commonest foot conditions among adults.

Skeleton of part of the leg and the foot.
1. Splint bone (fibula)
2. Shin bone (tibia)
3. Tarsal bones
4. Metatarsal bones
5. Phalanges

Foot pain

The feet are constantly exposed to shock and injury with every step, and when jumping or running are added, it is amazing that the feet do not suffer more injuries, as it is often only a small area on the ball of the foot that is taking the entire weight. Overweight people are more susceptible to foot injury because the pressure on their feet is so much greater.

A strain from overuse or sudden injury to the ligaments, tendons, bones or other tissues in the foot is the most common cause of pain in the foot. Ligaments and tendons may tear, or bones may break, when the tissue is suddenly stressed, or they may give way gradually over a period of time when the foot is over used. A march fracture is an example of the latter, when excessive unaccustomed use of the feet on a long march may cause some small bones in the forefoot to crack.

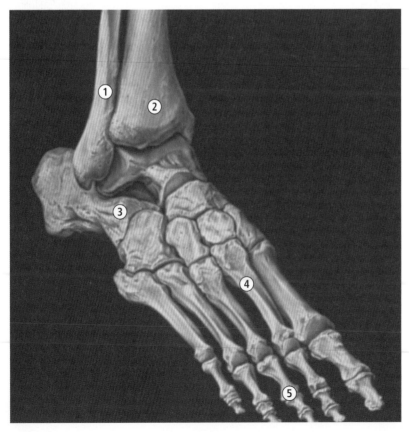

Osteoarthritis

Osteoarthritis is not, strictly speaking, a wear and tear injury to the joint, but can be considered as such without going into detailed physiology. The lining of a joint, often in the ball of the foot, degenerates with time, and becomes inflamed, resulting in pain with any movement or pressure on the joint.

Gout

Gout is a classic cause of foot pain. It is caused by a buildup of uric acid, a protein waste product, in the blood and in the lubricating synovial fluid inside joints. Joints put under greater pressure will usually be affected by gout when the excess uric acid forms microscopic double pointed needle shaped crystals in the synovial fluid. These crystals cause agonizingly sharp pain in the affected point.

The arch of the foot is maintained by a strong band of fibrous tissue that runs from the heel to the base of the toes along the outside edge of the foot under the sole. This is known as the plantar fascia, and it can be stretched or torn by injury, resulting in the disabling foot pain of plantar fasciitis, which is difficult to treat.

Summary of causes of foot pain

There are many other obvious causes of foot pain such as:

- ingrown toe nails;
- fungal infections of nails;
- bacterial infections of nails;
- corns;
- bunions;
- plantar warts;
- bruising.

Other causes of foot pain include:

- infection of the tissue and bones in the foot;
- developmental abnormalities;
- synovitis: inflammation of the synovial membrane;
- bursitis: excessive synovial fluid accumulation;
- tendinitis;
- poor blood supply to the foot;
- ulceration of the skin;
- Raynaud's phenomenon.

Any condition that can affect muscles, bone, tendons, ligaments, skin or even fat tissue can cause pain in the foot. Examples include:

- heel spurs;

- bone cancer;
- erythema nodosum;
- vasculitis;
- pernicious anemia;
- Morton's neuroma;
- Dupuytren contracture;
- Marfan syndrome;
- blood clots in veins;
- impingement syndromes, where ligaments, tendons and bones pinch each other.

Flat feet

When a child's foot does not have an arch, the foot is flat. An infant always

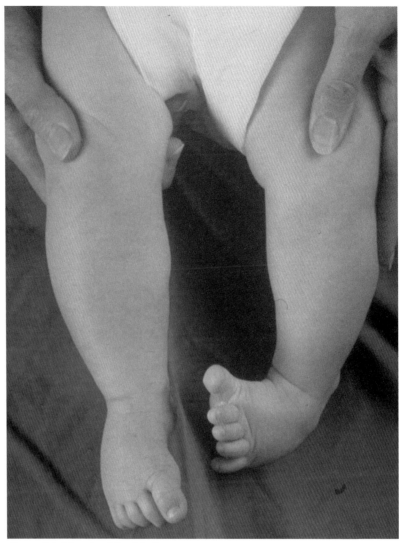

Congenital deformity of the right foot.

has flat feet because of a thick pad of fat present on the soles. Once a child begins to walk, fat pads begin to disappear.

Normal activity strengthens and shapes the ligaments, tendons, and bones of the feet into an arch. After several years of walking, the arch of the foot is fully formed, usually by the time a child is 3 or 4 years old.

Flat feet may result from bone or ligament problems present at birth that can persist into adulthood. Children usually outgrow mild flat feet. With effective treatment, severe flat feet can usually be corrected.

Flat feet not part of natural develop-

Foot conditions   Questions & Answers

What causes foot conditions?

Most foot conditions are due to poorly fitting or poor quality footwear. Corns are caused by pressure and friction on localised areas of the feet. Bunions can be due to pressure from narrow footwear squashing the toes out of shape, or wearing very high heels, or the tendency may be inherited. Most problems with smelly feet are due to excessive sweating and poor foot hygiene.

What are the symptoms?

- *Corns*
  These are small cone-shaped areas of thickened skin on the feet. They have a small central core. They can occur on the tops of the toes at sites of friction with does (hard corns), or under or between the toes (soft corns).
- *Calluses*
  These are larger areas of hard, toughened skin which form anywhere on the body in response to pressure or friction. They are particularly common on the hands, feet and knees.
- *Bunions*
  They are small, thickened, fluid-filled sacs overlying the joints at the base of the big toes. Osteoarthritis can also affect the big toe joints, making the toe rigid and painful.
- *Ingrown toenails*
  These are areas at the edges of the toenails where the nail digs into the surrounding skin or soft tissue. The tissue around the nail edge becomes overgrown, soft, red and infected.

What treatments are available?

- *Corns*
  These can be slowly softened by applying paints or other preparations containing salicylic acid. You need to take great care when applying these as they will damage the normal skin around the corn if they come into contact with it.
- *Calluses*
  Corns and calluses can be treated by soaking them and gently rubbing them down with emery board or a pumice stone. Never use scissors, razor blades or sharp instruments.
- *Bunions*
  These often do not need any treatment. However, if they become inflamed they will be tender and may be more comfortable if they are padded when you are walking around during the day.
- *Ingrown toenails*
  Start by soaking the nail to soften it, then try to pack a very small piece of cotton under the side edge of the nail to help it grow back out of the surrounding tissue. If there is obvious infection, see your doctor.

ment may be caused by loose ligaments. Loose ligaments cannot hold bones in position, and as a result, the rear of the heel and the front of the foot abnormally turn outward. This repositioning flattens the arch of the foot.

Signs and symptoms

When a flat-footed child stands, the entire sole of the foot touches the ground. Flat-footed children usually walk on the inside of the foot and break down the inner side, heel, and sole of their shoes.

Flat feet are obvious when a child stands.

A physician can make a diagnosis of flat feet by observing the presence of characteristic signs.

A physician also examines the feet for possible complications. The mobility of the foot joints and the strength of the tendons may be tested and X-ray films of the feet may be taken.

Flat feet that cause painful muscle spasms in the leg and interfere with a child's daily activities are known as symptomatic flat feet. This condition may develop when a child is between the ages of 3 and 5.

Treatment

Depending on the severity of the condition, a child's flat feet may or may not require treatment. Treatment is usually not needed if the foot is twisted only slightly at the heel but is otherwise normal, particularly if a child has reached adolescence.

Treatment of severe flat feet in a child involves repositioning the foot bones so that they develop into a normal arch.

A physician or physical therapist can prescribe walking exercises to be repeated at home that help straighten the foot bones and strengthen and tighten the ligaments. Children ages 4 to 6 years old with flat feet should walk barefoot on tiptoe for 5 to 10 minutes each day. An older flat-footed child should walk barefoot on the outer edge of the affected foot or feet with toes clenched for about 10 minutes each day.

If exercises are not sufficient to correct flat feet, a physician may recommend special shoes or appliances that help reposition bones and ligaments into an arch. All children's shoes should fit well in the heel and have room at the toes.

Orthopedic appliances such as plastic inserts that hold the foot straight, heel wedges, heel "seats" or cups, or sole wedges can be placed in regular shoes. These appliances work by gradually straightening the bones at the rear of the foot, eventually resulting in the formation of an arch. Arch supports may be recommended in cases of very severe flat feet.

If flat feet cannot be corrected through exercises or orthopedic appliances, and are troublesome and painful, a physician may recommend surgery.

Abnormalities

Some abnormal foot problems result from bone and muscle malformations in the foot and ankle that develop before birth.

Flat feet, pigeon toes, clubfoot, metatarsus adductus, and calcaneovalgus are the most common abnormal foot malformations

Metatarsus adductus

This is one of the most common foot malformations present at birth, a condition in which the front of the foot turns inward (unlike pigeon toes, in which the entire foot turns in toward the opposite foot).

This condition affects approximately 70 percent of newborns; the majority of problems correct themselves without treatment within the first few days of life.

The condition may persist, however, if an infant sleeps on his or her stomach with the feet turned inward.

If metatarsus adductus is not corrected, it may be difficult to find shoes that fit the child properly. Treatment is usually successful if begun before an infant is 8 months old.

Calcaneovalgus

This condition affects approximately 30 percent of infants. In this case the entire foot bends upward toward the knee, occasionally bending far enough so that the toes touch the front of the skin.

The heel of the foot turns outward. An infant cannot flex the foot downward because the muscles in the front of the foot are short and tight and restrict movement. The condition is usually corrected with plaster splinting.

Vertical talus

This is an uncommon foot malformation which, if uncorrected, interferes with an infant's ability to walk. The rear of an infant's foot is held off the ground and the front of the foot flexes upward toward the leg.

The center of the sole remains on the ground, resulting in a "rocker bottom," or upward bowing of the foot. An orthopedist should be consulted as soon as vertical talus is identified. In some cases a child's foot may be treated successfully through casting. Surgery, however, is usually required for complete correction.

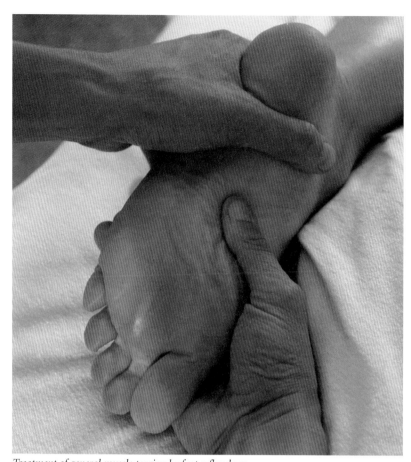

Treatment of general muscle tension by foot reflexology.

Foot dislocation

History
Force of violent nature upon plantar flexion of the foot; misstepping.
Pathology
May include a compound dislocation of the ankle. Slight to increased amount of trauma and strain upon all soft tissues of the foot.
Muscles
Marked tension of the muscles; swelling and discoloration
Complications
Fracture of the ankle. Weakness of the muscles of the plantar arch of the foot.
Treatment
Continuous application of cold for 24 hours to 48 hours. Then heat, massage, and passive and active exercises.
Strapping and support
Pillow splint or rigid splint as for fractures. The doctor will watch for swelling and cyanosis in the part.
Differentiation
Satisfactory reduction is made when the displaced astralagus (projecting on the back of the foot) has been levelled.

FRACTURES

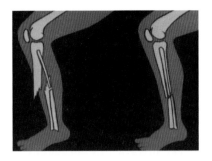

Description

A fracture is a broken of cracked bone. fractures are caused in several ways:

■ *Direct blow*
The bone is broken at the point of impact. For example, a person is hit in the leg by a piece of flying rock and the bone is broken at the point where the rock hit the leg.

■ *Indirect blow*
The bone is broken by forces travelling along the bone from the point of impact. Form example, a person who

falls and lands on the hands may suffer a broken arm.

■ *Twisting forces*
A severe twisting force can result in a fracture. For example, a person playing football or skiing is susceptible to this type of injury.

■ *Muscle contractions*
Violent muscle contractions can result in fracture. For example, a person who receives an electrical shock can experience muscle contractions so as to cause fractures.

■ *Pathological conditions*
Localized disease or aging can weaken bones to the point that the slightest stress may result in a fracture.
Broken bones, especially the long bones of the upper ad lower extremities, often have sharp,, sawtooth edges; even slight movement may cause the sharp edges to cut into the blood vessels, nerves, or muscles, and perhaps through the skin.
Careless or improper handling can convert a simple fracture into a compound fracture, and damage the surrounding blood vessels or nerves can make the injury much more serious.
A person handling a fracture should always bear this in mind. Damage due to careless handling of a simple fracture may greatly increase pain and shock, cause complications that will prolong the period of disability, and endanger life through hemorrhage of surrounding blood vessels.
The general signs and symptoms of a fracture are as follows:
- pain or tenderness in the region of the fracture;
- deformity or irregularity of the fracture;
- loss of function (disability) of the affected areas;

- moderate or severe swelling;
- discoloration;
- victim's information, if conscious.

Types of fractures

Fractures are nearly always the result of external forces but occasionally from violent muscular contractions as in tetanus and grand mal epilepsy. A closed fracture is one which does not communicate with the surface of the body. In a compound fractures, the broken bone pierces the skin and

Guidelines when splinting

- Gently remove all clothing from any suspected fracture or dislocation.
- Do not attempt to push bones back through an open wound.
- Do not attempt to straighten any fracture.
- Cover open wounds with a sterile dressing before splinting.
- Pad splints with soft material to prevent excessive pressure on the affected areas and to aid in supporting the injured part.
- Pad under all natural arches of the body such as the knee and wrist.
- Support the injured part while splint is being applied.
- Splint firmly, but not so tightly as to interfere with circulation or cause undue pain.
- Tie all knots on or near the splint.
- Do not transport the victim until the fracture or dislocation has been supported.
- Elevate the injured part and apply ice when possible.

Femur fracture

History
Usually sudden and severe trauma to the thigh.
Pathology
Bone and nerve injury; paralysis and permanent disability.
Complications
Deformity and shortening of the limb where an disturbance in bone continuity is present; severance of nerves and blood vessels; paralysis and gangrene.
Hemorrhage
The condition may or may not hemorrhage. Discoloration may be delayed.
Color of area
Slight or marked increase in ecchymosis.
Treatment
The doctor will apply a splint to the leg and the body. The patient will be kept flat. Traction is being provided and retained.
Transportation
A rigid stretcher will be used. The leg will be kept in traction until ready for reduction.

leaves an open wound.

The distinction is sometimes drawn between the fracture which is compound from without, i.e. the open wound results from the external violence, and one which is compound from within, i.e. a sharp spike of the fractured bone punctures the skin. The difference is of little importance as both are potentially infected and should be treated as any other open wound.

Spiral, transverse, oblique fractures are self-explanatory descriptive terms applied to the direction of the fracture. The pattern of fractures depends on the direction of the force applied and on the internal structure of the bone at the site of fracture.

In the long bones, the axial orientation of osteones make sharp transverse fractures rare. A broken bone, like a broken stick, and for similar reasons, usually splinters and shows minor irregularities in the fracture line; by their arrangement thy can contribute greatly to the stability of a reduction. Otherwise oblique and spiral fractures tend to override due to the pull of soft tissues.

Segmental and comminuted fractures, where the bone is broken in two or more places, mat heal slowly because of the poor blood supply of the smaller fragments. A compression fracture is a compaction of cancellous bone, as mar occur in the vertebral bodies. A greenstick fracture is an incomplete break occurring in tot pliable bones of a growing child.

An epiphyseal fracture separation, also confined to the growing period, takes place through the hypertrophic zone of epiphyseal cartilage which is a site of structural weakness. The cartilage plate retains its attachment to the epiphysis from which it gains its nutrition, and its growth is consequently not interrupted.

Avulsion fractures detach small fragments of bone at the sites of muscle insertions. In the growing period the entire epiphysis may become detached. A stress fracture is an undisplaced crack arising in a bone which has been subjected to repeated stresses, any one of which would be insufficient to produce a fracture.

The "march fracture" of the metatarsal bones in army recruits is

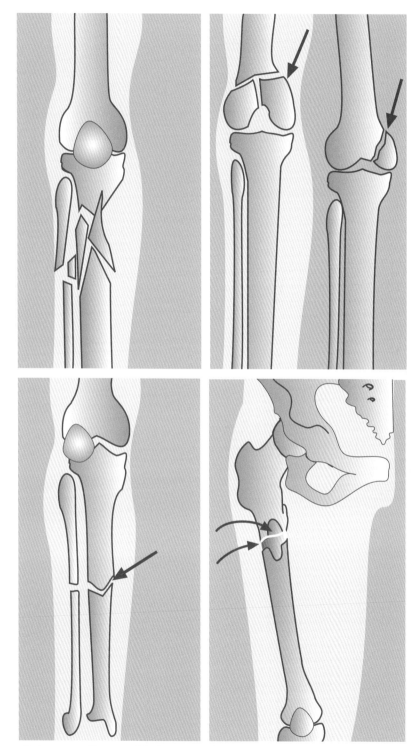

Various types of fractures of the lower extremity.
Upper left: complicated fracture of tibia and fibula.
Upper right: fractures of the condyle of the femur.
Lower left: fracture of the tibia and fibula caused by a direct blow.
Lower right: fracture of the femur caused by an indirect blow.

Forearm fracture

History
The fracture is the result of a twisting force upon the lower arm or wrist, or from violence exerted upon the arm in preventing the body from falling.
Pathology
Fracture and displacement of the distal end of the radius. The tip of the styloid process of the ulna is broken off. There is also backward dislocation.
Complications
Trauma and swelling of the tissues. Dislocations and sprains.
Hemorrhage
Slight; increased if the fracture is not immediately immobilized.
Color of area
Slight to marked.
Treatment
Rigid splint, arm support with a sling.
Transportation
The arm will be placed in a sling after splinting.

Humerus fracture

History
Fracture of the humerus results from a twisting force or blow upon the upper arm.
Pathology
Injury to the osseous structures. Trauma and lacerations of tissues, muscles, etc., if a compound fracture exists.
Complications
Severance of nerves and blood vessels; temporary deformity.
Hemorrhage
Slight; increased hemorrhage if a compound fracture exists.
Color of area
Slight or marked areas of discoloration.
Treatment
The doctor will immobilize the limb immediately by a splint or sling (weight of the forearm usually provides the necessary traction).
Transportation
Keep the arm in a sling or splint.

an example. These fractures may not be visible on the initial radiograph but may be recognized by a surrounding cuff of callus after a few days. Pathological fractures occur in bone which is weakened by disease. Common underlying causes are osteoporosis, primary and secondary bone tumors and bone cysts.

Factors affecting fracture healing

As with any other tissue, a fracture disrupts local blood vessels leading to a hematoma and local tissue death, resulting in the disappearance of the osteocytes in the fractured bone ends for a distance proportional to the disturbance of the blood supply.
Every fracture is associated with some injury to soft tissue, and this may involve periosteum, muscle, tendon, nerves, major vessels and viscera. The soft tissue injuries may be of more immediate significance than the fracture itself, and should always be looked for. It response to trauma, osteoblasts are stimulated top activity near the fracture and lay down a matrix of bone; this follows at the wake of the vascular granulation tissue until the bone ends are joined by a delicate network of bone which occupies the medullary cavity and surrounds the bone ends like a plumber's joint.

■ *Blood supply*
As is the case with wounds, an adequate blood supply is the most important factor and fractures through cancellous bone, which in general retain a good supply, heal more quickly that fractures through cortical bone in which the blood supply is more vulnerable.

■ *Bone apposition*
Callus can extend only a few millimetres from a fractured bone end and if there is a gap between bone ends which cannot be bridged in this way, non-union is likely. The size of the gap is critical and varies from individual to individual and from bone to bone, but in general is greater in a child than in an adult.

■ *Immobilization*
Immobility is not essential; fractures in wild animals may heal rapidly,

Fractures of the bone of the lower leg.

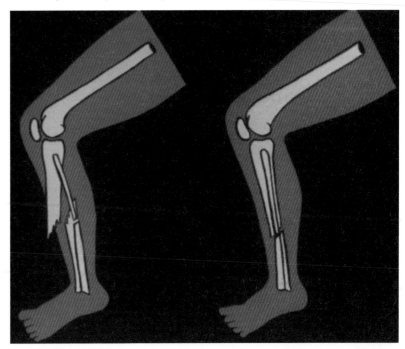

although usually with some deformity, and in man fractures of the ribs and clavicles are almost impossible to immobilize and yet non-union is rare. In general, however, fractures heal more certainly and more rapidly if immobilized, and the importance of good immobilization is increased in fractures where delayed healing may be expected, for example from a poor blood supply. In most fractures some degree of immobilization is necessary to prevent deformity arising during healing.

■ *Metabolic factors*
Healing of all tissues, including bone, is impaired in gross dietary deficiency. Vitamin D deficiency causes a marked impairment of mineralization of fracture callus so that fractures may remain painful and union unsound for months or years in patients with rickets or osteomalacia; elderly women are especially susceptible to vitamin D deficiency.
It might be supposed that calcium intake is important to fracture healing.
However, the reserves of calcium elsewhere in the skeleton are sufficient to meet any local requirement. Experiments have suggested that supplements of phosphates may accelerate healing of fractures, but this has not been confirmed. Hormonal influences on fracture healing are of little importance in the absence of endocrine disease.

■ *Infection*
Fracture healing may be inhibited by infection. Organisms gain access to a fracture site through a compound wound or may be introduced at operation on a fracture.
Meticulous surgical technique minimizes infection from these causes. The presence of dead bone or foreign material such as a metal plate favours the persistence of infection and healing the fracture may not occur until these are removed.

Splints and splinting

Splints are used to support, immobilize, and protect parts with injuries such as known or suspected fractures,

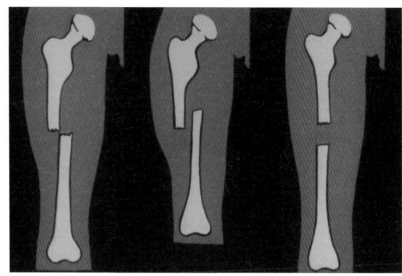

Fractures of the bone of the femur (thigh bone).

dislocations, or severe sprains. Many types of splints are available commercially. Plastic inflatable splints can be easily applied and quickly inflated, require minimum of dressing and give rigid support to injured limbs.

Ankle fracture
Potts fracture

History
Sudden or forceful wrenching of the lower end of the tibia and fibula.
Pathology
Fracture of the lower ends of the fibula and tibia. The foot is displaced outward. Impairment of tissues, vessels, etc., from the trauma.
Complications
Dislocation and sprains may occur simultaneously.
Hemorrhage
The condition may or may not cause a hemorrhage. Discoloration often occurs.
Color of area
Slight or marked areas of ecchymosis.
Treatment
Immobilize immediately by pillow splint or rigid splint.
Transportation
Keep limb well supported with slight elevation.

Improvised splints may be made from pieces of wood, broom handles, heavy cardboard, newspapers, magazines, or similar firm material.

Pelvis fracture

History
Fracture of the pelvis is caused by a blow or crushing force.
Pathology
Bone impairment; involvement of sacral nerves. Other pathological findings include: paralysis, torn ligaments, and lacerated muscles.
Complications
Rupture of the urinary bladder and rectum; deformity and shortening of the limb; sprain of pelvic joints.
Hemorrhage
Same as in a compound fracture. Discoloration may be delayed.
Color of area
Same as in a compound fracture if compound. Otherwise delayed.
Treatment
The patient will be kept in recumbent position; after reduction in prone position. Reduction of fragments; symptomatic treatment.
Transportation
On a rigid stretcher in dorsal recumbent position. The body should be kept extended.

GALLBLADDER DISEASES

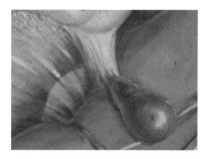

Description

The gallbladder is a pear-shaped sac that lies in its own depression, or fossa, under the liver. It is about 9 cm (3.5 inches) long, 2.5 cm (1 inch) wide and holds about 35 cubic centimetres of fluid.

It is covered on its free, exposed surface by peritoneum (the membrane that covers all the internal organs) and has a bare area on its upper surface where it is contact with the liver.

Arising from the gallbladder is the cystic duct, which is connected to the liver by the common hepatic duct, and to the first part of the small intestine - the duodenum - by the common bile duct.

The gallbladder functions as a storage place for the bile that is constantly being formed by the liver, and it may also concentrate it by extracting water. In the presence of fatty foods in the small intestine, a hormone - cholecystokinin - is produced by the cells of the small intestine and causes the gallbladder to contract and empty its contents into the duodenum.

No one knows why we need to store and concentrate bile in this way, for we can function perfectly well if our gallbladders are removed.

Gallstones

About 10 per cent of the general population and 20 per cent of those over 40 years of age have concretions in the gallbladder called gallstones, made up of bile pigment and/or cholesterol and ranging from the size of a tiny bead to that of a pigeon's egg.

The problem is commoner in women, in people who are obese and in those with cirrhosis of the liver or certain diseases of the small intestine.

Those with uncomplicated gallstones usually are without symptoms but may complain of:
▲ discomfort in the upper abdomen;
▲ bloating;
▲ belching;
▲ food intolerance.

Because these symptoms are also found in common conditions such as dyspepsia (i.e. indigestion), considerable controversy exists as to whether they should be attributed to the gallstones. Symptoms and signs depend upon the size, number and location of the gallstones. Multiple gallstones often cause intermittent episodes of abrupt, severe pain when a small stone passes into the common bile duct.

Large stones may cause pain by intermittent obstruction of the outlet of the gallbladder, the cystic duct. Despite the prevalence of gallstones, their natural history is not well understood or fully defined.

More than 60 per cent of those with gallstones will experience no pain, or only one attack; most of the remaining sufferers will have only episodic pain. Nevertheless, the incidence of serious complications is high enough that surgical removal of the gallbladder is often advocated as the treatment of choice, unless other serious illness contra-indicates surgery.

Multiple small stones are likely to

Bottom view of the liver and gallbladder.
1. Lobes of the liver
3. Gallbladder
3. Ducts of the gallbladder
4. Inferior caval vein

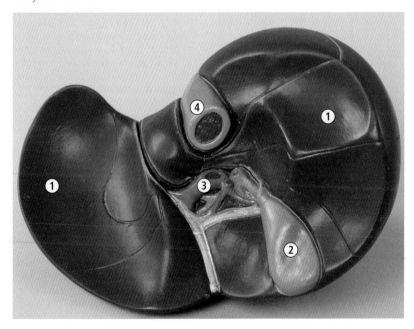

cause complications - for instance, obstruction of the cystic duct, inflammation of the pancreas and intestinal problems. Elderly and obese people require special consideration as to the threat of physical complications versus the increased risks of surgery.

Inflammation

Both acute and chronic cholecystitis (inflammation of the gallbladder resulting from infection by bacteria) exist. In most instances, acute cholecystitis is caused by a gallstone that blocks the cystic duct.

However, inflammation of the gallbladder can occur without stones and bacterial infection; chemical irritation and the digestive activities of certain enzymes may play a contributing role. In the acute condition, a sharp pain in the right upper part of the abdomen, often occurring at night or in the early morning, is a prominent symptom. Whether the onset is sudden or gradual, the pain reaches a plateau that is maintained with little fluctuation and is usually quite severe.

The diagnosis is usually based on the symptoms and physical examination of the person. In a few, X-rays or ultrasound examinations of the abdomen will reveal opaque gallstones. Most doctors recommend surgical removal of the gallbladder, but

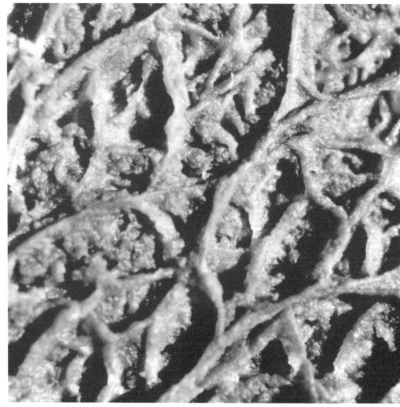

Microscopic view of the inner surface of the wall of the gallbladder. The many grooves increase the surface.

the decision must be based on each individual case. It is rarely necessary to rush someone to surgery because of an acute condition. When the diagnosis is in doubt and a surgical emergency is not indicated by severe irritation of the peritoneum or increasing signs of toxicity (poisoning), the person can be treated by other means.

If the acute stage subsides, surgery should be delayed for six weeks or two months. The chronic condition usually develops insidiously without a definite preceding attack of acute cholecystitis.

The symptoms and signs are ill-defined and are not unique to gallbladder diseases, as they vary with the extent of the disease, the presence and location of gallstones and the presence of complications. However, the surgical removal of the gallbladder is still the treatment of choice unless other serious illness contra-indicates surgery.

Cholesterol deposits

The cause of this condition is unknown. The appearance of yellow

Various types of gallstones

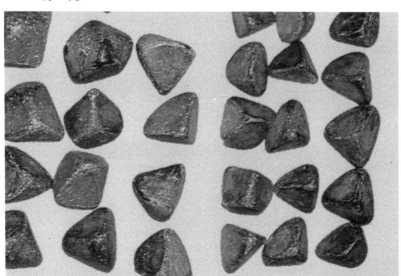

Gallbladder diseases   Questions & Answers

What is bile?
Bile is a viscous, dark green, alkaline fluid coloured by bilirubin, a breakdown product of hemoglobin, and containing quantities of cholesterol and bile salts. These salts have a detergent and emulsifying action, for their molecules have chemical grouping soluble both in watery and in fatty substances. This explains the ability of bile to enhance the absorption of fats from the intestines. When bile secretion is impaired, fat cannot be absorbed properly and is instead excreted in the faeces, and in addition the fat-soluble vitamins A, D and K are lost to the body.

What are the common causes of gallbladder disorders?
The most common causes of gallbladder disease are the following:
• Infection with bacteria.
• A functional disturbance in which the gallbladder fails to empty when it is called upon to secrete bile.
• A chemical disturbance causing stones to precipitate out from the bile. These stones may create an obstruction to the passage of bile along the ducts and into the intestinal tract.

What is the cause of gallbladder inflammation?
Both acute and chronic cholecystitis (inflammation of the gallbladder resulting from infection by bacteria) exist. In most instances, acute cholecystitis is caused by a gallstone that blocks the cystic duct.
However, inflammation of the gallbladder can occur without stones and bacterial infection; chemical irritation and the digestive activities of certain enzymes may play a contributing role.

What are the symptoms of gallbladder infection?
A sharp pain in the right upper part of the abdomen, often occurring at night or in the early morning, is a prominent symptom. Whether the onset is sudden or gradual, the pain reaches a plateau that is maintained with little fluctuation and is usually quite severe.

How is the diagnosis of a gallbladder disorder made?
The diagnosis is usually based on the symptoms and physical examination of the person. In a few, X-rays or ultrasound examinations of the abdomen will reveal opaque gallstones.

What is the best treatment of a gallbladder disorder?
Most doctors recommend surgical removal of the gallbladder, but the decision must be based on each individual case. It is also possible to remove the gallbladder by way of an endoscopic technique. When the diagnosis is in doubt and a surgical emergency is not indicated by severe irritation of the peritoneum or increasing signs of toxicity (poisoning), the person can be treated by other means. If the acute stage subsides, surgery will be delayed for six weeks or two months.

When does a chronic condition of the gallbladder develop?
The chronic condition usually develops insidiously without a definite preceding attack of acute cholecystitis. The symptoms and signs are ill-defined and are not unique to gallbladder disease, as they vary with the extent of the disease, the presence and location of gallstones, and the presence of complications. However, the surgical removal of the gallbladder is still the treatment of choice unless other serious illness contraindicates surgery.

What are gallstones?
Sometimes one or more of the constituents of bile are thrown out of solution and then they precipitate in crystalline form within the gall bladder or one of the ducts. These gallstones may consist of pure cholesterol, pure pigment or pure calcium but in the great majority they are mixed.

What is the incidence of gallstones?
Gallstones are exceedingly common. Probably 10 per cent of all people will form gallstones of one type or another sometimes in their lives, although not more than perhaps a quarter of these will ever develop symptoms. Precipitations of bile constituents may be caused by excessive formation as in hemolytic anemia when abnormal numbers of red blood cells are broken down to yield great amounts of pigment, or when excessive bone destruction releases abnormal amounts of calcium salts. If the common bile duct becomes obstructed by kinking, adhesions, inflammation extending from the duodenum or pressure from a mass in the abdomen, there is bile pile-up in the gall bladder, and its lining absorbs so much water that the bile is concentrated and its constituents precipitate as solids.

Are gallstones more common in men or women?
Gallstones are more common in women, and the incidence is proportional to the number of pregnancies. Obesity also predisposes to stone formation. Uncomplicated stones in the gall bladder usually cause no symptoms, unless they block one of the ducts. Most of them in the gall bladder remain "silent" for long periods, sometimes indefinitely. So-called "gallstone disease" is caused by the complication induced by the presence of these stones; this complication is cholecystitis (inflammation of the gall bladder).

What complications of gallstones may occur?
When a stone becomes lodged in the neck of the gall bladder or a duct, bile flow is obstructed. Flow stoppage results in over-concentration and then bile salts irritate the wall. An inflammatory reaction soon develops and, with lowering of resistance, infection is almost sure to follow. The gall bladder becomes distended, inflamed and exceedingly tender (painful to the touch). Because of the obstruction, the intestinal content is deprived of pigments and bile salts. The stools become light (clay-coloured). Fats are poorly digested. There are dyspepsia and flatulence whenever fried or fatty foods are ingested. Distention causes abdominal discomfort.

Cholecystostomy (creation of an opening into the gall bladder for drainage). Exposing the gall bladder (A); inserting two purse-string sutures (B); aspirating the infected bile (C); incising the gall bladder in the center of the areas enclosed by the purse-string sutures (D); suction (E); removing any loose stones (F). Introducing the tip of a Foley catheter into the gall bladder (G, H); tightening the purse-string sutures against the tube and using the ends to fix the catheter (I).

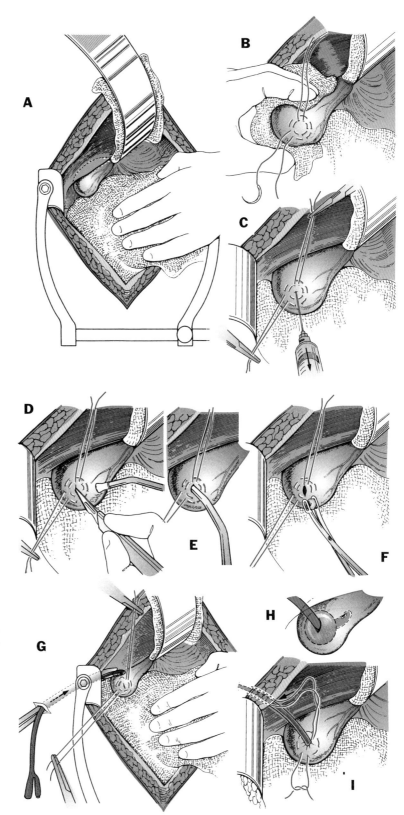

flecks of cholesterol on the reddish mucous membrane that lines the gallbladder has resulted in the name "strawberry gallbladder." There is no relationship to the cholesterol content of blood or to specific metabolic changes in the body.

Some authorities believe that the symptoms are like those of chronic inflammation and gallstones, while others state that this condition on its own produces no symptoms. Usually, the diagnosis is made by the pathologist after removal of the gallbladder.

Cancer

Cancer of the gallbladder has been found in 0.2 to 5.0 per cent of surgically removed gallbladders, and it ranks fifth among cancers of the gastro-intestinal system and allied glands. Most patients are women between the ages of 60 and 70.

The frequent association of gallstones and cancer of the gallbladder has been accepted by many as indicating a causal relationship, leading to the advice that early removal of the gallbladder from those with gallstones may prevent this particular type of cancer. Many patients with cancer of the gallbladder have intermittent pain and dyspepsia (similar to that seen in cholecystitis and gallstones) for several years.

Unfortunately, the symptoms of more severe pain, recent weight loss, and jaundice (yellowing of the skin due to a blockage of bile) appear only in the late stages of the disease, and only 30 per cent of cases of cancer of the gallbladder are suitable for a surgical operation.

GASTRITIS

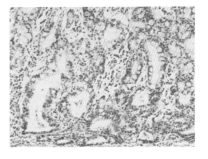

Description

Gastritis is defined as an inflammatory process of the stomach. It is characterized by pain or tenderness, nausea, vomiting and systemic electrolyte changes if vomiting persists. The mucosal lining of the stomach may be atrophic or hypertrophic.

On the basis of the clinical picture and the histological changes of the mucosal lining the following major types of gastritis can be distinguished:
- ▲ acute gastritis;
- ▲ corrosive gastritis;
- ▲ atrophic gastritis;
- ▲ hypertrophic gastritis.

Acute gastritis

This disorder of the stomach is characterized by superficial, mucosal lesions of the corpus of the stomach that occur very rapidly in relation to various stresses. The most common provocative stresses are:
- major burns;
- trauma with multiple injuries;
- shock;
- alcohol;
- corticosteroids;
- aspirin or other anti-inflammatory agents;
- food or drug allergens;
- toxins.

Most often there are no specific symptoms, but anorexia, nausea, vomiting and distress in the stomach region may occur. Hemorrhage (bleeding) causes the greatest concern. It occurs in about 10 percent of the patients, is usually mild and often follows the stressful event within 6 to 7 days.

Acute gastritis may account for as much as 30 percent of all gastrointestinal bleeding episodes. Presence of hemorrhage can be the only symptom of acute gastritis, although patients are commonly very ill as a result of the underlying disorder.

Prevention of hemorrhage is often possible. Treating the underlying disorder (for instance, shock) or withdrawing the offending agent prompts the disorder to subside spontaneously. The use of antacids not only relieves pain, but may prevent hemorrhage.

Their preventive use is recommended when predisposing conditions are apparent.

Corrosive gastritis

This disorder is caused by swallowing strong acids or alkalis, iodine, potassium permanganate or heavy metal salts. The degree of injury and the symptoms depend upon the nature and amount of the ingested substances.

Stomach damage may range from a mild hyperaemia (increased blood supply) and edema (accumulation of fluid) to severe necrosis (death of cells or tissue) of the mucosa, and a subsequent, possibly hemorrhagic, inflammatory reaction. Necrosis may extend to the deeper layers of the stomach wall and result in perforation. The treatment should be in the hands of a specialist familiar with the care of patients with poisonings.

Atrophic gastritis

Atrophy or wasting of tissue is a condition more common in the aged. The cause is unknown. Associations that are not fully explained have been noted between gastritis and stomach polyps, stomach cancer, peptic ulcer of the stomach and pernicious anemia.

No specific pattern of symptoms and/or signs have been identified. Some patients complain of nausea, pain and distress in the region of the stomach, especially after eating, but many have no symptoms at all.

Indirect evidence tends to corroborate the suggestion that there is a strong correlation between chronic gastritis and smoking. However, it is still not known whether smoking per se is a

Severe corrosive gastritis, microscopic picture.

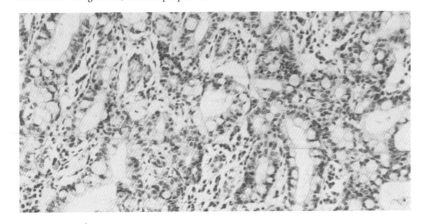

Anatomic model of the stomach.
1. Cardia
2. Fundus
3. Body (central portion)
4. Pyloric portion
5. Pylorus

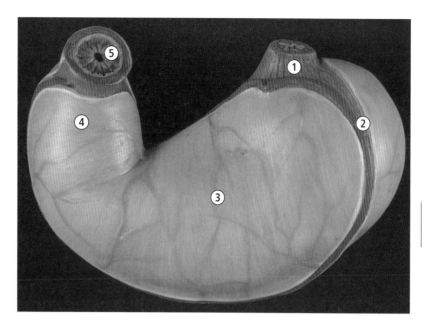

definite cause of chronic or atrophic gastritis.

Corticosteroids have been tried because some patients with atrophic gastritis have antibodies to certain glandular cells in the stomach. Patients with pernicious anemia (a type of anemia characterized by defective red blood cell production) may have antibodies to intrinsic factor as well.

However, the results of treatment with corticosteroids have generally been disappointing and their routine use is not recommended. Antacids may relieve distress.

Hypertrophic gastritis

In many patients the prominence of stomach folds seen with endoscopic examination disappear when air distends the stomach.

Although hyperaemia, turgidity and engorgement of the folds are visible with the endoscope in such patients, they may also be seen in patients with a normal stomach that shows an increase in secretion. Also chronic superficial gastritis may be observed. The cause is unknown, but increasing evidence has implicated bile salts in the pathogenesis in some cases.

Bile reflux in the stomach is commonly found in patients with peptic ulcer or prior stomach surgery, two conditions in which chronic gastritis is common. There is no consistent pattern of symptoms and the diagnosis may be suggested when endoscopy is performed to investigate nonspecific symptoms. No effective treatment is known.

Gastritis   Questions & Answers

What causes acute gastritis?
Acute gastritis is a inflammation of the lining of the stomach caused by bacteria, viruses, chemical irritants, or by eating spoiled foods. Acute gastritis is, in general, characterized by the following symptoms:
• nausea
• vomiting
• upper abdominal cramps
• fever

The condition is usually associated with a similar inflammation of the small intestine and is therefore often called gastroenteritis. The letter condition is accompanied by violent and mid-abdominal and lower abdominal cramps, with episodes of diarrhea. When only the stomach is involved, diarrhea is present.

I have been told to suffer from chronic gastritis; what are the symptoms and treatment?
Chronic gastritis is an inflammation of the lining of the stomach which persists over a long period of time. The cause is not

definitely known. It is thought that prolonged and excess use of spices, alcohol, and other irritants may eventually lead to a chronic inflammation of the stomach lining.
The most important symptoms are:
• upper abdominal discomfort
• abdominal pain
• heartburn
• a sense of fullness in the region
• loss of appetite
• loss of weight
• nausea
• vomiting
The basic treatment of the normal chronic gastritis is:
- stop smoking
- refrain from alcoholic beverages
- eat frequent, small, bland meals, with plenty of milk
- refrain from eating spicy foods
- if the chronic gastritis is associated with excess stomach acidity, take appropriate antacid medications
- if there is an absence of acid, then medications will be given

GENITAL HERPES

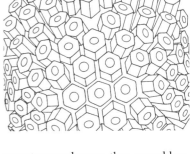

Description

Genital herpes is an infection of the genital and adjacent skin area with the herpes simplex virus (Type-2). It is now the commonest cause of genital ulceration. Blisters frequently develop four to seven days after contact and the condition tends to relapse. It is very painful, the initial attack lasting two to three weeks.

Babies can be infected in the womb or during delivery, and are at high risk of congenital eye abnormalities or damage to the central nervous system. In addition, women who have contracted genital herpes are more likely to get cervical cancer.

Herpetic ulcer of the penis.

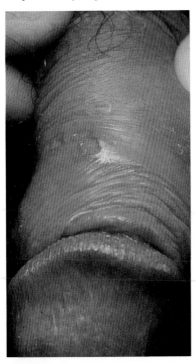

Incidence and Causes

Genital herpes is caused by the herpes simplex virus. It is related to but different from the varicella zoster virus, which causes chickenpox and shingles. Forms of herpes simplex also cause cold sores.

Herpes is actually a family of viruses that causes diseases you are probably familiar with, including fever blisters, mononucleosis and chickenpox. Most adults and children have been exposed to one or another of these viruses.

There are two different types of herpes simplex. usually, one affects the mouth while the other affects the genitals. Type-2 causes genital sores; Type-1 causes cold sores or fever blisters. Type-1 can be spread to the genitals through oral sex.

Conversely, a few cases of oral herpes are caused by Type-2. However, either type of virus can infect any sight of the body. About 90 per cent of genital herpes is due to Type-2, the remaining 10 per cent to Type-1.

The highly communicable virus newly infects half a million Americans a year; they join an estimated 23 million Americans who are already infected (1999 data). After the first infection, many people experience recurrences at rates that typically vary from once or twice a year to as much as once or twice a month.

In adults, genital herpes is primarily a sexually transmitted disease. It is acquired by direct exposure of the genitals to the infected genitals, or, sometimes to the infected mouth of another person. It can also be contracted through other forms of skin-to-skin contact.

Fifteen per cent of the people who get genital herpes get it from oral sex with partners with oral herpes. Because some people never recognize their symptoms as herpes, they spread herpes without knowing it. Other experience signs that a herpes outbreak is imminent. They notice itching or tingling before seeing a sore. These are called prodromal symptoms. With very rare exceptions, genital herpes is not acquired from infected toilet seats, moist towels or similar items.

Herpes can be spread whether people recognize symptoms or not-at any point that the virus is shed from the skin. For this reason using condoms and informing partners is important.

Shedding is the process by which the virus multiplies itself and is released from the skin. It takes place during initial outbreaks, recurrent outbreaks, and sometimes even between outbreaks when there are no prodromal signs or no noticeable sores.

Some people unknowingly transmit herpes to other parts of their body after touching their own sores. This is called "auto-inoculation" and almost always occurs during an initial outbreak. You can prevent auto-inoculation by simply washing your hands with soap and water.

Some people identify lack of sleep, poor diet, and menstruation as factors responsible for the infection or recurrent outbreaks. An increase in frequency and severity of outbreaks has been reported by people who abuse drugs, such as alcohol, cocaine or speed. In some people there are no clear patterns at all.

If you suspect that certain circumstances may contribute to your outbreaks, then adjusting your behavior accordingly may ease the problem.

Signs and Symptoms

The first episode usually occurs from 2 to 21 days after exposure. Symptoms may include swelling, pain, itching and burning at the site of the infection. They are followed by reddening and finally tiny blisters, which may then burst forming tender ulcers which crust and eventually heal.

Additional symptoms are often those experienced in any viral infection:

- fever;
- chills;
- muscle aches;
- lethargy;
- headaches.

Many people also experience burning during urination, vaginal or urethral discharge (release of a liquid-like substance), difficulty passing urine, and tender lymph nodes (small glands found under the arms, in the neck and in the groin area).

It is not uncommon, however, to have a first-time infection without any noticeable symptoms or with minimal symptoms. Herpes can come back. Eighty to ninety per cent of people who have genital herpes have recurrent outbreaks.

Generally, it reappears within three to six months of the first outbreak-though these subsequent occurrences are usually not as severe as once a month, in others rarely or not at all. For those who do have recurrent outbreaks, herpes recurs an average of four to six times a year.

After a number of years, however, outbreaks tend to become less frequent and less severe. It is likely, in about the fifth or sixth year, to see even further change in recurrence patterns.

Once a person has herpes, the virus remains in the body in a dormant or inactive state for that person's lifetime. Every so often the dormant infection reactivates and symptoms reappear.

But symptoms are usually much less severe than those experienced in an initial outbreak and generally do not last as long. Most people are unable to pinpoint what triggers a herpes outbreak, since outbreaks tend to occur randomly.

Treatment

At this time, there is no cure for herpes. However, the antiviral medication acyclovir (Zovirax) actually stops

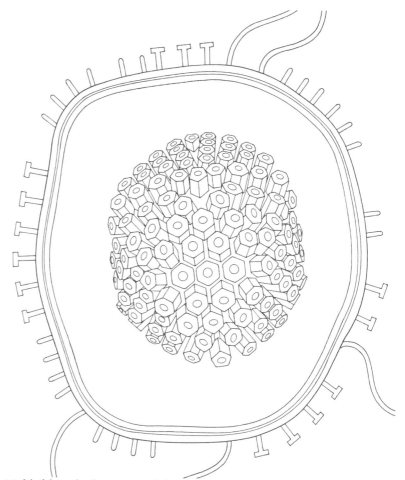

Model of the molecular structure of a herpesvirus.

the herpesvirus from making more virus. Researchers at 19 medical centers in the United States found that among 389 people who had been experiencing 12 or more recurrences of genital herpes outbreaks a year, daily doses of the drug acyclovir could reduce the number of flare-ups to an average of 1.7 a year in the first year of treatment and to an average of only 0.8 per year in the fifth year of treatment. Furthermore, 20 per cent of patients who took two 400-milligram tablets of acyclovir daily had no recurrences over the entire five-year test period. The most common side effects included nausea, diarrhea, headache, rash and vaginal yeast infection. Nearly all of these effects abated significantly after the first year and affected only a few per cent of patients during the fifth year.

Your doctor will recommend the treatment program best for you. After you have been treated for your first herpes outbreak, there are two different ways to treat future outbreaks with acyclovir: an episodic or daily treatment.

■ *Episodic treatment*
This means you take the medicine only when you have an episode or outbreak.

When taken correctly the drug helps to heal sores sooner and can shorten the length of time you have the outbreak.

■ *Daily treatment*
If your outbreaks are severe or frequent, you and your doctor may decide that taking the drug on a daily basis is the best course of action.

Genital herpes Questions & Answers

What is herpes simplex?

Herpes simplex is a common virus. It causes sores on or near the face (often called "cold sores" or "oral herpes"), and it causes the genital sores known as "genital herpes." There are two herpes simplex viruses - herpes simplex 1 (HSV-1) and herpes simplex type 2 (HSV-2). These viruses are very similar, and either type can infect the mouth or genitals. Most commonly, however, HSV-1 occurs above the waist, and HSV-2 below.

How do you get genital herpes?

Herpes is spread by direct skin-to-skin contact. Unlike a flu that you can get through the air, herpes spreads by direct contact - that is, directly from the site of infection to the site of contact. For example, if you have a cold sore and kiss someone, you can transfer the virus from your mouth to theirs. Similarly, if you have active genital herpes and have vaginal or anal intercourse, you can transfer the virus from your genitals to theirs. Finally, if you have a cold sore and put your mouth on your partner's genitals (oral sex), you can give your partner genital herpes.

When is genital herpes most likely to be spread?

Herpes is most easily spread when a sore is present, but it is often spread at other times, too. Some people notice itching, tingling, or other sensations before they see any sores on their skin. These are called "prodromal symptoms," and they warn that virus may be present on the skin. Herpes is most likely to be spread from the time these first symptoms are noticed until the area is completely healed and the skin looks normal again. Sexual contact - oral, vaginal, or anal - poses a very clear risk during this time.

Can genital herpes be transmitted when there are no symptoms?

Sometimes those who know they are infected spread the virus between recurrences, when no signs or symptoms are present. This is called "asymptomatic transmission." Research also shows that herpes simplex infections often are spread by people who do not know they are infected. These people might have symptoms so mild they do not notice them at all or else do not recognize them as herpes. Many genital herpes infections are spread from persons who are asymptomatic "shredders" of the virus. For those who recognize their symptoms, a sexual contact during asymptomatic periods is less likely to cause infection than a sexual contact when sores are present.

But people tend to have many more contacts when they have no sores, so the risk of asymptomatic transmission is very real. The best way to lower the risk is to use condoms in between recurrent episodes.

What are the typical symptoms of a first episode of genital herpes?

Symptoms of herpes usually develop within 2 to 20 days after contact with the virus, although it may take far longer. In some people, the herpes virus causes a first attack so mild that is unnoticed. In others, the first attack causes visible sores. But in either case the virus eventually retreats into the nervous system end lies dormant there. In a first episode the skin usually becomes inflamed, and soon afterward one or more blisters or bumps appear. The blisters first open and then heal as new skin tissue forms. During a first outbreak, the area is usually painful and may itch, burn, or tingle.

What are the characteristics of flu-like symptoms in case of genital herpes?

Flu-like symptoms include:

- swollen glands
- headache
- muscle aches
- fever

Herpes might also infect the urethra, and urinating might cause a burning sensation. The first outbreak might last up to several weeks. When the sores are completely healed, the active phase of infection is over. Symptoms may vary from one person to the next. In many people, the first infection is so mild that it goes unnoticed. Even so, subsequent recurrences of the disease might cause sores.

Are complications of herpes infections be possible?

One kind of complication involves moving the virus from the location of an outbreak to other places on the body by touching the sore(s). The fingers, eyes, and other body parts can accidentally become infected in this way. Preventing self-infection is simple: do not touch the area during an outbreak - especially the first outbreak. If you do, wash your hands as soon as possible. The herpes virus is easily killed with soap and water.

What should I do if I think I have genital herpes?

If you think you may have herpes, see a doctor while symptoms are still present. The doctor will look at the area, take a sample from the sore(s), and test to see if the herpes virus is present. The test you should request is a specific culture for HSV. The test will not work if the sores have healed and might not work if they are more than a few days old.

What else can I do after the diagnosis of a herpes infection?

Many people feel panicked when they first learn they have genital herpes. Partly as a result of these feelings, the first few outbreaks can cause a great deal of stress.

If maybe important, therefore, to take additional steps.

- First, get the information you need so you are not worrying unnecessarily. Understanding herpes gives you a positive way to deal with your concerns
- Second, seek emotional support when you need it. Keeping your feelings to yourself may to more harm than

Counselling

About 85 percent of cases of sexually transmitted diseases occur in persons aged between 15 and 29 years. In addition to syphilis and gonorrhea, the list of sexually transmitted diseases now includes:

- human immunodeficiency virus (HIV) infection
- Chlamydia trachomatis infection
- genital herpes virus infection
- human papilloma virus (HPV) infection
- chancroid
- genital mycoplasma
- cytomegalusvirus infection
- hepatitis B infection
- vaginitis
- enteric infections
- ectoparasitic diseases

Chlamydial infection is the most common sexually transmitted disease. Although the incidence of gonorrhea and syphilis decreased in the early 1990s, these sexually transmitted diseases remain a persistent public health problem. The consequences of sexually transmitted diseases are particularly troublesome for women and children. Apart from AIDS, the most serious complications of sexually transmitted diseases are:

- pelvic inflammatory disease
- an increased risk of cervical cancer
- ectopic pregnancy
- congenital infection
- congenital malformations
- delivery of premature infants
- delivery of low-birth-weight infants
- fetal death

Persons who are poor or medically under-served and racial and ethnic minorities also contract a disproportionate number of sexually transmitted diseases and the disabilities associated with them. Individuals who are at increased risk for sexually transmitted diseases and HIV infection include:

- ▲ those who are or were recently sexually active, especially persons with multiple sexual partners;
- ▲ those who use alcohol or illicit drugs;
- ▲ gay or bisexual men who have sex with other men;
- ▲ persons with a previous history of a documented sexually transmitted disease and their close contacts;

Genital herpes and pregnancy

If you and your partner want to have a child, even though you have recurrent herpes outbreaks, you can. Mothers with a history of recurrence have antibodies that will help protect the baby from infection.

Many women with herpes deliver healthy babies vaginally. However, if a woman has active herpes in the last stages of pregnancy, she may need a cesarean section to help avoid serious infection in the newborn.

A large majority of women with genital herpes do not have cesarean section. As a patient, you can help your doctor by reporting any symptoms of recurrence during your pregnancy.

After careful examination at the time of delivery, your doctor will determine whether a cesarean delivery is necessary.

- Tell your doctor if you or your partner have ever had herpes.
- Like most medications, acyclovir (Zovirax) is not routinely recommended for women who are pregnant.
- If a woman becomes pregnant while taking acyclovir, she should call her doctor.
- An expectant mother should be faithful about prenatal visits so her delivery date can be predicted if cesarean section will be necessary.
- To protect her pregnancy, a woman should follow her doctor's advice on diet and exercise.
- Use condoms and spermicides for protection throughout pregnancy, especially if the pregnant woman has no history of herpes.
- A woman should contact her doctor at any signs of an outbreak close to her delivery date. And she should be sure to have a careful herpes examination as soon as she starts labour or her water breaks.
- After the baby is born, be sure to wash your hands before you handle him or her.
- Your baby should not be kissed by you or anyone else with a cold sore.
- With the help of your doctor, your herpes should present few, if any, problems for you or your baby.

- ▲ persons involved in the exchange of sex for drugs or money;
- ▲ persons living in areas where the prevalence of human immunodeficiency virus infections and sexually transmitted diseases is high.

Health authorities state that all adolescent and adult patients should be advised about risk factors for sexually transmitted diseases and HIV infection and counseled appropriately about effective measures to reduce risk of infection.

The recommendation is based on the proven efficacy of risk reduction, although the effectiveness of clinical counseling in the primary health care setting is uncertain. Counseling should be tailored to the individual risk factors, needs, and abilities of each patient.

Assessment of risk should be based on the local epidemiology of sexually transmitted diseases and HIV infec-

tion. Patients at risk of sexually transmitted diseases should receive information on their risk and be advised about measures to reduce their risk. Effective measures include:

- ▲ abstaining from sex;
- ▲ maintaining a mutually faithful monogamous sexual relationship with a partner known to be uninfected;
- ▲ regular use of latex condoms;
- ▲ avoiding sexual contact with high-risk individuals (e.g., injection drug users, commercial sex workers, and persons with numerous sex partners).

Women at risk of sexually transmitted diseases should be advised of options to reduce their risk in situations when their male partner does not use a condom, including the female condom. Warnings should be provided that using alcohol and drugs can increase high-risk sexual behavior.

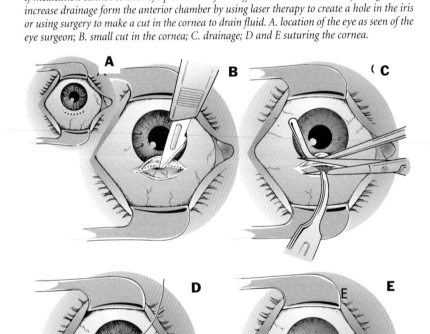

GLAUCOMA

Description

Glaucoma is optic nerve damage, often associated with increased eye pressure, that leads to progressive, irreversible loss of vision. The increased pressure in the eye can damage the optic nerve and blood vessels in the eye, resulting in blindness as early as 2 to 5 days after the beginning of the elevated pressure.

About 3 million people in the United States and 15 million people worldwide have glaucoma. Glaucoma is the third leading cause of blindness worldwide. About 90 percent of the victims of glaucoma have a long-term (chronic) condition.

Chronic glaucoma affects adults; it develops gradually as the flow of aqueous humor through the eye becomes obstructed, usually for unknown reasons. The aqueous humor is the watery fluid that fills the chambers between the iris and the lens, and between the cornea and the iris.

This fluid nourishes the cornea and the lens and regulates pressure within the eye. When flow of aqueous humor is obstructed, pressure within the eye increases and the eye receives insufficient blood, leading to glaucoma. Thus glaucoma occurs when an imbalance in production and drainage of fluid in the eye increases eye pressure to unhealthy levels.

Normally, the aqueous fluid, which nourishes the eye, is produced by the ciliary body behind the iris (in the posterior chamber) and flows to the front of the eye (anterior chamber), where it drains into drainage canals between the iris and the cornea (the "angle").

When functioning properly, the system works like a faucet (*ciliary body*) and sink (*drainage canals*). Balance between fluid production and drainage - between an open faucet and a properly drainage sink - keeps the fluid flowing freely and prevents pressure in the eye from building up.

If medication cannot control eye pressure or if side effects are intolerable, an eye surgeon can increase drainage form the anterior chamber by using laser therapy to create a hole in the iris or using surgery to make a cut in the cornea to drain fluid. A. location of the eye as seen of the eye surgeon; B. small cut in the cornea; C. drainage; D and E suturing the cornea.

Causes

The underlying cause of glaucoma is generally not known, although the condition tends to run in families. Sometimes, damage to the eye caused by infection, inflammation, tumor, large cataracts or surgery for cataracts, or other conditions keep the fluid from draining freely and leads to increased eye pressure and optic nerve damage.

Because the most common types of glaucoma can cause slow and silent loss of vision over years, early detection of the disease is extremely important.

All people at high risk (for instance, people who are very nearsighted or farsighted, relatives of people with glaucoma and people having diabetes, have used corticosteroids for a long time, or have had a previous eye injury) should have a comprehensive eye examination every 1 to 2 years.

Types of glaucoma

In glaucoma, the canals through which the fluid drains become clogged, blocked, or covered. Fluid cannot leave the eye even though new fluid is being produced in the posterior chamber.

Congenital and infantile glaucoma

Most children with this particular kind of eye disorder suffer from infantile glaucoma, which may be present at birth (congenital) or may develop during infancy or early childhood. Infantile glaucoma occurs when, for unknown reasons, the drainage area between the cornea and the iris is obstructed, and the aqueous humor cannot circulate through the eye. If glaucoma is diagnosed and treated immediately, the outlook is excellent and the child may retain normal vision.

The cause of infantile glaucoma is usually an abnormal development of the eye. Although the disease is usually an isolated abnormality, congenital and infantile glaucoma are occasionally associated with other disorders affecting a child's development.

For example, glaucoma may occur either with other eye disorders, such as retinoblastoma, or with diseases such as neurofibromatosis. It may occur with inflammatory conditions such as juvenile rheumatoid arthritis or with infections, such as congenital rubella. Severe eye injuries or eye tumors may also cause glaucoma among children.

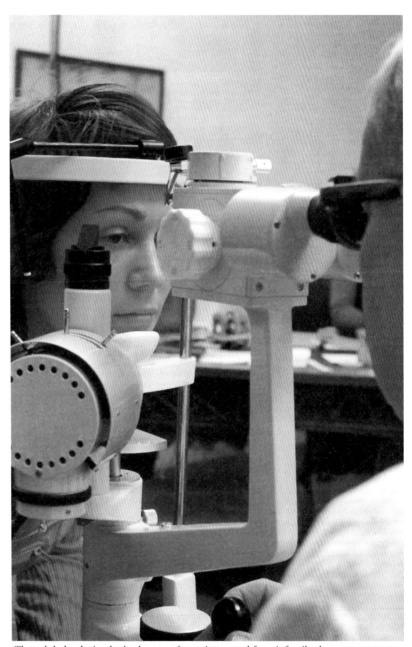

The ophthalmologist checks the eyes of a patient, cured from infantile glaucoma some years ago.

Major causes of blindness in percentage of total	
Senile macular degeneration	25%
Senile cataract	23%
Refractory errors	8%
Diabetic retinopathy	7%
All other causes	27%

Drugs used to treat glaucoma

Beta blockers

These drugs decrease the production of aqueous humor in the eye. The drugs are given as eye drops. Some side effects are worse in people with heart and blood vessel disease.

■ *Selected side effects*
- Shortness of breath
- Slow heart beat
- Cold fingers
- Cold toes
- Insomnia
- Fatigue
- Depression
- Vivid dreams
- Hallucinations
- Sexual dysfunction
- Hair loss

■ *Examples*
- Betaxolol
- Carteolol
- Levobetaxol
- Levobunolol
- Metipranolol
- Timolol

Prostaglandin-like compounds

These drugs increase the outflow of aqueous humor in the eye. The drugs are given as eye drops.

■ *Selected side effects*
- Increased eye pigmentation
- Increased skin pigmentation
- Elongated eyelashes
- Thickened eye lashes
- Muscle and joint pain
- Back pain
- Skin rash

■ *Examples*
- Bimatoprost
- Latanoprost
- Travoprost
- Unoprostone

Alpha-agonists

These drugs decrease the production of aqueous humor in the eye and increase the outflow of aqueous humor. The drugs are given as eye drops.

■ *Selected side effects*
- Blood pressure changes
- Abnormal heart rhythm
- Headache
- Fatigue
- Dry mouth
- Dry nose

■ *Examples*
- Apraclonidine
- Brimonidine
- Dipivefrin
- Epinephrine

Carbonic anhydrase inhibitors

These drugs decrease the production of aqueous humor in the eye. The drugs are given as eye drops and/or by mouth.

■ *Selected side effects*
- Blood pressure changes
- Depression
- Loss of appetite
- Nausea
- Erectile dysfunction
- Metallic or bitter taste
- Diarrhea
- Kidney stones
- Low blood counts

■ *Examples*
- Acetazolamide
- Brinzolamide
- Dorzolamide
- Methazolamide

Cholinergic agents

These drugs increase the outflow of aqueous humor in the eye and may widen "angle" of eye. The drugs are given as eye drops, physostigmine is given as ointment.

■ *Selected side effects*
- Pupil constriction
- Blurred vision
- Cataract formation
- Sweating
- Headache
- Tremor
- Excess saliva production
- Diarrhea
- Abdominal cramps
- Nausea

■ *Examples*
- Carbachol
- Demecarium
- Echothiophate
- Pilocarpine
- Physostigmine

Cholinergic agents

These drugs decrease the production of aqueous humor in the eye. The drugs are given as eye drops.

■ *Selected side effects*
- Shortness of breath
- Slow heart beat
- Shortness of breath
- Slow heart beat
- Shortness of breath
- Slow heart beat
- Shortness of breath
- Slow heart beat

n *Examples*
- Betaxolol
- Carteolol
- Levobunolol

■ *Symptoms and diagnosis*
The most common sign of both congenital and infantile glaucoma is enlargement and clouding of the cornea. Other signs include profuse tearing and extreme sensitivity to light. Glaucoma is usually suspected because of the characteristic symptoms. Positive diagnosis is made with an instrument called a tonometer, when placed on the eyeball, measures pressure within the eye.

■ *Treatment and prevention*
Surgery is required for childhood glaucoma. If surgery is performed very early, the outlook is excellent and the child may retain full vision.
Glaucoma cannot be prevented, but

Major signs and symptoms of acute angle-closure glaucoma	
Congestion	circumcorneal
Pupil	dilated
	oval
Pupil light reflex	reduced
Cornea	edema
Anterior chamber	clear
	shallow
Iris	edema
	gray
Tension	very high
Tenderness	marked
Pain	severe
Photophobia	moderate
Vision	impaired
Onset	abrupt

proper treatment prevents further, possibly permanent, damage.

Open-angle glaucoma

In this situation, the drainage canals in the eyes become clogged gradually over months or years. Pressure in the eye rises slowly because fluid is produced at a normal rate but drains sluggishly.

Closed-angle glaucoma

In this situation, the drainage canals in the eyes suddenly become blocked or covered. Pressure in the eye rises rapidly, because fluid drainage is abruptly blocked while production continues.

Treatment

Treatment of glaucoma is lifelong. It involves decreasing eye pressure by reducing the amount of fluid produced by the eye or by increasing fluid drainage. Eye drops and surgery are the main treatments for open-angle and closed-angle glaucoma.

The treatment of glaucoma caused by other disorders depends on the cause. For infection or inflammation, antibiotic, antiviral, or corticosteroid eye drops may provide a cure. A tumor

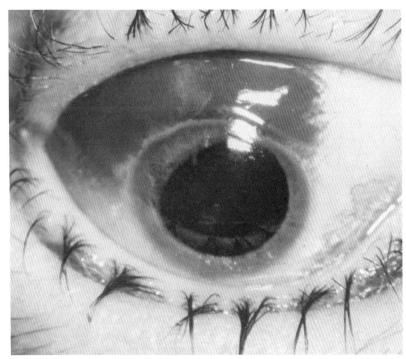

Hemorrhage in the choroid around the cornea due to an injury to the eyeball and socket. This condition may in some cases lead to glaucoma.

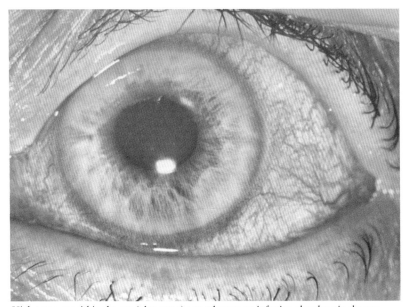

High pressure within the eye (glaucoma) secondary to an infection elsewhere in the eye.

obstructing fluid drainage should be treated, as should a cataract that is op large it causes eye pressure to rise.

High eye pressure that results from cataract surgery is treated with glau-coma eye drops that reduce eye pressure. If eye drops do not work, glaucoma infiltration surgery can be performed to create a new pathway for fluid to leave the eye.

GONORRHEA

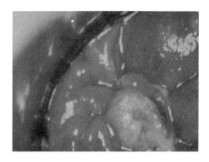

Description

The venereal diseases were previously thought of as a limited few such as syphilis, gonorrhea, and several other less common infections; a later concept expanded the field to include a more extensive group now identified as "sexually transmitted diseases" (STDs).

Gonorrhea is the second most common bacterial sexually transmitted disease in America and Europe. Approximately 1.2 million cases are reported each year in the United States and about 1.75 million cases in Europe between 25 and 50 per cent of women with gonorrhea also have Chlamydia. In addition, doctors report a tremendous increase in cases of penicillin-resistant gonorrhea, especially in big cities.

The gonorrhea germ (a bacterium, the gonococcus (Neisseria gonorrhea), requires warmth and moisture for survival. It does quickly on drying outside the human body; it would seem, therefore, unlikely to be acquired, as rumoured, from a toilet seat.

Transmitted usually by sex contact, possibly intimate bodily contact, with the surface of, or secretion (containing large numbers of gonococci) from an infected mucous membrane or gonococcal sore. The germ attacks and infects the mucous membranes, but can possibly cause a gonococcal lesion (sore) on contact with a break in the skin.

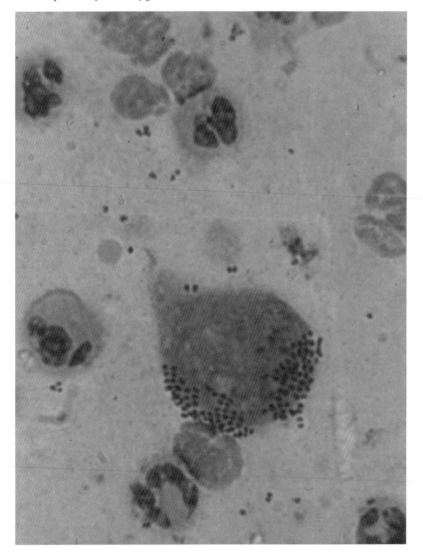

Microscopic view of clusters of gonococci.

Who is at risk

According to experts, most gonorrhea sufferers are 30 years old or younger. Having had gonorrhea does not provide immunity; reinfection is possible on exposure to the disease.

Dangers

When passed along to newborns, gonorrhea is associated with low birth weight, prematurity and eye infec-

Gonorrhea   Questions & Answers

What is the cause of gonorrhea?

Gonorrhea (the clap), is a sexually transmitted disease which is very common but which can be cured if treated properly. The disease is caused by bacteria which live on and in the mucous membrane.

Mucous membranes can be found in body openings such as the throat, vagina, penis and anus.In both men and women oral sex (penis in the mouth) can cause a gonorrhea infection in the throat. The mucous membrane of the mouth can turn red. One of more samples of blood, urine and pus are taken for examination. Treatment of gonorrhea consists of one or more injections or pills of antibiotics.

What are the most important symptoms of gonorrhea?

Women who are infected with gonorrhea usually have no symptoms. They may be slightly more vaginal discharge than usual. This may smell unpleasant and be green or yellow (pus). Urinating can be painful. Women who are infected with gonorrhea notice this usually between two and fourteen days after sexual contact.

There is discharge, often yellowish or greenish in colour. There may be a burning feeling or irritation when passing urine, or the tendency to frequently pass small amounts of urine. Sometimes men have no symptoms at all.

What are the possible complications of gonorrhea in women?

Without treatment gonorrhea can spread from the neck of the uterus (cervix) to the Fallopian tubes. This causes inflamma-

tion of the Fallopian tubes, which sometimes breaks through to the abdominal cavity. An inflammation of the Fallopian tubes caused by gonorrhea is often accompanied by fever; you feel ill and have pain in the lower and sometimes also upper part of the abdomen.

With swift and adequate treatment (i.e., antibiotics) the inflammation can be cured completely. However, the inflammation can become chronic and damage the Fallopian tubes. This can lead to infertility and ectopic pregnancy. During birth (not during pregnancy) the baby can be infected. The eyes of the child may come into contact with the bacteria in the vagina. But women can be treated adequately during pregnancy.

What are the possible complications of gonorrhea for men?

In man the inflammation of gonorrhea can spread further. This happens less often than in women. The bacteria can reach the seminal tubes via prostate and epididymis. This most commonly causes an inflammation of the epididymis. There is a fierce pain in the scrotum, sometimes expanding to the groin. You feel a swelling in the scrotum, and the spermatic cord (which passes to the abdominal cavity) can also be swollen and painful.

In some cases the inflammation causes infertility. Sometimes the inflammation of the epididymis can cause inflammation of the testicle. This also causes swelling and pain. An inflammation of the prostate gland can be accompanied by fever, trouble with urinating and pain in and around the genital organs. The inflammations are treated with drugs (antibiotics), sometimes special underwear is recommended.

G

tions. Gonorrhea is a major cause of PID, which can lead to infertility and ectopic pregnancy. Direct contact with the gonorrhea can cause blindness.

Some possible consequences of untreated gonorrhea are:
- infertility
- blindness
- arthritis
- heart disease
- meningitis
- prostatitis
- epididymitis
- pelvic inflammatory disease

Symptoms

Women may notice a vaginal discharge and burning while urinating. But gonorrhea, like Chlamydia, can also produce no symptoms at all. Incubation period is 1-14 days, usual-

ly 2-7 days. The diagnosis of gonorrhea is based on symptoms and/or specimens taken from those areas involved in sex activities such as the penis, rectum, throat and female genital organs including the cervix and urethra, and examined through smear and culture tests.

Gonococcal infection is systemic when it enters the bloodstream becoming disseminated gonococcal infection with such possible results as:
- skin lesions
- arthritis
- endocarditis
- meningitis

Complications

In a rare complication of gonorrhea, the infection spreads through the bloodstream to one or e few joints, which become swollen, tender, and

extremely painful, limiting movement. Bloodstream infection may also cause red pus-filled spots on the skin, fever, a general feeling of illness, or pain in many joints that moves from joint to joint (arthritis-dermatitis syndrome).

The interior of the heart may be infected (endocarditis), infection of the covering of the liver (perihepatitis) causes pain similar to that of gall bladder disease. These infections are treatable and rarely fatal, but recovery from arthritis or endocarditis may be slow.

Treatment

Cephalosporin-type antibiotics are used to treat penicillin-resistant gonorrhea. The use of a condom, germicidal preparations, and washing after sex contact help prevent gonorrhea.

GOUT

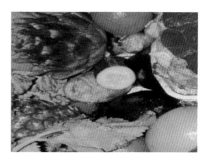

Description

Gout is a recurrent acute arthritis of peripheral joints which results from deposition, in and about the joints and tendons, of crystals of sodium urate from body fluids saturated with uric acid; the arthritis may become chronic and deforming.

The disease occurs predominantly in males. The incidence of gout varies widely throughout the world. Females do not suffer from gout until after the menopause and then only rarely. Eunuchs and prepubertal males very rarely suffer from gout. These and other fascinating observations remain to be explained.

The increased incidence of gout in stressful occupations and in higher intelligence groups may be in part related to higher dietary purine intake. That this is unlikely the sole factor is suggested by the relative unimportance of exogenous as opposed to endogenous purines in the metabolism of uric acid.

Acute gout

This occurs suddenly, commonly overnight, in a middle-aged male. Precipitating factors include the following:
- minor trauma;
- overindulgence of food;
- starvation diet;
- high alcohol intake;
- surgery;
- fatigue;
- emotional stress;
- infection;
- administration of penicillin, insulin, or mercurial diuretics;
- leukaemia.

Characteristically, the joint between the phalanx and metacarpal bone of the thumb or big toe is swollen, hot and excruciating painful. On rare occasions other joints may be involved leading to diagnostic confusion. The overlying skin is hot, dry, and purple in colour.

Systemic manifestations include:
▲ rise in temperature;
▲ chills;
▲ anorexia;
▲ elevated sedimentation rate of red blood cells;
▲ elevated count of white blood cells.

In the absence of therapy, this episode usually settles completely in one to two weeks. A remission than follows which may indeed be of sufficient duration to allow the patient to outlive his disease. More commonly, however, further episodes in this, and other joints, follow with diminishing time intervals and increasing residual joint damage. The diagnosis is suggested by the increased level of uric acid in the blood and confirmed by the finding of sodium urate crystals in the synovial fluid of the affected joint.

Chronic gout

Now that effective therapy is available this should become an increasingly rare phenomenon. Tophi (a tophus is a deposit of sodium urate in tissues) occur in the following locations:
- the helix of the ear;
- under the skin in relation to tendons or joints;
- in bone tissue around joints.

They consist of necrotic material surrounded by a zone of foreign body tissue reaction. Radiological examination reveals the tophus as a radiotranslucent clearly defined "punched out" lesion in bone around the joint.

A large proportion of gouty patients have minor degrees of kidney involvement due to deposition of uric acid crystals in the kidney tissue. Hopefully, with increasing use of effective therapy, their numbers will diminish. About 20 per cent of patients with gout suffer from kidney stones consisted of uric acid.

Prognosis

Current therapy permits most patients to live a normal life, if the diagnosis is made early and permanent medical supervision and preven-

---

Gout

Purine content of food
100 to 1000 mg of purine nitrogen per 100 g of food.
Foods in this list should be omitted from the diet of patients who have gout; some patients will solely rely on medicines to lower urate concentrations in the blood.
- anchovies
- bouillon
- brains
- broth
- goose
- gravy
- heart
- herring
- kidney
- liver
- mackerel
- mussels
- partridge
- roe
- sardines
- scallops
- sweetbreads
- yeast

tive medication are accepted by the patient.

For those with advanced disease, some reconstitution of joint structure can be achieved. Tophi can be resolved, joint function improved, and kidney dysfunction arrested. Gout is more severe in patients whose initial symptoms appear before age 30. Complications of kidney stones include obstruction and infection.

Treatment

Objectives of therapy are:
▲ termination of the acute attack with an anti-inflammatory drug;
▲ prevention of recurrent acute attacks by use of colchicine;
▲ prevention of further deposition of sodium urate crystals and resolution of existing tophi.

This can be achieved by blocking the production of uric acid, or by lowering the urate concentrations in body fluids. A preventive maintenance program will be aimed at averting both the disability resulting from erosion of bone and joint cartilage and the kidney damage. Specific treatment with medicines depends on the stage and severity of the disease and should be in the hands of a specialist.

Adjuncts to treatment

A high fluid intake of at least 3 litres per day is desirable for all gouty patients and especially those who are chronic uric acid stone formers. Drugs like allopurinol and probenecid are also effective in lowering the content of uric acid in the blood that rigid restriction of the purine content of the diet usually is unnecessary. Weight reduction in obese patients have to be undertaken during a quiescent phase of the disease. Surgical correction of severely damaged joints or removal of tophi or relieve tendon entrapment or for cosmetic reasons have to be referred until the disease and the blood concentration of uric acid has been controlled medically. Large tophi should be removed surgically; all others except those walled off by extensive fibrosis should resolve under adequate prophylactic therapy.

Pseudogout

Pseudogout (calcium pyrophosphate dihydrate crystal deposition disease) is a disorder characterized by intermittent attacks of painful arthritis caused by deposits of calcium pyrophosphate crystals.

The disorder usually occurs in older people and affects men and women equally. Ultimately, it causes degeneration of the affected joints.

Causes

The cause of pseudogout is un known. It may occur in people who have other diseases, such as an abnormal high calcium level in the blood caused by a high level of parathyroid hormone, an abnormally high iron level in the tissues, or an abnormally low magnesium level in the blood.

Symptoms

Symptoms vary widely. Some people have attacks of arthritis, usually in the knees, wrists, or other relatively large joints. Other people have lingering, chronic pain and stiffness in joints of arms and legs, which doctors may confuse with rheumatoid arthritis. Acute attacks are usually less severe than those in gout. Some people have no pain between attacks, and some have no pain at any time despite large deposits of crystals.

Diagnosis

Pseudogout is often confused with other joints disorders, especially gout. The diagnosis is made by taking fluid from an inflamed joint through a needle. Crystals composed of calcium pyrophosphate, rather than urate, are found in the joint fluid.

Treatment

Usually treatment can stop acute attacks and prevent new attacks but cannot prevent damage to the affected joints. Most often, nonsteroidal anti-inflammatory drugs (NSAIDs) such as ibuprofen are used to reduce the pain and inflammation. Occasionally, colchicine may be given intravenously to relieve the inflammation and pain during attacks and can be given orally in low doses daily to prevent attacks.

Foods rich in purine should be omitted by patients who have gout.

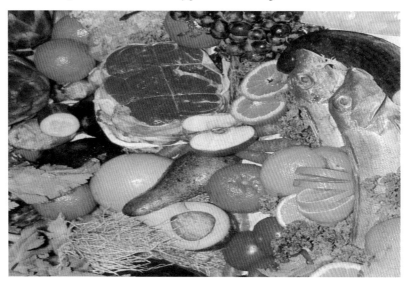

HAIR DISORDERS

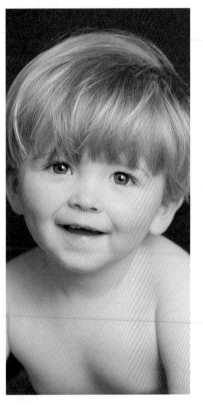

Normal hair

Threadlike, keratin-containing appendage of the outer layer of the skin present over most of the body surface except the palms, soles, lips, and a few other small areas. A hair develops inside a tubular hair follicle beneath the skin with the root of the hair expanded into a bulb. The part above the skin consists of an outer cuticle that covers the cortex, which contains pigment and gives the hair its colour, and an inner medulla.

Coarse and fine hair

The hairs on the head are continuously shed and replaced by new hairs growing from the follicle. Over 100 hairs are normally lost a day, the only obvious sign of which may be a clogged drain after washing. One hair takes about three years from the time it starts to grow to the time it drops off. Hair grows at the rate of twelve to sixteen centimetres a year. The type of hair on the scalp depends largely on the size and shape of the hair follicle. A hair follicle that is small in diameter will produce fine hair. Conversely, coarse hair grows from a large follicle. If the follicle is circular it will produce straight hair, and if it is oval it will produce curly hair. Whether hair is coarse or fine also depends on its structure. A single strand of hair consists of an outer scaly casing called the cuticle, and a soft fibrous inner cortex. In coarse hair the cuticle is up to four times as thick in proportion to the cortex as it is in fine hair.

Although all the hair follicles are present at birth, not all are functioning.

Men, women and children have approximately the same number of hair follicles, but in women and children the hairs in many parts of the body are more rudimentary.

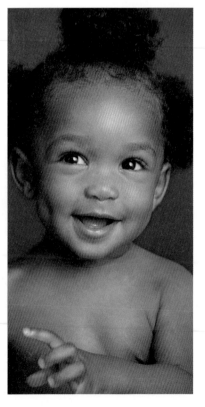

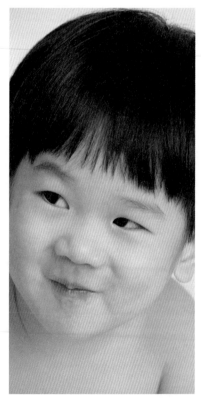

Some, such as those in the pubic area and under the arms, are inactive until puberty, when they are stimulated into production by the sex hormones. The production of hair in puberty increases far more in boys than it does in girls.

If a hair follicle is damaged, hair growth may continue, but once a follicle is destroyed, hair will not grow again in that spot.

Baldness

The common type of hair thinning that occurs in men is a normal process, not a disease, and so it's difficult to think of treatments in the conventional sense. There is no deficiency of vitamins or excess of hormones to be corrected, no infection to clear up. In women, on the other hand, thinning hair more often reflects a hormonal imbalance and can sometimes be influenced by medication.

Balding is fundamentally related to the growth cycles of hair follicles. Some follicles appear able and willing to continue these cycles indefinitely. But a certain group of them are included to shut down after a while. In men, these follicles are located predominantly on the temples and at the crown of the head. In women, they are distributed more diffusely across the top of the scalp.

As time goes on, each period of active growth gets shorter and shorter. the diameter of the hair diminished, and pigment is lost. Ultimately, a fine, short, colorless, nearly invisible hair remains. This process must overtake nearly half the follicles in any given area of the scalp before thinning becomes noticeable.

Known and unknown causes of hair loss

A healthy adult loses at least 100 hairs a day from their head, so only excessive hair loss above this level is abnormal. Hair may be lost in small patches (alopecia areata), large areas (alopecia totalis), or there may be diffuse loss of hair from all over the head (telogen effluvium). Alopecia areata causes a small area of the scalp to be completely hairless. There is often no apparent cause, but sometimes extreme stress, psychiatric disturbances and drugs may be found responsible.

The most common type of hair loss is male pattern baldness, which may start in the late teens and progress to total loss of all scalp hair. There is a strong hereditary tendency on this condition which cannot be reversed.

The hair density tends to decrease with age, and older persons will have fewer hair growing follicles on their scalp than when they were young. This occurs fare more after the menopause. Unfortunately there is nothing than can be done to reverse this process, but there are products available which will thicken the remaining hair to make it appear that more is present.

Drugs used to combat cancer are well known to cause serious hair loss, after involving the entire scalp, but other drugs may also cause the problem, although usually not as significantly. Examples include:

- anticoagulants that prevent blood clots;
- lithium;
- betablockers;
- oral contraceptive pill.

There are many rarer causes, some of which liver and kidney failure.

The myth of prevention

At present, there is no very satisfactory way to prevent baldness. Procedures to maintain a "healthy scalp" have no effect. For example, baldness does not result from poor circulation to the scalp, so there is no point in trying to stimulate blood flow.

Likewise, baldness does not result from excessive oiliness or from dryness of the scalp, and efforts to treat these conditions won't retard thinning. Vigorous brushing may cause resting hairs to fall out - but they would soon come out anyway, and brushing doesn't cause balding.

Nothing you eat or don't eat, short of malnutrition, will make a difference to the development of common bald-

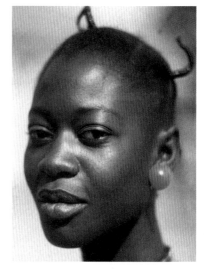

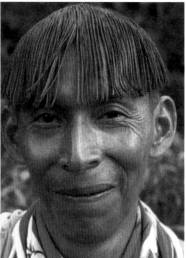

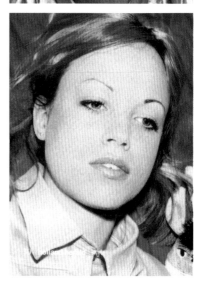

Hair color is determined by complex genetic factors.

ness. The vitamins and other products promoted for "healthy" hair are not effective.

Medical approaches

When medical attention is sought for hair thinning, the first thing to do is to make sure that the problem isn't something besides the common or pattern baldness that occurs all over the world.

At a hair clinic in an academic center, a lot of tests may be done - but at present most of these have more value as research tools than in direct application. The basic tests performed by a dermatologist or other physician are likely to include measurements of male and female hormones (more useful in women than men)(thyroid hormone (which markedly influences texture and abundance of hair), and iron stores (because thinning hair is occasionally associated with a deficiency).

A careful review of medications is worthwhile. Anticlotting agents, such as heparin and warfarin, cause some hair loss in about half the people who receive them, and amphetamines, oral gold, and propranolol have sometimes been linked to this side effect.

Minoxidil is a drug that has been approved as an anti-balding agent. Its effect on hair growth was first suspected because patients taking the drug to treat high blood pressure began to notice that their bodies were becoming hairier.

■ *Minoxidil*

Minoxidil is a drug that has been approved as an anti-balding agent. Its effect on hair growth was first suspected because patients taking the drug to treat high blood pressure began to notice that their bodies were becoming hairier.

It was then discovered that minoxidil would stimulate hair growth when rubbed on the skin. Since absorption into the system is minimal when it is applied this way, side effects (such as low blood pressure) do not appear to be an important problem for healthy adults. The striking fact about minoxidil has been its ability to reverse the balding process and not just to arrest it.

As soon as that is said, however, a number of qualifications are needed. Minoxidil is not a wonder drug. It works best for people who need it

Different types of alopecia areata.

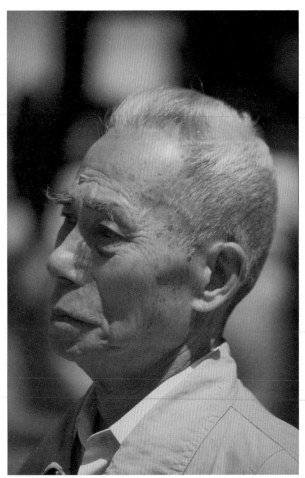
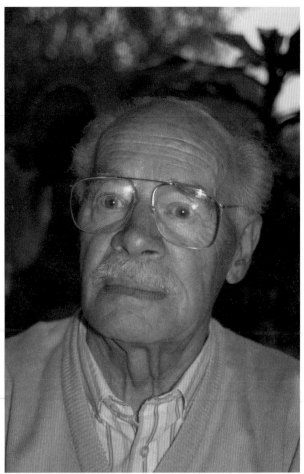

least - those who have been balding for less than 10 years and whose bald area is less than 4 inches in diameter - and it doesn't consistently work for all of those.

It is only effective as long as it is applied regularly, usually twice a day. The kind of hair growth produced is far from lush in most cases.

◼ Other routes

The majority of bald people will not benefit from any drug old or new. Their quest for a remedy can be very expensive. Some hair pieces look very good. The better they are, though, the more they cost. A related approach is to attach additional hairs to those still present in an area of thinning - but this procedure is time-consuming, expensive, and limited to the fact that the anchoring hair will grow, so the whole routine needs to be repeated at relatively frequent intervals.

Hair transplantation does work, and if skillfully done it can look quite natural. It succeeds because hair follicles that are removed to the top of then head don't become sensitive to male hormone. So if a small plug of skin, about 4 millimeters in diameter, is removed form the back of the head and placed in the bald area, its follicles will continue to produce full-sized hairs.

A very dangerous procedure, which has now been largely stopped, involved attaching bits of acrylic hair directly to the scalp with sutures. Infection and scarring were frequent complications of this procedure.

On the whole, medical ability to "treat" baldness is still pretty limited. For the present it may be more worthwhile to work on attitudes, as there is nothing unhealthy and shameful about hair loss.

Excessive hairiness

Different people have widely varying amounts of body hair. A person's age, sex, racial and ethnic origin, and hereditary factors determine the amount of body hair.

The definition of "excessive" hair is subjective.

In some cultures, hairy men are considered masculine; in others, hairiness is eschewed. Some women detest having any body hair, whereas others are not concerned with it. Rarely, excessive hairiness is present at birth (because of a hereditary disorder) but usually develops later in life.

In women and children, excessive hairiness can be caused by disorders of the pituitary gland, adrenal glands, or ovaries that result in overproduction of male hormones.

The condition may also result from the use of certain drugs, such as minoxidil, phenytoin, cyclosporine, and anabolic steroids.

◼ Hair removal

Excessive fine hair can be bleached to make it less obvious. The most common preparation is 6% hydrogen peroxide (commonly known as 20-volume peroxide). Adding about 10 drops of ammonia to an ounce of peroxide immediately before it is used will make the bleaching action more intense. There are several ways to remove hair. Plucking is painful but effective. Since each pluck starts another growing cycle in the hair root, this is not a permanent method.

Wax depilation is essentially widespread plucking. Warm wax is placed on the skin, allowed to dry, and then peeled off with the hairs attached. Shaving is quick, easy, and effective, and it does not cause hair to grow back more abundantly or rapidly. However, it does leave the cut shaft of hair in place. Rubbing with a pumice stone or some other mild abrasive also removes fine hair.

Depilatories cause hair to disintegrate though they leave the roots and thus permit regrowth. By disintegrating chemical bonds in the hair shaft, a depilatory turns it into a gelatinous mass, which is then wiped away. Because these agents dissolve protein, they also affect the skin and can irritate it left on too long.

Electrolysis is the only permanent method of hair removal. With this procedure, the hair bulb is destroyed by an electric current so that hair cannot regrow. However, electrolysis may be complicated by temporary irritation from the procedure or, later by pitlike scarring. Also, incomplete destruction may allow hair to grow back.

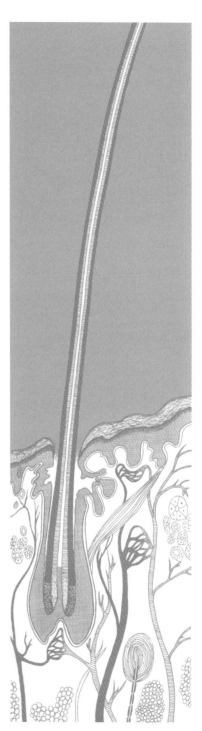

Microscopic view of a hair. A hair develops inside a tubular hair follicle beneath the skin with the root of the hair expanded into a bulb. Blood vessels, nerve terminals and sense organs surround the bulb. The part above the skin consists of an outer cuticle that covers the cortex.

HEADACHE

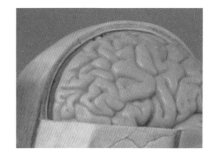

Description

Headache is a common manifestation of many diseases and disorders, involving the brain, eyes, nose, throat, teeth, and ears. However, such conditions account for only a few of the patients who consult doctors because of headache. The remainder usually suffer from muscle tension headache, migraine, or head pain for which no structural cause can be found.

The head has been invested with a significance that may partially explain why headache is one of the commonest symptoms, leading 70 per cent of the population to seek medical advice on its account at some stage in their lives. In a typical general physician's practice of 2500 patients, headaches account for about 400 consultations per year.

Such then is the dimension of the problem that demands that the practitioner distinguish the few that will require

further investigation or specific management from the many whose needs should be met with sympathy and reassurance.

Only a minority of headaches arise from disease within the skull. Brain tissue is insensitive, and pain most often arises from pressure upon, or displacement of, the arteries, veins or sinuses of the brain.

This sensitivity of the vessels to pain accounts for the throbbing quality of many headaches - due to the pulsing movement of blood - and the way in which this can be aggravated by the increase in the volume of blood within the skull because such things as stooping, coughing, and straining.

The major covering of the brain (the *dura mater*) also registers pain, which is then transmitted by the trigeminal nerve in the front and middle part of the skull and the tenth cranial nerve and cervical nerves in the back part of the skull.

Other headaches derive from the vessels outside the skull (extracranial vessels), the scalp and neck muscles and diseases of the upper part of the cervical spine. Even though the great majority of headaches are nothing to worry about, if they have come on abruptly without apparent reason and persist for more than a few days, they should be investigated.

"Eyestrain," contrary to popular belief, is not a common source of headache, although it can be. Another popular misconception is that high blood pressure always causes headache. Hypertension, although it can result in headache, usually produces no symptoms.

Signs and symptoms

The headaches due to increased pressure within the skull (raised intracranial pressure) generally take a person to a doctor in a matter of weeks or less, whereas headaches that have been present for years are unlikely to be due to a tumor or abscess.

The almost immediate onset of headache resulting from hemorrhage

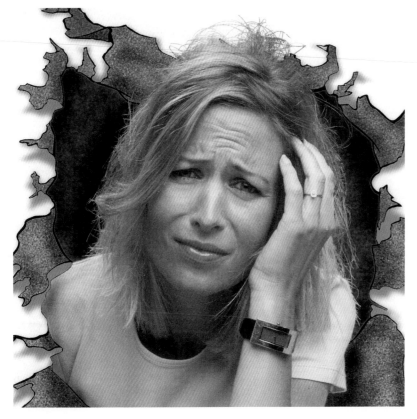

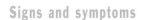

inside the coverings of the brain may be its only distinguishing feature. Periodicity - that is, the headaches recur with regularity - is the hallmark of migraine and reaches its most developed form in cluster headache (also called migrainous neuralgia). At the other end of the spectrum contin- uous discomfort over years is mostly psychological in origin; these are called psychogenic headaches.

Headaches arising from physical caus- es - called organic headaches - are more likely to waken the sufferer from sleep and to improve after rising; the reverse applies to tension headaches, which become worse as the day's stresses and strains progress. Although headaches resulting from stress or emotional disorders are often described with a graphic turn of phrase by their victims, this feature is less helpful for doctors than it might seem.

In common with pain elsewhere, peo- ple usually experience difficulty in expressing their discomfort in words, and their descriptions tend to mirror their personalities, intelligence and anxieties rather than the basic patho- logical condition of the disorder.

Quite often, people distinguish "headache" from "pain in the head" by which they mean assorted discom- forts including:
- fullness
- light-headedness
- dizziness
- unreality

These discomforts are less frequently associated with a structural disorder.

Relieving factors

Local pressure or the application of cold packs temporarily relieve headaches due to an increase in the volume of blood in the head, and occasionally this information is vol- unteered by the patient. Severe migraine drives the sufferer to seek refuge in a dim and quiet environ- ment where sleep may bring quiet relief.

However, response to treatment is for the doctor less helpful diagnostically than it might seem, since the headaches of about 30 per cent of patients in most migraine studies are improved by the taking of placebos (dummy pills), and organic headaches

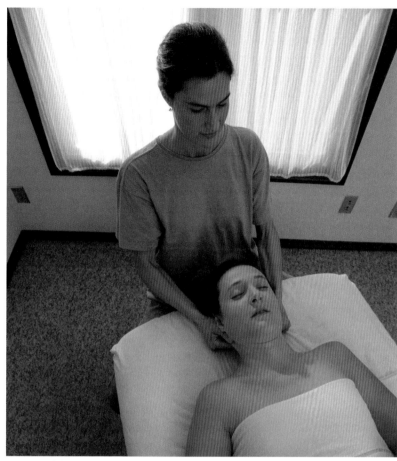

Massage of the neck muscle to relieve tension headache.

with true physical causes may be accompanied by anxiety, which can be relieved by the taking of psychoactive drugs.

Aggravating factors

As already mentioned, lying down, stooping, coughing and straining may intensify headache caused by raised blood pressure inside the skull. However, stooping and exertion also make vascular headaches (those caused by increased blood volume) worse, and the same is true during a bout of migraine.

Dietary factors, strobe lighting, glare, stress, relaxation and hormonal fluc- tuations are also well known for pre- cipitating migraine.

So striking is the relationship with certain precipitants that some headaches are named accordingly - for example, "ice cream" headache,

coital headache (after sexual inter- course) and "footballer's" migraine.

Associated features

Vomiting is unusual in those with psychogenic headache although it is a regular feature in those with raised pressure inside the skull, hematomas (bleeding into the brain) or migraine. The presence of nausea is much less significant.

Progressing neurological disability - that is, the development of tingling, numbness, paralysis, and other neu- ronal symptoms - strongly suggests the presence of a tumor. Neck stiffness indicates irritation of the coverings of the brain and spinal cord by infection or blood.

Lacrimation (eye-watering), infection of the conjunctiva (itching eye) and congestion of the nose are character- istic of cluster headache.

Headache   Questions & Answers

What causes headaches?

All the answers are not known. Some are caused by illness, allergies or stress. The three main types are related to traction, tension, and vascular problems. Even minor alterations in brain blood flow can lead to headaches.

Headaches can also be derived from changes in blood vessels in the head, due to hypertension, exposure to toxic substances (carbon monoxide, alcohol, certain drugs) and other causes.

Is there a difference between traction headache and tension headache?

Traction headache results from an injury (brain tumor, stroke, toothache, eye injury) or illness (cold, flue or allergies). The pain is caused by pressure on blood vessels or nerves. It can involve only a small area or the entire head. Identifying and treating the underlying injury or illness usually banishes the headache.

Tension headache is also known as muscle-contraction headache. Pain usually centers around the skull or in dull bands around the head. It is caused by tensing the muscles in the neck in response to some stimulus, such as:

- stress
- anger
- cold weather
- excessive noise
- air conditioning
- irritating light

Is migraine just a severe type of headache?

Some people call any severe headache a migraine, but that is a mistake. Classic migraine involves the following symptoms:

- seeing sparkles or stars
- a feeling of numbness
- dizziness
- a tingling sensation
- vision may blur
- severe headache may or may not occur
- skin may be pale
- nausea and vomiting may last for hours or days

Can migraine be treated effectively?

As far as treatment for headaches is concerned the following. For everyday headaches, aspirin or similar pain-relieving medicines still work best. Also, try massaging your temples and the back of your neck to improve blood flow.

Hot or cold compresses - or alternating temperatures - also stimulate blood circulation. More serious headaches merit a physician's attention, to identify the underlying problem and provide appropriate treatment. Migraine treatment can involve powerful drugs, as well as relaxation therapy and other life-style changes.

What is cluster headache?

A cluster headache is severe pain that is felt at the temple or around the eye on one side of the head, that lasts a relatively short time (less than 4 hours), and that usually occurs in groups for a 6- to 8-week period. Attacks may occur twice a week up to several times a day.

Other features of depression may accompany psychogenic headache and, in the very least, there is usually some irritability, excessive tiredness and other vague physical symptoms.

Causes of headache

The frequency, duration, nature, location and severity of the headache will help doctors to identify be related to

acute causes such as fatigue, fever or the drinking of alcohol ("hangover"). The cause of chronic or recurrent headache is often difficult to diagnose. Headache of recent origin especially requires careful attention.

Recurrent headaches associated with tissues inside or outside the skull are characterized by remissions lasting hours or days. Headaches from brain abscess or tumor are usually of recent origin. They tend to be intermittently persistent for several hours each day, and may be precipitated or relieved by a change of posture.

Irritation of the coverings of the brain

This type of headache is encountered most commonly in hemorrhage close to the coverings or in meningitis (inflammation of the coverings). The dramatically sudden onset of the former is one of the major features.

Vomiting is often present at the outset and may be profuse. Typically, there are few specific neurological features but consciousness may be impaired. It takes some hours for neck stiffness to appear, and if sufferers remain mobile, they may complain of back pain.

Cluster headache

This type of periodic migraine (also called migrainous neuralgia) often goes unrecognized. Most sufferers are men and it is rare for doctors to encounter a family history either of this disorder itself or of migraine.

The hallmark of the condition is that headaches occur in bouts, with months or years intervening between attacks during which the person is headache-free.

During attacks, headache occurs once or more daily, often at the same time each 24 hours. The throbbing pain, always located around the same eye, rapidly reaches a peak and is so intense that it disrupts work, sleep, and recreation - the common name "suicide headache" reflects its severity. It is often accompanied by the reddening and watering of the eye and by blockage of the nostril on the affected side. Precipitating factors are usually not identifiable. The condition is managed with the same preparations or measures as are used for migraine,

Differential diagnosis · Characteristics and diagnostic tests

Muscle tension

Characteristics
- Headaches occur frequently
- pain is intermittent, moderate
- felt on front and back of head
- or person has a general feeling of tightness or stiffness

Diagnostic tests
- Tests to rule out physical disease
- evaluation of psychologic factors
- personality tests

Migraine

Characteristics
- Pain begins in and around eye or temple
- spreads to one or both sides
- usually affects whole head but may be one-sided, throbs
- is accompanied by loss of appetite
- nausea and vomiting
- person has similar attacks over extended period
- attacks are often preceded by mood changes
- person may have weakness on one side of body
- disorder may run in families

Diagnostic tests
- MRI-scan
- CT-scan
- migraine drug to see if it works

Cluster headache

Characteristics
- Attacks are brief (1 hour)
- pain is severe and felt on one side of head
- attacks occur episodically in clusters
- periods of no headaches
- mainly in males
- person has the following symptoms on same side as pain:
  - swelling below eye
  - runny nose
  - watery eyes

Diagnostic tests
- Migraine drugs to see if they work
- oxygen inhalation

High blood pressure

Characteristics
- Rare cause of headache
- pain is throbbing, occurs in spasms
- pain is felt in back or top of head

Diagnostic tests
- Blood chemistry analysis
- kidney tests

Eye problems
- Iritis
- Glaucoma

Characteristics
- pain is at front of head
- or in or over eyes
- pain is moderate to severe
- often worse after using eyes

Diagnostic tests
- Eye examination

Sinus problems

Characteristics
- Pain is acute or subacute
- pain is felt in front of head
- dull or severe
- usually worse in morning, improved in afternoon
- worse in cold, damp weather
- history of upper respiratory infection

Diagnostic tests
- X-ray of sinuses

but generally cluster headaches prove more troublesome to control.

Migraine

Most people with migraine manage to deal satisfactorily with their headaches by taking painrelievers or drugs such as ergotamine tartrate that act more specifically on the blood vessels and chemical levels of serotonin in the brain. Some recently developed drugs have a similar effect but have less side effects.

Problems arise with those whose headaches are becoming increasingly frequent or who are resistant to treatment. Migraine is rarely continuous, and when this is encountered, tension headache is likely to be part of the mixture.

Intensification of migraine may be a manifestation of developing high blood pressure or, in a woman, may mean that she has to stop taking contraceptive pills. Migraine-like headaches that appear for the first time in middle age may be an important indicator of degenerative changes in the arterial blood vessels.

Tension headache

Although the term tension headache is frequently criticized as inadequate,

What to do and what not to do in case of headache or migraine

▲ Chronic and/or persistent headache demands a doctor's care. Mildness or severity is no indication, one war or the other, of the condition's seriousness.

▲ An "aura" - jagged streaks of light or flashes before the eyes as well as other unusual symptoms - probably indicates an oncoming migraine.

▲ Take the medication your doctor has prescribed and lie down in a quiet, dark place. Try to relax. This may forestall the actual pain.

▲ If you have a high blood pressure and have a headache, chances are you are not following your doctor's instructions.

▲ If you have been lax about taking the prescribed medication, blame yourself for the consequences.

▲ The "weekend headache" may result from rushing to get away on Friday. Try to taper off gradually. On weekends, avoid doing nothing.

▲ Lack of sleep or lack of food can cause headaches. The solution is obvious.

▲ Worry, stress and fatigue can bring on psychologically induced headache. Try to relax, especially if you discover that the muscles around your back and neck are becoming tense.

▲ Avoid nitrates and nitrites. Sodium nitrate is the culprit in the "hot dog headache." Nitrates and nitrites are used to preserve or cure meats - hot dogs, bacon, ham, salami, sausages, corned beef, etc.

▲ Avoid monosodium glutamate (MSG), a flavour enhancer. MSG, which is used exclusively in Chinese cookery and in many convenience foods, is probably the most famous headache-inducing chemical.

▲ It dilates blood vessels, and people who are susceptible to MSG get a headache 20 or 30 minutes after eating three grams of it on an empty stomach.

▲ Caffeine is a bloodvessel constrictor and, especially in combination with aspirin or ergotamine preparations, can help alleviate headache. But caffeine also does the opposite with some people - it can precipitate headaches.

▲ It is addictive, and if you are a heavy user (up to 15 cups of coffee a day and try to kick the habit, you can have a withdrawal headache, called a "rebound headache."

▲ Coffee is not the sole supplier of caffeine: cola drinks, tea, chocolate and some aspirin combinations and other -drugs also contain varying amounts of caffeine.

▲ Alcohol expands the blood vessels and is particularly a hazard for women who get vascular headaches. Many people have an intolerance to alcohol or to some of the substances in it.

▲ Different liquors have different chemicals (amines) to give them their distinctive flavours. Vodka is the purest type of alcoholic beverage and, from this point of view, the safest. You can have allergies to the corn in whisky, the hops in beers or the grapes in wine.

▲ Tyramine is a food chemical (an amine) that dilates blood vessels, and many people get headache from tyraminerich foods.

▲ To perform a valid tyramine test, eliminate all of the following foods at the same time for two to four weeks and see if your headaches go away:
  • Cheddar cheese
  • Stilton cheese
  • blue cheese
  • pickled herring
  • salted dry fish
  • broad beans
  • sauerkraut
  • citrus fruits
  • vanilla and chocolate
  • yeast and yeast extracts
  • beer, ale, red wines

▲ Drugs can contribute to the occurrence of headache. The medication you are taking to alleviate your headache, if abused, can contribute to the headache.

▲ Painkilling drugs blunt the more you incapacitate your own natural paininhibitory mechanisms, the more pain you feel.

▲ Nicotine is a strong vasoconstrictor. Not only can it be a headache trigger, but as with caffeine, you can get a rebound headache if you forego your habitual quota.

▲ Be careful with continuous use of drugs; some may be addictive.

H

no better alternative exists. Women between 25 and 55 years are predominantly affected, but why this should be is not understood.

The headaches are a common reaction to external stress and to unhappiness in marriage, work or social environment, yet by no means all sufferers have identifiable sources of tension or overt emotional illness.

Muscle contraction and vascular mechanisms probably conspire to cause the discomfort, which is more often described as pressure or fullness than actual pain. The location may be at the back of the head, the crown, in a tight band around the front and back of the head or shifting from place to place, and the pain may be intensified by exertion, stress or noise. The headache is continuous are rarely influenced for better by anything in particular except, sometimes, alcohol. Evenings are often the worst period of the day. Fatigue and mild depression are frequent associates, but other neurological features and vomiting are rare. There are no physical signs. The lack of any single satisfactory method of management is reflected in the wide variety of drugs prescribed for tension headaches.

Headache after injury

Headaches after a blow to the head naturally arouse the suspicion of a hematoma (bleeding) inside the skull. Much commoner, however, is the post-traumatic headache that afflicts around 60 per cent after a head injury but generally subsides over three months.

Although this headache tends to have the characteristics of tension headache, only vigilance and repeated examinations can clarify the issue in the early stages.

Children with headache

In general, children are less prone to headache than adults and, when present, the symptom is more likely to signify organic disease. Migraine in children is more likely to give rise to gastrointestinal symptoms than in adults so that the distinction between this and increased pressure inside the skull is made more difficult.

Children can also have emotional problems, which are usually centered

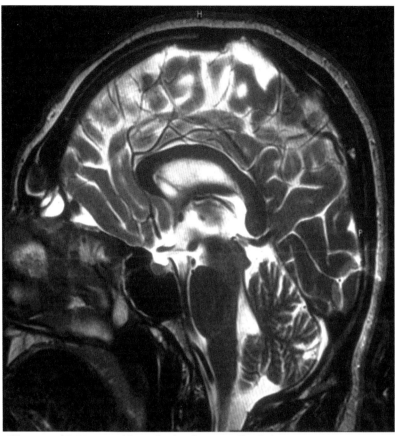

CT-scans and MRI are used for evaluating the cause of headache.

around school, and these may become manifest with tension headaches. A cornerstone for parents and doctors dealing with this is sympathy for the child and a mutual working out of his or her problems. In the meanwhile, the headaches should not be allowed to be a manipulative device and the child should be kept in school in all but exceptional circumstances.

Treatment

Besides attention to the cause, treatment with painrelievers is usually indicated. Many headaches are trivial, of short duration and require no further treatment.

Management of chronic headaches (psychogenic, post-traumatic or migrainous) is a common and more difficult problem. Both psychotherapy and pharmacotherapy (using drugs) are necessary.

Psychotherapy need not to be extensive in most cases. Understanding, reassuring doctors who accept the pain as real, not imaginary, can help greatly. Patients should see their doctors at frequent, regular intervals and be allowed to discuss their emotional difficulties.

Doctors should reassure them that no disease is present and should explain the emotional basis of the headache. Environmental readjustments, removal of irritants and stresses and reeducation may help.

The medicinal therapy of chronic headaches includes a variety of drugs. Many doctors supplement painrelievers with tranquillizers, and continuous use of a mild sedative for a short period is sometimes adequate.

The value of drug therapy depends not only on the particular medication, but on the emotional problems that may be present and the quality of the doctor-patient relationship.

HEART ATTACK

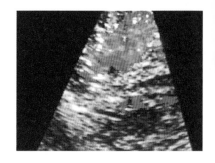

Introduction

A heart attack or myocardial infarction is a medical emergency in which some of the heart's blood supply is suddenly and severely reduced or cut off, causing the heart muscle (myocardium) to die because it is deprived of its oxygen supply.

In the United States about 1.25 million people have a heart attack each year; about two thirds of them are men. Almost all of them have underlying coronary artery disease.

A heart attack usually occurs when a blockage in a coronary artery greatly reduces or cuts off the blood supply to an area of the heart. It the supply is greatly reduced or cut off for more than a few minutes, heart tissue dies.

Causes

A blood cloth is the most common cause of a blocked coronary artery. Usually, the artery is already partially narrowed by atheromas. An atheroma may rupture or tear, narrowing the artery further and making blockage by a clot more likely. The ruptured atheroma not only reduces the flow of blood through an artery but also releases substances that make platelets stickier, further encouraging clots to form.

Coronary artery disease and its major consequence, myocardial infarction, has no one cause. Unlike many other medical conditions, coronary artery disease is a multifactorial disease. One risk factor, even optimally controlled, will not completely offset the impact of the other ones.

Risk factors are hereditary traits, personal habits or behaviors, or environmental factors that increase the chances of getting certain diseases - or, if those diseases are already present, the likelihood of disease progression.

The risk factors for coronary artery diseases fall into two categories, those one can control (for instance, high blood pressure, elevated lipid levels, obesity) and those one cannot control (for example, sex, age, heredity).

Although we cannot control our age, it is known that the incidence for diseases of heart and blood vessels rises significantly after the age of 35 and it

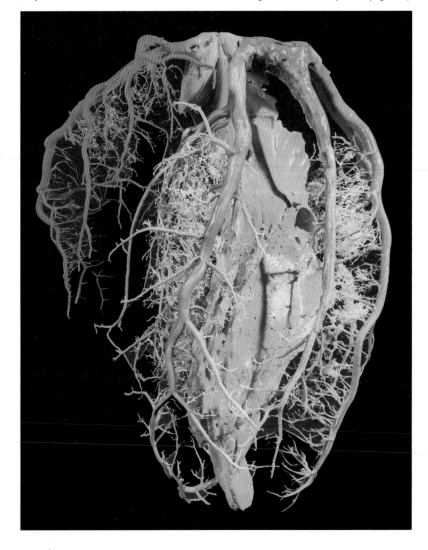

Coronary circulation of the heart; red: arteries; blue; veins.

is the major cause of death for those over this age.

For this reason, one is never too young to start taking preventive action before the process of coronary artery disease and other disorders of the heart and blood vessels become irreversible.

Like age, one's gender is not within control, but an interesting fact to note is that the incidence of coronary artery disease is significantly lower in women before the menopause than in men, but it soon catches up to the male incidence after the early menopause years.

It is believed that the female hormone estrogen causes lower lipid levels in the blood; during menopause the estrogen level drops, resulting in a greater tendency toward higher blood lipid levels and therefor, of disorders of the heart and blood vessels.

If a history of coronary artery disease exists in one's family, then the chances of that individual heart disease do increase if other factors are kept equal. However, the risk may be purely a function of similar life styles (smoking, exercise, eating habits), which can certainly be altered.

Symptoms

About two of three people who have heart attacks experience intermittent chest pain (angina), shortness of breath, or fatigue a few days or weeks beforehand. The episodes of pain may become more frequent and occur after less and less physical exertion. Such a change in the pattern of chest pain (unstable angina) may culminate in a heart attack.

Usually, the most recognizable symptom of a heart attack is pain in the middle of the chest that may spread to the back, jaw, or left arm. Less often, the pain spreads to the right arm. The pain may occur in one or more of these places and not in the chest at all. The pain of a heart attack is similar to the pain of angina but is generally more severe, lasts longer, and is not relieved by rest of nitroglycerin. Less often. pain is felt in the abdomen, where it may be mistaken for indigestion, especially because belching may bring partial or temporary relief.

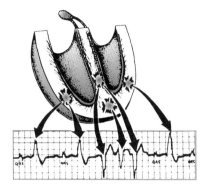

ECG: abnormal picture indicating ectopic foci in the ventricle.

ECG: abnormal picture indicating atrial flutter.

About one third of people who have a heart attack do not have chest pain. Such people are most likely to be women, people who are not white, those who are older than 75, those who have heart failure or diabetes or those who have had a stroke.

Other symptoms include:
- a feeling of faintness,
- sudden heavy sweating,
- nausea,
- shortness of breath,
- a heavy pounding of the heart.

Despite all the possible symptoms, as many as one of five people who have a heart attack have only mild symptoms or nonc at all. Such a silent heart attack may be recognized only when electrocardiography (ECG) is routinely performed some time afterward. During the early hours of a heart attack, heart murmurs and other abnormal heart sounds may be heard through a stethoscope.

Complications

The heart's ability to keep pumping after a heart attack is directly related

Measurement of an ECG in an emergency situation. The victim suddenly observed severe pain in the chest.

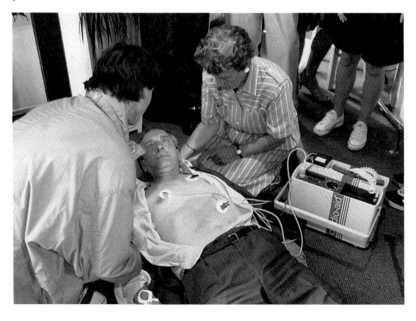

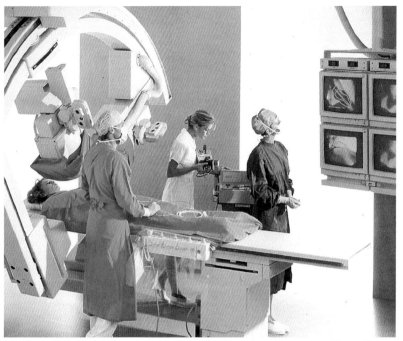

Cardiac catheterization is used extensively for the diagnosis and treatment of heart disease; the method can be used to measure how much blood the heart pumps out per minute and to detect birth defects of the heart and tumors.

In cardiac catheterization, a thin catheter (a tubular, flexible surgical instrument) is inserted into an artery or vein through a puncture made with a needle or a tiny incision. The catheter is then threaded through the major blood vessels and into the heart chambers. The cardiologist can follow the course of the catheter through the body on a number of monitors.

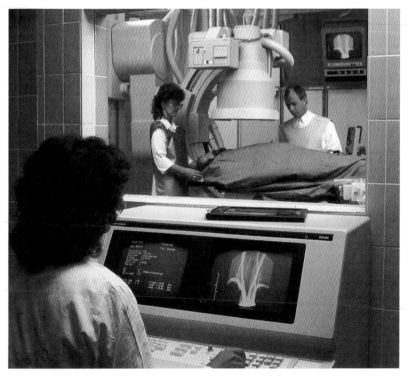

to the extent and location of the damaged or dead tissue. Dead tissue is eventually replaced by scar tissue, which does not contract.

Because each coronary artery supplies a specific area of the heart, the location of the damage is determined by which artery is blocked. If more than half of the heart tissue is damaged or dies, the heart generally cannot function, and severe disability or death is likely.

Even when damage is less extensive, the heart may be unable to pump adequately, resulting in heart failure or shock. The damaged heart may enlarge, partly to compensate for the decrease in pumping ability (a larger heart beats more forcefully). Enlargement of the heart makes abnormal heart rhythms more likely.

Pericarditis (inflammation of the membranes enveloping the heart) may develop in the first day or two after a heart attack or about 10 days to 2 months later. Symptoms of early developing pericarditis are seldom noticed, because symptoms of the heart attack are more prominent.

Other complications after a heart attack include:
- rupture of the heart muscle,
- a bulge in the wall of the ventricle,
- blood clots,
- low blood pressure.
- nervousness and depression.

Diagnosis

Whenever a man over age 35, or a woman over age 50 reports chest pain, doctors usually consider the possibility of a heart attack. But several other conditions can produce similar pain:
- pneumonia;
- a blood clot in the lung
- pericarditis
- pleuritis
- rib fracture
- spasm of the esophagus
- indigestion

Angiography of the aorta, used to detect abnormalities (such as an aneurysm or a dissection) in the aorta. It can also be used to detect leakage of the valve between the left ventricle and the aorta (aortic regurgitation).

- chest muscle tenderness of injury or exertion.

Electrocardiography (ECG) and certain blood tests can usually confirm the diagnosis of a heart attack within a few hours.

ECG is the most important initial diagnostic procedure when doctors suspect a heart attack. This procedure provides a graphic representation of the electrical current producing each heartbeat. In many instances, it immediately shows that a person is having a heart attack.

Several abnormalities may be detected by ECG, depending mainly on the size and location of the heart muscle damage. If a person has had previous heart problems, which can alter the ECG, the current muscle damage may be harder for doctors to detect.

Measuring levels of certain substances (called serum markers) in the blood also helps doctors diagnose a heart attack. The presence of these substances in the blood indicates damage to or death of heart muscle. These substances are normally found in heart muscle but are released into the bloodstream when heart muscle is damaged. When ECG and serum marker measurements do not provide enough information, echocardiography or radionuclide imaging may be performed. Echocardiography may show reduced motion in part of the wall of the left ventricle. This finding suggests damage to a heart attack.

Treatment

A heart attack is a medical emergency. Half of deaths due to a heart attack occur in the first 3 to 4 hours after symptoms begin. The sooner treatment begins, the better the chances of survival.

Anyone having symptoms that might indicate a heart attack should obtain prompt medical attention. Prompt transportation to a hospital's emergency department by an ambulance with trained personnel may save the person's life. Trying to contact the person's doctor, relatives, friends, or neighbors is a dangerous waste of time.

People who may be having a heart attack are usually admitted to a hospi-

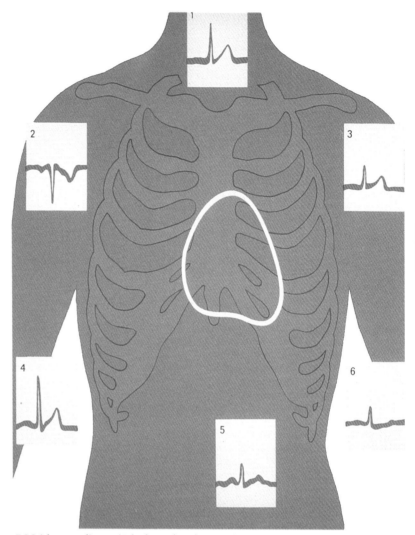

ECG (electrocardiogram) The form of an electrocardiogram is dependent on the sites at which the electrodes are attached to the body. In order to enable cardiologists around the world to compare data, a number of international agreements have been made. As a result of these, the electrodes have been given either number or letter combinations: I, II, III are bipolar leads, and aVR, aVL and avF are unipolar electrode leads.

1. Electrode lead I: difference in electrical potential, measured between the electrodes on the left and right arms.

2. Electrode lead aVR: measured with an electrode placed on the right arm; this electrode measures the difference in potential in that part of the heart that is directed towards the right shoulder.

3. Electrode lead aVL: measured with an electrode placed on the left arm; this electrode measures the difference in potential in that part of the heart that is directed towards the left shoulder.

4. Electrode lead II: difference in electrical potential, measured between the electrodes between the right arm and left leg.

5. Electrode lead aVF: measured with an electrode placed on the left leg; this electrode measures the difference in potential in that part of the heart that is directed towards the left hip.

6. Electrode lead III: difference in electrical potential, measured between the electrodes on the right arm and left leg.

5. Electrode lead I: difference in electrical potential between the electrodes on the left arm and left leg.

Heartattack   Questions & Answers

I was not doing anything unusual. Why should I have had a heart attack then?

Heart attacks can occur during rest or inactivity - just as they can occur during strenuous exercise. Physical exercise alone does not cause a coronary. Although it happens suddenly, a heart attack is the result of slowly developing disease (atherosclerosis) in the coronary arteries - the arteries that supply the heart with blood.

In atherosclerosis, the passageway through some of the coronary arteries is roughened and narrowed by deposits of cholesterol and other substances become embedded in the arterial walls. When a blood clot forms in a narrowed artery, the passageway is blocked, and blood cannot flow to the part of the heart muscle served by the artery.

Doctors sometimes call it coronary thrombosis or coronary occlusion. The injury that this produces in the heart muscle is the result of its decreased blood supply is called a myocardial infarction.

How was my heart injured in the myocardial infarction? How will this affect the way my heart works?

Atherosclerosis can go for many years without the appearance of any symptoms. This is largely due to the heart's own built-in repair system. When some of the coronary arteries become narrowed, nearby blood vessels get wider and even open up tiny new ones to carry blood around the narrowed artery to the heart muscle.

This is called collateral circulation and it explains why many people with atherosclerosis do not have heart attacks. Once a heart attack occurs, an increase in collateral circulation helps the heart to mend itself. In a heart attack, a small area of heart muscle dies because its supply of oxygen-carrying blood has been cut off.

However, the heart is a remarkably tough organ and goes on working in spite of the injury to one area. For a while, the heart is weakened and cannot pump a full quantity of blood, and so, during the first weeks after the attack, complete rest is usually recommended to give the heart time to mend itself.

This is similar to placing a broken leg in plaster, and keeping it there until the bone is firmly knit. As healing in the affected area of the heart takes place, a tough scar forms and collateral circulation develops to nourish the tissue around the scar.

What are my chances of leading a normal life again after a heart attack?

When convalescence is over, most people are able to take up life where they left off, with certain not-too-difficult modifications.

When the heart has healed, the scar is usually not large enough to interfere with the heart's ability to pump blood. It is reassuring to know that the great majority of heart attack victims survive their first attacks, and most recover fully to enjoy many years of productive activity.

Can I go back to mny old job?

Whether one is able to go back to the old job is a question that can only be answered by your doctor, in consultation, perhaps, with the medical department at your place of employment. Experience has shown that heart attack victims usually can return to their old jobs. This depends, of course, upon how much the heart has been damaged and upon the demands of the job.

Some people do change to different kinds of work, of a type that places less burden on the heart. Voluntary heart associations cooperate with community agencies on programs of vocational guidance, training and placement of heart patients.

Am I likely to have pain in coronary artery disease?

Not everyone has pain, but some people do have angina pectoris, a tight pain or pressure in the chest, usually brought on by physical exertion, intense emotion or eating a heavy meal. Angina pectoris is chest pain, often accompanied by a feeling of choking or impending death; the pain typically radiates down the left arm. It is usually caused by lack of oxygen to the heart muscle.

The pain does occur when a part of the heart muscle is receiving too little blood and oxygen for their work it is called upon to do at the moment. Doctors usually prescribe a blood vessel dilator, or a similar drug, to ease or prevent the pain, and will recommend care in avoiding situations that may bring on the pain.

Often, after a period of quiet living, collateral circulation develops by angina pectoris attacks. If your angina increases in severity or begins to come on after very little exertion, be sure to see your doctor immediately for an examination of the function of the heart.

What is a fat-controlled diet? Why is it recommended for some heart patients?

This is a diet that regulates both the amount and type of fat you eat. If your doctor should prescribe such a diet for you, the food you eat each day will differ from the average diet in two ways:
- you will eat somewhat less fat;
- more of the fat you eat will come from vegetable oils (polyunsaturated fats) and less from meat and dairy products (saturated fats).

The purpose of this diet is to reduce the amount of cholesterol and other fatty substances in blood. A lower cholesterol level tends to retard the process of atherosclerosis. Your doctor will advice a fat-controlled diet if he finds that the level of the cholesterol in your blood is too high, and may have you take additional tests from time to time.

These tests are aimed to discover whether the diet is bringing your cholesterol level closer to normal and to determine whether other dietary regimens or medications are required. If you are in your 60s or 70s, your doctor may permit you a more liberal diet.

tal that has a cardiac care unit. Heart rhythm, blood pressure, and the amount of oxygen in the blood are closely monitored so that heart damage can be assessed. Nurses in these units are specially trained to care for people with heart problems and to handle cardiac emergencies.

If no complications occur during the first few days, most people can safely leave the hospital within a few more dags. If complications such as abnormal heart rhythms develop or the heart can no longer pump adequately, hospitalization can be prolonged.

Initial treatment

People who think they may be having a heart attack should call an ambulance, then chew an aspirin tablet. If aspirin is not taken at home or given by emergency personnel, it is usually immediately given at the hospital. This therapy improves the chances of survival by reducing the size of the clot (if present) in the coronary artery.

Because decreasing the heart's workload also helps limit tissue damage, a beta-blocker is usually given to slow the heart rate, to enable the heart to work less hard, and to reduce the area of damaged tissue.

Prognosis

Most people who survive for a few days after a heart attack can expect a full recovery, but about 10 per cent die within a year. Most deaths occur in the first 3 or 4 months, typically in people who continue to have angina, abnormal heart rhythms originating in the ventricles, and heart failure.

Rehabilitation

Cardiac rehabilitation, an important part of recovery, begins in the hospital. Remaining in bed for longer than 2 or 3 days leads to physical deconditioning and sometimes to depression and a sense of helplessness.

Barring complications, people who have had a heart attack can usually progress to sitting in a chair, passive exercise, use of a commode chair, and reading on the first day. By the second or third day, people are encouraged to walk to the bathroom and engage in nonstressful activities, and they can perform more activities each day.

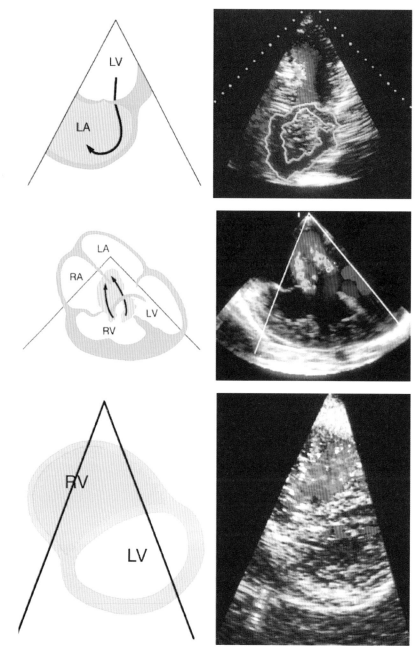

Echocardiography of the heart uses high-frequency (ultrasound) waves bounced off internal structures to produce a moving image. It uses no X-rays. Echocardiography of the heart is one of the most widely used procedures for diagnosing heart disorders because it is noninvasive, harmless, relatively inexpensive, and widely available and because it provides excellent images. The ECGs show a case of heart failure due to systolic dysfunction. This condition usually develops because the heart cannot contract normally. It may fill with blood it contains because the muscle is weaker. As a result, the amount of blood pumped to the body, particularly the left ventricle, usually enlarges.
LA: left atrium
LV: left ventricle
RA: right atrium
RV: right ventricle

Heartattack   Questions & Answers

What is catheterization of the heart?

There are a number of situations in the evaluation of a patient's heart in which routine methods such as ECG do not yield enough information. In such instances, catheterization of the heart may be performed. This method consists of passing and threading a long, narrow, hollow plastic tube into the blood vessel of one of the extremities until it reaches one or more chambers of the heart.

Pressure recordings are made through the tube and blood samples are withdrawn. This is not a routine procedure and requires the skill of a specially trained cardiologist. Catheterization of the heart is not usually undertaken unless it is that heart surgery may be indicated.

What is angioplasty and how is it being performed in patients with a coronary artery disease?

Angioplasty is a surgical procedure done on arteries, veins, or capillaries. It is a technique in which a balloon is inflated inside a blood vessel to flatten any plaque (patch) that obstructs it and causes it to become narrowed (used especially to open coronary arteries that supply the heart muscle).

Angioplasty is an alternative to a bypass operation in the patient with suitable anatomic lesions. The risk currently is comparable to bypass surgery. Mortality is about 1 per cent. Emergency bypass surgery is required in less than 5 per cent; the rate of success is greater than 90 per cent in highly experienced hands.

Why is coronary angiography needed before I can undergo an angioplasty or bypass operation for severe angina pectoris complaints?

The basic goal of an angioplasty or bypass surgery is the same: to foster myocardial revascularization, which means to establish an adequate blood supply to areas of the heart muscle that became deprived over the years due to the build-up of atherosclerotic plaques in the coronary arteries. An angioplasty achieves the goal of myocardial revascularization by dilating the coronary arteries at the sites where they have become narrowed by plaque. Bypass surgery can do this by detouring blood around the narrowed parts of the coronary arteries.

How will be decided whether I need an angioplasty or bypass surgery?

Your cardiologist will look at the pictures made during the angiography in order to pinpoint the exact spots where your coronary arteries are narrowed by plaque. Your doctor uses this information and the results of your left ventriculography - as well as everything else he or she knows about your case - to decide whether you are a suitable candidate for either angioplasty or bypass surgery.

Important considerations during this decision-making process are your symptoms, how well you are responding to medicine therapy, your age, the result of your exercise ECG, and the function of your left ventricle. Finally, your doctor notes the number of narrowed coronary arteries, and the sites and severity of the plaque build-up.

Will angiography or coronary bypass surgery be performed on everybody with a coronary artery disease?

Over the years, angioplasty's popularity has grown. During early years, the use of angioplasty was restricted to patients with partial blockage of the initial portion of a single coronary artery. Of all patients with a coronary artery disease, only 5 to 10 per cent were then considered for angioplasty. When it was performed, angioplasty was successfully performed in only about 60 per cent of cases. Today, angioplasty is routinely used in patients with more complex coronary artery disease, including those with narrowings farther down a coronary artery or in multiple arteries, with a totally blocked artery, or with bypassed vessels that have become obstructed.

When will, generally speaking, an angioplasty or a bypass operation be performed?

When the pros and cons of angioplasty versus bypass surgery are considered, a number of factors speak in favour of angioplasty. It requires a shorter hospital stay, there are fewer complications, and it is a less radical operation. It is important to understand that not all patients with coronary artery disease are candidates for angioplasty.

In fact, bypass surgery is the only revascularization procedure that will be used in patient who have arteriosclerotic obstructions in their left main coronary artery. This is because the left main coronary artery is the most dangerous spot at which to have a blockage, and angioplasty is unacceptably risky here.

What are the risks associated with angioplasty in a patient with coronary artery disease?

Overall, angioplasty is a relatively safe procedure. However, like most invasive procedures, angioplasty has some drawbacks. Although the initial success rate is now greater than 90 per cent, the dilated coronary arteries become obstructed again within about six months in about 25 to 30 per cent of cases.

According to statistics of large cardiology clinics in 1999, complications result in death, heart attack, or the immediate need for bypass surgery. Surgery is needed in about 4-5 per cent of patients undergoing angioplasty. It is because of this remote possibility that angioplasty should always be performed with an emergency heart surgery team on standby.

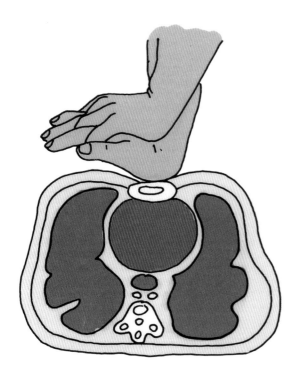 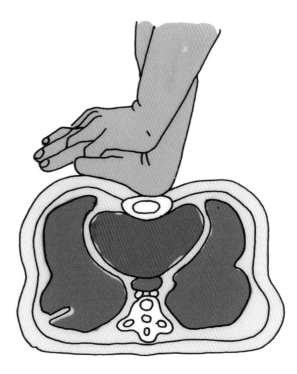

First aid for cardiac arrest.
Performing chest compressions: The rescuer kneels to one side and, with the arms held straight, leans over the person and places both hands, one on top of the other, on the lower part of the breastbone.
The rescuer compresses the chest to a depth of 1_ to 2 inches in an adult. Breaths are given about 15 to 20 times per minute (once every 3 to 4 seconds), and chest compressions are performed about 80 to 100 times per minute.
The illustrations show the position of the hands on a cross section of the thorax.

Risk factors

High blood pressure

Blood pressure measurement indicates the pressure behind the powerful left ventricle's contraction as it sends oxygenated blood to all parts of the body; this is followed by the pressure reading maintained during this chamber's relaxation period.

The first measurement is called the systolic blood pressure and the latter is the diastolic; they are written as a ratio, such as 120/90, a normal reading for a college age student. Normal systolic blood pressure for young adults ranges from 100 to 120 mm mercury (Hg) for older ages from 120 to 140 mm Hg. Diastolic pressure is usually below 90 mm Hg in healthy individuals.

High blood pressure or hypertension is a condition in which a continued reading above approximately 145/95 exists. About 85 per cent of persons with hypertension have essential hypertension, which is accompanied by constriction (narrowing) of the small arteries throughout the body.

This constriction decreases the amount of blood flow throughout the body, and therefore, the heart tries to pump harder to overcome this resistance. The cause of this arterial constriction is not yet known, although there seems to be an interrelationship between hypertension and atherosclerosis, each aggravating the other.

Hypertension is a predisposing factor to a number of heart diseases, kidney failure, stroke, eye complaints, and a number of other health problems. Although hypertension is difficult to prevent, it is readily controlled by medication and/or diet. According to medical practice guidelines, blood pressure should be recorded on any visit to a doctor, not just at periodic health examinations.

Elevated blood lipids (cholesterol)

Chronic high fat levels in the blood can lead to atherosclerosis. Lipids or fats are necessary for body functioning, and some, such as the unsaturated fat linoleic acid, must be obtained from the diet. The majority, however, are synthesized from other nutrients taken into the body.

Cholesterol is derived from the breakdown of fats in the liver and is manufactured by body cells in small amounts. It is essential to metabolism in all animals and therefore is found in all animal tissues.

When we eat animal products high in cholesterol, we are only adding to our own body's supply of cholesterol. Excessive amounts of cholesterol can be detected in the blood quite easily. This has now become a routine part of thorough physical examinations in conjunction with other blood analyses. Normal values range from 150 to 200 mg/dl depending on the individual's

Heartattack Questions & Answers

Will a bypass operation always prolong life?

Few topics in contemporary medicine have been more hotly debated. The reasons are obvious: although bypass surgery is a relatively safe operation, the operation is not without risk to life, it is expensive, and most important, there is still uncertainty concerning the effects of this surgery on long-term survival in some types of patients.

When patients have angina that does not respond to medical therapy, bypass surgery can be effective in alleviating these symptoms and thus improving their quality of life. Several major clinical trials comparing bypass surgery and drug therapy have documented better long-term survival after surgery for patients with either of these two conditions:

• obstructions in the left main coronary artery;
• in the case of patients with left ventricular dysfunction, obstructions in all three of the other major coronary arteries.

How is blood detoured around a blocked coronary artery during bypass surgery?

There are two major ways in which blood can be detoured around a blocked coronary artery. In the first, the detour is accomplished by sewing a section of the saphenous vein - a superficial vein that runs down the inside of your legs - to both the aorta and a portion of the blocked coronary artery just beyond the side of the atherosclerotic plaque. Because the saphenous vein is not a major vein, it does not need to be replaced and you won't miss it.

The second type of detour is created using an internal mammary artery. There are two internal mammary arteries (left and right) located just below the ribs and running down the chest about 1-2 cm from the margins of the breast bone. In most instances, the upper end of the internal mammary artery, which attaches to the subclavian artery, is not removed and the lower end is sewn onto the occluded coronary artery.

Which is preferable for bypass surgery: a saphenous vein graft or an internal mammary artery graft?

In contrast to the saphenous vein, the internal mammary artery appears to be a vessel that is relatively resistant to atherosclerotic plaque build-up. Because of this, internal mammary arteries have the potential to remain open longer than saphenous vein grafts.

Indeed, ten years after bypass surgery, 95 per cent of internal mammary artery grafts are still open, compared with 60 to 70 per cent of saphenous vein grafts. Moreover, a third of the saphenous vein grafts that remain open still become substantially narrowed by atherosclerosis, whereas internal mammary artery crafts usually remain unaffected.

Clinical studies reveal a few other tendencies: patients who receive internal mammary artery grafts have a lower death rate, fewer subsequent heart attacks, less angina pectoris, and a lower rate of repeat bypass surgery.

---

age and sex. Levels below 200 mg/dl are optimal. A blood cholesterol level over 240 mg/dl approximately doubles the risk of coronary heart disease. Restriction of foods high in cholesterol is valuable in reducing the cholesterol blood level. All animal products contain certain amounts of cholesterol, but the major culprits are egg yolks, shellfish, and organ meats such as liver, brain and kidney.

Triglycerides are a type of lipid synthesized by the liver from dietary or endogenous carbohydrates. Recently they have been considered equal to or more important than cholesterol in the etiology of atherosclerosis. Detection of triglycerides is also done through blood analyses; a normal range is 0.5 to 1.9 mmol/l, again depending on age and sex.

Reduction of triglyceride blood levels can be brought about by lowered carbohydrate and sugar intake in the diet. Saturated fats contribute to both atherosclerosis and diabetes. Saturated fats are usually those of animal origin, and in general are solid at room temperature.

The unsaturated fats are usually of vegetable origin and are produced from corn, peanuts, soybeans, seeds (for instance, safflower oil), or nuts. Linoleic acid is an unsaturated fatty acid that is necessary in diet, since it helps to break down saturated fats. The unsaturated fats do not produce high blood lipid levels, and in fact they usually cause a lowering of these levels.

■ Cigarette smoking

The risk of a heart attack among heavy smokers is almost three times that of nonsmokers; this risk increases with the number of cigarettes consumed daily; it also increases as the age at which one started smoking lowers. Interestingly enough, the death rate drops toward normal after the smoker stops smoking.

Nicotine, which is the active component in tobacco, acts as a stimulant on the central nervous system. In relation to the heart, it is manifested by:

▲ increased pulse rate (15 to 25 beats per minute faster);
▲ increased blood pressure (increased by 10 to 20 mm Hg systolic and 5 to 15 mm Hg diastolic);
▲ and lowering of the temperature in the extremities by as much as 5 to 7 degrees centigrade, experienced by many smokers as "cold feet" or "cold fingers."

Other detrimental effects of smoking on the heart include accelerated thrombosis (blood clot formation), which, if accompanied by atherosclerosis, can precipitate a heart attack, and decreased oxygen supply to the body cells and tissues due to the competition of carbon monoxide (in the smoke), which attaches to hemoglobin in the red blood cells instead of the needed oxygen.

■ Diabetes

A diabetic's pancreas produces inadequate amounts of insulin, resulting in abnormally high blood sugar levels. This high carbohydrate level stimulates lipid production, which in time, accelerates progress of atherosclerosis. Diabetics can control their carbohydrate metabolism through diet and/or medication; but early detection and treatment are essential to prevent disorders of the heart and blood vessels and other diseases.

The blood test for diabetes is a fairly simple test that should be part of one's yearly physical examination (see the description of diabetes in the section on the hormonal system).

■ Physical inactivity

The preceding risk factors have been statistically proved to contribute to diseases of the heart and blood vessels (cardiovascular system). That is, any one alone does not mean that you will develop heart disease, but it does increase the risk of developing such a condition. Exercise and the subsequent factors discussed have not been proved to be direct risk factors, but they can aggravate some conditions that have been proved to be risk factors. They do not directly contribute to heart or blood vessel disease, but their value is to be heeded, since they can help control or reduce the negative effects of other risk factors. The type of exercise that is most beneficial to the cardiovascular system is stamina or endurance training.

Using the heart and lungs to provide the maximum amount of oxygen to all body cells has also been called aerobic exercise, a term coined by Dr. Kenneth Cooper. As a result of regular and progressive aerobic or stamina training, one can expect to lower the resting pulse rate by as much as 15 beats per minute in a three-month period, to have the pulse and blood pressure return to normal more quickly after exertion, to lower blood cholesterol and triglyceride levels, and to increase vascularization (greater branching of capillaries).

All these results serve to produce a more efficient heart muscle and to counteract atherosclerosis. Overexertion can be just as detrimental as underexertion, so one must be careful to start out gradually and progress at a regular pace that is suitable to one's age and condition.

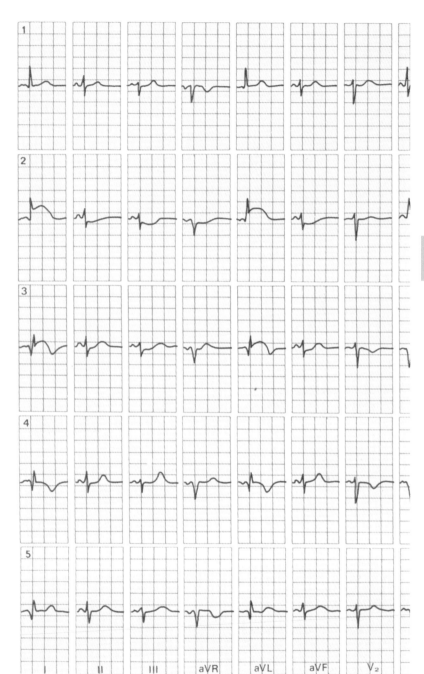

Electrocardiograms taken during the recovery from a heart attack. I, II, III and aVR, aVL, aVF are the standard electrode leads. V2, V4 and V6 are several extra leads that have been used because a disturbance in the front part of the ventricles of the heart is suspected.
V2: electrode placed in the space near the fourth rib, to the left of the breastbone;
V4: electrode placed in the space near the fifth rib, to the left of the breastbone;
V6: electrode placed a little more to one side of V4.
1. Normal ECG pattern.
2. An infarct on the front part of the heart.
3. ECG made several days later.
4. ECG made several weeks later.
5. ECG made several months later. The ECG is almost normal again (compare with 1).

Drugs used to treat coronary artery disease

Anticoagulants

These drugs prevent blood from clothing. They are used to treat people who have unstable angina or who have had a heart attack.

■ **Selected side effects**

Bleeding, especially when used with other drugs that have a similar effect (such as aspirin and other nonsteroidal anti-inflammatory drugs).

■ **Examples:**
- Enoxaparin
- Hirudin
- Heparin
- Warfarin

Antiplatelet drugs

These drugs prevent platelets from clumping and blood clots from forming. They also reduce the risk of a heart attack. They are used to treat people who have stable or instable angina or who have had a heart attack. Aspirin is taken as soon as a heart attack is suspected. People with an allergy to aspirin may take clopidogrel or ticlopidine as an alternative.

■ **Selected side effects**

Bleeding, especially when used with other drugs that have a similar effect (such as anticoagulants).

With aspirin, stomach irritation.

With ticlopidine and less so with clopidogrel, a small risk of reducing the white blood cell count.

■ **Examples:**
- Aspirin
- Ticlopidine
- Clopidogrel

Glycoprotein IIb/IIIa

These drugs prevent platelets from clumping and blood clots from forming. They are used to treat people who have unstable angina or who are undergoing percutaneous transluminal coronary angioplasty after a heart attack.

■ **Selected side effects**

Bleeding, especially when used with other drugs that have a similar effect (such as anticoagulants or thrombolytic drugs); reduction of the platelet count.

■ **Examples:**
- Alciximab
- Tirofiban
- Eptifibatide

Beta-blockers

These drugs reduce the workload of the heart and the risk of a heart attack and sudden death. They are used to treat people who have stable or instable angina or syndrome X or who have had a heart attack.

■ **Selected side effects**

Spasm of airways (bronchospasm), an abnormally slow heart rate (bradycardia), heart failure, insomnia, fatigue, shortness of breath, depression, Raynaud's phenomenon, vivid dreams, hallucinations, and sexual dysfunction. With some beta-blockers an increased triglyceride level.

■ **Examples:**
- Acebutolol
- Metoprolol
- Atenolol
- Nadolol
- Betaxolol
- Penbutolol
- Bisoprolol
- Propranolol
- Carteolol
- Timolol

Calcium channel blockers

These drugs prevent blood vessels from narrowing, and can counter artery spasm. Diltiazem and verapamil reduce the heart rate. Calcium channel blockers are used to treat people who have stable angina.

■ **Selected side effects**

Dizziness, fluid accumulation (edema) in the ankles, flushing, headache, heartburn, enlarged gums, and abnormal heart rhythms (arrhythmias).

With short-acting, but not long-acting, calcium channel blockers, possible increased risk of death, due to heart attack, especially in people who have had a heart attack recently.

■ **Examples:**
- Amlodipine
- Nicardipine
- Diltiazem
- Nifedipine
- Felodipine
- Nisoldipine
- Isradipine
- Verapamil

Nitrates

These drugs relieve angina, prevent episodes of angina, and reduce the risk of a heart attack, and sudden death. However, risk reduction is much less than with beta-blockers. They are used to treat people who have stable or instable angina or syndrome X.

8- to 12-hour periods without taking the drug are needed daily to maintain the long-term effectiveness of the drug.

■ **Selected side effects**

Flushing, headache, and a temporarily fast heart rate (tachycardia).

■ **Examples:**
- sosorbide dinitrate • Nitroglycerin
- sosorbide mononitrate

Opioids

In people who have had a heart attack, these drugs are used to relieve anxiety and pain if the pain persists despite use of other drugs.

■ **Selected side effects**

Low blood pressure when a person stands, constipation, nausea, vomiting, and confusion (especially in older people).

■ **Examples:**
- Morphine

Thrombolytic drugs

These drugs dissolve blood clots. They are used to treat people who have had a heart attack.

■ **Selected side effects**

Bleeding after injuries and, rarely, bleeding within the brain (intracerebral hemorrhage).

■ **Examples:**
- Anistreplase
- Streptokinase
- Alteplase
- Tenecteplase
- Reteplase

Obesity

The term obesity means that one has 20 per cent or more excess body fat. In terms of the heart, this means an extra load to pump blood and therefore oxygen. Although not really an independent risk factor in heart diseases, obesity does aggravate high blood pressure, sugar tolerance, and high blood lipid levels and increases the risk of diabetes.

Regarding a weight reduction program two principles should be kept in mind:
▲ in order to lose weight, more calories must be used than taken in (such as, smaller food portions and exercise);
▲ weight should be lost at the same rate it was gained (slowly);
▲ crash and fad diets, which initially appear to work because of the water weight loss, are unhealthy, as they rarely prescribe a well-balanced intake of food.

Stress

The relationship of emotional artery disease has been rather controversial in the past decade but recent research points to stress as a significant risk factor. Palpitation due to premature beats or to rapid heart rhythms is among the most widely recognized symptoms of emotional stress and therefore has been considered a precipitating factor in many heart rhythm disturbances.

Dr. J. Friedman described a relationship between the so-called type A personality and coronary artery disease.

This individual has intense ambition, competitive drive, and a sense of urgency; he is constantly preoccupied with deadlines and makes a sustained effort to achieve.

This type of stress has been shown to cause the following physiological effects which, if chronic, could aggravate coronary heart disease:
- increased pulse rate (heart rhythm);
- increase in blood pressure;
- increased fatty acids in the blood;
- increased coagulability of blood.

Other evidences suggest a correlation between stress and coronary heart disease: a greater incidence in urban versus rural areas, white collar versus agricultural and blue collar workers, persons with greater geographical mobility, and those with greater job mobility.

Stress can also aggravate symptoms in patients with advanced heart disease. A certain amount of stress is necessary for life functioning, but chronic, unrelieved emotional stress seems to take its toll on most body systems, including the heart. More direct evidence is needed, however, to define the degree of stress and determine its effects on individual personality types.

Some hidden risks

Lp(a)

Until now, the substance in the blood getting most of the blame for heart attack has been "bad" LDL cholesterol. But researchers have begun to recognize that one particular member of the LDL family, Lp(a), carries an additional heart risk.

A survey of women from the Framingham research showed that a very high Lp(a) level (generally 35 to 40) more than doubled the risk of heart attack. What seems to make lp(a) so troublesome is its unique design. Ordinary LDL is a ball of cholesterol wrapped by a strand of a protein,. As LDL travels through an artery, this protein can latch on to plaque and deliver the cholesterol cargo.

But Lp(a) has an extra protein strand that is shaped like a natural clotbuster in the blood. Since plaques are known to contain blood clots, scientists suspect this look-alike protein actually tricks blockage into soaking up more cholesterol instead of clotbuster.

Special blood tests can identify the problem, but neither a low-fat diet nor most drugs that lower LDL will budge drugs that lower LDL will budge high levels of Lp(a). Two exceptions are physician-supervised doses of the B vitamin niacin and, for women past menopause, estrogen.

Homocysteine

This amino acid, found in every's blood, is estimated to figure in 10 to 15 per cent of heart attacks, and 30 to 40 per cent of strokes. A high homocysteine level is considered to above 14. A major study at Harvard and Brigham and Woman's Hospital looked at nearly 15,000 male physicians over five years. In this health-conscious group, only 271 suffered heart attacks. But five per cent of the men with the highest homocysteines has a three-fold risk of having an attack. The good news about elevated homocysteine is that it is easily corrected in most people. However, there is no definite proof yet that lowered levels will reduce the chance of a heart attack. High homocysteine coincides with a deficiency of the B vitamin folic acid and, in some cases, vitamin B_6 and vitamin B_{12}.

People who have five daily servings of green leafy vegetables, beans and citrus fruits or juices can get the required 400 micrograms of folic acid. But doctors estimate that less than ten per cent of the population eats that much folic-acid-rich food.

Fibrinogen

This substance, a protein that helps form blood clots, gained much attention in 1990 when British researchers measured fibrinogen levels in the blood of male workers at a food-processing plant over a five-year period.

The scientists discovered that men with a fibrinogen level in the upper third has an 84-per cent increased risk of ischemic heart disease over those in the lower third. Since then other studies have added to this evidence.

Although high fibrinogen levels are linked to heart-attack risk, science has not yet demonstrated a cause-and-effect relationship. But one theory is that the more fibrinogen, the bigger the clots that form after an atherosclerotic plaque breaks.

Calcium deposits

Calcium accumulated in arterial blockages, which are made up of cholesterol and other substances. With ultrafast scanners doctors can capture sharper images of calcium. If a scan shows a lot of calcium in a patient's arteries, that person is at increased risk of having dangerous obstruction.

Ultrafast scanning of coronary arteries has been used clinically now for about seven years. Proponents say that scanners are capable of spotting trouble long before an angiogram. The test can also motivate people to lower their risk.

H

HEART DISORDERS

Introduction

Although disorders of the coronary arteries of the heart - angina pectoris, heart attack, myocardial infarction - comprise more than 95 per cent of all heart conditions, there are a number of other important heart diseases. A short survey is given below.

Bacterial endocarditis

Bacterial infection of the inner lining of the heart (endocardium), characterized by symptoms of systemic infection, clots (emboli) and the growth of material (vegetation) around the heart's valves.

The basic problem is the vegetation composed of fibrin (the substance intimately involved in the clotting of blood) in the form of masses and mesh, in which blood platelets, white blood cells and bacteria are entrapped. The heart valves are the usual primary site, but vegetations may start on or extend to the other parts of the endocardium, especially at a site of injury or anomaly. The onset of the bacterial endocarditis is insidious and may mimic many other diseases without early signs of involvement of the heart.

Untreated, the disease is fatal. Therapy with antibiotics has reduced death rates to about 15 per cent, but heart failure due to scarring and distortion of a valve may develop even after the infection is cured.

Cardiac arrhythmias

The normal heart rhythm (usually beating about 70 times a minute) originates within pacemaker cells of the sinu-atrial (SA) node in the right atrium, and is conducted via the atrioventricular (AV) node and the bundle of His to all cells of the heart muscle.

Cut-away view of the major structures of the heart. 1. myocard (heart muscle); 2. heart valve; 3. atrium; 4. ventricle. In the right picture more tissue is cut away to show sections of the myocard and valves.

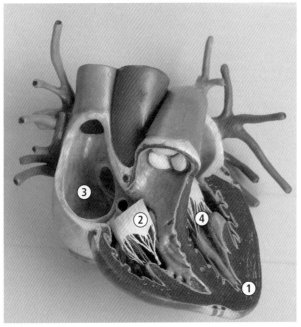
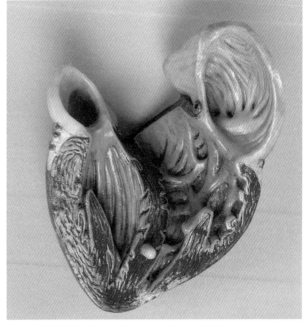

In the case of an arrhythmia - that is, an abnormal heartbeat - a disturbance occurs in one of these nodes or in the conduction system.

Most arrhythmias are accompanied by symptoms, and some can be detected and correctly diagnosed by physical examination: from characteristic changes in pulse rate, heartbeat or heart sounds, or from the relationship between the beats of the atria and ventricles. However, all arrhythmias are only diagnosed with any degree of accuracy with the use of an electrocardiogram. A number of different disorders may exist.

Sinus bradycardia

A slow sinus rhythm characterized on the electrocardiogram by a rate of less than 60 beats per minute.

This condition is most frequently the result of increased tone of the vagus nerve, is common in athletes and young persons in vigorous health, and often occurs normally during rest or sleep.

Sinus tachycardia

A rhythm of the atria of the heart of more than 100 beats per minute in an adult. Some nerve mechanism affects the rate of the pacemaker cells of the SA node.

Emotion, exercise, disorder of the thyroid gland, decreased blood pressure, hyperthermia (high body temperature), anemia, hemorrhage and infections are frequent causes.

Sinus arrhythmia

A common variant of regular sinus rhythm characterized by cyclic changes in heart rate due to periodic fluctuation in the discharge rate of the SA node. This condition is the result of alternate increases and decreases in the signals coming from the vagus and sympathetic nerves of the heart.

In the respiratory variety, the heart rate increases with inspiration and slows with expiration. Sinus arrhythmia produces no symptoms, and no treatment is required.

Sick sinus syndrome

A variety of syndromes associated with inadequate function of the SA node, most commonly resulting in manifestations of the brain, such as lightheadedness, dizziness and near or true blackouts (syncope). Coronary artery disease is the most common single cause for the malfunctioning of the SA node.

Paroxysmal supraventricular tachycardia

A condition in which the heart rate suddenly increases to 200 to 300 beats per minute, although a normal conduction between atria and ventricles is maintained.

The condition characteristically occurs in young persons with no evidence of organic heart disease, but may also occur in older persons with atherosclerosis of the coronary and other arteries.

H

Arterial and venous supply of the heart.
Left: frontal view; right: dorsal view. Like any other tissue in the body, the muscle of the heart must receive oxygen-rich blood and have waste products removed by the blood. The right and left coronary arteries, which branch off the aorta just after it leaves the heart, deliver oxygen-rich blood to the heart muscle. The cardiac veins empty the venous blood into a large vein on the back surface of the heart called the coronary sinus.

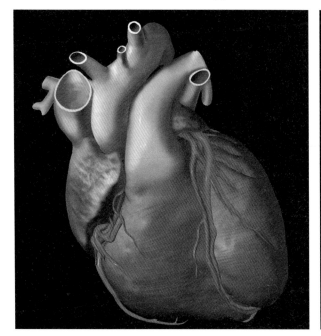
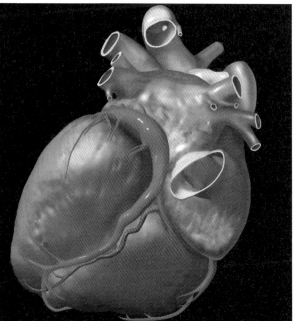

Heart disorders Questions & Answers

What is meant by the expression: a "strong heart" or a "weak heart?"

The doctor can evaluate the heart of a patient on the basis of the clinical history, the physical examination, and by other tests such as electrocardiography (ECG), ultra-sound scan or CT- or MRI-scan, which are carried out when additional investigation is indicated.

Any heart which is normal in structure and which functions efficiently can be called "strong." A heart which functions inefficiently because of underlying disease or defect in structure may be called a "weak heart."

What are some of the common causes of impaired heart function and heart disease?

The heart itself may be weakened so that it cannot contract with sufficient force. This may be caused by poor nourishment to the heart muscle (as in disease of the arteries supplying the heart); or infection, inflammation, toxins, hormonal disorders or blood-mineral imbalances may weaken the muscle tissue of the heart. The heart valves may not function properly - either because they do not open and close adequately or because they were defectively formed or absent as a result of a developmental birth deformity.

Heart valve disorders may be caused by acquired disease, the most common of which is rheumatic fever. Other less common causes of heart valve dysfunction are bacterial infection or syphilis.

Weakening of the heart muscle which has been overworked of high blood pressure, chronic lung disease, endocrine gland disorders, anemia, abnormal connections between arteries and veins, or the above-mentioned valvular disorders may occur in other groups of heart diseases.

Inflammatory diseases of the heart muscle and sheath of the heart are another group of heart diseases. These are most likely due to viral infections, known as myocarditis and pericarditis.

Disorders of the rhythmicity of the heart: instead of beating regularly, the heart may adopt any of a variety of disorderly or abnormal rhythm patterns. As a result of these rhythm disorders, the heart is sometimes unable to pump blood efficiently.

What is a condition called heart failure?

Heart failure, medically known as "cardiac decompensation," may be caused by pathological conditions of the internal lining (endocard), heart muscle (myocard), or surrounding membranes (pericard). The term is applied when the heart is no longer able to accommodate to the normal circulatory requirements of the body.

Ordinarily, the human heart has sufficient reserve strength to compensate for most ordinary handicaps in the course of one of the major heart disorders. However, as the disorder increases in severity and as the heart muscle becomes more and more fatigued, the heart becomes increasingly incapable of meeting its obligations.

What are the major symptoms and/or signs of a heart failure?

A heart failure is characterized by the following symptoms:
- easy fatiguability;
- shortness of breath, increased by mild exertion;
- swelling of the feet, ankles, and legs, usually increasing toward the end of the day and improving overnight;
- inability to lie flat in bed without becoming short of breath, thus requiring several cushions to prop up the head and chest;
- blueness of the lips, fingernails, and skin;
- accumulation of fluid in the abdomen, chest, and other areas of the body;
- sudden attacks of suffocation at night, forcing the patient to sit up or get out of bed and to gasp for air;
- distention of the veins in the neck.

How does a doctor evaluate the cardiac status of a patient?

After having taken a careful history of symptoms and past illnesses the doctor may perform the following examinations:
- listening to the heart through a stethoscope;
- X-raying the heart;
- taking an ECG (electrocardiogram);
- analyzing the heart with an ultrasound apparatus;
- performing other, more exhausting tests.

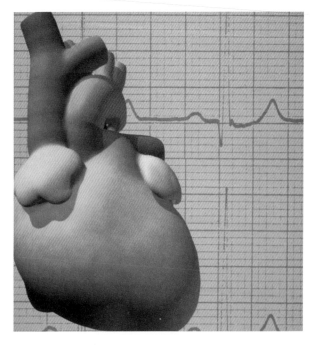

Model of the heart and large vessels. At the background an ECG is drawn.

H

Atrial flutter

An arrhythmia in which continuous electrical activity within the atrium is organized into regular cyclic waves, producing an atrial rate of between 240 and 400 (approximately 300) beats per minute.
This condition may occur in any organic heart disease, but particularly in atherosclerosis, heart attack, valvular heart disease and inflammation of the atrium.

Atrial fibrillation

An arrhythmia which results from the continuous and chaotic re-entry of electrical impulses within the muscle of the atrium.
Fibrillation is much more common than flutter, and occurs in the same diseases. In young people, the condition is most commonly the result of valvular heart disease.
In older persons, atherosclerosis of the arteries of the heart is the major cause.

Ventricular tachycardia

A regular rhythm of the ventricles at a rate of between 100 and 200 beats per minute.
The condition may occasionally occur in young people without other evidence of heart disease, but it occurs most commonly in those with atherosclerotic heart disease and in overdosages of the heart drug digitalis.

Ventricular fibrillation

An irregular and chaotic arrhythmia of the ventricles, with a rapid rate and disorganized spread of impulses through the muscle of the ventricles. Heart sounds become inaudible and syncope (a blackout) occurs, followed within minutes by death.
An acute myocardial infarction (heart attack) is the most common cause. Fibrillation of the ventricles is likely to occur within minutes and is probably the mechanism in most cases of sudden death.

Heart block

Conditions in which the spread of electrical impulses in the heart is slowed or interrupted in a portion of the normal conduction pathway.

Cardiac tumors

Primary tumors of the heart are rare, secondary tumors - that is, ones that have spread from other parts of the body - being 30 to 40 times more common. Tumors mimic other heart diseases and are frequently diagnosed either by chance or because of a strong suspicion.
Signs and symptoms may develop in someone with a tumor elsewhere in the body, which suggest that the initial disease has now involved the heart.

Congenital heart disease

Structural abnormalities of the heart and the large blood vessels attached to it, which are present from birth. The nature and severity of these anomalies are not static; some regress or disappear spontaneously, while others change in character or increase in severity with time. The disorders may result from single mutant genes, chromosomal aberrations, environmental factors or genetic-environmental interaction.
Exposure to a poisonous environmental agent can be deadly if it occurs

Cardiac catheterization of the left part of the heart is performed to obtain information about the heart chambers on the left side (left atrium and left ventricle), the mitral valve (located between the left atrium and left ventricle), and the aortic valve (located between the left ventricle and the aorta).
For catheterization of the left side of the heart, the catheter is inserted into an artery, usually in an arm or the groin.

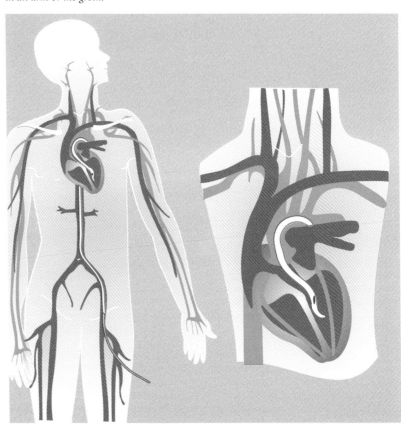

Heart disorders   Questions & Answers

What is an electrocardiogram (ECG)?

During contraction, electrical changes constantly take place in heart muscle. Active heart muscle fibers are electrically negative when resting.

The electrical differences in various parts of the heart, which occur constantly, can be detected on the surface of the body by electrodes placed on the extremities, or on the chest and abdomen, and connected to an electronic recording apparatus.

The standard leads used are:
- from right arm and left arm;
- from right arm and left leg;
- from left arm and left leg.

What is the meaning of P, Q, R, S and T in the electrocardiogram?

Each electrical heart cycle begins with a peaked elevation, called the P-wave, which is caused by the spread of excitation from the SA node.

The QRS-deflections are recorded as the electrical impulse spreads down the AV bundle and out over the ventricles (ventricular systole). The T-wave is recorded as ventricular excitation subsides.

What kind of information is yielded by the electrocardiogram?

The ECG is one of the most important methods yielding information about the heart in clinical medicine. It allows the following aspects of heart activity to be assessed:
- the heart rate at rest and during varying conditions;
- the rhythm, including the site of the pacemaker and any disturbances of the normal sequence of electrical events or disease of the conducting system;
- relative increase in muscle mass; for instance, hypertrophy (athlete's heart) or overdevelopment of one or more of the four heart chambers;
- damage to portions of the heart muscle, usually caused by cutting off of blood supply (myocardial infarction);
- inflammation of the pericardium or accumulation of fluid within the pericardial space.

What are heart sounds and murmurs?

If the ear is applied over the heart or one listens with the stethoscope, certain sounds are heard that recur with great regularity.

Two chief sounds can be heard during each cardiac cycle: the first is a comparatively long, booming sound; the second, a short, sharp one; the two sounds resembling the syllables lubb-dup.

What is the cause of heart sounds?

Heart sounds are caused by acceleration or deceleration of blood and turbulence developing during rapid blood flow.
The first sound occurs at the onset of ventricular contraction: blood is accelerating and surging towards the tricuspid

and bicuspid (mitral) valves. The acceleration occurs just before the valves are completely closed and taut, and at this time, vibrations of the first heart sound are heard.

The second sound is heard towards the end of systole (contraction) when blood decelerates, and ventricular and arterial pressures fall. Blood in the pulmonary artery and in the root of the aorta rushes back towards the ventricular chambers, but the flow is abruptly arrested by the closing of the semilunar valves. This causes much turbulence of the blood, and the second sound is heard.

In certain diseases of the heart these sounds become changed and are called murmurs. These are often due to failure of the valves to close properly, thus allowing a backflow of blood into the heart.

What can a chest X-ray tell about diseases of the heart?

The conventional chest X-ray is made with the patient close to and facing the film holder and with the X-ray source at least 2 metres behind. This arrangement slightly magnifies the heart outline on the film. In this way the doctor can measure the heart size.

Factors causing wide variations in normal size include the heart rate, the phases of the heart cycle, the depth and phase of respiration, blood volume, and body weight and build. Observation of chest X-rays will permit categorization of the heart size as follows:
- normal (which may not exclude significant heart disease);
- significantly abnormal (implying that heart disease is present);
- borderline (necessarily a large group).

What is an echocardiography of the heart?

This is a diagnostic procedure using ultrasound devices to study the heart, its structure and motions. Two-dimensional echocardiography provides correct images in space of the heart and this method has become the dominant echocardiographic modality.

The "real time" images are recorded on videotape. This method is particularly useful in assessing disorders of the valves of the heart, since all valvular abnormalities can be detected. It also provides an excellent opportunity to evaluate all heart chambers.

In addition, the method will enable the doctor to assess the location, size, shape, and motion of the septum between the ventricles. The motion of the various heart valves gives clues to alterations in both blood flow and pressure inside the heart.

Echocardiography is an excellent means of assessing regional wall motion of both left and right ventricles, making it helpful in assessing the presence and severity of coronary artery disease and in identifying the complications of myocardial infarction.

during the period when the heart and the large blood vessels are forming from the primitive vascular tube in the developing embryo.

Thalidomide is one agent that has proved to be teratogenic (defect-causing), and questions have been raised regarding the effects of other drugs such as antimetabolites and corticosteroids.

Congestive heart failure

A clinical syndrome in which the heart fails to propel blood forward normally, resulting in congestion of blood in the pulmonary (lung) and/or systemic (whole body) circulation and diminished blood flow to the tissues because of reduced output of the heart.

The condition, usually easily recognized by the doctor at the bedside, is caused by many different kinds of heart disease.

Cor pulmonale

Enlargement of the right ventricle of the heart secondary to disturbance in the function of the lungs that may be due to intrinsic lung disease, an abnormal chest bellows or a depressed ventilatory drive. The most common cause is chronic obstructive disease of the lungs such as chronic bronchitis or emphysema.

Other possible causes include extensive loss of lung tissue from surgery or injury, chronic recurrent pulmonary emboli (blood clots in the lungs), primary pulmonary hypertension (high blood pressure in the arteries of the lungs), some neuromuscular diseases and obesity.

Myocardial disease

A disease of the muscle of the heart itself is suspected when disorders of the heart valves, congenital diseases, hypertension (high blood pressure) and lung diseases are excluded. The major symptom is failure of the ventricle.

This condition includes myocarditis and cardiomyopathy.

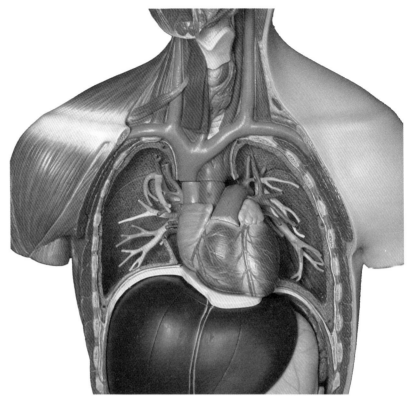

Location of the heart and large vessels in the thoracic cavity. The heart rests on the diaphragm.

Pericardial disease

The pericardium, or covering of the heart, may be damaged by inflammation, injury or tumors. An inflammation follows infection by virus, bacteria or fungi. Injury to the pericardium may be due to penetrating or non-penetrating chest wounds or may occur via the esophagus by swallowing foreign bodies.

Cardiac catheters (tubes placed into the heart) occasionally penetrate the heart muscle and enter the pericardial sac. Cancerous tumors affecting the pericardium include carcinomas (especially of the lung and breast) and sarcomas.

Valvular heart disease

Also called rheumatic heart disease. In the past, most cases of chronic valve disease either resulted from or were ascribed to previous rheumatic fever. With the declining incidence of acute rheumatic fever, other causes are increasingly recognized:
- congenital defects that may not become apparent until late childhood or during adult years;
- myxomatous degeneration (tumors of mucous tissue);
- infective endocarditis;
- syphilis;
- cancer;
- calcification (calcium deposits).

Whatever the cause, valve obstruction or back flow of blood causes characteristic clinical symptoms.

Treatment

Drugs
Because those suffering from heart disease often have more than one problem, several drugs may be prescribed at once. Many act directly on the heart to alter the rate and rhythm of the heartbeat. These are known as anti-arrhythmics and include beta blockers and digoxin.

Heart disorders   Questions & Answers

What is an exercise electrocardiogram of the heart?

Exercise or stress electrocardiography (ECG) is a way to find out whether an area of the heart begins to run out of blood during the stress of exercise. The exercise electrocardiogram may give additional information in cases where the doctor suspects problems in the blood flow to the heart muscle. The subject walks on a treadmill while the heart's electrical activity is measured by an ECG machine (attached by wires to electrodes pasted onto the arms, legs, and chest of the subject). Changes in the ECG tracing during exercise may reveal areas of deficient circulation or indicate that further diagnostic testing is worth considering.

Often today, a gentle form of this test is performed on heart disorder patients before they leave the hospital. This procedure promises to identify a group of patients who need special attention in the months after discharge.

When is thallium scanning used in the diagnosis of heart diseases?

Thallium scanning is sometimes used as a complement to exercise ECG, or it may be used alone. In this test, a small amount of radioactive material (thallium) is injected into a vein and, a few minutes later, a scanner to detect emitted radiation is used to measure how much of the material appears in various parts of the heart muscle.

A region that does not take up the thallium can be assumed to have deficient circulation. In general, adding a thallium scan to an exercise ECG increases the probability of detecting existing coronary artery disease from about 70 percent to about 90 percent.

What is the significance of coronary angiography for the diagnosis of heart diseases?

Catheterization or coronary angiography provides the most complete and accurate diagnostic information. In this proce- dure, a substance that demonstrates blood flow on X-ray pictures is injected into the coronary arteries while an X-ray movie is made of the heart. The resulting pictures give an excellent, detailed image of the coronary arteries and their larger branches.

The actual angiogram is performed in the catheterization laboratory of a hospital. The doctor inserts the catheter into either the groin or arm artery. While the doctor watches the X-ray monitor, he is threading the catheter up to the portion of the aorta from which the coronary arteries originate. Next, he inserts the catheter tip into the right and left coronary arteries and shoots radiopacque dye or contrast medium through the catheter and into these arteries while a series of X-ray pictures is made. The catheter is also placed inside the left ventricle and dye is injected there as well. This procedure is called left ventriculography, and is routinely performed during coronary angiography. It enables the cardiologist to accurately assess the functional capability of the left ventricle, a critical heart function.

What is an ischemic heart scan?

A device called the ischemic scan uses 30 electrodes to measure approximately 500 heart beats for evaluation. The analyzed by a high-speed array processing microcomputer, and the results indicate the overall amount of ischemic tissue (insufficient oxygen due to poor blood supply) present. The test is able to provide earlier detection of heart damage than ECGs, because it can test for as little as five grams of ischemic tissue, compared to an estimated 100 grams of tissue required to provide a positive reading with ECGs. Furthermore, the ischemic scan involves no risk of death, since no stress testing is involved.

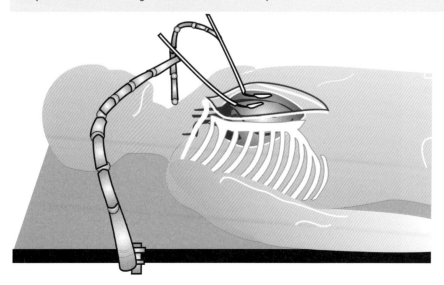

New method for bypass-operations. Such an operation is performed to detour blood around a blocked coronary artery.

Other drugs affect the blood vessel diameter, either dilating them (vasodilators) to improve blood flow and reduce blood pressure, or constricting them (vasoconstrictors). Drugs may also reduce blood volume and cholesterol levels, and alter clotting ability. Diuretics (used in the treatment of hypertension and heart failure) increase the body's excretion of water.

Lipid-lowering drugs reduce blood cholesterol levels, thereby minimizing the risk of atherosclerosis. Drugs to reduce blood clothing are administered when there is a risk of abnormal blood clots forming in the heart, veins, or arteries. Drugs that increase clotting are given when the body's natural clotting mechanism is defective.

Make sure you understand your medicines. You may have to take more than one type of medicine to help you recover or regulate your heart rhythm or avoid the occurrence of irregular heartbeats.

■ Positive approach to life

To prevent future problems it is vital that you improve certain aspects of your lifestyle to ensure that your heart stays in tip top condition. The most important steps you can take are:

▲ Stop smoking

By quitting now, you halve your chances of a further heart attack. You will also feel less breathless and better in shape yourself. Your pharmacist can advice you on how to stop smoking and will have a range of stop-smoking aids to help you.

▲ Watch your diet

A healthy diet (one with reduced amounts of salt, sugar, alcohol and saturated fat and more fiber, fresh fruit, lean meat and fish) with help:
- lower the amount of cholesterol in your blood;
- keep your weight within the normal range;
- lower your blood pressure.

▲ Take exercise

You may be frightened to put a strain on your heart by exercising, but your heart is a muscle and, like any others, needs exercise to keep it in good condition.

Start slowly with gentle exercises and build up to walking, swimming or cycling for 20 minutes three times a week.

▲ Relax and enjoy life

Being under stress can worsen your heart disease. It is important that you learn to recognise the symptoms of stress (headache, neck pain, indigestion). You may find the following approaches helpful:
- aromatherapy and massage;
- relaxation exercises;
- talking through your fears and problems with someone such as a friend, family member, religious leader or a support group.

▲ When diet is not enough

Changing your diet can only go so far in cutting cholesterol levels. And because of their genetic makeup, that is not far enough for millions. Happily, there are all sorts of cholesterol-lowering nostrums available to help make up the difference, from well-tested prescription drugs to newer alternative medicines.

▲ Statins

When combined with a low-fat diet, these cholesterol-lowering drugs can cut the risk of death from heart disease 40 per cent.

Statins interfere with the liver's ability to make cholesterol, keeping LDL levels to a minimum while boosting levels of HDL.

▲ Nicotinic acid

In large doses, this B vitamin cuts LDL 30 percent, triglyceride levels as much as 55 per cent and increases HDL 35 per cent.

The dosage that is needed, however, is up to 70 times the recommended daily allowance, and it comes at a price. Many patients experience flushing, itching and panic attacks. Adjusting the dose, taking an aspirin 30 minutes beforehand, or taking the medication on a full stomach alleviates some of the symptoms.

▲ Arginine

This amino acid is gaining popularity as a nonprescription treatment for high cholesterol.

Animal studies and preliminary studies in humans suggest that arginine may improve coronary blood flow and lower cholesterol levels by acting as an antioxidant and helping keep blood-vessel tissue elastic. Doctors have yet to show, however, that arginine can actually prevent heart disease.

▲ Coenzyme Q10

A powerful antioxidant, this natural compound has been studied as a treatment for heart failure - with mixed results.

Many Japanese and European practitioners prescribe coenzyme Q10 to keep arterial plaques at bay, but more rigorous studies are needed.

Birth defects of the heart

A major anomaly is apparent at birth in 3 to 4% of all newborns; by the age of five years, up to 7.5% of all children show a congenital defect. Individual defects - such common malformations as cleft palates and cleft lips - occur in one in every 1000 births.

The incidence of specific malformations varies because of a number of factors.

▲ The geographical area, because of factors such as differences in the genetic pool or the environment; for example, the occurrence of spina bifida is three to four times in every 1000 birth in areas in Ireland, but it is under two in every 1000 births in Scandinavian countries and the United States.

▲ Cultural practices; where marriages between relatives are frequent, the incidence of certain defects increases.

▲ Certain problems just before or just after birth. Certain factors associated with pregnancy and delivery can increase the likelihood of congenital malformation.

The specific cause of many congenital malformations is unknown. A variety of injuries to the developing fetus may produce the same defect if they occur at similar times during the development in the womb, when an organ system is susceptible.

Genetic factors are responsible for many single malformations as well as

429

Drugs used to treat arrhythmias of the heart

Sodium channel blockers

These drugs slow the conduction of electrical impulses through the heart. These drugs are used to treat ventricular premature beats, ventricular tachycardia, and ventricular fibrillation and to convert atrial fibrillation to normal rhythm (cardioversion).

■ Selected side effects

Arrhythmias (which can be fatal, particularly in people who have heart disease), digestive upset, dizziness, light-headedness, tremor, retention of urine, increased intraocular pressure in people who have glaucoma, and dry mouth.

■ Examples:
- Dysopyramide
- Flecainide
- Lidocaine
- Mexiletine
- Moricezine
- Phenytoin
- Procainamide
- Propafenone
- Quinidine
- Tocainide

Beta-blockers

These drugs are used to treat ventricular premature beats, ventricular tachycardia, ventricular fibrillation, and paroxysmal supraventricular tachycardia. They are also used to slow the ventricular rate in people with atrial fibrillation or atrial flutter. People who have asthma should not take these drugs.

■ Selected side effects

An abnormally slow heart rate (bradycardia); heart failure; spasm of the airways (bronchospasm); possible masking of low blood sugar levels; impaired circulation in the trunk, arms and legs; insomnia; shortness of breath; depression; Raynaud's phenomenon; hallucinations; sexual dysfunction; fatigue; and, with some beta-blockers, an increase in the triglyceride level.

■ Examples:
- Atenolol
- Metoprolol
- Nadololil
- Propranolol

Potassium channel blockers

These drugs are used to treat ventricular premature beats, ventricular tachycardia, ventricular fibrillation, atrial fibrillation, and atrial flutter. Because amiodarone can be toxic, it is used for long-term treatment only in some people who have serious arrhythmias. Bretylium is used only for short-term treatment of life-threatening ventricular tachycardia.

■ Selected side effects

Arrhythmias; scarring in the lungs (pulmonary fibrosis), and low blood pressure. For sotalol, which is also a beta-blocker, see above.

■ Examples:
- Amiodarone
- Bretylium
- Ibutilide
- Sotalol

Calcium channel blockers

Only certain calcium channel blockers, such as diltiazem and verapamil, are useful. They are used to slow the ventricular rate in people who have atrial fibrillation or atrial flutter and to treat paroxysmal supraventricular tachycardia. Diltiazem and verapamil slow the conduction of electrical impulses through the atrioventricular node.

■ Selected side effects

Constipation, diarrhea, low blood pressure and swollen feet.

■ Examples:
- Diltiazem
- Verapamil

Digoxin

Digoxin slows conduction of electrical impulses through the atrioventricular node. Digoxin is used to decrease the ventricular rate in people who have atrial fibrillation or atrial flutter and to treat paroxysmal supraventricular tachycardia.

■ Selected side effects

Rarely, weight loss; nausea, vomiting, and serious arrhythmias; if the dose is too high, xanthopsia (a condition in which objects appear greenish yellow).

■ Examples:
- Digoxin

Purine nucleoside

Adenosine slows conduction of electrical impulses through the atrioventricular node. Adenosine is used to end episodes of paroxysmal supraventricular tachycardia. People who have asthma are not given this drug.

■ Selected side effects

Spasm of the airway (bronchospasm) and flushing (for a short time).

■ Examples:
- Adenosine

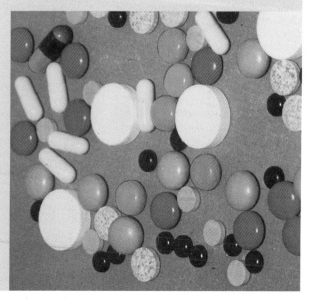

syndromes. When the inheritance is more complex, as in spina bifida, multiple factors are probably involved. These may include a genetic disposition or an increased susceptibility to certain environmental factors.

About six babies in every thousand are born with a heart abnormality. Some of the abnormalities are responsible for symptoms almost immediately after birth. Of the babies who die in the first month of life about 5% have a congenital malformation of the heart. Others die later in the first year but many survive childhood, sometimes with little or no disability.

Congenital heart disease rarely affects more than one member of a family, but it does so more often than is expected by chance. Furthermore, in many monozygotic twins, identical congenital lesions have been found.

Analysis of the role of genetics is made difficult by inadequate diagnosis and the tendency to group all congenital heart diseases as one, with the likely consequence of masking any specific lesion which might show a genetic basis.

In view of the reduced reproductive capability of many patients with congenital heart disease, it is unlikely that dominant inheritance is responsible for many lesions. However, some cases of atrial septal defect appear to be transmitted in the classical autosomal dominant fashion. Autosomal chromosomal aberrations are also often associated with a high frequency of congenital heart disease, for instance, Down's syndrome, and sex chromosome disorders (for instance, Turner's syndrome).

Possible causes

Congenital heart malformation may result from environmental factors such as an infection of the mother in early pregnancy by rubella and, possibly, the Coxsackie and other viruses; drugs taken during pregnancy may also be responsible. Epidemiological studies have established the importance of rubella infection. The possibility of greatest risk is the first trimester of pregnancy.

It is estimated that 4-6 per cent of cases of congenital heart disease owe their origin to this source; the whole range of abnormalities may ensue, patent ductus arteriosus and ventricular septal defect being most likely. Direct invasion of the causative agents in the fetal heart tissue appears to be responsible. These external factors have their greatest effect if they occur at a critical period in the development of the heart.

Congenital malformations usually take the form of either stenotic lesions of the heart valves or shunts between one part of the heart to another, or a combination of the two. In addition, relations between the heart chambers and the great vessels may be abnormal. Isolated stenotic lesions affecting the pulmonary and aortic valves and the aorta, although they may be present at birth, rarely produce symptoms before adolescence.

The same is true for left-to-right shunts, for instance, atrial and ventricular septal defects and persistent ductus arteriosus. However, when pulmonary stenosis is associated with a ventricular septal defect (the tetralogy of Fallot), breathlessness and cyanosis often develop within a few months of birth and may lead to death in early childhood. If the aorta and pulmonary artery are transposed and there is no large left-to-right shunt, severe cyanosis and death occurs within a few days of birth.

Stenotic lesions without shunts

The most common stenotic lesions without shunts are the following:
- congenital aortic stenosis
- pulmonary stenosis
- coarctation of the aorta

The congenital aortic stenosis may be valvular, or located below (subaortic) or rarely above the valve (supravalvular). In the former the aortic valves are thickened and rigid with a varying degree of commissural fusion; a congenital bicuspid aortic valve may lead to stenosis in later life. The majority of children with congenital aortic stenosis are free of symptoms and develop normally; attention is drawn to the abnormality when a murmur is detected on auscultation.

The symptoms and other physical signs of aortic stenosis may appear much later. Complete evaluation by echocardiography, heart catheterization, and angiocardiography may be necessary at any age if there is evidence of severe obstruction or if symptoms occur (for instance, exercise-induced chest pain or syncope), but this is usually delayed until adolescence.

Pulmonary stenosis may be an isolated lesion of the valve cusps or part of Fallot's tetralogy, in which case the stenosis is commonly below the valve (subvalvular). isolated lesions may be slight and give rise to a soft pulmonary systolic murmur. When more severe, they impose a load on the right ventricle, which shows hypertrophy in response. The symptoms are dyspnea and, less commonly, angina pectoris and syncope.

Cardiovascular shunts

In several types of congenital heart disease there are abnormal communications between the right and left sides of the heart or between the aorta and pulmonary arteries. These allow blood to shunt from one to the other, the direction depending upon the relative pressures.

During development the original single-tubed heart is partitioned and, when this fails, communications between the right and left heart may persist as an atrial or ventricular septal defect. Normally the pressures on the left side of the circulation are higher than those on the right, so oxygenated blood flows through the defect from left to right.

If in addition there is pulmonary stenosis or pulmonary hypertension, pressures on the right side may equal or exceed those on the left and venous blood flows into the systemic circulation.

▲ *Atrial septal defect*

This is the most common congenital abnormality found in adults, females especially being affected. Three types occur:
▲ a foramen secundum defect, which is the most common;
▲ a foramen primum defect near the atrioventricular valves, often present in Down's syndrome;
▲ a connection between the pulmonary veins and the right atrium in the heart.

The higher pressures on the left side of the heart and the greater compliance of the right ventricle cause a large flow of blood from the left to right and the output of the right ventricle into the pulmonary vessels may be two or three times normal. This high flow is responsible for the pulmonary systemic murmur, and for the delay in closure of the pulmonary valve producing a wide splitting of the second heart sound.

Patients with an atrial septal defect often have no symptoms before reaching 40 years. During adolescence the heart gradually increases in size and some patients develop irreversible pulmonary hypertension, which reduces or reverses the left to right shunt and so alters the physical signs. Surgical repair of a complete atrioventricular defect should be done early to prevent fixed pulmonary vascular, clearly under age 2 year, and possibly in the second half of the first year. The indication of surgical repair should be taken in the context of the patient's overall medical state, since many are severely retarded.

▲ *Ventricular septal defect*
This is one of the commonest of the congenital heart lesions and is an important cause of heart failure and death in infancy. The defect may be in any part of the septum but is most common in the membranous part. Septal defects often decrease in size or close during the early months of life.

If the patient survives infancy, there is a gradual improvement and most children over one year of age are not severely incapacitated, although stunting of growth and a limitation of exercise tolerance are sometimes present. Because of the pressure differences a left-to-right shunt at ventricular level imposes a greater work load on the left than on the right ventricle. A loud systolic murmur with a thrill at the lower left edge of the breast bone is produced by the jet of blood from the high-pressure left ventricle entering the low-pressure right ventricle. Patients with small defects often have loud murmurs, although the heart is of normal size and the prognosis excellent. If the defect is larger, there is a risk of increasing pulmonary high pressure and both right and left heart failure.

In all patients there is a potential complication of infective endocarditis,

which should be prevented by antibiotics. Infants with large shunts are liable to develop heart failure in the first few months of life. More commonly symptoms are gradual and later in onset. Dyspnea, fatigue and cyanosis develop during the second and third decades of life and hypertrophy of the right ventricle develops due to pulmonary hypertension.

X-ray studies of the chest show enlargement of the heart with prominence of the pulmonary vessels, left atrium and both ventricles. Heart catheterization usually shows that blood flow through the right ventricle is higher than through the right atrium. As is the case of severe atrial septal defects, deaths is likely before the age of 40 years.

Surgery is indicated if the defect is large, unless there is severe pulmonary hypertension. The operation carries some risk and the closure of small defects is not justifiable.

Cyanotic congenital heart disease
In the first few weeks of life this is most likely to be due to transposition of the great arteries. This is an anatomic abnormality where the aorta arises directly from the right ventricle and the pulmonary artery arises from the left ventricle, producing severe lack of oxygen in various organs and tissues. In later life, tetralogy of Fallot is the commonest cause, but Eisenmenger's syndrome becomes increasingly common in adolescence and early adult life.

In transposition of the great arteries, the position of the aorta and pulmonary arteries are reversed. There are many variations of this anomaly but in the commonest form, venous blood is directed via the right heart into the aorta, whilst oxygenated blood from the lungs flows to the left heart and into the pulmonary artery. Life can only be sustained by free communications between the two sides of the heart, i.e. an atrial or ventricular septal defect, patent foramen ovale or patent ductus arteriosus, but these are usually inadequate and death is liable to occur during the first few days or weeks of life.

The diagnosis will be suspected in any infant with cyanosis, but requires urgent confirmation by heart

catheterization and angiocardiography. This defect is the most frequent cause of heart failure in the first 2 months of life. Temporary relief, urgently required if the cyanosis is severe, is obtained by creating a large septal defect by rupturing the atrial septum. Eventually, total correction may be achieved by rechanneling the venous blood.

▲ *Tetralogy of Fallot*
This is an anatomic abnormality of the heart with severe or total right ventricular outflow tract obstruction and a ventricular septal defect allowing right ventricular unoxygenated blood to bypass the pulmonary artery and enter the aorta directly. The essential features of Fallot's tetralogy are a ventricular septal defect and pulmonary stenosis. In addition, there is right ventricular hypertrophy and displacement of the aortic route to the right with overriding aorta.

In most cases, the pulmonary stenosis is severe and the septal defect large so that blood flows from the right ventricle into the left ventricle and aorta. The progressively deepening cyanosis may appear at almost any time in the first year of life, depending probably upon the delay in closure of the ductus arteriosus.

It may be so gradual that suspicion by the parents is only slowly aroused, or swiftly precipitated perhaps by infection, when it provokes alarm. Patients with tetralogy of Fallot tend to become progressively more cyanosed and breathless during early childhood or adolescence, and die from lack of oxygen (hypoxia) before adult life is reached.

Affected children are small, show finger clubbing and squat after effort; the adoption of this position is believed to limit the amount of right to left shunt by increasing systemic vascular resistance. In infancy such patients are prone to dramatic attacks of deep cyanosis, gasping and possibly unconsciousness and convulsions.

Their cause is uncertain but the treatment is that of hypoxia and metabolic acidosis. Diagnosis depends on evidence of severe pulmonary stenosis and hypertrophy of the right ventricle of the heart. It is supported by the radiographic appearance of small pul-

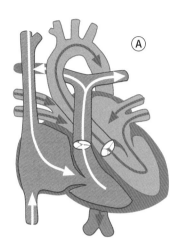 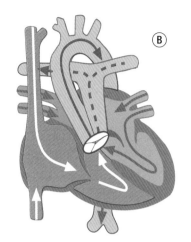 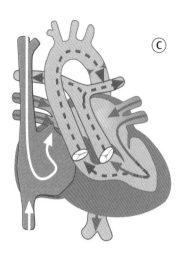

Congenital heart diseases
A. Cross section of a normal heart. B. Open connection between aorta and pulmonary artery. C. Open septum between left and right ventricle.

monary vessels, a prominent elevated apex of the heart, and the heart appearing "boot"-shaped; it may be confirmed by catheterization.
The lesion can be totally corrected by surgical means, but the operation is hazardous if there is severe cyanosis, especially in young children. It may be preferable, therefore, to perform a palliative operation in such cases.

▲ *Eisenmenger's syndrome*
This term describes the situation in which pulmonary hypertension leads to back pressure, causing a right to left shunt in defects which would otherwise permit left to right shunt.

In most cases there has been a left to right shunt during childhood but with an increasing and reversible pulmonary vascular resistance, pulmonary hypertension becomes so severe that the flood flow changes direction and flows from right to left. The patients usually do not show symptoms throughout childhood but develop cyanosis and finger clubbing in adolescence or early adult life.
The prominent signs are:
• cyanosis
• pulmonary hypertension
• hypertrophy of the right ventricle
• loud pulmonary second sound
The chest X-ray shows large main pul-

monary arteries, but the lesser pulmonary arteries are abnormally small. Right ventricular hypertrophy is confirmed both on the chest X-ray and on the electrocardiogram. The diagnosis will be established by heart catheterization. The prognosis is poor; death may occur very suddenly or follow heart failure. Surgical correction of all large septal defects and persistent ductus arteriosus in childhood will prevent the development of the Eisenmenger's syndrome in most instances.

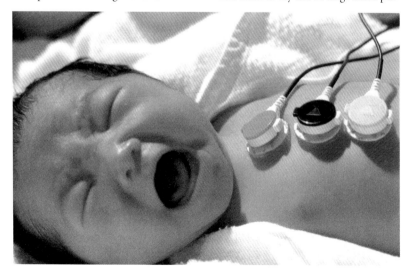

Location of ECG-leads in an infant

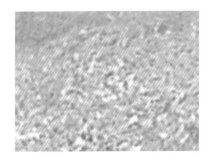

HEART FAILURE

Introduction

The heart is a hollow, muscular organ, situated in the chest between the lungs and above the central depression of the diaphragm. It is about the size of the closed fist, shaped like a blunt cone with the broader end, or base, directed upward, backward and to the right. The pointed end, or apex, points downward, forward and to the left. As placed in the body, it has an oblique position, and the right side is almost in front of the left.

The impact of the heart during contractions is felt against the chest wall in the space between the fifth and sixth ribs, a little below the left nipple, and about 8 cm (3 in) to the left of the median line. The wall of the heart is composed of:
- an outer layer, the pericard
- an inner layer, the endocard
- a middle layer, the myocard

Hypertrophy of the heart muscle due to severe atherosclerosis and hypertension. The condition causes marked heart failure.

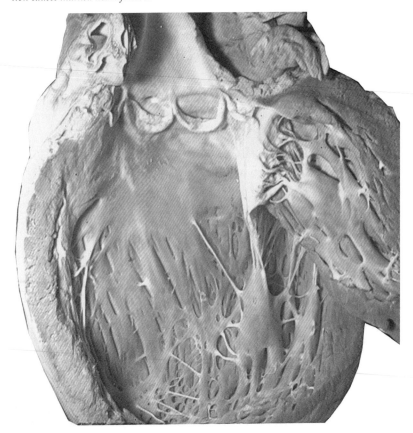

Cardiac output

At each systole (contraction), about 80 ml of blood (for an adult male at rest) moves from the left ventricle into the aorta. This is known as the stroke volume.

A similar amount is forced from the right ventricle into the pulmonary artery. The total cardiac output per beat is, therefore, 160 ml. Taking a pulse rate of 70 beats per minute, 5,6 litres - that is, 70 x 80 ml - of blood leave both the left and right ventricles every minute. This is known as the minute volume.

With an increase or decrease in stroke volume, in pulse rate or in both, the total output per minute would be increased or decreased. During exercise, the total cardiac output may be doubled. The heart muscle receives 10 per cent of cardiac output; the brain, 20 per cent; the liver, stomach and intestines, 25 per cent; the kidneys, 15 per cent; and the rest of the body, 25 per cent.

Blood supply to the brain is the most constantly maintained. In other organs the supply varies directly with activity - for example, during digestion the stomach and intestines receive far more blood than when at rest.

Heartbeat

The cause of the heartbeat is still unknown. General belief favours the myogenic theory - that is, the theory that the function of the nerve tissue in the heart is regulatory, that the contractions are due to the inherent power of contraction possessed by the muscle cells of the heart themselves.

It is believed that inorganic ions, neurohumoral substances and other factors still unknown are responsible for the innate rhythmic contractions of the heart muscle, but the exact role of each remains to be determined. Three ions are especially important - namely, calcium, potassium and sodium, which are always present in blood. There is a well-marked antagonism between the effects of calcium and the effects of potassium and sodium. Calcium has a direct stimulating effect and promotes contraction; potassium and sodium promote relaxation. Heart muscle becomes flaccid and heart rate slows in the presence of excess potassium ions in extracellular fluids.

The heart is not in a state of continuous contraction because of the long "refractory phase" of the cardiac muscle. From the time just before the contraction process begins in response to a stimulus until some time after relaxation begins, the heart muscle is unable to be further stimulated. Once the heart muscle begins to contract, it must relax (partially or completely) before it will contract again.

Congestive heart failure

Heart failure is a disorder in which the heart pumps blood inadequately, leading to reduced blood flow, backup (congestion) of blood in the veins and lungs, and other changes that may further weaken the heart. Because of the congestion of blood the condition is also called congestive heart failure. The heart is a pump with four chambers. Blood enters on one side and exits on the other. This pumping action maintains the circulation of blood throughout our bodies. When the heart is unable to expel sufficient blood to meet the body's needs, the blood backs up and congestive heart failure occurs. This results in diminished blood flow to all the body's tissues. Although heart failure can be acute, it most often develops slowly, with symptoms manifesting gradually.

Warning signs
The most important warning signs of congestive heart failure is edema - the retention of large amounts of fluid in the body. When the heart fails to do its pumping job correctly, blood is not properly circulated back through the veins.

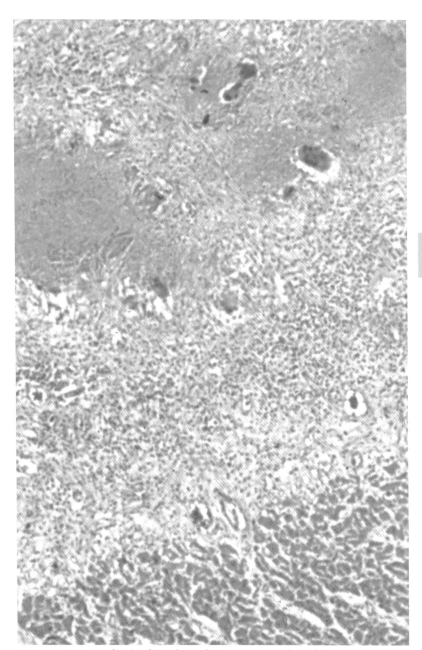

Microscopic picture of pericarditis. The condition causes severe heart failure.

Fluids also accumulate in the body tissues because of poor blood circulation. This is the "congestive" aspect of congestive heart failure. This extra fluid collects all over the body, causing puffiness of the extremities. The most noticeable swelling is in the legs after standing. However, if swelling only occurs in the ankles this may be an indication of some other, less serious condition. When a person with congestive heart failure lies down, fluid settles in the chest area, most noticeable in the lungs. There is difficulty in breathing that may sound like "rattling," especially during physical exertion. Coughing, shortness of breath, or a feeling of heaviness in the chest is also common. Because the circulatory system is not doing its job properly,

Drugs used to treat heart failure

Angiotensin-converting enzyme (ACE) inhibitors
ACE inhibitors cause blood vessels to widen (dilate), thus decreasing the amount of work the heart has to do; they also may have direct beneficial effects on the heart. These drugs are the mainstay of heart failure treatment. They reduce symptoms and the need for hospitalization, and they prolong life.
■ Examples:
- Benazepril
- Captopril
- Enalapril
- Fosinopril
- Lisinopril
- Moexipril
- Quinapril
- Ramipril
- Trandolapril

Angiotensin II receptor blockers
Angiotensin II receptor blockers have effects similar to those of ACE inhibitors and may be tolerated better. However, their effects are still being evaluated in people with heart failure. They may be used with an ACE inhibitor or used alone in people who cannot take an ACE inhibitor.
■ Examples:
- Candesartan
- Eprosartan
- Irbesartran
- Losartan
- Telmisartan
- Valsartan

Beta-blockers
Beta-blocking drugs slow the heart rate and block excessive stimulation of the heart. They are appropriate for some people with heart failure. These drugs are usually used with ACE-inhibitors and provide an added benefit. They may temporarily worsen symptoms but result in long-term improvement in heart function.
■ Examples:
- Bisoprolol
- Carvedilol
- Metoprolol

Other vasodilators
Vasodilators cause blood vessels to widen (dilate). These vasodilators are usually given to people who cannot take an ACE inhibitor or angiotensin II receptor blocker. Nitroglycerin is particularly useful in people who have heart failure and angina.
■ Examples:
- Hydralazine
- Isosorbide dinitrate
- Nitroglycerin

Cardiac glycosides
Cardiac glycosides increase the force of each heartbeat and slow a heart rate that is too fast.
■ Examples:
- Digotoxin
- Digoxin

Loop diuretics
These diuretics help the kidneys eliminate salt and water, thus decreasing the volume of fluid in the bloodstream.
■ Examples:
- Bumetanide
- Ethacrynic acid
- Furosemide

Potassium-sparing diuretics
Because these diuretics prevent potassium loss, they may be given in addition to thiazide or loop diuretics, which cause potassium to be lost. Spironolactone is particularly useful in the treatment of severe heart failure.
■ Examples:
- Amiloride
- Spironolactone
- Triamterene

Thiazide and thiazide-like diuretics
The effects of these diuretics are similar to but milder than those of loop diuretics. The two types of diuretics are particularly effective when used together.
■ Examples:
- Chlortalidone
- Hydrochlorothiazide
- Indapamide
- Metolazone

Anticoagulants
Anticoagulants may be given to prevent clots from forming in the heart chambers.
■ Examples:
- Heparin
- Warfarin

Opioids
Morphine is given to relieve the anxiety that usually accompanies acute pulmonary edema, which is a medical emergency.
■ Examples:
- Morphine

Positive inotropic drugs
For people who have severe symptoms, these drugs may be given intravenously to stimulate heart contractions and help keep blood circulating.
■ Examples:
- Inamrinone
- Dobutamine
- Dopamine
- Milrinone

What is catheterization of the heart?

There are a number of situations in the evaluation of a patient's heart in which routine methods such as ECG do not yield enough information. In such instances, catheterization of the heart may be performed. This method consists of passing and threading a long, narrow, hollow plastic tube into the blood vessel of one of the extremities until it reaches one or more chambers of the heart.

Pressure recordings are made through the tube and blood samples are withdrawn. This is not a routine procedure and requires the skill of a specially trained cardiologist. Catheterization of the heart is not usually undertaken unless it is that heart sur-gery may be indicated.

What is angioplasty and how is it being performed in patients with a coronary artery disease?

Angioplasty is a surgical procedure done on arteries, veins, or capillaries. It is a technique in which a balloon is inflated inside a blood vessel to flatten any plaque (patch) that obstructs it and causes it to become narrowed (used especially to open coronary arteries that supply the heart muscle). Angioplasty is an alternative to a bypass operation in the patient with suitable anatomic lesions. The risk currently is comparable to bypass surgery. Mortality is about 1 per cent. Emergency bypass surgery is required in less than 5 per cent; the rate of success is greater than 90 per cent in highly experienced hands.

Why is coronary angiography needed before I can undergo an angioplasty or bypass opera-tion for severe angina pectoris complaints?

The basic goal of an angioplasty or bypass surgery is the same: to foster myocardial revascularization, which means to establish an adequate blood supply to areas of the heart muscle that became deprived over the years due to the build-up of atherosclerotic plaques in the coronary arteries.

An angioplasty achieves the goal of myocardial revascularization by dilating the coronary arteries at the sites where they have become narrowed by plaque. Bypass surgery can do this by detouring blood around the narrowed parts of the coronary arteries.

How will be decided whether I need an angioplasty or bypass surgery?

Your cardiologist will look at the pictures made during the angiography in order to pinpoint the exact spots where your coronary arteries are narrowed by plaque. Your doctor uses this information and the results of your left ventriculography -as well as everything else he or she knows about your case- to decide whether you are a suitable candidate for either angioplasty or bypass surgery.

Important considerations during this decision-making process are your symptoms, how well you are responding to medicine therapy, your age, the result of your exercise ECG, and the function of your left ventricle. Finally, your doctor notes the number of narrowed coronary arteries, and the sites and severity of the plaque build-up.

Will angiography or coronary bypass surgery be performed on everybody with a coronary artery disease?

Over the years, angioplasty's popularity has grown. During early years, the use of angioplasty was restricted to patients with partial blockage of the initial portion of a single coronary artery. Of all patients with a coronary artery disease, only 5 to 10 per cent were then considered for angioplasty. When it was performed, angioplasty was successfully performed in only about 60 per cent of cases. Today, angioplasty is routinely used in patients with more complex coronary artery disease, including those with narrowings farther down a coronary artery or in multiple arteries, with a totally blocked artery, or with bypassed vessels that have become obstructed.

H

---

patients with congestive heart failure feel tired and weak.

Treatment

Treatment of congestive heart failure involves four important goals:
- Easing the strain on the heart.
- Improving the pumping action of the heart muscle.
- Controlling salt and water balance in the body.
- Identifying and treating the cause of the congestive heart failure.

Bed rest may be an important first aspect of treatment to reduce the heart's workload. Other treatment options include medications, such as ACE-inhibitors, and monitoring weight on a daily basis to ensure that excess fluid is not retained.

Obese patients are encouraged to lose weight to ease the strain on the heart. Once congestive heart failure is under control, the patient usually can return to normal activity, unless there are other complicating factors.

Medications are available to improve and strengthen the heart muscle and make its contractions more powerful. Digitalis increases the cardiac output and slows the heart rate.

Water and salt balance are controlled by changing the patient's diet and using diuretic medications. These help the kidneys excrete excess salt and water.

Finally, it is also important to identify the underlying cause of congestive heart failure.

There are many other diseases that can weaken the heart's pumping ability. Most common are arteriosclerosis - a hardening of the blood vessels, which may deprive the heart muscle of oxygen - and high blood pressure.

Other causes include abnmormnality of the heart valves, infection or congenital malformation of the heart. In many cases, treatment of the underlying cause can provide excellent relief from congestive heart failure.

HEART REHABILITATION

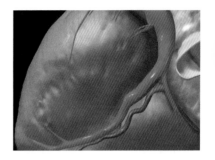

Introduction

Heart or cardiac rehabilitation is the restoration of an individual to normal function after myocardial infarction (heart attack). In the first few days in the coronary or intensive care unit a slight amount of activity, such as sitting in a chair for several hours each day, can limit the orthostatic intolerance that results from protracted bed rest.

Self care in matters of hygiene and selected exercises for the arms and legs help to maintain muscle tone and joint mobility. As the stay in the hospital progresses, physical activity will be increased gradually.

When he leaves the coronary unit, the patient will be helped to resume self care and home activities by the time he is discharged from the hospital.

The principal method of achieving this is through walking, with the pace and distance increasing gradually. Walking should be preceded by selected dynamic exercises of the arms, legs, and trunk.

Patients who have to climb stairs at home should practice before leaving the hospital, by walking down a flight of stairs one day and returning by lift, and walking slowly up a flight of stairs the next day. This will help the patient and his family to be less anxious when he first attempts to climb stairs at home.

Physical activity should not precipitate such symptoms as chest pain, dyspnea, undue fatigue, or palpitation; result in an inappropriate tachycardia or arrhythmia, or cause a fall in systolic blood pressure greater than 10-15 mm Hg, which usually indicates that heart output is inadequate to meet the demand. As a patient comes to tolerate one level of activity well he can be advanced to a slightly more intense workload.

In recent years, the period of bed confinement and hospitalization in the treatment of a myocardial infarction has been sharply curtailed. Patients without complications may be permitted chair rest, passive exercises and the use of the lavatory as soon as chest pain has faded (usually after three or four days).

By one week, walking to the lavatory and non-stressful paperwork or reading are allowed. Discharge from the hospital after two weeks is reasonable and without significant hazard.

Physical activity is gradually increased during the next weeks. Factors such as age, extent of injury, heart failure, occupation and personal ambition all influence the rehabilitation program. Resumption of sexual activity is often of great concern and may be encouraged in parallel with other moderate physical activities.

If cardiac function is well maintained six weeks after an acute attack, most patients are able to return to their full range of normal activity and some establish more regular exercise programs than prior to their heart attack.

System of rehabilitation programs

This 14-step program of exercises and other activities has been designed by cardiologists and specialists in rehabilitation medicine for patients who have suffered a cardiac infarction. The time-schedule of the steps is determined by the doctor.

■ STEP 1
1. Passive exercises to all extremities. You are taught bending of ankles to do several times per day.
2. Feeding self while sitting, with trunk and arms supported by overbed table.

■ STEP 2
1. Exercises of Step 1 to be repeated.
2. Feeding self, washing hands and face, brushing teeth in bed.
3. Light recreational activity, such as reading.

■ STEP 3
1. Active exercises in rotating shoulders and extending arms, hip bending, extending and rotating legs, knee bending, all with the assistance of a physiotherapist or other trained person.
2. Begin sitting in chair for short periods as tolerated.
3. Continuation of light recreation.

■ STEP 4
1. Exercises involving minimal resistance; stiffen all muscles to the count of two.
2. Increase sitting to three times per day.
3. Craft activities: leather lacing, hand sewing, embroidery, copper tooling.

■ STEP 5
1. Exercises with moderate resistance.
2. Sitting in chair at bedside for meals. Dressing, shaving, combing hair.
3. Continuation of craft activities.

■ STEP 6
1. Further resistive exercises while sitting on side of bed; manual resistance of knee extension and bending.
2. Walk to lavatory, if you can tolerate. Stand at sink to shave/brush hair.
3. You may attend group meetings in

a wheelchair for more than one hour.

■ *STEP 7*
1. Standing warm-up exercises. Rotation of arms together in circles. You may walk for a comfortable distance at average pace.
2. Bath in tub. Walk to telephone or sit in patients' lounge.
3. You may walk to group meetings on the same floor.

■ *STEP 8*
1. Warm-up exercises. Walk down one flight of stairs, taking the lift back up.
2. Walk to lounge twice a day. Stay sitting up most of the day.
3. Continuation of all previous craft and educational activities.

■ *STEP 9*
1. Exercises: side bending, five times each side; trunk twisting, five times each side; slight knee bends, ten times with hands on hips. Increase walking distance, walk down one flight of stairs.
2. Walk to lounge twice daily. Stay sitting up most of the day.
3. Discussion of work simplification techniques and pacing activities with occupational therapist.

■ *STEP 10*
1. Side bending with a ½ kg weight. Leg raising while leaning against wall. Increase walking distance and walk down one flight of stairs, taking lift back up.
2. Continuation of all of previous ward activities.
3. You may walk to occupational therapy department and work on craft projects.
4. Discussion of what exercises you will do at home.

■ *STEP 11*
1. Side bending with ½ kg weight while leaning against wall, ten times each side. Standing leg raising, five times. Trunk twisting

with a ½ kg weight, five times each side.
2. Continuation of all of previous ward activities.
3. Increase time in occupational therapy department to one hour.

■ *STEP 12*
1. Side bending with a 1 kg weight, ten times. Leg raising while leaning against wall, ten times each. Trunk twisting with ½ kg weight, ten times. Walk down two flights of stairs.
2. Continuation of all of previous ward activities.
3. Continuation of all craft activities.

■ *STEP 13*
1. Repetition of all exercises of step 12.
2. Continuation of all of previous ward activities.
3. Completion of all projects.

■ *STEP 14*
1. Side bending with 1 kg weight, ten times each side. Trunk twisting with 1 kg weight, ten times each side. Touch toes from sitting position ten times. Walk up flight of ten stairs and down.
2. Continuation of all of previous ward activities.
3. Final instructions about home activities. For exercise at home

Home activities

• Walk daily. Always include an adequate warm-up and cool-down period in each exercise session.

• Wait at least one hour after meals before exercising.

• Space exercise and activity periods evenly with adequate rest periods.

• Avoid steps, hills and strong winds when walking.

• Avoid situations and people who make you anxious or angry. Do not exercise when you feel tense. Instead, try to utilize relaxation techniques.

• If you get tired, or have chest pain, dizziness or shortness of breath, no matter what you are doing, stop and rest. Do not exceed your target heart rate.

• Take your medications as ordered. If you need to take a tablet before or during exercise, remember to do so. Any change (either a decrease or an increase) in certain medications may affect your exercise performance.

• Conserve your energy whenever possible: adapt your living situation for maximum convenience; eliminate unnecessary tasks; plan your day in advance.

• Pay attention to warning signs: call your doctor or go immediately to the nearest hospital casualty department if you have any of the following:
  - Pain or chest discomfort that does not go away with medication or with 15 minutes of rest
  - Shortness of breath that is not related to an activity
  - Dizziness
  - Fainting
  - Overly slow or very fast heartbeat that does not return to normal with a short period of rest

• Signs suggestive of developing congestive heart failure that would be important to discuss with your doctor include:
  - swelling of your feet and ankles
  - a sudden weight gain of 0.9 to 1.4 kg when you know you have not been overeating

439

HEMORRHOIDS

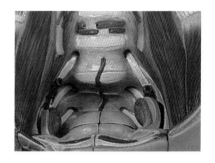

Introduction

Hemorrhoids (also known as "piles") are abnormally large or symptomatic conglomerates of blood vessels, supporting tissues, and overlying mucous membrane or skin of the anorectal area.

Hemorrhoidal disease appears with greatest frequency in subjects 20-50 years of age. Numerous etiologic factors give rise to the considerable confusion regarding the cause or cause of hemorrhoidal disease. Etiologic factors may be divided into predisposing and precipitating causes.

■ *Predisposing causes*
- erect posture;
- heredity;
- occupation;
- diet.

■ *Precipitating causes*
- constipation;
- diarrhea;
- pregnancy;
- anal infection;
- heart failure;
- high blood pressure in the portal circulation to the liver;
- tumors in the rectum or pelvis;
- coughing, sneezing, vomiting;
- physical exertion.

Symptoms

■ *Itching*

Itching, or pruritus, occurs as a manifestation of mild inflammation associated with many anorectal disorders. Pruritus ani refers to persistent itching in the anal and perianal area that may occur even with good hygiene.

Itching is one of the most common symptoms of anorectal disease and may be secondary to swelling, irritation due to dietary factors, or moisture in the anal area. Itching is not always symptomatic of hemorrhoidal disease. Sensitivity to fabric, dyes and perfumes in toilet tissue, detergents, and faecal contents may precipitate itching. Fungal infections, parasites, allergies, and associated anorectal pathologic lesions may also cause itching. Broad-spectrum antibiotic therapy may trigger itching as a result of infection secondary to overgrowth of nonsusceptible organisms. Sometimes

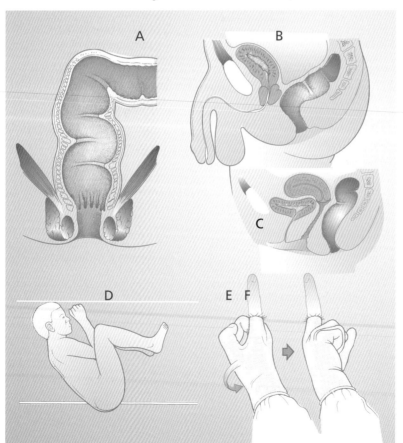

Manual examination of the anus and rectum. The anus and rectum are examined with a gloved finger, and a small sample of stool is sometimes tested for hidden blood.
A. Longitudinal section of the anus and rectum.
B. Location of the anus and rectum in the male pelvis.
C. Location of the anus and rectum in the female pelvis.
D. Position of the patient during manual; examination.
E/F. Movements of the gloved finger in the anus and rectum.

Anatomical site (A); site of hemorrhoidal masses as seen at proctoscopy (B); treatment by dilatation using no more than four fingers (C, D).

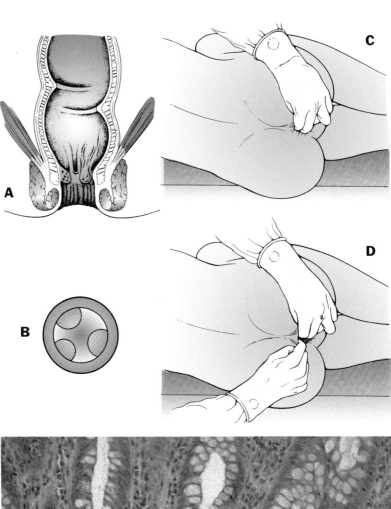

itching may be attributed to some psychologic cause.

■ Burning
Burning, a common symptom of anorectal disease, represents a somewhat greater degree of irritation of the anorectal sensory nerves than itching. The burning sensation may range from a feeling of warmth to a feeling of intense heat.

■ Pain
Acute inflammation of the anal tissue can cause pain. Hemorrhoidal pain has a steady and aching character that is usually not relieved by defecation. Pain is experienced in acute external hemorrhoids.

Chronic external hemorrhoids often exhibit no pain. In view of the absence of sensory nerve endings above the anorectal line, uncomplicated internal hemorrhoids rarely cause pain. When strangulation, thrombosis, or ulceration occur, however, the pain may be severe. Patients with severe persistent pain should consult a doctor.

■ Inflammation
Tissue reaction distinguished by redness, pain, and swelling characterizes inflammation. Inflammation often is caused by trauma, allergy, or infection. The inflammation itself, but not the underlying cause, may be relieved by self-medication.

■ Irritation, swelling and discomfort
Irritation is a response to stimulation of the nerve ending, and is characterized by the appearance of burning, itching, pain or swelling. Swelling represents accumulation of excess fluid associated with engorged hemorrhoids or hemorrhoidal tissue. Discomfort, a vague and generalized uneasiness, may result from any or all of these symptoms.

Microscopic view of the mucosal surface of the rectum, where histological changes may occur accompanying hemorrhoids.

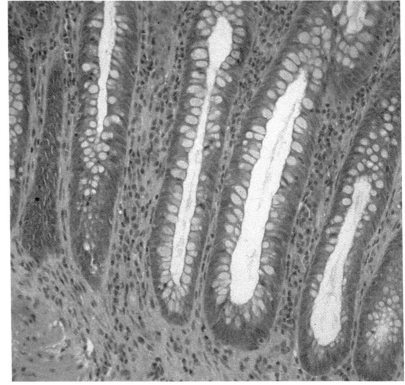

Hemorrhoids Questions & Answers

How can I tell if I have hemorrhoids?

There are one or more swellings or bulges about the anus, which become more pronounced on bowel vacuations. There is also a sense of fullness in the anal region, more pronounced on bowel evacuation. Hemorrhoids are frequently painful and may be accompanied by considerable rectal bleeding.

What are the major symptoms of hemorrhoids?

Hemorrhoids are varicose dilatations of the veins which drain the rectum and anus. It is felt that these veins break down and their valves become incompetent because of the strain placed upon them by irregular living habits.

Chronic constipation, irregularity of bowel evacuation, and prolonged sojourns on the toilet are thought to be conductive toward hemorrhoid formation. Pregnancy, because of the pressure of the baby's head in the pelvis, also leads toward hemorrhoid formation.

Hemorrhoids are the most common condition in the anal region and affects 10-15 percent of the population at one time or another. If hemorrhoids are not treated the following can happen:

- they may bleed severely and cause a marked anemia with all of its serious consequences;
- they may become thrombosed (clotted), producing extreme pain in the region;
- they may prolapse (drop out of the rectum and not go back again);
- they may become strangulated and gangrenous;

Are piles or hemorrhoids in all circumstances harmless conditions of the body?

Hemorrhoids are cushions of tissue that line the lower part of the rectum and may produce complete closure of the anal canal. Since hemorrhoids occur universally in adults and children, they should not be considered abnormal.

Symptoms due to hemorrhoids are:

- bleeding;
- protrusion;
- pain.

Rectal bleeding should be attributed to hemorrhoids only after other more serious conditions have been excluded. Hemorrhoidal bleeding, which typically occurs following defecation and is noted on toilet tissue, rarely leads to anemia; they are painful; only when they are ulcerated or thrombosed.

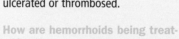

How are hemorrhoids being treated?

Correction of constipation and straining by means of stool softeners or psyllium seed may be effective. Bleeding hemorrhoids can be treated by injection of a sclerosing substance; this method is called sclerotherapy.

Larger hemorrhoids or those that fail to respond to injection sclerotherapy are treated by rubber-band ligation. Mucus discharge and a sensation of incomplete evacuation of the rectum are usually due to internal hemorrhoids, which are also ideally treated by rubber-band ligation.

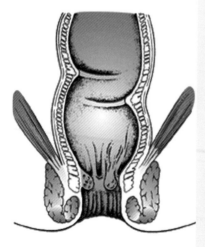

■ Bleeding

Bleeding is almost always associated with internal hemorrhoids and may occur before, during, or after defecation. The amount of bleeding experienced is often variable and is not related to the amount of hemorrhoidal tissue present.

When bleeding occurs from an external hemorrhoid, it is caused by an acute thrombosis accompanying rupture. Pain often accompanies the bleeding in this case, although a patient may experience some relief of the pain with the onset of the bleeding.

Blood from hemorrhoids is usually bright red and covers the faecal matter. Bleeding hemorrhoids infrequently produce severe anemias due to the chronic blood loss. Bleeding may indicate the presence of serious anorectal disease and should not be self-medicated.

■ Seepage and protrusion

Seepage is caused by an anal sphincter that cannot close completely and involves the involuntary passing of faecal material or mucus. This symptom cannot be self-medicated and the patient should consult a doctor.

Protrusion is an early symptom of uncomplicated internal and external hemorrhoids and is defined as the projection of hemorrhoidal tissue outside the anal canal. The rectal protrusion may vary in size and usually appears after defecation, prolonged standing, or unusual physical exertion. Self-treatment is not appropriate.

Treatment

Correction of constipation and straining by means of stool softeners or psyllium seed may be effective. Bleeding hemorrhoids, after other possible causes have been excluded, will be treated by injection sclerotherapy (injection of substances causing sclerosis or hardening of tissue).

Large hemorrhoids or those that fail to respond to injection sclerotherapy are treated by means of rubber-band ligation: a 0.6 cm diameter elastic band is dilated up to about 1.1 cm; the internal hemorrhoid is grasped in an

H

Banding hemorrhoids

- Some internal hemorrhoids are removed by tying them off with rubber bands in an out-patient procedure called rubber band ligation.

- The instrument used (ligator) consists of forceps surrounded by a cylinder with ½-inch rubber bands placed on one end.

- The ligator is inserted into the anus through an anoscope (a short, rigid viewing tube), and the hemorrhoid is grasped with the forceps.

- The cylinder is sled upward over the forceps and the hemorrhoid, pushing the rubber bands of the cylinder and around the base of the hemorrhoid.

- The rubber bands cut off the hemorrhoid's blood supply, causing it to wither and drop off painlessly in a few days.

- The treatment is usually applied to one hemorrhoid at a time at intervals of 2 weeks or longer.

- Internal hemorrhoids may also be destroyed with a laser (laser destruction), an artificial light (infrared photocoagulation), or en electrical current.

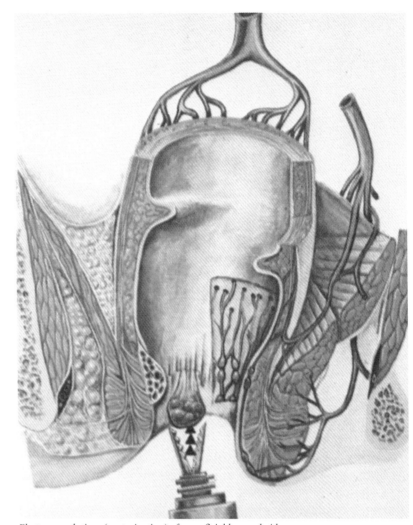

Electrocoagulation (cauterization) of superficial hemorrhoids.

area that is insensible to pain and withdrawn through the band, which is then released to ligate the hemorrhoid, resulting in its necrosis and sloughing.

One hemorrhoid is ligated every 2 weeks and a total of 3 to 6 treatments may be required. Operative hemorrhoidectomy is rarely performed for bleeding hemorrhoids.

If protruding hemorrhoids are internal, they are treated by rubber-band ligations. With mixed internal and external hemorrhoids, the internal component will be rubber-band ligated. If there is no significant internal component, an operative procedure or freezing is required.

HEPATITIS

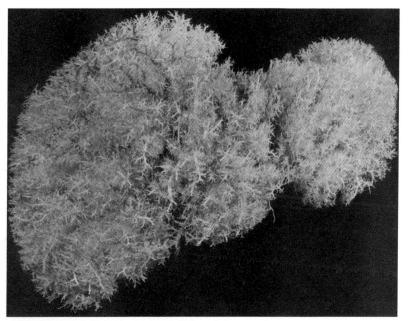

Description

Hepatitis is an inflammatory process in the liver characterized by diffuse or patchy degeneration of the liver tissue. The major causes of hepatitis are a number of viruses, alcohol and drugs. Viral hepatitis is the most common of the serious contagious diseases caused by several viruses that attack the liver.Hepatitis means inflammation of the liver, usually producing swelling and tenderness and sometimes permanent damage to the liver.

Hepatitis may also be caused by non-viral substances such as alcohol, chemicals and drugs. These types of hepatitis are known respectively as alcoholic, toxic and drug-induced hepatitis.

■ *Hepatitis and cancer*
A high incidence of liver cancer is found in some African and Asian countries where there are many hepatitis B carriers and appears to be related to the chronic hepatitis B carrier state. Research on this relationship is being actively pursued.

The number of cases of liver cancer in patients with chronic hepatitis C is unknown. About 15 per cent of hepatitis B carriers in the Orient are at risk of developing liver cancer, but the rate seems to be considerably less in the Western world.

■ *AIDS and hepatitis*
Any relation between AIDS and hepatitis is coincidental. Male homosexuals and intravenous drug users who are at high risk for infection with the HIV, the cause of AIDS, are at equally high risk for infection with the hepatitis B virus.

Types of viral hepatitis

At least five types of viral hepatitis are currently known, each caused by a different identified virus.

▲ *Hepatitis A*, formerly called infectious hepatitis, is most common in children in developing countries but is being seen more frequently in adults in the western world. Hepatitis A virus (HAV) spreads primarily by faecal-oral contact; blood and secretions are also possibly infectious.
Faecal shedding of the virus occurs during the incubation period and usually ceases a few days after symptoms begins; thus infectivity often has already passed when the diagnosis is made. Water- and food-borne epidemics are common, especially in underdeveloped countries. Eating of contaminated raw shellfish can be responsible.

▲ *Hepatitis B*, formerly called serum hepatitis, is the most serious form of hepatitis, with over 200 million carriers in the world. Hepatitis B virus (HBV) is the most thoroughly characterized. The infective particle consists of an inner core plus an outer surface coat. HBV is associated with a wide spectrum of liver disease such as:
- acute hepatitis;
- chronic hepatitis;
- cirrhosis;
- certain types of liver cancer.

▲ Hepatitis C, formerly called non-A, non-B hepatitis, is now the

The branching patterns of gallducts and blood vessels of the human liver. Yellow: gallducts; Blue: branches of the portal vein.

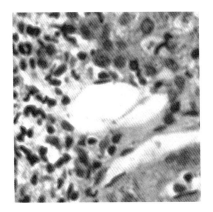

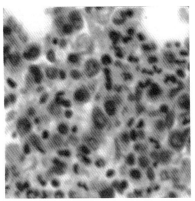

Characteristic changes in the blood smear of patients suffering from viral hepatitis. Above: peripheral blood smear; below: smear of the bone marrow.

most common cause of hepatitis after blood transfusion. More than one per cent of Americans are carriers of the virus.

▲ *Hepatitis D*, formerly called delta hepatitis, is found mainly in intravenous drug users who are carriers of the hepatitis B virus which is necessary for the hepatitis D virus to spread.

▲ *Hepatitis E*, formerly called enteric or epidemic non-A, non-B hepatitis, resembles hepatitis A, but is caused by a different virus commonly found in the Indian Ocean area.

Other viruses, especially members of the herpes virus family, including the cold sore virus, chicken pox virus, infectious mononucleosis virus and others can affect the liver as well as other organs they infect. This is particularly true when the immune system is impaired.

What is viral hepatitis?

Viral hepatitis is an inflammatory process in the liver characterized by diffuse or patchy degeneration of the liver tissue. The major causes of hepatitis are a number of viruses, alcohol and drugs.

Is viral hepatitis a common disease?

Viral hepatitis is the most common of the serious contagious diseases caused by several viruses that attack the liver.

What does hepatitis mean and what are the possible causes?

Hepatitis means inflammation of the liver, usually producing swelling and tenderness and sometimes permanent damage to the liver. Hepatitis may also be caused by non-viral substances such as alcohol, chemicals and drugs. These types of hepatitis are known respectively as alcoholic, toxic and drug-induced hepatitis.

Does viral hepatitis cause cancer?

A high incidence of liver cancer is found in some African and Asian countries where there are many hepatitis B carriers and appears to be related to the chronic hepatitis B carrier state. Research on this relationship is being actively pursued.

Is hepatitis related to AIDS?

Any relation between AIDS and hepatitis is coincidental. Male homosexuals and intravenous drug users who are at high risk for infection with the HIV, the cause of AIDS, are at equally high risk for infection with the hepatitis B virus.

Are there different types of viral hepatitis?

At least five types of viral hepatitis are currently known, each caused by a different identified virus. They are usually called hepatitis A, B, C, D and E, although other names such as infectious hepatitis, serum hepatitis are still being used.

What are the characteristics of hepatitis A?

Hepatitis A formerly called infectious hepatitis is most common in children in developing countries but is being seen more frequently in adults in the western world. Hepatitis A virus (HAV) spreads primarily by faecal-oral contact; blood and secretions are also possibly infectious.

Faecal shedding of the virus occurs during the incubation period and usually ceases a few days after symptoms begins; thus infectivity often has already passed when the diagnosis is made. Water- and food-borne epidemics are common, especially in underdeveloped countries. Eating of contaminated raw shellfish can be responsible.

What are the characteristics of hepatitis B?

Hepatitis B - formerly called serum hepatitis, is the most serious form of hepatitis, with over 200 million carriers in the world. Hepatitis B virus (HBV) is the most thoroughly characterized. The infective particle consists of an inner core plus an outer surface coat. HBV is associated with a wide spectrum of liver disease such as:
- acute hepatitis;
- chronic hepatitis;
- cirrhosis;
- certain types of liver cancer.

HEREDITARY DISEASES

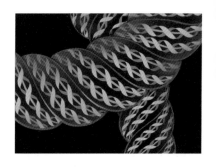

Introduction

Hereditary or genetic diseases involve disorders of the hereditary material - the genes and chromosomes. Genetic disorders are those with a clearly defined mechanism of inheritance, in which a genetic component always plays a substantial role or results from a chromosomal abnormality - one or mutant genes, or alterations in the number, size or arrangement of chromosomes.

They can cause disturbances in body chemistry, physiology or structure, often resulting in lifelong physical or mental impairment. The common tie among genetic diseases is that victims born with conditions or with the susceptibility to develop the disease in later life, and if the disease does not render them sterile, they can transmit it to their offspring.

Some genetic diseases are inherited in a complex manner in which several genes are involved, and some involve multiple genes plus certain environmental factors (for instance, dietary) for the condition to express itself. These factors make the problem of assessing the burden of genetic diseases in the nation today enormously difficult.

An estimated 70 million people worldwide (NIH data, 2000) today suffer the consequences of birth defects of varying severity. Not all these disorders are genetic: 20 per cent are estimated not to involve an inheritable component, but to represent the effects of agents such as infection, drugs and physical injury to the fetus. The remaining 80 per cent carry true genetic diseases due wholly or partly to defective genes or chromosomes.

Recognition

No comprehensive assessment of the number, variety and distribution of genetic and partially genetic diseases has yet been made, largely because all

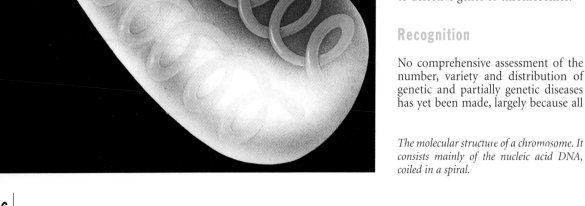

The molecular structure of a chromosome. It consists mainly of the nucleic acid DNA, coiled in a spiral.

data are not available. One reason is that the list of genetic diseases grows every year as "new" ones are recognized. The list of disorders, each of which is caused by a single defective gene (in single or double dosage), now numbers nearly 3000.

Another reason for the slow progress made in recognizing the real magnitude of the genetic disease problem is that, until recently, genetic diseases were considered extremely rare, each one, on the average, occurring only once in every 10,000 live births.

As the figure above shows, the total number of genetic diseases is extremely high - even considering only those recognized as purely genetic, which would exclude such widespread conditions as heart disease, arthritis, cancer, stroke, diabetes and mental illness.

And certain genetic disorders - such as sickle cell anemia, Tay-Sachs disease, cystic fibrosis and thalassaemia - have considerably greater impact upon particular ethnic or racial populations than the average 1-in-10,000 incidence reported for genetic diseases.

A third reason for the previous neglect of the genetic disease problem is that in only the past two decades have advances in basic sciences given the medical profession the technology for diagnosing precisely and undertaking the control and treatment of hereditary diseases.

Although strictly speaking, genetic defects are still incurable, much can be done toward detection, diagnosis, prevention and treatment of these difficult medical problems. It is now possible, for example, to diagnose some 450 serious genetic problems before

Gene pool

The total amount of information present at any one time in the genes of the reproductive members of a biological population. The frequency of any particular gene in the gene pool changes owing to natural selection, mutation and genetic drift. This change forms the basis of evolutionary change.

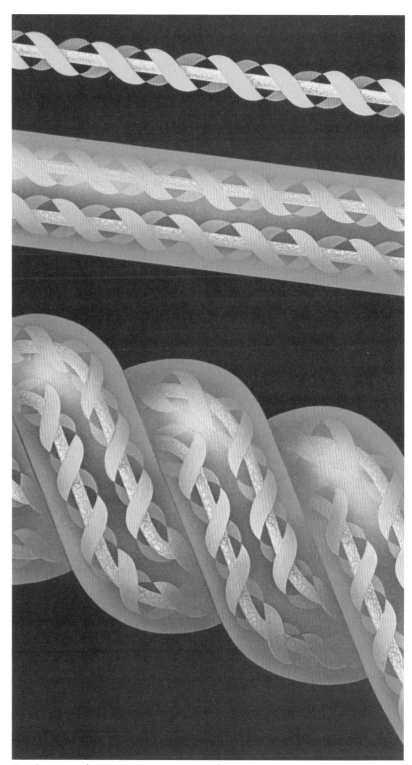

Proteins are an also an important component of the chromosome. Usually, protein molecules (green) are twisted around a nucleic acid (upper figure). All hereditary information is stored in this thread. The threads are usually found in pairs (middle figure) that, in turn, are twisted around each other in a specific manner (bottom figure).

Common screening tests for genetic diseases

PKU
An enzyme that processes the protein phenylalanine is missing.
Incidence
1 in 12,000
Prevention of:
- developmental delays
- seizures
- mental retardation

Congenital hypothyroidism
The thyroid gland does not produce enough of the hormone thyroxine.
Incidence
1 in 4,000
Prevention of:
- developmental delays
- lethargy
- mental retardation
- deafness

Galactosemia
The body is unable to break down galactose, a simple sugar found in milk products.
Incidence
1 in 60,000
Prevention of:
- lethargy
- feeding intolerance
- speech problems
- vision problems
- liver disorders

Sickle cell diseases
Deformed red blood cells reduce oxygen supply to organs.
Incidence
1 in 400 (people of African origin)
Prevention of:
- anemia
- pneumonia
- blood infections
- spleen disorders
- chronic pain

Maple syrup urine disease
The body does not process three proteins properly.
Incidence
1 in 225,000
Prevention of:
- sweet odour of urine
- lack of appetite
- poor sucking reflex
- severe physical disabilities
- severe mental disabilities

Homocystinuria
Certain parts of the protein homocystine cannot be broken down.
Incidence
1 in 150,000
Prevention of:
- developmental delays
- growth delays
- eye problems
- osteoporosis
- mental retardation

Congenital adrenal hyperplasia
The adrenal glands cannot make enough of their main hormones.
Incidence
1 in 12,000
Prevention of:
- drowsiness
- vomiting
- enlarged female genital organs
- growth problems
- reproductive disorders

Tyrosinaemia
A metabolic problem that causes tyrosine, an amino acid, to build up in the blood.
Incidence
1 in 100,000
Prevention of:
- lethargy
- difficulty swallowing
- impaired motor activity
- prolonged jaundice
- liver disease
- rickets

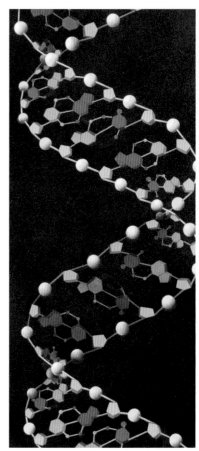

Model of DNA. Each strand of the double helix consists of a long chain of the sugar deoxyribose and phosphate residues. Four bases form the steps of the spirals.

birth, and to identify persons who carry the trait (but who do not actually have the disease) in man and these conditions.

These capabilities alone give physicians and patients alternatives they never had before to make informed decisions concerning the risk of genetic diseases. In addition, a dozen or more techniques for treating a number of genetic diseases have recently become available and more are being developed every year.

Transmission of hereditary diseases

The basis for all of genetic diseases is determined at conception and, when sterility does not result, can be passed

on to subsequent generations. Whereas many genetic diseases are immediately apparent or show signs early in life, some are not expressed until later years. Genetic diseases are transmitted in essentially three forms:
▲ as chromosomal abnormalities;
▲ as single-gene defects;
▲ as complex disorders (multi-gene disorders resulting from the combined action of multiple genes and/or environmental factors.

Chromosomal abnormalities

Few reliable estimates exists from the world as a whole. Reports of some populations indicate that 5-6 per cent of newborns are afflicted with serious disease in which genetic factors are significant. Surveys show that genetic factors contribute, directly or indirectly, to the hospitalization of a rather large proportion of children. Genetically determined conditions constitute the second most frequent death in children under the age of one year in the United States and Europe. Chromosome analysis should be obtained in all infants with multiple malformations. Fortunately, most syndromes associated with chromosome anomalies occur only once in a family, and an optimistic prognosis for future offspring can usually be given. The prime example is Down's syndrome, the results of a chromosomal abnormality called trisomy 21, in which there are three chromosomes of number 21 instead of two. In this, the age of the mother is an important factor.

Single-gene defects

Dominant single-gene defects occur in 1.8 to 2.0 per cent of all live births. These conditions fall into three general categories:
- dominant;
- recessive;
- sex-linked.

n *Dominant single-gene defects*
These can be transmitted by one affected parent. For each of the more than 1500 such disorders so far identified, each pregnancy involves a 50

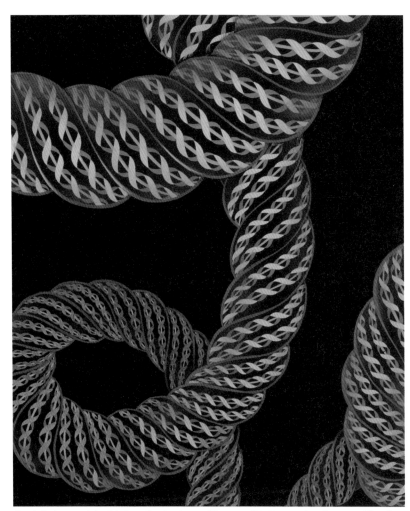

Spatial picture of the DNA molecule. One millimeter of DNA contains about 5 million base pairs. If you wanted to print the genetic code of such a piece of DNA in a book, you would need a volume of about 2,000 pages, with 5,000 letters to the page.

per cent risk of transmitting the defect if one parent is affected, and a 75 per cent risk if both parents carry the gene. Examples include some forms of dwarfism and other physical defects, and certain late-onset diseases, such as Huntington's chorea, a progressive degeneration of the brain.

n *Recessive single-gene defects*
Almost everyone is a carrier of deleterious recessive genes. The number of such genes per individual has been variously estimated as between one and ten. The usually minute probability that very rare recessive genes are expressed as disease is greatly increased by marriage between relatives.

Recessive single-gene defects can appear in the offspring if the recessive gene is received from each parent. If both parents are carriers of the particular trait, there is a 25 per cent chance in each pregnancy of producing an affected child.

Both parents, usually unaffected, carry a normal gene (N) which takes precedence over its faulty recessive counterpart (n). The odds for each child are:
• a 25 per cent risk of inheriting a double dose of n genes which may cause a serious birth defect;
• a 25 per cent chance of inheriting two N's, thus being free of the

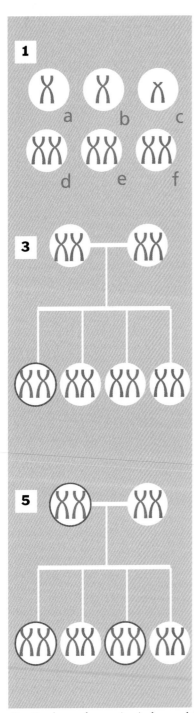

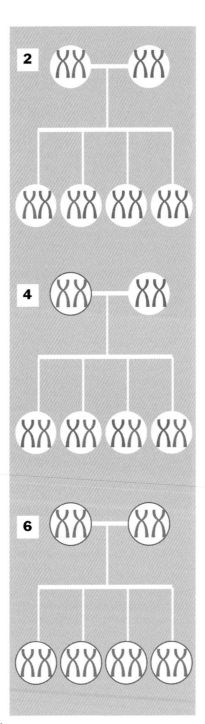

recessive gene;
• a 50 per cent chance of being a carrier like both parents.
Among the over 1000 recognized recessive single-gene disorders are:
- sickle cell anemia;
- Tay-Sachs disease;
- phenylketonuria (PKU);
- galactosaemia;
- cystic fibrosis.

n *Sex-linked single-gene disorders*
These are so named because the defect is carried on the X-chromosome. Women have two X-chromosomes (XX), while men have but one (which is paired with the dissimilar Y-chromosome, XY), and this leads to a different pattern of inheritance for those defective genes found on the X-chromosome.
This is based on the fact that men transmit their X-chromosome only to their daughters, never to their sons, who always receive the father's Y-chromosome. Thus, a female may carry the trait for such a recessive disorder but not the disease to balance the effect of the trait.
A male, however, must be affected if he receives from his mother an X-chromosome bearing the abnormal gene. The risk of affected offspring to a trait-carrying mother, then, is 50 per cent with each male birth.
Examples of X-linked recessive genetic disorders are:
- hemophilia;
- Hunter disease;
- muscular dystrophy;
- the Lesch-Nyhan syndrome;
- certain types of ataxia;
- diabetes insipidus.

Multiple gene defects

The third general category of genetic diseases (in addition to chromosomal and single-gene defects) consists of the complex or multi-gene disorders. There is as yet no complete estimate of the actual number of such multifactorial diseases, although an incidence of 1.7 to 2.5 per cent of all live birth has been suggested as reasonable.
There is no way of determining the potential risk of contracting a multifactorial disease; authorities tend to

Genetic schema of a recessive single-gene defect.
1a. normal chromosome; b. chromosome with gene defect; c. male Y-chromosome; d. single occurrence of defect; f. double occurrence of defect.
2. One parent is affected; 50 per cent of transmitting the defect.
3. Both parents carry the gene in a single dose.
4. One parent carries the gene in a double dose.
5. One parent carries a double dose, the other a single dose.
6. Both parents carry a double dose.

apply the "recurrence rule of thumb," which says that in a family with one affected offspring, the probably of having another is less than 5 per cent. The mode of transmission is at least as complex as is the action of the genes involved in each of these multiple gene diseases (for instance, club foot, congenital dislocation of the hip, certain forms of diabetes).

Altogether, the overall incidence of recognized genetic diseases is 4.8 to 5.0 per cent of all live births. And while this seems to be a high figure for a class of diseases once thought to be extremely rare, it is important to remember that the estimate does not include any of those disorders widely thought to be at least partly genetic in origin.

Prevention of genetic disorders

Effective prevention strategies have been devised for a number of specific conditions, and may prove applicable to other conditions as techniques for identifying families and pregnancies at risk become more refined. Secondary prevention of some inherited metabolic diseases is possible by the early finding of cases through screening either prior to or immediately after birth.

The condition that has been screened most extensively is phenylketonuria (PKU) - an inability to produce a specific enzyme that can lead to overaccumulation of an amino acid that, in turn can adversely affect the structure and function of the nervous system.

Many genetic diseases can be detected before birth by analysis of a small amount of amniotic fluid in which the fetus lies. Some cells of the placenta can also be used for this investigation. When testing reveals that a fetus will be afflicted by one of these diseases, parents can decide for themselves whether or not to continue the pregnancy.

For an increasing number of genetic disorders, there are screening tests that can identify parents who are carriers of defective genes. DNA-analysis shows the molecular basis of many

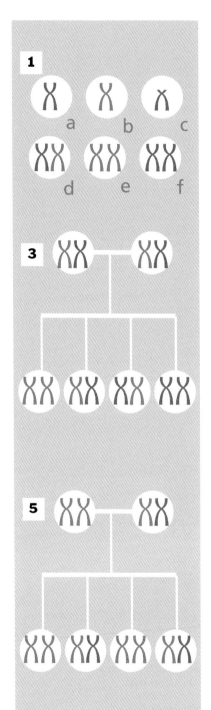
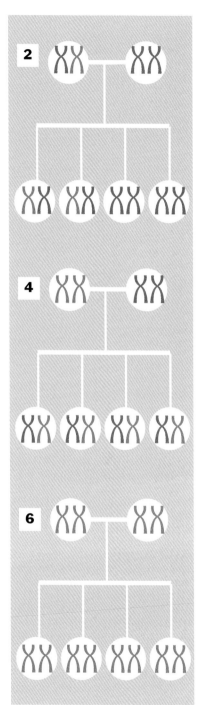

Genetic schema of a dominant single-gene defect.
1a. normal chromosome; b. chromosome with gene defect; c. male Y-chromosome; d. single occurrence of defect; f. double occurrence of defect.
2. One parent is affected; 50 per cent of transmitting the defect.
3. Both parents carry the gene.
4. One parent carries in a double dose.
5. One parent carries a double dose, the other a single dose.
6. Both parents carry a double dose.

genetic diseases. Some genetic disorders, such as hemophilia, affect primarily one sex, usually male. Because recessive sex-linked disorders are relatively rare, parents usually do not know they harbour the faulty genetic material until after the birth of the first affected child.

Today prenatal detection of the classic form of hemophilia has become possible, as is the case with cystic fibrosis. A revolution in the diagnosis of genetic disease is unfolding because of scientists' growing ability to find and interpret the messages of human genes (The Human Genome Project). Such diagnoses are becoming available for a every increasing roster of disorders caused by a fault in one or another single gene among the 80,000 to 100,000 that humans possess.

Individually, most of these diseases are quite rare, although cystic fibrosis occurs in about one per 1,000 live births and the Duchenne type of muscular dystrophy appears about once in every 5,000 males.

■ Detection of single-gene disorders

There are several ways of detecting a single-gene disorder in a fetus or of proving that a child or adult is a carrier. All are based on the fact that the messages of heredity in all living organisms are carried in the chemistry of DNA, deoxyribonucleic acid.

The long, twisted strands of this master chemical of heredity are made up of four different subunits repeated in various combinations thousands and even millions of times. The combinations constitute the universal code for the regulation and production of everything a cell makes.

The four subunits - adenine, guanine, cytosine and thymine - are usually identified by their initials. The sequence GAT (guanine-adenine-thymine), for example, is the code ordering a cell to add the amino acid leucine to a protein under construction. Other combinations are the codes for all the other 19 amino acids that make up the myriad of different proteins that are the main ingredients of living organisms.

The human genetic apparatus is an immense archive of about three billion subunits of DNA. Just one error among these can produce a disease such as muscular dystrophy or cystic fibrosis.

Even though a gene may contain several hundred to a few thousand subunits of genetic messages, scientists can sometimes detect the structure of a known gene from as few as 19 or 20 subunits.

The other main testing schema is useful even when the gene has not yet been found. It depends partly on the fact that genes close together on a chromosome are likely to be inherited together. Special chemical scalpels called restriction enzymes cut strands of DNA when they encounter particular sequences of the four subunits. More than 100 different restrictive enzymes that cut in different places are known. Using a large battery of these, scientists can chop up the complement of DNA from a person's cells into many thousands of fragments.

■ DNA-map of diseases

Though research is making important strides in detection of the estimated 3,000 or more different single-gene defects, major diseases such as heart disease and other widespread causes of human death and disability are far more complex in origin.

But the emergence of recombinant DNA technology in general, and the uses of restriction fragments in particular, seem capable of bringing even these complex diseases within reach of genetic analysis. The links between cigarette smoking and lung cancer are known, yet many smokers live their entire lives free of the disease. The less fortunate ones learn of their susceptibility too late.

A genetic linkage map could allow parents to know, sometimes even before a child is born, that he or she must be particularly careful to avoid smoking, for example, or should live on a diet that takes into account a risk of heart disease.

■ Genetic counselling

Genetic counselling is a part of all strategies for prevention of genetic diseases. Examples of situations where counselling can be h•elpful are:

- Couples in which the woman is over 35 years of age, and therefore has an increased risk of producing an infant with Down's syndrome (mongolism).
- Couples with a family history of certain inherited diseases.
- Couples in which the partners are blood relatives (their chances of passing a defective gene are much greater.
- Couples in which one or both parents has been exposed to powerful mutagenic agents, such as radiation or certain chemicals.
- Women with more than one unexplained miscarriage.

■ Environmental agents

Several environmental agents are probably important in such birth defects such as cleft palate, when the appropriate genetic make-up is present. Differing susceptibility to severe birth defects from infection during pregnancy by viruses such as rubella (German measles), cytomegalovirus and herpes, or other agents such as toxoplasmosis, may also have a genetic basis.

Once an infectious environmental agent is identified, the potential for prevention exists. This has been the case with the prevention of the congenital rubella syndrome through appropriate immunization and the prevention of congenital syphilis through early treatment of the mother-to-be.

Neural tube defects - when the spinal cord is not totally enclosed within the vertebral column - produce a range of serious impairments and often have associated abnormalities and complications. Infants that survive and undergo surgery to close the open lesions have severe handicaps:

- paralysis of the legs;
- incontinence;
- deformity;
- sometimes mental deterioration.

Caring for such a child puts a great strain on family members. One study revealed a divorce rate for families with a surviving spina bifida that was eight times the rate of a comparative population.

Lack of awareness by the general public and health professionals is particularly severe in the case of genetic disorders. At least one survey has revealed that genetic disease is not considered important by a majority of doctors, making them unlikely to take the steps necessary for prevention, or to inform the parents about the possibility of disease and the ways to avoid it.

Genetic disorders that can be tested before birth

The most common tests used to detect abnormalities in a fetus include ultrasonography, chorionic villus sampling, amniocentesis, and percutaneous umbilical blood sampling.

▲ Congenital adrenal hyperplasia
  Incidence 1 of 10,000
  Inheritance pattern Autosomal recessive

▲ Cystic fibrosis
  Incidence 1 of 3,300 (white people)
  Inheritance pattern Autosomal recessive

▲ Duchenne's muscular dystrophy
  Incidence 1 of 3,500 male births
  Inheritance pattern X-linked recessive

▲ Hemophilia A
  Incidence 1 of 8,500 male births
  Inheritance pattern X-linked recessive

▲ Huntington's disease
  Incidence 5 of 100,000
  Inheritance pattern Autosomal recessive

▲ Polycystic kidney disease
  Incidence 1 of 3,000
  Inheritance pattern Autosomal dominant

▲ Sickle cell anemia
  Incidence 1 of 400 black people in the US
  Inheritance pattern Autosomal recessive

▲ Tay-Sachs disease
  Incidence 1 of 3,600 Ashkenazi Jews
  Inheritance pattern Autosomal recessive

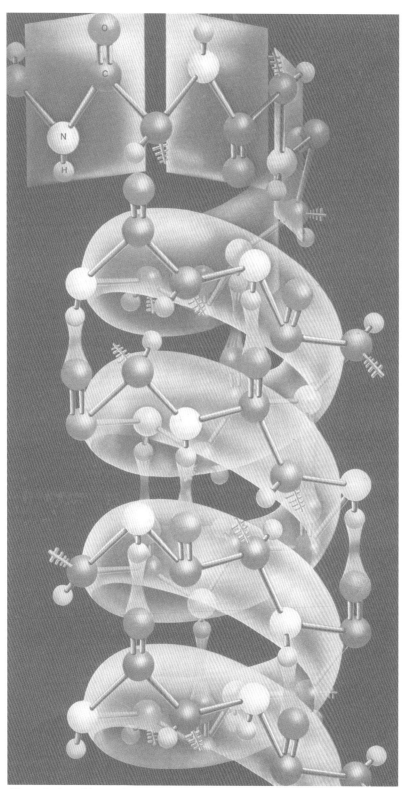

The methods used in genetic engineering are based on the possibility of changing the molecular structure of DNA (O = oxygen; C = carbon; H = hydrogen; N = nitrogen).

H

HIP DISORDERS

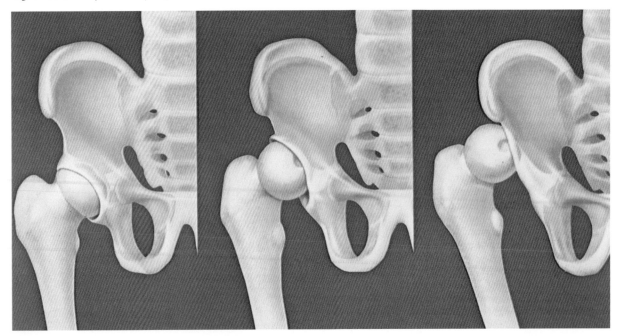

Description

The pelvis is made up of the sacral bone and the two hipbones. The latter are built up of the iliac bone, the pubic bone and the ischium (seat bone). The joint surfaces of the sacral bone and the hipbone have a cartilaginous mantle and are connected with collagen fibers. They have little mobility. The symphysis (the union of the two pubic bones) contains a cartilaginous disc supported from above and below by ligaments.

This is a ball-and-socket joint; the round head of the thighbone (femur) rests in the deep, cup-shaped cavity of the acetabulum of the hipbone. Both joint surfaces are coated with cartilage, that covering the head of the femur (about two-thirds of a sphere) being thicker above where it bears the weight of the body, and thinning out to an edge below at the margin of the femoral head.

The joint capsule is one of the strongest ligaments of the body. It is large and somewhat loose, so that in every position of the body, some portion of it is relaxed.

At the femur, the capsule is fixed above at the junction of the neck and greater trochanter and to the cervical tubercle. Added to the joint capsule, and strengthening it, are three auxiliary bands, whose fibers are intimately blended with and form part of the capsule.

The hip joint, like the shoulder joint, is a spheroidal joint, but differs in that it possesses a much more complete socket with a commensurable limitation of movement, since more than half of the spherical femoral head rests in the cavity of the acetabulum.

Each variety of movement of the thigh on the pelvis is permitted - namely, flexion, extension, abduction, adduction and rotation -and any two or more of these movements that are not

Congenital dislocation of the hip is a common defect found in newborn babies.
Left: Normal hip joint
Center: The head of the femur and hip joint do not meet properly
Right: Dislocation of the head of the femur

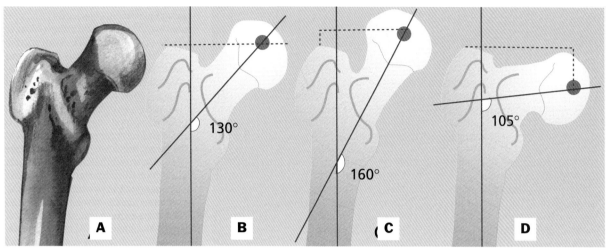

A. Upper part of the femur showing the caput, collum and part of the shaft. B. The normal angle between collum and shaft amount to 130°. C. In coxa valga the angle is much larger, for instance 160°. D. In coxa vara, the angle is much smaller, for instance 105°.

antagonistic can be combined - that is, flexion or extension can be associated with abduction, or adduction can be combined with rotation.

The most common disorders of the hip joint in children are congenital dislocation and Legg-Calve-Perthes disease, and in adults most often injuries and osteoarthritis occur.

Congenital dislocation

Congenital dislocation of a joint is the absence at birth of a correct of sufficiently snug and sturdy fit between the bones of a joint. A baby is diagnosed as having this condition whenever the structure of a joint allows for easy dislocation of a bone, regardless or whether the bone is actually dislocated at birth.

Most congenital dislocations are of the hip and involve an instability between the thighbone and hipbone socket in either or both legs. The rounded end of the thighbone may be totally or partially out of the socket or may simply have the potential to slip. It is common for the ligament connecting the hipbone socket to the head of the thighbone to be somewhat loose at birth.

In most cases congenital dislocation of the hip can be easly and entirely corrected within the first few months of life. Correction is possible because a newborn's bones are pliable at their ends. If poorly fitting bones are repositioned early enough during the development of the musculoskeletal system, tissues are likely to set in the correct position.

If the position is not corrected early enough or at all or if it is complicated by other congenital problems, congenital hip dislocation may lead to poor posture, walking difficulties, and persistent discomfort. Later in life a poorly treated case of congenital hip dislocation greatly increases a person's changes of developing osteoarthritis. About 1 out of every 100 newborns has some form of congenital hip problem, but the majority of these infants simply have unstable connections between the thighbone and socket that usually strengthen on their own during the first few days after birth. About 4 out of every 1,000 newborns have some form of hip dislocation requiring treatment.

Congenital hip dislocation is rarely obvious. It is painless to the infant and an affected joint may appear normal, since the musculoskeletal and nervous systems of all newborns are underdeveloped. To detect the condition as early as possible, physicians routinely examine newborns for hip dislocation. This procedure has dramatically reduced the need for surgery and the incidence of severe complications due to late diagnosis.

Approximately 70 percent of infants affected by congenital dislocation of the hip are girls. The left hip is affected about 60 percent of the time, the right hip about 20 percent and both around 20 percent. Approximately 20 percent of all congenital hip dislocations affect babies whose position in the uterus is abnormal and who are delivered in the breech position.

■ *Treatment*
Treatment of congenital hip dislocation varies with the age of the child at the time of diagnosis and with the nature of each case. As soon as congenital hip dislocation is suspected or diagnosed, a child should see an orthopedist for treatment. An orthopedist classifies a hip as "dislocated" if the thighbone is totally out of the hip socket; as "dislocatable" if the thighbobne tends to slip in and out of the socket; or as "subluxated" if the thighbone is partly but incorrectly attached to the socket.

In most cases a congenitally dislocated or subluxated hip discovered before a child is 3 months old can be corrected by having an orthopedist gently stretch the leg and ease the thighbone into place in the hip socket.

The hip bone is then held in position using a special harness, brace, splint, or pillow. If a child's hip joint is extremely loose, a plaster cast called a spica, which encompasses the child's lower trunk and upper legs, is used to prevent the hip from slipping as it sets.

H

Hip dislocation

History
If the dislocation of the hip is backward (posterior) than the condition is caused by violence upon the head of the femur. If the dislocation is forward (anterior) the cause is then violent hyperabduction.

Pathology
Injury to capsular and surrounding tissues of the capsule of the acetabulum.

Muscles
Posterior dislocation: hip is held rigidly flexed. Adduction, inward rotation and flexion of the thigh.
Anterior dislocation: hip is immovable in abduction and external rotation; the knee is flexed.

Complications
Torn tendons and ligaments. Fracture of the neck of the femur.

Treatment
Symptomatic treatment for discomfort. Splinting, since the fracture is frequently a sequel. Preparation for reduction of the dislocation.

Strapping and support
Board or rigid splint. The limb is kept in slight elevation unless a fracture is imminent.

Differentiation
Reduction will be complete when flexion with extension and adduction of the thigh are possible.

Hip fracture

History
Fracture of the hip is usually found in elderly people.

Pathology
Fracture through the neck or through the trochanter or both.

Complications
Loss of function; deformity and shortening.

Hemorrhage
Hemorrhage but not in large amounts.

Color of area
Ecchymosis but it may be delayed.

Treatment
Traction; Smith-Peterson nail.

Transportation
Place in Thomas splint as improvised.

Legg-Calve-Perthes disease

This disease (named for three physicians who identified it) is a non-infectious temporary disturbance in the blood supply to the ball in the hip socket. When this condition occurs, blood stops flowing into the rounded upper end of the thighbone, called the femoral head. Growth of the femoral head can become disturbed, and then the bone becomes misshapen.

The disease afflicts children between 3 and 11 years old, more often those from 4 to 8. Approximately 85 percent of the children affected are boys. In the United States the incidence of the problem for all children is 1 case in 2,200 (for boys 1 in 750, for girls 1 in 3,700). For 9 out of 10 children only 1 hip is involved.

The disease takes 1 to 5 years to run its cycle, depending on the age at onset (more rapid cycles occur among younger children). This cycle includes a short acute onset, followed by a lengthy period in which the bone tissue can soften and collapse without its blood supply, and finally a phase in which the bone repairs, rebuilds, and becomes solid once again.

Symptoms in the acute phase can last anywhere from 1 week to several months. The thrid phase can take several years for the bone to regenerate and the acetabulum (socket) to modify, if necessary, to accommodate the new shape of the femoral head.

The severity of Legg-Calve-Perthes disease depends on the child's age, the stage in which the disease is diagnosed, the treatment used, and the extent of disturbance in growth of the hip as the bone rebuilds.

Involvemnent can range anywhere from just the front third of the femoral head, in which case healing usually occurs quickly and independently, to situations where the entire femoral head deforms, often resulting in a severely arthritic joint in middle age.

Complete healing is likely for children younger than 4 years old because the femoral head has more time to reshape before maturity. For most children, who receive proper treatment, prospects for complete recovery are excellent, but again, much depends on how far the disease has progressed when diagnosed and the extent of bone degeneration. The disease is never fatal.

Injuries

Young children and older people are prone to suffer injuries to the hip, particularly fractures and dislocations. The major facts of hip dislocation and hip fracture are summarized in the tables.

Osteoarthritis

Osteoarthritis of the hip is a common disorder of elderly people, leading in many cases to disability. Hip replacement is now a routine operation being performed in more than 15,000 cases a year. Osteoarthritis is a chronic disorder of cartilage and surrounding tissues that is characterized by pain, stiffness, and loss of function. Osteoarthritis, the most common joint disorder, affects most people to some degree by age 70. Before the age of 40, men develop osteoarthritis more often than do women, because of injury. From age 40 to 70, women develop the disorder more often than do men. After age 70, the disorder develops in both sexes equally. Ostoarthritis is classified as primary when the cause is not known (the majority of cases)). It is classified as secondary when the cause is another disease or condition, such as Paget's disease, an infection, deformity, injury, or overuse of a joint or a group of joints, such as foundry workers, coal miners, and bus drivers, are particularly at risk. Obesity may be a major factor in the development of osteoarthritis, particularly of the knee and hip and especially in women.

Symptoms

Usually symptoms develop gradually and affect only one or a few joints at first. Pain, usually made worse by activity that involve weight bearing (such as standing) is the first symptom. In some people, the joint may be stiff after sleep or some particular activity, but the stiffness usually subsides within 30 minutes of moving the joint.
Osteoarthritis may be stable for many years or may progress very rapidly, but most often it progrsses slowly after symptoms develop. Many people develop some degree of disability.

Treatment

Appropriate exercises - including stretching, strengthening, and postural exercises - help maintain healthy cartilage, increase a joint's range of motion, and strengthen surrounding muscles so that they can absorb shock better.
Physical therapy, often with heat therapy, can be helpful. Heat improves mucles function by reducing stiffness and muscle spasm. Cold may be applied to reduce pain. Drugs are used to supplement exercise and physical

therapy. Drugs, which may be used in combination or individually, do not directly alter the course of osteoarthritis, they are used to reduce symptoms, and thus allow more appropriate exercise.

■ *Hip replacement*
If partial or total hip replacement is needed, special metallic implants are used that have a polished spherical surface to match with the joint socket and a strong stem to fit within the central marrow canal of the thighbone.
Some prosthetic implants are secured to the bone with a rapid-setting plastic cement. Others have special porous or ceramic coatings into which the surrounding lining bone can grow and bond directly.
After joint replacement surery, the person usually begins walking with crutches or a walker immediately and switches to a cane in 6 weeks. However, artificial joints do not last forever. The person especially someone who is active or heavy, may need to undergo another operation 10 or 20 years later.
Joint replacement is often advantageous for older people, because the likelihood that additional surgery will be needed is very low. In addition, older people benefit greatly from being able to walk almost immediately after surgery.
Sometimes the who joint needs to be replaced. This procedure is performed rarely for fractures, but most commonly for osteoarthritis.

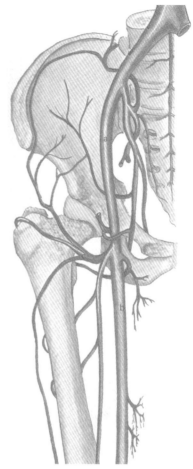

Hip dislocation
Front view of the hip joint between the head of the thighbone and the docket of the pelvis. The major arteries passing the hip joint are depicted.

How to live with osteoarthritis

▲ Exercise affected joints gently; in a pool, if possible.

▲ Massage at and around affected joints; this measure should preferably be performed by a trained therapist.

▲ Apply a heating pad or a damp and warm towel to affected joints.

▲ Maintain an appropriate weight; so as not to place extra stress on joints.

▲ Use special equipment as necessary; for example, cane, crutches, walker, neck collar.

▲ Wear well-supported shoes or athletic shoes.

HODGKIN DISEASE

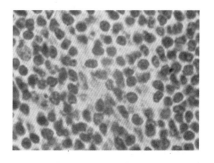

Description

A lymphoma is a growth of lymph cells involving the lymphatic system. It is one of the fastest rising cancers in the Western World, and no one knows precisely why. Lymphomas (the "oma" stands for tumor) affect the lymph system, which is a series of beady nodes spread throughout the body. The nodes are connected by tiny tubes much like veins in the separate circulatory system.

The lymph system plays a major role in the body's immune defenses against infection. A sore throat or boil often causes lymph nodes to swell in a local area. Doctors know little why lymphoma takes a more aggressive form in some people than in others, beyond the fact that sometimes it tends to become resistant to drugs

Types of lymphoma

Scientists have arbitrarily divided lymphomas into two types: Hodgkin's disease and a dozen other forms grouped as non-Hodgkin's lymphoma. Hodgkin's disease is named for Thomas Hodgkin, a 19th-century physician in London who distinguished the cancer from tuberculosis. Non-Hodgkin lymphoma appears in many types, and the prognosis varied tremendously according to the type. Many people live for decades hardly bothered by their lymphoma. Some may not need treatment for long peri-

Lymphomas

- ▲ Lymphomas are cancers of lymphocytes which reside in the lymphatic system and in blood-forming organs.
- ▲ Hodgkin's disease is a type of lymphoma distinguished by the presence of a particular kind of cancer cells called a Reed-Sternberg cell.
- ▲ Non-Hodgkin's lymphomas are a diverse group of cancers that develop in B or T lymphocytes.

ods. Yet many others die swiftly, even after responding to early therapy.

Non-Hodgkin's disease has been the third most rapidly rising cancer over the last 20 years, behind lung cancer in women (attributed to a surge in cigarette smoking several decades ago) and malignant melanomas in both sexes (attributed largely to sun exposure). More recently, a sharp rise in another kind of cancer, multiple myeloma, has challenged non-Hodgkin's lymphoma for third place.

Causes of lymphoma

Infectious agents have long been suspected to cause lymphomas. Speculation that lymphomas are a viral disease has been fueled by the identification of clustered cases of Hodgkin's disease that seemed to defy statistical chance. Yet extensive investigations have failed to turn un up a cause for the clusters. Nevertheless, the evidence suggesting that lymphomas are due to viruses is as strong as there is for any cancer. In recent years, HLTV-1, a member of the family of retroviruses that includes HIV

Characteristics of cells in Hodgkin disease.
Left: Microscopic picture of typical Hodgkin cells (Reed-Sternberg cells) in a lymph node.
Right: In comparison the blood smear of a patient with leukemia.
To make the diagnosis, a doctor must perform a biopsy of an affected lymph node to see if it is abnormal and if Reed-Sternberg cells are present. Reed-Sternberg cells are large cancerous cells that have more than one nucleus. Their distinctive appearance can be seen when a biopsy of lymph node tissue is examined under a microscope.

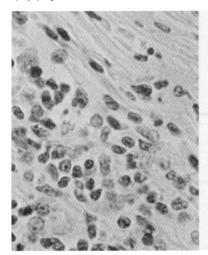
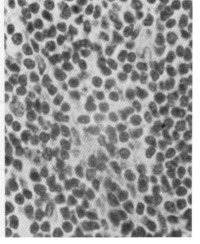

has been linked in Japan to one rare case of lymphoma. But even the discovery of viruses as causes of lymphoma may not explain how they are transmitted and why they have increased in number. Like many infectious diseases, the incidence of certain cancers goes through cycles, and the reasons are poorly understood.

An answer may come from further research into a recently identified link between a bacterium, Helicobacter pylori, and stomach cancer. Improved sanitation may have reduced the incidence of Helicobacter pylori, leading to a decline in stomach cancer. Additional research has linked Helicobacter pylori and a rare type of lymphoma of the stomach, which doctors recently begun treating with antibiotic therapy. Although the cancer has disappeared after antibiotic therapy, not enough time has passed to determine whether antibiotics will cure the cancer. Nevertheless, the initial favorable reports have intensified the search for microorganisms as the cause of lymphoma.

Possible causative factors

Since the incidence of lymphoma in this country is rising there is much debate why this should be. But three factors can explain part of the overall rise.
- One is HIV, the virus that causes AIDS, which somehow increases the risk of lymphoma.
- A second is the growing umber of people with transplanted organs, who are at increased risk for developing lymphoma because of the immunosuppressant drugs used to prevent rejection of donated organs.
- A third is improved diagnostic techniques.

Yet even in combination, the three can account at most for one-third of the rise in non-Hodgkin lymphoma. Among the reasons is that the rise has been greatest among people 60 years and older, a group least affected by AIDS and less likely to undergo organ transplant surgery.

One puzzle is why at least 3.5 per cent of AIDS patients develop lymphomas, often aggressive non-Hodgkin's tumors. Researchers of the US National Cancer Institute have estimated that at least 3,000 of the non-Hodgkin's lymphomas each year are associated with AIDS. The number of likely to increase as newer therapies extend the lives of AIDS patients. For unknown reasons, many HIV-associated AIDS cases tend to first develop in the intestines, spleen and brain rather than the lymph nodes.

Types of Hodgkin's disease

Lymphocyte pre-dominance

Microscopic appearance
- very few Reed-Sternberg cells
- many lymphocytes

Incidence
3 per cent of cases

Progression
Slow

Mixed cellularity

Microscopic appearance
- moderate number of Reed-Sternberg cells
- mixture opf otjher types of white blood cells

Incidence
25 per cent of cases

Progression
Somewhat rapid

Nodular sclerosis

Microscopic appearance
- small number of few Reed-Sternberg cells
- a mixture opf other types of whuite blood cells
- areas of fibrous connective tissue

Incidence
67 per cent of cases

Progression
Moderate

Lymphocyte depletione

Microscopic appearance
- numerous Reed-Sternberg cells
- few lymphocytes
- extensive strands of fibrous connective tissue

Incidence
5 per cent of cases

Progression
Rapid

Stages of Hodgkin's disease

Stage I
Extent of spread
- Limited to one lymph node
Likelihood of cure
- More than 95 %

Stage II
Extent of spread
- Involves two or more lymph nodes
- On same side of diaphragm
- Either above or below it
Likelihood of cure
- 90 %

Stage III
Extent of spread
- Involves lymph nodes above and below diaphragm
Likelihood of cure
- 80 %

Stage IV
Extent of spread
- Involves lymph nodes
- and other parts of the body
- such as bone marrow, lungs
Likelihood of cure
- 60 to 70 %

HYPERTENSION

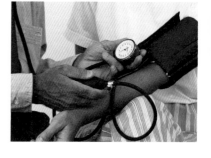

Description

Blood pressure is the pressure that the heart and arteries apply in order to squeeze the blood around the body. In a normal person, when sitting or lying quietly, the blood pressure stays at a steady, or resting level.

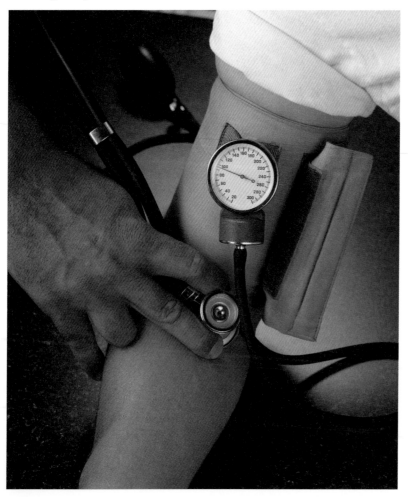

Measuring blood pressure.

In moments of exercise, excitement, anger or anxiety, the level of blood pressure is raised to increase the blood flow to the brain and muscles. When the moment has passed, the blood pressure drops again to its steady level. The sudden rise in blood pressure is brought about by the release of stress hormones such as adrenaline.

Hypertension, or high blood pressure, means that the resting blood pressure is higher than normal. Very few young people have high blood pressure, but after the age of 35 it becomes much more common, mainly because of the way we live our lives.

It is estimated that approximately one in ten people in the western world are hypertensive. This means that, when they have their blood pressure measured with a sphygmomanometer (the familiar cuff-type device), the pressure (measured in millimetres of mercury) is more than 160 mm at the highest (systolic) pressure during the heartbeat, and more than 95 mm at the lowest (diastolic) pressure. This is usually expressed as 160/95, and should be compared to a normal blood pressure level of about 120/70. About 25 per cent of these people do not know they are hypertensive, as hypertension often does not produce symptoms. Prevalence of the condition increases with age: nearly 25 per cent of people over the age of 65 are hypertensive.

■ *Primary and secondary hypertension*
Accounting for 90 per cent of all cases, primary or essential hypertension is not linked to a single cause, and may be only a slight deviation from the average. Heredity predisposes a person to hypertension, and can influence blood pressure to various extents. Most people with primary hypertension show heightened reactions of the blood vessels and heart to stress.

Secondary hypertension is associated with disorders of the kidneys or adrenal glands. It may also be associated with disorders of the thyroid gland, coarctation of the aorta (a congenital disorder in which the aorta is narrowed) or the use of oral contraceptive pills.

Causes

In primary hypertension, the basic cause is unknown. There are, however, a number of factors that are known to raise blood pressure in some people such as:
- being overweight;
- smoking;
- drinking too much alcohol;
- lack of regular exercise;
- eating too much salt;
- too much stress.

The trouble is that you may not even realize that your blood pressure is too high. By itself, high blood pressure does not feel any different, but it makes the heart work harder and speeds up the "furring up" of the arteries - atherosclerosis.

So people whose resting blood pressure is too high are more likely to suffer from angina or heart attack. They may be also in danger of having a stroke, when the blood supply to part of the brain is cut off by a blood clot or hemorrhage.

■ Stress

Most people would put stress at the top of their list of things that are bad for the heart. It seems obvious that worry and anxiety, or frequent crises and rows, can make your blood pressure go up and lead to a heart attack, but this is still difficult to prove, partly because stress is almost impossible to measure and define.

However, people who have a certain kind of personality - that is, those who are striving, ambitious, competitive, impatient and always pressed for time - seem to be more in danger of having a heart attack than more relaxed, easygoing types.

These high achievers have been called Type A personalities, and their relaxed counterparts are Type B. It seems that people who are more Type A are likely to have higher blood pressure and blood cholesterol levels than the calmer Type Bs. Type As also have more stress hormone circulating in the bloodstream, and this can lead, through high blood pressure and high blood cholesterol, to an increased risk

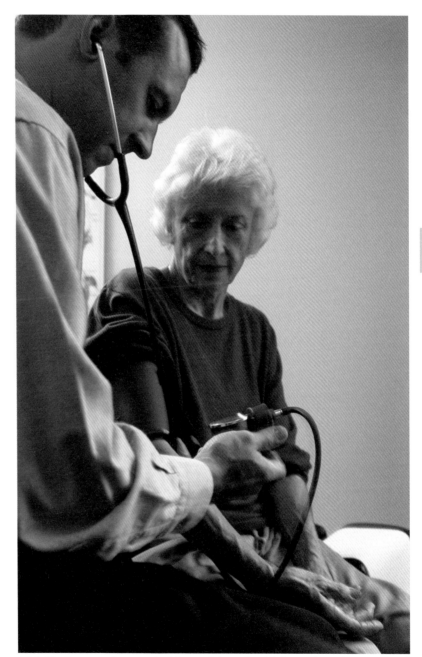

High blood pressure (hypertension) is one of the major risk factors for angina pectoris and myocardial infarction.

Several instruments can measure blood pressure quickly and with little discomfort. A sphyngomanometer is commonly used. It consists of a soft rubber cuff connected to a rubber bulb that is used to inflate the cuff and a meter that registers the pressure of the cuff.

A person sits with an arm bared (sleeves rolled up), bent and resting on a table, so that the arm is about the same level as the heart. The cuff is wrapped around the arm. Listening with a stethoscope placed over the artery below the cuff, a heath care practitioner inflates the cuff by squeezing the bulb until the cuff compresses the artery tightly enough to temporarily stop blood flow. Then the cuff is gradually deflated. The pressure at which the practitioner first hears a pulse in the artery is the systolic pressure. The cuff continues to be deflated, and at some point, the sound of blood flow stops. The pressure at this point is the diastolic pressure.

Hypertension   Questions & Answers

While there is usually no known cause for essential hypertension, it turns out that certain factors make some individuals more likely to develop it. These factors do not necessarily cause high blood pressure. But statistically, your chances of getting it are greater when one or more of the following factors apply to you.

Family history

High blood pressure tends to run in families. More than half the people with high blood pressure have other family members with it. This suggests that genetic factors may play a role.

Age

People of any age can get high blood pressure, but it is more common in older age groups. It affects close to half the population above the age of 64. Hypertension is usually first diagnosed between the ages of 35 and 50. However, some evidence suggests that the tendency may be present much earlier, perhaps in the first year or two of life.

Sex

Under the age of 50, high blood pressure is more common in men than in women. The rate becomes equal at about age 50, and by age 55 to 60, more women have it than men. Deaths resulting from its complications, however, occur twice as often among men.

Race

For both children and adults, blacks are twice as likely to have hypertension as whites. Furthermnore, blacks tend to develop it at younger ages and have higher blood pressure levels. Hypertension is the leading cause of death among blacks. For example, 100 times as many blacks die from its complications as they do from sickle-cell anemia, the well-publicized genetic disease.

Weight

High blood pressure is much more common in people who are overweight that in those whose weight is normal. Close to 40 per cent of all overweight people have hypertension. Weight loss tends to lower blood pressure.

Salt

Salt plays a part in the body's regulation of blood pressure, but the exact relationship between salt in the diet and hypertension is not clear. Apparently, those people who have a tendency to develop high blood pressure are more likely to get it if they eat foods with a great deal of salt. Meanwhile, others who do not have this underlying tendency may be able to eat salty foods without affecting their blood pressure. Again, genetic factors may be involved.

Stress

People with a particular type of personality (Type A) tend to have a higher risk for hypertension.

of heart disease.

It has also been suggested that some one who is normally calm but is frequently forced into stressful situations might eventually suffer the same effects as a person who is a born Type A. A certain amount of stress is an essential part of ordinary everyday life: it helps keep you on your toes and out of danger. Every time you cross a busy road or have an argument or watch an exciting program on television your stress level goes up for a while.

However, if anxiety or pressure of work continue for many months or years, your heart may suffer. This kind of chronic stress can be difficult to recognize and sometimes impossible to avoid. Family problems, money worries, difficulties at work may not be easy to solve.

However, you can help yourself by learning how to relax and trying to take things easy. When you have some free time, try to take up an activity, hobby or interest that helps keep your mind off your worries. It is difficult to worry about your problems when you are totally absorbed in doing some gardening, reading a book or watching a football of baseball match.

Symptoms and signs

Primary hypertension has no symptoms until complications develop. Symptoms and signs are non-specific and arise from complications in target organs. The following symptoms and signs can develop in hypertension:
- dizziness;
- flushed face;
- headache;
- fatigue;
- nose bleeding;
- nervousness.

Complications of high blood pressure include:
- heart failure;
- hemorrhage in the retina at the back of the eye;
- exudates (where constituents of the blood pass through a vessel wall and into tissue);
- swelling of the retina where the optic nerve emerges;
- bleeding in the brain;
- failure of the kidneys.

When doctors suspect that a person has mild or moderate hypertension (systolic pressure: 140-180; diastolic pressure: 90-115), they will conduct the following investigations:
- medical history;
- physical examination;
- complete blood count;
- routine analysis of the urine;
- chemical analysis of the blood.

Diagnosis and prognosis

The diagnosis of primary hypertension depends on demonstrating that the systolic and diastolic blood pressure are usually, but necessarily always, higher than normal, and on excluding secondary causes. The doctor should make at least two blood pressure determinations on three separate days before labelling a person hypertensive.

For those in the low hypertension range and especially for those with markedly unstable blood pressure, more than this minimum number of determinations are desirable. The upper limit of normal blood pressure in adults is 140/90; it is much lower for infants and children.

A somewhat higher limit, especially for systolic pressure, is acceptable (though probably not normal) for those over the age of 60. Sporadic high levels in those who have been resting for less than five minutes suggest an unusual instability for blood pressure that may precede sustained hypertension.

An untreated hypertensive person is at great risk of developing disability or fatal heart failure, heart attack, cerebral bleeding or kidney failure at an early stage. Hypertension is the most important risk factor predisposing a person to blood vessel disorders in the heart and brain. In addition, the higher the blood pressure, the more severe the changes in the retina, and the worse the prognosis.

Treatment

There is no cure for primary hypertension, but appropriate therapy can modify its course. Sedation, extra rest, prolonged holidays, admonitions not to worry and half-hearted attempts at weight reduction and restricting salt in the diet are poor substitutes for effective treatment with medicines.

Those with uncomplicated hypertension should live normal lives as long as they keep their blood pressure controlled with medication. Dietary restrictions should be imposed to control diabetes, obesity or abnormalities in the lipid content (e.g., cholesterol) of the blood. In mild hypertension, weight reduction to ideal levels and modest restriction of salt in the diet may make drug therapy unnecessary.

Foods to eat and to avoid

To eat
These foods are good for you. They have the perfect combination: high in potassium and low in salt:

Fruits
- apples
- apricots
- avocados
- bananas
- cantaloupes
- dates
- nectarines
- melons (casaba or honeydew)
- prunes
- raisins
- watermelon
- peaches

Vegetables
- asparagus
- beans (white, green, snap)
- brussels sprouts
- cabbage
- cauliflower
- mushrooms
- green peppers
- potatoes
- radishes
- squash
- tomatoes

Fruit juices
- apple
- grapefruit
- prune
- orange

Unsalted nuts
- peanuts
- pecan halves

Not to eat
Try to avoid these foods; they all have a great deal of salt or sodium.
- buttermilk
- cheese (except unsalted cottage or pot)
- dried, salted, smoked or canned meats
- canned tuna, or salmon
- mayonnaise
- sauces (soy, Worcestershire, ketchup)
- bottle dressings
- pretzels
- potato chips
- packed snack foods
- instant potatoes
- commercially prepared desserts
- frozen dinners

Any activity that gives you some exercise is especially good for your heart. Exercise helps to relieve tensions that have been building up inside you and your body gets a chance to let off steam. All kinds of exercise - from the gently stretching postures of yoga to the vigorous leaps and bounds of badminton - will help you to combat stress.

Exercise not only helps to reduce stress, but there is also good evidence to show that regular vigorous exercise can have a protective effect on the heart.

The heart will benefit most from the kind of exercise that builds up stamina. Stamina means staying power or the ability to keep going without gasping for breath. It depends on the efficiency of your muscles and circulation, and the most important "muscle" of all is exercise.

To build up your stamina you need to choose a form of exercise that gives your body plenty of movement, and is just energetic enough to make you fairly breathless (but not gasping for breath). This is called dynamic exercise.

The vigorous exercise of moving your muscles rhythmically creates a greater demand of oxygen in the blood, and more work for the heart and lungs.

Regular exercise of this kind improves the balance of fatty substances in the bloodstream, lowers resting blood pressure and strengthens the heart muscle.

At the simplest level, brisk walking is an excellent stamina-building exercise, but you could also try running up stairs, jogging, skipping, disco-dancing, cycling and swimming.

H

Drugs used to hypertension (high blood pressure)

Drugs that are used in the treatment of high blood pressure are called antihypertensives. With a wide variety of antihypertensives available, high blood pressure can be controlled in almost anyone, but treatment has to be tailored to the individual. Treatment is not effective when patient and doctor communicate well and collaborate on the treatment program.

Diuretics
Diuretics cause blood vessels to dilate. Diuretics also help the kidneys eliminate salt and water, decreasing fluid volume throughout the body and thus lowering blood pressure.

■ Loop diuretics
These diuretics help the kidneys eliminate salt and water, thus decreasing the volume of fluid in the bloodstream.
■ Selected side effects
Decreased levels of potassium and magnesium, temporarily increased levels of blood sugar and cholesterol, an increased level of uric acid, sexual dysfunction in men, and digestive upset.
■ Examples
• Bumetanide
• Ethacrynic acid
• Furosemide
• Torsemide

■ Potassium-sparing diuretics
Because these diuretics prevent potassium loss, they may be given in addition to thiazide or loop diuretics, which cause potassium to be lost. Spironolactone is particularly useful in the treatment of hypertension and severe heart failure.
■ Selected side effects
With all, a high potassium level and digestive upset. With spironolactone, breast enlargement in men and menstrual irregularities in women.
■ Examples
• Amiloride
• Spironolactone
• Triamterene
■ Thiazide and thiazide-like diuretics
The effects of these diuretics are similar to but milder than those of loop diuret-

ics. The two types of diuretics are particularly effective when used together.
■ Selected side effects
Decreased levels of potassium and magnesium, increased levels of calcium and uric acid, sexual dysfunction in men, and digestive upset.
■ Examples
• Chlortalidone
• Hydrochlorothiazide
• Indapamide
• Metolazone

Adrenergic blockers
These drugs block the effects of the sympathetic division, the part of the nervous system that can rapidly respond to stress by increasing blood pressure.

■ Alpha-blockers
These drugs block the alpha-receptors of the sympathetic nerves.
■ Selected side effects
Fainting (syncope) with the first dose, awareness of rapid heartbeats, dizziness, low blood pressure when the person stands, and fluid retention.
■ Examples
• Doxazosin
• Prazosin
• Terazosin

■ Beta-blockers
These drugs block the beta-receptors of the sympathetic nerves.
■ Selected side effects
Spasms of airways, an abnormally slow heart rate, heart failure, possible masking of low blood sugar levels after insulin injections, impaired peripheral circulation, insomnia, fatigue, shortness of breath, depression, vivid dreams, hallucinations, and sexual dysfunction.
■ Examples
• Acebutolol
• Atenolol
• Betaxolol
• Carteolol
• Metoprolol
• Nardolol
• Penbutolol
• Pimdolol

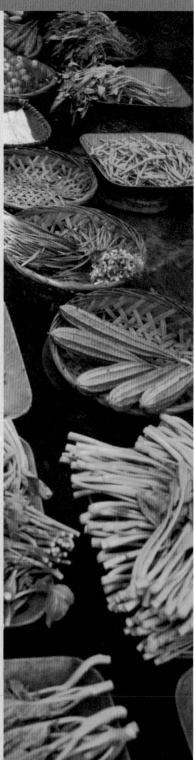

Drugs used to hypertension (high blood pressure)

■ Alpha-beta-blockers
These drugs block both alpha- and beta-receptors of the sympathetic nerves.
■ *Selected side effects*
Low blood pressure when the person stands and spasm of the airways.
■ *Examples*
• Carvedilol
• Labetalol

■ Peripherally acting adrenergic blockers
These drugs block the adrenergic receptors of the peripheral part of the sympathetic nervous system.
■ *Selected side effects*
With guanadrel and guanethidine, diarrhea, sexual dysfunction, low blood pressure when the person stands, and fluid retention
■ *Examples*
• Guanadrel
• Guanethidine
• Reserpine

Centrally acting alpha-antagonists
These drugs lower blood pressure through a mechanism that somewhat resembles that of adrenergic blockers. By stimulating certain receptors in the brain stem, these agonists inhibit the effects of the sympathetic division of the nervous system.
■ *Selected side effects*
Drowsiness, dry mouth, fatigue, an abnormal slow heart rate, rebound high blood pressure when the drug is withdrawn, sexual dysfunction.
■ *Examples*
• Clonidine
• Guanabenz
• Guanfacine
• Methyldopa

Angiotensin-converting enzyme (ACE) inhibitors
ACE inhibitors cause blood vessels to widen (dilate), thus decreasing the amount of work the heart has to do; they also may have direct beneficial effects on the heart.

■ *Selected side effects*
Cough, low blood pressure, an increased potassium level, rash, angioedema, and, in pregnant women, serious injury to the fetus
■ *Examples*
• Benazepril
• Captopril
• Enalapril
• Fosinopril
• Lisinopril
• Moexipril
• Perindopril
• Quinapril
• Ramipril
• Trandolapril

Angiotensin II blockers
These drugs directly block the action of angiotensin II, which causes arterioles to constrict. Because the mechanism is more direct, angiotensin II blockers may cause fewer side effects.
■ *Selected side effects*
Dizziness, an increased potassium level, angioedema, and, in pregnant women, serious injury to the fetus
■ *Examples*
• Candesartan
• Eprosartan
• Losartan
• Telmisartan
• Valsartan

Calcium channel blockers
Calcium channel blockers cause arterioles to dilate. They are particularly useful for older people and people who have angina pectoris.
■ *Selected side effects*
Dizziness, fluid retention in the ankles, flushing headache, heartburn, enlarged gums, and an abnormally fast heart rate
■ *Examples*
• Amlodipine
• Felodipine
• Isradipine
• Nicardipine
• Nifedipine
• Nisoldipine
• Diltiazem
• Verapamil

Direct vasodilators
Vasodilators cause blood vessels to widen (dilate). These vasodilators are usually given to people who cannot take an ACE inhibitor or angiotensin II receptor blocker.
■ *Selected side effects*
Headache, an abnormally fast heart rate, and fluid retention
■ *Examples*
• Hydralazine
• Minoxidil

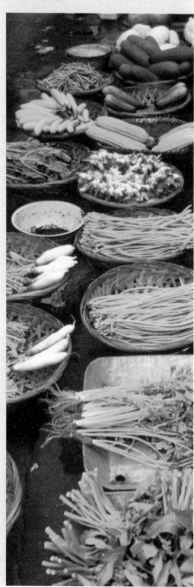

INFECTIOUS DISEASES

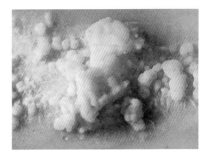

Description

Invasion and multiplication of microorganisms in body tissues, especially that causing local cellular injury due to competitive metabolism, toxins, intracellular replication, or antigen-antibody response. Most infectious diseases are caused by microorganisms that invade the body and multiply. Most bacteria and fungi are susceptible to antibiotics and antifungal agents, but most viral infections cannot be treated, although many can be prevented by vaccination, such as: chickenpox;, measles;, some types of hepatitis;, influenza, poliomyelitis. Some infectious disease have their reproduction slowed by antiviral medication (e.g. AIDS and a very small number may have their reproduction completely blocked by antiviral agents (e.g. herpes, influenza). Untreated infections may form abscesses or spread through the bloodstream to other organs or to the whole body (causing sepsis).

Electron microscopic view of a tetanus bacillus.

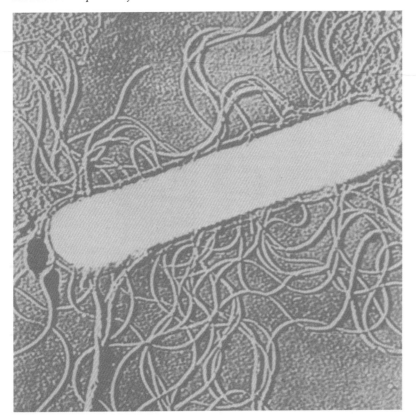

Commensal organisms

With many of the microorganisms that beset him man has with time come to terms. All of the outer surfaces of his body are covered with microorganisms that normally do him no harm and may in fact be useful to him.

Such organisms are called commensal. Those of the skin may help to break down dying skin cells or to use up debris secreted by the many minute glands and pores that open on the skin.

Many of the organisms in his intestinal tract break complex waste products into simple substances, and others help in the manufacture or synthesis of chemical compounds such as some of the vitamins that are essential to human life.

It should be understood in this connection that the gastrointestinal tract is one of the "outer" surfaces of the body. From its upper part, the stomach, duodenum and small intestine, food is absorbed into the body, and into its lower part, the large intestine or bowel, waste products are excreted from the inside of the body.

The mouth, the nose, and the sinuses, or spaces inside the bones of the face are in direct contact with the outside environment. These structures are heavily populated with microorganisms.

Some of these are true commensals; they live on man, deriving their sustenance from the surface cells of his body without doing him any harm. Others are disease germs, or indistinguishable from them; they live, like the true commensals, in the nose and throat of a human being and, in spite of their disease potential, may never occasion him inconvenience.

They are capable, however, when the

environment alters, of causing severe illness in their host, or, though not harming their host, they may, on spreading to another person, infect the second person with a serious disease. In this case the first host is the carrier of the microorganism, the second a victim of the microorganismal disease.

The microorganismal environment can be changed radically and obviously. If antibodies are given to a person, the commensal organisms in his body can be killed, and other organisms, less innocuous, may take their place.

In the mouth and throat, penicillin may eradicate pneumococci, streptococci, and other microorganisms that are sensitive to the drug, and microorganisms such as *Candida albicans*, insensitive to penicillin, may then proliferate in the absence of normal competitors and cause thrush, an inflammatory condition of the mouth and throat.

In the intestinal canal, an antibiotic may easily kill most of the microorganisms normally there and allow dangerous organisms, such as *Pseudomonas pyocyanea*, to multiply and perhaps invade the bloodstream and the tissues of the body.

If an infectious agent - for example a salmonella or food-poisoning germ - reaches the intestinal canal, the giving of an antibiotic may have an effect very different from what could be expected on theory; instead of attacking and destroying the salmonella, it kills the normal inhabitants of the bowel and allows the salmonella to flourish and persist. The balance between man and his normal commensal environment is delicate.

Organisms of disease

When a pathogenic microorganism assails the body for the first time, clinically the response of the body may vary from, nothing at all through various degrees of nonspecific reactions to a response recognized as a specific infectious disease.

Immunologically there is always a response, the purpose of which is defense, This defense may occur in three different ways:

▲ be completely successful, and in

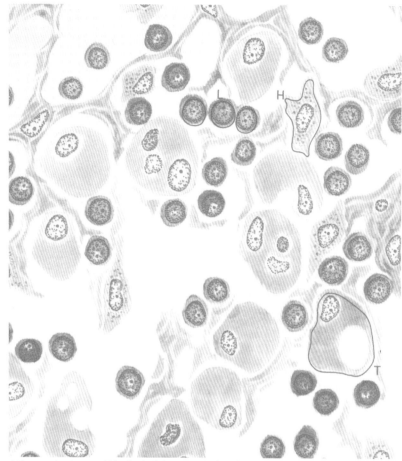

Microscopic picture of histological changes in a lymph node in the course of an infection by Salmonella (paratyphoid).

this case there is no obvious bodily reaction;

▲ partially successful, when the affected person suffers but recovers from an infectious disease;

▲ unsuccessful, when in spite of specific immune reactions, the patient is overwhelmed by the intensity of the infectious process and dies.

The types of infectious organisms pathogenic to men may be divided into four groups:

■ *Bacteria*
Bacteria are microscopic, single-celled organisms. Examples: *Streptococcus pyogenes* (strep throat); *Escherichia coli* (urinary tract infection).

■ *Viruses*
A virus is a small infectious organisms

- much smaller than a fungus or a bacterium - that cannot reproduce on its own; it must invade a living cell and use that cell's machinery to reproduce. Examples, HIV, varicella, herpes.

■ *Fungi*
Fungi are actually a type of plant. Yeasts, molds, and mushrooms are all types of fungi. Examples: *Candida albicans* (vaginal yeast infection); *Tinea pedis* (athlete's foot).

■ *Parasites*
A parasite is an organism, such as a worm or single-celled animal (protozoan) that survives by living inside another, usually much larger, organism (the host). Examples: *Enterobius vermicularis* (pinworm); *Plasmodium vivax* (malaria).

The world's deadliest infectious diseases

Australian bat lyssavirus

In November 1996, a women from Queensland who had recently become a bat handler became ill with numbness and weakness in her left arm, progressing to coma and death in three weeks. She was the first to die from the condition which affects the entire bat population of Australia. Another person died two years later. There us no treatment.

Bird flu

In May 1997 the world's flu experts feared the beginning of another pandemic on a scale of that seen in 1918 with Spanish Flu. In Hong Kong people caught chicken flu. Normally the flu virus mutates as it passes from birds to pigs, and then to human beings. But this strain had jumped the species barrier, causing a new strain in which humans have no natural resistance. Eighteen people contracted it, sex died (1997). In 2004 there was again an outbreak of chicken flu, an unknown number of people contracted it, 18 died.

Campylobacter jejuni

This is the leading cause of bacterial diarrhea in developed countries. It was identified in 1977. Although anyone can have a Campylobacter jejuni infection, children under five and young adults are most at risk. Raw chicken and raw milk are sources of infection.

Creutzfeldt-Jakob disease

This disease was first discovered in the 1920s as a rare condition affecting the elderly. But in 1996 a previously unrecognised disease pattern was identified, with the average age of victims 29. It was strongly linked to exposure, probably through food, to a similar disease in cattle called bovine spongiform encephalopathy (BSE). The disease is caused by a prion. So far some 120 people have contracted the new disease. It is fatal and there is no cure.

Cryptosporidium parvum

A bacterial cause of diarrhea, probably affecting one in 50 people in the UK.

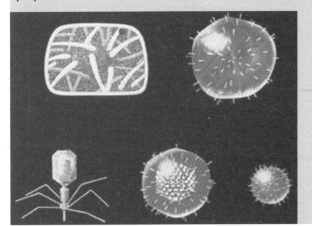

Ebola

Ebola hemorrhagic fever is a severe, often-fatal disease in human beings and monkeys that has appeared sporadically since its recognition in 1976. The ebola virus is named after a river in Congo. It is highly infectious through contact with bodily fluids, causing high fever and vomiting. Most victims die through internal collapse within one week of becoming infected. There is no cure.

Guanarito virus

In September 1989, doctors in Venezuela became aware of an outbreak of a severe feverish illness among young adults in the countryside. More than 100 cases have been confirmed, and a third have died. It is probably spread by rats.

Hantavirus pulmonary syndrome

This disease was first recognised in 1993 after the investigation of an outbreak of sudden fatal respiratory illness in the south-western United States. Since then, some 100 cases of the disease have been recognised in 20 states, mostly in the western part of the US. The disease is caught from rodents, especially deer mouse. The major symptoms are: fever, muscle aches, shortness of breath, lungoedema. Death may occur from suffocation.

Hendra virus

This virus is very similar to the Nipah virus, carried by the fruit bat, but it is prevalent in Australia. So far there have been three outbreaks in Australia, and three human cases, all acquiring it through close contact with horses. Two of them died.

Hepatitis C

A viral infection of the liver which is a major cause of liver cancer, jaundice and death through blood poisoning. In 1989, it is spread by direct contact with human blood, such as through sex or blood transfusion. Globally, an estimated 170 million persons are chronically infected and up to four million people are infected each year. No vaccine is available to prevent hepatitis C.

Hepatitis E

Discovered in 1988 it is similar to hepatitis C, except that it can be transferred through food and is less likely to be fatal.

HIV/AIDS

In 1983 HIV was discovered to be responsible for acquired immune deficiency syndrome, a disease first identified among homosexual men in America. Sine then the spread of the disease has become more virulent among heterosexual people, especially in Africa and Asia. A combitherapy of antiviral drugs slows the progress of the disease.

The world's deadliest infectious diseases

Kaposi sarcoma virus

In 1997 doctors noticed purplish-black lesions on the skin or internal organs of AIDS patients. It was a new and rare form of skin cancer, which is actually caused by a variant of the herpes virus, and in those with damaged immune system it can spread to the lymph nodes and lungs, with fatal consequences.

Legionnaires' disease

Legionnaires' disease acquired its name in 1976 when an outbreak of pneumonia occurred among people attending a convention of the American Legion in Philadelphia. Hundreds of people get it every year in the UK, mostly the elderly; between five and 30 per cent of them die. It is normally spread through air-conditioning systems. It can be treated if caught early.

Lyme disease

Named in 1977 when arthritis was observed in children around Lyme, Connecticut. It is caused by the bacteria Borrelia burgdorferi transmitted by ticks. It is rarely fatal but if the initial rash is left untreated it can be disabling through joint disease and chronic fatigue.

Nipa virus

This virus was discovered in Nipah, Malaysia, in 1999. Although it has so fare caused only a few outbreaks, its ability to switch between animals and human beings and its high death rate makes it one of the newest and greatest fears for public-health experts.

Rota virus

This is endemic worldwide, accounting for half of all cases of hospital admissions for diarrhea in children. Discovered in 1973, it is caused by preparing food with unwashed hands, often at home. About one million children die of it every year.

Sabia virus

This new form of virus was first identified in South America. Only two cases have been reported; one died after bleeding from internal organs, the other survived after a horrific illness. The virus is little understood.

SARS

Abbreviation of Severe Acute Respiratory Syndrome, a new viral infection that attacks the lungs of humans. It is probably a mutated coronavirus, that has been transferred form animals to humans by close contact between them, and the virus has mutated during the transfer. First identified in southern China, Hang Kong and northern Vietnam in early 2003, it has spread rapidly with infected air travellers. Some 5000 people contracted the disease in 2003, 840 died. In 2004 some 20 cases have been reported.

Vibrio cholera 0130

This is the bacteria responsible for Asiatic cholera, first isolated in 1991 in Peru. Outbreaks spread quickly in polluted water to reach epidemic proportions: 1,099,882 cases and 10,453 deaths were reported in the western hemisphere between January 1991 and July 1995. Death is caused by dehydration. Antibiotics can help to shorten the illness.

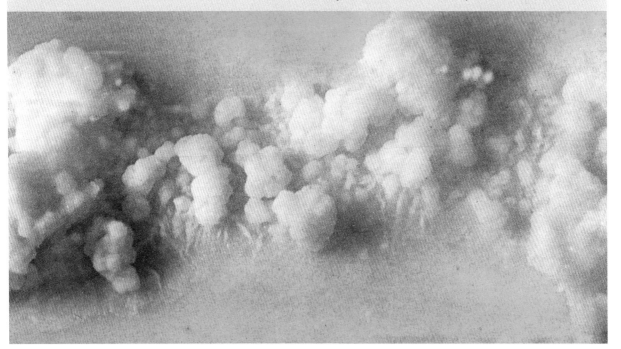

INFLAMMATORY BOWEL DISEASES

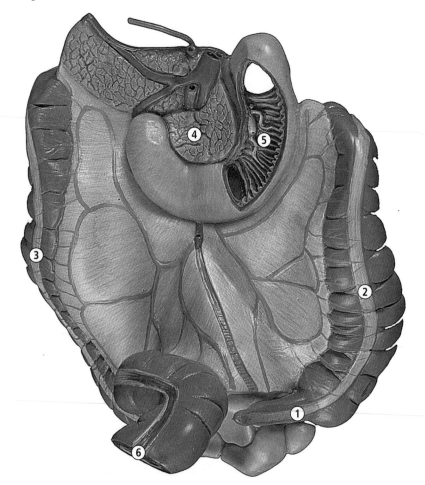

Introduction

Disorders of the intestines are fairly common. Almost everyone has had some degree of difficulty in this area at one time or another. These disorders can be functional, because of the extensive nerve connections in the digestive system; fear, anger, and other nervous upsets may set off attacks of nausea, cramps, or diarrhea.

Organic diseases such as colorectal cancer, Crohn's disease and ulcerative colitis can also affect these organs, as do contagious diseases, such as salmonellosis (eating food contaminated with Salmonella bacteria) and virus infections, as well as constipation, dyspepsia, allergies - and a list almost as long as the digestive tract itself.

Inflammatory disorders are now grouped together as inflammatory bowel diseases, in which the intestine (bowel) becomes inflamed, often causing recurring cramps and diarrhea

The two primary types of inflammatory bowel disease are Crohn's disease and ulcerative colitis. These two diseases have many similarities and sometimes are difficult to distinguish from each other.

However, there are several differences. For example, Crohn's disease can affect almost any part of the digestive tract, whereas ulcerative colitis almost always affects only the large intestine.

The cause of these diseases are not known. More recently recognized inflammatory bowel diseases include:
- collagenous colitis
- lymphocytic colitis
- diversion colitis

The chronic inflammatory diseases of the bowel comprise a spectrum of disorders with overlapping signs and symptoms, but without a definite cause. The two representative diseases of this group - regional enteritis and ulcerative colitis - are characterized by chronic inflammation at various sites of the gastrointestinal system.

Crohn's disease

Crohn's disease or regional enteritis is a chronic inflammatory condition affecting the colon and/or terminal part of the small intestine (ileum) and produces symptoms of frequent episodes of diarrhea (the faeces are

Position and structure of the large intestine.
View from behind.
1. Ileocolic transition
2. Ascending colon
3. Descending colon
4. Liver
5. Stomach
6. Sigmoid and rectum

non-bloody and semisoft), abdominal symptoms and general disorders.

The cause is still unknown, although extensive research has been performed on immunological factors, infectious agents, and dietary factors. Regional enteritis has been reported with increasing frequency in Europe and the United States. The disease occurs about equally in both sexes, and shows a familial tendency that frequently overlaps with the occurrence of ulcerative colitis (see below). Most cases begin before age 40, with the peak incidence in the 20s. It involves the small bowel only in thirty per cent of patients; the colon only in fifteen per cent and both the colon and small bowel in fifty-five per cent. The term regional denotes that some parts of the colon are severely affected, while other parts are normal. The affected parts show multiple ulcerations, involving all layers of the intestinal wall.

Symptoms and signs

The disease is characterized by the following symptoms and signs:

Common patterns of Crohn's disease

Symptoms differ among people with Crohn's disease, but there are four common patterns:

▲ Inflammation with pain and tenderness in the right lower part of the abdomen.

▲ Recurring acute intestinal obstructions that cause severe painful spasms of the intestinal wall, swelling of the abdomen, constipation, and vomiting.

▲ Inflammation and chronic partial intestinal obstruction causing malnutrition and chronic debility.

▲ Abnormal channels and pus-filled pockets of infection (abscesses) that often cause fever, painful masses in the abdomen, and severe weight loss.

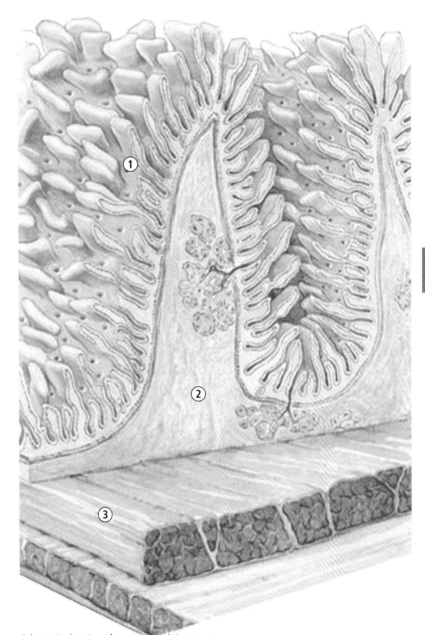

Schematic drawing of a segment of the intestine.
1. Mucous membrane
2. Submucosa with blood vessels and lymph nodes
3. Circular and longitudinal muscle layer

- chronic diarrhea
- pain in the abdomen
- fever
- anorexia
- weight loss

The disease shows a number of peculiarities: the disorders of the intestine other organs may be affected such as joints, part of the eye, inner lining of the mouth, skin, kidneys.

Treatment

No specific therapy is known. Some medicines may relieve cramps and

Inflammatory diseases Questions & Answers

What are ileitis and colitis for types of diseases?
Ileitis and colitis are inflammatory diseases of the intestines. In colitis, all or part of the large intestine or colon is involved.
In ileitis, the small intestine is affected, most commonly the lower part. Collectively, ileitis and colitis may be referred to as inflammatory bowel disease (IBD).
This term includes ulcerative colitis, ulcerative proctitis and the various distributions of Crohn's disease, encompassing enteritis and granulomatous colitis but excluding the irritable colon syndrome.

Is inflammatory bowel disease limited to the intestines?
Not always. Crohn's disease and ulcerative colitis, for example, are systemic diseases. In addition to an inflamed colon, patients may have the following conditions:
• skin lesions
• liver disorders
• arthritis
• eye inflammation

What are the symptoms of inflammatory bowel disease?
The gastrointestinal system has a comparatively small "vocabulary," so symptoms may be similar for any disorder affecting it, even though the underlying problem may be different.
Irritable colon (also called spastic colon or mucous colitis) usually causes abdominal cramps and pain, as well as abdominal distention, more frequent bowel movements, diarrhea and constipation or alternating bouts of the two. The typical symptoms of Crohn's disease also known as regional ileitis) are cramps, abdominal pain, diarrhea, and a generalized feeling of illness; weight loss and low fever also may occur and, occasionally bowel obstruction and bleeding.

What is the cause of inflammatory bowel disease?
The causes of these diseases remain unknown. There is some tendency of these diseases to occur in families, usually the relative develops the same disease, but sometimes the other.
There may be a genetic predisposition, which can be triggered by some environmental insult, such as an infection. Scientists now suspect that ileitis and colitis may be linked to body's immune system because normal defense mechanisms seem to be confused and attacking its own tissue in the intestines.

What is collagenous colitis?
Collagenous colitis is a chronic disease in which certain kinds of white blood cells infiltrate the lining of the large intestine, leading to watery diarrhea.
This disease can affect the entire length of the large intestine, including the sigmoid colon and the rectum but often in a patchy distribution.

What is diversion colitis?
Diversion colitis is inflammation that develops in a lower part of the large intestine after the passage of stool above this part has been surgically diverted. Most people do not require treatment because the symptoms remain mild.

diarrhea. Antibiotic medicines are given in case of bacterial complications. Corticosteroids are useful in acute stages of the disease. They may dramatically reduce fever and diarrhea, relieve abdominal pain and tenderness, and improve appetite and sense of well-being.
Striking responses have been reported with the use of some new immuno-suppressive medicines, but their exact role in therapy is not established. Some patients have improved on elemental diets, at least over a short term, and some children have achieved increased rates of growth with one of the above-mentioned therapeutic measures.
Surgical procedures are usually necessary when recurrent obstruction of the intestine or abscesses are present. Several authorities are of the opinion, that surgery should not be performed unless specific complications or failure of medical therapy makes it necessary.
When operations have been required, however, most patients consider their quality of life to have been improved by surgery.

Lifestyle

Avoidance of raw fruits and vegetables to limit mechanical trauma to the inflamed mucosa of the colon may result in improvement of the symptoms. A milk-free diet may decrease symptoms in one-third of patients, but need not be continued if no benefit is noted.
Mild to moderate disease may respond to sulfasalazine or related compounds. Long-term therapy with this medicine may help to maintain remissions and reduce the frequency of elapses. In some cases the doctor will discuss with the patient operative procedures, particularly in cases of bleeding or threatening perforation.

Ulcerative colitis

Ulcerative colitis is a chronic disease in which the large intestine becomes inflamed and ulcerated (pitted or eroded), leading to flare-ups (bouts or attacks) of bloody diarrhea, abdominal cramps, and fever.
The disease may start at any age but

Drugs that reduce bowel inflammation

Aminosalicylates

These drugs are used to reduce the inflammation of ulcerative colitis and prevent flare-ups of symptoms. Abdominal pain, dizziness and fatigue are related to dose.

- *Selected side effects*
- Nausea
- Headache
- Dizziness
- Fatigue
- Hepatitis
- Pancreatitis
- *Examples*
- Balsalazide
- Mesalamine
- Olsalazine
- Sulfasalazine

Corticosteroids

These drugs may dramatically reduce fever and diarrhea, relieve abdominal pain and tenderness, and improve appetite and sense of well-being. However, long-term corticosteroid therapy invariably results in side effects. Diabetes and high blood pressure more likely to occur in people with other risk factors.

- *Selected side effects*
- Diabetes
- High blood pressure
- Cataracts
- Osteoporosis
- Thinning of skin
- Mental problems
- *Examples*
- Prednisone
- Budesonide

Immunomodulators

Drugs such as azathioprine and mercaptopurine, which modify the actions of the immune system, are effective for people with Crohn's disesase who do not respond to other drugs and are especially effective for maintaining long periods of remission.

- *Selected side effects*
- Allergic reactions
- Low white blood cell count
- High blood pressure
- Cirrhosis
- Kidney failure
- Abdominal pain
- *Examples*
- Azathioprine
- Mercaptopurine
- Cyclosporine
- Methotrexate
- Infliximab

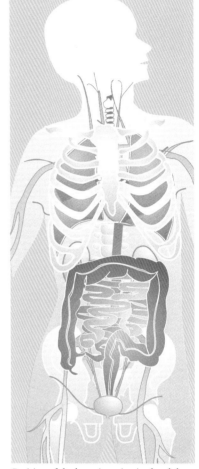

Position of the large intestine in the abdominal cavity.

usually begins between the ages 15 and 30. A small group of people have their first attack between the ages of 50 and 70.

Ulcerative colitis usually does not affect the full thickness of the wall of the large intestine and rarely affects the small intestine. The condition usually begins in the rectum or the sigmoid colon and eventually spreads along the partial or entire length of the large intestine.

The cause of ulcerative colitis is not known, but heredity and an overactive immune response in the intestine may be contributing factors.

Signs and symptoms

The symptoms of the colitis occur in flare-ups. A flare-up may be sudden and severe, producing the following signs and symptoms

- violent diarrhea
- high fever
- abdominal pain
- peritonitis

More often, a flare-up begins gradually, and the person has an urgency to have a bowel movement, mild cramps in the lower abdomen, and visible blood and mucus in the stool.

The major complications of ulcerative colitis are:

- bleeding
- toxic colitis
- toxic megacolon
- colon cancer

Prognosis and treatment

Usually, ulcerative colitis is chronic, with repeated flare-ups and remissions. A rapidly progressive initial attack results in serious complications in about 10 percent of people.

Complete recovery after a single attack may occur in another 10 percent. However, some people who have only a single attack may actually have ulcerations from an undetected infection rather than true ulcerative colitis. Treatment aims to control the inflammation, reduce symptoms, and replace any lost fluid and nutrients. Basic treatment consists of:

- dietary restrictions
- antidiarrheal drugs
- anti-inflammatory drugs
- immunomudulating drugs
- surgery

Surgery may be necessary for unremitting chronic disease that would otherwise make the person an invalid or chronically dependent on high doses of corticosteroids.

INFLUENZA

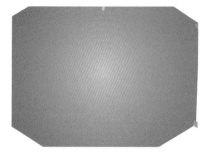

Introduction

Influenza is an acute, epidemic, viral infection, marked by fever, chills, and a generalized feeling of weakness and pain in muscles, together with varying signs of soreness in the respiratory tract, head and abdomen. Influenza is caused by several types of myxoviruses, categorized as group A, B, and C. In these groups many subgroups can be distinguished.

These various types of influenza viruses generally produce similar symptoms but are completely unrelated as far as their antigens are concerned; so that infection with one type confers no immunity against another. Influenza is caused in wavelike epidemics, throughout the world. Influenza A tends to reappear in cycles of two to three years and influenza B in cycles of four to five years.

Every so often, a strain of influenza unfamiliar in humans suddenly begins passing from person to person. Because the virus is so unusual, few if any people have built-in immunity from past exposures.

Even the vaccinated have no defence; flu shots shield against influenza variants that health experts have anticipated will be active in a given flu season, not against other, unforeseen kinds. Finding no deterrent, the new strain spreads unabated, causing illness - and death - on a global scale.

The worst worldwide epidemic, or pandemic, on record struck in 1918 and killed more than 20 million people, sometimes within hours after the first symptoms appeared. This disaster, traced to the so-called Spanish influenza virus, was followed by epidemics of Asian flu in 1957, Hong Kong flu in 1968 and Russian flu in 1977. The names reflect popular impressions of where the pandemics began, although all four episodes, and perhaps most others, are now thought to have originated in China.

Public health experts warn that another pandemic can strike any time now and that it could well be as vicious as the 1918 episode. In 1997, when a lethal influenza virus variant afflicted 18 people in Hong Kong, contributing to the death of six, officials feared the next wave had begun.

Authorities in the region managed to contain the problem quickly, however, by finding the source - infected chickens, ducks and geese - and then destroying all the poultry in Hong Kong.

Next time, humankind may not be so fortunate. If a virus as deadly as that Hong Kong strain tore through the world's crowded communities today, 30 per cent of the earth's population could conceivably be dead (from the virus itself or from secondary bacterial infections) before a vaccine became

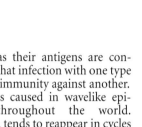

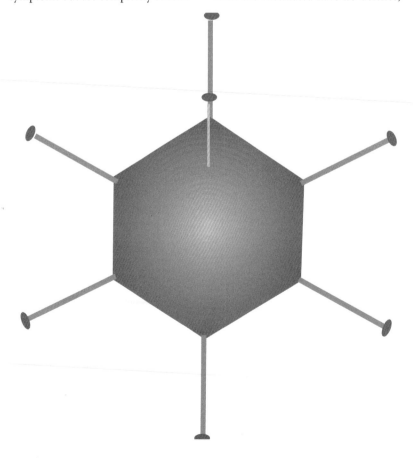

Reconstruction of the molecular structure of a adenovirus, the causative agent of influenza.

available to protect those who initially managed to escape infection.

Vaccines against any given influenza variant take about six months to produce, test for safety and distribute - too long to do much good in the face of a fast-moving pandemic.

If the feared pandemic does not materialize until next year or beyond, though, new methods for limiting sickness and death could be available. Two drugs have been approved for sale as new missiles in the fight against influenza.

The agents - called Tamiflu and Relenza - are being able to prevent infections and reduce the duration and severity of symptoms in people who begin treatment after they start to feel sick.

Unlike vaccines (which prime the immune system to prevent viruses from gaining a foothold in the body) and unlike standard home remedies (which ease symptoms but have no effect on the infection itself), these drugs have been designed to attack the influenza virus directly.

They hobble a critical viral enzyme, called neuraminidase, and in so doing markedly reduce proliferation of the virus in the body. Additional neuraminidase inhibitors, not yet evaluated in humans, are under study as well. Influenza may affect individuals of all ages and is generally more frequent during the colder months of the year. The infection is transmitted from person to person through the respiratory tract, by such means as inhalation of infected droplets resulting from coughing and sneezing.

Mechanism of viral infection

The life cycle of the influenza virus often involves transmission from one person's airways to another's via water droplets emitted during as sneeze.

An individual virus enters a cell lining the respiratory tract after a molecule called hemagglutinin on the virus binds to sialic acid on the cell. This binding induces the cell to take up the virus, which soon dispatches its genetic material, made of RNA, and its internal proteins to the nucleus. Some of those proteins then help to duplicate the RNA and to produce

messenger RNA, which the cell's protein-making machinery uses as a template for making viral proteins. Next, the viral genes and proteins assemble into new viral copies, or particles, and bud from the cell.

The particles emerge coated with sialic acid. If that substance remained on the virus and on the cell, the hemagglutinin molecules on one particle would soon attach to the sialic acid on other particles and on the cell, causing new viruses to clump together and stick to the cell.

But neuraminidase on the virus clips sialic acid from the offending surfaces, leaving the new particles free to travel on and invade other cells.

Symptoms and diagnosis

Symptoms start 24 to 48 hours after infection and can begin suddenly.

How to cope with influenza

■ Rest is important, so go to bed.

■ Drink plenty of liquids to replace those lost in fever.

■ Take aspirin or ibuprofen (adults only) or paracetamol to relive pain and lower your temperature. Sponge children with cool water if they are very hot.

■ Call the doctor if
- Your temperature stays above 103 degrees Fahrenheit.
- Symptoms include dislike of light plus severe headache an a stiff neck.
- You are not feeling any better within three days (fewer for the young, frail or elderly).
- You start to wheeze and cough green or brown mucus, a sign of infection.
- Anyone elderly or suffering from lung or heart disease catches influenza. Anti-viral drugs called amantadine and rimantadine can help if given in the first 24 hours.

Various types of influenza

Type A
This type is responsible for much shivering, aching misery, and is constantly changing. Major shifts in its make-up cause epidemics.

Symptoms include:
- cough
- sore throat
- runny nose followed by
- fever and aching joints.

The worst should be over in 2-5 days, and you should be better in 7-10 days, though a cough and depression may persist.

Type B
This type is usually milder but can still, like Type A, cause stomach pain and lead to secondary bacterial infection.

Type C
This type is virtually indistinguishable from a heavy cold. One attack gives immunity for life.

Influenza Questions & Answers

What is the flu?
It is a viral infection that attacks through the respiratory system. There are three basic types of flu virus - A, B and C - but only A and B are responsible for flu epidemics.

What are the basic symptoms of an influenza as compared to those of a common cold?
Influenza is a viral respiratory tract infection that may mimic a cold is called influenza, or the flu. Flu is usually distinguishable from the common cold by its epidemic occurrence and by:
• fever
• dry cough
• joint and muscle pain
• significant general malaise
Although treatment is symptomatic, it usually is more vigorous than cold treatment, and complications, especially secondary bacterial infections, are more likely to develop.

How do I get the flu?
It spreads like a cold, primarily moving from person to person via virus-contaminated airborne droplets released by coughs, sneezes and even normal conversation. The illness can be spread, as well, through contaminated hands and inanimate objects.
Moreover, like colds, flu can be transmitted by people who have not yet developed symptoms. The incubation period - the time between becoming infected with the virus and knowing you are ill - is one to three days, and during that time you can spread the virus to someone else.

Is it possible to protect myself from the flu?
Yes, getting an annual vaccination weeks before the flu season helps significantly reduce your risk of catching the flu.

Why to I need a flu shot every year?
The viruses that cause influenza are genetically unstable. They change both gradually and abruptly, and each change may enable the virus to skirt around your hard-won immunity from a previous viral bout, invade your respiratory tract and cause the flu. This genetic instability is why people get influenza over and over again, why they get it some years and not others, why some attacks made them much sicker, and why it is necessary to get a new flu shot every year for maximum protection.

Who should be immunized?
The following people have the greatest chance of suffering serious complications from the flu:
• Anyone over six months old with cancer or an immunosuppressed disorder.
• Any child or adult with chronic heart or lung disease, cystic fibrosis, diabetes, kidney disease, anemia or severe asthma.
• Anyone 65 years and older.
• Residents of nursing homes and other chronic-care facilities, particularly those with long-term health problems.
• Anyone who works in a hospital, outpatient facility, nursing home or chronic-care facility.
• Health-care workers who provide in-home care to high-risk patients.

Chills or a chilly sensation are often the first indication of influenza. Fever is common during the first few dags, and the temperature may rise to 39° C.
Many people feel sufficiently ill to remain in bed for days, they have aches and pains throughout the body, most pronounced in the back and legs. Headache is often severe, with aching around and behind the eyes. Bright light may make the headache worse.
At first, the respiratory symptoms may be relatively mild, with a scratchy sore throat, a burning sensation in the chest, a dry cough and a runny nose. Later, the cough can become severe and bring up sputum.
The skin may be warm and flushed, especially on the face. The mouth and throat may redden, the eyes may water, and the whites of the eyes may become bloodshot.
The ill person, especially a child, may have nausea and vomiting. A small percentage of people with influenza lose their sense of smell for a few days or weeks, rarely the loss is permanent. Most symptoms subside after 2 or 3 days. However, fever sometimes lasts up to 5 days, cough may persist for 10 days or longer, and airway irritation may take 6 to 8 weeks to completely resolve. Weakness and fatigue may persist for several days or occasionally for weeks.
Because most people are familiar with the symptoms of influenza, and because influenza occurs in epidemics, the illness is often correctly diagnosed by the person who has it or by family members.
The severity of the illness and the presence of a high fever and body aches help distinguish influenza from a cold. Tests on samples of blood or respiratory secretions can identify the influenza virus but are useful only in special circumstances.

Complications

The most common complication of influenza is pneumonia. This can be viral pneumonia, in which the influenza virus itself spreads into the lungs, or bacterial pneumonia, in which unrelated bacteria (such as pneumococci) attack the person's weakened defenses.

In both cases, the person may have a worsened cough, difficulty breathing, persistent or recurring fever, and sometimes bloody sputum.

Pneumonia is more common in older people and in people with heart or lung disease. As many as 7 percent of older people in long-term care facilities who develop influenza have to be hospitalized, and 1 to 4 percent die. Younger people with chronic illnesses are also at risk of developing severe complications.

Prevention

Influenza is a significant cause of mortality and morbidity in most industrialized countries.

Approximately 90 percent of influenza-related deaths occur in persons aged 65 years and older.

Older adults with underlying health problems, such a pulmonary or cardiovascular disorders, are at particularly high risk of death and serious illness from influenza. Nonelderly adults and children with certain chronic medical problems are at increased risk for influenza-related complications. Influenza vaccine is approximately 50% to 60% effective in preventing hospitalizations and pneumonia and 80% effective in preventing death in older adults.

Approximately 55% of noninstitutionalized older adults receive immunization annually. The antiviral agents amantadine and rimantadine are 70% to 90% effective for preventing influenza type A illness in adults, but these medications do not prevent influenza type B.

Health authorities recommend that influenza immunization should be provided annually to all individuals 65 years of age or older. Immunization should also be provided to adults and children at least 6 months of age who are at increased risk for influenza-related complications due to certain medical conditions, such as chronic pulmonary and cardiovascular disorders, or who may transmit influenza to individuals at increased risk, such as health care workers and household members.

Basics of influenza immunization

Vaccine types

Two basic types of influenza vaccine are available; one is prepared from whole-virus particles, and the other is prepared from split-virus particles. Either type of vaccine is equally appropriate for use in adults and children older than age 12 years. The split-virus preparation is used in children aged 12 years or younger.

The vaccines are trivalent - containing viruses or virus particles from three strains: two type A and one type B. The mixture of viruses used is updated annually according to antigenic change in the viruses causing infection.

Schedule

The influenza vaccine is administered annually, preferably shortly before the onset of the influenza season. Because antibody levels decline with time, one should not give immunizations too early in the season. Immunization programs may begin as soon as the current vaccine is available.

Dose and administration

The recommended dose in adults and children aged 3 years older is 0.5 mL administered intramuscularly. The recommended dose for children aged 6 to 35 months is 0.25 mL. Two doses of vaccine are administered, at least 1 month apart, to children younger than age 9 years who have not previously been vaccinated; this approach minimizes the chance of a satisfactory antibody response.

The vaccine may be given concurrently with pneumococcal vaccine and all routine childhood vaccines, including diphtheria-tetanus-pertussis vaccines.

Contraindications/Precautions

Inactivated influenza vaccine should not be administered to persons known to have anaphylactic hypersensitivity to eggs or other components of the influenza vaccine. Use of an antiviral agent (e.g., amantadine or rimantadine) is an option for preventing influenza type A in such persons. Persons who have a history of anaphylactic hypersensitivity to vaccine com-

ponents but who are also at high risk for complications to vaccine components may benefit from vaccination after appropriate allergy evaluation and desensitization.

People with acute febrile illness should not be vaccinated until their symptoms have abated. The presence of minor illness, with or without fever, is not a contraindication to use of influenza vaccine, particularly in children with mild upper respiratory tract infection or allergic rhinitis.

Adverse reactions

Because influenza vaccine contains only noninfectious viruses, it cannot cause influenza. Respiratory disease that occurs after vaccination represents coincidental illness unrelated to influenza vaccination.

Adverse reactions to vaccination generally are mild. Soreness at the site of injection persisting up to 2 days is the most common side effect. Fever, malaise, myalgia, and other systemic symptoms occur infrequently; these symptoms may occur as early as 6 hours after immunization and can persist for as long as 48 hours. Rarely, an immediate allergic reaction can occur.

How can I help myself

- Keep warm, but do not let the room get stuffy. A little fresh air will help.
- Get plenty of rest. If you try to soldier on, you will probably just make the flu last longer, and you may infect other people.
- Drink plenty of liquids to make up for fluids lost in sweating, and to help soothe your throat. Hot drinks containing lemon or blackcurrant are particularly helpful. Keep tea and coffee to a minimum.
- Do not smoke. If you are a smoker, this could be a good time to give up.
- Try to eat, even if you do not really feel like it. Light meals will help keep your strength up.

Tamiflu

What is Tamiflu?

This medicine contains as active ingredient oxeltamivir phosphate used in de treatment of symptoms of influenza (flu). Tamiflu is one of a new class of antiviral drugs called neuraminidase inhibitors.

Why is this drug prescribed?

This medicine speeds recovery from the flu. When started during the first 2 days of the illness, it hastens improvement by at least a day. Il also can prevent the flu if treatment is started within 2 days after exposure to a flu victim.

As the flu virus takes hold in the body, it forms new copies of itself and spreads from cell to cell. Neuraminidase inhibitors fight the virus by preventing the release of new copies from infected cells. Tamiflu is taken in liquid or capsule form.

What are the most important facts about this drug?

Tamiflu can prevent the flu as long as you continue taking this medication, but getting a yearly flu shot is still the best way of avoiding the disease entirely. For older adults, those in high-risk situations such as health-care work, and people with an immune deficiency or respiratory disease, vaccination remains a must.

How should you take this medication?

- To provide any benefit, Tamiflu must be started within two days of the onset of symptoms, or exposure to the flu. If you have the flu, continue taking it twice daily for 5 days, even if you start to feel better.
- To prevent the flu, take it once a day for at least 7 days. Protection lasts as you take the medicine.
- Unless otherwise directed by your doctor or pharmacist take this medication as directed. Do not take more of them and do not take them more often than recommended on the label.
- If Tamiflu upsets your stomach, try taking it with food. Shake the liquid suspension before each use.

- If you miss a dose: take Tamiflu as soon as possible. If it is within two hours of your next dose, skip the missed dose and go back to your regular schedule.

What side effects may occur?

Along with the needed effects, a medicine may cause some unwanted effects. Most problems noted during tests of Tamiflu were indistinguishable from the symptoms of flu. Here are the reactions that showed up more frequently in patients taking the drug.

- More common side effects may include:
  - Abdominal pain
  - Diarrhea
  - Headache
  - Nausea
  - Vomiting
- Less common side effects may include:
  - Bronchitis
  - Insomnia
  - Vertigo

The effectiveness of Tamiflu has not been established for people with weakened immune systems. The medicine has not been studied in people with liver disease. Tamiflu works only on the flu virus. It won't stop bacterial infections that may have flu-like symptoms or bacterial infections that may develop while you have the flu. If your symptoms persist, check with your doctor.

Why should this medicine not be prescribed?

If this medicine gives you an allergic reaction, avoid it in the future.

Are there any special warnings about this medication?

- The effectiveness of Tamiflu has not been established for people with weakened immune systems.
- The medicine has not been studied in people with liver disease.
- Tamiflu works only on the flu virus. It won't stop bacterial infections that may have flu-like symptoms or bacterial infections that may develop while you have the flu. If your symptoms persist, check with your doctor.

What about the use of the medicine during pregnancy or while breastfeeding?

It is not known whether Tamiflu is completely safe during pregnancy. If you are pregnant of plan to become pregnant, inform your doctor before taking this medication. Tamiflu may appear in breast milk and should affect a nursing infant. Taking it while breastfeeding is usually not recommended.

What is the recommended dosage?

Adults and children 13 and older

- Treatment of influenza

The usual dosage is 75 milligrams taken twice daily (morning and evening) for 5 days. If you have kidney disease, take a 75-milligram dose once a day.

- Prevention of influenza

The usual dosage is 75 milligrams taken one a day for at least 7 days. If the is a general outbreak of the flu in your community, your doctor may recommend that you continue taking this medication for up to 6 weeks.

If you have kidney disease take a 75-milligram capsule every other day, or 30 milligrams of liquid once a day.

Children 1 to 12

- Treatment of influenza

Doses should be given twice daily for 5 days using the dispenser that comes with the liquid suspension. Each dose is determined by the child's weight:

- Under 35 pounds: 30 milligrams
- 33 to 55 pounds: 45 milligrams
- 51 to 88 pounds: 60 milligrams
- Over 88 pounds: 75 milligrams
- Prevention of influenza

Tamiflu's ability to prevent the flu in children under age 13 has not been established.

What happens in case of overdosage?

High doses of Tamiflu can cause nausea and vomiting. As with any medication, if you suspect an overdose, seek emergency medical treatment immediately.

Amantidine

What is Amantidine?
This medicine contains as active ingredient zanamivir used in de treatment of symptoms of influenza (flu). Amantidine is one of a new class of antiviral drugs called neuraminidase inhibitors. This medicine is believed to work by interfering with the spread of virus particles inside the respiratory tract.

Why is this drug prescribed?
This medicine speeds recovery from the flu. When started during the first 2 days of the illness, it hastens improvement by at least a day. Il also can prevent the flu if treatment is started within 2 days after exposure to a flu victim. As the flu virus takes hold in the body, it forms new copies of itself and spreads from cell to cell. Neuraminidase inhibitors fight the virus by preventing the release of new copies from infected cells. Amantidine is taken in liquid or capsule form.

What are the most important facts about this drug?
Amantidine can prevent some of the symptoms of influenza as long as you continue taking this medication. There is no evidence that Amantidine protects you from catching the flu, and it will not prevent you from spreading the flu virus to others. Getting a yearly flu shot is still the best way of avoiding the disease entirely. For older adults, those in high-risk situations such as health-care work, and people with an immune deficiency or respiratory disease, vaccination remains a must.

How should you take this medication?
■ Amantidine is delivered directly to the lungs by oral inhalation from a Diskhaler device.
■ To provide any benefit, Amantidine must be started two days of the onset of symptoms, or exposure to the flu. If you have the flu, continue taking it for 5 days, even if you start to feel better.
■ Unless otherwise directed by your doctor or pharmacist take this medication as directed. Do not take more of them and do not take them more often than recommended on the label.
■ Be sure to take two doses on the first day, allowing at least 2 hours between them. On the following day, take a dose every 12 hours (morning and evening).
■ Do not puncture a blister containing the medicine until you are ready to use it.
■ Children should use this medication only under the supervision of an adult.
■ If you miss a dose: take Amantidine as soon as possible. If it is within two hours of your next dose, skip the missed dose and go back to your regular schedule. Do not take 2 doses at the same time.

What side effects may occur?
Along with the needed effects, a medicine may cause some unwanted effects. Most problems noted during tests of Amantidine were indistinguishable from the symptoms of flu. Problems reported during clinical tests are listed below.
■ More common side effects may include: Headache, Difficulty in concentrating, Insomnia, Irritability, Dizziness, Nervousness, Nightmares
■ Inffrequent side effects may include: Blurred vision, Changed vision, Confusion, Difficult urination, Hallucinations, Fainting
■ Rare side effects may include: Swelling of the eyes, Irritated eyes, Depression, Swelling of the hands or legs, Skin rash, Heartbeat irregularities, Seizure
Amantidine works only on the flu virus. It won't stop bacterial infections that may have flu-like symptoms or bacterial infections that may develop while you have the flu. If your symptoms persist, check with your doctor.

Why should this medicine not be prescribed?
If this medicine gives you an allergic reaction, avoid it in the future. Amantidine can cause serious allergic reactions. If you experience swelling of the face, tongue, or throat, or develop a skin rash, stop taking this medication and contact your doctor.

Are there any special warnings about this medication?
■ Amantidine is generally not recommended for anyone with a chronic pulmonary disease. If you do use it under these circumstances, be extremely cautious, and make sure that you have a fast-acting inhaled bronchodilator available and ready to use whenever you take it.
■ If you use an inhaled bronchodilator regularly and have a dose scheduled at the same time as Amantidine, use the bronchodilator first.
■ The effectiveness of Amantidine has not been established for people with weakened immune systems.
■ The medicine has not been studied in people with liver disease.
■ The medicine has not been tested in people with medical conditions severe enough for possible hospitalization. Use it with caution if you have any kind of serious health problem in addition to the flu.
■ Amantidine works only on the flu virus. It won't stop bacterial infections that may have flu-like symptoms or bacterial infections that may develop while you have the flu. If your symptoms persist, check with your doctor.

What about the use of the medicine during pregnancy or while breastfeeding?
The effects of Amantidine during pregnancy have not been adequately studied. If you are pregnant of plan to become pregnant, inform your doctor before taking this medication. It is not known whether Amantidine appears in breast milk. Caution is recommended if you are breastfeeding.

What is the recommended dosage?
The recommended dose for adults and children 7 years and older is 2 inhalations (one 5-milligram blister per inhalation) twice a day, approximately 12 hours apart, for 5 days. Safety and efficacy have not been established for children under 7.

IRRITABLE BOWEL DISEASE

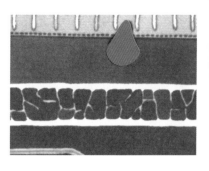

Introduction

Disorders of the intestines are fairly common. Almost everyone has had some degree of difficulty in this area at one time or another. These disorders can be functional, because of the extensive nerve connections in the digestive system; fear, anger, and other nervous upsets may set off attacks of nausea, cramps, or diarrhea.

Organic diseases such as peptic ulcers and cancer can also affect these organs, as do contagious diseases, such as salmonellosis (eating food contaminated with Salmonella bacteria) and virus infections, as well as constipation, dyspepsia, allergies - and a list almost as long as the digestive tract itself.

The irritable bowel syndrome is a condition characterized by recurrent abdominal pain, constipation, and/or diarrhea. Occurring most often in young adults, it has no known organic cause and is often associated with emotional stress.

It is a motility disorder involving the small and large bowel associated with variable degrees of abdominal pain, largely as a reaction to stress in a susceptible individual. The disorder is also known as spastic colon or mucous colitis.

The syndrome represents about half of all gastrointestinal referrals or initial gastro-intestinal complaints in private and institutional care facilities. Women are more commonly affected than men, in a 3:1 ratio.

Causes and physiological aspects

No anatomic cause can be found. The following factors may precipitate or aggravate an inherent heightened sensitivity to motility of the intestines:
· emotional factors
· diet
· medicines
· hormones
Patients with an irritable bowel syn-

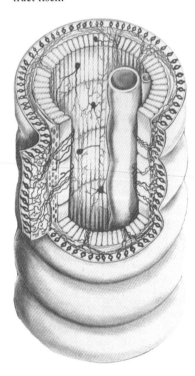

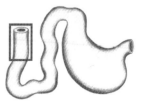

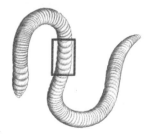

Microscopic structure of the wall of the duodenum (left) and ileum (right). The smooth muscles (innervated by plexus of the autonomic nervous system) serve in mixing the chyme as well as its transport by means of peristaltic movements. This double function is brought about by a layer of longitudinal and circular smooth muscles. The intestinal wall further shows a large number of tubular sacs (Lieberkühn's crypts), in which the intestinal juices are excreted.

drome are more often neurotic, anxious, or depressed than comparable patients. Periods of stress and emotional conflict, particularly those resulting in depression, frequently coincide with onset and recurrences, such as:
- marital discord
- anxiety related to children
- loss of a loved one
- obsessional worries over trivial everyday problems

In addition it appears that patients suffering from irritable bowel syndrome are more prone to chronic illness behavior and that this behavior is learned. The circulatory and longitudinal muscles of the small bowel and sigmoid colon are particularly susceptible to motor abnormalities.

The proximal small bowel and the colon appear to be hyperactive to ingestion of food and medicines that mimic the function of the parasympathetic part of the autonomic nervous system. Patients are more aware of normal amounts of intestinal gas and also have a heightened perception of pain in the presence of normal intestinal gas.

The pain of irritable bowel syndrome seems to be due to abnormally strong contractions of the intestinal smooth muscle or to undue sensitivity to distention of the intestine. Some patients may be intolerant to wheat, dairy products, coffee, tea, or citrus fruits.

Symptoms and signs

Symptoms can be listed as follows:
- abdominal distress
- erratic frequency of bowel action
- variation in stool consistency

Disagreeable abdominal sensations may also be associated with nonspecific symptoms, such as:
- bloating
- flatulence
- nausea
- headache
- fatigue
- lassitude
- depression
- anxiety
- difficulty with mental concentration

Two major groups or clinical types of irritable bowel syndrome are recog-

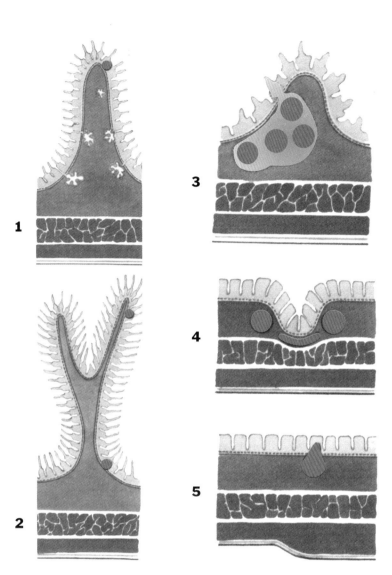

Differences in structure of the various parts of the small and large intestine.
1. Duodenum; 2. jejunum; 3. ileum; 4. appendix; 5. colon.
The following layers of tissue may be recognized (from top to bottom);
- mucosa;
- connective tissue with blood vessels and nerve plexus;
- muscular layer consisting of longitudinally and circularly arranged fibers;
- peritoneum.
Red: system of lymph nodes.

nized.
▲ In the first group the spastic colon type, bowel movements are variable. Symptoms are commonly triggered by eating. Most patients have pain of colonic origin over one or more areas of the colon in association with either periodic constipation or diarrheas; in some patients, the two alternate. Headache and backache are commonly present.

The most common location of the pain or discomfort is over the course of the sigmoid colon. The pain is either colicky and comes in

Irritable bowel disease   Questions & Answers

What is irritable bowel syndrome?
Irritable bowel syndrome is a disorder of motility of the entire digestive tract that causes a number of major symptoms:
- pain
- constipation
- diarrhea

What is the mechanism of origin of irritable bowel syndrome?
In irritable bowel syndrome, the digestive tract is especially sensitive to many stimuli, such as
- stress
- diet
- drugs
- hormones
- minor irritants

These stimuli may cause the digestive tract to contract abnormally, usually leading to diarrhea.

What is the course of irritable bowel syndrome?
Irritable bowel syndrome may show periods of constipation between bouts of diarrhea. If an emotional disorder is identified as the cause, treatment of the disorder may relieve irritable bowel syndrome symptoms.

Are men more affected than women?
No. Women are three times more affected than men.

Does the brain have anything to do with irritable bowel syndrome?
The brain has major control over the digestive system. Many psychological conditions can lead to diarrhea, constipation, and other changes in bowel function. To name a few:
- stress
- anxiety
- depression
- anger
- neurotic obsession

How is irritable bowel syndrome treated?
The treatment for irritable bowel syndrome differs from person to person. People who can identify particular foods or types of stress that bring on the problem should avoid them if possible. For most people, especially those who tend to be constipated, regular physical activity helps keep the digestive tract functioning normally.

Are men more affected than women?
No. Women are three times more affected than men.

bouts or is a continuous dull ache. It may be relieved by a bowel movement.
▲ The second group primarily manifests painless diarrhea that is usually urgent and precipitous. It occurs immediately upon rising or, more typically, during or immediately after a meal. Incontinence may occur, but nocturnal diarrhea is unusual.

Diagnosis

The diagnosis of irritable bowel syndrome is based upon identification of the clinical syndromes described above and exclusion of other disease processes. In general, the manifestations characteristic for a given patient remain consistent; variations or deviations from the usual symptoms suggest the possibility of intercurrent organic disease and will be thoroughly investigated by the medical specialist.

On physical examination, the doctor finds patients with either variant of irritable bowel syndrome generally to be in good health without evidence of significant organic disease. Palpation of the abdomen may reveal tenderness, at times associated with a contracted, tender colon.

A major problem for the doctor in the differential diagnosis of irritable bowel syndrome is the similarity of its manifestations to organic bowel disease. A diagnosis of irritable bowel syndrome will never preclude suspicion of an intercurrent disease, particularly in patients over age 40.

Symptoms indicative of organic diseases requiring investigation include the following:
- fresh blood mixed with the stool
- weight loss
- steady progressing worsening of symptoms
- very severe abdominal pain
- unusual abdominal distention
- steatorrhea (excessive fat in stool)
- noticeably foul-smelling stools
- fever and/or chills
- persistent vomiting
- hematemesis
- symptoms that awaken the patient from sleep

In patients over 40 years of age, par-

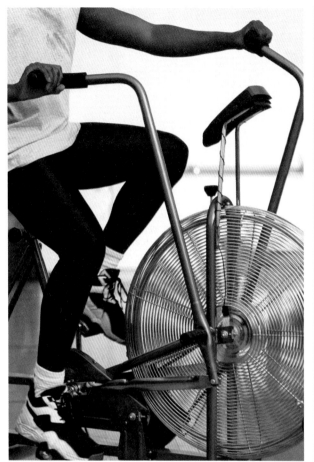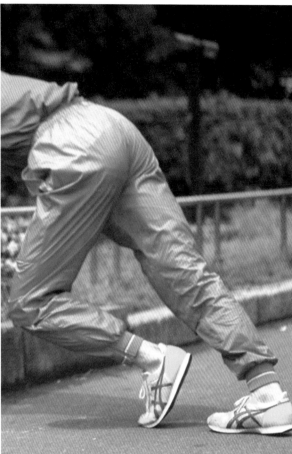

For most people with irritable bowel syndrome, especially those who tend to be constipated, regular physical activity helps keep the digestive tract functioning normally.

ticularly those with no previous history of irritable bowel syndrome symptoms, polyps in the colon and cancer must be excluded.

Treatment

The treatment for irritable bowel syndrome differs from person to person. People who can identify particular foods or types of stress that bring on the problem should avoid them if possible.

Therapy is supportive and palliative. The doctor's sympathetic understanding and guidance are of overriding importance. Both patient and doctor must be assured that no organic disease is present. The doctor shall explain the nature of the underlying condition and convincingly demonstrate to the patient that no organic disease is present.

This requires time for listening and explaining and includes a discussion of normal bowel physiology and the bowel's hypersensitivity to stress, food, drugs, or hormones. These explanations will form the foundation for attempting to reestablish regular bowel routine and the selection of individualized therapy.

The prevalence and chronicity of the syndrome will be emphasized, and the need for regular follow-up evaluation mandated (both for symptom control and early detection of possible intercurrent organic disease).

Psychological stress, particularly a depressive reaction, will be sought, evaluated, and treated. Informed awareness will help the patient avoid stressful situations. Regular physical therapy helps to relieve stress and assists in bowel function, particularly in patients who present with constipation. In those patients with spastic colon and constipation, a blend bulk-producing agent may be helpful (for instance, raw bran starting with a dose of 15 ml (a spoonful) with each meal, supplemented with increased fluid intake).

Alternatively, psyllium hydrophillic mucilloid taken with two glasses of water tends to stabilize the water content of the bowel and provide bulk. Sometimes a mild sedative is useful in combination with bulk-producing agents.

For the small group of patients totally refractory to the therapeutic modalities noted above, hypnotherapy or psychotherapy may be indicated.

JUVENILE RHEUMATOID ARTHRITIS

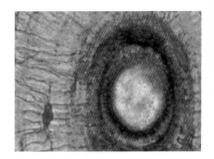

Introduction

Juvenile rheumatoid arthritis is a serious condition in young children. The word, arthritis, means inflammation (that is, swelling, heat, and pain) in a joint. According to estimates of the WHO, as many as 425,000 children in Europe and as many as 165,000 children in the United States may have some form of arthritis.

In fact, arthritis can be a feature of many different childhood illnesses. For example, ankylosing spondylitis, lupus, and juvenile rheumatoid arthritis are all childhood illnesses which may have arthritis as a feature. Juvenile rheumatoid arthritis affects about 185,000 children in Europe and about 72,000 children in the United States. It is often a mild condition which causes few problems - but it can also be quite serious. Its signs and symptoms can change from day to day, even from morning to afternoon. Joint stiffness and pain may be mild one day and then so severe the next that the child cannot move without great difficulty.

There are at least three forms of juvenile rheumatoid arthritis. Each form begins in a different way and has different signs and symptoms. The three forms are:

▲ polyarticular juvenile rheumatoid arthritis ("poly" means several or many and "articular" means joint: many joints);
▲ pauciarticular juvenile rheumatoid arthritis ("pauci" means few and "articular" means joint: few joints);
▲ systemic juvenile rheumatoid arthritis ("systemic" means internal organs and other body parts).

In addition, boys can develop a form of arthritis (called B-27 arthritis) that is closely related to ankylosing spondylitis in adults. Most children with juvenile rheumatoid arthritis do well in the long run. As a parent, you may feel discouraged because the disease seems to go on and on.

But permanent damage to joints by arthritis is much less common in children than in adults. Children with juvenile rheumatoid arthritis can usually keep up with school and social activities. Some changes will need to be made when the child is in a flare (a period during which the arthritis is particular troublesome) or if there has been joint damage.

Causes

Doctors and scientists are not sure what causes any of the forms of juvenile rheumatoid arthritis. It is certain that juvenile rheumatoid arthritis is not contagious, so the child can't "catch" it from anyone and can't five it to anyone.

It is also known that heredity plays some part in the development of some forms of juvenile rheumatoid arthritis. However, the inherited trait alone does not cause the illness. Investigators think that this trait along with some other unknown factor triggers the disease. It is unusual for more than one child in a family to have juvenile rheumatoid arthritis.

There is a great deal of research going on to find the cause or causes of juvenile rheumatoid arthritis. Once these are found, it should be possible to cure this illness or to prevent it from starting.

General signs and symptoms

Juvenile rheumatoid arthritis is a chronic disease - one that lasts for many years, or throughout the child's entire life. Eventually, the child will most likely to get well and experience no serious permanent disability. But "eventually" can mean months, or years.

Sometimes, the signs and symptoms of juvenile rheumatoid arthritis may go away. When this happens, it is called a remission. A remission may last for months, or years, or even forever.

Juvenile rheumatoid arthritis can usually be controlled, even though there is no cure for it right now.

To control your child's juvenile rheumatoid arthritis, you and your family have to make some adjustments in your lives. The most important thing you can do is work with your doctor and other health professionals to manage the disease and keep it under control.

There are four major features which can occur in each form of juvenile rheumatoid arthritis. Remember; juvenile rheumatoid arthritis affects every child differently, so your child may not have all these features, and may have only mild problems with others.

Features which may occur in any of the three forms of juvenile rheumatoid arthritis are:

• joint inflammation
• joint deformity
• joint damage
• altered growth

Joint inflammation

Joint inflammation is the most common symptom of juvenile rheumatoid arthritis. It causes the heat, pain, swelling, and stiffness in joints that most people think of as arthritis.

The lining of the joint, called synovium, becomes swollen and overgrown and produces too much fluid. This causes stiffness, swelling, pain, warmth, and sometimes redness of the skin over the affected joints.

Joint deformity

Since it usually hurts to move an inflamed joint, a child will often hold it still. If the child holds a sore joint in one place for a long time, the muscles around the joint will become stiff and weak. After a while, the tendons (tissues which connects the muscles to the bone) may tighten up and shorten, causing a deformity called a joint contracture.

Joint damage

In some children with severe disease, long-lasting inflammation damages the joint surfaces. This is called joint erosion, and can result in the kinds of crippling you have seen in adults with rheumatoid arthritis. Fortunately, this does not happen in many children.

Altered growth

Sometimes joint inflammation either speeds up or slows down the growth centers in bones. This can make the affected bones longer or shorter than normal. If the growth centers have been damaged by inflammation, a child may stop growing entirely.

If no damage had occurred, however, the child will usually continue to grow once the juvenile rheumatoid arthritis is under control. These features ate common to all forms of juvenile rheumatoid arthritis, but there are differences in the types of joint problems and other features in each form of juvenile rheumatoid arthritis.

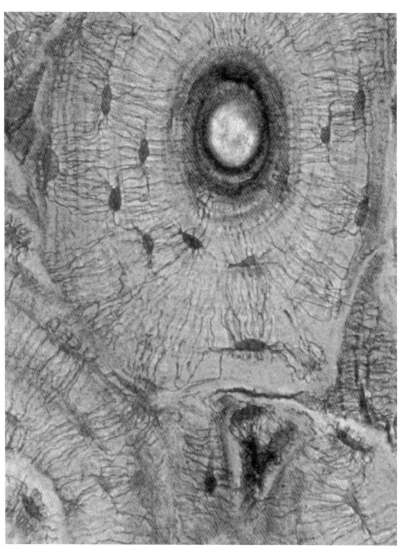

Microscopic picture of bone of a patient not only showing joint inflammation and deformity but also altered growth of bone (lower part of figure).

Diagnosis

The signs and symptoms of juvenile rheumatoid arthritis vary from child to child and there may be many steps involved in finding out if your child really does have juvenile rheumatoid arthritis. However, your child may not have to go through all the steps listed here to be diagnosed. The main steps involved in diagnosis are:

- child's health history
- physical examination
- laboratory tests
- X-ray examinations
- joint fluid and tissue tests

Health history

To make a correct diagnosis, the doctor will ask questions such as:
- Hoe has your child been feeling?
- What has happened during his or her lifetime and in the present illness?
- How long has the present illness lasted?

Many infections can lead to joint problems in children, but in these cases the arthritis usually goes away rapidly. In order to make a diagnosis of juvenile rheumatoid arthritis, the arthritis must have been present for six or more consecutive weeks. The doctor may also want to know if other members of the family have had any other form of arthritis, since some forms may be inherited.

Physical examination

During the physical examination, the doctor will look for:
- joint inflammation
- rash
- nodules
- eye problems

The doctor must be able to find evidence of joint inflammation to be sure juvenile rheumatoid arthritis is the problem.

Juvenile rheumatoid arthritis   Questions & Answers

What is juvenile rheumatoid arthritis?

Juvenile rheumatoid arthritis is a serious condition in young children. The word, arthritis, means inflammation (that is, swelling, heat, and pain) in a joint. According to estimates of the WHO, as many as 1,400,000 children in the world may have some form of arthritis.

Does arthritis in children always mean juvenile rheumatoid arthritis?

No, in fact, arthritis can be a feature of many different childhood illnesses. For example, ankylosing spondylitis, lupus, and juvenile rheumatoid arthritis are all childhood illnesses which may have arthritis as a feature.

Are many children affected by juvenile rheumatoid arthritis?

Juvenile rheumatoid arthritis affects about 570,000 children in the world. It is often a mild condition which causes few problems - but it can also be quite serious. Its signs and symptoms can change from day to day, even from morning to afternoon. Joint stiffness and pain may be mild one day and then so severe the next that the child cannot move without great difficulty.

What are the features of the various types of juvenile rheumatoid arthritis?

There are at least three forms of juvenile rheumatoid arthritis. Each form begins in a different way and has different signs and symptoms.
The three forms are:
- polyarticular juvenile rheumatoid arthritis ("poly" means several or many and "articular" means joint: many joints);
- pauciarticular juvenile rheumatoid arthritis ("pauci" means few and "articular" means joint: few joints);
- systemic juvenile rheumatoid arthritis ("systemic" means internal organs and other body parts).

In addition, boys can develop a form of arthritis (called B-27 arthritis) that is closely related to ankylosing spondylitis in adults.

What is the prognosis of children with juvenile rheumatoid arthritis?

Most children with juvenile rheumatoid arthritis do well in the long run. As a parent, you may feel discouraged because the disease seems to go on and on. But permanent damage to joints by arthritis is much less common in children than in adults.
Children with juvenile rheumatoid arthritis can usually keep up with school and social activities. Some changes will need to be made when the child is in a flare (a period during which the arthritis is particular troublesome) or if there has been joint damage.

What are the causes of juvenile rheumatoid arthritis?

Doctors and scientists are not sure what causes any of the forms of juvenile rheumatoid arthritis. It is certain that juvenile rheumatoid arthritis is not contagious, so the child cannot "catch" it from anyone and cannot five it to anyone.
It is also known that heredity plays some part in the development of some forms of juvenile rheumatoid arthritis. However, the inherited trait alone does not cause the illness. Investigators think that this trait along with some other unknown factor triggers the disease. It is unusual for more than one child in a family to have juvenile rheumatoid arthritis.

What are the major signs and symptoms of juvenile rheumatoid arthritis?

Juvenile rheumatoid arthritis is a chronic disease - one that lasts for many years, or throughout the child's entire life. Eventually, the child will most likely to get well and experience no serious permanent disability. But "eventually" can mean months, or years. Sometimes, the signs and symptoms of juvenile rheumatoid arthritis may go away. When this happens, it is called a remission. A remission may last for months, or years, or even forever.

Can juvenile rheumatoid arthritis be controlled?

Juvenile rheumatoid arthritis can usually be controlled, even though there is no cure for it right now. To control your child's juvenile rheumatoid arthritis, you and your family have to make some adjustments in your lives. The most important thing you can do is work with your doctor and other health professionals to manage the disease and keep it under control.

What are the features of juvenile rheumatoid arthritis?

There are four major features which can occur in each form of juvenile rheumatoid arthritis. Remember: juvenile rheumatoid arthritis affects every child differently, so your child may not have all these features, and may have only mild problems with others.
Features which may occur in any of the three forms of juvenile rheumatoid arthritis are:
- joint inflammation
- joint deformity
- joint damage
- altered growth

Can juvenile rheumatoid arthritis alter the growth of joints?

Sometimes joint inflammation either speeds up or slows down the growth centers in bones. This can make the affected bones longer or shorter than normal. If the growth centers have been damaged by inflammation, a child may stop growing entirely. If no damage had occurred, however, the child will usually continue to grow once the juvenile rheumatoid arthritis is under control.

A child who complains of aches and pains, but who shows no joint changes, may not have juvenile rheumatoid arthritis. If the doctor finds an eye problem, an ophthalmologist may also need to examine your child's eyes.

Laboratory tests
Although there are several laboratory tests that may point to juvenile rheumatoid arthritis, there is no single test that provides positive proof one way or another.
The most common blood tests are:
• erythrocyte sedimentation rate
• rheumatoid factor test
• antinuclear antibody test
• HLA B-27 typing
• hemoglobin test.
If the diagnosis is particularly hard to make, the doctor may be additional tests to rule out other diseases.

X-ray examinations
X-ray examinations of joints may be helpful early in the course of the illness to find out if another condition such as bone infection, tumor, or fracture is causing the problem. Later on, X-rays may be used to check on joint damage, or changes in bones. X-rays of the spine help the doctor till if ankylosing spondylitis is present.

Joints fluid
A sample of fluid from one or more joints may be withdrawn by a needle and examined to find out if there is an infection in the joint. Sometimes the doctor will take a small bit of tissue from a joint or a nodule for examination in the laboratory. This is called a biopsy. Other diseases such as psoriasis (a chronic skin condition) and colitis (inflammation of the large intestine) can cause arthritis. All these must be ruled out before the doctor can diagnose juvenile rheumatoid arthritis. It may seem to take a long time to pinpoint the problem. But it is necessary to be as specific as possible about your child's problems so that treatment can be tailored to fit the condition.

Treatment

If the child's doctor is well-informed about juvenile rheumatoid arthritis, then this person may be able to treat the child. The doctor who already knows the child's medical history is usually the best person to see first.
Pediatric rheumatologists are doctors who specialize in childhood juvenile rheumatoid arthritis. If your child's disease is severe or puzzling, your regular doctor may refer you to one of these specialists either for a consultation, or for continuous care. If there is no paediatric rheumatologist in your area, your doctor may refer you to a rheumatologist who also treats adults. The child's treatment program will be based on the kind of arthritis she had and on her specific symptoms.
The goals of any treatment program for juvenile rheumatoid arthritis are to:
• control inflammation
• relieve pain
• prevent or control joint damage
To reach these goals, the treatment program for juvenile rheumatoid arthritis usually includes:
• medications
• rest
• exercises
• eye care
• a balanced diet
Other types of treatment, such as surgery, may be necessary for special long-term problems. There is no simple, rapid solution to juvenile rheumatoid arthritis. Treatment is likely to last for a long time, and will probably change as your child's symptoms change.
However, it is important to continue the treatment chosen by the physician so that you can help prevent serious joint damage and other problems in your child.

Psychological aspects

Your child may feel angry or sad about having juvenile rheumatoid arthritis. But be aware that you as parents, and other family members may also have troubling feelings about the disease and its effect on the family.

When you are first told your child has juvenile rheumatoid arthritis, you might feel shocked, numbed, or disbelieving. You might also feel guilty, and ask yourself if something you did or did not caused your child's juvenile rheumatoid arthritis.

■ *The child with juvenile rheumatoid arthritis*
▲ The child with arthritis may feel many different emotions. Children can feel "hurt" by an illness that is not their fault, blame parents for the illness, adopt a "why me?" attitude, and indulge in self-pity or anger because of restrictions on activities. They may also resent other children who are well, including brothers and sisters.
▲ The key to dealing with all these emotions is to talk about them with one another. How does each family member feel about their role in the child's illness?
▲ What attitudes does your child learn from you about the disease? While juvenile rheumatoid arthritis will cause some changes in your family's life, try to accept those changes as part of your new life with juvenile rheumatoid arthritis.

■ *Help for your child with juvenile rheumatoid arthritis*
▲ Talk to your child about how he or she feels about the illness. Allow your child to express his anger about arthritis from time to time.
▲ Encourage your child to develop her special talents - if she or he likes to paint, for example, help him to improve his painting skills.
▲ Expect your child to behave as well as other children - do not give him "special allowances" just because he or she has arthritis.
▲ Encourage your child to learn as much as he can about arthritis and about the treatment program.

■ *Help for brothers and sisters in case of a child with other family members juvenile rheumatoid arthritis*
▲ Talk to your child's brothers and sisters about juvenile rheumatoid arthritis - let them express their feelings about the disease.
▲ Encourage the family to treat the ill child as they did before he became ill - but at the same time, do remember that he or she will need some special attention.

KIDNEY CANCER

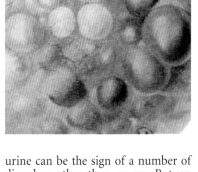

Description

The kidneys do not only help to remove wastes from the body but are also glands that manufacture and secrete a variety of hormones. These hormonal and endocrine functions are important in the diagnosis and treatment of kidney cancer because the cells of a kidney cancer are off-springs of normal kidney cells and secrete the same hormones.

Childhood kidney cancer is very different from kidney cancer in adults. The most common type of childhood kidney cancer is the Wilms' tumor.

Symptoms

The most common symptom of kidney cancer is visible blood in the urine. The blood may be present one day and absent the next. Blood in the urine can be the sign of a number of disorders other than cancer. But no matter what the cause, the condition should be brought to the attention of the physician. Other common symptoms of kidney cancer are the presence of a lump mass in the abdomen, and pain in the side. You may have felt a mass when you touched your abdomen. It probably felt smooth, hard and "fixed."

Like all cancers, kidney cancer can cause fatigue, loss of appetite, weight loss and anemia. You may have been told recently that you have high blood pressure. There also may be other symptoms that seem entirely unrelated to the kidneys. When you see your physician, you should report all aches or pains, or any other way in which you do not "feel like yourself." These may be important clues.

Diagnosis

Diagnosis begins with a physical examination by your physician. Diagnostic radiology (pictures taken with X-rays) is always used to confirm a suspected diagnosis of kidney cancer. Your physician will probably arrange for a special kind of X-ray test called a nephrotomography.

Tomography is a series of pictures of the kidney. When the pictures are put together, they can give a three-dimensional picture of an abnormal growth in the kidney. Another type of special X-ray examination is the CT-scan or MRI-scan. While you lie still, a narrow X-ray beam directed by a computer revolves around you.

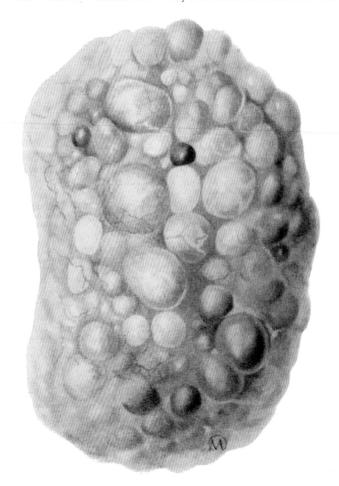

Polycystic kidney disease characterized by many fluid-filled sacs (cysts). In some cases, this condition is accompanied by malignant degeneration of kidney tissue.

K

In a matter of seconds, the machine registers thousands of bits of information that are translated into a cross-sectional picture on a viewing screen. At the same time that a tomogram is made, you may have a "sound-picture" made of your kidney. Ultrasound is an experimental technique that is based on the principles of sonar. Ultrasound is used only as a supplement to nephrotomography. Tomography (both CT and MRI scans) and ultrasound can tell your physician with a high degree of accuracy whether a suspected mass is a cyst (a fluid-filled sac) or a tumor.

If the first tests indicate the mass is a tumor, another kind of X-ray test called selective renal arteriography can tell the doctor whether the tumor is likely to be cancerous. Selective renal arteriography permits the direct visualization of the veins and arteries that crisscross the kidney and mass. The veins and arteries are made visible by the introduction of a harmless dye into the bloodstream through a catheter placed in the femoral artery. This is not a painful procedure, but it requires a few hours of hospitalization and a mild local sedative.

If the various radiological examinations confirm a diagnosis of kidney cancer, your physician will want to perform other tests that will tell him whether the cancer has spread. Chest X-rays and radioisotope bone scans are always easy included among these tests, because the lungs and the long bones are the areas to which kidney cancer cells most often travel.

When a diagnosis of kidney cancer is confirmed by your physician, it is best to begin treatment in a hospital that has an expert staff and the resources available to apply all forms of effective treatment right from the beginning. You may wish to request a second opinion from another physician to confirm the first diagnosis and recommendations for therapy.

Cell types are the basis for classification of kidney cancers. More than 8 out of 10 kidney cancers are renal adenocarcinomas, sometimes called renal cell carcinomas or Grawitz tumor. Renal adenocarcinomas start in the cells that form the lining of a renal tubule. The most prevalent of kidney cancers appear most often after age 40

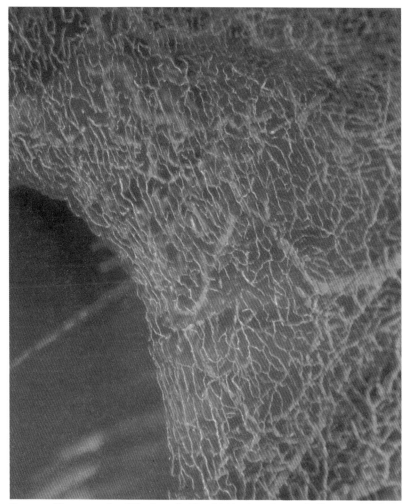

Dense capillary networks of blood vessels. The rich blood supply may facilitate spread of cancer cells.

and are twice as likely to occur in a man as in a woman. Other kidney cancers may be fibrocarcinomas, which are cancers of the renal capsule.

Treatment

Your medical history, your general health, the type and location of the cancer or cancers, and many other factors are considered in determining the treatment needed. Your treatment must be tailored to your individual needs.

Surgery
Surgery is the treatment for most cases of adult kidney cancers that have

not spread to distant areas of the body. Radiation therapy may be used as a supplement to surgery. The surgery procedure used in the treatment of kidney cancers is called radical nephrectomy. The word "nephrectomy" means removal of a kidney.

In the operation called "radical nephrectomy," large portions of the tissue surrounding the kidney and the neighboring lymph nodes are also removed. The remaining kidney will generally be able to do the work normally shared by two.

In recent years, advances in surgical techniques and medical care have made extensive surgery possible for persons previously considered too old for this form of treatment. Today sur-

Kidney cancer   Questions & Answers

What types of tumors may occur in the kidneys?
The kidneys may be the site of primary or secondary malignant tumors. Malignant cells may invade the kidney tissue in leukaemia.

What is a Wilms tumor of the kidneys?
This growth is also called nephroblastoma. It is an adenosarcoma with mixed cancer elements that occurs in the fetus and may lie dormant for years.
The tumor is second only to neuroblastoma in frequency of solid tumors of childhood. The most frequent finding is an abdominal mass, discovered by parent or doctor. Other findings include:
• pain
• blood in the urine
• fever
• loss of appetite
• nausea and vomiting
With early diagnosis and prompt treatment (surgery, medicines and radiation) up to 80 per cent of children with this tumor survive for two years, and more than 50 per cent for more than five years. Prompt surgical intervention is indicated.

What are the symptoms of carcinoma of the kidneys?
Carcinoma of the kidney accounts for 1 to 2 per cent of adult cancers, with two-thirds of cases occurring in males. Blood in the urine is the most common sign, followed by flank pain, a mass that can be felt and high blood pressure.
In many cases the involvement of the interstitial tissue may be quite extensive in the early stages, contrary to minimal involvement of the function of the kidneys. The doctor will always ask the specialist for an X-ray of the chest, since lung metastases occur frequently.
Increasingly, kidney cell carcinoma is being incidentally detected as a result of the increased use of ultrasound and computer scan techniques of the abdomen.

What is the best therapy for cancer of the kidneys?
Radical removal of the kidney and the lymph nodes in the same area offers the best chance for cure. Removal of the primary tumor may rarely cause regression of the carcinoma that has spread elsewhere.
Metastases of kidney cancers are usually resistant to radiotherapy and also the effect of chemotherapeutic agents is minimal. The role of immunotherapy in the treatment of kidney cancer is being investigated.

geons have the help of highly competent teams of nurses, therapists, technicians and other professionals to support patients throughout their postoperative period.

Radiation therapy
Radiation therapy may be used before or after surgery. When radiation is used before nephrectomy, the purpose is to shrink the cancer or change it in other ways that will make it easier for the surgeon to operate. Preoperative radiation requires a waiting period of up to four weeks between irradiation and surgery. When surgery is used after nephrectomy, its purpose is to guard against recurrence of the cancer where the kidney was removed. Radiation also may be used to relieve pain in the bones caused by metastatic cancer. The basic principle of radiation therapy is to focus the beam of radiation on the cancer at doses that will destroy cancerous cells without damaging surrounding normal tissue. Radiation therapy uses X-rays, cobalt, or other sources of ionizing radiation.

Chemotherapy
If you have widespread kidney cancer, your physician may recommend anticancer drugs. Chemotherapy for adult kidney cancer is in an early developmental phase, but drugs have been found effective in some cases. Anticancer drugs kill cancer cells. Because the drug can act on normal cells as well as cancerous ones, your physician must maintain a delicate balance of enough drugs to kill cancer cells without destroying too many healthy cells.
Some anticancer drugs may make you feel sick temporarily, but your physician tries to work out a treatment schedule that disrupts your daily routine as little as possible. The length and frequency of chemotherapy depend upon a number of factors. These include your type of cancer, the type of anticancer drugs prescribed, how long it takes you to respond to these drugs, and how well you tolerate side effects of the drugs. Most chemotherapy are carried out in the outpatient department of a hospital. However, sometimes short periods of hospitalization may be necessary in order to monitor the drug treatment very closely.
After treatment you should continue to have medical examinations regularly so that your physician can check your progress. If rehabilitation is needed, your physician will make recommendations to you. Staff at your hospital and other community organizations are ready to give you many kinds of help.
The social service department of the hospital can advice you about many local organizations that offer help for cancer patients and their families. Many organizations provide services that may include transportation to and from the hospital for medical care, person-to-person assistance, patient group meetings, as well as other services.

Psychological aspects

You may feel many different emotional reactions from the time cancer is diagnosed "Why me?" is a question every patient asks. This is a normal reaction to the diagnosis of cancer. You may also have periods of anxiety or depression. You may need to go through these feelings before you can accept the diagnosis and learn to live with it.

K

Talking to your physician, other health professionals, your family, and even other cancer patients can give you emotional support during and after treatment. Because your physician knows your condition, he is in the best position to answer questions about your individual case.

Making a list of questions before you see the physician can help you remember to ask him everything you want to know. You may be assured that your physician and other health professionals will continue to offer you the best care that medicine has to offer.

Wilms' tumor

This type of tumor is a malignant growth of the kidney, occurring mostly in young children. Almost without exception, cases of kidney cancer in children are Wilms' tumors. Scientists think this type of cancer starts in immature cells that normally become mature kidney cells. Wilms' tumor occur in children from birth to age 15. It is rare in older patients and is very different from adult kidney cancer.

Symptoms
Wilms' tumor has a unique symptom to reveal its presence. The most common sign is a lump in the belly, or a swollen abdomen. Blood in the urine occurs in about 25 per cent of Wilms' tumors when viewed through a microscope.

It may be present constantly, or it may be seen only from time to time. Blood in the urine can also be a sign of disorders other than cancer. But no matter what the cause, blood in the urine should be brought to the attention of a physician.

Like all cancers, kidney cancers in some children can cause the following symptoms:
- low grade fever
- fatigue
- loss of appetite
- weight loss
- anemia

Most Wilms' tumor patients will begin treatment very soon after their visit to the physician, with diagnostic and preoperative tests scheduled on a first-priority basis.

Important questions to ask your physician about kidney cancer

- Is the tumor benign or malignant?
- If it is benign, has it been cured?
- If it is cancer, what kind do I have?
- If it is cancer, has it spread?
- Can you predict how successful an operation or additional treatment would be?
- What are the risks?
- Should I get an opinion from another physician?
- If an operation is done, will I need other treatment?
- How helpful will this be in resuming no-mal activities afterward?
- If I take anticancer drugs, what will the side effects be?
- How often will I need medical checkups?
- What should I tell my relatives and friends?

Treatment
Wilms' tumor is one of some 25 cancers for which treatments have been developed combining surgery, radiation therapy and chemotherapy. Overall, more than 8 out of 10 youngsters with Wilms' tumor can expect to achieve the long-term disease-free status that, for this cancer, is the equivalent of cure.

The way in which the three treatments methods will be used in your child's treatment depends upon his medical history and general health, but above all on the stage of his disease. Radiation therapy, for example, is not used in children under the age of 2 when they have localized tumors.

The medical specialist will discharge your child from the hospital as soon as possible. most often he will be well enough to lead a normal life at home and school. It is important to discuss with the physician just how active the child can be so that he will not be overly limited in his play or attendance at school.

To overprotect a child in this situation may unnecessarily keep him from many of the activities that he enjoys the most. Also, to alter disciplinary measures or to overindulge the child with toys and other gifts may lead to a situation that is unrealistic from the child's point of view.

Children need certain limits and boundaries and are usually happiest when treated in a normal and consistent manner. On the other hand, the physician may feel that the child needs special care and consideration. If these are necessary, the overall program may be briefly explained to him so that he does not view these limitations as punishment.

It should be made clear to the child that if he becomes ill and has to return to the hospital, that it is not because he did anything "bad." The hospital and the child's physician should always be pictured as a source of help. If there are other children in the family, they will want to know what is wrong with their brother or sister. They will sense from the actions of their parents that something serious has happened. It is important to answer their questions honestly.

While younger children may be satisfied with simple explanations, older children will want more detailed information. It is important to indicate that Wilms' tumor is serious and not "just a cold." Children can be assured, however, that the disease is not contagious and that they need not worry about their own health.

When children understand the illness, they are less likely to resent special treatment which is invariably given to the ill child. In addition, older children welcome the opportunity to be taken into the family confidence and will often respond in helpful ways. In fact, the opportunity to participate in some manner in the care of their brother or sister gives them a sense of belonging which tend to promote family solidarity.

K

491

KIDNEY DISEASES

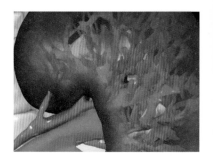

Introduction

The description of kidney, or renal, diseases has for long been plagued by confused classification or vague jargon. Such terms as nephrotic nephritis or type II nephritis may have had some meaning to their originators but now serve only to obscure proper understanding of the major features of renal disease.

Advances in the chemical analysis of urine and the wide use of kidney biopsies have greatly improved the knowledge of the various manifestations of disorders of the structure and/or function of the kidneys.

Signs and symptoms

Kidney disease is often accompanied by fever, weight loss and malaise. The presence of fever together with symptoms of infection of the urinary tract is helpful in evaluating the site of the infection.

Simple infection of the urinary bladder usually does not cause fever, whereas an acute infection of the pelvis of the kidney or an acute infection of the prostate gland produces high fever.

Occasionally, a malignant tumor of the kidney is associated with fever. Weight loss is to be expected in the advanced stages of cancer. The following important symptoms and signs are indicative for disorders and diseases of the kidney and urinary tract:

- changes in urination
- changes in urinary output
- changes in the appearance of urine
- pain
- edema (swelling)
- non-specific symptoms and signs

Changes in urination

Most people urinate four to six times per day, mostly in the daytime. Frequency (medically called frequent micturition) not associated with an increase in the volume of the urine is a symptom of diminution in effective filling capacity of the urinary bladder. A functional decrease, pain and a compelling urgency to urinate may be caused by the following disorders:

- infection
- foreign bodies
- stones, causing injury to the bladder
- tumors, causing damage to the bladder

Involuntary urination may even occur, if voiding is not immediate. Voidings are usually small in volume and the desire to urinate may be felt as

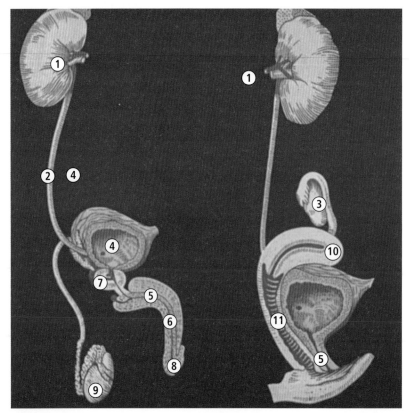

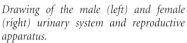

Drawing of the male (left) and female (right) urinary system and reproductive apparatus.
1. Kidneys
2. Ureter
3. Ovary
4. Urinary bladder
5. Penis
6. Urethra
7. Prostate gland
8. Glans penis
9. Testis
10. Uterus
11. Vagina

almost constant urinary tenesmus (ineffectual and painful straining) until the irritation resolves.

Painful urination, or dysuria, suggests irritation or inflammation in the bladder neck or urethra, usually due to bacterial infection. Persistent symptoms in the absence of such infection require careful evaluation of the bladder and urethra. Voiding during the night (nocturia) is an abnormal but non-specific symptom, which may reflect early renal disease with a decrease in concentrating capacity, but is more commonly associated with failure of the heart or liver without evidence of a specific disorder of the kidney. Nocturia may also occur without diseases, for instance, as a result of excessive fluid intake in the late evening. Bedwetting at night (enuresis nocturna) is physiological during the first three or four years of life, but becomes a decreasing problem after that age. Hesitancy, straining and a decrease in the force and caliber of the urinary system are common symptoms of obstructions outside the bladder. In men, these are most commonly associated with obstruction by the prostate gland, less often with stricture in the urethra.

Incontinence, or a loss of urine without warning, is associated with various bladder dysfunctions, as well as injuries sustained during a prostate operation or childbirth. In women, incontinence due to mild physical stress such as coughing, laughing, running or lifting is commonly associated with a cystocele (protrusion of the bladder into the vagina).

Loss of urine due to bladder outlet obstruction or a flaccid bladder may produce overflow incontinence. The passage of intestinal gas in the urine (pneumaturia) is a rare symptom, usually indicative of a fistula (connection) between the urinary tract and the bowel.

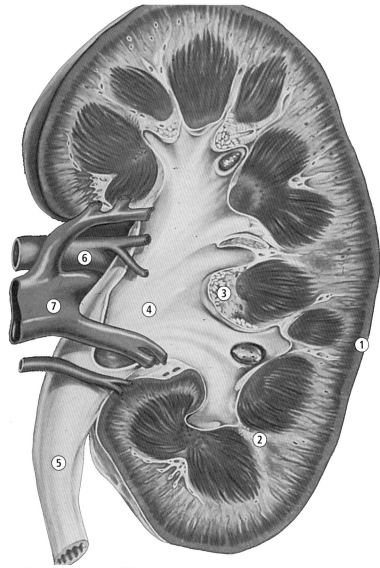

Sagittal view of the cut-open kidney.
1. Cortex
2. Medulla
3. Pyramid
4. Pelvis
5. Ureter
6. Renal artery
7. Renal vein

Changes in urinary output

Normally, adults void between 700 and 2000 ml daily. Impairment in the concentrating capacity of the kidneys may occur with many forms of kidney diseases and may produce a daily volume of more than 2500 ml, a condition called polyuria. Oliguria, a daily urine volume of less than 500 mL per day, tends to be an acute condition that may be due to decreased renal perfusion, outlet obstruction of the urethra or bladder, or primary diseases of the kidneys.

Anuria, a daily urine volume of less than 100 mL, is most often associated with uraemia (when toxic wastes usually excreted accumulate in the blood) and may signal acute renal failure or the end stage of chronic progressive renal insufficiency.

Appearance of urine

Urine may be clear when mostly water is being voided or may be a deep yel-

Kidney diseases   Questions & Answers

What is meant by the urinary apparatus?

The organs forming the urinary apparatus are the kidneys that produce the urine; the ureters that convey the urine to the bladder; the urinary bladder that serves as a reservoir for the urine and from which a single duct, the urethra, the urine is carried to the exterior.

Where are the kidneys located?

The kidneys are paired organs in the back part of the abdomen, on each side of the vertebral column (spine) immediately behind the peritoneum (serious membrane that covers the abdominal wall and envelops most of the abdominal organs). The right kidney is normally lower than the left, probably because of the presence of the liver on the right side.

How does a kidney look like?

Each kidney is somewhat bean-shaped and is slightly tilted. The upper extremity of the kidney is usually larger than the lower extremity, and is about 1 cm nearer to the spine. The part of the kidney nearest the side of the trunk (lateral border) is narrow and convex, while the part closest to the spine (medial border) is concave and, within its middle third, has a slit-like aperture, the hilus.
This is the orifice of a cavity called renal sinus that is about 2.5 cm in depth and is occupied by the pelvis and calyces (sing. = calyx) of the kidney, by the blood vessels and nerves, and by small amounts of fat tissue. Except for the sinus, the kidneys are solid organs, moderately elastic and, because of the high number of blood vessels, of a dark, reddish-brown colour.

How are the kidneys fixed in the abdomen?

The surface of the kidney is covered with a thin but strong fibrous capsule. It may be peeled off readily from a healthy kidney, except at the bottom of the sinus, where it is adherent to the blood vessels entering the kidney substance.
External to the capsule is a quantity of fat tissue - the adipose capsule - that completely covers the organ. The peritoneum that covers the front of the adipose capsule has usually been regarded as the principal means of fixation of the kidney, but in reality this is accomplished by means of a special fascia. A fascia is a fibrous connective tissue that supports soft organs and sheaths structures such as muscles.

Where are the kidneys located in the abdominal cavity?

The kidneys lie in the lumbar (lower back) region. Its vertical extent may be said to correspond to the last thoracic and upper two lumbar vertebrae of the spine, the right lying from 8 to 12 mm lower than the left in most cases; exceptions to this rule, however, are not infrequent.
The back surface of the kidney rests upon the back part of the abdominal wall, overlying the 11th and 12th ribs and the tips of the transverse processes of the first, second and, occasionally, the third lumbar vertebrae.

Are there differences between the kidneys of men and women?

There is considerable variation in the relation of the kidneys to ribs and vertebrae. In women, the kidneys are usually one-half vertebra lower; moreover they are normally lower on inspiration (breathing in) than on expiration (breathing out), and while standing than while lying down.
In males, the left kidney may reach the lower border of the tenth rib while the right kidney seldom extends above the 11th rib. In females, the top of the left kidney usually lies slightly above the 11th rib while the right barely reaches its lower border.
The upper portion of the back of the kidney rests on the diaphragm, and is near a number of muscles in the back portion of the abdomen, such as the psoas major, the quadratus lumborum and the tendon of the transverse abdominal muscle.

low color due to the presence of chromogens, such as urobilin, when maximally concentrated. If the excretion of food pigments (usually red) or drugs (brown, black, blue, green or red) can be excluded, colors other than yellow suggest the presence of diseases such as:

- hematuria (blood in the urine)
- myoglobinuria (presence of the muscle protein myoglobin in the urine)
- pyuria (presence of pus in the urine)
- porphyria (presence of porphyrins in the urine)
- melanoma (tumor consisting of melanin-containing cells).

Urine frequently appears cloudy, suggesting pyuria due to a urinary tract inflammation, but this is more commonly due to precipitated phosphate salts in an alkaline urine.
Hematuria can produce red to brown discoloration depending on the amount of blood present and the acidity of the urine. Slight hematuria may cause no discoloration and may only be detected by chemical testing or microscopic examination.
When hematuria is noted, the presence or absence of pain related to the urinary system is important. Hematuria without pain is usually due to disorders of the kidneys, urinary bladder or prostate gland.

Pain

Pain related to disease of the kidney usually occurs in the flank or in the back between the 12th rib and the top of the ilium (haunch bone). The stretching of the pain-sensitive capsule of the kidney is the probable cause and may occur in any condition producing swelling of the kidney tissue.
There is often marked tenderness over the kidney in the costovertebral angle formed by the 12th rib and the lumbar (lower back) spine. Inflammation or distention of the pelvis of the kidney or ureter causes pain in the flank, with radiation into the iliac fossa (lower corner of the abdomen) and often into the upper thigh, testicle or labium.
The pain is intermittent but does not completely remit between waves of colic. The most common cause of

K

bladder pain is a bacterial infection of the bladder, and the discomfort is commonly above the pubic bone.

Acute urinary retention causes agonizing pain in the same area, but chronic urinary retention due to obstruction of the neck of the urinary bladder usually causes little discomfort.

Edema

Edema usually represents excessive amounts of water and sodium due to abnormal excretion, but it may be caused by disorders of the heart, liver or kidneys. Initially, the problem is evident only by an increase in weight, but, later, it becomes obvious to the eye.

Edema associated with disease of the kidney may be noted first as puffiness in the face rather than swelling in dependent or lower parts of the body, but this characteristic is neither essential nor specific.

If fluid retention continues, generalized oedema with fluid transudates (effusions) in the pleural and peritoneal cavities may be seen. It is most frequently associated with continuous, heavy proteinuria (presence of excessive amounts of proteins in the urine).

Diagnostic procedures

The major diagnostic procedures are:
- analysis of the urine
- X-rays and scans
- biopsy of the kidney
- cytology of urine

Analysis of the urine

The chemical and structural analysis of urine (also called urinalysis) is the best guide to diseases of the kidney and urinary tract. It includes a qualitative analysis for the presence of
- protein
- glucose
- ketones
- blood
- nitrites
- urinary pH
- sediments

■ Protein

The presence of protein in the urine (proteinuria) can be determined with

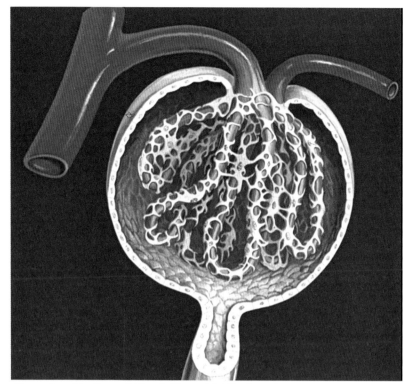

Glomerulus with afferent (left) and efferent right) blood vessel.

the dipstick method. The major mechanisms producing proteins in the urine are:
- elevated plasma concentrations of normal or abnormal proteins;
- increased secretion by the tubular cells of the kidney;
- decreased resorption by the tubular cells of normal filtered proteins;
- an increase of filtered proteins caused by altered permeability of the capillaries in the glomerulus.

In most adults with protein in their urine, the abnormality is first observed as an isolated finding during a routine physical examination in a someone without symptoms who appears healthy and exhibits no evidence of systemic or kidney disease.

■ Glucose

The presence of glucose in the urine - glucosuria - can also be determined by dip-sticks. The most common cause of glucosuria is hyperglycemia (high blood sugar, or diabetic coma) with normal transport of glucose in the kidneys.

■ Ketones

The dipstick method is much more sensitive to aceto-acetic acid than to acetone. The presence of ketones in the urine (ketonuria) offers clues to the causes of metabolic acidosis. It is present in starvation, uncontrolled diabetes and, occasionally, in alcohol intoxication. It is not specific for intrinsic diseases of the urinary system.

■ Blood

The presence of blood in the urine (hematuria) can also be detected by dipsticks, as this method is sensitive to free hemoglobin and to myoglobin, the protein that provides the red color in muscle. The presence of hemoglobin or myoglobin in the urine is an important clue to the presence of acute failure of the kidney function.

■ Nitrites

The presence of nitrites in the urine (nitrituria) is determined by a dipstick test. Normally, no detectable nitrite is present. However, when there is a significant amount of bacte-

Kidney diseases   Questions & Answers

What are the relations of the kidneys to the intestines?
The front part of the kidneys is close to the ascending and descending parts of the large intestine and to the duodenum and pancreas.
Just as there may be variation in the position of the kidneys, so too there may be considerable variation in the extent to which they are in relation to these various structures.
This is especially true for the ascending and descending parts of the large intestine.
The top of each kidney is partially crowned by an adrenal gland that also encroaches upon the front part and the medial border, and is fixed to the capsule of the kidney by fibers.
The bottom of the right kidney lies in contact with the ascending part of the large intestine, the jejunum and the duodenum, while the left is near to the descending part of the large intestine and the jejunum.

How does kidney tissue looks under the microscope?
A cross-section through the kidney shows its substance to be composed of an internal medulla (marrow) and an external cortex (bark).
The medulla consists of a variable number (8 to 18) of conical segments called pyramids, the tops of which project into the bottom or sides of the sinus of the kidney and are received into the various minor calyces of the pelvis, while their bases are turned towards the surface, but are separated from it and from each other by the cortex.
The pyramids are smooth and somewhat glistening in cross-section and are marked with delicate stripes that converge from the base to the apex and indicate the course of the tubules of the kidney.

What is the significance of a nephron for the functioning of the kidney?
Principally, the basic functional unit of the kidney is the nephron, a long tubular structure made up of successive segments of diverse structure and transport functions.
Each nephron commences in a spherical Bowman's capsule, the wall of which covers a small glomerulus of blood vessels, comprising an afferent arteriole (through which blood flows into the capsule) and an efferent arteriole (through which blood leaves the capsule).
Together the glomerulus and the capsule form what is termed a kidney corpuscle.
Arising from each capsule is the proximal convoluted tubule, which passes into a straight tubule (Henle's loop), which has an ascending and a descending portion.
The tubule than becomes convoluted again (distal convoluted tubule), finally to descend into the pyramid where it unites with other collecting tubules and, as a papillary duct, opens in the calyx at the summit of a papilla.

What are the major functions of the kidneys?
The kidneys are concerned in a number of activities, which include:
▲ the removal of nitrogenous waste, mostly in the form of urea
▲ the maintenance of electrolyte balance
▲ the maintenance of water balance
▲ the regulation of the acid-base balance
In addition, a number of chemical substances (acting as hormones) are released into the blood. Urine is formed in the kidneys as an aqueous solution containing metabolic waste products, foreign substances and water-soluble constituents of the body in quantities depending upon homeostatic needs - that is, the balance of water and other essential substances in the body.

ria in the urine, the test will be positive in 80 per cent of cases when the urine has been retained for at least five hours in the bladder, because enzymes from the bacteria can produce nitrites.
Thus, a positive test is a reliable index of significant bacteriuria (presence of bacteria in the urine). However, a negative test should never be interpreted as indicating the absence of bacteriuria.

■ Urinary pH
Here also a dipstick method is used, to discover the acidity or alkalinity of the urine. Although this test is routinely done, it neither identifies nor excludes those with a disease of the urinary system.

■ Sediment
Normal urine contains a small number of cells and other elements shed from the whole length of the urinary system. With disease, these cells are increased and may help to localize the site and type of injury. Particles of various elements in urine can be separated and concentrated by forcing urine through a membrane filter.
The following elements may be found:
▲ Cells from blood: erythrocytes, leukocytes.
▲ Cells from genito-urinary system: epithelial cells, sperm.
▲ Foreign cells: bacteria, fungi, parasites, malignant cells.
▲ Crystals: oxalate, phosphate, uric acid, various drugs.
The finding of casts - cylindrical masses of mucoprotein in which cellular elements, protein or fat droplets may be entrapped - in urine sediment is most important in distinguishing primary kidney disease from diseases of the lower urinary tract.

■ Measurement of kidney function
Functional tests of the kidney are useful in evaluating the severity of kidney disease and in following its progress.

■ X-rays and scans
A simple X-ray or scan of the abdomen is performed first to demonstrate the size and location of the kidneys. However, the outline of the kidneys can be obscured by bowel

content, hematoma (collection of blood) or abscess, but this difficulty can be overcome by tomography, where the X-ray tube is moved in such a way that only structures in a selected plane cast clear shadows.

Congenital absence of a kidney may be suggested, and if both kidneys are unusually large, polycystic kidney disease, tumors or hydronephrosis may be present.

■ *Biopsy of the kidney*
A biopsy is the removal and examination, usually microscopic, of tissue from the living body, performed to establish precise diagnosis.
Biopsy of kidney tissue is performed for four reasons:
▲ to help establish a diagnosis;
▲ to help estimate prognosis and the potential reversibility or progression of the lesion of the kidney;
▲ to estimate the value of therapeutic methods;
▲ to determine the natural history of diseases of the kidney.
There are two methods - the open surgical and the percutaneous - the latter being much more common. For the percutaneous method, the patient is sedated, and the kidney is visualized by ultrasound methods.

■ *Cytology of urine*
This method - in which cells in the urine are microscopically examined - is useful for possible urinary tract tumors in high-risk populations such as industrial dye workers and those with painless hematuria.
A sample from the second urination of the morning is best, since the cells in the initial morning specimen often show extensive deterioration.

Glomerular diseases

The glomerular diseases of the kidney are a group of diverse conditions including, but not limited to, glomerulonephritis, in which the disease process appears mainly to affect the glomeruli of the kidney.
Due to the limited number of ways that a tissue can respond to injury and that these injuries can be expressed as symptoms and signs, there are structural, functional and clinical similari-

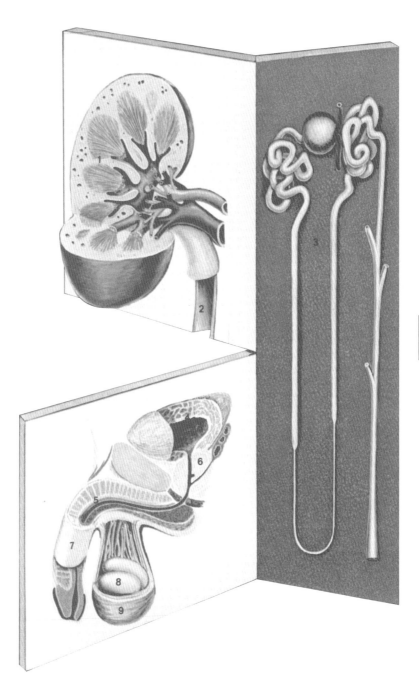

Schematic drawing of the male urogenital system.
Upper left: longitudinal section of the kidney.
Upper right: basic unit of the kidney, the nephron.
Below: urinary bladder and the reproductive system.
The urinary system includes the organs that convert the soluble waste products of cellular metabolism into urine and eliminate the urine from the body. These organs are two kidneys, two ureters, the urinary bladder, and the urethra.
1. Kidney; 2. ureter; 3. nephron; 4. bladder; 5. urethra; 6. prostate gland; 7. penis; 8. testis; 6. scrotum.

Kidney diseases   Questions & Answers

What are general symptoms of kidney disease?

Disease of the kidney is often accompanied by fever, weight loss and malaise. The presence of fever together with symptoms of infection of the urinary tract is helpful for the doctor in evaluating the site of the infection.

Simple infection of the urinary bladder usually does not cause fever, whereas an acute infection of the pelvis of the kidney or an acute infection of the prostate gland produces high fever.

The following important symptoms and signs are indicative for disorders and diseases of the kidney and urinary tract:

- changes in urination
- changes in urinary output
- changes in the appearance of urine
- pain and edema
- non-specific symptoms and signs

How can the diagnosis of a urinary tract disorder be confirmed?

The diagnosis of urinary tract disorders may be confirmed by analysis of the urine (urinalysis), or with radiographic methods, including ultrasonography and computer scans. In a small number of cases a biopsy may be taken from the kidney in order to clarify the findings of other methods.

What is the cause of frequent urination or micturition?

Most people void about four to six times per day, mostly in the daytime. Frequent urination or micturition, not associated with an increase in urine volume, is a symptom of lessened effective filling capacity of the bladder. A functional decrease, pain and a compelling urgency to urinate may be caused by the following disorders:

- infection
- foreign bodies
- stones, causing injury to the mucous membrane lining of the bladder
- tumors causing damage to the inner surface of the urinary bladder

Involuntary urination may occur if voiding is not immediate. Voidings usually are small in volume and the desire to urinate may be felt as almost constant painful straining (urinary tenesmus) until the irritative process resolves.

What is the major cause of painful urination?

Painful urination (dysuria) suggests irritation or inflammation in the bladder neck or urethra, usually due to bacterial infection.

What is the major cause of voiding urine during the night?

Voiding urine during the night (nocturia) is an abnormal, but non-specific, symptom, which may reflect early kidney disease with a decrease in concentrating capacity but is sometimes associated with heart and liver failure without evidence of a real kidney disease.

Nocturia may also occur without disease; for instance, as a result of excessive fluid intake in the late evening or from retention of urine secondary to obstruction in the region of the bladder neck, as in hypertrophy (overgrowth) of the prostate gland.

What is a normal urinary output?

Normally, adults void between 700 and 2000 mL daily. Impairment in kidney concentration capacity may occur in many forms of kidney disease and may cause polyuria (a daily volume of more than 2500 mL urine per day).

Oliguria (less than 500 mL urine per day) tends to be acute and may be due to decreased kidney perfusion or obstruction of the outlet of the ureter or bladder. Persistent anuria (less than 100 mL urine per day) is always associated with the presence of excessive amounts of urea in the blood (uremia).

ties within the group. Clear-cut differentiation may be impossible.

Examination of kidney biopsies has shown a wide variety of glomerular lesions, especially when the biopsy has been examined by electronmicroscopy or by fluorescent microscopy.

Unfortunately, this variation in the appearances of the glomeruli has led to a confusion of terms, which has not contributed to clear understanding of these modern developments.

The glomerulus, like many other tissues in the body, can only react to injury in a limited number of ways. The major changes seen in biopsies in various forms of disorders of the kidney are:

▲ an increase in the number of capillary epithelial or endothelial cells lining the capsule (so-called proliferative glomerulonephritis);

▲ an increase in the mesangial cells between the capillary loops;

▲ an increase in the thickness or other abnormality of the capillary basement membrane (so-called membranous nephropathy);

▲ a combination of both of these variables (membranoproliferative nephritis);

▲ normal glomerular appearance on light microscopy and fluorescent microscopy with abnormality of the epithelial cell foot processes on electronmicroscopy (so-called minimal change disease or lipoid nephrosis).

All these lesions can result in the appearance of proteins in the urine but no other symptoms, or can lead to heavy protein loss and the nephrotic syndrome. On the basis of the above mentioned data, the following disease entities can be distinguished:

- glomerular disease of acute onset
- rapidly progressive glomerular disease
- slowly progressive glomerular disease
- nephrotic syndrome

Tubulo-interstitial disorders

Abnormalities of the tubules and the tissues that surround them - the interstitial tissue - occur in all kidney diseases. There may be an acute or

K

chronic condition or a disease, and there may also be a kidney disorder characterized by toxic damage to the tubules.

Acute tubulo-interstitial nephritis

This is a syndrome of acute renal failure most commonly due to hypersensitivity to a drug affecting the tubules and interstitial tissue. This disorder was previously often associated with severe systemic infections, but with the advent of antibiotics, the dominant cause now is a reaction to drugs. Among the most commonly incriminated are methicillin, anticonvulsants, penicillin, ampicillin, rifampicin and diuretics. The initial presentation may be that of acute failure of the kidney, with or without decreased urinary output.

Helpful clinical clues include a medical history of exposure to suspect drugs and signs of hypersensitivity, such as fever, skin rash and eosinophilia (abnormal increase of a certain type of white blood cell).

The urine usually contains proteins, and the kidneys are often large because of oedema. The interval between exposure to the drug and development of kidney damage varies between five days and five weeks.

If severe, prolonged oliguria (minimal urination) is present, patients are treated for acute failure of the kidneys. On withdrawal of the offending drug, they usually recover as far as the function of the kidney is concerned but some irreversible cases have been reported.

Chronic tubulo-interstitial nephropathy

This term includes all those chronic kidney disorders in which generalized or localized changes in the tubules or interstitial tissues predominate over the lesions in the glomeruli or blood vessels.

Although the causes and pathological changes are variable, certain features are consistent. Toxins, metabolic diseases and inherited disorders may all cause this disease.

The kidneys are small and, generally, symptoms indicating progression of kidney disease are absent, and edema, excessive loss of protein in the urine and presence of blood in the urine do

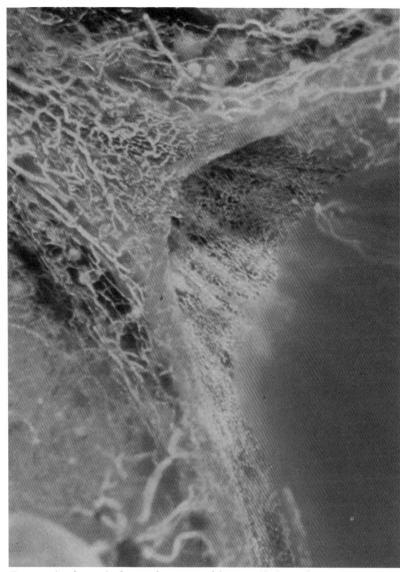

Degenerative changes in the vascular pattern of the pyramids due to chronic glomerular disease.

not appear in the early stages. High blood pressure is a common finding. Additional signs and symptoms are:

· increased amount of urine
· acidosis due to tubular disorders
· inability to conserve sodium

These functional defects result from a loss of function of the tubules and interstitial tissue.

Toxic syndromes of the kidney

This refers to any functional or structural change in the kidney produced by a drug or a chemical or biological agent that is ingested, injected, inhaled or absorbed.

General measures include:
▲ withdrawal of the offending agent;
▲ induction of vomiting;
▲ enhancing excretion while function remains;
▲ direct removal of the agent from the bloodstream by the most efficient method.

Kidney infections

Infections usually occur when the offending micro-organism ascends

K

Kidney diseases Questions & Answers

What treatment methods are available for severe failure of the kidneys?
When disease causes failure of the kidneys, or otherwise compromises the ability of the kidneys to remove toxic materials from the blood and maintain fluid, electrolyte, and acid-base balance, a number of special treatment methods can be used:
- dialysis
- hemoperfusion
- hemofiltration
- transplantation

These measures may be required urgently in acute failure of the kidneys, as in certain types of poisoning, or when the kidneys of a person with progressive disease are unable to work well enough to maintain health at an acceptable level.

What is dialysis of the blood for severe kidney diseases?
Dialysis is the process of separating elements in a solution by diffusing it across a semi-permeable membrane. Either the person's own peritoneum (the membrane lining the abdominal cavity) or a machine using a synthetic semi-permeable membrane such as cellophane may be used. These procedures are called peritoneal dialysis and hemodialysis, respectively.
Dialysis requires special dietary care and medications, as well as awareness and support regarding the psychological aspects of dialysis. Generally, patients eat a protein-restricted diet containing 1 to 1.2 g or protein per kilogram of body weight per day. This diet generally emphasizes, but is not limited to, high biological value proteins, and also contains only 2 g sodium and 2 g potassium.

What types of maintenance dialysis programs are available for severe kidney diseases?
Five types of maintenance dialysis programs are available for management of chronic kidney failure:
- home hemodialysis;
- home peritoneal dialysis
- self-care (performed at a kidney dialysis center by patients themselves, with limited supervision)
- passive-care analysis
- continuous ambulatory peritoneal dialysis

Home dialysis is generally the least expensive and promotes the greatest independence. About 50 per cent of kidney patients are suitable candidates for home dialysis.

What treatment methods are available for children with failure of the kidneys?
A number of special treatment methods can be used:- dialysis;
- hemoperfusion
- hemofiltration
- transplantation

These measures may be required urgently in acute failure of the kidneys, as in certain types of poisoning, or when the kidneys of a person with progressive disease are unable to work well enough to maintain health at an acceptable level.

What is the significance of dialysis?
Dialysis is the process of separating elements in a solution by diffusing it across a semi-permeable membrane. Either the person's own peritoneum (the membrane lining the abdominal cavity) or a machine using a synthetic semi-permeable membrane such as cellophane may be used. Dialysis will restore the imbalance of water and electrolytes in the body.

the urethra. Obstruction (strictures, stones, tumors, hypertrophy of the prostate gland) makes a person more predisposed to develop an infection. The role of obstruction in predisposing to infection cannot be overemphasized: obstruction causes stasis (when urine ceases to flow and becomes stagnant), stasis invites bacterial invasion and infection is established.

Acute bacterial pyelonephritis
Pyelonephritis is especially likely in females during childhood or pregnancy, and after catheterization of the urethra, but is uncommon in males free from urinary tract abnormalities. Coli bacilli (Escherichia coli) are the most common bacteria and account for about 85 per cent of uncomplicated infections. Spread via the bloodstream to the kidney may occur from any systemic infection but is commonest with staphylococci in the blood. Those subjected to instrumentation or with catheters in place, or who become infected while in hospital, are on chronic antibiotic therapy or are being treated with corticosteroids are particularly likely to have unusual micro-organisms set up colonies in their urinary tracts.
Typically, the onset of this disease is rapid and characterized by the following signs and symptoms:
- chills
- fever
- flank pain
- nausea and vomiting

Bladder irritation from infected urine may result in frequency and urgency. The diagnosis is established on the basis of the signs and symptoms and analysis of the urine.
Antibiotics will be instituted as soon as the doctor has established the diagnosis; thorough analysis of the urine and even a culture of a urine sample is usually necessary. Treatment should be continued for a minimum of 10 to 14 days and, in some instances, for four weeks. Urine culture should be repeated during therapy and after its completion. If obstruction is present, surgery may be required.

Chronic bacterial pyelonephritis
This is a chronic, patchy infection of the kidney, often occurring in both of

them at the same time, that produces severe damage to the kidney tissues.

The disorder causes complete failure of the kidneys in about 10 to 15 per cent of those who are treated by dialysis or transplantation.

Clinical clues, such as fever and flank or abdominal pain, are often vague and inconsistent. A medical history of urinary tract infection and recurrent pyelonephritis and a typical pattern of dysfunction of the kidneys occasionally occurs and strongly suggests the diagnosis.

There is no protein in the urine at first, and it is only minimal or intermittent until scarring of the kidneys is far advanced. Even than proteinuria is usually less than 3 g per day.

The course of the disease is extremely variable but, typically, it progresses extremely slowly, with sufferers having adequate function of the kidneys for 20 years or more after the onset.

Two important factors influence the outcome of the disorder: if there is recurrent pyelonephritis, and which type of urinary obstruction there is.

Frequent exacerbations of acute pyelonephritis, even though controlled, usually produce some further deterioration of the structure and function of the kidney.

Continued obstruction acts both by predisposing to or perpetuating infection of the kidneys, and by increasing the pelvic pressure, which damages the kidney directly. The most important therapeutic measures are the elimination of obstruction and eradication of bacteria in the urine.

Where obstruction cannot be eliminated and recurrent infections are common, the specialist will propose long-term antibiotic therapy. The use of methenamine salts (commonly prescribed for chronic and recurrent urinary infections) will be avoided because they are not effective in suppressing bacterial infections in the kidney.

In the absence of demonstrable obstruction or dysfunction of the kidneys, it has not been clearly established that the presence of non-symptom-producing bacteria in the urine is deleterious.

Therefore, according to the opinion of kidney specialists, it is nowadays not indicated to repeat courses of antibi-

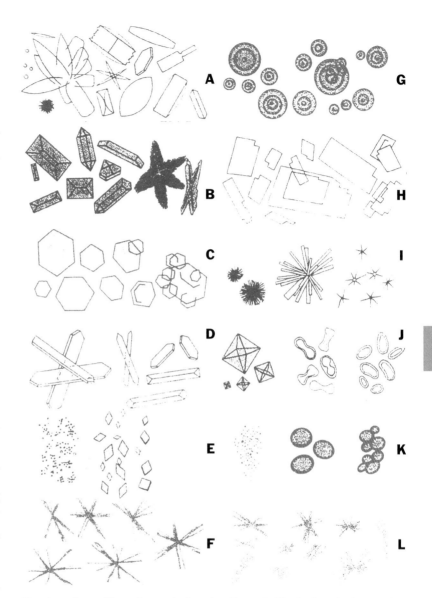

Drawings of crystalline sediments in the urine. Except for blood cells and microorganisms, crystals of various kinds may be found in the urine.
A. uric acid; B. ammonium magnesium phosphate; C. cysteine; D. hippuric acid; E. bilirubin; F. tyrosine;
G. leucine; H. cholesterol; I. calcium oxalate; J. calcium phosphate; K. urate; L. sulphonamide.

otics or immunosuppressive drugs. If uraemia or high blood pressure are appropriate treatments will be started.

Vascular disease

Five major vascular diseases produce kidney syndromes:
- malignant hypertension
- renal infarction
- athero-embolic renal disease
- renal cortical necrosis
- renal veinous thrombosis

Malignant hypertension

Most of these diseases appear as accelerated cardiovascular disease in the course of high blood pressure of unknown origin, especially in untreated cases. Although no more than 1 per cent of individuals with high blood pressure of unknown origin have been reported to develop this complication, the incidence is not exactly known.

However, about 20 per cent of those with this condition have hypertension in which the kidneys play a major role. The peak incidence in men occurs during their 40s and 50s, and in women about a decade earlier.

Those affected have symptoms representing varying degrees of involvement of the brain, the heart and the kidneys. Headaches, blurring of vision, and varying degrees of numbness are usually present at some time during the disease. Functional disturbance of the kidneys also varies.

The urinary findings include:
- protein in the urine
- blood in the urine
- casts of red blood corpuscles
- problems in the clotting of blood
- high levels of renin and aldosterone in the blood

Untreated sufferers die in a relatively short period of time - about 50 per cent within six months, and most of the remainder within one year. Death usually results from uraemia (40 per cent), stroke (40 per cent) or heart attack (15 per cent).

Although some have spontaneous remissions, aggressive lowering of the blood pressure and management of the failure of the kidney function significantly reduce the effects of the condition. With therapy, fewer die, especially from the failure of the kidney function and brain disease, but the proportion developing heart attack increases.

Those without significant failure of kidney function improve most, and if the high blood pressure can be reduced satisfactorily with dietary and drug therapy, most will be alive after three to five years.

Renal infarction

Renal infarction (i.e. death of kidney tissue due to lack of blood) is caused by blockage (occlusion) of an artery or vein. Occlusion of the renal artery is most frequently due to embolism (e.g. blood clot), narrowing as the

result of atherosclerosis, and injury. Small occlusions of the renal artery frequently occur without any symptoms or signs. Typically, however, a steady, aching pain in the flank develops that becomes concentrated in the affected kidney area. Fever, nausea and vomiting may occur.

When infarction is a result of occlusion of an artery, the kidney becomes small and cannot be felt by the doctor. However, with thrombosis of the renal veins, the kidney is usually tender and enlarged enough to be felt by the doctor.

When renal infarction is suspected, the doctor will ask the specialist for X-rays. A combination of medical history (atrial fibrillation, recent heart attack or injury), symptoms and signs, virtual absence of excretory function on the involved side, and a normal collecting system is strong evidence for renal infarction.

Arteriography, CT-scan or MRI-scan can provide a is definite diagnosis, but is done only if a surgical attempt to relieve the obstruction is being considered.

Although surgical removal of the embolus may cause reversal of the functional disturbance of the kidney up to six weeks after the occurrence of the embolus, conservative medical therapy with anti-coagulant drugs is usually indicated, especially in those with serious heart disease.

Athero-embolic renal disease

This condition is defined as a clinical syndrome involving either rapid deterioration of kidney function or a more slowly progressive kidney failure, depending on the amount of atheromatous material obstructing the renal arteries.

This syndrome may occur spontaneously or as a result of vascular surgery or arteriography, when atheromatous plaque from an artery breaks off to form an embolus and travels via the bloodstream to block a renal artery.

In those with severe erosive disease of the main artery of the body - the aorta - the frequency of this disease is approximately 15 to 30 per cent; in those with mild atherosclerosis, peripheral embolism (i.e. occurring on the outer parts of the body) has an

incidence of only about 1 per cent. Emboli in the kidney occur most commonly in the elderly and the incidence increases with age. Most people with this disorder and failure of the kidney function have high blood pressure.

Signs of peripheral embolism such as painful muscle nodules or overt gangrene strongly suggest the diagnosis, but these are not often present. There are no distinctive laboratory findings or abnormalities of the urine sediment. Diagnosis is confirmed only by biopsy of the kidney.

No treatment reverses the failure of the kidney function. Those with athero-embolic renal disease and advanced insufficiency of the kidney do not regain normal kidney function even transiently. Surgical experience involving severe atherosclerosis of the aorta has shown that careful technique can minimize the likelihood of athero-embolism of the renal arteries.

Renal cortical necrosis

This condition is defined as a form of arterial infarction (changes in tissue due to lack of blood because of a blocked artery), characterized by necrosis (tissue death) of part of the cortex of the kidney while sparing the medulla.

This disease can occur at any age; for example, about 10 per cent occurs in infancy and childhood. Over 50 per cent of reported cases are associated with childbirth; the next most common association is bacterial sepsis, in which the body becomes poisoned as a result of a bacterial infection. In children, causes include infections, dehydration, shock and hemolysis (blood breakdown).

Fever and leucocytosis (increase of a certain type of white blood cell that indicates a weakness in the body's resistance) are common even in the absence of sepsis. The urine contains much protein and red blood corpuscles. In the early stages, mildly raised blood pressure, or even lowered blood pressure, is common.

However, in surviving patients who regain some residual kidney function, accelerated or malignant high blood pressure is typical. Treatment does not differ from other forms of acute kidney failure, although more problems may be encountered because of the prolonged lack of urine production and the precipitating causes.

All appropriate means, including maintenance dialysis, are used to allow recovery of any residual function.

After several months, a few may regain enough function to discontinue maintenance dialysis, but for the majority, chronic dialysis or kidney transplantation is the usual solution.

Renal vein thrombosis

Conditions associated with renal vein thrombosis, in which the renal vein becomes blocked by a blood clot, are:

▲ retroperitoneal conditions, such as abscess, tumor, injury;
▲ thrombo-embolic disease;
▲ depletion of the extracellular volume (i.e. the amount of fluid bathing the cells), mostly in infants;
▲ various degenerative conditions of the kidneys (amyloidosis, systemic lupus erythematosus, diabetes).

The frequency of this disease is difficult to determine because, aside from the acute forms usually seen in children, most cases induce only mild symptoms that often go unnoticed. Clinically, two different pictures are seen. With children, the signs and symptoms are:

• loin pain
• blood in the urine
• oliguria (drastically reduced urination)
• edema
• leucocytosis
• kidney failure

Treatment

In the course of the descriptions of the various diseases, several therapeutic measures (drugs, diet, fluid) have already been discussed.

When disease causes failure of the kidneys, or otherwise compromises the ability of the kidneys to remove toxic materials from the blood and maintain fluid, electrolyte and acid-base balance, a number of special therapeutic methods can be used:

• dialysis
• hemoperfusion
• hemofiltration
• transplantation

These measures may be required urgently in acute failure of the kidneys, as in certain types of poisoning, or when the kidneys of a person with progressive disease are unable to work well enough to maintain health at an acceptable level.

Dialysis

Dialysis is defined as the process of separating elements in a solution by diffusing it across a semi-permeable membrane.

Either the person's own peritoneum (the membrane lining the abdominal cavity) or a machine using a synthetic semi-permeable membrane such as cellophane may be used.

These procedures are called peritoneal dialysis and hemodialysis, respectively. Dialysis requires special dietary care and medications, as well as awareness and support regarding the psychological aspects of dialysis.

Generally, patients eat a protein-restricted diet containing 1 to 1.2 g of protein per kilogram of body weight per day. This diet generally emphasizes, but is not limited to, high biological value proteins, and also contains only 2 g sodium and 2 g potassium.

Limitation of phosphorus intake may also be required. Daily fluid intake is limited to 500 to 1000 cc plus measured urinary output, and must be monitored by weight gain.

Hemoperfusion and hemofiltration

In hemoperfusion (perfusion of blood through a device that absorbs waste products instead of a hemodialyser), the absorbent materials (called sorbents) employed are either activated coal or resin beads.

This technique is particularly useful in the treatment of drug overdose, especially where the drug involved is poorly soluble in water, and has also been used to treat liver failure and as an adjunct in treating uraemia.

While these sorbents are effective in removing solutes such as potassium, creatinine and uric acid from uraemic blood, urea removal remains a problem.

Hemofiltration, a similar technique used in uraemia, differs from hemodialysis in that it uses convective transport of solutes through ultrafiltration across the membrane rather than diffusion.

The theoretical rationale is that convective transport is more effective than diffuse transport.

The principle clinical advantage is better control of high blood pressure. Although this technique is very expensive, it can sustain the life of an uraemic patient as the sole form of therapy.

Transplantation

Despite surgical techniques making transplantation of almost any tissue feasible, the clinical use of transplantation to remedy disease is still limited for most organ systems.

The greatest obstacle is the rejection reaction, which generally destroys the tissue shortly after transplantation (except in special circumstances, such as corneal grafts or transplants between identical twins).

Nevertheless, with improved understanding of immune mechanisms and methods for preventing rejection, organ transplantation may save many people with otherwise fatal diseases.

Since long-term success can be expected in 75 to 90 per cent of kidney transplants, all those with terminal renal failure will be considered for transplantation except those at risk from another life-threatening condition.

In addition, rehabilitation following successful transplantation is generally much more complete than that achieved with hemodialysis, not only because of the freedom from the requirement of prolonged treatment three times weekly but also because of the beneficial metabolic functions of the kidney.

Over 95 per cent of those who have received a transplant from a living relative survive for one year, with approximately 75 to 80 per cent of these transplanted kidneys still functioning. Subsequently, an annual patient or graft loss of 3 to 5 per cent is observed.

K

KIDNEY FAILURE

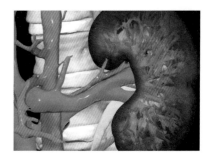

Introduction

Kidney disease is often accompanied by fever, weight loss and malaise. The presence of fever together with symptoms of infection of the urinary tract is helpful in evaluating the site of the infection. Simple infection of the urinary bladder usually does not cause fever, whereas an acute infection of the pelvis of the kidney or an acute infection of the prostate gland produces high fever. Occasionally, a malignant tumor of the kidney is associated with fever. Weight loss is to be expected in the advanced stages of cancer. The following important symptoms and signs are indicative for disorders and diseases of the kidney and urinary tract:

Major causes of acute

Insufficient blood supply to the kidneys
- Not enough blood because of blood loss
- Heart pumping too weakly
- Extremely low blood pressure
- Liver failure

Obstructed urine flow
- Enlarged prostate
- Tumor pressing on the urinary tract

Injuries within the kidneys
- Allergic reactions
- Toxic substances
- Conditions affecting the filtering units
- Blocked arteries or veins
- Crystals, protein, or other substances in the kidneys

- changes in urination
- changes in urinary output
- changes in the appearance of urine
- pain
- oedema (swelling)
- non-specific symptoms and signs

Diagnostic procedures

The major diagnostic procedures are:
- analysis of the urine
- X-rays and scans
- biopsy of the kidney
- cytology of urine

Acute renal failure

Acute renal failure (acute failure of the kidneys) is the clinical condition associated with rapid, steadily increasing excess urea in the blood, with or without oliguria, a daily urine volume of less than 500 mL.
The causes of acute failure of the kidneys can be grouped into three diagnostic categories:
- inadequate perfusion of the kidneys
- obstruction
- kidney diseases

Chronic renal failure

Chronic renal failure (chronic failure of the kidneys) is the clinical condition resulting from a multitude of pathological processes that lead to the derangement and insufficiency of the excretory and regulatory functions of the kidneys.
Chronic renal failure may result from any cause of dysfunction of sufficient magnitude. The functional effects of chronic renal failure can be grouped into three stages:

- diminished reserve of the kidneys
- failure of the kidneys
- excess amounts of urea in the blood

Those with just a diminished reserve of the kidneys do not show specific symptoms, and dysfunction of the kidneys can only be detected by careful testing. Those with insufficiency of the kidneys have only vague symptoms, principally due to a failure to concentrate the urine during the night. Lassitude, fatigue and decreased mental acuity are often the first manifestations of uraemia.
In advanced diseases, the following symptoms may be noted:
- coarse muscular twitching
- peripheral neuropathies
- muscle cramps
- convulsions
- loss of appetite
- nausea and vomiting

Localization of the kidneys in the back part of the abdominal cavity. The kidneys are located just below the diaphragm.

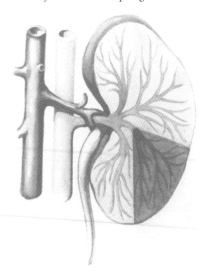

K

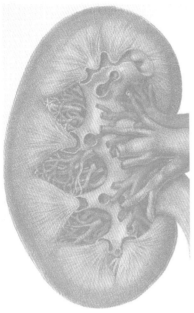 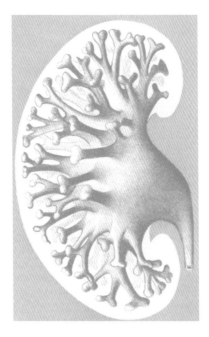 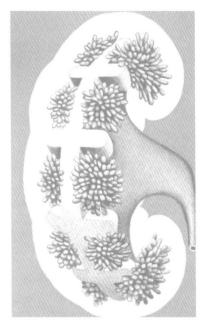

Vertical section through a kidney.
Left: the outer peripheral portion, called cortex, lies immediately beneath the capsule. An inner zone of tissue between the cortex and the renal sinus is called the medulla.
Middle: prolongations that lie between the renal pyramids are called the renal columns.
Right: small branches of the medullary pyramids.

K

- stomatitis (inflammation of the mucous membrane of the mouth)
- unpleasant taste in the mouth

The skin may develop a yellow-brown discoloration and, occasionally, urea from sweat may crystallize on the skin as so-called "uraemic frost." Pruritus, or itching, is an especially uncomfortable feature of chronic uraemia in some. High blood pressure (hypertension) is often present in advanced insufficiency of the kidneys. Hypertension and retention of sodium and water may lead to congestive heart failure.

The outcome depends on the nature of the underlying disorder and superimposed complications, especially since the latter may cause acute reductions in the function of the kidneys that are reversible with therapy.

In any case, underlying chronic diseases of the kidneys are generally not susceptible to specific treatment, and low urine output, increased amounts of potassium in the blood and pericarditis are often manifestations of an early death. Even in these situations, however, if no other major organ failure exists, dialysis or transplantation will improve the outlook.

A uraemic death is not pleasant, but an easy and gentle exit from this world, with full support from relatives, nurses and doctors may still be best for many of the elderly, in particular those with severe atherosclerosis and/or brain disease, and for those who are unlikely to be able to come to terms with a major change in their pattern of life. Of course, the burning question in this respect is: what is meant by elderly? Opinions vary everywhere, but generally kidney specialists tend to include anyone over the age of 40 who fits the above criteria, but would, on the other hand, not include an otherwise sound and adaptable person of 60 plus.

Generalized systemic disease is no longer an absolute contra-indication to dialysis or transplantation, but if the person has advanced diabetic complications, severe and widespread systemic lupus erythematosus or even gross osteodystrophy with multiple skeletal distortions and fractures, it must be pointed out that staving off inevitable death for a few months, or even a year or two, is not necessarily a kindness to either the sufferer nor his/her family. Each case must be considered on its own merits.

Factors aggravating or producing failure of the kidney (for instance, salt and water depletion, toxins, congestive heart failure, infection, high amounts of calcium in the blood, obstruction) must be treated specifically. When it has been established that uraemia is the result of a progressive and untreatable disorder, conservative management will often prolong useful, comfortable life until dialysis or transplantation is required.

When the limits of effectiveness of conventional treatment have been reached, long-term dialysis or transplantation should be considered. When chronic dialysis is used to treat irreversible uraemia, anemia and high blood pressure may still persist and require transfusions and restrictions of fluid and salt intake, respectively.

Occasionally, peripheral neuropathy may progress and become disabling despite frequent dialysis. Fatigue and lassitude may be major problems in the days just prior to each dialysis.

KNEE DISORDERS

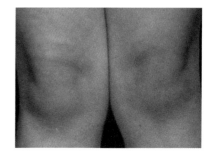

Introduction

The knee is defined as the front of the leg where the femur (thighbone) and tibia (shinbone) meet, and the joint itself, covered in front by the patella, or kneecap. The knee joint is the largest joint in the body and, because the bony surfaces do not exactly match, one of the weakest joints; in no position are the bones in more than partial contact.

Its strength lies in the number, size and arrangement of the ligaments, and the powerful muscles and fascia (fibrous membranes) that pass over the joint and enable it to withstand the leverage of the two longest bones in the body. It consists of two articulations (making it a compound joint) with a common joint cavity.

Joint surfaces and cartilage

The articular surfaces involved in the knee joint are the condyles (heads) and patellar surface of the femur, the upper articular surface of the tibia, and the articular surface of the patella. The condyles are in the form of rollers or thick wheels, not exactly parallel but diverging backward and downward. The curves change gradually from a circle of larger radius in front to one of smaller radius in the back, giving a spiral curve. The spiral curves of the two condyles differ, in that the medial is of smaller radius than the lateral; also the medial condylar surface is longer than the lateral.

The patellar articular surface projects more to the side than to the middle and is demarcated from the condylar surface by the frontal margins of the grooves of the menisci.

On the tibia, the articular surface is divided into two quite separate, cartilage-covered surfaces by a groove. The medial surface is slightly concave and approximates an oval outline, whereas the lateral is slightly convex and circular.

The contour of the articular surface of the patella is faceted in adaptation to the contour of the articular surface of the femur. The articular cartilage is between 2.5 and 6.5 mm thick, thinnest on the femoral condyles, 3.5 mm in the middle of the patellar surface, but 5.5 to 6.5 mm deep at the longitudinal ridge of the articular surface of the patella. The cartilage of the lateral articular surface on the tibia is thicker than that of the medial surface (4 to 5 mm in the central part).

Menisci

Injuries to the knee often involve the menisci, crescent-shaped cartilages on each side of the joint, wedged between and moving with the two bones. The menisci serve as buffer-bonds and cushions between the contiguous bones, as well as an important apparatus in the mechanism of movement of the joint.

The more frequent displacement of the medial meniscus (on the inner side of the knee) is explained by its greater fixity and, therefore, its greater reaction to strains. Thus, in addition to the weaker attachments of this

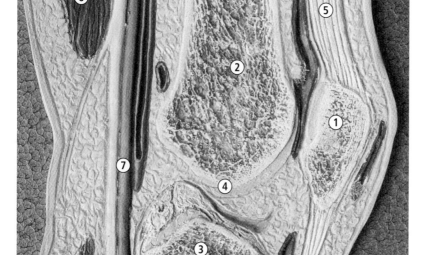

Longitudinal section of the knee joint.
1. Kneecap (patella)
2. Thigh bone (femur)
3. Shin bone (tibia)
4. Joint space
5. Tendon of quadriceps muscle
6. Posterior thigh muscle
7. Knee artery

meniscus to the transverse ligament, it is connected all along its outer, convex border with the capsule, and strongly with the tibial collateral ligament.

On the other hand, the lateral meniscus (on the outer side of the knee) is less firmly attached to the capsule, especially opposite the popliteus tendon, and has no tie to the collateral ligament of the fibula.

When, in the erect position, the femur is rotated to one side slightly bent (a common position), an especial strain is thrown upon the very important tibial collateral ligament and also on the medial meniscus.

Ligaments

The ligaments uniting the bones of the knee may be divided into an external and internal set. Superficial to the fibrous expansion of the quadriceps extensor tendons, the fascia lata of the thigh covers the front and sides of the knee joint.

The deep fascia of the thigh, as it descends to its attachment with the tibia, not only overlies but blends with the fibrous expansion of the extensor tendons. The ligamentum patellae is the continuation of the central portion of the quadriceps tendon, some fibers of which are prolonged over the front of the patella into the ligament. It is an extremely strong, flat band, attached, above, to the lower margin of the patella; below, it is inserted into the tibia. For movement and stability of the knee joint, the collateral ligaments are very important. The tibial collateral ligament is a strong, flat band that extends from the side of the femur to the side of the shaft of the tibia, about 4 cm (1½ in) away from the condyle.

The fibular collateral ligament is a strong, rounded cord, about 5 cm (2 in) long, attached above to the femur, just below and in front of the origin of the lateral head of the gastrocnemius muscle, above and behind the groove from which the popliteus muscle arises. Below, it is fixed to the middle of the side of the head of the fibula.

The internal ligaments comprise the anterior and posterior cruciate ligaments. The anterior cruciate ligament is strong and cord-like. It is attached in the groove of the tibia, and to the lateral margin of the medial articular

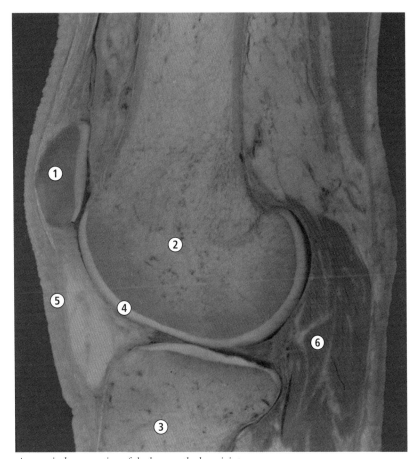

Anatomical preparation of the human the knee joint.
1. *Kneecap (patella)*
2. *Thigh bone (femur)*
3. *Shin bone (tibia)*
4. *Joint space*
5. *Tendon of quadriceps muscle*
6. *Posterior thigh muscles*

surface. It passes upward, backward and to one side of the posterior part of the medial surface of the lateral condyle of the femur.

The posterior cruciate ligament is stronger and less angled than the anterior. It is fixed below to the greater portion of the groove. It ascends to the anterior part of the lateral surface of the medial condyle of the femur, having a wide crescent-shaped attachment, just above the articular surface.

Movements

The movements that occur at the knee joint are flexion (bending) and extension (stretching), with a certain

amount of rotation in the bent position. These movements are not simple rolling on a transverse axis and rotating on a vertical axis for, in addition to and complicating these movements, there is the shifting or gliding motion of the joint surfaces upon each other. The transverse axis of hinge movement is affected in its position by the spiral contour of the condylar surfaces. The vertical axis of rotation passes near the middle of the joint, but in a plane nearer the medial condyle.

Holding the tibia fixed and moving the femur from a position of half flexion to one of complete extension - that is, with the tibia and femur in a

Knee disorders   Questions & Answers

What is arthroscopy?

The word arthroscopy comes from two Greek words, "arthro" (joint) and "skopein" (to look). The term literally means, "to look within the joint." Arthroscopy is a surgical procedure used to visualize, diagnose and treat problems inside a joint.

In an arthroscopic examination, the surgeon makes a small incision in the patient's skin and then inserts pencil-size instruments. These instruments contain a small lens and lighting system to magnify and illuminate the structures inside the joint. By attaching the arthroscope to a miniature camera, the surgeon is able to see the interior of the joint through a very small incision rather than the larger incision needed for surgery.

The arthroscope displays the image of the joint on a television screen, allowing the surgeon to look, for example, throughout the knee and under the kneecap.

What are the goals of arthroscopy?

Initially, arthroscopy was a diagnostic tool for planning standard open surgery. Today, many disorders are treated with arthroscopy alone or in combination with standard surgery. For example, meniscal tears in the knee and some problems related to arthritis are successfully treated arthroscopically.

What are some conditions found by arthroscopy?

Different diseases and injuries can damage bones, cartilage, ligaments, muscles and tendons. Some conditions found during arthroscopic exams include:

- ▲ Synovitis, an inflammation of the lining in the knee, shoulder, elbow, wrist or ankle.
- ▲ Shoulder injuries such as rotator cuff tendon tears, impingement syndrome and recurrent dislocations.
- ▲ Knee injuries such as meniscal (cartilage) tears, chondromalacia (wearing or injury of cartilage cushion).
- ▲ Wrist injuries involving cartilage and ligaments.

How is arthroscopy performed?

Arthroscopic surgery requires the use of anesthetics and special equipment in a hospital operating room or outpatient surgical suite. Depending on the problem, you will be given a general, spinal or local anesthetic. The arthroscope is inserted after a small incision is made. Corrective surgery may then be performed with specially designed instruments that are inserted into the joint.

After surgery, the incisions will be covered with a dressing and you will be moved to a recovery room. Some patients may need pain medication. During a visit with your doctor you will be given instructions on care for your incisions, exercises, and what to do to aid your recovery.

What are the advantages?

Arthroscopy is a valuable tool for orthopedic patients. Most patients have the procedure done on an outpatient basis and are home within hours following surgery.

straight line - and observing the movement of the femoral condyles, the following will be seen, explaining the entire system of complex movements of the knee joint.

First, there is a rolling forward, accompanied by a gliding backward of the condyles on the upper articular surfaces of the tibia. As the femur is nearly in the extended position, it undergoes medial rotation, and when extension is complete, no further excursion of the bone is possible.

Further observation reveals that the lateral meniscus moves forward, adjusting itself to the larger curve of the lateral condyle as it glides and rolls to the close of extension. At this moment, the cartilage becomes wedged between the tibial surface and the condylopatellar groove of the lateral condyle. Rotation now takes place on the vertical axis, in which the medial condyle moves backward until its oblique part next to the patellar surface is pressed in contact with the tibial articular surface, and the condylopatellar groove of the medial condyle is pressed against the edge of the medial meniscus.

■ Ligaments

Regarding the ligaments, in the semi-flexed joint it will be found that both collateral ligaments are relaxed. As extension proceeds, they tighten because the greater curves of the forepart of the condyles are exerting leverage upon the posteriorly located attachments of these ligaments.

The cruciate ligaments in the semi-flexed position are moderately stretched, but as the knee is bent, the anterior cruciate ligament tightens towards the close of extension and terminates the rolling of the lateral condyle.

■ Rotation

It remains stretched during the rotation of the femur, but is slightly relaxed at the end of rotation. From their attachments and directions, the cruciate ligaments in the fully extended joint prevent further rotation of the condyles.

With the femur fixed and the tibia movable, the latter rotates laterally at the close of extension. The beginning of flexion is marked by an unwinding of the knee joint, the femur rotating laterally or the tibia medially.

It has been observed that rotation in the fully extended joint is brought to an end; rotatory movement to a range of 50 degrees is permitted in the semi-flexed knee. When the knee joint is extended, all the ligaments are stretched with the exception of the ligamentum patellae and front of the capsule.

■ *Flexion and extension*

Extension is checked by both the cruciate ligaments and the collateral ligaments. In flexion, the ligamentum patellae and anterior portion of the capsule are stretched; so, also, is the posterior cruciate in extreme flexion, though it is not quite taut in the semi-flexed state of the joint.

All the other ligaments are relaxed, although the relaxation of the anterior cruciate ligament is slight in extreme flexion. Flexion is checked only by the contact of the soft parts - that is, the calf with the back of the thigh.

Rotation of the leg medially (towards the inside) is checked by the anterior cruciate ligament; the collateral ligaments being loose. Rotation laterally (towards the outside) is checked by the collateral ligaments; the cruciate ligaments have no controlling effect on it, as they are untwisted by it.

Sliding movements of the patella are checked by the cruciate and collateral ligaments, sliding forward especially by the anterior, and sliding backward by the posterior cruciate ligament.

Examination of the knee

Such gross deformities as swelling, quadriceps muscle atrophy (wasting) and joint instability may be more obvious when the person stands and walks. Careful palpation of the knee, especially noting the presence of joint fluid, synovial thickening and local tenderness, will help the doctor to detect arthritis.

Detection of small knee effusions (in which the cavities within the knee become fluid-filled) is a common problem in joint evaluation and is best done using the "bulge sign." The knee is extended and the leg is slightly

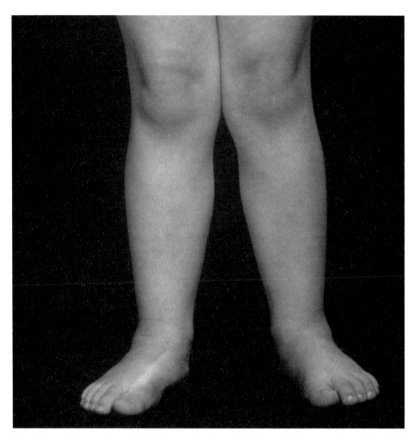

Knock knees (genu valgum). The knees point inward. This condition most often affects children ages 3 to 5 years. Usually the condition corrects itself by the age of 10 without treatment.

externally rotated while the person is lying down with muscles relaxed.

The inner side of the knee is stroked to express any fluid away from this area. The doctor places one hand on the suprapatellar pouch just above the kneecap and then strokes or presses gently on the outer side of the knee, creating a fluid wave or bulge that is visible on the inner side. Full 180° extension of the knee will be attempted by the doctor to see if the knee can be bent.

With meniscus tears or collateral ligament injuries, forceful bending of the knee to either side while extending the leg produces pain by compressing the meniscus and simultaneously stretching the opposite collateral ligament.

The joint line can be located by gently pressing on both sides while slowly flexing and extending the knee. A displaced meniscus is painful on firm pressure; a collateral ligament injury is tender in a longitudinal direction.

The state of the cruciate ligaments can be determined by grasping the leg with the knee at 90° (best done with the person sitting on a table edge with his/her legs dangling) and estimating the amount of front-to-back movement (which should be minimal).

The kneecap can be tested for free, painless motion. To gauge excess mobility of the joint, especially lateral instability, the thigh is firmly fixed and an attempt is made to rock the relaxed, almost extended, knee from side to side. If necessary, arthroscopy (direct visualization by means of an arthroscope, a fiber-optic telescope) can be performed, and special X-ray techniques are also available.

Disorders and diseases

Dislocation

Dislocations of the knee are, in themselves, unusual. The so-called disloca-

Knee disorders   Questions & Answers

What is total joint replacement?

Total joint replacement is a surgical procedure in which a diseased or damaged joint such as in a knee, hip, shoulder, ankle, foot, elbow, or finger, is removed and replaced by an artificial joint.

How does a healthy joint work?

A joint is an area of the body where two or more bones are connected by thick tissue. The ends of the bones are covered by a smooth layer called cartilage, which allows the bones to move smoothly. The tissue that encloses a joint produced a fluid, which reduces friction and wear.

Why is total joint replacement sometimes necessary?

The cartilage of a joint can become damaged by arthritis or injury, which can cause pain, inflammation, and stiffness. Treatment for arthritis or injury includes medications, injections, and physical therapy. Your physician may ask you to change your everyday activities, or in some cases, use a cane. Even after taking these steps, some people will experience severe pain, which may make total joint replacement necessary.

What is the goal of the surgery?

The goal of total joint replacement is to relieve pain and restore function in the joint caused by damage to the cartilage.

How is the procedure performed?

While you are under anesthesia, your orthopedic surgeon will replace the damaged part of the joint. For example, if you having surgery on your knee, your surgeon will replace the damaged ends of your thigh and shin bones and cartilage by metal and plastic materials so that your bones will move smoothly and painlessly. A grout-like cement may be used to attach the materials to your bones.

What can I expect after surgery?

Shortly after surgery, your orthopedist will encourage you to exercise your new joint, often with the assistance of a walker, crutches, or cane if you have had your knee or hip joint replaced. You will feel some pain in the new joint and nearby muscles after surgery and will receive medications to relieve it. Pain usually passes in a few weeks or months.

Exercise is critical to your recovery. Your orthopedic surgeon will recommend a plan and discuss it with you. Strenuous sports, such as tennis or running, however, may be discouraged, since they can cause too much wear and damage to the artificial joint.

Is an artificial joint permanent?

Most older people can expect their artificial joint to last ten or more years. Younger people may eventually need a second surgery, as loosening of the artificial joint does happen over time. Improvements in technology, however, have extended the life of artificial joints.

What are the advantages?

Total joint replacement can provide tremendous relief from the pain, stiffness, and inflammation of damaged or deceased joints. It can greatly improve your quality of life and enable you to return to all but the most strenuous activities of life.

tion of the knee is usually due to various injuries of the joint and of the complicated structures of the knee, such as the tearing of tendons or ligaments, or slipping of the cartilages.

They should be treated either by a straight splint, as in a fracture of the kneecap, or two splints, one on either side of the knee, as in a fracture. The person should then be transported to hospital as quickly as possible. A true dislocation of the knee is fortunately, an uncommon injury and is usually the result of severe violence.

It is important first to exclude any damage to the main blood vessels running behind the knee. This injury involves disruption of ligaments and these should be treated as soon as possible after the joint has been properly realigned.

Lateral dislocation of the patella (kneecap) may result from a direct blow to the inner side of the bone as part of a twisting injury when the knee is slightly bent. Diagnosis is easy when the dislocation persists but may be difficult when it goes back into place spontaneously.

When there has not been a direct blow on the knee, the injury is identical to that of a tear of the medial cartilage of the knee. In severe cases, the limb should be immobilized in a plaster cylinder from the groin to above the ankle for three weeks. During this period, the injured person gradually puts more and more weight on the limb, and performs quadriceps exercises from the start.

Housemaid's knee

The so-called housemaid's knee is an inflamed condition of the bursa (a cushioning bag of fluid) in front of the patella resulting in an increased accumulation of fluid within the bursa.

It may be seen in those who have to kneel frequently or continually while working. It is treated by removing the excess fluid via a syringe inserted into the bursa.

The knee is then bandaged tightly until pain and tenderness disappear. Kneeling must be avoided until the bandage comes off.

Chronic bursitis of this type may necessitate the surgical removal of the affected bursa.

K

K

Fractures

Indirect violence usually causes a clean break of the patella with separation of the fragments and tearing of the quadriceps expansion on both sides of the patella.

Direct violence results in either a crack fracture without displacement or a comminuted fracture, in which the bone shatters. Under the age of 45, the fracture is treated by surgically opening up the knee and aligning the various parts of the joint, the fragments being fixed by a vertical screw.

The torn extensor expansion on both sides of the patella should be repaired at the same time. A plastic cylinder is than worn for six to ten weeks but the person can walk as soon as his/her stitches are removed. Over the age of 45, or if the kneecap is too badly damaged, it is removed. If only the proximal or distal pole is involved it alone is excised.

Injuries to ligaments

The collateral ligament can be injured by forced abduction (moving away from the body) or adduction (moving towards the body) of the tibia on the femur when the knee is completely straight.

The way that the cruciate ligaments inside the knee can be damaged is often more complex, but, luckily, serious injury to one ligament amounting to rupture is uncommon. If a collateral ligament is torn, the corresponding cruciate ligament is usually also damaged.

A ligament may be ruptured by the application of some external force to the leg, such as occurs when a car or an opponent at sport strikes it. If this happens, the swelling is reduced by removing excess fluid or blood via a syringe, and then a compression bandage is applied.

The injured person begins quadriceps exercises immediately and is allowed to walk on the affected leg as soon as he/she can comfortably do so. The compression bandage is worn for at least three weeks or until the swelling of the joint has subsided, whichever is the longer period. If the ligaments are ruptured, the ligament should be repaired surgically within seven-to-ten days of injury, at the latest.

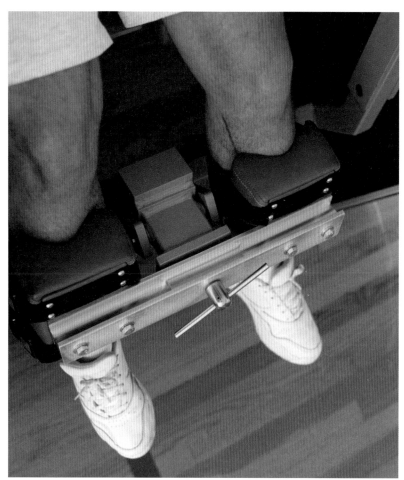

Exercises for strengthening the quadriceps muscles after a knee injury.

Injuries to the menisci

These structures are injured by a combination of flexion and rotation of the tibia on the femur and without any external force being applied to the knee.

This occurs when a person turns with the knee bent or when in the kneeling or squatting position. Classically, a "bucket-handle tear" occurs, the handle portion of the meniscus coming to lie within the groove of the tibia.

This causes pain on the injured side of the knee and the person has to stop whatever he or she is doing - for example, playing a game or working on his/her knees. The knee swells and cannot be extended, although it can be bent. This is known as "locking" of the knee.

The knee may spontaneously unlock and there may thereafter be episodes of recurrence of kneelock, usually due to a similar mechanism of rotation of the flexed knee. Later, one or other end of the meniscus may become torn and a "parrot beak" tear results. The person then finds that the knee does not lock but suddenly gives way with pain as the parrot beak is nipped between the tibia and femur.

In older people, a horizontal cleavage may develop in the substance of the cartilage without injury. As soon as convenient after the diagnosis is established, the damaged meniscus should be removed. After operation, a compression bandage is applied and intensive quadriceps exercises practised. The person is not allowed to walk until the stitches are removed on the tenth day. She or he should be fit for sedentary work within four weeks of the operation.

LARYNGEAL CANCER

Description

Laryngeal cancer is a malignant tumor of the larynx, or voice box. While not a common disease, it does account for from 2 to 5 per cent of all cancer cases. The outcome of this form of cancer is almost entirely dependent on how early it is discovered and treatment begun.

If diagnosed early, when the cancer is commonly limited to one vocal cord, the disease can be cured. In the great majority of such cases, a normal voice will still be possible. In the disease's later stages, however, when the cancer has spread to other areas of the larynx and throat, treatment often involves laryngectomy, the surgical removal of the larynx.

Cancer of the larynx, like other cancers, is characterized by an unchecked multiplication of cells, which build up into an invasive tumor. As the tumor develops, the cancer spreads, not only to adjacent tissue areas, but to distant parts of the body as well, using the lymph ducts and blood vessels for passage. These new, related growths are called metastases and the spreading cancer is said to have metastasized. Eventually, the tumors interfere with vital body functions and, if left uncontrolled, will kill.

Cancer of the larynx is primarily a disease of men in their 50s and 60s; it is rarely seen before the age of 40 and the frequency with which it occurs levels off after the age of 65. The ratio of male to female sufferers is about 7 to 1. The death rate for cancer of the larynx varies widely from country to country: France has the highest mortality rate for cancer of the larynx, and Norway the lowest. The United States and the United Kingdom are about midway in this list, with (respectively) 9500 new cases of laryngeal cancer each year.

Several environmental or occupational factors have been linked with laryngeal cancer, and habitual smoking and heavy drinking are among the most important of these. A British study showed that bartenders and tobacconists, when compared with the general population in England and Wales, have a significantly higher death rate for laryngeal cancer.

The disease keratosis, which produces wart-like growths on the larynx, is believed to be a pre-cancerous condition and those with the disease should be examined regularly by a doctor.

Diagnosis and symptoms

An important reason for the encouraging prognosis that can be made for many cases of laryngeal cancer is the fact that symptoms usually occur at a stage of the disease when the tumor is small and localized (i.e. it has not metastasized). However, the relative mildness of most of those symptoms is often misleading and frequently the warning signs are not heeded until much later.

One of the most common early symptoms of laryngeal cancer is a prolonged hoarseness. Any hoarseness lasting for more than two weeks should be investigated by a doctor. Hoarseness in cancer of the larynx is a direct result of a tumor on the vocal cords, the most common early site of the disease.

However, early growths often occur elsewhere on the larynx, causing such symptoms as a change in voice pitch, lump in the throat, coughing, difficulty and pain on breathing or swallowing, and even earache. In these instances, hoarseness may not develop until much later, if at all. A relatively simple preliminary examination for laryngeal cancer can be made by doctors in the office using a laryngoscope, a device that resembles a dentist's mir-

---

Rehabilitation

If laryngectomy - the removal of the larynx - is the necessary form of treatment, most patients can learn to speak again through a technique known as 'oesophageal speech.' This 'substitute' speech is produced by expelling swallowed air from the oesophagus. A well-trained and practised oesophageal voice produces intelligible speech of surprisingly good quality.

The method is best learned from a qualified speech therapist and often the person will work in group sessions with others who are learning, as well as with those who have already mastered the technique. Although oesophageal speech produces the best quality of voice and is the most convenient non-laryngeal speech method, there are mechanical devices available for those persons who are unable to learn it.

Artificial larynxes, both mechanical and electric, and a device that is attached to the upper dental plate are among the aids that may produce an intelligible voice. So generally successful are the means of rehabilitation that the great majority of persons who have undergone laryngectomy are able to return to full employment activity and lead relatively normal lives.

ror with a long handle. Doctors using this can detect most tumors of the larynx, but further direct examination under local anesthesia may be necessary.

If they suspect cancer, doctors will need to take a biopsy or specimen of the suspected tumor to be examined under a microscope to confirm the presence of cancer cells. X-ray and fluoroscopic examination are also often used to determine the actual size, extent and effect of the tumor. The discovery of the exact site of the primary and metastasizing lesions in laryngeal cancer is of great importance to the scheduling of a treatment program.

Treatment

In selecting a course of treatment for laryngeal cancer, the aim of doctors is to cure the cancer while preserving the maximum degree of speech. As in most other cancers, the two main types of treatment are radiation and surgery. Most investigators and clinicians in the field agree that radiation is probably the best treatment for the early, confined laryngeal lesion and produces a minimum of after-effects. Surgery, or a combination of surgery and radiation, is generally used for the more advanced laryngeal cancers. It must be emphasized that the correct treatment for the individual is dictated by the particular characteristics of his or her case, especially the site, size and extent of the tumor as well as the person's general health.

A collaboration between radiotherapist and surgeon is desirable to evaluate these factors and prescribe the proper program of treatment. In two-thirds of cases of laryngeal cancer, the person is able to retain the larynx but, again, early treatment is essential. In addition, there is a definite need for regular follow-up examinations to check for recurrence or metastases.

During the past 15 years there has been an upward trend in the survival of those with cancer of the larynx: more than half of these now live five years or more after diagnosis. This improvement in survival rates seems

to be the result of earlier detection and more effective treatment. Over 80 per cent of those whose cancer was detected early and treated surgically survived five years after diagnosis, and nearly three out of four survived ten years.

Left: front view of the larynx. From top to bottom: hyoid bone, thyroid gland, thyroid cartilage, cricoid cartilage, trachea
Middle: back view of the larynx. From top to bottom: epiglottis, vocal cords, arytenoid cartilage, cricoid cartilage, trachea
Right: medial view of the larynx. From top to bottom: epiglottis, vocal cord, arytenoid cartilage, inner surface of the trachea.
Middle: back view of the larynx.

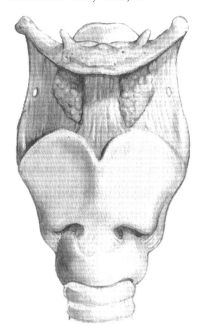 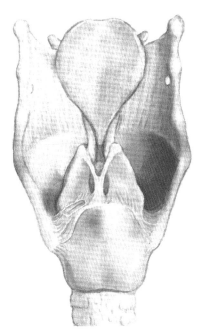 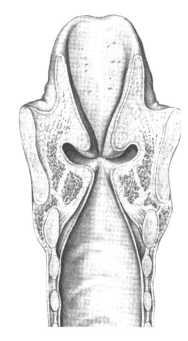

LARYNGITIS

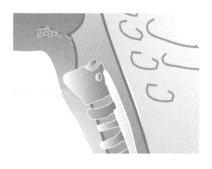

Introduction

Inflammation of the larynx can be caused by bacteria or viruses, and may occur in the course of bronchitis, pneumonia, influenza, pertussis (whooping cough), measles, and diphtheria.

Excessive use of the voice, allergic reactions and inhalation of irritating substances such as cigarette smoke can cause an acute or chronic inflammation of the pharynx.

Symptoms

An unnatural change of voice is usually the most prominent symptom. Hoarseness and even aphonia (loss of voice), together with a sensation of tickling, rawness and a constant urge to clear the throat, may occur.

Symptoms vary with the severity of the inflammation: fever, malaise, difficulty in swallowing and a sore throat may occur in the more severe infections; shortness of breath may be apparent if there is swelling of the larynx.

Treatment

There is no specific treatment for laryngitis caused by viruses. Penicillin is the drug of choice for bacterial infections caused by streptococci and pneumococci. Treatment of acute or chronic bronchitis may improve the condition of the larynx. Voice rest and steam inhalation will relieve symptoms and promote resolution of the acute condition.

Other conditions resembling laryngitis

■ *Polyps*
Polyps may show similar symptoms as laryngitis in the beginning. Polyps usually develop from voice abuse, chronic allergic reactions and chronic inhalation or irritants such as industrial fumes and cigarette smoke.

They occur when a small blood vessel on one of the vocal cods ruptures, and a small, berry-like swelling (the polyp) appears. This results in hoarseness and a breathy voice quality.

Treatment involves surgical removal of the polyp to restore the voice, and attention to the underlying cause to prevent recurrence, including voice therapy if voice abuse is the cause.

■ *Vocal cord nodules*
Nodules on a vocal cord - also called singer's, teacher's or screamer's nod-

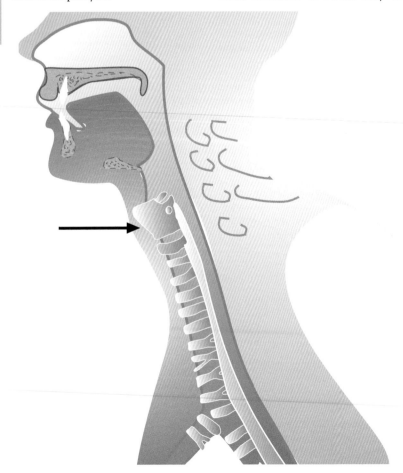

Median section of part of the head and neck. The arrow indicated the external prominence of the larynx.

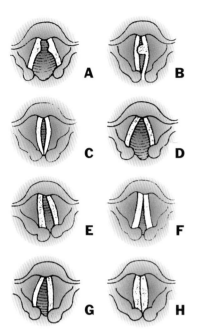

Vocal cord nodules
Schematic representation of characteristic disorders of the vocal cords.
A. vocal cord nodules; B. presence of a polyp on the vocal cord; C. paralysis of vocal cords; D. flaccid paralysis of the left vocal cord; E. complete paralysis of the vocal cords; F. spastic paralysis of the recurrence nerve; G. phonation disorder due to nerve paralysis.

Laryngitis Questions & Answers

The respiratory tract or system consists of the organs and structures associated with breathing, gaseous exchange, and the entrance of air into the body.
It includes organs and structures of the upper respiratory tract: the nasal cavity (nose), pharynx (throat), larynx (voice box), and trachea (windpipe), and those of the lower respiratory tract: bronchi, bronchioles (small branches of the bronchial system), alveoli and associated muscles.

What is the pharynx?
The pharynx (throat) is the muscular tube extending from the base of the skull to the esophagus (foodpipe) that serves as a passageway for food from the mouth to the esophagus and for air from the nose and mouth to the larynx. It is divided into the nasopharynx (part behind the nose), oropharynx (part behind the mouth), and laryngopharynx (part connected to the voice box).

What is the structure of the larynx?
The larynx or voice box connects the pharynx to the windpipe. It is here that the vocal cords are found and where speech is made possible. The whole organ is made up of a number of bones, cartilages, and muscles, which are connected to each other in a complicated manner and which can be moved with respect to each other. The thyroid cartilage and below it the ring-shaped cartilage are the most important. The entrance to the larynx is closed by the epiglottis, which moves upward when swallowing takes place, closing off this area, so that no food can enter the windpipe.

Where are the vocal cords located?
Between the thyroid cartilage and the cup-shaped cartilage of the larynx or voice box, the elastic vocal cords are stretched and can vibrate when air is expired. These cords run horizontally in a front-to-back direction. Between them is a slitlike opening, the glottis, located. The opening can be narrowed or widened by muscular contraction and relaxation. Chest, lips, tongue and palate (roof of the mouth) also play important roles in sound (voice) production.

What is the structure of the trachea?
The trachea or windpipe is the tube extending from the larynx to the bronchi that conveys air to the lungs. It is about 11 centimetres long, covered in front by the isthmus of the thyroid gland, and is in contact in the back with the esophagus.
The trachea has a pseudostratified ciliated columnar epithelium with so-called globet cells and numerous mucous and serous glands with duct openings through the epithelium. The mucous secretions provide a sticky slimy layer which traps the particles; the mucus and its contents are moved upwards by the action of the cilia, pass through the larynx and are swallowed.

ules -are caused by chronic abuse of the voice, such as screaming or shouting, or speaking or singing unnaturally low. The nodules are condensations of hyaline connective tissue on the sides of the vocal cords.
Hoarseness and a breathy voice quality result.
Treatment involves surgical removal of the nodules and correction of the underlying voice abuse. Vocal nodules in children usually regress with voice therapy alone.

■ *Contact ulcers*
Ulcers of the mucous membrane over the arytenoid cartilage may result from voice abuse, and can cause mild pain on swallowing and varying degrees of hoarseness. Prolonged ulceration leads to formation of nonspecific granulomas (growths made up of granulation tissue), which pro-

duce varying degrees of hoarseness.
Treatment consists of prolonged resting of the voice (six weeks maximum) to heal the ulcers. Sufferers must recognize the limitations of their voices and learn to adjust their activities to avoid recurrent ulcers. Granulomas tend to recur after surgical removal but respond to extensive voice therapy.

■ *Tumors*
Benign tumors of various histological types may occur at all ages. Removal restores the voice, the functional integrity of the laryngeal sphincter, and the airway.
For malignant tumors see: Laryngeal cancer.

LEGIONNAIRES' DISEASE

Description

Legionnaires disease made a dramatic appearance on the medical scene in 1976 when 182 delegates attending an annual convention of the American Legion in Philadelphia contracted a severe respiratory infection. Of 147 of those hospitalized, 90 per cent developed pneumonia and 29 died. All had stayed in, or visited, the same hotel during the four-day convention.

The outbreak attracted wide publicity, and considerable scientific effort was made to define the nature of the disease. Five months later, the organism responsible - a small Gram-negative, non-acid-fast bacillus - was isolated in guinea pigs from the lung tissues of four fatal cases, and was subsequently named Legionella pneumophila.

A great deal of knowledge has been acquired since 1976 and it is now clear that the organism is a significant respiratory pathogen, both in the US and in Western Europe.

Signs and symptoms

After an incubation period of two to ten days, the illness begins with the non-specific symptoms of malaise, headache and muscular aches and pains, succeeded in a few hours by high fever and shivering.

A dry cough, or a cough producing of small amounts of bloodstained sputum, begins on the second or third day, with pleurisy (inflammation of the pleura, the membrane covering the lungs) a common occurrence. Watery diarrhea with abdominal distention, occurring in around 50 per cent of sufferers, may precede the onset of fever.

The main pathological changes are found in the lungs which on X-ray show patchy areas of consolidated tissue. Samples of this tissue reveal large numbers of L. pneumophila, seen as small rods which do not take up Gram's stain. This picture is uncommon except in Legionnaires' pneumo-nia. Although biochemical abnormalities seem to imply that many of the organ systems of the body are involved, there are few findings to support a specific process outside the lungs. There is no gross change in the liver or the brain and, despite the occasional prominence of kidney failure, L. pneumophila has been shown to be a fastidious organism, early attempts to isolate it having been met with failure until the development of an enriched agar in which it could be cultured. In practice, the diagnosis and the selection of appropriate treatment are decided by the clinical picture. The combination of a severe pneumonia, unproductive cough, or a cough productive of small amounts of sputum, clouding of consciousness, diarrhea, a normal or modestly elevated white blood cell count, and the absence of common bacterial pathogens, should alert doctors to the possibility of Legionnaires disease and help them to distinguish it from other pneumonias.

Treatment

Cephalothin, aminoglycosides, chloramphenicol, ampicillin penicillin, tetracycline and erythromycin were all used to treat the patients in the Philadelphia epidemic, and while no antibiotic was found to be clearly effective, the mortality rate was lowest when erythromycin and tetracycline were used.

Accumulated experience has since confirmed these findings, but the consensus of opinion is that erythromycin is more effective than tetracycline. When faced by a patient seriously ill with pneumonia, it is incumbent on the doctor to choose an antibiotic regimen that is effective against several

Patient hospitalized for Legionnaire's disease.

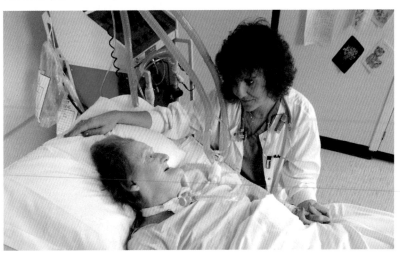

possible pathogens. A combination of rifampicin and erythromycin, or rifampicin and tetracycline, meets most requirements.

How the disease spreads

An accumulation of indirect evidence supports the theory that Legionnaires' disease is spread by the airborne route, but the reservoirs of infection and mode of dissemination remain largely undetermined. Person-to-person transmission is certainly unimportant, if it occurs at all.

The majority of recorded epidemics have originated in hotels and institutions and it has been postulated, largely on circumstantial evidence, that air-conditioning equipment has provided both the source of infection and the means of dispersal.

In support of this view, there have been several isolations of the organism from air-cooling systems at the site of epidemics. It has also been shown that L. pneumophila can survive in tap water for up to 370 days.

While air conditioning systems may be important in some geographical areas, they clearly play no part in the dissemination of disease in others. There is a great deal still to be learned about the ecology and epidemiology of Legionnaires' disease.

X-ray examination for Legionnaire's disease.

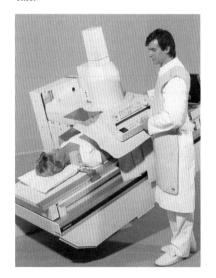

Erythromycin

This antibiotic medicine is prescribed for Legionnaires' disease. Generally, erythromycin as active ingredient. This antibiotic is prescribed to treat infections caused by bacteria. They will not work for colds, flu, or other virus infections. Erythromycins are available only with your doctor's prescription.

Before using this medicine
Before you use this medicine check with your doctor, or pharmacist:
- if you ever had any unusual or allergic reaction to any of the erythromycins.
- if you are on a low-salt, low-sugar, or any other special diet, or if you are allergic to any substance, such as sulfites or other preservatives or dyes.
- if you are pregnant or intend to become pregnant while using this medicine. Although erythromycins have not been shown to cause birth defects or other problems in humans, the chance always exists.
- if you are breast-feeding an infant. Most erythromycins pass into the breast milk. Although erythromycins have not been shown to cause problems in humans, the chance always exists.
- if you have liver disease.

Treatment
This medication belongs to the general family of medicines called antibiotics. It is used to treat a wide variety of bacterial infections. It is also used to treat infections in persons who are allergic to penicillin. Erythromycins are also used to prevent strep infections in patients with a history of rheumatic heart disease. They may also be used in Legionnaires' disease and for other problems as determined by your doctor.
- Keep taking this medicine for the full time of treatment even if you begin to feel better after a few days; do not miss any doses. This is especially important if you have a strep infection since serious heart problems could develop later if your infection is not cleared up completely.
- If you do miss a dose of this medicine, take it as soon as possible. This will help to keep a constant amount of medicine in the blood. However, if it is almost time for your next dose, skip the missed dose and go back to your regular dosing schedule.
- This medication has been prescribed for your current infection only. Another infection later on, or one that someone else has, may require a different medicine. You should not give your medicine to other people or use it for other infections, unless your doctor specifically directs you to do so.

Side effects
Along with the needed effects, a medicine may cause some unwanted effects. Side effects that usually do not require medical attention: abdominal cramps, black tongue, cough, diarrhea, fatigue, irritation of the mouth, loss of appetite, nausea, or vomiting. These side effects should disappear as your body adjusts to the medication.
- Other side effects that should be reported to your doctor immediately are: Fever, Hearing loss, Hives or rash, Rectal or vaginal itching, Yellowing of the eyes or skin

Interactions
This medicine may interact with several other drugs such as anticoagulants, theophylline preparations, carbamazepine, etc.
- Be sure to tell your doctor about any medications you are currently taking.

Storage
Tablets, capsules, etc. should be stored at room temperature in tightly closed, light-resistant containers as directed by your pharmacist.

LEUKEMIA

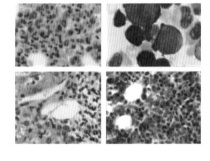

Description

Leukemia is a cancer-like disease characterized by a great degree of uncontrolled proliferation of one of the types of white blood cells. The leukemias cause an estimated 45,000 deaths each year throughout the world. Acute leukemia is the most common form of cancer in children, but actually affects many more adults. Chronic leukemia usually appears after the age of 40.

Leukemia, whether acute or chronic, occurs as one of two major types, depending on the kind of white cell affected. Lymphocytic leukemia affects the lymphocytes (made in the lymph nodes and bone marrow); myelocytic leukemia (myelocyte = immature white blood cell), also known as granulocytic or myelogenous leukemia, affects the granulocytes (made exclusively in the bone marrow). In leukemia, the bone marrow begins to produce damaged white cells, which do not mature properly and, unlike normal mature white cells, are able to multiply uncontrollable and then rapidly displace the normal cells. Because they do not mature, they are unable to perform their usual function of fighting foreign invaders, and so sufferers are at a far greater risk of infection.

In addition, the abnormal functioning of the bone marrow also reduces the amount of red blood cells and platelets formed there, and sufferers become greatly anaemic and their blood does not clot correctly, leaving them open to the risk of hemorrhage. In fact, infection and hemorrhage are the two major causes of death in leukaemic patients.

The causes of most cases of human leukemia are unknown but certain specific factors have been identified, such as excessive exposure to radiation and possibly to certain chemicals, chiefly benzene, a constituent of petroleum. The possibility that viruses may cause leukemia in humans is being intensively investigated. These

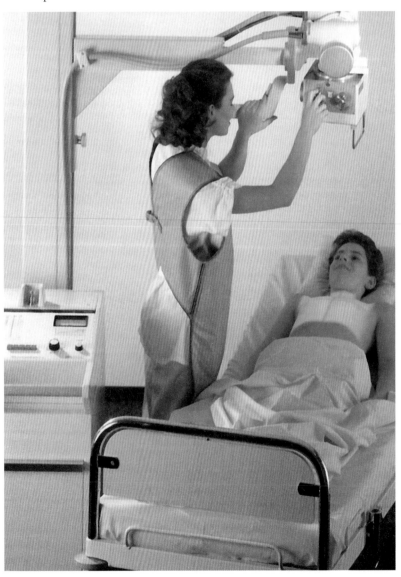

X-ray examination of a young patient suspected of leukemia.

studies are an outgrowth of laboratory experiments in which leukemia is induced in animals by viruses.

Similar pathological changes have been seen in tissues from patients with leukemia and lymphoma studied with the electron microscope, but have not been positively identified as viruses. In addition to environment factors such as radiation, chemicals and possibly viruses, genetic abnormalities also appear involved in the development of leukemia in laboratory animals. Several of such factors working together may ultimately be found to cause the disease in humans.

Acute leukemia

Acute leukemia in children usually appears suddenly with symptoms similar to those of a cold, and the disease progresses rapidly. The lymph nodes, spleen and liver become infiltrated with white blood cells and may become enlarged. Bone pain, paleness, a tendency to bleed or bruise easily and frequent infections are all associated symptoms. In adults, acute leukemia may come on more slowly after a chronic phase.

Leukemia can be diagnosed only by microscopic examination of the blood and bone marrow. If abnormal white cells characteristic of leukemia are present in these tissues, they can be identified and the diagnosis made.

■ Treatment

Much progress has been made in extending the survival of acute leukemia patients. This improvement is due to chemotherapy (the use of drugs), radiotherapy (in small doses, not the large ones that can cause the disease) and the development of better methods of patient care. A variety of anti-cancer drugs, used singly and in combination, can achieve remissions in a high percentage of patients with acute leukemia.

In some centers, combinations of

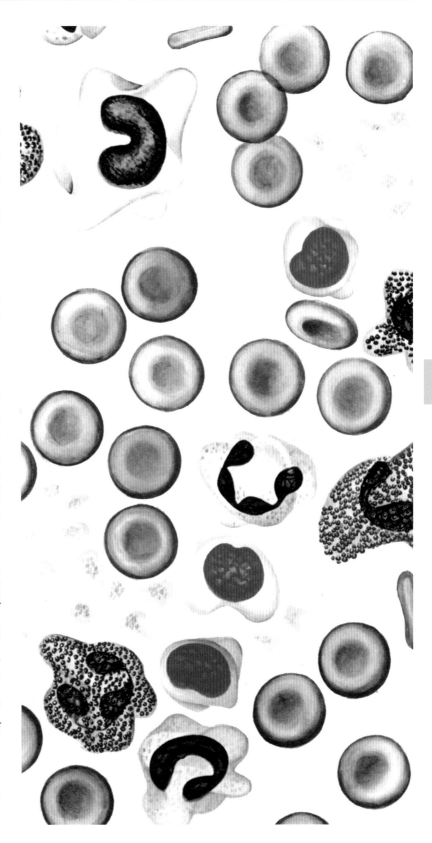

In leukemia the white blood cells or leucocytes may increase in number and thus cause pathological changes in the blood-forming organs. The leucocytes are colored.

Leukemia   Questions & Answers

What is leukemia?
Leukemia is cancer of white blood cells or of cells that develop into white blood cells.

What is acute lymphocytic leukemia?
Acute lymphocytic leukemia is a life-threatening disease in which the cells that normally develop into lymphocytes become cancerous and rapidly replace normal cells in the bone marrow.

What is acute myelocytic leukemia?
Acute myelocytic (myeloid, myelogenous, myeloblastic, myelomonocytic) leukemia is a life-threatening disease in which the cells that normally develop into neutrophils become cancerous and rapidly replace normal cells in the bone marrow.

What is a myelodysplastic syndrome?
In myelodysplastic syndromes, a line of identical cells develops and occupies the bone marrow. These abnormal cells do not grow and mature normally, resulting in deficits of red blood cells, white blood cells, and platelets. The cause is usually not known. However, in some people, exposure of bone marrow to radiation therapy or certain types of chemotherapy drugs may play a role.

What is chronic lymphocytic leukemia?
Chronic lymphocytic leukemia is a disease in which mature lymphocytes become cancerous and gradually replace normal cells in lymph nodes.

What is chronic myelocytic leukemia?
Chronic myelocytic leukemia is a disease in which cells that normally would develop into neutrophils, basophils, eosinophils, and monocytes become cancerous.

Is the treatment with stem cells in chronic myelocytic leukemia beneficial for the patient?
Chronic myelocytic leukemia may be treated with a transplantation of stem cells, which must come from a donor who has a competitive type, usually a sibling. It is the most effective treatment during the early stages of the disease but is considerably less effective during the accelerated phase or blast crisis.

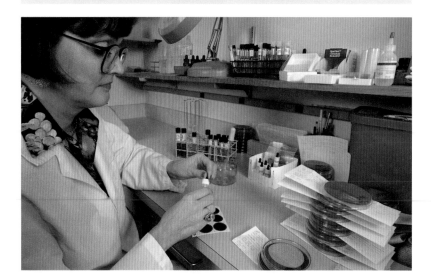

Laboratory research of blood preparations.

these drugs plus radiotherapy or chemotherapy to destroy leukaemic cells have resulted in five-year disease-free remissions for more than 50 per cent of the persons so treated, and many of these are undoubtedly cured. Since the drugs used to treat acute leukemia interfere, like the leukaemic process itself, with the production of normal blood elements, hemorrhage and infection are serious problems. However, transfusions of platelets have proved very effective in preventing or stopping hemorrhage, the use of antibiotics helps prevent infections, and the use of transfusions of granulocytes (infection-fighting white cells) is being explored.

Chronic leukemia

Chronic leukemia, the most common form of the disease in adults, comes on slowly and without warning. Many cases are discovered during routine examinations and, even after changes in the blood are noticed, several years may pass before significant symptoms appear.

The symptoms of the chronic leukemias are like those of the acute forms of the disease: fatigue, a tendency to bruise and bleed easily and an increased susceptibility to infections. The doctor may be able to feel an enlarged spleen or lymph nodes. Diagnosis is established by microscopic examination of the circulating blood and of the bone marrow, which show increased numbers of white cells.

In most cases these cells are mature in chronic leukemias and can thus be distinguished from the acute leukemias which are characterized by large numbers of immature white blood cells.

■ *Treatment*
Although treatment is effective in lessening symptoms and temporarily controlling progress of the disease, it has not substantially increased life expectancy, which is about three to four years following diagnosis. Better ways to control this disease are under

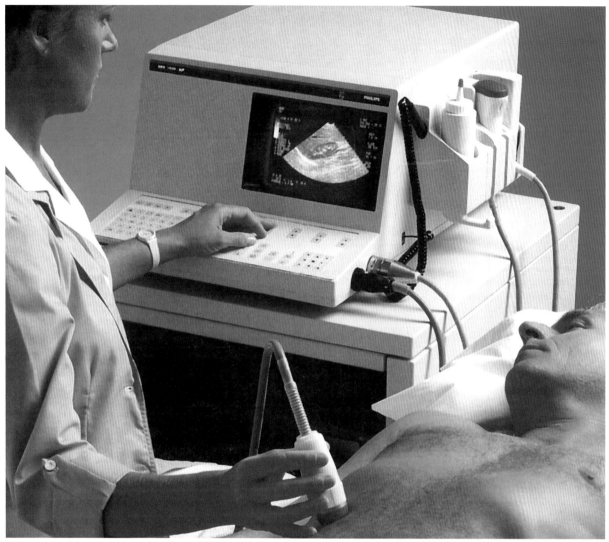

Ultrasonographic examination of the liver to look for pathological changes in the liver

intensive study. Chronic myelocytic leukemia is usually treated by drugs, but X-ray therapy to the spleen may bring about remission in early stages of the disease.

In its symptoms, course and response to treatment, chronic lymphocytic leukemia is much more variable than the myelocytic form of the disease. However, drugs are also used in treating chronic lymphocytic leukemia and, when the disease is localized, irradiation helps reduce lymph node size.

Total body irradiation and radioactive phosphorus P32, may also be used with benefit.

Types of leukaemia

Acute lymphocytic (lymphoblastic) leukaemia
- Progression: Rapid
- White blood cells affected: Lymphocytes

Acute myeloid (myelocytic, myelogenous, myeloblastic, myelomonocytic) leukaemia
- Progression: Rapid
- White blood cells affected: Myelocytes

Chronic lymphocytic leukaemia
- Progression: Slow
- White blood cells affected: Lymphocytes

Chronic myelocytic (myeloid, myelogenous, granulocytic) leukaemia
- Progression: Slow
- White blood cells affected: Myelocytes

LIVER CANCER

Description

Tumors of the liver may be benign or malignant. Benign tumors do not spread. Cancerous tumors or malignant hepatoma may originate in the liver, or they spread (metastasize) to the liver from other parts of the body. Cancer originating in the liver is called primary liver cancer or hepatoma; cancer originating elsewhere in the body is called metastatic cancer. The vast majority of liver cancers are metastatic.

Benign tumors are relatively common but usually cause no symptoms. Most are detected when people have a scanning test - such as ultrasound, computed tomography (CT-scan) or magnetic resonance imaging (MRI-scan).

In certain areas of Africa and Southeast Asia, primary liver cancers are more common than metastatic liver cancer, and they are a prominent cause of death. In these areas, there is a high prevalence of chronic infection with hepatitis B virus, which increases the risk of malignant liver tumors more than 100-fold.

In subtropical regions where primary liver cancers are common, food is often contaminated by carcinogens called aflatoxins, substances that are produced by certain types of fungi. Aflatoxins are known to be carcinogenic. In Europe, United States and Canada, and other areas of the world where primary liver cancers are less common, most people with hepatomas are alcoholics with longstanding liver cirrhosis.

Symptoms

The first symptoms of liver cancer are the following:
- abdominal pain;
- fever;
- weight loss;
- a large mass of the abdomen that can be felt in the upper right part of the abdomen.

In some cases, a person who had had cirrhosis for a long time may unexpectedly become much more ill. Occasionally, the first symptoms are acute abdominal pain and shock, caused by a rupture or bleeding of the tumor. In case of a metastatic liver cancer, the first symptoms include weight loss and poor appetite. Typically, the liver is enlarged and hard and may be tender. Fever may be present. The abdominal cavity may become distended with fluid, a condition called ascites. At first, jaundice is absent or mild, unless the cancer is blocking the bile ducts. In the weeks before the person dies,

Relation of the liver to the gallbladder and the various ducts. After leaving the liver, the right and left hepatic ducts join to form the common hepatic duct. This is a relatively short duct (4 cm long) lying between the layers of the lesser omentum. Extending downward, it joins the cystic duct from the gallbladder to form the common bile duct (about 7.5 cm long) that empties into the second part of the duodenum.

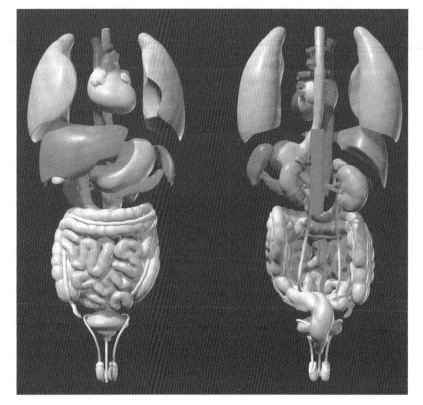

jaundice progressively worsens. Also, the person may become confused and drowsy as toxins accumulate in the brain, a condition called liver encephalopathy.

Diagnosis

At first, the symptoms do not provide many clues to the diagnosis, However, once the liver enlarges enough to be felt, a doctor may suspect the diagnosis, especially if the person has long-standing cirrhosis.

Abdominal ultrasound and computed tomography (CT-scans) or magnetic resonance imaging (MRI-scans) sometimes detect cancers that have not yet caused symptoms.

Hepatic arteriography (X-rays taken after a radiopacque substance is injected into the hepatic artery) may reveal liver cancer. Hepatic arteriography is particularly useful before surgical removal of the tumor because it shows the surgeon the precise location of the liver blood vessels.

A liver biopsy, in which a small sample of liver tissue is removed by needle for examination under a microscope, can confirm the diagnosis. To improve the chances of obtaining cancerous tissue, ultrasound can be used to guide the insertion of the biopsy needle.

Treatment

Usually, the prognosis for people with primary liver cancer is poor because the tumor is detected too late. Occasionally, a person with a small tumor may do very well after the tumor is surgically removed. In case of a metastatic liver cancer, depending on the type of cancer, anticancer drugs may temporarily shrink the tumor and prolong life, but they do not cure the cancer.

Anticancer drugs may be injected into the hepatic artery, which then delivers a high concentration of the drugs directly to the cancer cells in the liver. This technique is more likely to shrink the tumor and to produce fewer side effects, but it has not been proved to prolong life. Radiation therapy to the liver can sometimes reduce severe pain, but it has little other benefit.

Liver cancer   Questions & Answers

What kind of liver tumors may occur?
Liver tumors may be noncancerous (benign) or cancerous (malignant). Cancerous liver tumor are classified as primary (originating in the liver) or metastatic (spreading from elsewhere in the body). Most liver tumors are metastatic because of the large volume of blood that it filters form the heart and the digestive tract.

What are the major symptoms or signs of noncancerous liver tumors?
Noncancerous liver tumors are relatively common and usually cause no symptoms. Most are detected only when people happen to undergo a scanning test - such as ultrasonography, computed tomography (CT) or magnetic resonance imaging (MRI) - for an unrelated reason.
Generally, there are no specific signs or symptoms. The liver functions normally even when a noncancerous tumor is present, and results of liver function tests are usually within normal limits.

What is the common treatment for metastatic liver cancer?
Depending on the type of cancer, chemotherapy drugs may be used to temporarily shrink the tumor and prolong life, but they do not cure the cancer. If only a single tumor is found in the liver, it may be surgically removed, especially if it originated in the intestines.

What is hemangioma?
Hemangioma is a noncancerous liver tumor composed of a mass of abnormal blood vessels.

What is hepatocellular adenoma?
Hepatocellular adenoma is a common noncancerous liver tumor that may be mistaken for a cancerous tumor and that in rare cases may rupture and bleed.

What is hepatoma?
Hepatoma in a cancer that begins in the liver cells; a primary liver cancer.

Microscopic section of the liver, showing the hepatic lobules, small structural units of the liver. Where several lobules join, the connective tissue is more abundant and encloses a blood vessel, vein, nerves, lymphatic vessels, and small bile ducts.

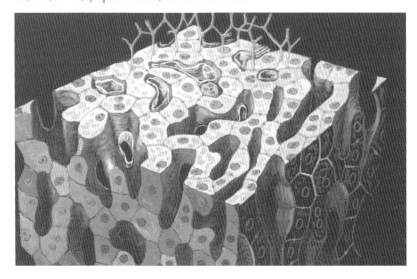

LIVER DISEASES

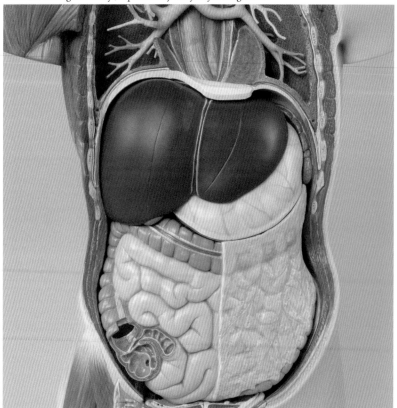

Description

Signs and symptoms of diseases and disorders of the liver are numerous. Some abnormalities occur only in chronic disease; others are seen in either acute or chronic disorders. Interference with the blood supply of the liver is common in cirrhosis and other chronic diseases and is usually manifested by raised blood pressure in the portal vein.

The most characteristic sign of a disturbance in liver function is jaundice. This is a yellow discoloration of the skin, whites of the eyes and other tissues due to excess circulating bilirubin, a major constituent of bile.

Increased formation, impaired uptake by the liver or decreased conjugation in the liver may all cause jaundice. The different reasons for the appearance of jaundice means that doctors must find the answers to specific questions to narrow the possibilities.

The first question should be whether the jaundice is due to hemolysis (breakdown of the blood, an uncommon occurrence), dysfunction of the liver (common) or obstruction of bile in the system of ducts (intermediate). If a disease of the liver and/or gallbladder is present, other important questions follow:

- ▲ Is the condition acute or chronic?
- ▲ Is it due to primary liver disease or to a general disorder involving the liver?
- ▲ Are alcohol or other drugs responsible?
- ▲ Will surgery be needed?
- ▲ Are complications present?

The answers to these questions will be approached by the family doctor or specialist by clinical, structural and functional assessment.

Fatty liver

The abnormal accumulation of fat in liver cells (hepatocytes) is said to occur in 25 per cent of individuals and to be the commonest response of the liver to injury.

Diffuse fatty change of the liver, often zonal in distribution, is associated with many clinical situations. Fatty change in specific areas is much less common and less well recognized.

Occurring in nodular form and usually located beneath the capsule, focal fatty change can be important in determining the diagnosis of space-occupying lesions of the liver. If the deposit of lipids in the liver is marked, the organ tends to be grossly enlarged, smooth and pale.

Under the microscope, the general architecture of the cells can be normal but the fat (in the form of triglycerides) tends to appear as large

The liver is the largest organ in the body and is located in the upper part of the abdominal cavity under the dome of the diaphragm. The liver is demarcated into four loves; the two main lobes are the right and left, separated by the falciform ligament.

droplets that coalesce and shift the cell nucleus to the periphery.

Free fatty acids collect in acute fatty liver of pregnancy and probably in Rey's syndrome. Cholesterol esters gather in familial high-density lipoprotein deficiency, cholesterol ester storage disease and Wolman's disease.

Phospholipids accumulate under the influence of certain drugs and in several inborn errors of phospholipid metabolism. The condition is most often discovered on physical examination as non-tender enlargement of the liver and is usually without specific symptoms.

However, it can be present with pain in the upper quadrant and jaundice, or can be the only physical abnormality found after sudden, unexpected death that is presumably due to a damaged metabolism.

There is a poor association between fatty liver and abnormalities found in the commonly used biochemical tests for liver disease; thus the positive diagnosis of fatty liver can be made only on examination of tissue.

Fatty liver is potentially reversible and usually is not in itself harmful. However, since it may indicate the action of a toxic substance or the presence of an unrecognized disease or metabolic abnormality, the diagnosis calls for further evaluation of the person. No specific therapy is known except to eliminate the cause or treat the underlying disorder.

Fibrosis

This condition is defined as excess fibrous tissue in the liver resulting either from the collapse and condensation of pre-existing fibers or from the synthesis of new fibers by fibroblasts.

Fibrosis is a common response to cell injury induced by a wide variety of agents, including numerous chemicals and drugs such as:
- alcohol
- methotrexate
- arsenicals
- isoniazid
- methyldopa

In addition, various infections of the liver can cause fibrosis, as can chronic

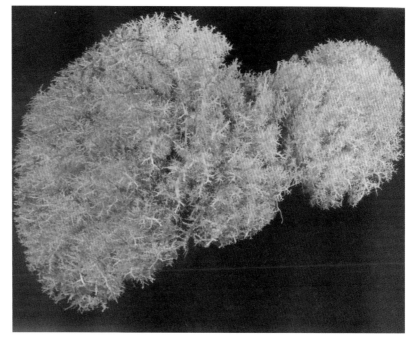

The rich blood supply of the liver is shown in this preparation of the human liver.

obstruction of bile flow and various disturbances of the hepatic circulation of blood in the liver. The influence of fibrosis on the structure and function of the liver depends upon its location.

Extensive fibrosis can result in the formation of septa (fibrous partitions), which can interfere significantly with the circulation in the liver; however, the fibrosis that accompanies many liver disorders is rarely the main characteristic of the disease.

The diagnosis depends upon examination of a tissue sample from the liver. Treatment includes overcoming the underlying cause and dealing with complications - for instance, portal hypertension (raised pressure in the portal vein.

Cirrhosis

This liver disorder is defined as the disorganization of liver architecture by widespread fibrosis and nodule formation. The nodules are portions of secreting cells demarcated by connective tissue. In cirrhosis, all parts of the liver must be involved, but large nodules can contain intact tissue.

Cirrhosis is exceeded only by heart disease, cancer and cerebrovascular disease ("stroke") as a cause of death in the 45 to 65 age group in this country, and the vast majority of cases are a result of chronic alcohol abuse. In many parts of Asia and Africa, cirrhosis due to chronic hepatitis (caused by virus) is a major cause of death.

The structural classification of cirrhosis is difficult because each cirrhotic liver has a different configuration, the end result of the interplay of many independent factors; furthermore, cirrhosis is not a static lesion.

A current tendency avoids classifying cirrhosis and accepts instead a description of how it becomes diseased. Much more important than its classification are the activity, stage of development, and complications of the disease process. Many of those with cirrhosis are without specific symptoms and are well-nourished, making the diagnosis difficult and somewhat surprising.

Generalized weakness, loss of appetite, malaise, weight loss and loss of sex drive are common. In those who are malnourished, other problems may exist, for instance paraesthesia (numbness, tingling, etc.) and

525

Liver diseases   Questions & Answers

How is the liver supplied with blood?

One remarkable feature is its double blood supply; besides receiving fresh arterial blood from the hepatic artery, which arises from the aorta, it is also fed with blood from the portal vein, carrying the products of digestion from the intestines. Its spent blood drains into the inferior vena cava via the hepatic vein. The portal vein conveys blood from the stomach, intestines, pancreas and spleen to the liver.

What are the basic functions of the liver?

As well as being the largest the liver is also the body's most versatile organ, having an extraordinarily wide range of functions. These include production, destruction and storage, and its cells contain enzymes for many chemical processes as well as vital stores of essential materials.
The substances stored by the liver include carbohydrates, fats and proteins, and the metabolism of each of these three groups of food material takes place there.

How is glycogen stored in the liver?

Glycogen, which is a condensed, readily available derivative of glucose, is deposited as granules inside the liver cells and is broken down and its products released into the blood to supply energy needs.

How is fat treated in the liver?

Fat is split up in the liver and also manufactured and laid down in the cells.

How are nitrogenous waste products handled by the liver?

Many nitrogenous waste products are rendered harmless in the liver by combination with other substances; urea, the chief nitrogen-containing product of protein metabolism, is formed there from ammonia (which is toxic to the body) and carbon dioxide.

What is the involvement of the liver in protein synthesis?

The liver cells also synthesize proteins. They make the albumin and part of the globulin in the blood plasma, and the fibrinogen and prothrombin essential for blood clotting.

What is bile?

Bile is a viscous, dark green, alkaline fluid coloured by bilirubin, a breakdown product of hemoglobin, and containing quantities of cholesterol and bile salts. These salts have a detergent and emulsifying action, for their molecules have chemical grouping soluble both in watery and in fatty substances.
This explains the ability of bile to enhance the absorption of fats from the intestines. When bile secretion is impaired, fat cannot be absorbed properly and is instead excreted in the faeces, and in addition the fat-soluble vitamins A, D and K are lost to the body.

What is the involvement of the liver in vitamin storage?

Storage of certain vitamins is another function of the liver. Vitamin A is present in large quantities in liver fat, and vitamin D is also found (hence the value of cod-liver oil). The liver contains vitamin B_{12}, enabling the maturation of red blood cells to continue for many months, after deficient diet or stomach disease deprives the body of fresh supplies.

glossitis (inflammation of the tongue).

A palpable, firm, smooth liver with a blunt edge is characteristic. Ordinary cirrhotic nodules are rarely if ever present. Other signs of chronic liver disease include:
- muscular wasting
- palmar erythema (rash on the palms)
- gynecomastia (abnormal enlargement of the male breasts)
- enlargement of parotid glands
- hair loss
- atrophy of the testicles
- peripheral neuropathy (damage to nerves on the outer parts of the body)

If the person has experienced major complications, such as hematemesis (vomiting blood), hepatic coma, ascites (swelling of the abdomen) and jaundice, the prognosis is grave - for instance, a one-year survival of less than 50 per cent can be expected in such a person with alcohol-induced liver disease who continues to consume excess alcohol.

However, even with severe signs, a sufferer may respond to treatment, especially if the offending agent (alcohol, copper, etc.) can be removed. Treatment of cirrhosis is based upon the cause and the management of specific complications.

Abstinence from alcohol, a nutritious diet containing protein (as tolerated), reasonable rest and therapeutic multivitamins are indicated for those with alcohol-induced liver disease.

The use of corticosteroids remains controversial but may aid the treatment of chronic active hepatitis when cirrhosis has developed.

Alcoholic liver disease

In general, a correlation exists between the severity of liver damage and the intensity of alcohol abuse as measured by duration and dose. However, the mechanisms by which alcohol actually damages the liver have not yet been adequately defined. By providing calories without essential nutrients, decreasing appetite and causing malabsorption through its toxic effects on the gut and pancreas, alcohol promotes malnutrition. It is also a toxin to the liver cells whose metabolism then creates profound derangements of the cellular constituents.

Apparent variations in the susceptibility of individuals and the greater susceptibility of females to alcoholic liver disease suggest that other factors are also significant. The fact that alcoholic liver disease frequently runs in families means that the influence of genetic factors cannot be dismissed.

Although the data are controversial, and many abnormalities are no doubt secondary rather than primary, various immunological abnormalities in those with alcoholic liver disease suggest that a person's immunological status may play a major role in determining susceptibility to alcohol.

The spectrum of changes associated with prolonged alcohol consumption range from the simple accumulation of neutral fat in liver cells to cirrhosis and cancer. The findings usually overlap and many present features of the entire spectrum. The key lesions may well be fibrosis around the small veins.

Fatty liver appears to be the initial change associated with alcoholic liver disease and is the most common liver abnormality in hospitalized alcoholics. Hydropic change (i.e. swelling due to excess fluid in the body) is prevalent in the early stages of alcoholic liver injury.

Although insufficiently explained, alcohol does affect the transport of certain substances through the membranes of cells, thus increasing the amount of sodium and water in the cells. It can also be associated with the accumulation of excess protein in the cells.

About 20 per cent of heavy drinkers will develop cirrhosis in which the liver is finely nodular with its architecture is organized by thin fibrous septa and nodules.

If drinking stops and the liver undergoes a constructive regenerative response, the picture can be that of a mixed cirrhosis.

Increased amounts of iron in the liver are seen in alcoholics with normal, fatty or cirrhotic livers, but the incidence is less than 10 per cent. The underlying mechanisms are obscure, but there appears to be no relation-

Major clinical features of liver diseases

Specific features
- jaundice
- enlarged liver
- fluid in the abdomen
- gastrointestinal bleeding from varices
- portal hypertension

Skin
- spiderlike blood vessels
- red palms
- florid complexion
- itching

Blood
- anemia
- leukopenia
- thrombocytopenia
- a tendency to bleed

Hormones
- high levels of insulin
- cessation of menstrual cycles
- impotence

Heart and blood vessels
- increased heart rate
- low blood pressure

General features
- fatigue
- weakness
- weight loss
- poor appetite
- nausea
- fever

Schematic drawing of a liver lobulus.
1. gall capillaries
2. central vein
3. liver cell
4. gall duct
5. liver artery
6. lymph vessel
7. portal vein

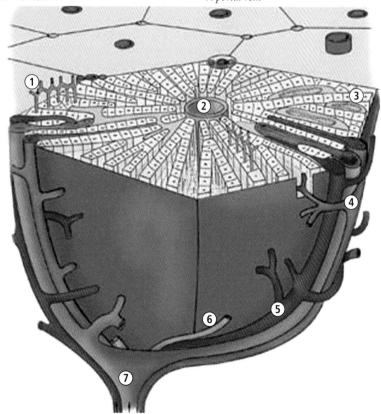

L

Liver diseases   Questions & Answers

What is cirrhosis of the liver?

Cirrhosis is a general term meant to signify generalized destruction and scarring of liver tissue, with impairment of liver function to a slight or greater degree. Any disease process which involves the liver may eventually lead to cirrhosis, that is, destruction of liver cells and replacement by scar tissue.

Has abuse of alcohol something to do with cirrhosis of the liver?

Abuse of alcohol is a serious cause of cirr-hosis. The association between people who drink alcoholic beverages excessively and the occurrence of cirrhosis is well known.

It is thought that the liver damage results from the combined effect of the toxic action of the alcohol upon the liver and the poor nutritional intake usually associated with those whom drink excessively.

What are the major symptoms of cirrhosis?

The symptoms of cirrhosis vary with the degree of liver destruction and liver reserve. Many cases remain undetected and without symptoms for years.

As liver function deteriorates, it may be accompanied by loss of appetite, nausea, vomiting, and weight loss. There may be abdominal discomfort, fullness in the upper abdomen, and indigestion. When the disease progresses, there may be a listlessness and weakness, with loss of energy.

How is the diagnose oi cirrhosis made?

The diagnosis of cirrhosis is generally made on the basis of the symptoms and physical examination, together with a history of risk factors such as alcohol abuse. On physical examination, a doctor may feel a small, firm liver, occasionally, small lumps (nodules) on the surface of the liver are felt as well.

Liver function tests often are normal because of the tremendous reserve of the liver and the relative insensitivity of these biochemical tests. An ultrasound or CT scan may show that the liver is shrunken or abnormally patterned, suggesting cirrhosis.

Is there a relationship between liver cancer and cirrhosis?

There may be a primary cancer, in which the cells of the liver themselves originate the cancer; or there may be metastatic involvement of the liver, in which the cancer cells have originated elsewhere in the body. The cause of primary cancer of the liver is not really known, but it has been found that a considerable number of cases develop in those livers that have been previously cirrhotic.

In addition, certain chemical toxins and infections have been incriminated in a small percentage of these cases. It is common for the liver to be involved in cancer which has originated elsewhere (metastatic spread of a primary cancer).

The liver is the organ most commonly involved by cancer which has spread from another organ, such as the stomach, pancreas, gallbladder, breast, kidney, or intestines. The symptoms vary widely, depending upon the extent and nature of the involvement as well as upon how the other organs of the body are involved.

The most common symptoms are:
- loss of weight
- weakness
- loss of appetite
- nodular enlargement of the liver

Eventually, all the symptoms of typical severe liver damage ensue such as:
- jaundice
- hemorrhage
- swelling of the legs
- coma

ship with the amount of iron consumed in the alcohol or with the length of the drinking history.

Variations in drinking pattern, individual susceptibility to the toxic effects of alcohol and the many kinds of damage means that there is a highly variable clinical picture. For a long time, there may be no symptoms and no signs referable to the liver. In general, symptoms can be related to the amount of alcohol drunk and the overall duration of alcohol ingestion.

Thus, symptoms usually become apparent when a person is in his/her 30s and severe problems tend to appear in the 40s.

Those with only a fatty liver are usually without specific symptoms, but may have an enlarged, smooth and occasionally tender liver. In theory, the treatment of this condition is simple and straightforward; in practice, it is difficult: the person must stop drinking alcohol.

However, following severe bouts of illness, major adverse social consequences and a review of the facts by a doctor who establishes rapport, many will stop drinking. It also helps to point out that much of alcoholic liver disease is reversible.

Although still controversial, it is unlikely that corticosteroids have any role to play in the treatment of alcoholic liver disease. The survival rate of those with alcoholic hepatitis, fibrosis and cirrhosis improves if drinking stops.

Disorders of the blood circulation

Occlusion (blockage) of the hepatic artery is usually caused by thrombosis or embolism or by its circulation being somehow cut off during surgery. The occlusion may cause damage or death to the tissue whose blood supply has been stopped, but results are unpredictable because of individual differences in the system of arteries and veins in the liver and the extent of collateral circulation (where new blood vessels develop to take over from damaged ones).

The underlying problem is usually part of a disease involving the whole body. The hepatic artery and its branches are involved in approximately 60 per cent of cases of polyarteritis nodosa, a disease involving inflammation along areas of the arteries, giving rise to nodules in their walls.

Lesions of the portal vein

Thrombosis of the portal vein may occur at any point in its course. In less than 50 per cent of causes, no cause can be identified, but it may be associated with inflammation. The condition is rare in cirrhosis without cancer, but it frequently complicates cancer of the liver. Portal vein thrombosis infrequently occurs in pregnancy, especially in eclampsia.

What this does to the body, depends on the location and extent of the thrombosis and the nature of the underlying liver disease. It may lead to infarction (damage and death of a part) of the liver or to segmental atrophy (where a segment becomes wasted). In general, portal hypertension is the end result.

Portal hypertension

This condition is defined as increased blood pressure in the portal vein caused by:
- obstruction of the portal vein outside the liver;
- increased blood flow through the liver;
- increased resistance to liver blood outflow.

The veins of the portal venous system carry all blood from the gastro-intestinal tract, spleen, pancreas and gall bladder to the liver. The portal vein itself carries about 1000 to 1200 mL (35-42 fl. oz) of blood per minute and 70 per cent of the oxygen supplied to the liver.

The portal venous system is valveless; its pressure, produced and maintained by the volume of inflow and resistance to outflow, is normally less than 14 mm of mercury seen on a blood pressure measuring device.

It is controlled by the sympathetic nervous system and is therefore responsive to certain vasoactive drugs and hormones (i.e. those that affect the diameter of the blood vessels). The venous outflow tracts - the venules and veins - are passive con-

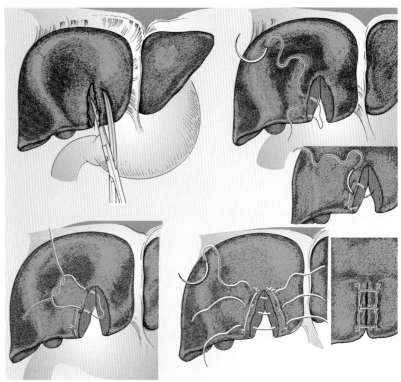

Suture of a laceration of the liver. Excising non-viable liver tissue (A); inserting overlapping mattress stitches on both sides of the wound, B, C, D, E) and stitching the two sides together (E, F).

duits do not react to nervous or other stimulation.

The normal portal vein pressure is therefore chiefly controlled by variations in inflow. Furthermore, it is limited, and the portal vein pressure does not usually rise above 25 mm of mercury.

Therefore, most cases of portal hypertension not caused by obstruction to the portal vein outside the liver are thought to be caused by increased resistance to blood outflow.

The creation of artery-to-vein or vein-to-vein connections (anastomoses), the creation of abnormal and conflicting inflow currents and mechanical compression are sufficient to explain the portal hypertension in cirrhosis.

Clinically, portal hypertension is most often associated with cirrhosis and is present with enlargement of the liver, ascites (swelling of the abdomen) and bleeding in the gastro-intestinal tract. The disorder needs treatment by a specialist in a hospital.

Benign and malignant tumors

Benign tumors are relatively uncommon. Many show no symptoms and are only detected incidentally. Metastatic carcinoma - that is, a cancer that has spread from another site - is by far the most common form of liver tumor.

The liver provides a fertile bed for metastases: lung, breast, colon, pancreas and stomach are the most frequent original sites, though virtually any source may be responsible.

Spread to the liver is not uncommonly the initial clinical manifestation of cancer elsewhere. In terms of symptoms, non-specific evidence of malignancy is frequent, such as weight loss, loss of appetite and fever.

The liver is characteristically enlarged and hard, and may be tender; massive enlargement with easily felt lumps signifies advanced disease. Liver involvement in leukaemia and related disorders is common, due to infiltration with the abnormal cells.

529

LUNG CANCER

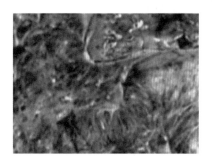

Introduction

Lung cancer is the leading cause of deaths from cancer in males in more than 35 countries, and the death rate for females is increasing. In both developed and developing countries, it is already a serious health problem or is rapidly becoming one. About 80-90 per cent of all cases of lung cancer in developed countries are caused by tobacco - chiefly by the smoking of manufactured cigarettes.

The risk of lung cancer has increased among women in recent years in most countries of the world; a slight decrease in men has been observed in a small number of countries. In those countries in which studies of the "geography" of the disease have been conducted, the risk is particularly high among cigarette smokers and a clear-cut relationship has been observed. Further, the risk has been found to be greater among those who started smoking at a young age and among those who smoke "high-yield" cigarettes. The association with smoking is strongest for the squamous and small-cell types of the disease.

An increased risk of lung cancer has also been observed among individuals exposed to occupational and environmental carcinogens (cancer-causing agents) such as asbestos dust and radiation.

This risk is enhanced by cigarette smoking. After several years, the risk of lung cancer for persons who have stopped smoking approaches that for persons who have always been non-smokers. A regular daily intake of certain foods such as green and yellow vegetables (rich in beta-carotene) has, in certain studies, also been observed to lower the risk.

Diagnosis

A classification of lung cancer that discriminates between small-cell and non-small-cell cancers (squamous cell carcinoma, adenocarcinoma, large-cell carcinoma) is essential. The following diagnostic tests are generally considered to be the most appropriate.

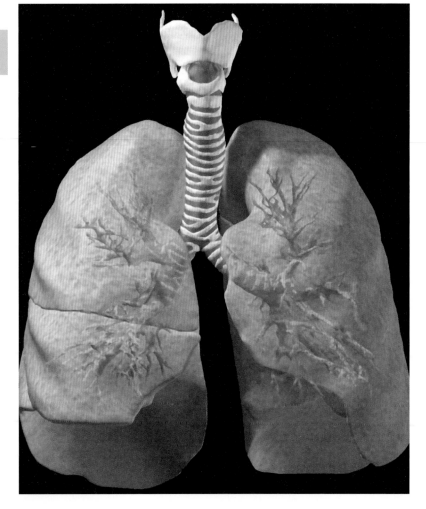

The lungs are cone-shaped organs which completely fill the pleural space, extending from the diaphragm to about 1½ inches above the clavicle. The adult lung is a spongy mass, frequently blue-gray in color because of inhaled dust and soot in the respiratory lymphatics.

Small-cell carcinoma

Small-cell carcinoma is now recognized as a specific entity among the various types of lung cancer, and has its own biological characteristics. In the majority of cases, unfortunately small-cell cancer has already spread to other parts of the body by the time it is diagnosed. For the diagnosis of small-cell cancer, the following minimum investigations are recommended:

- medical history and physical examination;
- chest X-ray or chest CT-scan;
- kidney function tests;
- liver function tests.

The following tests may assist in discovering whether the disease is "limited" or "extensive," which has implications for the prognosis and may influence treatment:

▲ scans of bone and brain (even if the patient has no adverse symptoms);

▲ samples taken from bone marrow and a biopsy performed.

CT scans (computerized axial tomography) are not felt to be necessary in these investigations.

Non-small-cell carcinoma

Non-small-cell carcinoma includes squamous cell carcinoma, adenocarcinoma and large-cell carcinoma. For the diagnosis of this form of the disease, the following minimum investigations are recommended:

▲ medical history and physical examination;

▲ chest X-ray or CT chest scan;

▲ mediastinoscopy (the investigation of the mediastinum, the space between the lungs and the heart, using an endoscope;

▲ liver function tests;

▲ CT scans of bone or brain, which should be carried out if abnormalities are suggested in the medical history or detected on physical examination or laboratory investigation;

▲ pulmonary arteriography (special X-rays of the pulmonary artery).

The following additional investigations are recommended to assess whether surgery is possible:

- lung function tests;
- electrocardiogram (ECG);
- hemogram (a special type of blood count).

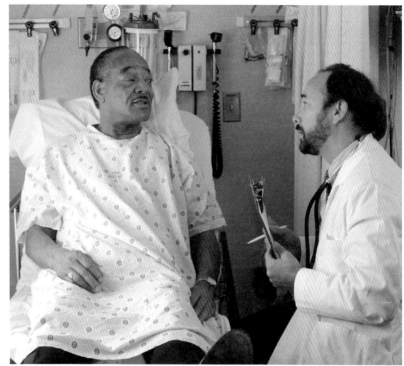

Patient being prepared for surgery for lung cancer. Lung cancer is the most common cause of death from cancer in both men and women, It occurs most commonly between the ages of 45 and 70.

Surgery for lung cancer. Surgery is the treatment of choice for lung cancer that has not spread beyond the lung. Older people should not be excluded from surgery based solely on their age.

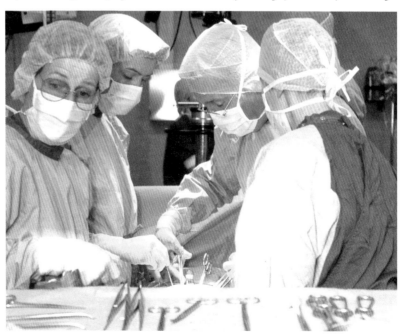

Lung cancer   Questions & Answers

What is the difference between lung cancer and bronchial cancer?

Lung cancer (since the bronchi are primarily affected, doctors often speak of bronchial carcinoma, but universally) is the leading cause of death from cancer in males in more than 35 countries, and the death rate for females is increasing. About 80-90 per cent of all cases of lung cancer in Western countries are caused by tobacco - chiefly by smoking of manufactured cigarettes.

What is the risk of getting lung cancer?

The risk of lung cancer has increased in recent years in most countries of the world. In those countries in which studies of the "geography" of the disease have been conducted, the risk is particularly high among cigarette smokers and a clear-cut relationship has been observed. Further, the risk has been found to be greater among those who started smoking at a young age and among those who smoke "high-yield" cigarettes. The association with smoking is strongest for the squamous (characterized by plate-like cells) and small-cell types of the disease. After several years, the risk of lung cancer for persons who have stopped smoking approaches that for persons who have always been non-smokers. A regular daily intake of certain foods such as green and yellow vegetables (rich in beta-carotene) has, in certain studies, also been observed to lower the risk.

What types of cancer may occur in the lungs?

Tumors of the lungs can be one of two types:
- Tumors that are not cancers are called benign. They do not spread to other parts of the body and are seldom a threat to life. Often, benign tumors can be removed by surgery, and they are not likely to return.
- Cancerous tumors are called malignant. They invade and destroy nearby healthy tissues and organs. Cancers can also metastasize, or spread, to other parts of the body causing new tumors.

What is a small-cell carcinoma?

Small-cell carcinoma is now recognized as a specific entity among the various types of lung cancer, and has its own biological characteristics. In the majority of cases, unfortunately small-cell cancer has already spread to other parts of the body by the time it is diagnosed.

For the diagnosis of small-cell cancer, the following minimum investigations are recommended:
- medical history and physical examination;
- chest X-ray and lung scans;
- kidney function tests;
- liver function tests.

What tests are being performed to detect lung cancer?

The following tests may assist in discovering whether the disease is a cancer and whether the disorder is "limited" or "extensive", which has implications for the prognosis and may influence treatment:
- scans of bones and brain (even if the patient has no adverse symptoms);
- samples taken from bone marrow and a biopsy (removal of a small amount of tissue) performed; bronchoscopy is routinely performed on patients with severe lung problems.

Treatment

Small-cell cancer

The main mode of treatment is systemic - that is, it aims to treat the whole body - and comprises the giving of a number of drugs (combination chemotherapy). This technique is constantly being modified and improved as more research is done and new and more effective anti-cancer drugs come on the market.

For example, in 1990, the survival rate two years after diagnosis was about 12 per cent, but ten years later (2000), it was 23-26 per cent. However, the disease is still usually fatal, with the median survival period being two to three months for untreated patients, and 20-26 months for those receiving combination chemotherapy.

The most active cytostatic drugs (those that stop the growth of cancer cells) include cyclophosphamide, etoposide, doxorubicin, vincristine, lomustine, methotrexate and their derivatives, and most treatment schedules now include three or four of these drugs. It has been demonstrated in controlled clinical trials that treatment with a combination of three or four drugs is superior to treatment with a single one.

Drug dosage should be chosen so as to produce an optimal therapeutic response. As well as adversely affecting the cancer cells, other toxic manifestations may occur, depending upon the nature of the drugs employed.

Response to treatment is usually associated with prolonged maintenance of both activity ("performance status") and comfort ("quality of life"), or a considerable improvement in these respects. This form of treatment does not usually require hospitalization.

If progression of the disease is noted within two months of treatment, the initial drug combination will be discontinued; "second-line chemotherapy" is usually unsuccessful. However, if the patient responds to the initial treatment, it will be maintained for at least six months. There is not yet sufficient information to permit the establishment of an upper limit beyond six months for the duration of treatment.

Radiotherapy, which has been used in

the past as a single treatment, usually produces a tumor response. Yet, at present, there are no unequivocal data that demonstrate improvement in survival when radiotherapy is given to those with disease confined to one side of the chest. n addition, recent improvements in combination chemotherapy pose the question of the need for radiotherapy.

Current data from a limited number of studies suggest no advantage in short-term survival resulting from the addition of radiotherapy, but it should be stressed that improvement in controlling the tumor itself has yet to be evaluated with respect to long-term survival.

The energy of megavoltage irradiation is of lesser importance than the precision with which it is delivered to its target, the tumor. However, if combined chemo- and radiotherapy is used, an increase in adverse effects on the body can be anticipated. There are considerable data indicating that the use of preventive irradiation of the brain reduces the incidence of cancer spreading to that area (cranial metastases).

However, several controlled trials have also shown that it does not alter the overall short-term survival rate. Those who, for medical reasons, cannot tolerate surgery despite having resectable tumors may be considered for potentially "curative" radiotherapy. Further research in this form of therapy is needed.

For those with disease confined to one lung with the cancer extending elsewhere in the same region but who are deemed inoperable, there are no unequivocal data supporting the value of radiotherapy as "curative" treatment, although some studies have reported long-term survival following radiotherapy.

However, in the absence of controlled clinical trials, it is uncertain that these were due to the irradiation. It is conceivable that one or more of the currently utilized combination chemotherapeutic regimens do have a beneficial effect on both the quality and duration of survival. Yet it still remains to be proved that any chemotherapy is superior to supportive care or changes the ultimate, usually fatal, outcome in this form of the

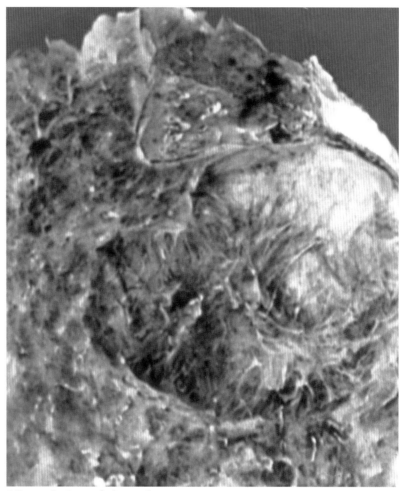

Microscopic picture of a large pulmonary cancer.

disease.

Non-small-cell cancer

Surgery is the preferred form of treatment for non-small-cell lung cancer, provided the tumor is resectable (meaning that all apparent cancer can be removed) and the patient is medically fit and accepts the operation. So-called "palliative" surgery -that is, surgery that relieves symptoms but does not attempt a cure - is not recommended as a routine procedure.

Prior to surgery, a careful evaluation of the patient should be carried out by a multidisciplinary team.

At present, additional treatment such as post-operative irradiation, chemotherapy or immunotherapy is under consideration. Although they are not essential for decisions con-

cerning primary treatment, specimens of the tumor, the area around the site of the tumor, the pleural fluid and the lymph nodes should be obtained and submitted for pathological examination.

Other measures

Many people with lung cancer experience a substantial decrease in lung function, whether or not they undergo treatment. Oxygen therapy and drugs that widen the airways may ease breathing difficulties. Many people with advanced lung cancer develop such pain and difficulty in breathing that they require large doses of narcotics in the weeks or months before their death. Fortunately, narcotics can help substantially if used in adequate doses.

LUNG DISEASES

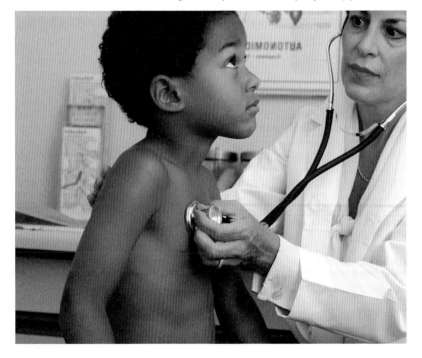

Introduction

The proper approach to diagnosis and treatment of lung disorders requires:
- a medical history;
- a physical examination;
- chest imaging
  chest X-rays
  computed tomography (CT) scanning
  magnetic resonance imaging (MRI)
  ultrasound scanning
  nuclear lung scanning
- bronchoscopy
  direct visual examination of the voice box and airways through a fiber-optic viewing tube
- an estimate of whether the disorder is acute or chronic
- a judgement as to whether the disorder is active or inactive

The relative importance of each of these elements in the appraisal varies from patient to patient. For instance, the detection of an occupational lung disease, such as asbestosis, often requires a more detailed medical (and occupational) history to uncover the offending agent. In contrast, the physical examination may be most helpful in following the course of someone with acute pneumonia.

Chest imaging is an essential supplement to the medical history and physical examination. Certain symptoms and signs that direct attention to the lungs as the focus of a clinical disorder are cough, dyspnea (difficulty in breathing) and hemoptysis (spitting of blood).

Physical examination of a patient with a lung disorder will consist of inspection, palpation, percussion and auscultation.

Signs and symptoms

As already mentioned above the major signs and symptoms of a lung disorder are cough, difficulty in breathing (dyspnoea) and spitting of blood (hemoptysis).

■ Cough

This is an explosive expiration required for the self-cleaning of the lungs, and it is a reflex generally arising from stimulation of the mucous membrane lining the airways. Many different stimuli can elicit a cough. The sudden onset of a distressing cough that is part of acute bronchitis or pneumonia is difficult for the sufferer to ignore, but commonly, the person with chronic cough either fails to notice the cough or takes it for granted.

This is particularly true for the "smoker's cough" that many individuals come to accept as part of the waking-up process each morning. Indeed, the person with chronic bronchitis often denies that he or she has a cough until pressed for details. None the less, the disregarded cough may have disease implications. Coughs should be characterized in terms of when and under what circumstances they occur. For example, a cough may occur only when the person is at work, when it is triggered by noxious or allergenic

Using a stethoscope, a doctor listens to the breath sounds to determine whether airflow is normal or obstructed and whether the lungs contain fluid as a result of respiratory failure.

materials, or it may occur in relation to changes in posture, as commonly seen in those with chronic bronchitis or bronchiectasis when they lie down at night or get up in the morning. Coughs should also be characterized with regard to whether it is non-productive (dry) or productive (i.e. it brings up sputum). A productive cough that persists for months and tends to recur year after year is characteristic of chronic bronchitis.

■ *Difficulty in breathing*

This condition is defined as breathlessness, shortness of breath, the sensation of difficult, laboured or uncomfortable breathing. Dyspnoea is a subjective complaint and represents the person's perception that breathing is excessive, difficult or uncomfortable; usually, it signifies an unpleasant sensation.

Dyspnoea is an important manifestation of disease when it occurs at a less strenuous level of activity than the individual normally tolerates. Dyspnoea may refer to one or more sensations and may represent the subjective response to one or more mechanisms. Among the different sensations encompassed by the word "dyspnoea" are:

▲ the profound overbreathing (hyperpnoea) that occurs during and after severe exercise;

▲ the sensation arising from obstruction in the bronchi in those with asthma and bronchitis;

▲ the inappropriate breathlessness that may occur with only slight exertion in those with heart disease or severe enemia;

▲ the sensation that compels the person to take the next breath after a period of breath-holding.

Dyspnoea from lung causes is usually either restrictive or obstructive. Those with restrictive dyspnoea (for instance, due to lung fibrosis or chest deformities) are usually comfortable at rest but become intensely dyspneic when exertion causes lung ventilation to approach their greatly limited breathing capacity.

In obstructive dyspnoea (for instance, as in obstructive emphysema or asthma), increased ventilatory effort induces dyspnoea even at rest, and breathing is laboured and retarded, especially during expiration.

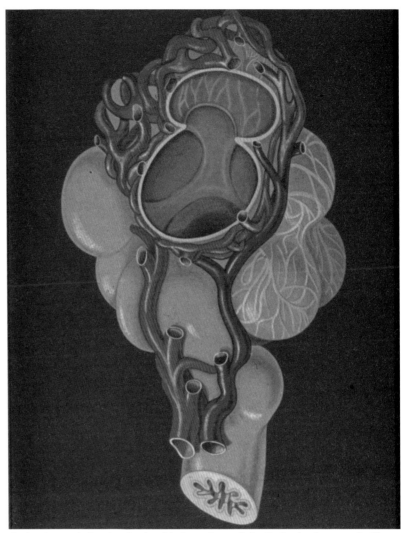

Basic microscopic functional units of the lung. Group of alveoli, alveolar ducts, terminal bronchioli, and arterial and venous capillaries.

There is also a possibility of a heart condition causing dyspnoea. In the early stages of heart failure, cardiac output fails to keep pace with increased metabolic need during exercise. As a result, the respiratory drive is increased largely because of increased acid content of the blood. The shortness of breath is often accompanied by lassitude or a feeling of smothering or oppression of the breastbone. In later stages of congestive heart failure, the lungs are congested and swollen with excess fluid, the ventilatory capacity of the stiff lungs is reduced, and ventilatory effort is increased.

■ *Spitting of blood (hemoptysis)*

This condition is characterized by the coughing up of blood as a result of bleeding from the respiratory tract. The source of hemoptysis may be either the mucous membrane of the airways or granulation tissue that contains blood vessels. Blood-streaked sputum is a rather common complaint but is usually non-threatening.

Inflammation accounts for 70 to 80 per cent of cases of hemoptysis. Acute or chronic bronchitis is probably the commonest cause, bronchitis and bronchiectasis together causing about half of all cases. Tuberculosis accounts

Lung diseases Questions & Answers

How are disorders of the respiratory system being diagnosed?

Diagnosis of disorders of the respiratory system require a medical history and physical examination, X-rays, and lung function tests. Some special procedures (for example, bronchoscopy) will almost always be necessary. History-taking provides for the family doctor or medical specialist essential information and it initiates understanding of the patient as a person, of the patient's environment, expectations and fears, and is the best way for the doctor to develop understanding and collaboration with the patient. Data desired include those related to occupational or other exposures; family, travel, and contact history; an account of previous illnesses and medications. Most important, however, are the clear definition of the present complaint, and both general symptoms (for example, lassitude, weight loss, or fever) and the major respiratory symptoms of cough, sputum, chest pain, wheeze, and spitting of blood.

What are the important diagnostic tools to detect disorders of the respiratory system?

The diagnosis and treatment of lung disorders and other diseases of the respiratory system require the following methods and procedures:
- physical examination;
- radiological procedures such as chest X-rays and lung scans;
- lung function tests.

In most cases of severe lung disease, the sputum will also be examined for cells and micro-organisms. The relative importance of each of the elements of the diagnostic procedures in the appraisal varies from patient to patient. The chest X-ray or lung scan is an essential supplement to the medical history and physical examination. Certain symptoms and signs that direct attention to the lungs as focus of a clinical disorder are cough, dyspnea (difficulty in breathing) and hemoptysis (spitting of blood).

What methods are used in physical examination of the respiratory system?

Physical examination of a patient with a lung disorder will consist of inspection, palpation, percussion, and auscultation. The doctor will generally perform these procedures during the first visit.

How is inspection of the chest performed?

The shape of the chest on inspection is usually fairly symmetrical, moving relatively little during normal breathing. Full expansion usually amounts to 5 cm or so. Respiratory movement in men is chiefly-seen in the abdomen, but in women, it is usually seen as the chest itself is moving.

Over-inflation of the chest may be visible in those with chronic airways obstruction; this is characterized by prominence of the breastbone and a barrel-shaped chest that appears to be held in a state of full inspiration. In those with restrictive defects of the lung, as opposed to airways obstruction, breathing may be rapid and shallow and the so-called "doorstop" sign may be seen, where inspiration is topped abruptly by a restriction of some kind.

What is a "frozen" chest?

Where there are underlying abnormalities of the lung such as fibrosis (an increase in the formation of fibrous connective tissue), consolidation (hardening), collapse or pleural effusion (in which the spaces of the pleural cavity are filled with fluid), movement of the chest wall at that site may be sizably reduced.

A "frozen" chest may reflect fibrosis after injury for instance. The person may also be obviously breathing rapidly, the normal rate of respiration averaging between 12 and 16 per minute. This may be due to anxiety, chest disease or heart disease, and its origin usually becomes clearer as the examination proceeds.

What is the commonest cause of difficult breathing?

The commonest cause of difficult breathing is heart disease, especially incipient failure of the left ventricle or left atrium of the heart, leading to an increase in fluid in the lungs, chiefly at the bases of the lungs when the person is in an upright position. Less often, particularly difficult breathing (in lying down) may be the feature of chronic obstructive bronchitis, where redistribution of bronchial secretion and postural changes in the airways in lying flat may account for irritability of the bronchi, coughing and the difficult breathing.

What is the commonest cause of hyperventilation?

Hyperventilation, or hyperpnoea, is usually due to anxiety, though it may also be induced by metabolic disturbances (acidosis). Where it is voluntary, the person complains of tingling and other unusual sensations, muscle cramp and, rarely, seizures ("fits") due to the blowing off of too much carbon dioxide.

What information can the doctor obtain from palpation of the chest?

The doctor will attempt to confirm by palpation - gentle feeling and pressing - any abnormalities of shape or movement first noticed at inspection. Measurement of chest movement will be made by applying the flat of the hands to the chest wall with the thumbs placed centrally and the fingers lightly spread and gripping laterally (sidewards); full inspiration will then shift the thumbs and give an indication of general and local expansion.

for 10 to 20 per cent of cases. Tumors (especially cancer), supplied primarily by bronchial blood vessels, account for about 20 per cent of cases.

Special procedures

Lung function testing has progressed from simple measurement of lung volumes to sophisticated applications of special procedures.

■ *Chest imaging*
The chest X-ray (and other chest imaging methods such as CT-scan and MRI-scan) is an integral part of the examination of any person with persisting chest symptoms. There is general agreement on how the specialist should read a chest X-ray. In clinical practice, the changes seen on the X-ray usually concur with those suspected on examination, although there are some important exceptions. These include early adult tuberculosis in which the upper part of the lung is infiltrated, and the hilar mass or coin lesion in the periphery of the lungs with bronchial cancer.
Collapse or consolidation of various lobes of the lung give specific shadows. In bronchiectasis, there may be ring shadows indicating bronchial wall thickening. In pneumothorax (where an injury to the chest opens the pleural cavity), the lung edge can be seen displaced from the thoracic wall and this may be exaggerated if an X-ray is taken when the person is breathing in.
In the diseases characterized by diffuse air-flow obstruction - namely, chronic obstructive bronchitis, emphysema and asthma - the characteristic features seen are hyperinflation with horizontal ribs, hyperlucent lung fields and flat diaphragm.

■ *Sputum examination*
Sputum will be collected carefully, and an adequate fresh sample, uncontaminated by saliva, will be sent to the laboratory. Often an early morning sample is best. The first step is inspection of its characteristics by eye.
Thereafter, smear, culture and test for antibiotic sensitivities are indicated. The sputum may show asbestos bodies in asbestosis and eosinophilia

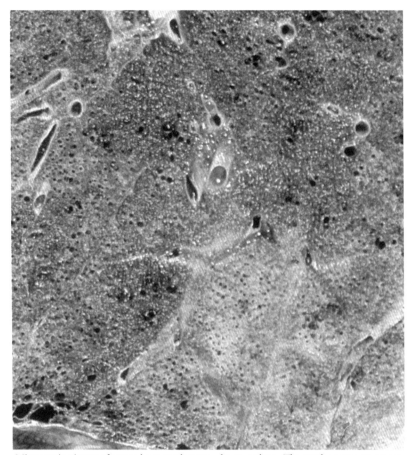
Microscopic picture of severe lung emphysema, due to asthma. The emphysema was accompanied by a cancerous growth.

(excess numbers of a certain type of white blood cell) in asthma.
Sputum cytology (the microscopic examination of cells) is an important technique for diagnosing lung cancer. At least three specimens of sputum should be examined; this gives a positive result in over 50 per cent of cases.

■ *Bronchoscopy*
This is the direct visual examination of the interior of the body using an endoscope, a flexible tube containing light-transmitting glass fibers that return a magnified image. Those used to examine the bronchi are called fiberbronchoscopes, and they range in external diameter from 3 to 6 mm; the proper diameter depends on the size of the patient.
The small calibre (internal diameter) of the instrument makes it possible to enter fairly small parts of the bronchi.

The central channel of the bronchoscope is 2 to 2.5 mm in diameter and is used to suck out secretions, to give anesthetic agents, to obtain tissue samples using brush or forceps and to introduce contrast material used for X-rays.
The method is used to explore the cause of an unexplained persistent cough, wheeze, spitting up blood (hemoptysis) or unresolved pneumonia or atelectasis (shrunken and airless part of the lung), especially in a male smoker about the age of 30. The flexible bronchoscope is also used to obtain samples of blood-tinged sputum or small quantities of blood.
In thoracoscopy, the specialist examines the pleural cavity with an endoscope, mainly to obtain a sample from a lesion on the outer edge of the lung or pleura. Under general anesthesia, the location for the incision is chosen

537

Lung diseases   Questions & Answers

What is an occupational lung disease?

Injury to the lungs occurring at work may be caused by inhalation of gases, fumes, vapours, dusts, or micro-organisms.

The site and degree of the lung reaction is determined by a number of factors:
- the physical and chemical properties of the substance inhaled
- the intensity and duration of exposure
- the presence of pre-existing lung disease
- individual differences in susceptibility

The occupational diseases of the respiratory system are usually divided into three categories:
- those due to inorganic or mineral dusts
- those due to organic dusts
- those due to irritant gases and chemicals

What are the types of injury that may cause occupational lung disease?

The type of injury sustained by inhalation of gases is in part dependent on their solubility. Thus sulphur dioxide which is readily soluble produces an acute exudative reaction. Exudation is the slow escape (oozing) of fluids and cellular matter from blood vessels or cells through small pores or breaks in the cell membranes, sometimes the result of inflammation.

Other substances, like toluene di-isocyanate is without immediate clinical effect so that affected individuals may be subjected to repeated exposure before symptoms are noticed. Only those substances with a particle size in the range of 0.5-3 micrometer can penetrate to the alveoli, larger particles being deposited within the airways are rapidly removed by ciliary transport and coughing.

How may dust particles affect lung tissue?

Dust particles which have penetrated beyond the inner lining of the respiratory system (epithelium with cilia) are engulfed by alveolar macrophages and there then be transported by the ciliary mechanism or pass into the lymph vessels around the alveoli.

What effect then follow depends both upon the quality of dust inhaled and its

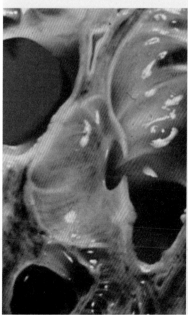

physical and chemical properties. If the quantity inhaled overwhelms the clearance mechanisms of the lung, dust-laden macrophages will accumulate.

How can inert substances, such as iron and carbon, affect lung tissue?

Inert substances such as iron, tin and carbon will have little injurious effect and although the accumulation of macrophages laden with these substances may produce dramatic abnormalities on chest X-rays, there is little or no fibrosis.

Fibrosis is an increase in the formation of fibrous connective tissue, either normally as a scar formation, or abnormally to replace normal tissues, especially in the lungs. This mechanism can also occur in other organs, such as the heart or uterus. Silica and asbestos cause severe reactions of the macrophages and strong fibrotic reactions.

in the chest wall according to the location of the lesion. A small incision is made through the skin and the intercostal muscles, the instrument is introduced to explore the pleura and the lung and a sample is taken with forceps that are part of the instrument.

The lung, having collapsed from the change in air pressure during the procedure, is then reinflated. Usually, a tube for drainage is left in after the procedure.

With mediastinoscopy, the specialist is able to investigate the mediastinum (the space in the chest between the lungs and the heart) with an endoscope. It is mainly used to obtain a tissue sample from a tumor of the upper mediastinum or to determine whether cancer has spread into lymph nodes.

Under general anesthesia, the patient is laid on his/her back with the neck extended. A transverse incision is made in the notch at the top of the breastbone. Because of anatomic limitations imposed by the presence of the aortic arch, the surgeon has easiest access to structures on the right side, particularly those in the same plane as the trachea (windpipe).

The endoscope is introduced into the chest, and under direct sight of the lymph nodes in the region, the sample is obtained. At the end of the procedure, the fascia and skin are sewn back together without a drainage tube being left in.

■ *Ultrasound*

Ultrasonography is the use of very high frequency sounds to create echoes; these are reproduced on a machine and the resulting "picture" will show (among other things) differences in tissue density within the body and thus display disease processes that are not adequately seen by other diagnostic procedures.

However, since air in the lungs is a poor conductor of high-frequency sound waves, deep structures do not show up well by this method. With ultrasound, three conditions may be identified as fluid-containing or solid tissue:
- thickening of the pleura;
- masses close to the chest wall;
- masses in the mediastinum.

■ Lung biopsy

Biopsy is the cutting off of a small piece of tissue for microscopic examination. Either open lung biopsy (when the structures covering the lung are cut away) or closed biopsy (when an endoscope is used) may be helpful in dealing with an unexplained diffuse process that primarily affects the lung air sacs; with a lung process that inexplicably worsens under treatment; and with solitary or multiple nodules when the diagnosis is uncertain.

Since lung biopsy is an invasive procedure, the decision to perform the biopsy is influenced by the general condition of the patient and by the likelihood that the information obtained may modify the outcome. Open biopsy permits the surgeon to see the surface of the lung, to select the optimum area for biopsy and to obtain adequate tissue for the required studies. A small incision is made and the pleura is opened. Most of the biopsies are taken from the lingula on the left or from the middle lobe on the right side. After the biopsy, the lung is re-expanded and the chest is closed.

A drainage tube is left in place for one to two days, if the surgeon is concerned with the possibility of a pneumothorax (collection of air on the outside of the lung, causing it to collapse inwards. Repeated X-rays of the chest are used to check that the lung is fully expanded.

■ Tracheal aspiration

Aspiration is the method whereby fluid or tissue is withdrawn from a cavity by suction using an instrument called an aspirator. Diagnostic tracheal aspiration is performed to obtain, for laboratory examination, secretions that are relatively uncontaminated by mouth, nose and throat secretions, and is used when there is inadequate or absent cough.

The situations most often associated with this are:

▲ deep coma with absence of protective reflexes;
▲ neuromuscular disorders;
▲ chronic airway obstruction;
▲ bronchiectases (dilation of the bronchioles) and cachexia (serious general feebleness);

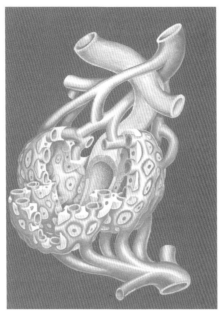
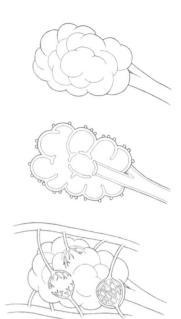

Left: microscopic structure of the alveoli. The alveoli are surrounded by numerous capillaries for the exchange of oxygen and carbon dioxide.
Right: schematic drawings of a small bronchiole with alveoli. From top to bottom: outer surface; cross section; presence of capillaries.

▲ situations in which instability of the chest wall or severe pain prevents effective coughing - for instance, chest injury, postoperative pain from surgery or rib fractures.

Those from whom secretion samples are apt to be required for laboratory examination, especially special staining and cultures, include individuals with lung infection who fail to respond to treatment or have a relapse while on previously effective antibiotic therapy, and the critically ill with lung infiltrates whose lives seem imminently threatened by the infection.

Acute respiratory distress syndrome

This condition - also known as "shock lung," "wet lung" and "pump lung" - is respiratory failure with life-threatening respiratory distress and lowered oxygen-content in the blood, associated with various acute injuries to the lungs. This important and common medical emergency is precipitated by

an acute illness or injury that directly affects the lungs, including such conditions as:

• direct injury to the chest trauma
• prolonged or profound shock
• fat embolism
• massive blood transfusion
• oxygen toxicity
• sepsis
• hemorrhagic inflammatory process of the pancreas

The following signs and symptoms are indicative for this lung condition. Twelve to 24 hours following the initial injury or illness or, more commonly, five to ten days later, following the onset of sepsis, convalescence is interrupted by progressive respiratory distress and failure. Dyspnea (difficulty in breathing) occurs initially, accompanied by hyperventilation, grunting when breathing out and decreased content of oxygen in the blood.

Secondary bacterial invasion of the lung and persistent lung sepsis, the most common complications, are frequently fatal, and prompt recognition of the emergency and correct treatment are necessary to prevent sudden death.

539

Lung diseases   Questions & Answers

What is silicosis?

Silicosis is the oldest known occupational lung disease. The disorder usually follows long-term inhalation of small particles of free crystalline silica in such industries as mining, foundries, pottery making, and sandstone and granite cutting.

Usually, 20 to 30 years of exposure are necessary before the disease becomes apparent, though it may also develop in less than 10 years when the dust-dose is extremely high, as in industries such as tunnelling, and sandblasting.

Patients with simple silicosis have no respiratory symptoms and usually no impairment of respiration. They may cough and raise sputum, but these symptoms are due to industrial bronchitis and occur often in persons with normal X-rays.

Conglomerate silicosis, in contrast, may lead to severe shortness of breath, cough, and sputum. The severity of the shortness of breath is related to the size of the conglomerate masses in the lungs; when they are extensive, the patient becomes severely disabled.

How can silicosis be diagnosed?

The disorder is diagnosed from characteristic chest X-ray changes and a medical history of exposure to free silica. Effective dust control can prevent silicosis. Since dust suppression cannot reduce the risk in sandblasting, external-air supplied hoods should be used. No effective treatment is known.

What is asbestosis?

This disease is a consequence of long-term inhalation of asbestos fibers in the mining, milling, manufacturing, or application (for instance, of insulation) of asbestos products. Most of these products are now forbidden by law, but many cases still exist of previous exposure and exposure in other countries.

The risk of developing asbestosis is related to the dose of asbestos due to which the worker has been exposed. The incidence of lung cancer is also increased in asbestos-exposed persons. The risk of lung cancer is usually less for non-smokers. Certain malignant tumors of the pleural membranes (mesotheliomas), have been associated with asbestos exposure, although the exposure may have occurred many years earlier and may have been brief.

What are the symptoms of asbestosis?

The patient with asbestosis characteristically notices the insidious onset of exertional dyspnea and reduced exercise tolerance. Symptoms of airways disease (cough, wheezing) are not usual but may occur in heavy smokers with associated chronic bronchitis.

How is asbestosis diagnosed?

The diagnosis of asbestosis is made on the basis of the medical history, and X-ray examination. The presence of a malignant mesothelioma may be confirmed only by biopsy. Asbestosis is preventable, primarily by effective dust suppression in the work environment. No specific therapy is available and the treatment is symptomatic.

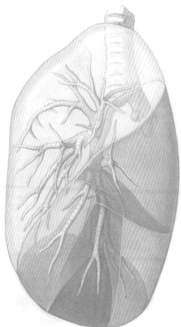

Pneumothorax (air pressure from outside the chest collapsing a lung inwards) occurring late in acute respiratory distress syndrome is an ominous sign, since it is usually associated with severe lung damage and a need for high ventilatory pressures.

The survival rate is 60 to 70 per cent with prompt early treatment; only 10 to 20 per cent survive without treatment. Victims who respond quickly to treatment have little or no residual disturbance of lung function or disability.

Those requiring prolonged treatment, however, may develop restrictive lung disease.

Despite different causes, the principles of treatment are similar. Ventilation must be improved and the underlying cause of the acute lung injury corrected.

Obstruction of the airways

The major conditions causing airways obstruction are:
- bronchial asthma
- acute bronchitis
- cystic fibrosis
- chronic obstructive pulmonary disease

Here, special attention will be paid to the chronic obstructive pulmonary disease.

This is irreversible, generalized airway obstruction associated with varying degrees of chronic bronchitis, abnormalities in the small airways and emphysema.

The term "chronic obstructive pulmonary disease" was introduced because chronic bronchitis, small airways abnormalities and emphysema often co-exist and it may be difficult for doctors to decide in an individual case which is the major factor producing the airways obstruction.

The development of this condition appears to be determined by a balance between individual susceptibility and exposure to provocative agents. The basic damage caused by emphysema apparently results from the effect of certain enzymes on the walls of the small alveoli of the lungs and such enzymes can be released from leucocytes (white blood cells) in the course of inflammation. Thus, any factor leading to a chronic inflammatory reaction encourages development of such lesions. Smoking presumably plays a role due to its adverse effects on lung defence mechanisms, which permit a low-grade inflammatory reactions to develop with consequent recurrent or chronic release of the above-mentioned enzymes.

Fortunately, most people can neutralize these enzymes, but in those who are unable to do so, emphysema may develop by middle age even in the absence of exposure to substances that interfere with lung defense mechanisms. It is uncertain why persons with similar degrees of emphysema may have considerably varying degrees of severity of airway obstruction.

With sufficient exposure to bronchial irritants, particularly cigarette smoke, most persons develop some degree of chronic bronchitis. The damage essential to the development of severe airway obstruction is apparently located in the small airways and may be basically different from the ordinary abnormalities of the large airways that lead to hypersecretion in most smokers.

The reason why abnormalities in the small airways develop in some people with chronic bronchitis is uncertain, but infections in childhood, unidentified immunological mechanisms or unidentified genetic characteristics could be predisposing factors.

Prevalence

Chronic obstructive pulmonary disease is a major cause of disability and death. In western Europe and the United States, it is second only to heart disease as a cause of disability in health statistics, and reported mortality rates have been doubling about every five years.

Its true death rate probably exceeds that of lung cancer. Some of this increase reflects the longer survival of people who previously have died of pneumonia caused by bacteria before the chronic obstructive pulmonary disease became known.

Overall, it has been estimated that this disease affects as many as 15 per cent of older men. It affects men about eight times more often that women, presumably because of the more frequent, prolonged, and heavier smoking in men; however, the incidence in women is now increasing.

Signs and symptoms

This disease is thought to begin early in life, though significant symptoms and disability usually do not occur until middle age. Mild ventilatory abnormalities may be discernible long before the onset of significant clinical symptoms. A mild "smoker's cough" is often present many years before the appearance of breathing difficulties on exertion, called exertional dyspnea. Gradually progressive exertional dyspnea is the most common complaint.

Sufferers may date the onset of dyspnea to an acute respiratory illness, but the acute infection may only unmask a pre-existing chronic respiratory disorder.

Cough, wheezing, recurrent respiratory infections and occasionally, weakness, weight loss or lack of libido (sex drive) may also be initial manifestations. Cough and sputum production are extremely variable. The person may admit only to `clearing his/her chest' on awakening in the morning or after smoking the first cigarette of the day.

Others may have a severely disabling cough. Wheezing also varies in character and intensity. Asthma-like episodes may occur with acute infections, and a mild chronic wheeze that is most obvious on reclining may be noted. Many deny having any wheeze.

Course and prognosis

Some reversal of airways obstruction and considerable improvement of symptoms can often be obtained initially, but the long-term prognosis is less favourable in those with a persistent obstructive abnormality. After initial improvement, the forced expiratory volume (a measure of lung volume) generally falls by 50 to 75 ml per year, which is two to three times the rate of decline expected from aging alone.

There is a concomitant slow progression of exertional dyspnea and disability. The course is punctuated by

Various stages in the development of lung emphysema.

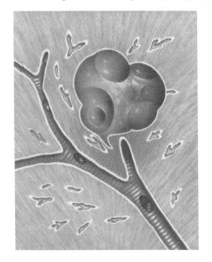
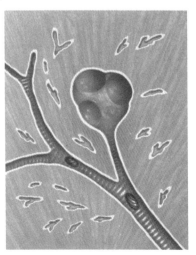
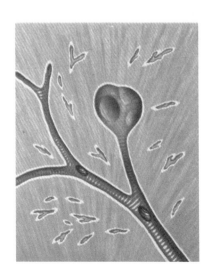

Categories of chronic lung diseases

Airways obstruction
- chronic bronchitis
- emphysema
- cystic fibrosis
- asthma

Abnormal lung tissue
- sarcoidosis
- pneumoconiosis
- rheumatoid lung
- idiopathic fibrosis
- Hodgkin's disease
- systemic lupus erythematosus
- radiation
- leukemia

Disturbance in the regulation of ventilation
- chronic exposure of carbon dioxide
- metabolic diseases
- myasthenia gravis
- polyneuritis
- muscular dystrophy
- poliomyelitis
- obesity
- decreased function of the thyroid gland

acute worsening of symptoms generally related to superimposed infections of the bronchi.

Prognosis of this disease is closely related to the severity of expiratory slowing. When the forced expiratory volume exceeds 1.25 litre, the ten-year survival rate is about 50 per cent; when the forced expiratory volume is only 1 litre, the average patient survives about five year. When there is very severe expiratory slowing (about 0.5 litre), survival for more than two years is unusual, particularly if the person has also a chronic heart condition.

Treatment

Treatment does not result in cure, but provides relief of symptoms and controls potentially fatal exacerbations; it may also slow the progression of the disorder, though this is unproved.

Treatment is directed at alleviating conditions that cause symptoms and exacerbations, such as:
- infection
- bronchospasm
- bronchial hypersecretion
- low oxygen content of the blood
- unnecessary limitation of physical activity.

Bronchiectasis and atelectasis

These conditions are both severe lung disorders. Bronchiectasis is a chronic congenital or acquired disease characterized by irreversible dilation widening of the bronchi, with secondary infection. Atelectasis is a shrunken and airless state of part or all of the lung; the disorder may be acute or chronic, complete or incomplete.

Bronchiectasis

This condition can develop at any age, but most often begins in early childhood. It usually follows bronchial infection, most often a severe childhood pneumonia, which destroys the supporting elastic and muscular components of the walls of the bronchi.

The bronchi in areas of lung that have been extensively affected by fibrosing lung diseases (those that result in the production of fibers - for instance, tuberculosis and silicosis) usually are shortened, widened and sometimes chronically inflamed. They are unable to get rid of secretions effectively, which then form an increasingly large deposit of infected material.

The severity and characteristics of symptoms vary widely from patient to patient and in some patients from time to time, depending largely on the extent of the disease and the amount of complicating chronic infection present.

Chronic cough and sputum production are the most characteristic and common symptoms. These often begin insidiously, usually following a respiratory infection, and tend to worsen gradually over a period of years. A severe pneumonia with incomplete clearing of symptoms and residual persistence of cough and sputum production is a common mode of onset.

Causes of bronchiectasis

Respiratory infections
- measles
- whooping cough
- adenoviral infection
- influenza
- tuberculosis
- fungal infection
- mycoplasma infection

Bronchial obstruction
- inhaled object
- enlarged lymph glands
- lung tumor
- mucus plug

Inhalation injuries
- injury from noxious fumes
- gases
- injury from particles
- aspiration of stomach acid
- aspiration of food particles

Genetic conditions
- cystic fibrosis
- ciliary dyskinesia
- antitrypsin deficiency

Immunological conditions
- immunoglobin deficiency syndrome
- white blood cell dysfunctions
- complement deficiencies
- autoimmune disorders
- hyperimmune disorders

Other conditions
- drug abuse
- human immunodeficiency virus
- Young's syndrome
- Marfan's syndrome
- whooping cough

542

As the condition progresses, the cough tends to become more productive and has a typical regularity, occurring in the morning on arising, late in the afternoon and on retiring; many patients are relatively free of cough during the intervening hours. The sputum is usually similar to that of bronchitis. Physical findings are not specific, but persistent rales (sounds additional to those of normal breathing) over any portion of the lung suggest bronchiectasis. Clubbing of the fingers sometimes occurs when disease is advanced, and there is persistent chronic infection.

Treatment in most cases is directed at controlling infection with appropriate antibiotics, and postural drainage - where the person lies on the affected side over the edge of a bed with the head well down so that the infected secretions can drain into the windpipe and can be coughed up.

Postural drainage at least twice a day should be continued indefinitely, even when minimal or no secretions are produced. Some may also have diffuse chronic bronchitis, and this must be treated accordingly.

The cutting out of the affected part of the lung is seldom necessary due to the effectiveness of antibiotics, but is indicated when the diseased area is limited and non-progressive, or when medical treatment is inadequate, as demonstrated by recurrent pneumonia or bronchial infection.

Atelectasis

The chief cause of acute or chronic atelectasis in adults is bronchial obstruction, although small areas of atelectasis may occur because of inadequate ventilation in a particular region of the lung.

After the oxygen in the peripheral air sacs has been absorbed by the circulating blood, the lung contracts because no more air can reach it due to the obstruction.

This produces the airless state within a few hours. Lung shrinkage or collapse may be complete in the absence of an infection and in the early stages, blood perfuses the airless lung, with consequent decrease of oxygen in the blood of the arteries.

Hyperventilation and dyspnea are common. If the obstruction is

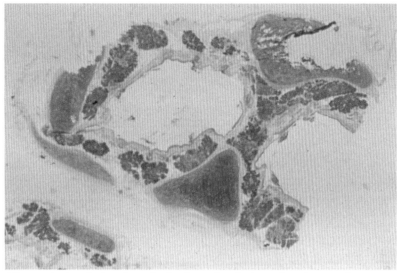

Microscopic view of a large lung alveolus due to chronic obstructive pulmonary disease.

removed, air will enter the affected area, any complicating infection will subside and the lung will return to normal in a variable length of time, depending how much infection is present. If the obstruction is not removed and infection is present, airlessness and lack of circulation initiate changes that lead to the development of fibrosis.

Most of the symptoms and signs of atelectasis are determined by the rapidity with which the bronchial occlusion (blockage) occurs, by the size of the area of lung affected and by the presence or absence or complicating infection.

Rapid occlusion with massive collapse, particularly if infection is present, causes the following symptoms:
- pain on the affected side
- sudden onset of dyspnea
- cyanosis (a bluish tint to the skin)
- a drop in blood pressure
- increased heart rate
- elevated temperature
- shock

Chest percussion reveals dull-to-flat sounds over the involved area, and auscultation shows diminished or absent breath sounds. The trachea (windpipe) and heart are deviated towards the affected side. Slowly developing atelectasis may be without symptoms or cause only minor lung symptoms. Acute atelectasis requires removal of the underlying cause.

Acute massive atelectasis is best combated by prevention.

When an obstructed bronchus is suspected but relief is not obtained by cough or suction, the doctor will perform bronchoscopy. Once bronchial obstruction is established, treatment is directed at the obstruction and at the infection invariably present.

The following measures will be taken:
- the patient is so placed that the uninvolved side is lower, to promote increased drainage of the affected area;
- the patient is given vigorous chest physiotherapy;
- the patient is encouraged to cough.

If improvement is not evident in one to two hours, bronchoscopy is repeated to suck up as much secretion as possible. Chest physiotherapy is then continued and the patient is encouraged to cough, move from side to side, and breathe deeply.

Chronic atelectasis is treated by the surgical removal of the affected segment or lobe. Since atelectasis usually becomes infected regardless of the cause of obstruction, a broad-spectrum antibiotic is given.

Obstruction of a major bronchus may cause a severe hacking or spasmodic cough. Treatment resulting in too great reduction in the cough reflex may produce further obstruction and should be avoided.

LUPUS

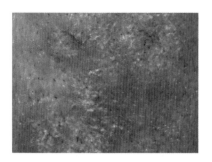

Description

Lupus is a chronic superficial inflammation of the skin marked by red macules covered with scanty adherent scales which fall off, leaving scars. The lesions typically form a butterfly pattern over the bridge of the nose and cheek, but other areas may be involved.

■ *Disseminated lupus erythematosus*
Form of lupus erythematosus that may affect any organ or structure of the body, especially the skin, the joints, the kidneys, the heart, the serous membranes (membranes that moisture, such as those of the joints and those lining the abdomen), and the lymph nodes.

■ *Systemic lupus erythematosus*
A chronic generalized connective tissue disorder, ranging from mild to fulminating, marked by the following signs and symptoms:
- skin eruptions;
- arthralgia, pain in joints;
- arthritis, inflammation of joints;
- leucopenia, decrease in leucocytes in the peripheral blood;
- enemia;
- visceral lesions;
- neurological manifestations;
- lymphadenopathy;
- fever;
- other constitutional symptoms. Typically there are many abnormal immunological phenomena.

■ *Lupus erythematosus profundus*
A form of lupus erythematosus in which deep browny indurations or subcutaneous nodules occur under normal or less often involved skin; the overlying skin may be erythematous, atrophic, and ulcerated and on healing may leave a depressed scar.

■ *Lupus hypertrophicus*
A variant of lupus vulgaris in which the lesions consist of a warty vegetative growth, often crushed or slightly exudative, usually occurring on most areas near body orifices.

■ *Lupus vulgaris*
The most common and severe form of tuberculosis of the skin, most often affecting the face, marked by the formation of reddish-brown patches of nodules in a specific part of the skin (corium), which progressively spread peripherally with central atrophy, causing ulceration and scarring and destruction of cartilage in involved sites.

■ *Lupus syndrome*
Closely resembling systemic lupus erythematosus, precipitated by prolonged use of certain drugs, most commonly hydralazine, isoniazid, various anticonvulsants, and procainamide.

Complications

Some complications can be fatal. Severe kidney damage, severe infection (often resulting from immune system malfunctioning), or central nervous involvement are the most

Characteristics of lupus

- ▲ At least four of the following symptoms are generally present for a diagnosis to be made.
- ▲ Red, butterfly-shaped rash on the face, affecting the cheeks, across the nose (malar butterfly erythema).
- ▲ Typical skin rash on other parts of the body, such as red, flat or raised areas on the face and sun-exposed areas of the neck, upper chest, and elbows.
- ▲ Sensitivity to sunlight over the whole body, causing blisters and in rare cases ulcers.
- ▲ Mouth sores; ulcers may occur on mucous membranes, particularly on the roof of the mouth, on the inside of the cheeks, and on the gums.
- ▲ Inflammation of one of more joints (arthritis); the joints are often swollen and painful when moved.
- ▲ Fluid around the lungs, heart, or other organs (serositis). The person feels pain when breathing deeply. The pain is due to recurring inflammation of the sac around the lung (pleurisy), with or without fluid inside this sac. Chest pain is due to inflammation of the sac around the heart (pericarditis).
- ▲ Kidney dysfunction; the most common result of this impairment is protein in the urine.
- ▲ Low white blood cell count, low red blood cell count due to hemolytic anemia, or low platelet count.
- ▲ Positive results of a blood test for antinuclear antibodies; the immune response may result in connective tissue damage.
- ▲ Positive results of a blood test for antibodies to double-stranded DNA. This test is very accurate and can be performed by a specialist in an academic hospital.

common causes of death associated with lupus.

Other complications of lupus include inflammation of the membrane around the heart, of the membrane lining the abdominal cavity, or of the membrane surrounding the lungs.

Treatment

Treatment focuses on relieving and controlling symptoms. Treatment varies according to the severity of the disorder. In general, treatment of lupus includes:

- plenty of rest
- good nutrition
- avoidance of stress
- avoidance of exposure to sunlight

If no symptoms are present, treatment is usually not required. Treatment of mild cases of systemic lupus often includes only over-the-counter medications to reduce inflammation and pain, and sunscreen (containing PABA) to limit exposure to the sun's rays.

Discoid lupus sometimes disappears spontaneously. Treatment for persistent cases includes the application of cortisone ointment (an anti-inflammatory steroid) to the skin to control the rash, and the use of mild soaps and body lotions to avoid further irritation of the skin.

Treatment of more severe cases of lupus involving the kidneys, heart, or central nervous system may include anti-inflammatory medications, such as steroids. A physician may also recommend blood transfusion and immunosuppressant medications to control the most serious lupus crisis.

Spasms of the fingertips and toes can be prevented by avoiding exposure to extreme cold and heat. Women who are severely affected by lupus often decide against pregnancy because lupus may become worse after childbirth.

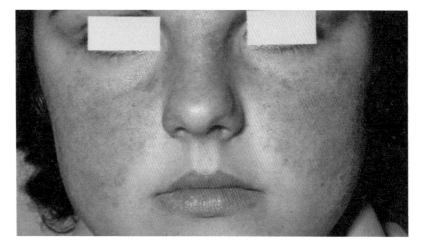
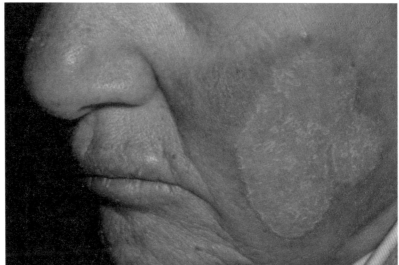
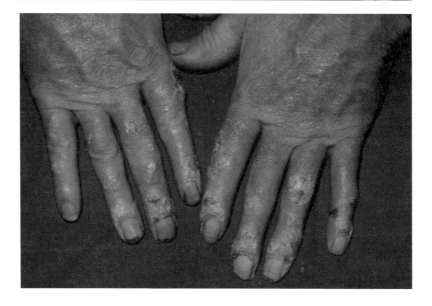

Typical skin rashes on the face (above and center) and on the fingers in lupus erythematosus. In this condition, raised round bumps occur, with scaling and sometimes with scarring and hair loss in affected areas. The patients also show a red, butterfly-shaped rash on the face, affecting the cheeks.

LYME DISEASE

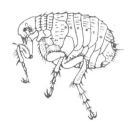

Lyme disease   Questions & Answers

What is lyme disease, and how does a person get it?

Lyme disease is a bacterial infection transmitted to humans by ticks - usually deer ticks - which lash on to the skin in order to feed on blood. Most people who contract the disease get it after being outdoors in the summer months.

If caught early, Lyme disease is generally a minor ailment that is easily cured with antibiotics. Left untreated, however, it can cause serious health problems, including severe fatigue, chronic headaches, arthritis, and an irregular heartbeat.

How can I reduce my child's chances to getting Lyme disease?

Teach children to avoid places where ticks live: Rock walls, wood piles, and wooded areas are favourites. Other ways to keep kids tick-free include dressing them in long pants and long-sleeved shirts that fit snugly around the wrists, neck, and ankles; applying tick repellent before they go outside and in high-risk areas, having yards professionally sprayed with insecticide each spring.

What can I do in preventing Lyme disease?

Daily body checks are important in high-risk areas, especially during tick season, which is May through August. Look carefully: Mature deer ticks are roughly the size of an apple seed, but early in their life cycle, when they are most likely to transmit Lyme disease, they are no bigger than a poppy seed.

They usually attach themselves to arms, legs, and torsos, but can also hide on the scalp or neck, in the armpits, or behind the ears, where they can feed unnoticed for several days.

If my child is bitten by a tick, should she automatically be treated with antibiotics?

Probably not, since the risk of infection with any given bite is fairly low. If a tick is found, it is important to remove it quickly. The best way is to grasp the tick close to the skin with a pair of fine-tipped tweezers, and slowly pull it straight out. After removing the tick, sterilize the bite with alcohol or an antibiotic ointment.

How can I tell if my child is beginning to develop Lyme disease?

The early symptoms are usually easy to recognize. Within a few weeks after being bitten, most infected people develop a red, bull's-eye-shaped rash near the bite, which gradually expands to an inch or more in diameter, and experience aches, chills, and a fever. Sometimes there's a secondary rash that shows up far from the bite. Neither rash typically causes itching or pain. Occasionally, though, the symptoms are so mild they go unnoticed - low fever, headache, aching joints.

For that reason, if a parent suspects exposure to ticks, the child should see a physician. Blood tests can help determine whether she actually has Lyme disease. If she does, a two- to three-week course of antibiotics should quickly clear up the infection.

Description

Lyme disease is a relatively common blood infection caused by the bacterium Borrelia burgdorferi that occurs in the northeast United States. It is spread by the bite of the tick Ixodes from infected mice or deer to humans. The tic may lie dormant for up to a year before passing on the infection with a bite.

The disease has three stages:

▲ In stage one the patient has a flat or slightly raised red patchy rash, fever, muscle aches and headache.

▲ Stage two comes two to four weeks later with a stiff neck, severe headache, meningitis and possibly Bell's palsy.

▲ In stage three, which may come three to twelve months later, the patient has muscle pains, and most seriously a long lasting severe form of arthritis that may move from joint to joint.

The diagnosis is confirmed by specific blood tests, then a prolonged course of antibiotics is prescribed.

Diagnosis

A physician should be consulted if the characteristic rash of Lyme disease is accompanied by its typical signs and symptoms. After recording the history of the illness, the physician examines the child, adolescent or adult, paying particular attention to the rash and its pattern.

Since infected ticks are most often found in certain parts of the United States (coastal areas of New England, Middle Atlantic states, Minnesota, Wisconsin, and the West Coast), the physician may ask if the person has been in any of these areas recently.

The presence of Lyme disease sometimes can be diagnosed by analysis of a blood sample or some fluid extracted from the rash. If the disease has developed into meningitis, a diagnosis can be made in some cases by specialized laboratory analysis of a sample of cerebrospinal fluid.

Treatment

Lyme disease can be successfully treated at home with antibiotics prescribed by a physician. Typical signs and symptoms can be treated at home, as necessary, until the antibiotics eliminate the spirochete and end the infection.

The period of convalescence of a very sick person can last 2 to 3 weeks. If complications such as arthritis, cardiomyopathy, or meningitis develop, they must be treated promptly by the physician, often in a hospital.

Prevention

The most effective prevention against acquiring tick bites in brush or woodlands during the summer tick season is wearing protective clothing (long-sleeved shirts, turtleneck jerseys, long trousers, hats, and gloves) and using insect repellent.

If a tick is discovered on any skin surface, it should be removed slowly and carefully, preferably with gloves and tweezers. The tick should be grasped as close to the head as possible and pulled straight out with tweezers. The tick should not be crushed because infection through unbroken skin is possible. The skin should be washed with water and soap.

Since deer ticks are so tiny, it is important to search for them with care, perhaps using a flashlight to aid in detection. Because pets often pick up ticks, their coats should be examined after they have been outdoors during tick seasons.

Doxycycline

This antibiotic belongs to the tetracycline group of drugs, prescribed for the treatment of infections susceptible to this antibiotic, such as the spirochete Borrelia burgforferi, transmitted by ticks. The drug will not treat viral infections such as cold or flu. The drug prevents bacteria from growing and reproducing. The drug is prescribed for:

- ▲ Treatment for acne (topical application).
- ▲ Treatment for lyme disease (systemic application).
- ▲ Treatment for infections susceptible to any tetracycline.
- ▲ Treatment for ulcer (Helicobacter pylori infection).

Before using this medicine

Before you use this medicine check with your doctor, or pharmacist:

- if you ever had any unusual or allergic reaction to tetracyclines or any other antibiotic.
- if you have lupus erythematosus.
- if you have myasthenia gravis.
- if you are pregnant or intend to become pregnant while using this medicine. Although this antibiotic has not been shown to cause problems in humans, the chance always exists.
- if you are breast-feeding an infant. The drug passes into the breast milk; avoid drug or discontinue nursing until you finish the medicine.

Treatment

This medication is used to treat numerous infections susceptible to this antibiotic

- ▲ Tablet or capsule: take on empty stomach, 1 hour before or 2 hours after eating.
- ▲ Delayed-release capsule: swallow whole with liquid (do not take with milk).
- ▲ Liquid: shake well; take with measuring spoon.
- ▲ Keep taking this medicine for the full time of treatment even if you begin to feel better after a few days; do not miss any doses. This is especially important if you have a strep infection since serious heart problems could develop later if your infection is not cleared up completely.
- ▲ If you do miss a dose of this medicine, take it as soon as possible. However, if it is almost time for your next dose, skip the missed dose and go back to your regular dosing schedule.

Side effects

Along with the needed effects, a medicine may cause some unwanted effects.

- ▲ Stop taking this medicine and get emergency help immediately if you notice: Rash, Hives, Intense itching, Faintness soon after a dose, Swollen face or extremities, Diarrhea, Nausea and vomiting, Numbness or tingling in hands , Unusual bleeding or bruising, Blurred vision, Possible vision loss, Delirium

Overdose

Major symptoms of overdose are: nausea, vomiting, diarrhea. An overdose is unlikely to threaten life. If a person takes a much larger amount than prescribed call a doctor or hospital emergency room for instructions.

Interactions

This medicine may interact with several other drugs such as antacids, anticoagulants, oral antidiabetics, anticonvulsants, antivirals, etc.

- ▲ Be sure to tell your doctor about any medications you are currently taking.

Driving or hazardous work

Do not drive until you learn how the medicine affects you. Do not work around dangerous machinery. Do not climb ladders or work in high places. Danger increases if you drink alcohol.

Storage

The drug should be stored in a cool, dry place out of the reach of children. Protect from light.

547

LYMPHOMA

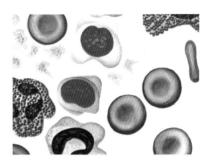

Introduction

A lymphoma is a growth of lymph cells involving the lymphatic system. It is one of the fastest rising cancers in the Western World, and no one knows precisely why. Lymphomas (the "oma" stands for tumor) affect the lymph system, which is a series of beady nodes spread throughout the body. The nodes are connected by tiny tubes

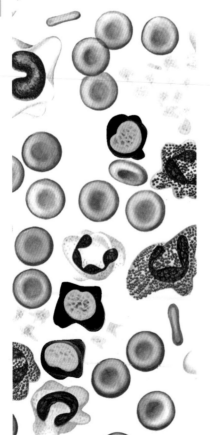

Drawing of a blood picture. Three lymphocytes are coloured.

much like veins in the separate circulatory system.

The lymph system plays a major role in the body's immune defenses against infection. A sore throat or boil often causes lymph nodes to swell in a local area. Doctors know little why lymphoma takes a more aggressive form in some people than in others, beyond the fact that sometimes it tends to become resistant to drugs

Types of lymphoma

Scientists have arbitrarily divided lymphomas into two types: Hodgkin's disease and a dozen other forms grouped as non-Hodgkin's lymphoma. Hodgkin's disease is named for Thomas Hodgkin, a 19th-century physician in London who distinguished the cancer from tuberculosis. Non-Hodgkin lymphoma appears in many types, and the prognosis varied tremendously according to the type. Many people live for decades hardly bothered by their lymphoma. Some may not need treatment for long periods. Yet many others die swiftly, even after responding to early therapy.

Non-Hodgkin's disease has been the third most rapidly rising cancer over the last 20 years, behind lung cancer in women (attributed to a surge in cigarette smoking several decades ago) and malignant melanomas in both sexes (attributed largely to sun exposure). More recently, a sharp rise in another kind of cancer, multiple myeloma, has challenged non-Hodgkin's lymphoma for third place.

Causes

Infectious agents have long been suspected to cause lymphomas.

Speculation that lymphomas are a viral disease has been fueled by the identification of clustered cases of Hodgkin's disease that seemed to defy statistical chance. Yet extensive investigations have failed to turn un up a cause for the clusters.

Nevertheless, the evidence suggesting that lymphomas are due to viruses is as strong as there is for any cancer. In recent years, HLTV-1, a member of the family of retroviruses that includes HIV has been linked in Japan to one rare case of lymphoma.

But even the discovery of viruses as causes of lymphoma may not explain how they are transmitted and why they have increased in number. Like many infectious diseases, the incidence of certain cancers goes through cycles, and the reasons are poorly understood.

An answer may come from further research into a recently identified link between a bacterium, *Helicobacter pylori*, and stomach cancer. Improved sanitation may have reduced the incidence of *Helicobacter pylori*, leading to a decline in stomach cancer. Additional research has linked *Helicobacter pylori* and a rare type of lymphoma of the stomach, which doctors recently begun treating with antibiotic therapy.

Although the cancer has disappeared after antibiotic therapy, not enough time has passed to determine whether antibiotics will cure the cancer. Nevertheless, the initial favorable reports have intensified the search for microorganisms as the cause of lymphoma.

Possible causative factors

Since the incidence of lymphoma in this country is rising there is much debate why this should be. But three factors can explain part of the overall rise.

- One is HIV, the virus that causes AIDS, which somehow increases the risk of lymphoma.
- A second is the growing umber of people with transplanted organs, who are at increased risk for developing lymphoma because of the immunosuppressant drugs used to prevent rejection of donated organs.
- A third is improved diagnostic techniques.

Symptoms

The possibly infectious nature of lymphomas is reflected in their symptoms, including:

- fever
- fatigue
- anemia
- weight loss

Most lymphomas are symptomless in their early stages. Usually, it is a painless swollen lymph node that leads a person to seek medical attention for a lymphoma. Generally, when nodes swell as a result of an infection, they are tender, yet when they enlarge because of cancer they are painless.

Diagnosis

In diagnosing lymphomas, a doctor performs a biopsy on the largest lymph node detected and then sends the specimens to a pathologist. Chemicals are added to the tissue to highlight the architecture of the cells when they are examined under a microscope. Similar tests can be made of the bone marrow.

As lymph cells mature to manufacture the immunoglobulins that fight infections and substances that are foreign to the body, they permanently rearrange their genes. A number of now standard monoclonal antibody and other sophisticated laboratory tests are used to identify the rearrangements and to further classify lymphomas by characterizing dozens of proteins that protrude from the surface of the cell. From such tests, a cell can be determined to be normal

or malignant, which type it is and whether all daughter and son cells are derived from a single abnormal type.

Treatment

Radiation, cytotoxic agents, and bone marrow transplants are among the therapeutic possibilities. The overall cure rate for Hodgkin's disease now approaches 85 per cent, thanks to steady improvement in the radiation and chemotherapy regimens that were

first developed about 40 years ago. But the cure rate depends in part on the age of the patient, with younger patients faring better than older ones. Hodgkin's disease has two main peaks of incidence. The larger is from 15 to 40 years old, and a smaller second peak occurs around 50. Non-Hodgkin's lymphoma can occur at any age, but most cases occur after the age of 50. The overall cure rate is about 40 to 45 per cent, aided by newer therapies like bone marrow transplants.

Combination chemotherapy regimens for non-Hodgkin's lymphomas

CVP (COP) regimen
■ *Drugs*
- Cyclophosphamide or
- Chlorambucil

■ *Comments*
Used in low-grade lymphomas to decrease size of lymph nodes and relieve symptoms.

CHOP regimen
■ *Drugs*
- Cyclophosphamide
- Vincristine (Oncovin)
- Prednisone

■ *Comments*
Used in low-grade lymphomas and some intermediate-grade lymphomas to decrease size of lymph nodes and relieve symptoms; produces a faster response than single agents.

C-MOPP regimen
■ *Drugs*
- Cyclophosphamide
- Vincristine (Oncovin)
- Prednisone
- Procarbazine

■ *Comments*
Used for intermediate-grade and high-grade lymphomas; also used in people with heart problems and cannot tolerate Doxorubicin.

M-BACOD regimen
■ *Drugs*
- Cyclophosphamide
- Vincristine (Oncovin)
- Dexamethasone
- Doxorubicin (Adriamycin)
- Methotreate
- Bleomycin

■ *Comments*
Has more toxic effects that CHOP and requires monitoring of lung and kidney function; overall benefits simuilar to CHOP.

ProMACE-CytaBOM regimen
■ *Drugs*
- Cyclophosphamide
- Vincristine (Oncovin)
- Etoposide
- Doxorubicin (Adriamycin)
- Methotrexate
- Procarbazine
- Cytarabine
- Bleomycin

■ *Comments*
Benefits similar to CHOP.

MAMOP-B regimen
■ *Drugs*
- Cyclophosphamide
- Vincristine (Oncovin)
- Prednisone
- Doxorubicin (Adriamycin)
- Methotrexate
- Bleomycine

■ *Comments*
Main advantage in therapy duration (only 12 weeks), but weekly treatments are required (most other regimens are given every 3 to 4 weeks for 6 cycles); overall benefits similar to CHOP.

MALARIA

Introduction

Tropical parasitic disease causing malaise and intermittent fever, violent shivering, and sweating, either on alternate days or every third day; bouts often reoccur over many years. One form, cerebral malaria, develops rapidly with encephalitis, coma and shock. Malaria is due to infection with the Plasmodium protozoa carried by mosquitos of the genus Anopheles from the blood of infected persons.

The cyclic fever is due to the parasite's life cycle in the blood and liver; diagnosis is by examination of blood. Derivatives of quinine especially chloroquine and primaquine, are used both in prevention and treatment but other drugs may also be used.

■ *Malarial cachexia*
A generalized state of debility that is marked by:
- anemia;
- jaundice;
- splenomegaly;
- emaciation.

The condition results from long-continued chronic malarial infection.

■ *Malaria parasite*
A protozoan of the sporozoan genus Plasmodium that is transmitted to man or to certain other mammals by the bite of a mosquito in which its sexual reproduction takes place, that multiplies asexually in the vertebrate host by schizogony in the red blood cells or in certain tissue cells, and that causes destruction of the red blood cells and the febrile disease malaria or produces gametocytes by sporogony which if taken up by a suitable mosquito initiate a new sexual cycle.

In severe cases, brain infections, extremely high fevers that may cause brain damage, and gut infections may occur. Blackwater fever is a complication in which large amounts of blood are passed in the urine ("black water") due to the massive breakdown of red blood cells, and the patients become anaemic, a deep yellow colour, feverish and desperately ill. With good treatment, 95 per cent of patients recover, but the disease still kills over a million people in poor tropical countries every year.

Prevention and treatment

Mosquito control measures, which include eliminating breeding areas and killing larvae in the standing

Drawings of developmental stages of Plasmodium protozoa, responsible for the occurrence of malaria.
1. Plasmodium vivax; 2. Plasmodium malariae; 3. Plasmodium falciparum; 4. Plasmodium ovale.

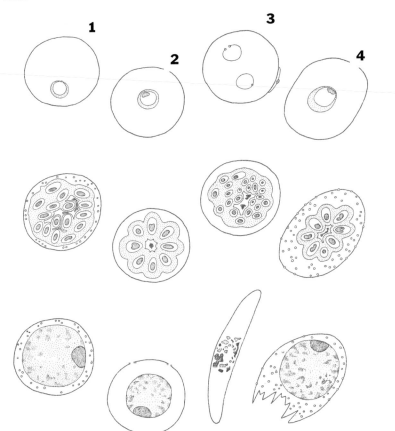

M

Chloroquine

Chloroquine is the drug of choice for:
▲ Treatment for protozoal infections such as malaria.
▲ Treatment for protozoal infections such amebiasis.
▲ Treatment for some forms of arthritis.
▲ Treatment for some forms of lupus.

Before using this medicine
Before you use this medicine check with your doctor, or pharmacist:
- if you ever had any unusual or allergic reaction to chloroquine or any other such preparation.
- if you are breast-feeding an infant. The drug passes into the breast milk; avoid drug or discontinue nursing until you finish the medicine
- if you have blood disease.
- if you have eye or vision problems.
- if you have liver disease.
- if you have porphyria.
- if you have psoriasis.
- if you have stomach or intestinal disease.

Treatment
This medication is used to treat malaria and other protozoal infections.

▲ Tablet: Swallow tith food or milk to lessen stomach irritation.
▲ Malaria prevention: Begin taking medicine 2 weeks before travelling to areas where malaria is present and until 8 weeks after return.
▲ If you do miss a dose of this medicine, take it as soon as possible. However, if it is almost time for your next dose, skip the missed dose and go back to your regular dosing schedule.

Side effects
Along with the needed effects, a medicine may cause some unwanted effects.
▲ Stop taking this medicine and get emergency help immediately if you notice: Severe breathing difficulty, Drowsiness, Faintness soon after a dose, Headache, Nausea and vomiting, Numbness or tingling in hands, Seizures, Blurred vision, Possible vision loss, Delirium
▲ Common side effects include: Headache, Appetite loss, Abdominal pain, Rash or itch, Diarrhea, Vomiting, Nervousness

Overdose

Major symptoms of overdose are: severe breathing difficulty, drowsiness, faintness, seizures. An overdose is unlikely to threaten life. If a person takes a much larger amount than prescribed call a doctor or hospital emergency room for instructions. Dial 911 (emergency) for medical help or call poison control center 1-800-222-1222 for instructions.

Interactions
This medicine may interact with several other drugs such as penicillamine.
n Be sure to tell your doctor about any medications you are currently taking.

Driving or hazardous work
Do not drive until you learn how the medicine affects you. Do not work around dangerous machinery. Do not climb ladders or work in high places. Danger increases if you drink alcohol.

M

water where they live, are very important. People who live in or travel to malaria-infested areas can also take precautions to limit mosquito exposure, such as using insecticide sprays in homes and outbuildings, placing screens on doors and windows, using permethrin-impregnated mosquito netting over beds, and applying mosquito repellents containing DEET on exposed areas of the skin.

People can wear long pants and long-sleeved shirts, particularly between dusk and dawn, to protect against mosquito bites. People subject to intense mosquito exposure can spray permethrin on their clothing before it is worn.

Drugs should be taken to prevent malaria during travel in areas where malaria is prevalent. The preventive drug is started before travel begins, continued throughout the stay, and extended for a period of time that

varies for each drug but is usually 4 weeks after the person leaves the high-risk area. Many drugs are used to prevent and treat malaria. Drug resistance is a serious problem, particularly with the dangerous *Plasmodium falciparum* species.

Chloroquine is the drug of choice for treatment in a person who has malaria caused by *Plasmodium vivax*, *Plasmodium ovale*, or *Plasmodium malariae* - except in a very few cases where resistance to chloroquine in people with *Plasmodium vivax* has been reported.

Chloroquine is relatively save and is approved for use in children and pregnant women.

Male and female mosquitos of the genus Anopheles.

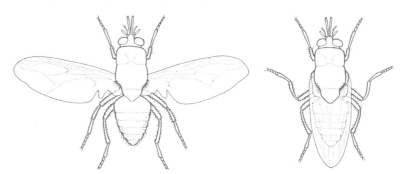

MANIC-DEPRESSIVE ILLNESS

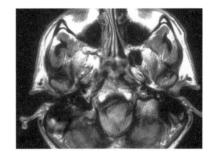

Description

In manic-depressive illness, also called bipolar disorder, episodes of depression alternate with episodes of mania or lesser degree of joyousness or elation. Manic-depressive illness affects slightly less that two percent of the U.S. population to some degree. The disease is believed to be hereditary, although the exact genetic defect is still unknown.

Signs and symptoms

Manic-depressive psychoses are characterized by profound disturbance of affect, for instance, feelings and emotions. The illness usually appears unprovoked but may occasionally follow some stress. The psychosis has a

strong tendency to recur and be self-limiting. Attacks are often repetitious, alternating and cyclical, with depression and elation.

Associated with depression may be symptoms such as:
* insomnia
* anorexia
* weight loss
* feelings of guilt
* self-reproach
* feelings of futility
* suicidal thoughts

Associated with elation may be hyperactivity, flight of ideas, marked overtalkativiness and pressure of thought. In serious manic-depression, the patient often exhibits delusions and hallucinations, the content of which can be understood as arising out of the primary disturbance of mood. Such symptoms occurring in the setting of a profound mood disorder do not justify a diagnosis of schizophrenia.

As with schizophrenia, whenever a causal rather than an incidental physical factor can be found, the condition passes over into the category of organic psychoses. It is often thought convenient to differentiate so-called "endogenous" cases of affective disorder from psychogenic or reactive cases.

However, it is more likely that depressive illnesses are best regarded as continually extending between the classical psychotic archetype, manic-depressive psychosis, and the neurotic archetype, neurotic depression.

Manic-depressive psychosis carries a high risk of suicide. Official statistics

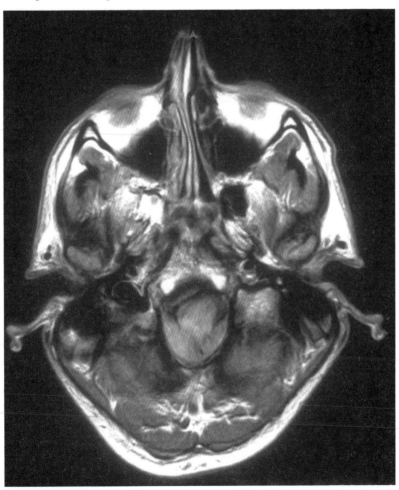

MRI-scan of the base of the skull and brain. The nose is located at the top of the illustration, the occiput or occipital lobe at the bottom.

M

Manic-depressive Illness

Major characteristics of the manic syndrome

Mood
- Elated, irritable or hostile.
- Momentary tearfulness (as part of mixed state.

Associated psychic manifestations
- Inflated self-esteem; boasting; grandiosity.
- Racing thoughts; clang associations (new thoughts triggered by word sounds rather than meaning);
- Distractibility.
- Heightened interest in new activities, people, creative pursuits; increased involvement with people (who are often alienated because of the patient's intrusive and meddlesome behavior); buying sprees; sexual indiscretions; foolish business investments.

Somatic manifestations
- Psychomotor acceleration; eutonia (increased sense of psychical well-being).
- Possible weight loss from increased activity and inattention to proper dietary habits.
- Decreased need for sleep.
- Increased sexual desire.

Psychotic symptoms
- Grandiose delusions of exceptional talent.
- Delusions of assistance; delusions of reference and persecution.
- Delusions of exceptional mental and physical fitness.
- Delusions of wealth, aristocratic ancestry or other grandiose identity.
- Fleeting auditory or visual hallucinations.

Major characteristics of the depressive syndrome

Mood
- Depressed, irritable or anxious. The patient may, however, smile or deny subjective mood change.
- Crying spells. The patient may, however, complain of inability to cry or to experience emotions.

Associated psychic manifestations
- Lack of self-confidence; low self-esteem; self-reproach.
- Poor concentration; indeciveness.
- Reduction in gratification; loss of interest in usual activities; loss of attachments; social withdrawal.
- Recurrent thought of death and suicide.

Somatic manifestations
- Diurnal variations in mood and activity.
- Psychomotor retardation; fatigue.
- Pain; agitation.
- Anorexia and weight loss, or weight gain.
- Insomnia or hypersomnia.
- Menstrual irregularities; amenorrhoea.
- Anhedonia; loss of sexual desire.

Psychotic symptoms
- Delusions of worthlessness and sinfulness.
- Delusions of reference and persecution.
- Delusions of ill health (nihilistic, somatic or hypochondriacal).
- Delusions of poverty.
- Depressive hallucinations in the auditory, visual and olfactory spheres.

M

and epidemiological studies indicate those individuals who are most at risk and hence provide possible clues to causes and prevention.

It has been emphasized that a substantial proportion of suicides could be prevented if general practitioners were as well trained in their recognition and management of depression and of other psychiatric conditions associated with high rates of suicide as there are in the diagnosis and treatment of basic medical conditions.

Symptoms in children

Many children with manic-depressive illness exhibit a mixture od depression and of mania characterized by:
· a state of elation
· excitation
· racing thoughts
· irritability
· grandiosity

The mania and depression occur simultaneously or in rapid alteration. During manic episodes, sleep is disturbed, the child may become aggressive, and school performance often deteriorates.

Children with manic-depressive illness appear normal between episodes, in contract to children with hyperactivity, who have a constant state of increased activity. Because ADHD can produce some similar symptoms, differentiating between the two conditions is important.

Treatment

The treatment of the more severe forms of manic-depressive illness usually requires the diagnostic and treatment resources of the specialized psychiatric services.

The use of lithium salts in the treatment of mania in patients whose mood has been stabilized after treatment of an affective illness necessitates the family physician being informed concerning the side effects and the toxic effects which can be anticipated.

In the majority of cases of moderate and serious depression, anti-depressants and psychotherapy in combination restore the mood to its premorbid level.

MENOPAUSE

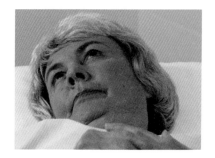

Description

Once a woman passes her menopause, her ovaries will no longer produce eggs, her monthly periods will cease and no more female hormones will be manufactured. The process usually occurs gradually over several years, between the early forties and the mid-fifties, but it may occur as early as thirty-five or as late as fifty-eight. It is therefore not unusual for a woman to

In the United States, the average age at which menopause occurs is about 51 to 52. No smoking, avoiding stress, and exercising regularly may help overcome the negative aspects of menopause.

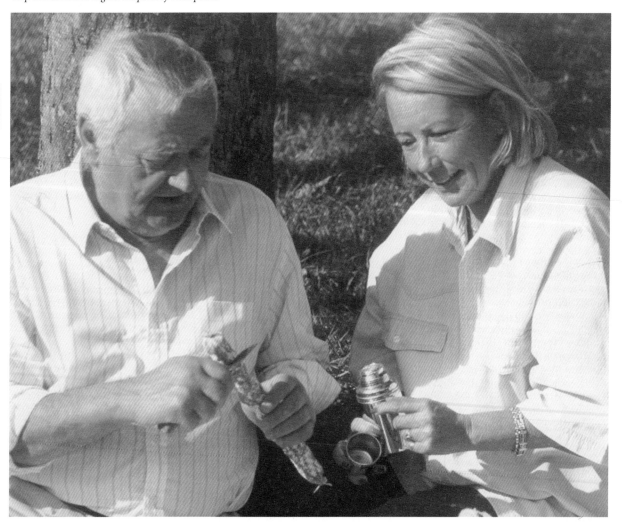

Checklist of menopausal signs

- Flushes
- Night sweats
- Vaginal dryness
- Irregular periods
- Frequency in passing urine
- Stress incontinence
- Forgetfulness
- Depression
- Loss of confidence
- Sleeplessness
- Aches in bones and joints
- Palpitations
- Panic attacks
- Headaches
- Loss of sex drive

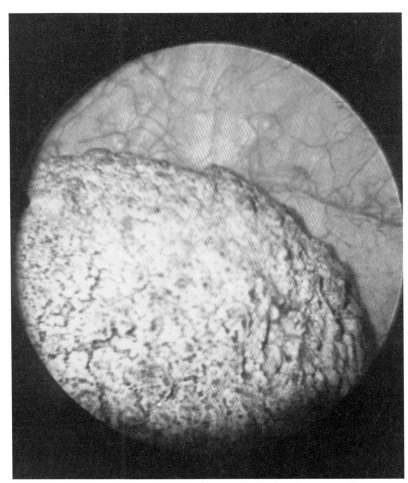

Some women report also in menopause problems in bladder function. In a small percentage of women the formation of bladder stones has increased. Cystoscopic view of a bladder stone in a 57-year old woman, who never reported before of bladder problems.

spend more of her life after the menopause (or change of life) than she spends being fertile, but this does not mean that she loses her femininity. Many women treat the end of their periods as a blessing and lead very active lives for many years afterwards (active sexually as well as physically and mentally).

The menopause is a natural event, and psychologically most women take it in their stride, as simply another stage of life, but it is wrong to dismiss the unpleasant physical symptoms without seeking medical assistance.

Menopause cannot be cured, because it is a natural occurrence, but doctors can relieve most of the symptoms. Sex hormone tablets are the mainstay of treatment. They can be taken constantly after the change has finished, but during the menopause they are usually taken cyclically. One hormone (estrogen) is taken for three weeks per month, and a different one (progestogen) is added on for the last ten to fourteen days. This maintains a near normal hormonal balance, and the woman will keep having periods, while underneath the artificial hormones, her natural menopause is occurring, so that when the tablets are stopped after a year or two the menopausal symptoms will have gone. Hormones may also be given as skin patches, vaginal creams and by injection.

After the menopause, women should continue the hormones for many years to prevent osteoporosis, skin thinning and to slow ageing.

Minor symptoms can be controlled individually. Fluid tablets can help bloating and headaches; other agents can help uterine cramps and heavy bleeding. Depression can be treated with specific medications. An obvious problem faced by a woman passing through the menopause is when to stop using contraceptives. As a rule of thumb, doctors advise that contraception should be continued for six months after the last period, or for a year if the women is under fifty. Taking the contraceptive pill may actually mask many of the menopausal symptoms and cause the periods to continue. It may be necessary to use another form of contraception to determine whether the woman has gone through menopause.

Signs and symptoms

When your menopause is beginning, there will be signs you can see and signs you cannot. You can use a checklist to record any signs, this will be useful to take to your general physician if you suspect the menopause has started for you.

■ *Irregular and infrequent periods*
The most obvious sign is irregular and unpredictable periods, often with increased premenstrual symptoms.

M

Menopause Questions & Answers

How will the menopause affect my long-term wellbeing?
The reduced amount of estrogen in your body during and after the menopause has a big impact on more than just your periods.

■ *Appearance*
Estrogen plays an important part in keeping your skin looking fresh and young, helping in the production of collagen. With less estrogen your skin can become thin, causing facial wrinkles, brittle nails and dry hair. A shift in the balance of your hormones can also lead to unwanted hair growth on your body and face.

■ *Osteoporosis*
Aches and pains in your joints during the menopause may be a reaction to the changing levels of hormones within your body. However, the menopause brings with it an increased risk of the serious bone disorder, osteoporosis. This is a condition in which bones become thin and prone to fracture.

■ *Heart condition*
Heart attack is the most common cause of death for women over the age of 50. At the menopause, the falling level of estrogen in your body removes the natural protection younger women have against chronic heart disease. This is probably due to the fact that estrogen helps keep the arteries supple, produces "good" blood fats, reduced harmful forms of cholesterol and tackles damaging free radical chemicals. Along with family history, raised blood pressure, high cholesterol levels and smoking, this lack of estrogen can put you at risk of chronic heart disease and it is important to pay attention to your diet and fitness to reduce the risk.

■ *Forgetfulness and lapses in concentration*
Reduced estrogen levels also have an effect on the activity of the brain and can lead to forgetfulness, short-term memory loss and lapses in concentration, although in many cases this improves over time. More seriously, a lack of estrogen has been linked to a slowing down of the neural connections in the brain and an increase in the risk of Alzheimer's disease.

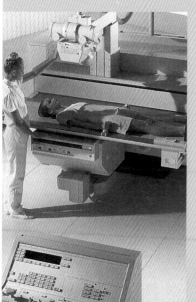

How can I help myself to stay healthy?
Improving your general health will help your body cope with both the short-term and long-term effects of the menopause.

Should I change the way I eat?
As you age, your metabolic rate slows, so your body needs fewer calories to produce the same amount of energy. If you continue to eat in the same way as before, it is likely that you will put on excess weight.
Your body shape will also change, as failing hormone levels lead to weight being distributed differently. Instead of putting excess weight on your breasts, hips and thighs, after the menopause your will store it on your tummy, just like men do. This can increase your risk of heart disease.

Your cycle may initially become shorter, then longer with infrequent periods. Your flow may also vary considerably.
If you recognise these symptoms and you are in your late 40s or early 50s, it is likely that your menopause is starting. However, whatever your age, you should talk to your physician about these changes as he will be able to check that there are no underlying problems and offer you advise and support.

■ *Hot flushes*
Three out of four women experience hot flushes during the menopause, and these usually last for two to three years. While this can be uncomfortable and annoying, most women find that things return to normal eventually, though an unlucky few will suffer for live to ten years and one in fifty will continue having flushes for life.
Most women describe hot flushes as beginning with pressure in the head, followed by a wave of heat passing over the body, sometimes accompanied by redness, tingling of sweating.

■ *Disturbed sleep*
Night sweats, anxiety and feeling of depression can often prevent you sleeping properly during the menopause.

■ *Vaginal dryness*
Lots of women experience vaginal dryness during the menopause. This is because the tissue of your vagina can become finer and thinner, causing dryness and increasing the risk of infection.

■ *Bladder problems*
In a similar way to the tissue of the vagina, the bladder lining can become thinner, increasing your risk of cystitis and other infections. Estrogen loss can also aggravate pelvic floor muscles already weakened by childbirth, and lead to problems in controlling the urge to pass urine.
The medical term for this condition is stress incontinence, and it can cause small amounts of urine to leak out of your body when you sneeze, cough or run.
Pelvic floor exercises can help to relieve this embarrassing problem, so

M

there is no need to suffer, simply ask your doctor for advice.

Diagnosis

In about three fourth of women, menopause is obvious. If menopause needs to be confirmed (particularly in younger women) blood tests are performed to measure levels of estrogen and follicle-stimulating hormone (which stimulates the ovaries to produce estrogen and progesterone).

Before any treatment is started, doctors ask women about their medical and family history and perform a physical examination, including breast and pelvic examinations and measurement of blood pressure. Mammography is also performed. Blood tests may be performed and bone density may be measured.

The information thus obtained helps doctors determine the woman's risk of developing disorders after menopause. For women with a history of abnormal bleeding from the vagina, an endometrial biopsy may be performed to check for signs of cancer.

A small sample of tissue is removed from the lining of the uterus (endometrium) and is examined under a microscope.

Treatment

Not consuming spicy foods, hot beverages, caffeine, and alcohol may help prevent hot flashes, because these substances can trigger hot flashes. Eating foods rich in B vitamins or vitamin E or foods rich in plant estrogens may also help.

Not smoking, avoiding stress, and exercising regularly may help improve sleep as well as relieve hot flashes. Wearing layers of clothing which can be taken off when a woman feels hot and put on when she feels cold, can help her cope with hot flashes. Wearing clothes that breath, such as cotton underwear and sleepwear, may enhance comfort.

■ *The benefits and risk and also the alternatives of hormone replacement therapy are summarized in the table.*

Hormone replacement therapy (HRT) and alternatives

Benefits of HRT

- For many women, hormone replacement therapy (HRT) is the treatment that gets them through a difficult time and greatly improves their quality of life.
- HRT restores your estrogen levels to their natural, premenopausal levels, helping you to deal with the short-term symptoms of the menopause and reducing your risk of developing longer-term health problems associated with depleted estrogen levels.
- It is not just an option for women currently going through the menopause. Even those who left the menopause behind many years ago can start taking HRT and enjoy similar benefits. HRT is not always the best solution for everybody, and your physician will be able to give your further information and advice on whether it is suitable for you.

Alternatives

There are no natural substitutes for HRT, but the following ideas about dietary supplements, herbs and minerals may help to alleviate your symptoms and boost your long-term health.

- Vitamin D, calcium, boron and magnesium are important for bone health and advisable for women at risk for osteoporosis.
- Isoflavones, derived from either red clover or soya can help maintain general health and wellbeing through the menopause.
- Evening primrose oil can help to maintain hormonal levels.
- Garlic tablets can help maintain a healthy immune system as well as energy and vitality.
- Ginkgo biloba supplements can maintain the flow of blood to the brain and therefore is good for short-term memory.
- Vitamin B_3, B_6 and folic acid have beneficial effects during the menopause.
- Antioxidants, such as betacarotene, selenium, zinc, vitamins A, C and E can help your body to fight free radicals, which attack healthy cells thereby maintaining healthy skin, hair and nails.
- Hypericum, St. John's Wort and the Chinese herb Dong Quai can help to lift your spirits and alleviate the stresses and strains of everyday life.
- Sage, drunk in tea form, can help with hot flushes.
- Alfalfa is rich in calcium and has estrogenic properties.
- Vervain, drunk in tea form, can help to relieve emotional symptoms.

Nutritional therapists believe that plant compounds which occur naturally in some foods can help to compensate for the body's loss of this important hormone. Soya is one of the richest sources, but phyto-estrogens are also found in fortified breads, broccoli, rhubarb and members of the cabbage family like Chinese leaves or kohl rabi.

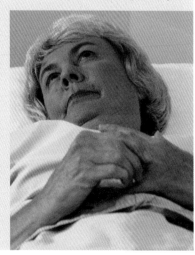

M

MEN'S DISEASES

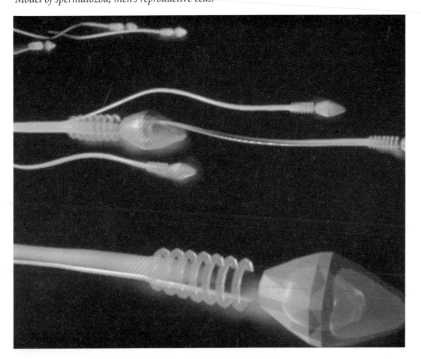

Introduction

Studies by the National Institute of Aging show that being born male is a disadvantage with regard to health and life expectancy. Baby boys are more frequent victims of Sudden Infant Death Syndrome than girls and the average life expectancy for men is only 74 compared with 79 for women. In the most senior age groups, over 80 years old, women outnumber men by 4 to 1. Men are far more likely to die prematurely before reaching old age than women, falling victim to strokes, heart diseases and cancer. In addition, males are more likely to commit suicide or die as a result of violence or aggression. Nowadays young men are much more aware of the benefits of a healthy lifestyle and are more likely to be concerned about their personal wellbeing. There are indications that entrenched and ingrained male attitudes towards, for example, the open discussion of potentially embarrassing health topics, are changing.

Disorders of the penis

Inflammation
Balanitis is inflammation of the sensitive glans of the penis which results in itching, heat, redness, and some swelling, usually due to a bacterial or fungal infection. Infections may be contracted by sexual intercourse or result from poor personal hygiene. Occasionally, balanitis is an allergic reaction to a spermicide, soap of detergent. Treatment is by means of antibiotic, antifungal or other creams depending upon cause.

In a case of balanoposthitis the inflammation concerns the glans penis and foreskin. The condition is characterized by redness, irritation, pain and discharge resulting from a bacterial or fungal infection. Treatment is by means of antifungal or antibacterial creams or drugs.

Growths
Growths on the penis are sometimes caused by infections, such as may be the case in syphilis, which causes flat or gray growths. Also, certain viral infections can produce one or more small, firm, raised skin growths (genital warts, or *condylomata acuminata*) or small, firm dimpled growths (*molluscum contagiosum*).

Skin cancer can occur anywhere on the penis, most commonly at the glans penis, especially its base. The cause of this type of cancer may be longstanding irritation, usually under the foreskin.

Squamous cell carcinoma, occurring most commonly, first appears as a painless, reddened area with sores that do not heal for weeks. To treat the cancer, a surgeon removes it and some normal surrounding tissue, sparing as much of the penis as possible. Most men with small cancers that have not spread survive for many years after treatment.

Disorders of the testes

Testes
The testes or testicles are a pair of male gonads, or sex glands, that produce sperm and secrete androgens.

Model of spermatozoa, men's reproductive cells.

M

Injury

The location of the scrotum makes it susceptible to injury. Blunt forces cause most injuries. However, occasionally gunshot or stab wounds penetrate the scrotum or testes. Testicular injury causes sudden, severe pain, usually with nausea and vomiting. Ultrasound may show whether the testes have ruptured.

Ice packs, a jockstrap, and drugs for pain and nausea usually effectively treat internal bleeding in or around the testes. Ruptured testes require surgical repair.

Testicular torsion

This condition concerns the twisting of a testis on its spermatic cord so that the testis's blood supply is blocked. Testicular torsion usually occurs in men between puberty and about 25 years; however, it can occur at any age. Abnormal development of the spermatic cord or the membrane covering the testis makes testicular torsion possible in later life. With torsion, the testis usually dies within 6 to 12 hours after the blood supply is cut off unless it is treated.

Severe pain and swelling develop suddenly in the testis The pain may seem to come from the abdomen, and nausea and vomiting may develop.

Because the testis may die rapidly, emergency surgery to untwist the spermatic cord is required. Urologists usually secure both testes during surgery to prevent future episodes of torsion.

Testicular cancer

Malignant growth of one or both testes. Testicular cancer may cause an enlarged testis or a lump in the scrotum. Most lumps in the scrotum are not caused by testicular cancer, but most lumps in the testes are. The initial treatment for testicular cancer is surgical removal of the entire testis. Treatment may also include radiation therapy.

Prostate disorders

The prostate gland is situated immediately below the bladder and internal urethral orifice. It surrounds the first portion of the urethra, referred to as

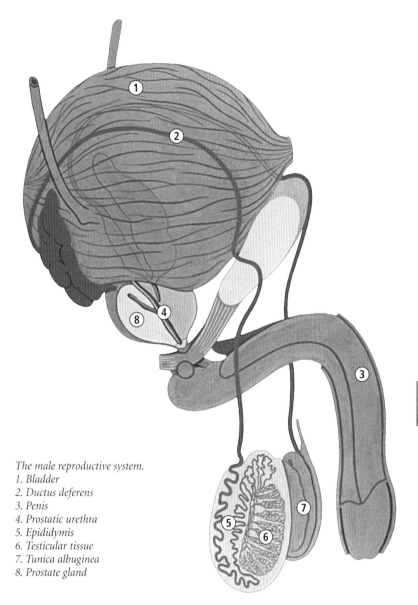

The male reproductive system.
1. Bladder
2. Ductus deferens
3. Penis
4. Prostatic urethra
5. Epididymis
6. Testicular tissue
7. Tunica albuginea
8. Prostate gland

the prostatic urethra, and is comparable to a chestnut in shape, size, and consistency.

The major disorders of the prostate gland concern age changes and cancer. The prostate enlarges during adolescence along with the other reproductive organs owing to the effect of androgens secreted by the interstitial cells of the testes. It attains full size during the twenties.

In older age, for reasons not yet understood, frequently the prostate increases in size so that two out of three man reaching the age of 70 suffer from some degree of obstruction

to urination. This can be serious because of the obstructive effect on urethral pressure.

Benign prostatic hyperplasia (BPH)

Description

Benign prostatic hyperplasia (BPH) is an enlargement of the prostate gland. The symptoms of BPH, however, can be caused by an increase in the tightness of muscles in the prostate. If the muscle inside the prostate tighten,

M

Prostate cancer Questions & Answers

What is the incidence of prostate cancer?
The incidence of prostate cancer is less than 1 per cent. An estimated 35,000 American men and 59,000 Europeans will have died of the disease in 2000.

Who gets prostate cancer?
Most men who get prostate cancer are 65 years of age or older, and the risk increases with age. Incidence rates are higher among blacks, and men with a family history of prostate cancer.

What are the symptoms of prostate cancer?
Cancer of the prostate usually involves enlargement of the gland. However, some enlargement occurs in about 50 per cent or more of males. While this enlargement should be investigated, it does not in itself mean cancer.
Any prostate enlargement can lead to a variety of urinary problems, such as difficulty in urinating or controlling urination, the need to urinate frequently, painful or burning urination, or blood in the urine.

How is prostate cancer found?
The American Cancer Society recommends that every man 40 and over should include a digital rectal examination in his annual health check-up. A new technique, prostate ultrasound, may reveal cancers too small to be detected by physical examination.
This new approach may be of special benefit to men who are at high risk. If a suspicious area is found, you will receive more extensive tests, including X-rays and an analysis of urine and blood. The physician makes a final diagnosis from a biopsy - the removal of a small piece of tissue from the area for examination under a microscope.

How is prostate cancer treated?
Your doctor may use one or more of the following methods:
- surgery;
- hormone treatments;

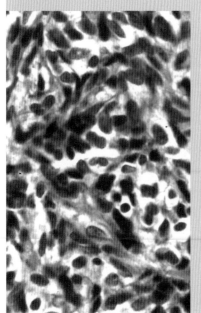

- radiation;
- anticancer drugs.
The choice depends on the stage of the cancer and your age and health. Surgery or radiation therapy may be the treatment chosen to cure prostate cancer if it is found in an early localized stage. Hormone treatment and anticancer drugs also may control this cancer for long periods by shrinking the size of the tumor and greatly relieving pain.

What is the hope for the future in case of prostate cancer?
Currently, men diagnosed with localized prostate cancer have a five-year survival rate of 90 per cent. Because it is important that this form of cancer is discovered early, cancer specialists are nor working to improve methods for early detection and to develop more effective combinations of treatments.

they can squeeze the urethra and slow the flow of urine.
This can lead to symptoms such as:
- a weak or interrupted stream when urinating;
- a feeling that you cannot empty your bladder completely;
- a feeling of delay when you start to urinate;
- a need to urinate often, especially at night, or
- a feeling that you must urinate right away.

Treatment options
There are three main treatment options for benign prostate hyperplasia:

■ *Program or monitoring or "watchful waiting"*
Some men have an enlarged prostate gland, but no symptoms, or symptoms that are not bothersome. If this applies, you and your doctor may decide on a program of monitoring including regular checkups, instead of medication or surgery.

■ *Medication*
There are different kinds of medication used to treat benign prostate hyperplasia, e.g., terazocin HCl (Hytrin).

■ *Surgery*
Some patients may need surgery. Your doctor can describe several different surgical operations to treat benign prostate hyperplasia. Which procedure is best depends on your symptoms and medical condition.

■ *Medication*
TerazocineHCl (Hytrin) is one of s series of newly developed medicines for the treatment of benign prostate hyperplasia. It relaxes the tightness of a certain type of muscle in the prostate and at the opening of the bladder. This may increase the rate of urine flow and/or decrease the symptoms of benign prostate hyperplasia.
▲ This medication helps relieve the symptoms of benign prostate hyperplasia. It does not change the size of the prostate, which may continue to grow. However, a larger prostate does not necessarily cause more or worse symptoms.

- If this medication is helping you, you should notice an effect on your particular symptoms in 2 to 4 weeks of starting to take the medication.
- Even though you take this medication and it may help you, this medication may not prevent the need for surgery in the future.
- Your doctor has prescribed this medication for your benign prostate hyperplasia and not for prostate cancer. However, a man can have benign prostate hyperplasia and prostate cancer at the same time.

Doctors usually recommend that men be checked for prostate cancer once a year when they turn 50 (or 40 if a family member has had prostate cancer). These checks should continue even if you are taking terazocinHCl. This medication is not a treatment for prostate cancer.

Prostate cancer

Description

The prostate - a gland just below the bladder in the male genital tract - has the third highest incidence of cancer in man, next to skin cancer and lung cancer. Most men who get prostate cancer are 55 years of age or older, and the risk increases with age. Rates are higher among blacks than whites, and more married men than singles develop it. The etiology is unknown, but appears to be related to hormones.

The usual prostate cancer is glandular, not unlike the histological configuration of normal prostate gland. Large nuclei, mitoses, stromal invasion, and involvement of lymphatic vessels are the principal histological criteria of diagnosis.

Symptoms and diagnosis

In the very early stage of prostate cancer, there usually are no symptoms. When symptoms do come up, they vary according to the size and location of the tumor, and are often the same as those for benign prostate conditions.

In fact, it is more likely that any of these symptoms would indicate enlargement known as benign prostatic hypertrophy, infection, or other

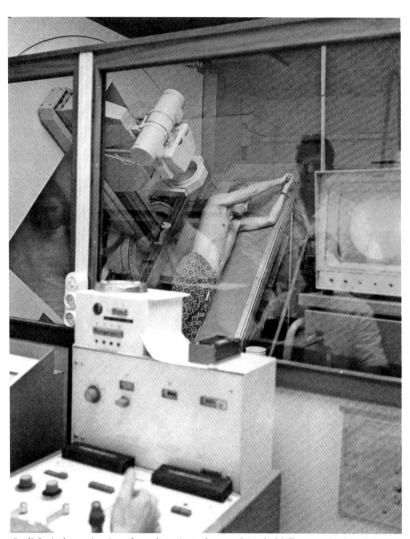

Radiological examination of a male patient who complained of diffuse pain in the pelvic area.

Prostate test

Answer the following questions:

Do you urine often, especially during the night?	YES/NO
Do you have trouble starting your urine stream?	YES/NO
Do you have a weak or interrupted urine stream?	YES/NO
Does it feel like your bladder is not emptying completely?	YES/NO

If you answered "yes" to any question, you should see your doctor. You may be experiencing the symptoms of a condition called benign prostatic hyperplasia, which is an enlargement of the prostate gland.

Prostate gland   Questions & Answers

What is the prostate gland?
The prostate is a gland possessed only by men. It is a walnut-sized gland located in the lower pelvis, just below the bladder, where it is wrapped around the urethra, the canal that carries urine from the bladder into he penis.

What does the prostate do?
The prostate is responsible for producing most of the seminal fluid which is the tick whitish fluid that carries sperm from the testes.

Why does the prostate gland enlarge?
Doctors do not know yet. The size of the gland is relatively unimportant - which is important is whether or not the gland impedes the flow of urine.

What happens when the prostate gland enlarges?
As the gland enlarges, it applies pressure to the urethra. This places a strain on the bladder, which has the added burden of forcing urine past the partial obstruction. In turn, this leads to bladder enlargement, which can lessen the flow of urine and lead to urinary infection. Pressure can also force urine back up the ureters into the kidneys, damaging those organs. Impaired kidney function can produce uraemia and/or high blood pressure.

What are the symptoms of prostate enlargement?
One of the first symptoms is the need to urinate frequently and often urgently. The affected man also may experience difficulty in starting or stopping the urinary stream and usually always notices a decrease in the flow or calibre of his urinary stream. Symptoms range from mild to severe and may require urological evaluation and treatment.

How is prostate enlargement diagnosed?
Usually by the patient's history. Initially, the physician can diagnose an enlarged prostate by inserting a finger into the rectum and feeling the gland. All men over age 50 should have such a checkup every year.
If enlargement is suspected, the physician may insert a rubber catheter into the bladder after the man has urinated to determine whether "residual urine" is present. A significant amount is a sign of severe and long-standing obstruction.

Are most enlarged prostate glands cancerous?
No. For most men, it is just benign prostatic hypertrophy.

How are enlarged prostates treated?
Treatment of mild enlargement usually just requires reassurance on he part of the physician and education for the patient to be on he look-out for more significant

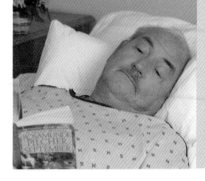

signs and/or symptoms.
When this does occur the anatomical problem is dealt with surgically to relieve the obstruction. Since 1995 there a number of drugs that will decrease the size of the prostate gland.

Does prostate surgery make you impotent?
When prostate surgery is done for presumed benign prostatic hypertrophy the incidence of impotency following surgery is less than 1 per cent.

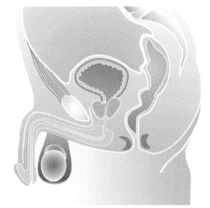

Side view of the lower abdomen and pelvis. Localization of the prostate gland immediately below the bladder and internal urethral orifice.

conditions, rather than cancer. Still, any symptom should be checked by a physician.
Any prostate enlargement can lead to a variety of urinary problems, such as difficulty in urinating or controlling urination, the need to urinate frequently, painful or burning urination, or blood in the urine. Metastases to the pelvis, ribs, and vertebral bodies may cause bone pain. Only a physician conducting the proper tests can determine for sure whether the condition is cancer or benign.
Many prostate cancers can be felt by your doctor during a digital rectal examination. This examination should be a part of your regular health checkup every year after the age of 40. If a suspicious area is found, you may receive more extensive tests, such as special X-rays and blood tests. The physician makes a final diagnosis from a biopsy - the removal of a small piece of tissue from the area for examination under a microscope.
In blood tests, an elevated serum acid phosphatase indicates local extension or metastases. Radioimmunoassay methods for determination of prostate acid phosphatase may give added information regarding the detection of localized prostatic cancer as well as later stages of the disease. The acid phosphatase level declines after successful treatment and rises again with recurrence.
A prostate-specific antigen (PSA) blood test can signal the presence of

M

prostate abnormalities at an early stage. Examination of the amount of DNA in abnormal cells can indicate how aggressive a cancer may be.

Prognosis

Ten-year cure rates approaching 65 per cent with localized prostate cancer treated by radical removal of the prostate gland (prostatectomy) or radiation therapy. Five-year survival rate for all stages of prostate cancer amounts to over 85 per cent. If distant spread of metastases is involved the five-year survival rate is about 30 per cent.

Prostate cancer not amenable to radical surgery or radiation therapy may respond for several years to adequate hormonal control and/or removal of the genital glands. This is particularly true in older men and when the cancer is well differentiated. The presence of metastases at the time of initial diagnosis obviously worsens the prognosis, but therapy may yield significant long-term palliation without cure.

Various new methods are under study, such as radiation therapy with beams that are controlled so as to maximize radiation dose to the tumor with the smallest amount of collateral exposure. Another development is the combination of radiation therapy with hormones.

Treatment

Your doctor may use one or more of the following methods:
- surgery
- hormone treatments
- radiation
- anticancer drugs
- combination of radiation therapy with hormones

The choice depends on the stage of the cancer and your age and health. Surgery or radiation therapy may be the treatment chosen to cure prostate cancer in advanced stages for long periods by shrinking the size of the tumor and greatly relieving pain.

Because it is important that this form of cancer is discovered early, cancer specialists are now working to improve methods for early detection and develop more effective combinations of treatments. Extensive local disease, age or general health of the

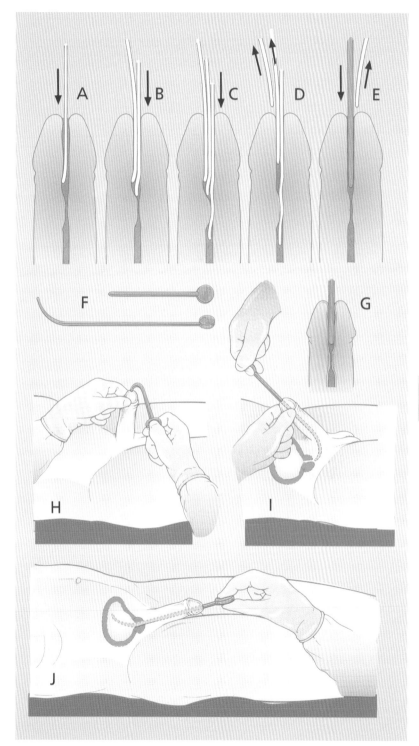

Constricture of the urethra in the penis. Urethral dilatation in the male patient. Dilatation of an irregular stricture using filiform bougies (A, B); once a filiform bougie passes through the stricture (C, D), progressive dilatation can be started (E).
A straight and a curved bougie (F); dilatation of an anterior stricture with a straight bougie (G); dilatation with a curved bougie (H, I, J).

M

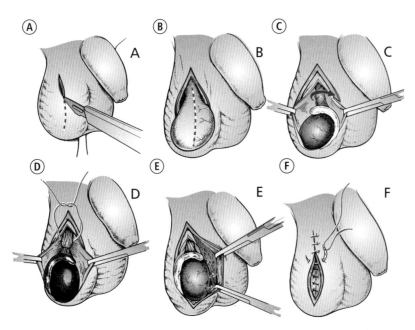

Treatment of torsion of the testis. Making the first incision (A); site of incision in the tunica vaginalis (B); torsion of the testis, to be untwisted in the direction of the arrow (C); excising a gangrenous (black) testis and doubly ligating the cord (D); fixing the tunica albuginea of a non-gangrenous testis to the scrotal septum (E); and closing the wound in two layers (F).

M

Testicular cancer   Questions & Answers

How common is testes cancer?
Cancer of the testes - the male reproductive glands - is one of the most common cancers in men 15 to 34 years of age. It accounts for 3 per cent of all cancer deaths in this group. If discovered in the early stages, testicular cancer can be treated promptly and effectively.

Who are at risk of developing testes cancer?
Men who have an undescended or partially descended testicle are at a much higher risk of developing testicular cancer than others. However, it is a simple procedure to correct the undescended testicle condition.

What are the symptoms of testicular cancer?
The first sign of testicular cancer is usually a slight enlarged testis and a change it its consistency. Pain may be absent, but often there is a dull ache in the lower abdomen and groin, together with a sensation of dragging and heaviness.

Can testicular cancer be prevented?
Your best hope for early detection of testicular cancer is a minute monthly self-examination. The best time is after a warm bath or shower, when the scrotal skin is most relaxed. Roll each testicle gently between the thumb and fingers of both hands.

What is the treatment for testicular cancer?
Surgery is usually the preferred treatment, and in certain cases it may be used together with radiation therapy or chemotherapy.

patient, or the presence of metastases may preclude cure of these modalities. In these situations, palliation may result from hormone control therapy. Short term high dose intravenous injection of the hormone diethyl-stilbestrol may provide dramatic symptomatic relief in a few days. Local radiation therapy provides relief of pain due to bony metastases refractory to other treatment and also may be effective in controlling local disease in the prostatic area. Chemotherapy after hormone failure has not been effective. Finasteride, a drug used to relieve symptoms caused by benign enlargement of the prostate, may prevent cancer.

Impotence

Impotence is the inability to have sexual intercourse due to failure in achieving or maintaining an erection. The cause may be organic, i.e. due to a condition or disease, such as diabetes, or an endocrine gland disorder.
More commonly, it is psychogenic and caused by psychological or emotional factors. Stress and anxiety relat-

Ways by which prostate cancer may spread to neighboring organs and tissues.

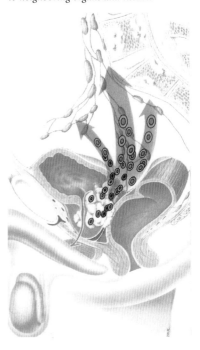

ing to some other aspect of life can cause impotence, as may excess consumption of alcohol, or drug abuse. Obesity and smoking may contribute to the problem which can also arise as an side effect of some prescription drugs. In older age, many men find that they require more prolonged stimulation to achieve an erection than was the cause when they were younger, but this is not true impotence.

In men aged over 65 years, some cases of impotence are caused by low levels of testosterone, a condition which can be corrected by hormone replacement therapy.

Treatment

Treatment of impotence depends upon the underlying cause and a combination of approaches may be recommended. These may include measures to combat stress, counselling and sexual therapy to help resolve relationship problems, changes in lifestyle, weight control, alternation in prescribed medication and pelvic floor exercises.

Viagra (active ingredient: sildenafil citrate) and analogous drugs work by enhancing the effects of one of the chemicals the body normally releases into the penis during sexual arousal. This results in an increased blood flow into the penis, which in turn increases the man's ability to achieve and maintain an erection.

This drug may only be prescribed by a doctor after a complete medical history has been taken and an examination made to determine the cause of impotence.

Also there are various other devices which can help, particularly the use of special condoms. A recently-developed therapy, particularly helpful for diabetic men, is self-injection of the drug papaverine into the penis which produces an erection. There is a slight risk of side effects, particularly uncomfortable scarring and priapism (painful, persistent erections unaccompanied by sexual desire or excitement).

For those men whose impotence has resulted from injury to nerves and blood vessels supplying the penis, two forms of penile implant can be inserted by means of a surgical operation.

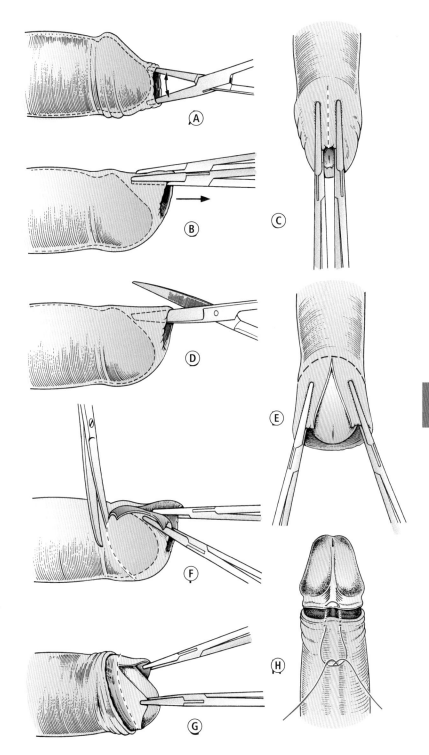

Stretching the opening of the prepuce (A); holding the prepuce (A); holding the prepuce with two pairs of forceps ((B) and cutting down the midline dorsally (C, D, E); excising the prepuce (F); inner layer of the prepuce to be trimmed (G, dottel line); ligating the artery of the frenulum (H).

M

MENSTRUAL DISORDERS

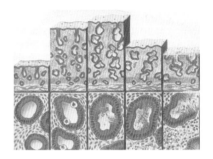

Menstruation

Once a month, just after a woman releases the egg (at ovulation) from her ovary, the lining (endometrium) of the womb (uterus) as at its peak to allow the embedding of a fertilised egg.

If pregnancy does not occur, the endometrium starts to deteriorate as the hormones that sustain it in peak condition alter. After a few days, the lining breaks down completely, sloughs off the wall of the uterus, and is washed away by the blood released from the arteries that supply it - a process known as menstruation. Contraction of the uterus help remove the debris. After three to five days, the bleeding stops, and a new lining starts to develop ready for the next month's ovulation.

Failure to start menstruation

Normally, a young woman starts her menstrual periods between eleven and thirteen years of age, but some commence earlier or later, without any subsequent problems.

If a girl fails to start her periods by the age of sixteen, investigation is appropriate.

If the breasts have not developed, and there is no sign of pubic hair by the age of fourteen, investigation may be commence earlier.

A number of uncommon medical conditions may be responsible for the problem, which is medically known as primary amenorrhoea.

In some girls, the hymen completely covers the vaginal opening and has no hole, so that menstrual blood accumulates in the vagina with no way to escape. The periods are occurring, but no blood appears.

If there is damage to the hypothalamus or pituitary gland from a tumor, cancer, abscess, infection, poor blood supply or other disease, the appropriate signals may not be received by the ovary to activate the production of the sex hormone estrogen, which is essential for the transformation of a girl into a woman at puberty.

The ovaries may not develop normally in some girls due to a birth defect, or chromosomal abnormalities such as Turner syndrome.

Menstrual irregularities

If menstrual (or other vaginal) bleeding is unusually profuse, or if bleeding lasts for more than 10 days, and is accompanied by signs and symptoms of excess blood loss (such as dizziness, fainting, and nausea) consult a physician promptly.

Amenorrhea

If periods stop for more than 3 months or do not start by the time a young woman is 16, a condition called amenorrhea is present. Amenorrhea is not an illness but always represents a symptom of some underlying problem. A very thin or active girl may experience delay in reaching puberty and starting to menstruate. Most disorders causing amenorrhea can be cured or controlled so that menstruation begins or resumes.

Menorrhagia

Prolonged periods (more than 10 days) with heavy flow or periods that occur frequently (such as every 2 weeks) are usually signs of anovulatory cycles but occasionally indicate disorders of the reproductive system. In these cases medical evaluation is necessary. Most menstrual irregularities

disappear as an adolescent's body matures and produces sufficient amounts of reproductive hormones.

Menstrual pain

Menstrual cramps are often described as a dull ache or a sense of pressure in the lower abdomen. Sometimes they come and go, growing stronger and then fading. Sometimes they are a constant, dull ache. The discomfort may spread to the hips, the lower back, and the inner thighs.

The vagina and/or the uterus may ache and feel heavy. When cramps are severe, nausea, vomiting, diarrhea, or general achiness can occur along with the pain. Sometimes these symptoms can occur even if cramps are mild.

Why and how

The uterus is a muscle. Like all muscles, it contracts and relaxes. Must uterine contractions are not even noticed, but strong ones are painful. During menstruation, the uterus contracts more strongly than at other times of the month. This can produce the uncomfortable feeling of menstrual cramps.

These contractions are caused by prostaglandins, natural substances made by cells in the wall of the uterus and other parts of the body for many purposes. The prostaglandins made in the uterus make the muscle of the uterus contract. During strong contractions, the uterus may begin to contract too strongly or too frequently. The blood supply to the uterus is cut off temporarily. This deprives the muscle of oxygen, causing pain.

Many women experience the pain and aggravation of dysmenorrhea. Severe menstrual cramps, in all but rare cases, can and should be treated. If severe or unusual menstrual cramps are a problem for you, talk with your doctor about treatments that are now available. You will most likely to be able to stay active every day of the month, free from distress and disruption of painful menstrual cramps.

Primary dysmenorrhea

The more common type of dysmenorrhea, primary dysmenorrhea, is due to the normal production of prostaglandins by the inner lining of the uterus. It is not a sign that something is wrong with a woman's reproductive organs.

Primary dysmenorrhea is usually noticed by women during cycles in which ovulation has occurred (an egg has been released). It can begin during adolescence, or it can begin later in life. It often disappears after a full-term pregnancy but may sometimes return. As a woman gets older, the pain usually lessens but may become worse or remain unchanged.

Secondary dysmenorrhea

Menstrual pain may also result when there are abnormalities, such as a tumor, infection, or bleeding in the pelvic area - any of these are called secondary dysmenorrhea.

Secondary dysmenorrhea usually occurs after a woman has had normal menstrual periods for some time, but it may occur in teenagers. If differs from primary dysmenorrhea in that the pain is caused by disease of the uterus, tubes, or ovaries.

However, sometimes the pain lasts longer than the usual 2-3 days during the monthly flow. Pelvic pain may also occur at other times of the month or during sexual intercourse. Often, but not always, one of the following problems is present:
- endometriosis
- pelvic inflammatory disease
- leiomyomas
- intrauterine device

■ *Endometriosis*

Endometriosis is a condition in which tissue that looks and acts like the inner lining of the uterus is found outside of the uterus in the lower abdomen. It may be attached to the ovaries, the intestines, or some other part of the lower abdomen.

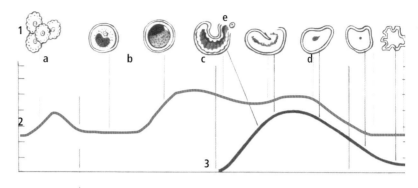

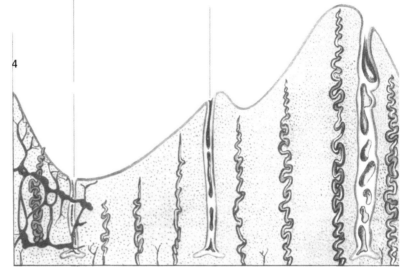

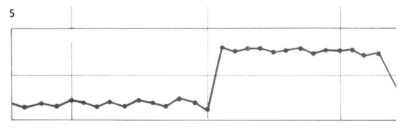

Graphical summary of changes in the ovary (1), hormone content of the blood (2 and 3) uterine endometrium (4) and body temperature (5).

The time scale equals the length of a menstrual cycle.

1. Summary of changes in the ovary. a. Primordial follicle; b. follicle of De Graaf; c. rupture of the follicle under the influence of luteinizing hormone (LH); d. yellow body; e. ovulation.

2. Changes in the blood content of estrogen during the menstrual cycle.

3. Changes in the blood content of progestogen during the menstrual cycle.

4. Changes in the endometrium of the uterus.

During the proliferative phase (days 4-16) the basal layer repairs and its surface is re-epithelialized by cells from the basal ends of the uterine glands. This takes about two days and is followed by a period of rapid growth of a new functional layer. This phase is controlled by estrogen, a hormone secreted by the ovary as a Graafian follicle is maturing.

The secretory phase (days 16-30) follows the rupture of the mature follicle and ovulation, when a corpus luteum forms within the ruptured follicle and begins to secrete a second hormone, progestogen. About two days elapse before enough progestogen is available to affect the endometrium, and this is why the proliferative phase extends two days beyond ovulation.

Causes of irregular vaginal bleeding

The major causes of irregular vaginal bleeding are:

- Stress or illness
- Weight change (particularly if its is abrupt, such as that caused by crash dieting) or anorexia nervosa
- Strenuous endurance activities (such as ballet, gymnastics, and track)
- Infection or injury to part of the reproductive system, such as the cervix or uterus
- Ovarian cysts, benign (not cancerous) tumors, and rarely, cancerous tumors
- Birth defects of the reproductive system
- Overgrowth of the lining of the uterus
- Exposure to drugs before birth (e.g. DES exposure)
- A foreign object in the vagina (such as a forgotten tampon)
- Diseases such as tuberculosis, cystic fibrosis, and diabetes
- A hormonal imbalance resulting from disorders such as adrenal problems and thyroid problems
- Blood disorders such as clotting problems and leukemia
- The use of birth control pills (which may make menstrual flow lighter than normal or irregular
- The use of IUD (intrauterine device), which may cause heavy menstrual flow
- Hormonal imbalances such as polycystic ovary syndrome (numerous cysts in the ovaries associated with an imbalance in the pituitary hormone levels and sometimes excess body hair growth)

M

The tissue is affected by female hormones as if it were in the uterus. At the end of each month, this tissue bleeds, but since the fluid cannot be flushed freely out of the body, it builds up inside.

Nearby tissues become red, swollen, and painful. Often, endometriosis causes pain that begins several days before the beginning of menstrual bleeding, sometimes accompanied by spotting (slight bleeding).

■ *Pelvic inflammatory diseases (PID)*
This condition, belonging to the group of secondary dysmenorrheas, is a chronic infection that involves some of the reproductive organs. PID, usually caused by sexually transmitted diseases, causes menstrual pain that usually lasts longer than ,menstrual bleeding. The pain may begin early or late in the period and usually lasts for several days.

■ *Leiomyomas*
Leiomyomas, also called fibroids, are tumors of the uterine wall that may be linked with menstrual cramping when they involve the inner cavity of the uterus.

■ *Intrauterine device (IUD)*
Such a device may be placed in the uterus to prevent pregnancy. It can cause pelvic pain and cramping. It may intensify normal menstrual cramps and may cause cramps at other times, too.

Diagnosis of secondary dysmenorrhea
If menstrual pain is not caused by normal prostaglandins, what is causing it? Before your doctor can answer this question, there are many questions he or she may need to ask:
- Do you have regular menstrual cycles?
- How long have you had regular menstrual periods?
- On which days of the cycle to you have pain?
- How long have you had menstrual cramps?
- Do you have pain when you have intercourse?
- Do you have pain with a bowel movement?
- Where is the pain?
- Have you ever had an infection of the uterus, tubes, or ovaries?
- Have you ever had endometriosis?

- Is your flow heavy?
- What types of birth control have you used?
- Have you ever been pregnant?
- Do other women in your family have severe menstrual cramps?
- Have you ever had surgery in the pelvic area?

To check for problems in the reproductive system a pelvic exam is done. This is a method of examining the uterus, tubes, and ovaries for any abnormalities.

It is usually not uncomfortable and it does not take very long. The doctor inserts the index and middle fingers of one hand into the patient's vagina. With the fingers of the other hand, pressure is applied gently on the abdomen. By using both hands together, it is possible to feel the size and contours of the reproductive organs. The doctor will usually also examine the rectum during the pelvic exam.

When there is a chance that menstrual pain is caused by a disease, a special test called laparoscopy may be needed. this test involves surgery and requires an anesthetic that either numbs the area being examined or puts you to sleep.

A laparoscope, which is like a slender telescope with a light, is inserted through a tiny cut in the lower abdomen. During the operation, the doctor looks through an eyepiece and with the aid of a light is able to see the organs inside.

Treatment
Before medicines for dysmenorrhea were available, women tried home remedies, which seldom worked well. Fortunately, today there are more effective means of treating primary and secondary dysmenorrhea. If a woman's pain is mild and does not bother her, she may not need any treatment.

■ *Antiprostaglandins*
These are new drugs that help women with primary dysmenorrhea. They prevent the formation of the prostaglandins that cause menstrual cramps. They usually also prevent the other unpleasant menstrual symptoms caused by prostaglandins, such

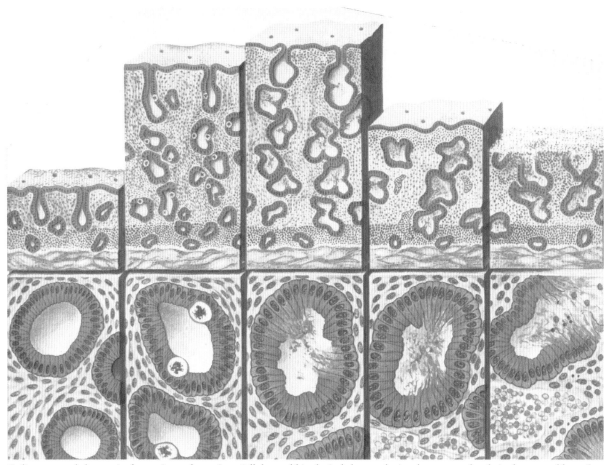

Cyclic menstrual changes in the uterine endometrium Cellular and histological changes during the menstrual cycle in the mucosal layer (top row of figures) and submucosal tissue (bottom row of figures). Compare the legend of the illustration on page 567.

as nausea, vomiting, diarrhea, and general achiness.

Aspirin prevents prostaglandin formation too, but the newer drugs are more powerful and effective. In some cases, aspirin may be enough to relieve the pain.

Antiprostaglandins are started on the day the menstrual period or the pain starts, and they are usually needed for only a day or two.

These drugs are safe, although they can upset the stomach and are best taken with at least a small amount of food in the stomach. If you think you might be pregnant, do not use any drug until after your period starts.

If at the first cycle or two there is no improvement in your pain, tell your doctor. An increase in the dose may bring a change. If that fails, one of the other antiprostaglandin drugs, of which there are several, may be more helpful.

■ *Oral contraceptives*

Oral contraceptives (birth control pills) often relieve or reduce the pain of primary dysmenorrhea. The pill prevents ovulation and alters the normal hormone changes of the menstrual cycle. As a result, fewer prostaglandins are made. This may explain why women using the pill have less or no menstrual pain.

One drawback to birth control pills is that they must be taken for most of the month for a problem that lasts only 1-3 days. This is not an inconvenience to women who are using the pill for contraception, in which case relief from menstrual cramps may provide an added bonus. With the advice of your doctor, you can decide if this is a good choice for you.

Some side effects such as nausea or breast tenderness may keep some women from using the pill. These side effects are very uncommon among women who are taking the low-dose pill available today.

Because of the small risk of blood clotting, some women may be unable to use the pill or may simply decide not to use it. Women who smoke have an increased clotting risk and are advised not to use the pill.

For secondary dysmenorrhea, the specific cause of the pain may require medical or surgical treatment. A woman with fibroids is helped in a different way from a women who has cramps because of an IUD. Treatment may relieve the pain, although how much relief it will bring is different for each woman.

MENTAL RETARDATION

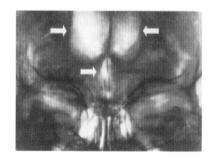

Description

Mental retardation is defined as a predominant disturbance in the acquisition of cognitive, language, motor, or social skills. The disorder is characterized by three major features:

▲ significantly subaverage general intellectual functioning, accompanied by
▲ significant deficits or impairments in adaptive functioning, with
▲ onset before age 18.

General intellectual functioning is defined as an intelligence quotient obtained by assessment with one or more of the individually administered general intelligence tests (e.g., Wechsler Intelligence Scale for Children). Significantly subaverage intellectual functioning is defined as an IQ of 70 or below on an individually administered IQ test.

Adaptive functioning refers to the person's effectiveness in areas such as social skills, communication, and daily living skills, and how well the person meets the standards of personal independence and social responsibility expected of his or her age by his or her cultural group.

Adaptive functioning in people with mental retardation is influenced by personality characteristics, motivation, and social and vocational opportunities. Adaptive behavior is more likely to improve with remedial efforts than is IQ, which tends to remain more stable.

Behavioral symptoms commonly seen in mental retardation include:

· passivity
· dependency
· low self-esteem
· low frustration tolerance
· aggressiveness
· poor impulse control
· stereotyped self-stimulation
· self-injurious behavior

The prevalence of other mental disorders is at least three or four times

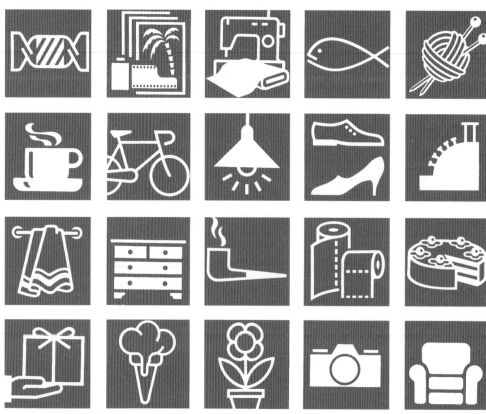

Example of a modern intelligence test to evaluate certain memory mechanisms. The person looks for some time at the pictures which he later has to memorize. In the second part of the test the person is asked to give alternative descriptions of the pictures.

greater among people with mental retardation than in the general population. Particularly common are:

- ▲ pervasive developmental disorders;
- ▲ attention-deficit hyperactivity disorder;
- ▲ stereotypy/habit disorder.

The course of mental retardation is a function of both biologic factors, such as an underlying etiologic physical disorder, and environmental factors, such as educational and other opportunities, environmental stimulation, and appropriateness of management. If the underlying physical abnormality is static, the course of the disorder is variable; with good environmental influences, functioning may improve; with poor environmental influences, it may deteriorate.

If the underlying physical abnormality is progressive (as in lipid storage disorder), functioning will tend to deteriorate, although with good environmental influences, the deterioration may proceed more slowly.

Causes and familial patterns

Etiologic factors may be primarily biologic, psychosocial, or a combination of both. In approximately 30-40 per cent of the cases seen in clinical settings, no clear etiology can be determined despite extensive evaluation efforts.

The following are the major causative factors in the remaining cases:

- ▲ hereditary factors (in approximately 5 per cent of cases), such as inborn errors of metabolism (e.g., Tay Sachs disease), other single-gene abnormalities (e.g., tuberous sclerosis), and chromosomal aberrations (e.g., translocation Down syndrome);
- ▲ early alterations of embryonic development (in approximately 30 per cent), such as chromosomal changes (e.g., trisomy 21 syndrome), prenatal damage due to toxins (e.g., maternal alcohol consumption, infections) or unknown causes;
- ▲ pregnancy and perinatal problems (in approximately 10 per cent), such as fetal malnutrition, prematurity, hypoxia, trauma;
- ▲ physical disorders acquired in childhood (in approximately 5 per cent), such as infections, traumas, and lead poisoning;
- ▲ environmental influences and mental disorders (in approximately 15-20 per cent), such as deprivation of nurturance and of social, linguistic, and other stimulation, and complications of severe mental disorders (e.g., a drop in adaptive functioning in a person with borderline-level IQ following early-onset schizophrenia).

Prevalence and age of onset

The prevalence of mental retardation due to known biologic factors is similar among children of upper and lower socioeconomic classes, except that certain etiologic factors are linked to lower socioeconomic status, such as lead poisoning and premature births. In cases in which no specific biologic causation can be identified, lower socioeconomic classes are over-represented, and the mental retardation is usually milder (but all degrees of severity are present).

The age at which a diagnosis of mental retardation is first made in a person depends on the degree of its severity and whether a physical disor-

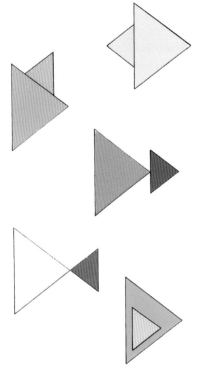

Test to help determine the level of mental retardation.

M

Test to help determine the level of mental retardation.

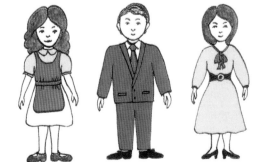
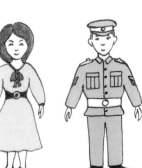
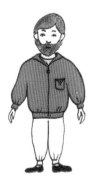
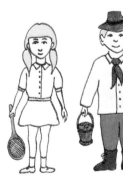

M

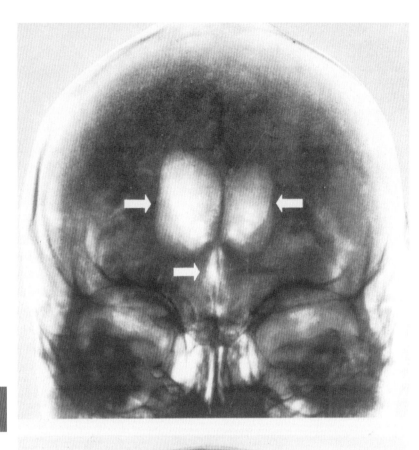

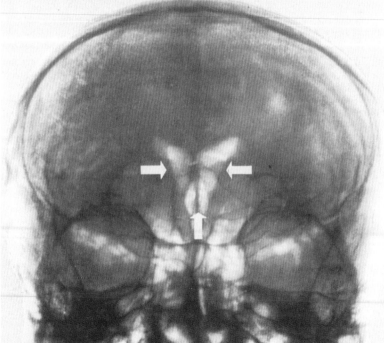

In these X-rays of the brain, the arrows indicate widening of the cerebral ventricles, which is typical of certain types of severe mental retardation.

der with characteristic phenotypic features is present. Thus, children with severe mental retardation and children with Down syndrome are diagnosed earlier than children with mild retardation of unknown cause.

Degrees of severity

There are four degrees of severity, reflecting the degree of intellectual impairment: mild, moderate, severe, and profound. IQ levels to be used as guides in distinguishing the four degrees of severity are:

Mild IQ	:	50-55 to approx. 70
Moderate IQ	:	35-40 to 50-55
Severe IQ	:	20-25 to 35-40
Profound IQ	:	below 20 or 25

■ *Mild mental retardation*

Mild mental retardation is roughly equivalent to what used to be referred to as the educational category of "educable." This group constitutes the largest segment of those with the disorder - about 85 per cent.

People with this level of mental retardation typically develop social and communication skills during the preschool years (ages 0-5), have minimal impairment in sensorimotor areas, and often are not distinguishable from normal children until a later age. By their late teens they can acquire academic skills up to approximately sixth-grade level; during their adult years, they usually achieve social and vocational skills adequate for minimum self-support, but may need guidance and assistance when under unusual social or economic stress.

At the present time, virtually all people with mild mental retardation can live successfully in the community, independently or in supervised apartments or group homes (unless there is an associated disorder that makes this impossible).

■ *Moderate mental retardation*

This disorder is roughly equivalent to what used to be referred to as the educational category or "trainable." This former term should not be used since it wrongly implies that people with moderate mental retardation cannot benefit from educational programs. This group constitutes 10 per cent of the entire population of people with mental retardation. Those with this level of mental retardation can talk or learn to communicate during the preschool years. They may profit from vocational training and, with moderate supervision, can take care of themselves. They can profit from training in social and occupational skills, but are unlikely to progress beyond the second grade level in academic subjects. They may learn to travel independently in familiar places. During adolescence, their difficulties in recognizing social conventions may interfere with peer relationships.

In their adult years, they may be able to contribute to their own support by performing unskilled or semiskilled work under close supervision in sheltered workshops or in the competitive job market. They need supervision and guidance when under stress. They adapt well to life in the community, but usually in supervised group homes.

■ Severe mental retardation

This group constitutes 3 per cent to 4 per cent of people with mental retardation. During the preschool period, they display poor motor development, and they acquire little or no communicative speech. During the school-age period, they may learn to talk, and can be trained in elementary hygiene skills. They profit to only a limited extent from instruction in pre-academic subjects, such as familiarity with the alphabet and simple counting, but can master skills such as learning sight-reading of some "survival" words, such as "men" and "women" and "stop."

In their adult years, they may be able to perform simple tasks under close

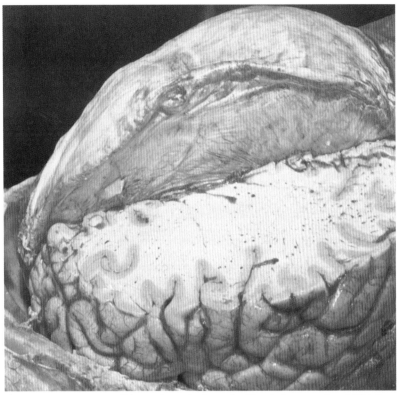

At autopsy, numerous small hemorrhages in the cerebral hemisphere were found. This have been one of the causative factors in mental retardation.

supervision. Most adapt well to life in the community, in group homes or with their families, unless they have an associated handicap that requires specialized nursing or other care.

■ Profound mental retardation

This group constitutes approximately 1%-2% of people with mental retardation. During the early years, these children display minimal capacity for sensorimotor functioning. A highly structured environment, with constant aid and supervision, and an individualized relationship with a caregiver are required for optimal development.

Motor development and self-care and communication skills may improve if appropriate training is provided. Currently, many of these people live in the community, in group homes, intermediate care facilities, or with their families. Most attend day programs, and some can perform simple tasks under close supervision in a sheltered workshop.

Mental capacity

Sufficient memory and understanding to comprehend in a general way the situation in which pone finds himself and the nature, purpose, and consequence of any act or transaction into which one proposes to enter. The term is also used to designate the degree of understanding and memory the law requires to uphold validity of or to charge one with responsibility for a particular act or transaction.

Mental disorder

Condition characterized by abnormal function of the higher centers of the brain responsible for thought, perception, mood and behavior, in which organic disease has been eliminated as a possible cause.
The borderline between disease and the range of normal variability is indistinct and may be determined by cultural factors.

Mental age

Measure used in psychological testing that expresses an individual's mental attainment in terms of the number of years it takes an average child to reach the same level.

M

MULTIPLE SCLEROSE

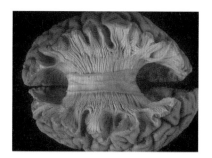

Description

Multiple sclerosis is defined as a diseased condition marked by patches of hardened tissue in the brain or the spinal cord and associated especially with partial or complete paralysis and jerking muscle tremor. Multiple sclerosis is a neurological disorder in which the nerves of the eye, brain, and spinal cord lose patches of myelin.

In most cases the early manifestations of the disease are followed by conspicuous improvement, so that remissions and relapses are a striking feature of the disorder, the course of which may thus be prolonged for many years.

The early symptoms are often those of focal lesions of the nervous system, while the later clinical picture is one of progressive dissemination tending to produce the classical features of nystagmus, dysarthria, intention tremor, and ataxic paraplegia. The disease principally attacks young adults. In two-thirds of all cases it begins between 20 and 40, rather more often in the third than in the fourth decade. Its occurrence below the age of 10 is doubtful, but it is occasionally seen in children between the ages of 12 and 15. During recent years the proportion of patients in whom the disease begins after the age of 50 has increased, but it is almost unknown after 60. In most published series males have been reported more often than females, but in Great Britain the reverse is the case, female patients outnumbering males in the ratio of 3 to 2.

Causes

The cause of multiple sclerosis is unknown, but a likely explanation is that a virus or some unknown antibody or small protein (prion) somehow triggers an autoimmune process, usually early in life. Then the body, for some reason, produces antibodies against its own myelin (major constituent of the protecting sheaths of nerve fibers); the antibodies provoke inflammation and damage the myelin sheath.

Heredity seems to have a role in multiple sclerosis. About 5 per cent of the people with the disease have a brother or sister who is also affected, and about 15 per cent have a close relative who is affected.

Environment also plays a role; multiple sclerosis occurs in 1 out of every 2,000 people who spend their first decade of life in a temperate climate but in only 1 out of every 10,000 people born in a tropical climate.

Signs and symptoms

■ *The clinical picture*
The natural history of the disease produces a very varied picture. In the early stages it is often that of a single focal lesion, acute or, during a remission, quiescent. As times goes on, cumulative effects of earlier lesions constitute a persistent background of incapacity upon which fresh disabilities due to new lesions are superimposed.

The early stages thus usually show long and often remarkably complete remissions, while later the patient's condition fluctuates only to the small extent that fresh lesions temporarily regress.

Multiple sclerosis is a disease of the central nervous system. Particularly, the motor parts of the spinal cord and cerebellum (shown here) are affected.

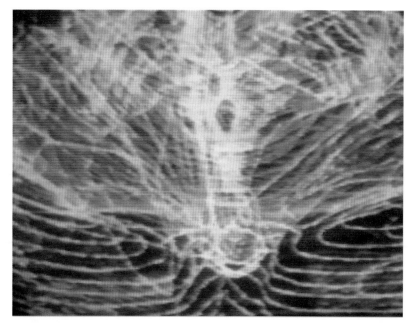

◼ Motor symptoms

Loss of power in the lower limbs is first manifested as fatigability or a feeling of heaviness, and later as spastic paraplegia. Sometimes sudden weakness of one upper limb occurs, often associated with loss of postural sensibility in the fingers. Facial weakness and hemiplegia occur occasionally.

Muscular wasting is very rare owing to the infrequency of involvement of the anterior horn cells in the patches, but an amyotrophic form has been described, and wasting may occur in any group, but most often in the forearms and hands.

Incoordination is frequently present. In the upper limbs it usually takes the form of intention tremor occurring only on voluntary movement and increasing in intensity the greater the accuracy demanded of the movement. In touching the nose with the finger the tremor increases in amplitude as the finger approaches the nose. The same phenomenon is shown if the patient be asked to touch his own nose and the observer's finger alternately, and also in lifting a glass of water to the lips. In the lower limbs incoordination is evident in an ataxic gait. Tremor of the head is common in the late stages.

A speech disorder (dysarthria) may be due to spastic weakness or to ataxia of the muscles of articulation or to a combination of these factors. In the early stages articulation may be slurred, later it may become explosive and almost unintelligible. The syllabic or scanning speech, sometimes regarded as typical, is exceptional.

◼ Sensory symptoms

Paraesthesia (strange feelings or sensation) occurs at some period of the disease in most cases, commonly in the form of numbness and formication over one side of the face or one upper or both lower limbs.

Pain is uncommon except in the back, but typical trigeminal neuralgia, which is sometimes bilateral, is occasionally encountered. Defect of postural sensibility and of appreciation of vibration is the commonest disturbance.

Diseases causing symptoms similar to those of multiple sclerosis

- Viral or bacterial infections of the brain:
  lyme disease;
  AIDS;
  syphilis.

- Structural abnormalities of the base of the skull and spine:
  severe arthritis of the neck;
  ruptured spinal disc.

- Tumors or cysts of the brain and spinal cord
  syringomyelia;
  syringobulbia.

- Spinocerebellar degeneration and the hereditary ataxias; disorders in which muscle action is irregular or muscles fail to coordinate.

- Small strokes; especially in people with diabetes or hypertension who are prone to such strokes.

- Amyotrophic lateral sclerosis.

- Inflammation of the blood vessels inn the brain or spinal cord:
  lupus;
  arteritis.

M

Degeneration of motoneurons in the spinal cord; one of the major characteristics of multiple sclerosis.

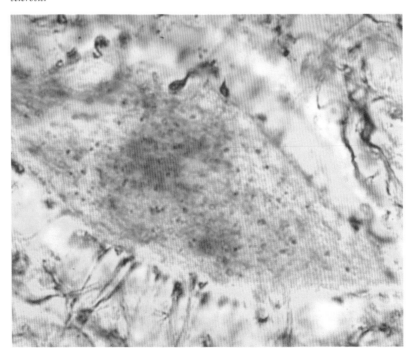

Multiple sclerose   Questions & Answers

How does multiple sclerosis (MS) damage the nervous system?
The nervous system initiates and regulates all our activities, such as walking, talking, seeing, hearing, and eating. To do this, the nervous system acts as a communications center receiving and sensing messages - which are conveyed as impulses travelling along nerve fibers from the brain, through the spinal cord and peripheral nerves throughout the body.
Nerve fibers are protected with a substance called myelin, just as a rubber coating protects a telephone wire. Multiple sclerosis attacks the myelin and causes it to wear away, leaving bare scar tissue, in a process called demyelinization.
This short circuits the signals that travel to and from the brain. What actually causes multiple sclerosis in a particular patient is not exactly known - although physicians know it is not contagious. An immunological abnormality, possibly triggered by a virus, is suspected.
Some environmental factor may also be involved because MS is far more common in temperate climates than in the tropics.

When does multiple sclerosis occur?
Multiple sclerosis usually attacks those between the ages of 20 and 40 but can occur at any age. Six out of every 10 victims are women.

What are the symptoms of multiple sclerosis (MS) and how is the disease being treated?
Symptoms vary widely from person to person and may come and go. These may include:
- partial or complete paralysis of parts of the body, which includes difficulty in walking and coordination;
- numbness or a prickling 'pins and needles' sensation in parts of the body;
- noticeable dragging of one or both feet;
- loss of control over urinary or bowel habits;
- staggering or loss of balance;
- extreme weakness or fatigue;
- trembling of the hands;
- blurred or double vision;
- temporary blindness or pain in one or both eyes;
- dizziness;
- pain in one or both sides of the face;
- difficulty speaking or slurred speech.
If you experience three or more of these symptoms see your doctor right away.

How is multiple sclerosis treated?
There is no cure for multiple sclerosis. Spontaneous remissions make experimental treatments difficult to assess. Many physicians believe that short-term therapy with corticosteroids can hasten recovery from acute attacks. Generally, treatment is aimed to maintaining strength so that patients can best withstand attacks. This may include extra rest, special exercises and brace.

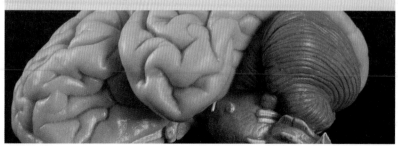

■ *Ocular symptoms*
Acute unilateral retrobulbar neuritis (inflammation of the optic nerve on one side) is one of the most important early symptoms of the disease. It occurs most often between the ages of 20 and 390.
The vision of one eye becomes misty and in 24 or 48 hours is reduced to a perception of hand movement or of light only. The eye is painful on movement and tender on pressure, and there is a central scotoma larger for red and green than white.
The optic disc is usually normal in appearance during the acute stage, but if the lesion is near the disc papillitis may occur, though the swelling is usually light.
In a few weeks vision improves, but the residual damage to the nerve manifests itself in some degree of optic atrophy - pallor of the disc, especially in its temporal half - and often a persistent though smaller central scotoma. Permanent blindness is very rare.

■ *Reflex changes*
The length of the corticospinal tracts exposes them to a great chance of injury by some of the multiple lesions, hence the reflex signs of corticospinal tract damage are frequent. The tendon reflexes are exaggerated.
The abdominal reflexes are absent in at least two-thirds of all cases and may be lost at an early stage, and extensor plantar reflexes occur in from 80 to 90 percent of cases in the later stages.

Diagnosis

No single test is diagnostic, but laboratory tests can distinguish between multiple sclerosis and other conditions with similar symptoms.
Doctors may take a sample of cerebrospinal fluid by spinal tap. People with multiple sclerosis may have a few more white blood cells and slightly more protein than normal in the fluid.
The concentration of antibodies in the cerebrospinal fluid may be high, and specific types of antibody and other substances are present in up to 90 per cent of the people with multiple sclerosis.

M

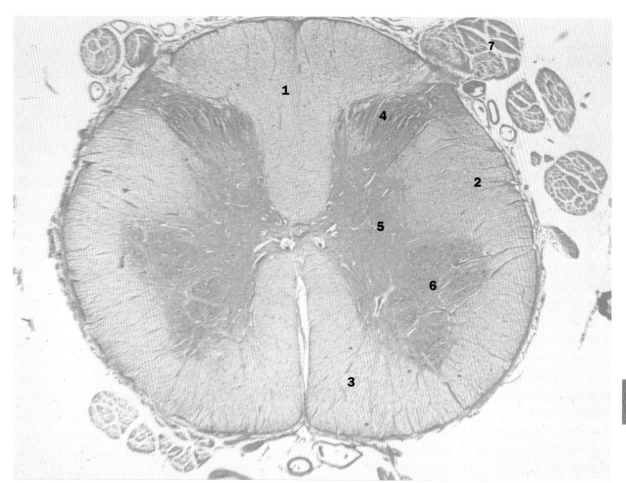

Cross section of the spinal cord.
1. posterior tract system; 2. lateral tract system; 3. anterior tract system; 4. posterior horn; 5. lateral horn; 6. anterior horn; 7. roots of the spinal nerves.

Magnetic resonance imaging (MRI-scans) is the most sensitive diagnostic imaging technique, possibly revealing areas of the brain or spinal cord that have lost myelin.

Treatment

Corticosteroid to relieve acute symptoms have been the main form of therapy for decades. Although corticosteroids may shorten the duration of attacks, they do not stop progressive disability over the long term.

Some new drugs, such as beta-interferon, have been shown in some patients to reduce the frequency of relapses. Other promising drugs still under investigation include other interferons, oral myelin, and glatiramer to help keep the body from attacking its own myelin.

Patients can often maintain an active lifestyle, though they may tire easily and may nog be able to keep up with a demanding schedule. Regular exercise reduces spasticity and helps maintain cardiovascular, muscular, and psychologic health.

M

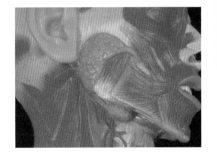

Muscle pain

Pain can develop in any muscle because of injury, cramping, or inflammation. Pain may be present in a small part of a muscle, such as at the point of injury, or may extend throughout a muscle. Muscle pain itself is a symptom of an underlying condition or illness.

Severity of muscle injury ranges from mild to quite severe, Mildly injured muscles retain their elasticity and ability to function, usually healing with rest. More severely damaged muscles are partially or completely torn and may require surgery for full recovery.

■ Cramps

Cramps, which are painful contractions of muscle fibers, frequently occur in growing and physically active children. Cramps may last from a few seconds to a few hours and may occur in any muscle of the body.

They may vary from mild to strong enough to wake a child during the night (such as a charley horse).

Cramps can be severe and violent enough to break the bone.

■ Myositis

Myositis or muscle inflammation, frequently associated with common illnesses such as colds and influenza, may affect children of all ages. Myositis-induced pain frequently occurs as a dull ache in the large muscles of the body, such as those of the neck, back, shoulders and arms.

Causes

The most common injuries causing muscle pain are muscle strain (stretching or partial tearing of muscles) or damage to muscle nerves and blood vessels (usually resulting in formation of a bruise) caused by forceful blow.

These injuries frequently occur during participation in contact sports or other vigorous physical activity. Such pain may be confused with pain caused by injuries such as sprains and mild fractures.

Pain due to cramps often occurs as a child's muscles grow and develop. These cramps usually develop when a growing child is at rest, often during the night. Cramps may also develop when a child participates in vigorous physical activity involving previously inactive muscles. Vigorous movement can also result in cramps if large amounts of the body's salts and minerals, such as potassium and magnesium, are lost through heavy sweating. Hyperventilating and restriction of blood flow to muscles may also result in cramps.

Because of their size and the frequency with which they are used, large muscles such as those of the calf and upper arm tend to cramp more frequently than others.

Muscle inflammation often results from viral infections such as influenza. Other less common causes of inflammation are infestations b‌   mus-

quires

M

Microscopic pictures of a myoblastoma.

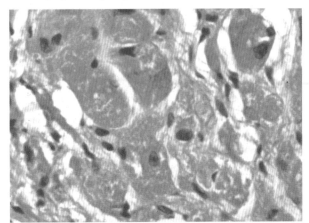

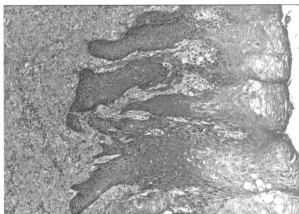

treatment of underlying causes. Minor muscle injuries usually heal with home treatment. Rest is essential, because the more an injured muscle is exercised, the more slowly it heals.

Treatment of inflammation should begin with reduction of swelling. Rest is essential, as it helps reduce or prevent muscle contractions that can interfere with healing. Once swelling is significantly reduced, an affected muscle should be relaxed by applying heat, either through warm water soaks or warm compresses. Muscles should then be gently massaged and exercised to prevent stiffening during healing.

If muscle pain is not reduced significantly within 24 to 48 hours and a muscle cannot be used, medical attention is required. A physician's care or, in some cases, surgery may be recommended to avoid permanent muscle weakness.

Muscle weakness

Weakness can occur when any part of the musculoskeletal system (muscles, joints, ligaments, tendons, and bursas) is abnormal. If the muscle itself cannot contract, weakness occurs. If a nerve does not adequately stimulate the muscle, the muscle contractions are weak. If a joint is frozen and unable to move normally, the muscle may not be adequately able to cause movement. Even pain, due to inflammation, prevents normal movement, causing weakness.

Weakness may be limited to one joint or limb, as is typically the case when a nerve, joint, or single muscle is deceased, or diffuse, as occurs in widespread neurological or muscular diseases. Muscle strength may also be limited by pain in the muscles, tendons, bones, or joints, giving the impression of weakness.

Weakness is a common symptom of muscle injury or disease. Muscle weakness can also result from many diseases affecting the whole body. Although many people complain of muscle weakness when they feel tired or run down, true muscle weakness means that full effort does not generate normal strength.

True muscle weakness can be caused by problems in the muscle itself (such

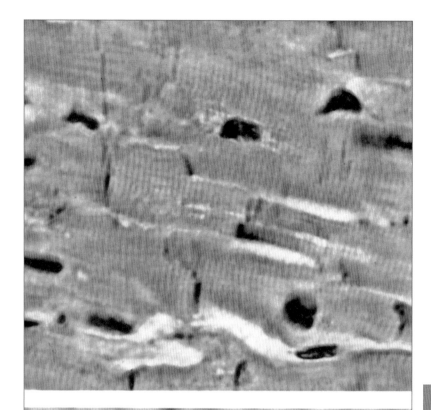

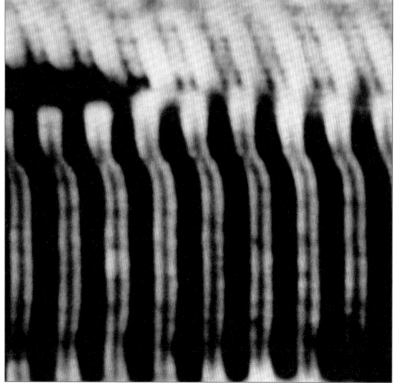

Top figure: Microscopic picture of normal muscle tissue.
Bottom figure: Electron microscopic picture of muscle tissue.

Muscle weakness classification

Muscle disease
■ *Examples*
- Muscular dystrophy
- Viral myositis
- Viral polymyositis

Muscular dystrophies are a group of muscle disorders that lead to muscle weakness of varying severity. In case of infection the muscles are tender or painful and weak.

Neuromuscular junction disorder
■ *Examples*
- Myasthenia gravis
- Curare toxicity
- Insecticide poisoning
- Botulism
- Diphtheria

The major signs and symptoms are weakness or paralysis of many muscles.

Spinal cord damage
■ *Examples*
- Trauma to the neck or back
- Spinal cord tumors
- Spinal stenosis
- Multiple sclerosis
- Transverse myelitis
- Vitamin B$_{12}$ deficiency

Weakness or paralysis of the arms and legs below the level of injury, progressive loss of sensation below the level of injury, back pain. Bowel, bladder, and sexual function may be affected.

Degeneration of spinal cord neurons
■ *Examples*
- Amyotrophic lateral sclerosis
- Slow hereditary degeneration of spinal cord

Progressive loss of muscle bulk and strength, not no loss of sensation.

Spinal nerve root damage
■ *Examples*
- Ruptured disk in the neck
- Ruptured disk in the lower spine
- Severe spinal injury

Pain in the neck and weakness or numbness in an arm, low back pain, shooting down the leg, and the injured nerve.

Damage to a single nerve (mononeuropathy)
■ *Examples*
- Diabetic neuropathy
- Local pressure

Weakness or paralysis of muscles and loss of sensation in the area served by the injured nerve.

Damage to a many nerve (polyneuropathy)
■ *Examples*
- Diabetic neuropathy
- Guillain-Barré syndrome
- Folate deficiency
- Other metabolic disorders

Weakness or paralysis of muscles and loss of sensation in the area served by the affected nerves.

Use of corticosteroid drugs
■ *Example*
- Corticosteroid myopathy

Muscle weakness usually begins at the hips and gradually spreads to all muscles.

Low blood levels of potassium
■ *Example*
- Hypokalemic myopathy

The person experiences periods of weakness throughout the body that begins rapidly.

Abnormal levels of thyroid hormone
■ *Examples*
- Hypothyroidism
- Hyperthyroidism

High levels of thyroid hormone produced weakness that is usually more pronounced in the shoulders than in the legs. Low levels of thyroid hormone produces weakness that is usually more pronounced in the legs.

as in muscular dystrophy or polymyositis); by problems in the nervous system, which helps to control movements (such as following a stroke or after a spinal cord injury); or by disease affecting the connection between the nerve and the muscles, called the neuromuscular junction (such as myasthenia gravis).

Muscle weakness can occur in old age because of an age-related reduction in muscle mass called sarcopenia. The word "asthenia" is sometimes used by doctors to describe weakness, but in the sense of feebleness or infirmity rather than simple weakness.

Muscular dystrophy

Muscular dystrophy is the term applied to any inherited muscle disorder that is characterized by progressive degeneration of the nervous system. The heart and the respiratory system may be affected. In general, these muscle disorders are uncommon.

Duchenne muscular dystrophy
This type of dystrophy is the most devastating one. It is a progressive disease that usually ends in death before age 20, although a few individuals survive into their 20s. Children do not die because of the muscle disorder itself but because of complications caused by it. In most cases death results from respiratory infection, which initially may be mild but progresses rapidly; death may also be caused by heart failure.

Only male children develop Duchenne muscular dystrophy. It is usually inherited and occurs in 1 of every 3,500 live male births. The genetic factor, a defective gene, involved is passed on to children by mothers who carry it but do not develop the disorder themselves.

In most cases signs and symptoms of Duchenne muscular dystrophy do not appear until a child begins to walk. Half of the children with the disease begin to walk after 18 months of age. Onset of symptoms usually occurs between ages 2 and 5, with muscles of the lower body areas and spine affected first. Symptoms of Duchenne muscular dystrophy include:

- reluctance to walk;
- delay in walking;
- abnormal walk, most often a wad-
  dling or swaying gait;
- walking on the toes;
- inability to hop or run normally;
- difficulty in climbing stairs;
- difficulty in getting in and out of
  cars;
- frequent falls.

A child with Duchenne muscular dystrophy tires easily and has difficulty
supporting body weight in one leg.
Muscle enlargement is usually present, particularly in the calves; the legs
are usually affected symmetrically.

The arms are not usually affected
until the disease is advanced. Dental
problems, including widening of the
jaw and widening of the spaces
between the teeth, often develop.

Treatment

Because no cure exists for muscular
dystrophy, treatment focuses on
maintaining the child's ability to walk
and use affected muscles as long as
possible. Children should be encouraged to use involved muscles as much
as possible to delay stiffening and
deterioration. Even during periods of
illness, children should be encouraged
to move. In addition to using their
muscles, children should perform
stretching exercises recommended by
a physician or physical therapist.

These exercises are designed to take
the joints through a full range of
movement and to prevent muscle and
tendon contractions that may reduce
walking ability,

When not moving about or exercising, the child should be encouraged to
lie on his or her stomach in an effort
to extend the hips and reduce muscle
contractions. In addition to exercising
and wearing braces, walking may be
prolonged through surgical release of
contracted muscles and tendons.
Once the child loses the ability to
walk, posture supports are essential to
control bone deformities.

No matter what type of muscular dystrophy is present, affected individuals
need constant encouragement and emotional support from family and friends.
Muscular dystrophy can be a devastating
disease for all concerned and an especially difficult battle for a child to fight,
even with all kinds of help.

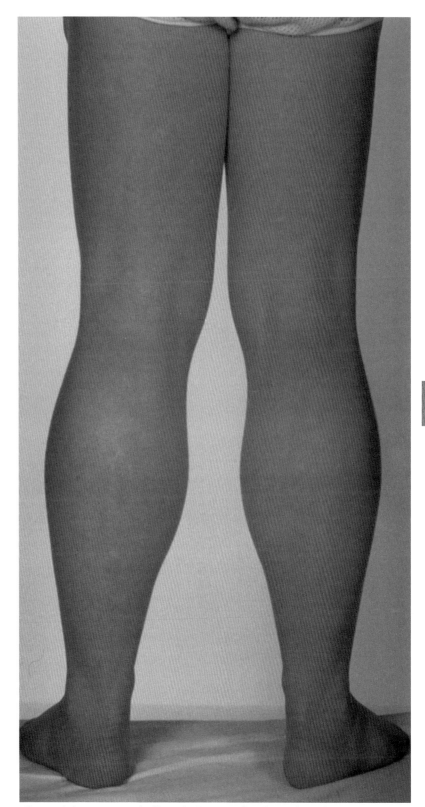

Characteristic appearance of calf muscles in a case of Duchenne-dystrophy.

M

NARCOLEPSY

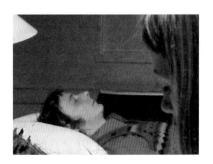

Description

Narcolepsy is a sleep which is abnormal by reason of its onset's being irresistible, though the circumstances may be inappropriate and excessive fatigue is absent. The patient can be aroused from the narcoleptic attack as from normal sleep.

The irresistible attacks of sleep characteristic of narcolepsy may be very numerous, occurring many times a day. In the attacks the patient suddenly becomes unconscious and the condition resembles normal in that he can be aroused immediately by appropriate stimuli. The attacks are most likely to occur in circumstances normally conducive of drowsiness, such as after a heavy meal or during a monotonous occupation, especially when driving a car.

They are usually worse in the afternoon and are occasionally precipitated by strong emotion. The sleep is usually brief, lasting only for seconds or minutes, but if the patient remains undisturbed he may sleep for hours.

Narcolepsy is surprising in its wide range of incidence.

It affects between one in 1,000 and one in 2,000 people in the western world. Rates in other countries range from one in 600 in Japan and one in 500,000 in Israel. Genetic factors linked to ethnicity or possibly environmental conditions may be responsible for this variation.

Pathophysiology

It is necessary to consider with narcolepsy four other forms of sleep disturbance which, since they may be associated with narcolepsy or with each other in the same patient, are closely related to one another.

■ Cataplexy

By cataplexy is understood an attack to which sufferers from narcolepsy are liable, but which differs from sleep in that, though the patient suddenly loses all power of movement and of maintaining posture, consciousness is preserved.

Sometimes tremor of the head or muscular twitching occurs at the onset, but these may be absent. The patient sinks limply to the ground with the eyes closed.

The muscles are hypotonic, the pupils may fail to react to light, the tendon reflexes may be diminished or lost, and during attacks the plantar reflexes may be extensor.

Though completely unable to move or to utter a sound, the patient is fully aware of all that is happening. Cataplectic attacks usually last less than a minute and recovery is rapid.

The cataplectic attacks of narcolepsy are frequently prompted by laughter; other times, embarrassment, social interactions, sudden anger, athletic exertion or sexual intercourse may trigger an episode.

■ Sleep paralysis

Sleep paralysis resembles cataplexy except that instead of being precipitated during the day of emotion, it usually occurs during the period of falling asleep or of awakening. The patient, though fully conscious, is unable to move hand or foot and often experiences intense anxiety. A touch will rapidly disperse the paralysis.

■ Hallucinatory states associated with sleep

Sufferers from narcolepsy sometimes experience vivid hallucinations. These, which are more often visual than auditory, may occur as the patient is falling asleep, when they are termed hypnagogic hallucinations. Sometimes, however, they occur during the night, when the patient is apparently awake. These hallucinations are often elaborate and terrifying, and though they seem real at the time their true character is readily recognized during normal waking life. The night-terrors of childhood appear to be of a similar nature.

■ Somnambulism

Somnambulism may be regarded as the reciprocal of cataplexy in that the patient, though partly asleep, is able to stand and walk in an automatic fashion. It is occasionally associated with narcolepsy, but usually occurs in adolescents of a neurotic disposition but otherwise normal.

Causes

Narcolepsy may be symptomatic or idiopathic. Symptomatic narcolepsy may follow head injury or may be due to cerebral atherosclerosis, neurosyphilis, encephalitis, or intracranial tumor involving the posterior part of the hypothalamus. In such cases it is probably due to disturbance of function of the sleep center of the brain.

More often no cause can be found, and the disorder is then designated idiopathic narcolepsy. Males are more subject to this than females and the onset usually occurs during adolescence or, at any rate, under the age of thirty. Idiopathic narcolepsy is probably in many instances in the true sense a functional disorder, that is, disturbance of function consisting of an exaggeration of a normal tendency to drowsiness.

Physical abnormalities indicative of disorder of other functions of the hypothalamus may be present, espe-

N

cially obesity, with or without genital atrophy.

Narcolepsy is linked to a disruption of the sleep control mechanisms. People who are not narcoleptic begin their nighttime rest with non-REM sleep, with REM sleep following roughly 90 minutes later.

But narcoleptics frequently go straight into REM sleep. Because of this trait - and because narcoleptics experience loss of muscle tone and dreamlike hallucinations that normally occur only during REM sleep - researchers have hypothesized that these symptoms of narcolepsy result from the inappropriate triggering of some aspects of REM sleep.

Some scientists have proposed that narcolepsy arises when unknown agents in the environment spur an autoimmune reaction that winds up damaging neurones in the brain circuit that control arousal and muscle tone.

Diagnosis

Both narcolepsy and cataplexy are so distinctive that diagnosis usually prevents no difficulty. Narcolepsy is distinguished from both epilepsy and syncope in the circumstances in which the attacks occur and in that when consciousness is lost the patient can be immediately aroused.

Cataplexy is distinguished from these disorders by the preservation of consciousness. Careful investigation should be made for evidence of organic disease involving the hypothalamus.

Prognosis and treatment

The disorder does not threaten life unless the patient should be unfortunate enough to have an attack in a dangerous situation.

Stimulant drugs, such as ephedrine, amphetamine, dextroamphetamine, and methylphenidate, may help, relieve narcolepsy. The dose may need to be adjusted to prevent side effects such as jitteriness, overactivity, or weight loss, so doctors monitor patients closely when they begin drug treatment.

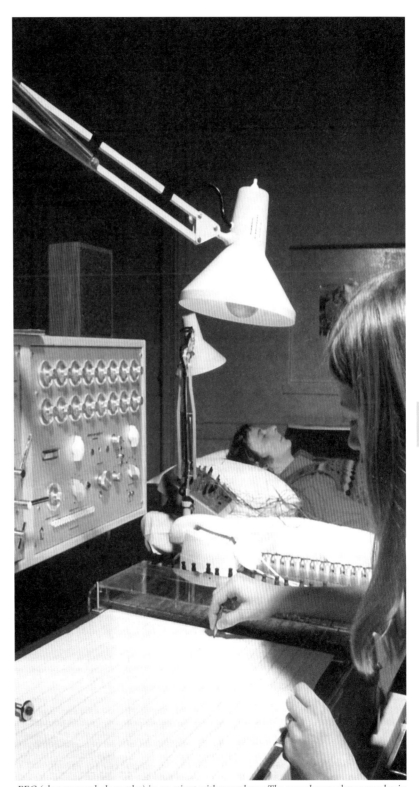

EEG (electroencephalography) in a patient with narcolepsy. The records may show some brain abnormalities.

NARCOTIC DRUGS

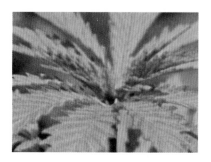

Description

Narcotics are strong, addictive and effective painkillers that are derived from the opium poppy. They are available as injections, tablets, suppositories (for anal use), patches and mixtures. They are highly restricted in their use, and must be kept in safes by chemists and doctors. If used appropriately, they give relief from severe pain to patients with acute injuries, and pain from diseases such as cancer and kidney stones. They are often used before, during and after operations to ease the pain of the procedure. If used this way, it is unlikely that addiction will occur. If used excessively, a psychological and physical addiction can rapidly develop.

Narcotic drugs not only relieve pain, they also reduce anxiety, stop cough, slow diarrhea, sedate and cause euphoria. They should be used with caution in asthma and other lung diseases, liver diseases and after head injury. Examples include codeine, dextropropoxyphene, fentanyl, morphine and pethidine.

Drug abuse

Drug abuse is the use of a mind-altering drug without medical need, in an amount large enough or over a period long enough to threaten the quality of life or health and safety of the user or others. Many people use drugs without medical need but keep that use under control so that it does not threaten their health or adversely affect their functioning.

If opium were the only drug of abuse, and the only kind of abuse were one of habitual, compulsive use, discussion of addiction might be a simple matter.

But opium or heroin is not the only drug of abuse, and there are probably as many kinds of abuse as there are drugs of abuse, or, indeed, as maybe there are persons who abuse.

Various substances are used in many different ways by so many different people for so many different purposes that no one view or one definition could possibly embrace all the medical, psychological, psychiatric, sociological and cultural considerations that have been an important bearing on addiction.

Prejudice and ignorance have led to the labelling of all use of nonsanctioned drugs as addiction and of all drugs, when misused, as narcotics. The continued practice of treating addiction as a single entity is dictated by custom and law, not by the facts of addiction.

The tradition of equating drug abuse with narcotic addiction originally had some basis in fact. Until recent times, questions of addiction centered on the misuse of opiates, the various concoctions prepared from powdered opium. The various alkaloids of opium, such as morphine and heroin, were isolated and introduced into use. Being the more active principles of opium, their addictions were simply more severe.

More recently, new drugs such as methadone and demarol were synthesized but their effects were still sufficiently similar to those of opium and its derivatives to be included in the older concept of addiction. With the introduction of various barbiturates in the form of sedatives and sleeping pills, the homogeneity of addictions began to break down. Then came various tranquilizers. stimulants, new and old hallucinogens, and the various combinations of each.

At this point, the unitary consideration of addiction became untenable.

Legal attempts at control often forced the inclusion of some nonaddicting drugs into old, established categories - such as the practice of calling marihuana a narcotic. Problems also arose in attempting to broaden addiction to include habituation and, finally, drug dependence. Unitary conceptions cannot embrace the diverse and heterogeneous drugs current in use (See the data in the tables).

Physical dependence

The condition popularly known as drug addiction is more appropriate described as physical dependence upon a narcotic drug. Physical dependence is closely related to drug tolerance, a condition in which standard doses of the drug produce progressively less effect.

Dependence has been attributed to various factors, including delayed or incomplete absorption, altered tissue distribution in the central nervous system, or increased rate of metabolism or excretion; it is generally agreed that psychologic dependence develops initially at the cellular level.

Cells of the central nervous system that initially acquire the ability to function in the presence of relatively high levels of narcotics soon become unable to function normally in their absence. The blood plasma levels of narcotics that prevent the onset of withdrawal symptoms, however, may be substantially below the peak levels that follow injection.

Because of tolerance, the euphoria initially produced by the drug diminishes with chronic exposure and progressive physical dependence. The resulting paradox in established addiction is the absence of euphoria and the need for increasing dosage.

Narcotic drugs

What are narcotic drugs?

The term narcotic refers to opium and to pain-relieving drugs made from opium, such as morphine, paregoric and codeine. These and other opiates are obtained from the juice of the opium poppy (Papaver somniferum). Heroin and perdocan are derivatives of morphine. Several synthetic drugs such as demerol and methadone are also classed as analgesics which relieve pain and induce sleep. Heroin is morphine chemically altered to make it some three to six times stronger.

What are the effects of abuse of a narcotic drug?

Typically, the first emotional reaction to heroin is reduction of tension, easing of fears and relief from worry. Feeling "high" may be followed by a period of inactivity bordering a stupor. Heroin is usually sold heavily "cut" or adulterated with milk sugar, quinine or other materials. Typically it is mixed into a liquid solution and injected into a vein ("main-lining") although it can also be injected just under the skin ("skin popping"), or sniffed through the nose.

Taken in any way, the drug appears to dull the edges of reality. Addicts will relate that heroin "makes my troubles roll off my mind," and "it makes me more sure of myself." The drug depresses certain areas of the brain, and may reduce hunger, thirst and the sex drive. Because addicts do not usually feel hungry, and spend their money for heroin, they can become malnourished and physically depleted.

Who take narcotic drugs?

Studies of the National Institutes of Health show that heroin addiction today is found generally among young men of minority groups in ghetto areas. However, heroin usage is spreading to young people of both sexes from more fortunate backgrounds. All narcotic addiction is not limited to the hero-in users. Some middle-aged and older people who take narcotic drugs regularly to relieve pain can also become addict-ed. So do some people who can obtain opiates easily, such as doctors and nurses. They take injections to keep going under pressure, and eventually find themselves locked into narcotic addiction. The addict will admit that, once "hooked" obtain-ing a continued supply becomes the main goal of his life. His concentration on getting money and drugs frequently pre-vents the addict from continuing either his educa-tion or his job. His health is often bad. He may be sick one day from an overdose. Statistics indicate that his life span may be short-ened by 15 to 20 years. He is usually in trouble with his fam-ily and in constant threat of trouble with the law. He lives to support his addiction.

What is the treatment for narcotic addicti-on?

Medical authorities say that the addict is a sick person. He needs treatment for his personality problems, physical addic-tion and withdrawal sickness. Then, he needs considerable help to keep him from going back to drugs after his with-drawal. The most difficult part of his treatment comes after he is out of the hospital. Doc-tors can help him off the drug and help to restore his health. But it is harder to keep him from picking up the habit again, for many reasons.

Drug-taking may have become his career. His friends may all be addicted. He may have no job skills and his work record is gene-rally poor. He will have great difficul-ty making a fresh start in life and learning to enjoy existence without drugs. A number of reha-bilitation approaches to the problem of addicti-on are being tested including ex-addict self-help groups and narcotic substitutes. Rehabilitation means to rebuild - physi-cal, mental, emotional, social and vocational reconstruction.

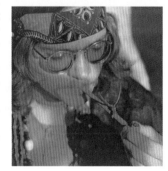

Withdrawal effects

Upon withdrawal the following signs and symptoms of physiological dependence in man appear:

- yawning
- tearing
- perspiration
- running of the nose
- dilation of the pupils
- tremors
- restlessness
- abdominal cramps
- gooseflesh
- defecation
- vomiting
- increase in systolic blood pressure
- raised rectal temperature
- increase in respiratory rate

Subjects who are excessively depend-ent may experience convulsions, res-piratory failure, and death. Dependence develops more rapidly to heroin that to morphine, and more rapidly to morphine than to oxymor-phone, or meperidine. The adminis-tration of a narcotic antagonist can precipitate signs of physiological dependence.

Methadone therapy

A new approach to the rehabilitation of heroin and other opiate is termed methadone therapy. Methadone is a narcotic with analgesic and other effects similar to morphine. Unlike most other narcotics, it is effective upon oral administration.

It is used in the management of hero-in addicts because of its ability to block the euphorogenic effects and cravings for heroin without, appar-ently, duplicating the physical and mental debilitation produced by that drug. Because of its relatively long duration of effect,. a single, daily oral dose of methadone may suffice in most cases of heroin dependence. Methadone itself is addicting, though less so than heroin. In methadone therapy, methadone addiction is sub-stituted for heroin addiction because it is believed that the former allows the patient to function more normal-ly in a social matrix.

Table Narcotic Drugs

Amphetamines

To this category belong not only the original group of amphetamines but also a group of newly synthesized products (one well-known product is called "ice").

Pharmacological category
- Central nervous system stimulants.

Mode of action
- Amphetamines increase the release of norepinephrine from nerve endings and neurosynaptic junctions in the central nervous system and sympathetic part of the autonomic nervous system, yielding a generalized increase in nerve activity.

Source
- Synthesized primarily by the drug industry and illegal laboratories.

Dosage forms abused
- Capsules (time-released)
- tablets
- crystalline powder for injection in solution

Routes of administration
- oral
- intravenous injection

Slang terminology
- speed
- hearts
- bennys
- footballs
- crystal
- uppers
- meth
- copiots
- ice

Medical uses (with a prescription)
- for narcolepsy
- to reduce mental depression
- to control appetite and obesity
- for hyperkinetic or hyperactive children

Short-term effects
- transient sense of alertness, wakefulness
- feeling of well-being and mental clarity
- hunger is diminished
- increased heart rate
- increased blood pressure
- dilation of pupils
- dryness in mouth and throat
- sweating

Long-term effects
- damage to heart and brain
- general exhaustion
- nutritional deficiencies
- psychotic episodes
- infections due to unsanitary injections

Unique problems
- Amphetamine abuse causes overexertion of normal body function, yielding such symptoms as nausea, exhaustion and cramps.
- Depressants (alcohol, heroin, tranquillizers and barbiturates) are often taken to relieve these symptoms.

Tolerance potential
- Yes

Psychological dependence potential
- Yes

Physical dependence potential
- Questionable

Barbiturates

Pharmacological category
- Central nervous system depressants which act as sedatives and hypnotics.

Mode of action
- The drugs interfere with the transmission of impulses to the cortex of the brain.

Examples
- amobarbital (blue heavens, blue birds)
- pentobarbital (yellow jackets, membies)
- secobarbital (reds, pinks, red devils)
- amobarbital + secobarbital

Source
- Manufactured by the drug industry.

Dosage form
- capsules
- tablets

Route of administration
- oral
- parenteral

Table Narcotic Drugs

Medical indications
- preoperative sedation
- insomnia
- epilepsy
- anxiety
- tension

Short-term effects
Low dosage (30 mg)
- depression of sensory function
- sedation without analgesia
- drowsiness

High dosage (100 mg)
- depression of motor function
- depression of brain stem function
- depression of circulation
- sleep
- anesthesia

Long-term effects with overdose
- mental confusion
- venous system damage
- dermatitis
- liver damage

Unique problems
- Death due overdosage is common because the fatal dose for an individual does not increase with tolerance to the psychoactive effects of the drug. There is also a narrower range between toxic and therapeutic levels than with other depressants.
- Withdrawal effects from barbiturates are more severe than those from heroin.

Tolerance potential
- Yes

Psychological dependence potential
- Yes; with withdrawal symptoms such as
- weakness
- increased blood pressure
- anxiety
- motor incoordination
- behavior problems
- apprehension
- agitation
- dehydration
- weight loss
- psychosis (similar to delirium tremens)

Cocaine - Crack

Pharmacological category
- Stimulant and local; anesthetic

Mode of action
- Cocaine elevates the threshold of inhibitory nerve excitability and thus enhances normal stimulation of the central nervous system.

Slang terminology
- coke
- snow
- stardust
- flade
- speedball (combination with heroin)
- crack (new synthetic preparation)

Source
- Cocaine is an odourless, white fluffy powder derived from the coca tree, grown in Bolivia, Colombia, Peru and Chili.

Route of administration
- through nasal mucous membranes
- intravenous injection

Medical use
- None; has been used as local anesthetic.

Short-term effects
- euphoria
- energetic sensations
- possible hallucinations
- possible delusions
- dilated pupils
- loss of appetite

Long-term effects
- digestive disorders
- loss of weight
- insomnia
- occasional convulsions
- sometimes heart troubles
- memory disturbances
- social disorders
- possible perforation of the septum of the nose

Tolerance potential
- None

Psychological dependence potential
- Yes, very strong

Physical dependence potential
- No

N

Table Narcotic Drugs

Hallucinogens

To this category of drugs belong such substances as:
- STP, DOM
- Mescaline
- Phenyclydine
- DMT

These drugs have short-term activity comparable to that of LSD, but even less is known about their long term effects

Characteristics of STP (DOIMN; di-methoxy-methyl amphetamine)
- one-tenth as potent as LSD
- synthetic
- taken orally in tablet or capsule form

Characteristics of mescaline
- 1/200 as potent as LSD
- active ingredient of the peyote cactus
- taken orally

Characteristics of phencyclidine
- taken by injection or orally
- sometimes smoked in tobacco
- once used as a general anesthetic
- used in counterfeit drugs

Characteristics of DMT (dimethyltryptamine)
- short-acting
- taken by injection
- smoked in tobacco
- causes more pronounced rise in blood pressure

LSD

Pharmacological category
- LSD belongs to the group of hallucinogens. The hallucinogens represent a broad group of drugs, both natural and synthetic, which have the ability to induce hallucinations and illusions through alterations of sensory perception.

Mode of action
- LSD may alter the levels of certain natural chemicals in the brain, including serotonin, which could produce changes in the brain's electrical; activity.

Source
- LSD is a modified form of lysergic acid, a chemical obtained from a fungus that grows on rye and wheat.

Routes of administration
- oral
- injection

Common dosage forms
- LSD in pure form is a white powder that is easily dissolved and may be incorporated into numerous substances for oral administration:
- sugar cubes
- cookies
- tablets
- capsules
- beverages
- glycerin wafers

Medical uses
- LSD has no specific medical use. Sometimes LSD is being used in special cases such as:
- alcoholism
- emotional disorders
- terminal illnesses
- concentration camp syndrome

Short-term physical effects (lasting 8-10 hours)
- slight increase in heart rate
- slight increase in blood pressure
- slight increase in temperature
- dilated pupils
- shaking of hands and feet
- cold, sweaty palms
- loss of appetite and nausea
- irregular breathing

Short-term psychological effects
- sudden changes in sensory perception
- synaesthesia (scrambling of sensory input)
- feeling of detachment from reality
- alteration of mood
- altered perception of time
- altered perception of space
- alteration of thinking and feelings
- disorders of perception
- depersonalization
- loss of identity

Long-term effects
- severe mental illness is the only documented long-term effect of LSD.

Unique problems
- severe panic may accompany LSD trips
- paranoia may persist up to 72 hours
- accidental deaths
- the drug state may recur days
- or even months after using LSD.

Tolerance potential
- Possible

Table Narcotic Drugs

Psychological dependence potential
- Possible

Physical dependence potential
- No

Marijuana and its derivatives

Pharmacological category
- marijuana: intoxicant
- hashish: intoxicant to hallucinogen
- THC: intoxicant to hallucinogen

Mode of action
- The active ingredient in marijuana is 9-THC tetrahydro-cannabinol); and its mode of action is unknown. Research has shown that it affects the brain and nervous system.

Slang terminology
- pot
- tea
- grass
- mary jane
- weed

Abused dosage forms
- crude plant material
- hashish (resin)
- oil concentrates

Routes of administration
- smoked
- added top food and taken orally

Medical uses
- none

Short-term physical effects (2-4 hours)
- enters blood stream quickly
- increased heart rate
- reddening of the eyes
- increased hunger
- irritation of mucous membranes of nose
- irritation of bronchioles from smoke

Short-term psychological effects
- alteration of thinking process
- tranquillizing effect
- alteration of spatial sense
- alteration of time perception
- uncontrollable hilarity
- illusions (in high doses)
- paranoia

Long-term effects
- bronchitis
- alienation from society

Tolerance potential
- mild to none

Psychological dependence potential
- Yes

Physical dependence potential
- No

Ecstasy

Pharmacological category
- psychoactive drug
- serotonin activating substance
- methylenedioxymethamphetamine

Mode of action
- Ecstasy primarily affects nerve cells that produce serotonin, one of several brain chemicals that transmit signals from one nerve to the next. Serotonin neurones originate in the raphe nucleus, near the base of the brain and, with long, threadlike extensions known as axons, reach more distant regions.
- Release of serotonin by these nerve cells may be responsible for feelings of empathy, bliss and perceived insight.
- Ecstasy causes the nerve cells to release all the stored serotonin at once, even without an electrical signal. The chemical floods the synapse, overwhelming the serotonin receptors.

Slang terminology
- MDMA

Abused dosage forms
- pill

Routes of administration
- oral

Medical uses
- none

Short-term physical effects (2-4 hours)
- enters blood stream quickly
- aims at brain cells that release serotonin
- causes mood changes
- changes in body temperature

N

Table Narcotic Drugs

Short-term psychological effects
- alteration of thinking process
- feeling of well-being
- feeling of mental clarity
- strong feeling of empathy
- alteration of time perception
- uncontrollable hilarity

Long-term effects
- damage to serotonergic nerve cells
- psychotic episodes

Tolerance potential
- Yes

Psychological dependence potential
- Yes

Physical dependence potential
- Questionable

Minor tranquillizers

Pharmacological category
- Central nervous system depressants

Mode of action
- Tranquillizers generally act at a subcortical level by central nervous system depression.

Examples
- meprobamate
- chlordiazepoxide
- diazepam (Valium)
- other benzodiazepines

Sources
- The drug industry manufactures tranquillizers from natural of synthetic products.

Dosage forms abused
- capsules
- tablets

Route of administration
- generally, oral

Medical use (with prescription)
- muscle relaxants
- anticonvulsants
- relief of anxiety
- decrease of vomiting
- adjuvant in treatment of alcoholism

Short-term effects
- reduction in motor activity
- mild drowsiness
- blockage of conditioned reflexes
- reduction of anxiety
- dermatitis
- disorientation
- blurred vision
- coordination problems

Long-term effects
- obstructive hepatitis
- bone marrow depression
- induced nervous disorders

Tolerance potential
- Yes

Physical dependence potential
- Yes

Psychological dependence potential
- Yes

Opiates and their derivatives

Pharmacological category
- Central nervous system depressants which act as analgesics, sedatives, and cough depressants.

Mode of action
- Narcotics depress the following centers in the brain and spinal cord:
- pain perception center
- respiratory center
- smooth muscle stimulating center
- vasomotor center

Examples
OPIUM DERIVATIVES
- morphine
- codeine
- paregoric
- heroin
SYNTHETIC FORMS
- hydromorphine
- meperidine
- oxymorphone
- methadone

Sources
- Opium poppy
- Synthesized by drug industry

Table Narcotic Drugs

Dosage forms abused
- capsules
- tablets
- powder for injections
- cough preparations

Routes of administration
- oral
- nasal (sniffing)
- parental (intradermal or intravenous)

Medical use (with a prescription)
- morphine and morphine derivatives are used for the treatment of severe pain
- codeine is used to depress coughing and relieve pain
- paregoric is used to control diarrhea and to relieve pain of teething

Short-term effects
- reduction in sensitivity to pain
- drowsiness
- induced sleep
- reduction in physical activity
- constipation
- constriction or pupils
- respiratory depression

Long-term effects
- physical dependence
- tolerance
- psychological dependence

Medical problems
- hepatitis due to septic administration
- death from overdosage
- skin infections due to septic administration
- AIDS due to use of dirty syringes

Social problems
- Heroin eventually will most likely to be injected ("mainlined"), and the addict may resort to crude instruments for administration.
- The craving for heroin leads most addicts to commit crimes in order to obtain a substantial amount of money per day support the habit.
- Heroin is diluted, or cut, by dealers, who add lactose, quinine, or other material until the concentration of heroin is only about 3 to 10 per cent.
- Therapy for the addict is often unsuccessful because of the strong psychological dependence.

Tolerance [potential
- Yes

Volatile solvents

Mode of action
- The solvents are extremely soluble in the mucous membranes of the respiratory tract and quickly depress the central nervous system and motor activity because they reach high concentrations in the blood shortly after inhalation.

Examples
- glue
- fingernail polish and remover
- paint thinners
- freon and other aerosol propellants
- gasoline
- ether

Source
- Most of the solvents listed above may be found in the home.

Route of administration
- Inhalation, often with the aid of a paper or plastic bag, which concentrates the vapours of the solvent.

Medicinal uses
- None. It should be noted, however, that these solvents are similar in action to general anesthetics used during surgery.

Short-term effects
- feeling of drunkenness
- slurring of speech
- dizziness
- impaired sensory perception
- disorganized behavior
- uncoordinated muscular activity
- unconsciousness, which can even lead to death

Long-term effects
- damage to heart and lungs
- malfunctioning of kidneys and liver
- impaired perception
- impaired coordination and judgment

Tolerance potential
- Unknown

Psychological dependence potential
- Yes

Physical dependence potential
- No

N

NEPHROTIC SYNDROME

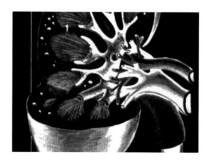

Description

A nephrotic syndrome is a predictable complex of signs and symptoms that follows a severe and prolonged increase in the ability of protein to permeate the glomeruli of the kidney. The major features are:

*   edema
*   low content of sodium in the urine
*   low content of albumin (a protein) in the blood
*   presence of lipids (e.g. fats) in the urine
*   increase of lipid content in the blood

These symptoms are all of variable relative severity. New cases of nephrotic syndrome average two per 100,000 per year in the western world.

This syndrome may result from many different lesions in the kidney, but in all cases, the underlying abnormality is an increase in the permeability of the capillaries of the glomeruli, which allows an increase of the protein leak into the glomerular filtrate. The changes in the kidney tubules are usually secondary to this increased protein load. Causes of the nephrotic syndrome are listed in the table.

Causes

Major causes of the nephrotic syndrome in children and adults are listed in the table.

Metabolic complications

A wide variety of severe metabolic complications may be seen in prolonged nephrotic syndrome in children and adults. These include:

*   nutritional deficiencies

*   brittle hair and nails
*   alopecia (hair loss)
*   stunted growth
*   demineralization of bone
*   presence of glucose in urine
*   presence of amino acids in urine
*   depletion of potassium
*   muscular disorders
*   tetany (muscle spasm)
*   decreased metabolism

Peritonitis and an increase in opportunistic infections are also seen.

Prognosis and treatment

The prognosis of the nephrotic syndrome varies with the specific cause.

Many sufferers of the diseases mentioned in the table have spontaneous remissions, and this can also happen to those with the nephrotic syndrome, even after six or seven years. On the other hand, prognosis may be altered drastically by infections or by thrombosis in the veins. Supportive treatment includes salt restriction, moderately high-protein diets, graded exercise and sparing, judicious use of diuretics to control oedema.

High blood pressure will be treated appropriately. Nutritional guidance is essential. Counselling for parents is important to avoid the "deprived sibling" syndrome, in which a nephrotic child dominates parental energies.

Major causes of nephrotic syndrome

Metabolic diseases
-   diabetes
-   amyloidosis
-   systemic lupus erythematosus
-   polyarteritis nodosa
-   Goodpasture's syndrome

Malignant diseases
-   multiple myeloma
-   Hodgkin's disease
-   various carcinomas

Circulatory disorders
-   renal vein thrombosis
-   congestive heart failure
-   constrictive pericarditis
-   sickle cell anemia
-   renal artery stenosis
-   pulmonary artery thrombosis
-   inferior vena cava stenosis
-   tricuspid valvular insufficiency
-   inferior vena cava thrombosis

Toxins
-   organic mercurial diuretics
-   mercury ointments
-   bismuth
-   gold

Infectious diseases
-   malaria
-   subacute bacterial endocarditis
-   syphilis
-   typhus
-   chronic jejunoileitis
-   herpes zoster

Allergens and drugs
-   pollen
-   bee stings
-   poison oak
-   troxidone
-   insect repellents
-   insect bites
-   snake bites
-   probenecid
-   penicillamine

Simple medical treatment can do much to alleviate the physical problems in many of those with the nephrotic syndrome; however, specific treatment is still rarely available except in certain well-defined types of nephritis. High-protein diets remain essential in the treatment of those with heavy protein losses in the urine. When it is realized that some may lose up to 20 g or more of albumin per day, replacement is obviously of vital importance. Unfortunately, intravenous albumin (i.e. albumin injected into a vein) is quite useless as up to 75 per cent of the infused protein is lost in the urine within 24 hours of treatment.

An increase of protein intake from meat, fish or milk product sources is usually impossibly expensive and also results in an unacceptable increase in the sodium chloride intake, with consequent worsening of edema, so that low-salt protein supplements have to be used, even though these are often regarded as somewhat unpalatable and some may resist taking them.

When it is realized that after several months of heavy loss of proteins, body protein stores may be depleted by over 40 per cent, the importance of adequate replacement becomes more obvious.

Modern diuretic therapy has also improved the effectiveness of the treatment of symptoms in the nephrotic syndrome.

As the increased sodium retention that causes the oedema is largely the result of aldosterone secretion, drugs that specifically antagonize the action of this hormone should theoretically be the most effective.

However, this is often not the case in practice and those substances that block sodium transport in the tubules of the kidney often appear to produce more effective urine production.

Immunosuppressive therapy

It has been shown that most types of nephritis leading to the nephrotic syndrome are the result of some immunological reaction occurring at the level of the blood capillary of the glomerulus. Therefore, corticosteroids or other immunosuppressive drugs would be expected to be effective.

What is a nephrotic syndrome?

This is a predictable complex of signs and symptoms that follows a severe and prolonged increase in the ability of protein to permeate the glomeruli of the kidney.

The major features are:

- oedema;
- low content of sodium in the urine;
- low content of albumin (a protein) in the blood;
- presence of lipids (e.g., fats) in the urine;
- increase of lipid content in the blood.

These symptoms are all of variable relative severity. New cases of nephrotic syndrome average two per 100,000 per year.

What are the causes of a nephrotic syndrome?

A nephrotic syndrome may result from many different lesions in the kidney, but in all cases, the underlying abnormality is an increase in the permeability of the capillaries of the glomeruli, which allow protein leak into the glomerular filtrate. The changes in the kidney tubules are usually secondary to this increased protein load.

What types of complications may occur in the course of the development of a nephrotic syndrome?

A wide variety of severe metabolic complications may be seen in prolonged nephrotic syndrome in children and adults. These include:

- nutritional deficiencies;
- brittle hair and nails;
- alopecia (hair loss);
- stunted growth;
- demineralization of bone;
- presence of glucose in urine;
- presence of amino acids in urine;
- depletion of potassium;
- muscular disorders;
- tetany (muscle spasm);
- decreased metabolism.

What is the prognosis of a nephrotic syndrome?

The prognosis of the nephrotic syndrome varies with the specific cause.

Many sufferers of the diseases mentioned in the table have spontaneous remissions, and this can also happen to those with the nephrotic syndrome, even after six or seven years. On the other hand, prognosis may be altered drastically by infections or by thrombosis in the veins.

How is a nephrotic syndrome treated?

Supportive treatment includes:

- salt restriction;
- moderately high-protein diets;
- graded exercise;
- judicious use of diuretics to control edema.

High blood pressure will be treated appropriately. Nutritional guidance is essential. Counselling for parents is important to avoid the "deprived sibling" syndrome, in which a nephrotic child dominates parental energies.

Simple medical treatment can do much to alleviate the physical problems in many of those with the nephrotic syndrome; however, specific treatment is still rarely available except in certain well-defined types of kidney infection.

What is the significance of immunosuppressive therapy in the treatment of nephrotic syndrome?

It has been shown that most types of kidney infection leading to the nephrotic syndrome are the result of some immunological reaction occurring at the level of the blood capillary of the glomerulus.

Therefore, corticosteroids or other immunosuppressive medicines would be expected to be effective. The paradox remains that the only condition that almost invariably responds to corticosteroid medicines is minimal change disease characterized by heavy loss of protein in the urine. The objective of treatment will clearly be the disappearance of loss of protein in the urine and the healing of the kidney lesion.

N

ORAL CANCER

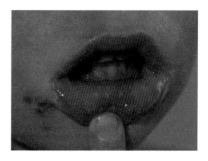

Description

Benign and malignant tumors may develop in any part of the oral cavity. Most often, cancer is found on the lips, the lining of the cheeks, the gums, and the floor of the mouth. The tongue, the area directly behind the wisdom teeth, the pharynx, and the tonsils are other common sites. Cancers of the hard and soft palate are less common.

When oral cancer spreads, it usually travels through the lymphatic system. This system is made up of a network of thin tubes that branch like blood vessels, into tissues throughout the body. Cancer cells that enter the lymphatic system are carried by lymph, a

The oral cavity.
1. Upper jaw
2. Lower jaw
3. Hard and soft palate
4. Tongue
5. Uvula

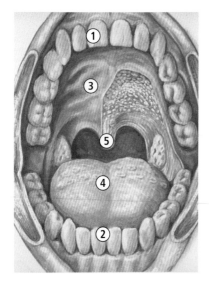

colourless, watery fluid containing cells that help the body fight infection and disease. Along the lymphatic system are groups of small, bean-shaped organs called lymph nodes. Cancer cells are carried by the lymph to the lymph nodes and from there further in the body. The disease is still called oral cancer, even when it spreads to the lymph nodes or another part of the body.

Symptoms

More than 90 per cent of all oral cancers are found in people over the age of 45, but oral cancer can occur at any age. Individuals can spot symptoms by doing a monthly oral self-examination. This examination should include a check for these symptoms, which are some of the warning signs of oral cancer:

▲ a sore in the mouth that bleeds easily and does not heal;
▲ a lump or thickening in the cheek that can be felt with the tongue;
▲ a white or red patch on the gums, tongue, or lining of the mouth;
▲ soreness or a feeling that something is caught in the throat;
▲ difficulty in chewing or swallowing;
▲ difficulty moving the jaw or tongue;
▲ numbness of the tongue or other areas of the mouth;
▲ swelling of the jaw that causes dentures to fit poorly or become uncomfortable.

These symptoms are not sure signs of cancer. They can also be caused by many other conditions. However, it is important to see a dentist or physician if any of these problems lasts more than two weeks. Pain is usually not a symptom of oral cancer.

Diagnosis

To diagnose oral cancer, a dentist or physician carefully checks the mouth for lumps, swelling, or abnormal-looking areas. When a problem is found, a biopsy is the only sure way to know whether cancer is present. Usually, an oral surgeon removes part or all of a lump or abnormal-looking area. A pathologist examines the tissue under a microscope to see whether cancer cells are present and, if so, what type they are.

Almost all oral cancers are squamous cell carcinomas (cancers that begin in the flat, scale-like cells that line the oral cavity). When oral cancer is found, the physician needs to know whether it has spread. This process is called staging. Staging generally includes dental X-rays and X-rays of the head and chest. The physician feels the lymph nodes in the front and back of the neck to check for swelling or other changes.

Sometimes, the physician uses an endoscope, a flexible, lighted instrument, to look for tumors in the throat. The physician may also want the patient to have a CT-scan; this is a series of X-rays put together by a computer to form a detailed picture.

Ultrasound is another scan that creates pictures of the inside of the body. High-frequency sound waves, which cannot be heard by humans, and bounces off organs and tissues. Their echoes make an image on a video screen that is much like a television screen. Sometimes the physician asks for magnetic resonance imaging (MRI). In this scan, a cross-sectional image (like a CT-scan) is produced with a powerful magnet instead of radiation.

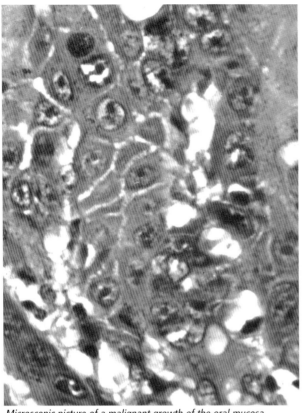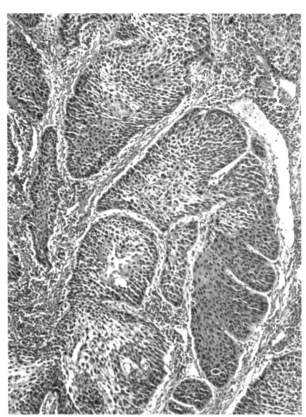

Microscopic picture of a malignant growth of the oral mucosa.

Treatment

Treatment for oral cancer depends on the size, location, and extent (stage) of the disease. The physician also takes into account the patient's age and general health. Treatment may be surgery, radiation therapy, or a combination of the two. Treatment may cause damage in a patient's appearance and may lead to problems with chewing, swallowing, or talking. For these important reasons, the patient and the physician should carefully review treatment choices.

Before starting treatment, the patient might want a second physician to review the diagnosis and treatment plan. Patients with oral cancer may be treated by a team of specialists. The medical team may include an oral surgeon; ear, nose and throat surgeon; medical oncologist (cancer specialist); radiation therapist; plastic surgeon; dietician; and speech therapist.

Most patients with oral cancer have surgery to remove the tumor in the mouth. If there is evidence that the cancer may have spread, the surgeon may remove lymph nodes in the neck. The surgeon will attempt to take out only cancerous lymph nodes and a small amount of tissue close to them. If the disease involves muscles and other tissues in the neck, the operation may be more extensive.

Radiation therapy uses high-energy rays to destroy cancer cells' ability to grow and multiply. Radiation therapy may be used instead of surgery for small tumors in the mouth. Patients with larger tumors may need both surgery and radiation. The radiation may be given before or after surgery. Before surgery, radiation helps shrink the tumor so that it can be removed. Radiation after surgery is used to destroy cancer cells that may remain.

The radiation may come from a machine outside the body (external radiation), or the physician may put materials that give off radiation into the tissues of the mouth (implant radiation). Implant radiation puts cancer-killing rays as close as possible to the tumor. A small capsule containing radioactive material is placed into the tissues of the mouth or put directly into the tumor.

Generally, an implant is left in place for several days, and the patient needs to stay in the hospital. To keep from moving the implant, the patient is put on a special liquid diet given in small portions through a tiny straw. The patient gets most nutrition and fluids during the treatment period through an intravenous tube in a vein.

Sometimes an implant is left in place permanently. It loses a little radiation each day. The patient stays in the hospital while the radiation is most active. After a few days, the patient can go home, because the amount of radiation left in the implant is not dangerous. Chemotherapy uses drugs to kill cancer cells. To date, chemotherapy has not been very effective in treating oral cancers. Researchers are still looking for effective drugs or drug combinations.

O

OSTEOARTHRITIS

Description

Osteoarthritis is a condition in which the cartilage that normally cushions a joint begins to deteriorate, causing pain and stiffness. Only rarely does inflammation become a problem in osteoarthritis.

The traditional wisdom was that this form of arthritis (once called rheumatism) was an inevitable "wear-and-tear" condition that would be visited upon us all if we lived long enough. However, many people live long lives without ever suffering stiff and creaky joints. Osteoarthritis does take time to develop - usually dozens of years - so that most of the people who have it are at least middle-aged. And since women outlive men, more women are ultimately plagued with the condition.

Causes

Hundreds of researchers have spent years investigating the process of degeneration.

Just about anything that subjects a joint to unnatural stress can lead to osteoarthritis:

▲ being overweight (that can cause strain on the knee and hip joints as well as the spine);
▲ congenital misalignment of bones (such as scoliosis);
▲ repeated occupational strain (the knees of auto mechanics who work in a squatting position, for example);
▲ poor posture that places continual strain on the joints;
▲ sports injuries that involve torn ligaments and cartilage.

Although more than one joint in the body can be affected, osteoarthritis rarely attacks several joints simultaneously, unlike some of the other forms of arthritis, nor does it roam from one joint to another.

Osteoarthritis attacks joints on an individual basis. Eventually, changes occur in and around the joint, and overgrowth of bone ends and thickening of surrounding tissues may change its size and appearance. Sometimes, if a person avoids using the painful joint, nearby muscles may be affected - typically, weakening from disuse.

Treatment

The warning signs of a variety of arthritic conditions are often quite similar, so it's important to consult a doctor to determine if you have osteoarthritis and not some other kind of joint condition.

Treatment at an early stage is important, so don't ignore the signals your body may be sending. If any of the following symptoms persists for more than two weeks, consult your family physician:

▲ swelling in one or more joints;
▲ recurring pain or tenderness in any joint of your body;
▲ inability to move a joint properly or do normal activities;
▲ obvious redness and warmth in one or more joints;
▲ persistent early morning pain and stiffness in joints;

Aspiration of fluid from the knee joint for investigation of the nature of the process of osteoarthritis.

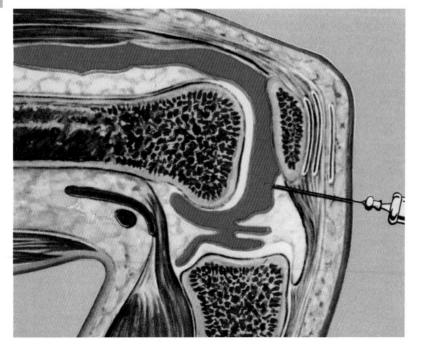

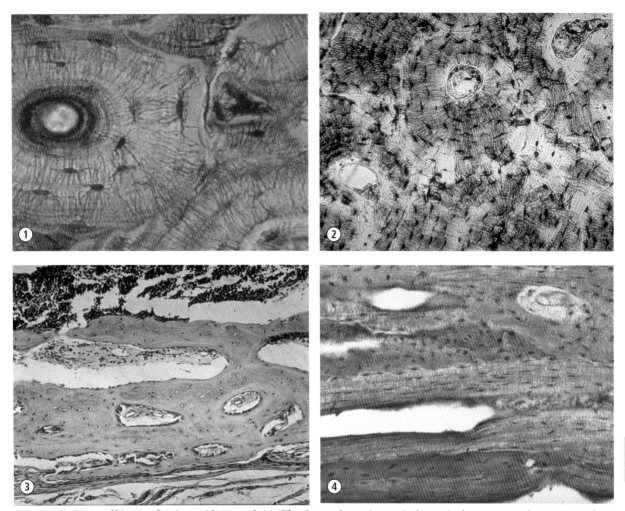

Microscopic pictures of biopsies of patients with osteoarthritis. The pictures show microscopic changes in the structure and composition of cartilage and bone tissue close to the cartilage.

▲ unexplained weight loss, fever, weakness or fatigue combined with joint pain.

The aim of treatment is twofold: to relieve pain or discomfort, and to keep the affected joint operating as well as possible.

Once a diagnosis has been made, simple do-it-yourself measures often suffice, and continued professional care is not required.

Ordinary over-the-counter painkillers, such as paracetamol, ibuprofen or aspirin, are frequently enough to relieve discomfort.

Occasionally, stronger prescription painkillers may be needed, but doctors caution that these should not be used too often, since "masking" of discomfort can lead to overuse of the joint. Moist heat helps some people, but others find that cold packs are more effective. While stress and strain are obviously not advisable, neither is prolonged immobilization. Research has shown that lack of use can encourage further breakdown of cartilage.

Apparently, some degree of movement is needed to sustain lubrication within the joint, allowing it to work smoothly. If a weight-bearing joint is affected, losing excess weight is a good idea. Special exercises can help to strengthen muscles around the joint but these should be undertaken with professional guidance from a physiotherapist.

If cartilage has deteriorated to the point of causing constant pain, joint replacement surgery is another alternative. Known as arthroplasty, this procedure involves the complete replacement of joints by mechanical constructions using metals, plastics and other materials.

Thus therapy may include regular exercises, particularly activities that involve smooth rather than jerky movement - swimming or walking in preference to tennis or jogging - and can be increased gradually. Aspirin and other drugs are used in moderation.

Osteoarthritis can be helped, but the keys to controlling it are early diagnosis and prompt treatment.

OSTEOPOROSIS

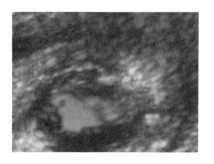

Introduction

Osteoporosis is a generalized, progressive diminution of bone tissue mass (a reduced amount of bone), even though the ratio of mineral to organic elements is unchanged in the remaining morphologically normal bone.

Osteoporosis is a disease characterized by insufficient production of bone matrix, the basic material from which bone develops, or by serious reduction in bone calcium content. In acute osteoporosis, large amounts of calcium are excreted in the urine and may lead to grave kidney complications.

This disease is most commonly associated with the postmenopausal state in women, when decreased secretion of estrogen (female sex hormone) changes normal metabolic function; but it is also attributed to malnutrition, simple disuse (immobilization in bed) and treatment with corticosteroids.

In osteoporosis, the calcified mass of all bones decreases because bone resorption (normal loss of substance) continue at a regular rate, while formation practically ceases, and thus demand exceeds supply. The body responses to depletion by stimulating osteoblastic (boneproducing) cell activity so that bone mass is restored to some extent but seldom in sufficient quantity. In malnutrition often associated with eating habits of the elderly, all protein tissues are depleted, and lack of certain vitamins results in deficient protoplasm production, thus adding to the natural atrophy, or wasting away, of bone and other tissue that occurs in older persons. Sometimes hyperthyroidism (overactivity of the thyroid gland) will cause osteoporosis in younger people because it increases the rate of metabolism and promotes excessive activity that in turn places added stress on the bones and increases bone tissue depletion. Only rarely is osteoporosis seen in children, and when it appears it is usually the result of serious metabolic disorder.

Symptoms

The disease is most common in women over the age of fifty. The severity of symptoms has little correlation to the amount of osteoporosis seen on X-ray examination. About 50 per cent of those patients X-rayed will show grossly decreased bone mass; 30 per cent will reveal previously undetected fractures of the vertebrae in the spine, but only 10 per cent will have experienced pain or signs related to these fractures.

Artificial or surgically induced menopause leads to a more severe degree of bone destruction, in which spontaneous fractures of the spine and pelvis are fairly common. Only occasionally are bones of the skull and extremities (arms and legs) involved. Sometimes the disease causes repeated formation of kidney stones.

Causes

The cause of primary osteoporosis probably is multifactorial. Important factors include:

- ▲ failure to develop sufficient bone mass during young adult life;
- ▲ accentuation of age-related bone loss;
- ▲ increased sensitivity to the hormone from the parathyroid glands;
- ▲ defective absorption of calcium in the intestinal system;
- ▲ menopause.

Possible environmental factors include the following:

- ▲ smoking;
- ▲ excessive alcohol consumption;
- ▲ decreased exercise.

Treatment and prevention

Treatment is preventive as well as symptomatic and inhibitory. Preventive treatment comprises recognition of high-risk patients plus

---

Living with osteoarthritis

- ▲ oint pain should not be ignored. Exercise affected joints gently; in a pool if possible.
- ▲ Do special exercises recommended by your physician or physical therapist, to help keep joints mobile.
- ▲ Massage at or around affected joint by a trained physical therapist.
- ▲ Apply a heating pad or a damp and warm towel to affected joints.
- ▲ Maintain an appropriate weight, so as not to place extra stress on joints.
- ▲ Use special equipment as necessary, for example, crutches, cane, walker.
- ▲ A fixed seat in a bathtub will enable you less stretching while washing.
- ▲ Your physical therapist will also provide tips on how to make living with arthritis easier and suggest well-supported shoes.
- ▲ Stiffness and pain in joints may be osteoarthritis - or it may be a much more severe type of arthritis or perhaps some other disease. See a physician promptly.

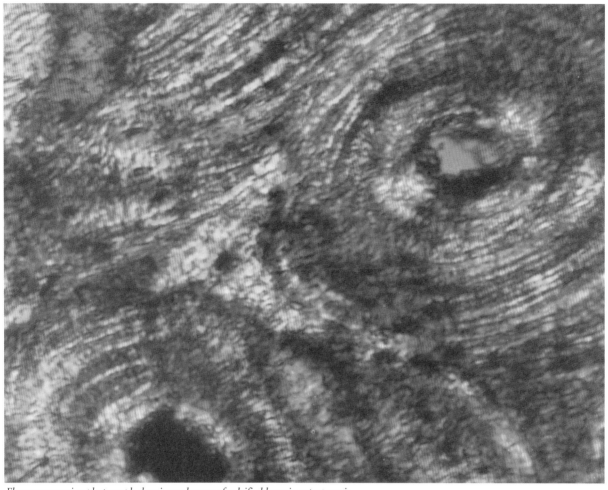

Fluorescence microphotograph showing a decease of calcified bone in osteoporosis.

exercise and supplementary calcium and, in selected postmenopausal women, estrogen replacement therapy. A number of studies now suggest that osteoporosis can be prevented to a large extent by relatively simple nutritional and other means.

Particularly useful preventive measurements include:

■ Calcium supplementation
Calcium supplements to increase bone strength and reduce the risk of osteoporosis have been tried in a number of studies and form the mainstay of the nonhormonal treatment of osteoporosis. It has been shown that a certain percentage of older women have calcium intakes below the recommended daily allowance and thus may be at risk of

losing calcium from their bones. Ensuring calcium absorption. A number of processes inhibit calcium absorption from the digestive tract. These include:
- poor acid production by the stomach;
- the removal of the stomach at an operation;
- the ingestion of bran and wholemeal bread;
- gastrointestinal diseases that result in fat and calcium malabsorption;
- a deficiency of vitamin D.

■ Other supplements
With advancing years, deficiencies of vitamins and minerals become increasingly common. Though calcium has been extensively studied in

osteoporosis, it is almost certain that other minerals, especially magnesium and zinc, will prove to be important. A magnesium supplement giving 0.5-0.75 g per day in conjunction with a calcium supplement is also recommended.

■ Stop smoking
It appears that smokers have thinner bones than nonsmokers.

■ Get regular exercises
Weightbearing exercise such as walking, running, simple gymnastics or jogging, can help reduce calcium losses from the skeleton.

■ Avoid salt, sugar and coffee
All these may have an adverse effect upon mineral balance.

Osteoporosis   Questions & Answers

What is osteoporosis?

Osteoporosis is a condition in which your bones lose the supporting structure that keeps them strong. They become thin, weak or porous, making them susceptible to fracture.

When does osteoporosis starts?

When we are younger, our bones, like other parts of our bodies, are constantly being renewed as old cells are worn out and replaced by new ones. But after the age of 35 our bones begin to lose density, with old cells wearing out faster than new ones can replace them.

What causes osteoporosis?

A decrease in estrogen at the menopause causes this loss of bone density to become more rapid and leaves many women at risk of a broken hip, spine or wrist, often after even a very minor fall.

What are the effects?

As the spine begins to compress, some sufferers experience back pain. In severe cases this can lead to breathing problems, loss of height, a hunched back and, if internal organs begin to press on the bladder, incontinence.

Who is at risk from osteoporosis?

The menopause puts women at a far greater risk of developing osteoporosis than men. However, other medical hereditary and lifestyle factors can also increase risk:

- Early menopause (before the age of 45).
- Hysterectomy - particularly if both ovaries are removed before the age of 40.
- A break in periods for reasons other than pregnancy, e.g. anorexia or excessive exercising.
- High dose or long-term oral corticosteroids (drugs to treat asthma, arthritis and other inflammatory conditions).
- A close family history of osteoporosis.
- Smoking.
- Drinking excessive alcohol.
- Not getting enough exercise.
- An unbalanced diet - particularly if it is low in calcium.
- Medical conditions such as hyperthyroidism, hyperparathyroidism, diabetes, some kidney and liver disorders and Cushing's syndrome.
- A low body weight in proportion to your height.

If one or more of these risk factors applies to you, it does not necessarily mean you will end up with a fractured hip or spine in your old age. There is lots you can do to help yourself, even if you have already been diagnosed with this condition.

How is osteoporosis diagnosed?

Sadly, most women do not realise they have osteoporosis until they suffer a fracture after a minor trip or fall. If you have already broken a bone in these circumstances, you should talk to your doctor about the possibility of osteoporosis. Taking action now could reduce your likelihood of suffering further fractures in the future. Your doctor may gibe you an X-ray or a bone scan called Dual X-Ray Absorptiometer (DXA). These will give a clearer picture of your bone density, enabling your doctor to determine whether or not you have osteoporosis.

How can I relieve the pain of osteoporosis?

If you are diagnosed with osteoporosis, your doctor will discuss treatment options with you. In the meantime, you will probably want some form of pain relief.

All fractures are painful, but if you are suffering from osteoporosis it is important to get relief from your pain so you can regain your mobility and get out and about again. Exercise will help to prevent further deterioration of your bones.

■ Painkillers

Most over-the-counter painkillers, such as paracetamol, aspirin and ibuprofen will be helpful in relieving your pain. Take care not to exceed the recommended dose, and ask your doctor or pharmacist if you are not sure. If this does not help, talk to your doctor about taking something stronger.

■ TENS

A TENS (Transcutaneous Electric Nerve Stimulation) machine can help by sending electrical impulses to the painful area.

■ Physiotherapy

Many people find physiotherapy very helpful in relieving pain and increasing mobility. Your physiotherapist will help you to do beneficial exercises during treatment sessions and give you a programme to work on at home.

■ Heat

Try applying a hot water bottle to the effected area, or alternating this with an ice pack if this works for you.

How can my diet help?

The most important requirement for building and maintaining healthy bones is calcium. A good intake of this throughout your life will help to reduce your risk of developing osteoporosis in old age. At different stages in your life you will require different intakes of calcium.

Calcium rich foods

Full fat milk - third of a pint	225 mg
Semi-skimmed milk - third of a pint	231 mg
Skimmed milk- third of a pint	235 mg
Small pot of yoghurt	240 mg
Parmesan cheese - in 30 g	360 mg
Cheddar cheese - in 30 g	216 mg
Sardines (canned) in 100 g	540 mg
Spinach - in 100 g	170 mg
Tofy - in 50 g	750 mg

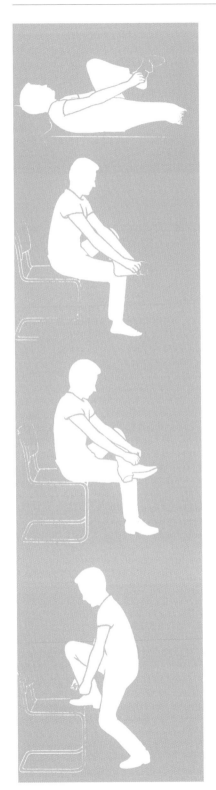

The progression in osteoporosis may be slowed down by certain exercises and adaptations to daily activities.

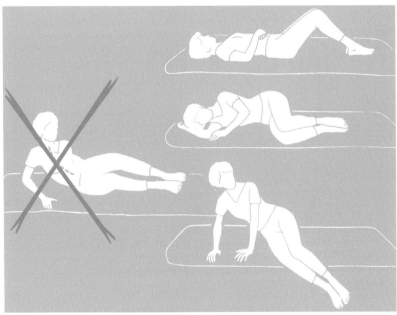

The development of osteoporosis may be slowed down by certain exercises and adaptations to daily activities. Left: wrong way of standing up. Right: right way of standing up.

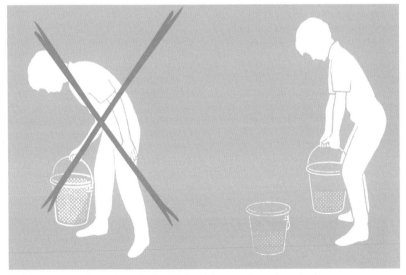

Left: wrong way of carrying a bucket. Right: right way of carrying a bucket.

Recommended daily intake of calcium

Women 20-45	1000 mg
Pregnant and nursing women	1200 mg
Pregnant and nursing teenagers	1500 mg
Women over 45	1500 mg
Women over 45 on HRT	1000 mg

O

OVARIAN DISORDERS

Introduction

The ovaries, located in the lower abdomen, are a pair of very delicate and important female gonads. They store the potential eggs throughout a woman's life and develop each month into a mature egg or ovum.

The ovaries also produce hormones such as estrogen and progesterone, which develop and maintain a woman's secondary sexual characteristics. These hormones prepare the uterus for pregnancy and regulate the menstrual cycle.

An ovarian cyst is a fluid-filled sac in or on an ovary. Such cysts are relatively common. Most are noncancerous cysts and disappear on their own. Cancerous cysts are more likely to occur in women older than 40.

Cancer of the ovaries develops most often in women aged 50 to 70. This cancer eventually develops in about 1 of 50 women. It is the second most common gynecologic cancer. However, more women die of ovarian cancer than of any other gynecologic cancer.

Ovarian cysts

Ovarian cysts are growths that form on the ovaries, the two small organs on either side of a woman's uterus that produce an egg each month.

Each month when an ovary produces an egg, a small, cyst-like structure - the follicle - begins to grow inside the ovary. When it is mature, the follicle ruptures at ovulation, when an egg is released. After ovulation, the empty follicle becomes the corpus luteum. If pregnancy does not occur, the corpus luteum eventually dissolves.

Ovarian cysts are very common in women during their reproductive years. Some types of ovarian cysts are normal and usually harmless, often going away without any treatment. Other cysts are abnormal and may cause problems.

Since ovarian cysts are often first found during a pelvic exam, it is important to have regular checkups by your doctor. This is especially important if you have symptoms of ovarian cysts, if you have had abnormal ovarian cysts before, or if you are over age 40, when the risk of ovarian cancer is greater. If ovarian cysts are found early, many of the problems caused by them can be prevented.

Because ovarian cysts rarely cause symptoms, it is important to have regular pelvic exams if you have ever had abnormal ovarian cysts. If you have had ovarian cysts in the past, you are more likely to develop them again at some point than someone who has never had them at all.

If cysts are found early, they may be less likely to cause more serious problems.

▲ Severe pain may result from an infected, ruptured, or bleeding cyst, or from torsion.
▲ If present, endometriosis can worsen, requiring removal of one or both ovaries.
▲ If a cyst turns out to be cancerous, chances for successful treatment are greatly improved if it is found at an early stage.

Types and causes of ovarian cysts

A cyst is a fluid-filled sac, similar to a blister. Some types of ovarian cysts are formed as a result of the normal process of ovulation - the monthly release of an egg from an ovary.

Cysts that are abnormal often occur as a result of an imbalance in the female hormones estrogen and progesterone, which are produced in the ovaries.

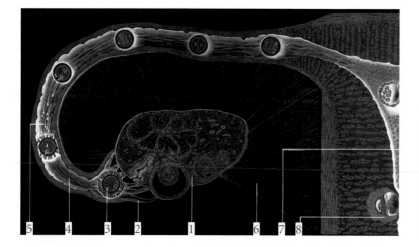

Cross section of part of the internal female sexual organs. 1. Ovary with follicles; 2. fimbriae of the tube; 3. ovum; 4. uterine tube; 5. sperm; 6. broad ligament; 7. uterus; 8. fertilized ovum in uterine wall.

■ *Functional cysts*

The most common type of ovarian cyst is called a functional cyst. It is formed from a cyst-like structure normally produced in an ovary during the course of ovulation. If this structure does not go through its normal cycle and eventually dissolve, a functional cyst may be formed.

Functional cysts usually do not cause symptoms or require treatment. Normally they stop growing, shrink, and disappear within one, or at the most three, menstrual cycles.

These cysts are common in women who menstruate, but they are rare in women who have reached menopause (when menstrual period ends), because no more eggs are being produced.

■ *Other types of cysts*

Functional cysts are normal and must be distinguished by a doctor from abnormal cysts. These other, abnormal ovarian cysts are more likely to cause problems and usually require treatment:

▲ *Dermoid*: A cystic growth filled with various types of tissue, such as hair and skin tissue.

▲ *Cystadenoma*: Cysts that develop from cells on the outer surface of the ovary.

▲ *Endometrioma*: A cyst formed when tissue similar to that lining the uterus is attached to the ovaries, a condition known as endometriosis; sometimes called endometrial cysts or chocolate cysts (because of the dark, reddish-brown blood inside the cyst).

▲ *Polycystic ovarian disease*: A build-up of follicle cysts that causes the ovaries to become enlarged and form a think outer covering, preventing ovulation.

These types of cysts are usually benign, or noncancerous. Although benign cysts may cause problems or symptoms that require treatment, they usually do not spread to other parts of the body. A few cysts, though, may turn out to be malignant, or cancerous tumors. For this reason, all cysts must be evaluated carefully.

Symptoms

Although most ovarian cysts do not cause any symptoms, when symptoms do occur there may be a dull ache or a sense of pressure or fullness in the abdomen.

Ovarian cysts may cause pain during intercourse or at other times. Severe pain sometimes requires hospitalization. Pain or pressure may be caused by a number of factors:

▲ a cyst bleeding or breaking open, irritating the tissues inside the abdomen;

▲ the large size of a cyst;

▲ torsion (twisting of a cyst), which blocks blood flow to the cyst.

Delayed, irregular, or unusually painful periods may also be a symptom of ovarian cysts. Enlargement or swelling of the lower abdomen is another possible symptom of ovarian cysts. If you have any of these symptoms, you should report them to your doctor.

Diagnosis

Ovarian cysts are often first found during a pelvic exam performed routinely, as a regular part of a woman's health care, or for some other unrelated reason.

Through a pelvic exam, a cyst can be found before it becomes so large that it ruptures or undergoes torsion, causing pain or other symptoms. If your doctor detects what may be an abnormal ovarian growth during a pelvic exam, other tests may be performed to confirm the diagnosis.

Ultrasound is a test in which sound waves are used to create pictures of the internal organs. An electronic device is moved over the abdomen or placed in the vagina, creating echoes that are then turned into images that can be viewed on a TV-like screen.

Ultrasound may be used to determine whether an ovary is enlarged and whether a growth on an ovary is solid or filled with fluid.

Laparoscopy is a surgical procedure that allows a doctor to look inside the abdomen at the ovaries and other pelvic organs. The laparoscope, a slender instrument somewhat like a telescope, is inserted into the abdomen through a small incision made through or just below the navel.

Using a light attached to this instrument, the doctor looks through an eyepiece to examine the ovaries, uterus, and Fallopian tubes. With a

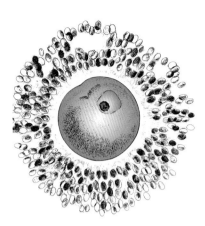

Human ovum with surrounding satellite cells.

laparoscope, a doctor can sometimes stop bleeding from a cyst, test for an infection, drain the fluid from a cyst, or take a sample of the tissue so that it can be examined in the laboratory.

Treatment

Treatment of ovarian cysts will depend on several factors, including the size and type of the cyst, the woman's age and overall state of health, her plans to have children, and whether she is having any symptoms. If a cyst is found early, less extensive treatment may be needed.

If a young woman has a small cyst that is not causing any symptoms, a doctor may decide to wait two or three menstrual cycles before treating it to see if it goes away. Most functional cysts will go away without any treatment after 1-3 months. In some cases a doctor may prescribe hormones (such as birth control pills) to "shrink" the cysts. Since oral contraceptives prevent ovulation, functional cysts are very rare in women taking the pill.

Although the pill does not prevent other types of benign cysts, it does offer some protection against malignant, or cancerous, ovarian cysts.

The chances of new cysts forming are also decreased when oral contraceptives are taken, because ovulation is prevented.

Some types of ovarian cysts do not respond well to treatment with oral contraceptives. in these cases surgery may be needed to remove the cysts. Surgery may be needed if:

Ovarian cancer   Questions & Answers

What is ovarian cancer?

Malignant growth and multiplication of the cells of the female reproductive gland (ovary).

What is the incidence of ovarian cancer?

Cancer of the ovary is the fourth most common cancer in women in the UK, with over 6,800 cases diagnosed annually. Each year, 4,480 women die from the disease, more than from any other cancer of the reproductive system. The reason for this is the lack of detectable symptoms in its early, and most treatable, stages so it remains undiagnosed and untreated.

Who is most at risk from ovarian cancer?

- Women with one or more ovarian cysts.
- Women who go through their menopause after the age of 52.
- Women who have never had children.
- Women with a close relative who developed the condition before the age of 50.

If you have a close relative with ovarian cancer, it is advisable to ask your physician about screening for this condition. Early detection could help to insure that, should you be diagnosed with this type of cancer, you receive the most effective treatment and the best chances of recovery.

What are the symptoms?

While ovarian cancer is usually without symptoms in the early stages, some women may notice signs similar to those of an ovarian cyst, such as irregular periods. In most cases, symptoms only appear when the cancer has spread to other parts of the body, and may include:

- Pain in the lower abdomen.
- Swelling in the abdomen caused by excess fluid.
- Frequent need to pass urine.
- Abnormal vaginal bleeding (in rare cases).

If you recognise any of these symptoms, or you are experiencing the general symptoms of cancer, such as loss of body weight, nausea and vomiting, it is important to see your physician as soon as possible.

How will my general physician know I have ovarian cancer?

- Whether you have asked your general physician to screen you for ovarian cancer due to the illness of a close relative, or due to the appearance of the symptoms listed above, you may be offered ultrasound scanning as the first in a series of checks for the condition.
- This scanning will be carried out through the vagina, and will look for signs of a tumor in the ovaries.
- Blood tests may also be carried out to look for a specific protein which is produced by this type of cancer.

Your physician may also examine your abdomen for swellings and lumps and perhaps recommend that you have an ultrasound scan of your ovaries and a laparoscopy.

How can I protect myself?

Looking out for the symptoms and adopting a healthy lifestyle will help to reduce your risk of developing cancer. Try to cut down the amount of fat and increase the amount of fiber in your diet, making sure you eat at least five portions of fruit or vegetables a day. Exercise regularly, drink a sensible amount of alcohol (two or three units per day or less) and stop smoking.

What is the most common form of treatment?

The most common form of treatment is surgery to remove the affected ovary and surrounding tissue, followed by drug treatment (chemotherapy) with cytotoxics.

How is the prognosis after treatment?

The prognosis varies widely depending on the degree of spread at the time of treatment. The overall five year survival rate is only 35 per cent, usually due to the early spread of the cancer to other parts of the body.

▲ A cyst does not go away after a few menstrual periods.

▲ Cysts do not go away after treatment with oral contraceptives.

▲ Cysts are very large.

▲ A cyst is found in a woman past the menopause.

▲ Symptoms, such as severe pain or bleeding, are present.

▲ A cyst becomes twisted (torsion).

The extent and type of surgery that is needed will depend on several factors. If a cyst is found early, chances are that surgery will be less extensive. Sometimes a cyst can be removed while leaving the ovary intact. In other cases, one or both ovaries may have to be removed. In still other situations, more extensive surgery, such as hysterectomy (removal of the uterus) may be needed.

Your doctor will give you as much information as possible before any proposed surgery. Occasionally, though, the extent of the necessary surgery cannot be know until the actual time of the operation. You should discuss this with your doctor.

Polycystic ovary syndrome

The formation of small cysts in one or both ovaries. The cause is unknown. but the cysts interfere with the production of hormones by the ovaries and the patient develops such symptoms as:

- facial hairs
- excess weight
- menstrual problems
- infertility

Abnormal levels of hormones can be measured in the bloodstream, but the syndrome is often discovered on an ultrasound scan while investigating infertility. Treatment involves surgically cutting away part of the affected ovarian tissue, and using hormones to stimulate the ovary to restart its correct function.

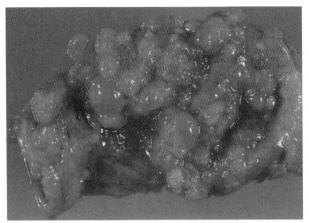

Although the outer surface of this ovarian cystic tumor was smooth, the inside wall had multiple small cysts and yellow papillary nodules.

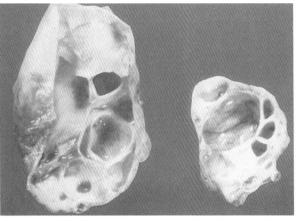

A benign multicystic serous ovarian tumor with different-sized cystic spaces with smooth walls.

Ovarian cancer

Cancer of the ovaries is a severe malignant growth, causing more deaths than any cancer of the female reproductive system. The ovaries are situated in the pelvis one on each side of the uterus and in close relation to the Fallopian tube. Each ovary is attached to the back of the broad ligament by a peritoneal fold called the mesovarium; the blood supply, venous and lymphatic drainage of the ovary and its nerve supply pass through the mesovarium.

A fibromuscular cord, the round ligament of the ovary, attaches it to the back of the uterus.

The ovary is an extremely pale, wrinkled organ about the size of the end joint of a thumb. The ovaries vary much in size in different women and even in the same woman; the approximate dimensions are 3.5 to 5 cm long, 2.5 cm wide and 1.5 cm thick. Each ovary weighs 5 to 10 grams.

Incidence of ovarian cancer

The chances of contracting ovarian cancer in your lifetime are slim - about one in 70, compared with one in nine for breast cancer. But women with strong family histories of breast, ovarian, and colon cancers may face a somewhat higher risk - about one in 25.

Chances of surviving

To cut the risk, several measures could be taken. Researchers believe ovarian cancer is tied to ovulation. And the less you ovulate, the lower your risk. Experts say women who take the pill for 10 years can cut their risk from one in 70 to one in 350. Pregnancies, during which you do not ovulate, also help. Those who ovulate more may be at a higher risk. Using fertility drugs may triple a woman's risk of developing ovarian cancer. Only 39 per cent of ovarian cancer victims survive more than five years following diagnosis, compared with a 90 per cent five-year survival rate for breast cancer victims. The survival rate rises to about 90 per cent if the cancer is diagnosed and treated when malignant growth are still limited to the ovaries. Unfortunately, fewer that one in four cases are detected at this early stage. The majority of women who have ovarian cancer first see their doctors after the disease is widespread and metastatic. The problem with ovarian cancer is that it is a silent killer.

Symptoms

In its early stages, ovarian cancer has no real symptoms. In latter stages, women may suffer from persistent bloating, constipation, urinary frequency, and a heavy feeling in the abdomen. An uncomplicated ovarian tumor generally causes no symptoms until it reaches a size large enough to be appreciated by the patient or to be discovered accidentally at routine examination or during pregnancy. The growth of ovarian tumors whether innocent or malignant is notoriously insidious and this accounts for the reports of removal of very large cysts. Menstruation is not affected except in the case of hormone-producing tumors.

The physical signs depend on the size of the tumor, on its mobility and on its relation to surrounding organs. A small tumor, up to the size of a large egg, tends to remain located in one or other lateral fornix and is felt bimanually to one side of the uterus. A large cyst tends to be displaced above the pelvic brim when there is no longer room in the pelvis and thus to present as a central abdominal tumor.

Diagnosis

Ultrasound examination of the pelvis demonstrates the size of the ovaries, the presence of Graafian follicles and makes it possible to give a size to tumors.

Furthermore, doctors can detect the cancer by one of several means; gynaecologists feel for tumors during routine pelvic examinations, a blood test can seek out heightened levels of a protein called CA-125 (80 per cent of women with ovarian cancer have elevated levels of the protein), and doctors use transvaginal ultrasound and Doppler imaging to detect any internal abnormalities in the patient's ovaries.

Complications of ovarian tumors

The most important complications of ovarian tumors are: torsion, hemorrhage, rupture, infection, incarceration, malignant change, pregnancy

O

Polycystic ovary syndrome Questions & Answers

What is polycystic ovary syndrome?

The syndrome is an inherited disorder affecting the functioning of the ovaries, which produce eggs, and the hormones estrogen and progestogen. Numerous tiny cysts are usually present in the ovaries.

What are the major symptoms of this disorder?

Sufferers have raised levels of the hormone insulin, which stimulates the ovaries to produce too much testosterone. Other imbalances include elevated levels of luteinizing hormone (LH) and relative deficiency of follicle-stimulating hormone (FSH), both of which control the release of eggs from the ovaries. As the ovaries are not working properly, eggs may not be released in a regular monthly cycle.
High levels of testosterone can cause acne and an increase in body hair. It also builds up body tissue's resistance to insulin, which regulates blood sugar levels, so food metabolism becomes inefficient.

Who is at risk?

As the medical condition is inherited, it can develop from birth. Having polycystic ovaries is very common, affecting about 20 per cent of women, of who three-quarters will have symptoms. Being overweight increases your risk of developing symptoms.

How is the condition diagnosed?

Your physician can refer you to a gynaecologist, who will arrange for an ultrasound scan of your ovaries end blood tests to check levels of FSH, LH and testosterone.

Is infertility inevitable?

Not at all. Many women conceive spontaneously, although about half of those with symptoms suffer from infertility as a result of not ovulating.

How is the condition treated?

The hormonal imbalance is being treated with various specific drugs. The first treatment for infertility that is usually tried is stimulation of the ovaries with the drug clomiphene. This induces ovulation in about 70 per cent of women, and about half of these women will become pregnant within six months. If this fails, injections of FSH may be tried, which triggers ovulation in around 80 per cent of women treated, of which about 60 per cent will conceive within six months.
If drug treatment does not work surgery that involves cauterising the ovary is very successful in triggering ovulation. It is vital, however, that ovarian stimulation is monitored by ultrasound in a fertility unit as women with this syndrome have a tendency to develop a high number of eggs.

■ Torsion

Torsion of the pedicle occurs most often in the small more mobile tumors and is commonest in dermoid cysts but it may affect any adnexal mass such as hydrosalpinx. Initially it causes unilateral lower abdominal pain, but it is sufficient to obstruct the circulation, and especially the venous return, the tumor becomes filled with blood and an acute abdominal emergency results.
There is great pain, fever, rapid pulse, shock and eventually leucocytosis.

Vomiting and diarrhea may be seen also.

■ Hemorrhage

Hemorrhage into an ovarian tumor causes pain similar to but generally less severe than that of torsion. The tumor enlarges and becomes tender. rarely rupture of a surface vessel leads to intraperitoneal bleeding with collapse as in ruptured ectopic pregnancy.

■ Rupture

An ovarian cyst may rupture sponta-neously or by trauma as a blow on the abdomen or coitus. The woman may feel something give way and there may be pain and vomiting with signs of peritoneal irritation.

■ Infection

Invasion with organisms from the bowel or in association with salpingitis may cause infection.

■ Incarceration

Incarceration of an ovarian tumor in the pelvis behind the uterus, sometimes occurs and leads to retention of urine. The condition may be distinguished from impaction of a fibroid or retroverted gravid uterus.

■ Very large tumor

A very large tumor causes symptoms of abdominal distension and pressure. These include indigestion, loss of appetite, breathlessness and swelling of the legs.

■ Malignant change

This can occur at any age but is commonest after the menopause, except that tumors in young children are often malignant. The symptoms of malignant change include rapid growth of the tumor, abdominal distension indicating ascites, pain of an aching character and tenderness. Swelling of the legs is always an indication of malignant change except with very large benign tumors.

■ Pregnancy

An ovarian tumor may be revealed for the first time at routine examination during pregnancy. Torsion of the pedicle may occur either during pregnancy or in the puerperium. The tumor generally has little effect on pregnancy unless it becomes incarcerated. In most cases the tumor rises into the abdomen as the uterus enlarges, but occasionally an ovarian tumor in the pelvis below the presenting part may cause a malpresentation, may obstruct labour or may be ruptured in the course of labour.

Treatment

Aggressive chemotherapy may prolong survival. And experimental drugs, such as Taxol, have shown some promise in trials. But these

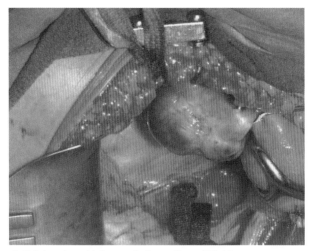

A slightly enlarged left ovary is shown. Several bluish cysts are present under the ovarian surface. The irregular bluish-brown areas on the ovarian surface closer to the uterus suggest endometriosis.

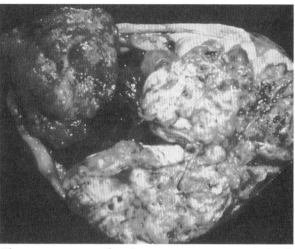

The cross appearance of an immature teratoma on cut section is shown. It is solid, fleshy, and yellow with multiple areas of hemorrhage.

drugs are currently being used only for latter-stage patients. Genentech companies have engineered a series of specific antibodies designed to prevent the growth of cancerous cells in humans. The antibodies are now being tested in trials on ovarian cancer patients. Cancer of the ovary will be treated initially by surgery which will involve total hysterectomy and bilateral removal of the Fallopian tubes, though in young women a normal, uninvolved ovary might be left.

In advanced cases, as much pelvic peritoneum as possible will be removed; if there is spread beyond the ovary the greater omentum will also be excised. A search will be made for peritoneal metastases, including those on the under surface of the diaphragm. A further second look laparotomy or laparoscopy to ensure that the peritoneal cavity is free from secondary deposits may be carried out three to six months after the original operation. Even in apparently

advanced disease the ultimate prognosis appears to be improved by operative removal of the main tumor masses. Radiotherapy in the form of abdominal radiation has given doubtful results in the treatment of advanced disease; the same may be said for the use of intraperitoneal isotopes - usually radioactive gold. Chemotherapy with cytotoxic agents seems to give more hopeful results and a variety have been or are under trial.

O

Trabecular pattern of a carcinoid tumor. The ovary is seen. The cells are similar to those of the granulosa cell tumor, but the nuclei are more round and uniform.

This ovarian endometrioid carcinoma is both solid and cystic. A large hemorrhagic area is seen.

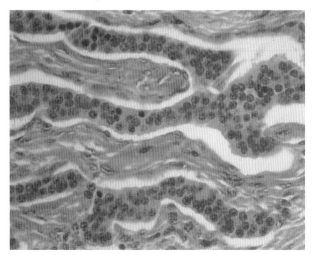

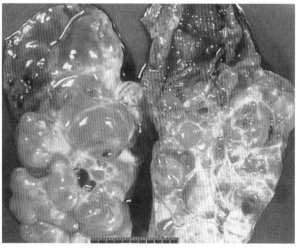

PAIN

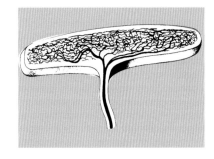

Description

Pain is usually a protective mechanism, occurring when tissue is damaged or when cells are altered by pain stimuli that threaten to produce tissue damage. Pain resulting from a functional disturbance or pathology is called "organic" pain. In contrast, "psychogenic" pain is a symptom of an underlying emotional disturbance and is not a consequence of organic pathology.

Even though pain is a common experience, it is not a simple condition to define. Pain is a sensation, but it is also an interpretation of that sensation that can be influenced by many factors. Fatigue, anxiety, fear, and the anticipation of more pain all affect the perception of and reaction to pain. Studies show that various personality types may experience pain differently; the introverted personality has a lower pain threshold that the extrovert.

In addition the perception of pain may be modified significantly by suggestion. Studies indicate that approximately 35 per cent of patients suffering pain from a variety of causes report their pain as being "satisfactorily relieved" by placebo.

Origin and perception of pain

Pain is categorized, according to its origin, as either somatic or visceral. Somatic pain arises from the musculoskeletal system or skin; visceral pain originates from the organs or viscera of the thorax and abdomen.

Free nerve endings serve as pain receptors to initiate nerve impulses which travel through specialized pain fibers through the spinal cord and/or brainstem to specific receiving areas of the brain.

These receptors are found throughout the superficial skin layers and in certain deeper tissues such as membranous bone covering, arterial walls, muscles, tendons, joint surfaces, and membranes lining the skull.

Pain-evoking stimuli have in common the ability to injure cells and to release proteolytic enzymes and polypeptides that stimulate nerve endings and initiate the pain impulse. Pain fibers enter the dorsal roots of the sinal cord and interconnect with the other nerve cells that cross to the opposite side of the cord and ascend to the brain.

A pain impulse terminates in the thalamus, where the conscious perception of pain is localized, or in well-defined areas of the cerebral cortex, where recognition and interpretation of the nature and location of the pain impulse occurs.

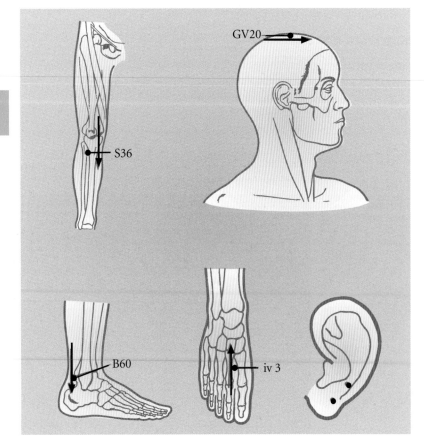

Pain may be treated by pain-relieving medicines, but also acupuncture may be of great benefit in the treatment of certain pain syndromes. The illustrations show various important acupuncture points used in the local treatment of pain.

Pain initiation, transmission, and perception are essentially the same for both visceral and somatic pain. One important distinction, however, is that highly localized visceral damage rarely causes severe pain. Diffuse stimulation of nerve endings throughout an organ is required to produce significant visceral pain. Conditions producing visceral pain include:

▲ ischemia of organ tissue
▲ chemical destruction of visceral tissue
▲ spasm of visceral smooth muscle
▲ physical distention of an organ
▲ stretching of its associated mesentery

A special category of pain is distinguished as referred pain. Referred pain is perceived as coming from a part of the body other than that part actually initiating the pain signal.

Unlike somatic pain, visceral pain cannot be localized by the brain as coming from a specific organ. Instead, moist visceral pain is interpreted by the brain as coming from various skin or muscle segments (it is "referred" to various body surface areas.

Failure to recognize the possibility of referred visceral pain could mean that a serious visceral pathology might go undiagnosed and untreated while ineffective self-medication with non-prescription pain-relievers is attempted.

Evaluation of patients with pain

Though the etiology of chronic pain in individual patients varies remarkably, the rigorous evaluation each deserves has many elements in common. In all cases, a detailed history of pain should assess:

▲ severity
▲ location
▲ quality
▲ duration and course
▲ timing
▲ associated symptoms (with emphasis on psychologic state and vegetative symptoms)

A personal or family history of chronic pain can often illuminate the current problem and will be evaluated by the general physician of medical specialist. Finally, a detailed assessment of the patient's level of function is necessary.]V should focus on family life (including sexual relationships), social network, and employment or avocations.

In all spheres, the doctor will attempt to clarify the role played by the patient.s pain in his or her interactions with others and attempts at normal living. Through this comprehensive interview, the issue of secondary gain is assessed, an evaluation is made of current and premorbid psychopathology, the role of family pathology is clarified, and a sense of the overall degree of abnormal illness behavior is obtained.

The pain history should also try to identify the meaning of pain descriptors to the patient. It is more socially acceptable to report pain that anxiety or depression, and proper therapy often depends on sorting out these similarly described, but divergently experienced, perceptions.

Similarly, the distinction between pain and suffering should be clarified. This is especially salient in the cancer patient, whose suffering may be due as much to loss of function and fear of impending death as to pain. Physical examination is used to assist in identifying underlying causes and to further evaluate the degree of functional impairment.

Treatment

Regardless of the underlying disease mechanism, pain management depends on the understanding that the perception of pain can represent more than the pathology intrinsic to the disease. On the basis of careful patient history evaluation, the physician will decide whether the pain can be self-medicated or if specialist referral is necessary. Most difficult to treat are psychogenic pain syndromes.

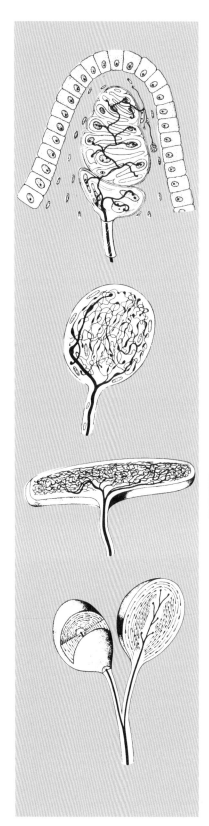

Many sensory organs in the skin and subcutaneous tissue play an important role in the reception of pain stimuli. The illustration shows various types of sensory organs that, upon strong stimulation, show a pain sensation.

Quick and simple ways to erase pain naturally

Breathe into the pain

Resisting pain can sometimes aggravate it, just like trying to untie a knot by pulling it tighter. Taking a deep, abdominal breath into and through the pain can be relaxing and healing.

Focus your attention on the pain and imagine you are inhaling and exhaling through the primary site of the pain. Breathing into the pain while during yoga exercises can provide additional effects.

Get to the point

There are acupressure points all over your body that can be effective in educing the pain and beginning healing.

The best points are never immediately on the primary source of the pain. Seek out trigger points, that is, points that seem hypersensitive to the tough.

Sometimes good points are around joints that are near the pain; sometimes they are on the other side of the body parallel to where the pain is. Press the point firmly with your thumb for five seconds and then repeat the pressure several times.

Laying on of hands

Ask a friend to practice laying on of hands, which is an ancient healing practice that has been used in numerous cultures and is used today by thousands of nurses and other health professionals in hospitals.

The person doing it should concentrate, imagining loving and healing energies emitting from his hands into your body. he may choose to hold his hands near the area of pain, though you should encourage him to use intuition to determine where to apply the energy. While your friend is there, perhaps he can also give you a massage, which can be wonderfully relaxing and pain-relieving.

Pain diary

Keep a pain journal. By observing carefully when and where you experience pain, you can sometimes find certain patterns to it, and then try to break these patterns.

You may, for instance, discover that you develop your symptoms when you do not get enough sleep, do inadequate physical exercise, miss a meal, eat certain foods or visit relatives.

Describe the pain in as much detail as possible including shape and colour; then draw it with crayons or coloured pens or pencils. Imagine and draw the shapes and colours you feel may soothe it; then visualize these colours and shapes in your body.

Mental methods

Research on biofeedback has not only shown its value in teaching people to relax but also its influence on many bodily functions. Biofeedback is very valuable in teaching people to have greater control and direction over their bodies and thus over their pain. Learn how to use it.

Meditation and hypnosis

Meditation not only helps you achieve greater relaxation, it encourages more focused concentration, giving you greater control of your mind, and thus greater control over your sense of pain. Auto-hypnosis is a popular technique for relaxation and can be used effectively for healing and pain control. One hypnosis strategy, called glove anesthesia, is to put yourself in a trance and imagine your hand to the numb, heavy and wooden.

Then, move your hand to the part or parts of the body that feel pain and imagine those parts feeling similarly relaxed, heavy and numb.

Stimulate the endorphins

Research has found that exercise increases endorphin levels in the blood. The increase in these opiate-like substances is one reason that athletes sometimes feel high when they are exercising.

Likewise, exercise may help reduce your pain. However, this strategy should not be considered if the exercise causes pain.

Foot massage

Your feet, especially their soles, have thousands of nerve endings. By massaging them, you are stimulating various parts of the body, that the nerves feed, thus reducing pain. The joy and relaxation that massaging the feet creates is good for the sole and for the soul.

Believe in a good result

Whatever you do to relieve your pain, believe in it and it will work better. research has shown that approximately 33 per cent of people with pain experience relief of symptoms from a placebo.

Try not to let pain interfere with your life. Keep busy with activities that require concentration so that you can forget about your pain for a while.

Consider joining a support group of people who experience chronic pain. It is best to avoid groups which simply complain about their problems; instead, seek out a group that shares information about strategies that are helpful in dealing with pain.

A sense of control over your life is therapeutic in itself. The decision to utilize strategies to help yourself may be almost as helpful as actually doing them.

Chronic pain with either insufficient of o organic explanation is a common problem. Typical syndromes include chronic headache, failed low back pain, atypical facial pain, and abdominal or pelvic pain of unknown etiology. The experience of pain for most of these patients is like that of organic disease, i.e. the pain is not factitious. However, whole accepting that the pain is real, it is better understood as a psychologic, rather than physical, disorder. These patients often develop a pattern of inactivity, social withdrawal, rumination about physical health, and inappropriate utilization of health care which has been described as abnormal illness behavior.

Though the degree of physical disease contributing to the patient's disability should be clearly identified, and peri-

Pain in the thoracic or abdominal cavity can be an indication of problems of the respiratory system heart and major blood vessels, digestive tract, or a condition elsewhere in the abdomen. Elderly people tend to have less abdominal pain than younger adults, and the pain develops more gradually.

Pain can arise from several causes, including infection, inflammation, angina pectoris, formation of ulcers, perforation or rupture of organs, and lack of oxygen needed by digestive tract muscles.

The description of the pain's location may vary, from a vague sense of being present everywhere to being felt in one specific spot.

Location of abdominal pain, and probable causes

A. Colic in the small intestine
B. Acute dyspepsia
C. Kidney colic
D. Gallstones

E. Appendicitis
F. Peritonitis
G. Intestinal obstruction
H. Intussusception

I. Perforation of a peptic ulcer
J. Ectopic of abdominal pregnancy
K. Miscarriage
L. Cystitis (bladder infection)

odic reevaluation should be done when this factor is not static, primary therapy must be directed at maintaining and improving function and in treating the psychologic disorder.

Therapy with pain-relieving drugs can be pursued, but if used exclusively, will undoubtedly fail, because pain per se is not the only, or even the major, cause of disability. Nonpharmacologic methods of pain control should be stressed, including TENS and counterirritation, trigger point injection and spray and stretch, and physical therapy.

Reputable pain clinics provide a multidisciplinary, comprehensive approach to patients with pain, which is most appropriate for the patient with chronic nonmalignant functional impairment or failure to respond to a reasonable attempt at management by the individual physician.

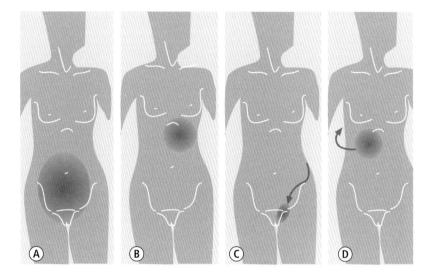

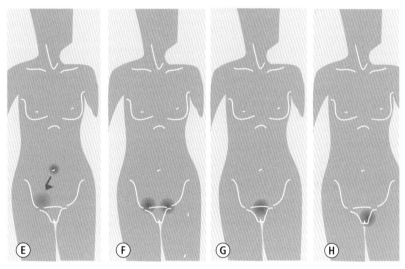

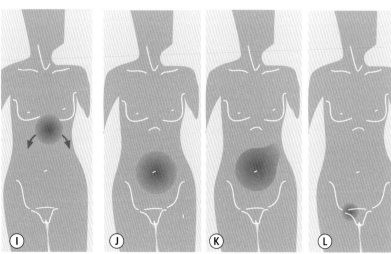

PANCREAS DISORDERS

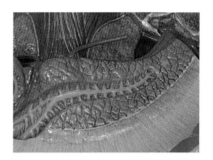

Introduction

The pancreas is an organ consisting partly of exocrine gland tissue, secreting into the duodenum, and partly of endocrine gland tissue (the islets of Langerhans), whose principal hormones include insulin and glucagon. The pancreas lies on the back wall of the upper abdomen, much of it within the duodenal loop. Powerful digestive enzymes (pepsin, trypsin, lipase, amylase) are secreted into the gut; this secretion is in part controlled by intestinal hormones (secretin) and in part by nerve reflexes. Insulin and glucagon have important roles in glucose and fat metabolism; other pancreatic hormones affect gastrointestinal tract secretion and activity.

Pancreas cancer

Tumors of the pancreas may be benign or malignant. Benign tumors do not spread. About 95 per cent of the malignant tumors of the pancreas are adenocarcinomas. These tumors are nearly twice as common in men as in women and two to three times more common in heavy smokers than in nonsmokers. People with chronic pancreatitis have a higher risk of acquiring it.

The disease has become increasingly common in Western Europe, Japan and the United States as life expectancy has increased. It rarely develops before age 50; the average age at diagnosis is 55. Little is known about the cause.

Symptoms

Cancer of the pancreas typically causes no symptoms until the tumor has grown large. Thus, at the time of diagnosis, the tumor has already spread (metastasize) beyond the pancreas to the neighbouring lymph nodes or to the liver or lung in 80 percent of the cases.

Typically, the first symptoms are pain and weight loss. At the time of diagnosis, 90 per cent of people have abdominal pain - usually severe pain in the upper abdomen, that penetrates to the back - and weight loss at least 10 per cent of their ideal weight.

Jaundice caused by obstruction of the common bile duct is typically an early symptom, because the majority to pancreas cancers occur in the head of the pancreas, the part nearest the duodenum and common bile duct.

Tumors in the body and tail of the pancreas (the middle part and the part farthest from the duodenum) may obstruct the vein draining the spleen, resulting in an enlargement of the spleen and varices (enlarged, tortuous, swollen varicose veins) around the stomach and esophagus.

Diagnosis

When a malignant tumor of the pancreas is suspected, the most commonly used diagnostic tests are:
- ultrasound scans
- computed tomography (CT-scan)
- endoscopic retrograde pancreatography (an X-ray technique that shows the structure of the pancreatic duct)

To confirm the diagnosis, a doctor may obtain a sample of the pancreas (by a biopsy needle) for microscopic examination. The sample is obtained by inserting a needle through the skin while using a CT or ultrasound scan as a guide.

Treatment

The prognosis is poor. Fewer than 2 per cent of the people with adenocarcinoma of the pancreas survive for 5 years after the diagnosis. The only hope for cure is surgery, which is performed on patients whose cancer has not spread. Either the pancreas alone

Location of the pancreas in the upper part of the abdominal cavity, next to the spleen and the duodenum.

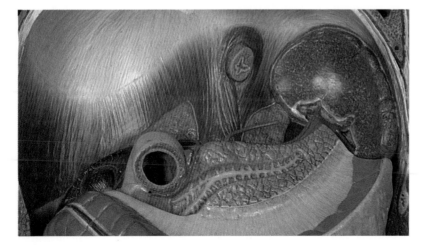

or the pancreas and the duodenum are removed. Even after such surgery, only 10 percent of patients live for 5 years, regardless of further treatment. Another type of pancreatic cancer, cyst-adenocarcinoma has a much better prognosis than adenocarcinoma. Only 20 percent of these cancers have spread by the time surgery is performed. If the cancer has not spread and the whole pancreas is removed surgically, the person has a 65 percent chance of survival for at least 5 years. In other, rare, tumors of the pancreas, anticancer drugs (chemotherapy) may help reduce the number of tumor cells.

Pancreatitis

In general, acute pancreatitis is a self-limited disease in 80 per cent of cases associated with minimal morbidity and mortality. However, complications do increase in severity, making it important to identify high-risk patients. The diagnosis of acute pancreatitis is made on clinical grounds, by confirmation of laboratory and radiological studies.
The most common causes are:
- alcohol abuse
- common duct gallstone passage
- surgical procedures
- medicines
The diagnosis is considered when patients present complaints of relatively severe pain in the middle part of the abdomen. The pain is constant and boring in nature, usually radiating to the back and associated with nausea, vomiting, and abdominal tenderness.
Analysis of the blood shows an elevation of the enzyme amylase. However, a normal amylase content of the blood does not exclude the diagnosis of pancreatitis. Special diagnostic methods such as abdominal sonography (using ultrasound) and CT-scan or MRI-scan may show the inflammatory process of the pancreas.
There is no specific treatment of proved value for pancreatitis. Care is supportive and aimed at the management of complications. Patients with initial presentations of pancreatitis will be admitted to the hospital for observation.

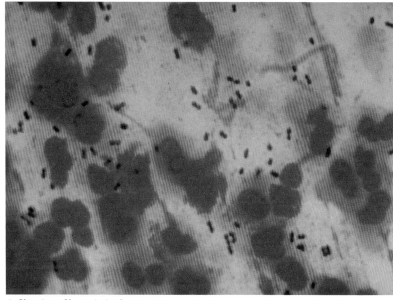

Infiltration of bacteria in the pancreas.

Chronic pancreatitis
The presence of irreversible inflammatory changes in the tissue of the pancreas is clinically characterized by chronic severe abdominal pain or findings of insufficiency of the pancreas such as:
▲ steatorrhoea (increased amount of fat in the faeces);
▲ weight loss;
▲ glucose intolerance.
The most common cause is alcohol abuse. Less common causes include:
- trauma
- hereditary pancreatitis
- cystic fibrosis
- cancer
Abdominal pain is characteristic of early disease and tends to resolve within 2 years of calcification of the pancreas.

Degenerative process in pancreatic tissue.

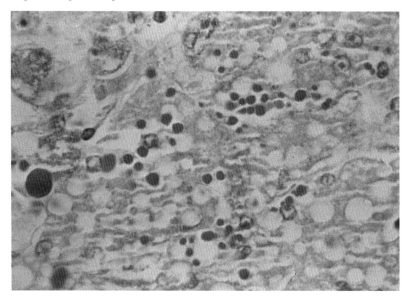

Pancreas Questions & Answers

What is the pancreas?

The pancreas is an oblong organ, located in the curve of the duodenum, behind the peritoneum. This gland releases the pancreatic juice via the pancreatic duct; the enzyme-rich juice is important for the breakdown of proteins, fats and carbohydrates.

What are the hormones of the pancreas?

Two hormones, insulin and glucagon (see the Section on the Hormonal system), are also pancreatic products and both are delivered into the blood stream. They play an important role in the metabolism of carbohydrates.

Diseases of the pancreas are difficult to evaluate and manage because of the organ's unusual anatomy, and complex physiological functions.

What are the major disorders of the pancreas?

Acute and chronic inflammation of the pancreas (pancreatitis) are the major diseases afflicting the pancreas, and their presentations often overlap.

There is no treatment for pancreatitis as such, and management is therefore based on the recognition and management of complications. Malignant tumors are also difficult to detect and almost impossible to treat.

What are the characteristics of acute pancreatitis?

In general, acute pancreatitis is a self-limited disease in 80 per cent of cases associated with minimal morbidity and mortality. However, complications do increase in severity, making it important to identify high-risk patients. The diagnosis of acute pancreatitis is made on clinical grounds, by confirmation of laboratory and radiological studies.

What are the causes of acute pancreatitis?

The most common causes are:
- alcohol abuse;
- common duct gallstone passage;
- surgical procedures;
- medicines.

How is the diagnosis made of acute pancreatitis?

The diagnosis is considered when patients present complaints of relatively severe pain in the middle part of the abdomen. The pain is constant and boring in nature, usually radiating to the back and associated with nausea, vomiting, and abdominal tenderness.

Analysis of the blood shows an elevation of the enzyme amylase. However, a normal amylase content of the blood does not exclude the diagnosis of pancreatitis. Special diagnostic methods such as abdominal sonography (using ultrasound) and CT-scan or MRI-scan may show the inflammatory process of the pancreas.

What is the best treatment of acute pancreatitis?

There is no specific treatment of proved value for pancreatitis. Care is supportive and aimed at the management of complications. Patients with initial presentations of pancreatitis will be admitted to the hospital for observation.

What are the characteristics of chronic pancreatitis?

The presence of irreversible inflammatory changes in the tissue of the pancreas is clinically characterized by chronic severe abdominal pain or findings of insufficiency of the pancreas such as:
- teatorrhoea (increased amount of fat in the faeces);
- weight loss;
- glucose intolerance.

What is the common cause of chronic pancreatitis?

The most common cause is alcohol abuse. Less common causes include:
- trauma;
- hereditary pancreatitis;
- cystic fibrosis;
- cancer.

What are the symptoms of chronic pancreatitis?

Abdominal pain is characteristic of early disease and tends to resolve within 2 years of calcification of the pancreas. Patients must observe strict alcohol abstinence and should be withdrawn from narcotic medicines. Surgical procedures are reserved for patients wit intractable pain, and significant obstruction of the pancreatic duct.

What types of cancer occur in the pancreas?

Adenocarcinoma of the exocrine part of the pancreas occurs in eighty percent in the head of the gland and may produce jaundice. Tumors located in the body and tail may produce enlargement of the spleen, varices in the stomach and esophagus, and bleeding in the gastrointestinal tract. Otherwise, symptoms are similar, regardless of the location of the cancer. Cancers appear at the mean age of 55 years and occur about two times oftener in men. At diagnosis, weight loss and abdominal pain are present in 90 per cent of patients. Severe pain usually radiates to the back. Relief may be obtained by bending forward, or using aspirin. Symptoms occur late; by the time of diagnosis, in about 90 per cent of the patients the tumor has spread beyond the gland or has metastasized.

P

Causes of acute pancreatitis

- Gallstones

- Alcoholism

- Drugs such as furosemide and azathioprine

- Mumps

- High blood levels of lipids, especially triglycerides

- Damage to the pancreas from surgery or endoscopy

- Damage to the pancreas from blunt or penetrating injuries

- Cancer of the pancreas

- Reduced blood supply to the pancreas, for example, from severely low blood pressure

- Hereditary pancreatitis

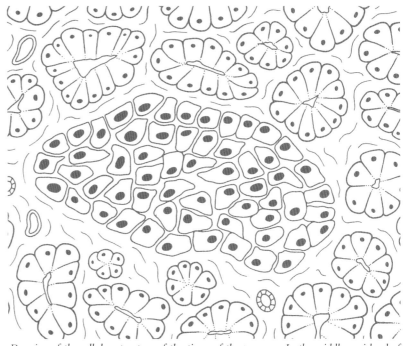

Drawing of the cellular structure of the tissue of the pancreas. In the middle an island of Langerhans.

Patients must observe strict alcohol abstinence and should be withdrawn from narcotic medicines. Surgical procedures are reserved for patients wit intractable pain, and significant obstruction of the pancreatic duct.

Insulinoma

This tumor - as the name indicates - is characterized by a high secretion of insulin.
Symptoms and signs of hypoglycaemia secondary to an insulinoma appear during fasting. Disturbances of the central nervous system are characteristic:

- headache and confusion;
- visual disturbances;
- motor weakness;
- palsy and ataxia;
- marked personality changes.

A small, single tumor at or near the surface of the pancreas can usually be removed; in other cases part or all of the pancreas may be removed.

Topography and vascular supply (left: arteries; right: veins) of the pancreas. The pancreas is a long, elongated racemose gland situated between the spleen and the duodenum.

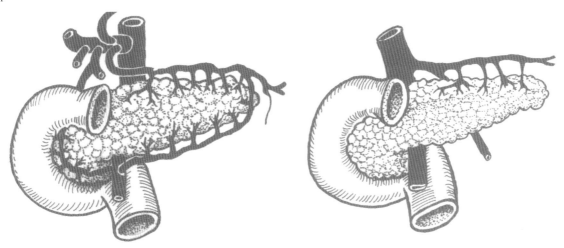

PARKINSON'S DISEASE

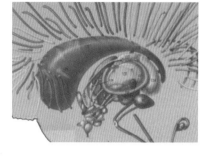

Description

Parkinson's disease is a chronic progressive nervous disease of later life that is marked by tremor and weakness of resting muscles and by a peculiar gait. In Parkinson's disease there is an increased incidence of dementia and of depression.

Parkinson's disease affects about 1 in every 250 people over 40 years old and about 1 in every 100 people over 65 years old. Parkinsonism is a general term used to indicate a chronic neurological disorder that is marked by muscle rigidity but without tremor of resting muscles.

Causes

Parkinson's disease has a variety of causes, but the most common is degeneration of the dopamine-producing cells in the brain. These cells are located in many areas of the brain, particularly in the basal ganglia.

The neurological disorder is caused by an imbalance between the neurotransmitters dopamine and acetylcholine in the brain. These chemicals are responsible for the transmission of nerve signals in the part of the brain that coordinates movement. They have opposing actions and are normally finely balanced.

Other causes, particularly of parkinsonism include the side effects of certain drugs, notably antipsychotics, brain damage, and narrowing of the blood vessels in the brain.

In Parkinson's disease, nerve cells in the basal ganglia degenerate, resulting in lower production of dopamine and fewer connections with other nerve cells and muscles. The cause of the nerve cell degeneration and dopamine loss usually is not known.

Genetics does not appear to play a major role, although the disease tends to occur in some families. Sometimes the cause is known, Parkinson's disease is a very late complication of viral encephalitis, a relatively rare but severe, flulike infection that causes brain inflammation.

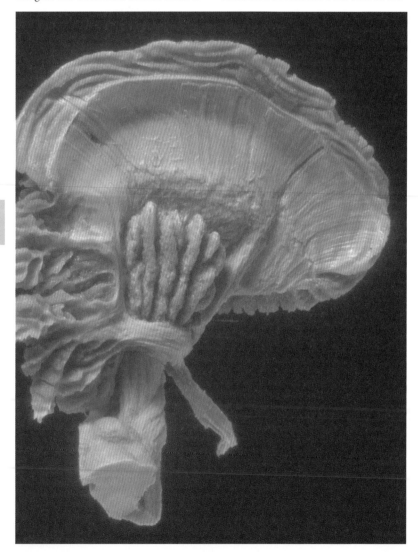

Macroscopic view of part of the nuclei of the cerebellum. In some Parkinson patients part of the cerebellar nuclei tend to degenerate.

Basic exercises for the facial muscles.
1. Upward movement of the upper lip.
2. Movement of the lips to the left.
3. Movement of the lips to the right.
4. Downward movement of the lower lip.
5. Movement of the lower lip to the left.
6. Closing of the left eyelids.
7. Closing of both eyelids
8. Blowing of the left cheek.
9. Closing of the right eyelids.

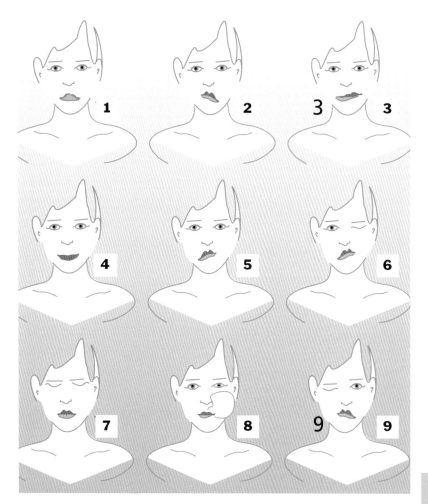

Signs and symptoms

Parkinson's disease begins subtle and progresses gradually. In many people, it begins with a tremor in the hand while the hand is at rest; the tremor decreases when the hand is moving purposefully and disappears completely during sleep.

Facies and attitude

The Parkinsonian facies is characteristic. The palpebral fissures are usually wider than normal, and blinking is infrequent.

The eyes have a staring appearance, due partly to these features and partly to the fact that spontaneous ocular movements are lacking or seldom occur.

The facial muscles exhibit an unnatural immobility.

The attitude of the limbs and trunk is one of moderate flexion. The spine is usually somewhat flexed, but is occasionally extended. There is little rotatory movement of the cervical spine. The limbs are moderately flexed and adducted, but the wrist is usually slightly extended.

The fingers are flexed at the metacarpophalangeal, and extended or only slightly flexed at the interphalangeal, joints, and adducted. The thumb is usually adducted, and extended at the metacarpo- and interphalangeal joints.

Disorders of movement

Voluntary movement exhibits some impairment of power, but more striking is the slowness with which it is performed.

Hence the patient shows weakness of the ocular movements, especially convergence of the facial movements, associated with tremor of the eyelids on closure of the eyes; and in move-

ments concerned in mastication, deglutition, and articulation.

The speech in severe cases is slurred and monotonous, owing to defective pronunciation of consonants and lack of variation in pitch.

Emotional movements of the face are also reduced in amplitude, slow in developing, and unduly contracted.

Movements of the small muscles of the hands are also markedly affected, with resulting clumsiness and inability to perform fine movements, such as those in needlework, dealing cards, and taking money from a pocket.

Certain associated and synergic movements suffer conspicuously. Swinging of the arms in walking is early diminished and later lost, and the synergic extension of the wrist, which is normally associated with flexion of the fingers, is also impaired.

Muscular rigidity

Muscular rigidity differs from the hypertonia associated with corticospinal lesions in that it is present to an equal extent in opposing musclegroups, for example, the flexors and extensors of the elbow; it is uniform throughout the whole angle of movement at a joint.

When tremor also is present the rigidity exhibits an interrupted character when tested by passive movement, the muscles yielding to tension in a series of jerks, hence the term "cog-wheel rigidity." When tremor is absent the rigidity is smooth and is of the so-called "lead-pipe" variety.

Gait

The Parkinsonian gait is in part at least the outcome of the patient's attitude and rigidity. It is usually slow, shuffling, and composed of small

617

Parkinson's disease   Questions & Answers

Who gets Parkinson's disease?

Parkinson's disease is a slowly progressive degenerative disorder affecting special groups of nerve cells in the brain. It may cause any combination of:

- slowed movement;

- muscular rigidity;

- postural changes;

- tremors;

- balance problems.

When does Parkinson's disease start?

Parkinson's disease (also known as Parkinsonism and paralysis agitans) usually begins in middle aged or older people. Men are at slightly greater risk than women. In most cases, it is idiopathic, that is, the cause is unknown. In a small percentage of cases, it may occur secondarily to some other problem, such as brain infection or tumors, carbon monoxide poisoning, or use of certain drugs.

What are the possible causes of Parkinson's disease?

Whatever the cause, it is known that the loss of dopamine, an important brain chemical, is involved in the development of symptoms. Some doctors believe that psychological factors may be involved in the cause of the disease. About half of all victims develop moderate to severe depression, which may be a result of the symptoms rather than a symptom itself. Further, tremors may be more severe when the patient is fatigued or under stress.

What are the major symptoms of Parkinson's disease and can it be treated?

It usually begins with mild tremors of the hand, which are more marked at rest than when alert. Progressive involvement usually extends to the muscle of the hands, face, arms, and legs. The face may become expressionless and head tremor may be noticed.

Muscle rigidity makes it harder to initiate and maintain movement, so walking becomes difficult. Posture tends to become stooped. With the loss of postural reflexes, there is a greater risk of falling. Salivation may increase. In the latest stages of the disease, memory loss and dementia may occur.

Can Parkinson's disease be treated effectively?

The sooner treatment begins, the better. The primary drug used to treat Parkinson's disease is levodopa, also known as L-dopa. A metabolic precursor of dopamine, it replaces the missing substance in the brain.

This medicine can completely eliminate symptoms in some patients and sharply decrease them in others. However, levodopa does not halt the underlying progression of disease and increasing doses usually are needed to prevent symptoms. Other drugs also may be used to supplement or replace levodopa, if its action alone is insufficient.

steps. The patient is often unable to stop quickly when pushed forwards or backwards - propulsion and retropulsion.

When propulsion occurs spontaneously during walking, the patient exhibits a "festinating" gait, hurrying with small steps in a bent attitude as if trying to catch up his center of gravity.

Some patients find their gait arrested, especially if they try to change direction, or when attempting to begin to walk.

A striking feature of Parkinsonism is the frequent ability of the patient to carry out rapid movements requiring considerable exertion better than slower and less energetic movements. Thus a patient who can walk only very slowly may be able to run quite fast.

■ Tremor

Tremor is the characteristic involuntary movement. Tremor, rigidity, and slowness and weakness of movements are, however, to a large extent independent variables. Tremor may be the first symptom, as it frequently is in Parkinson's disease, and may precede rigidity by months or years.

The tremor consists of rhythmic alternating movements of opposing muscle-groups. In the upper limb the hand is most affected. Movements of the fingers occur at the metacarpophalangeal joints and may be combined with movements of the thumb - the "pill-rolling movement."

Movements at the wrist may be flexion and extension, lateral displacement, or pronation and supination. Often the tremor shifts from one to another group of muscles while the patient is under observation.

■ Sensory symptoms

There is no loss of sensibility in Parkinson's disease. Pain, however, is common, especially in the later stages, when most patients complain of cramp-like pains in the limbs and spine due to the muscular rigidity and the changes induced in the joints and ligaments by the abnormal posture. Extreme restlessness is also a common symptom, the patient suffering great discomfort unless his position is changed every few minutes.

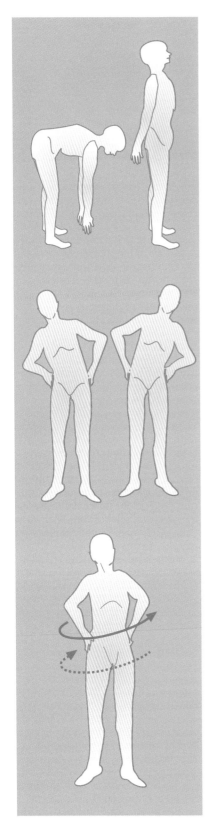

Basic exercises for the arms. Arms sidewards.
1. Flexion and extension in the elbow joint.
2. 90 degrees movement of the arms.
3. 180 degrees movement of the arms.

Treatment

■ Drugs

Physical therapy and drugs can help to relieve the symptoms of the Parkinson's disease; they cannot cure the underlying cause of the chemical imbalance. In particular, the degeneration of brain cells in Parkinson's disease cannot be halted, although drugs can minimize symptoms of the disease for many years.

Drugs restore the imbalance between dopamine and acetylcholine. They fall into two main categories: those that act by reducing the effect of acetylcholine (anticholinergic drugs), and those that act by boosting the effect of dopamine.

The particular drug that is prescribed depends on both the severity of the disease and the potential adverse effects of the drug, Anticholinergic drugs are often effective in the early stages of Parkinson's disease when they may control symptoms adequately without any other antiparkinson drugs.

■ Physical therapy

Continuing to perform as many daily activities as possible and following a program of regular exercise can help people with Parkinson's disease maintain mobility. Physical therapy and mechanical aids, such as wheeled walkers, can also help them maintain independence.

A nutritious diet rich in high-fiber foods can help counteract the constipation that may result from inactivity, dehydration, and some drugs. Dietary supplements and stool softeners can help keep bowel movements regular.

Basic exercises for the hip joints.
1. Flexion and extension in the hip joint.
2. Moving sideward; abduction and adduction in the hip.
3. Move the hips round and round in circles.

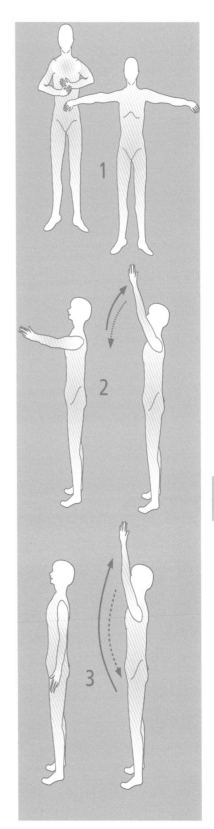

PELVIC DISORDERS

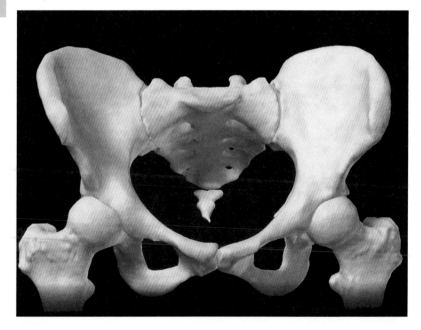

Pelvic nerve syndromes

Nerves for the pelvis are derived from the lumbar and sacral plexus. The lumbar nerves are derived from lumbar spinal cord segments located between the ninth and eleventh chest (thoracic) vertebrae.
The following nerves emerge from this plexus:
• iliohypogastric nerve
• ilioinguinal nerve
• genitofemoral nerve
• obturator nerve
• femoral nerve
• lateral cutaneous femoral nerve
The sacral nerves are derived from the sacral part of the spinal cord located

opposite the twelfth thoracic and first lumbar nerves.
The following nerves are part of this plexus or network:
• tibial nerve
• common peroneal nerve
• superior gluteal nerve
• inferior gluteal nerve
• pudendal nerve

Ilioinguinal nerve
The components of the ilioinguinal nerve (*nervus ilioinguinalis*) originate from the first lumbar spinal segment. It runs slightly below the iliohypogastric nerve.
The nerve encircles the trunk of the psoas muscle and goes across the

quadratus lumborum muscle. It runs between the internal oblique and transverse muscles and then runs along the inguinal ligament in the inguinal canal. En route it gives off a number of motor branches to the internal oblique and transverse muscles of the abdomen. The anterior cutaneous branches of this nerve supply the root of the penis and scrotum or the mons pubis and the greater lip.

Iliohypogastric nerve
The components of the iliohypogastric nerve (*nervus iliohypogastricus*) originate from the twelfth thoracic segment and the first lumbar segment; it is uppermost in the lumbar plexus.
The nerve traverses the lateral border of the psoas muscle and descends in front of the quadratus lumborum muscle and behind the colon. It pierces the aponeurosis of the transverse muscle of the abdomen and then runs between the internal oblique and transverse muscles of the abdomen. A number of small motor branches are given off to these muscles.
A number of small motor branches are given off into a cutaneous branch to the skin of the upper and lateral aspect of the gluteal region and a cutaneous branch to the skin over the symphysis.

Genitofemoral nerve
The components of the genitofemoral nerve (*nervus genitofemoralis*) originate from the first and second lumbar spinal segments. It passes obliquely downward and forward through the psoas muscle and emerges at the lower level of the third lumbar vertebra.
The main nerve divides into two branches:
• the femoral branch which passes behind the inguinal ligament to the thigh. After penetrating the

Skeleton of the adult female pelvic girdle, formed by the two pelvic bones, the sacrum and the coccyx. The paired os coxae (pelvic bone) originally consists of three separate bones, the ilium, ischium and pubis. These names are retained for descriptive regions for areas of the fused adult pelvic bone.

P

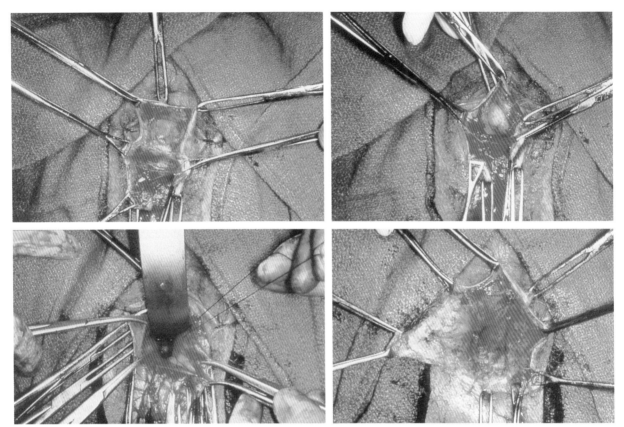

Surgical repair of an enterocele causing a severe pelvic floor disorder.
Upper left: Completed vaginal incision.
Upper right: Identification of enterocele.
Lower left: Placement of permanent suture high in enterocele.
Lower right: Completed enterocele closure.

fascia lata it supplies the skin of the middle upper part of the thigh
- the second branch traverses the inguinal canal to supply the cremaster muscle and the skin of the scrotum and the adjacent part of the thigh

Clinal aspects

Lesions of the spinal cord or lumbar plexus involve the femoral nerve. Rheumatic arthritis, particularly in patients over 50 years of age, causes frequently disorders of the nerve. Furthermore compression or injury of the femoral nerve may result from pelvis fractures and tumors, stab and bullet wounds, etc.

The clinical symptoms depend upon the level of involvement. If the lesion is high enough the iliopsoas muscle is involved. The patient is unable to extend the leg at the knee joint and the flexion of the thigh is severely impaired. However, the patient is able to stand and to walk. The knee jerk is lost. In lesions at a lower level the quadriceps muscle is only paralysed. Sensory disturbances are encountered in the cutaneous distribution of the femoral nerve. In isolated lesions of the saphenus nerve the sensory disturbance extends to inner side of the leg from knee to ankle.

Pelvic inflammatory disease (pid)

The venereal diseases were previously thought of as a limited few such as syphilis, gonorrhoea, and several other less common infections; a later concept expanded the field to include a more extensive group now identified as "sexually transmitted diseases" (STDs).

Past efforts to treat STDs out of existence have failed and we must use all available methods for prevention, in conjunction with treatment, to combat the present epidemic. People are beginning to realize that sexually transmitted diseases are dangerous illnesses that affect men and women of all ages, races and life-styles.

Many of these diseases lead to infertility, birth defects and an increased risk of cancer. The advice for women from doctors in every area of research regarding venereal diseases is simple and blunt: the most important treatment is prevention. And an important part of prevention is knowing your partner's sexual history.

Pelvic inflammatory disease is a bacterial infection, which can involve inflammation of the Fallopian tubes, ovaries and other structures in the pelvic cavity. It has been estimated, there are about 1,300,000 cases in Europe and some 750,000 cases of PID in the United States this year, one third of them requiring hospitalization.

Women who are sexually active at an early age, have multiple sex partners, engage in unprotected sexual activity or use an intrauterine device are at risk for PID.

Dangers

One of the major dangers is infertility. With a really bad infection, it can take as little as a few weeks to become sterile. PID can cause the formation of scar tissue inside the Fallopian tubes, blocking eggs from entering the uterus. Such scarring also increases the risk of tubal pregnancies.

Symptoms

Pelvic inflammatory disease includes the following symptoms:
- abdominal pain or tenderness;
- sudden increase in the severity of menstrual cramps;
- lower back pain;
- painful intercourse;
- a burning sensation during urination;
- vaginal discharge;
- chills;
- fever.

Vaginitis and bladder infection, as well as a series of irregular periods, can also signal pelvic infection.

Treatment

Antibiotics. Conventional or laser surgery may be used to try to open blocked Fallopian tubes.

Pelvic floor problems

Description

Many women notice changes in the lower pelvis as they get older and have had children. They may have a feeling of pelvic pressure or heaviness. These symptoms may be caused by problems with pelvic support. These problems occur most often as the result of childbirth or aging.

Many women suffer from pelvic support problems when they might not have to. If you have any of the symptoms described below, tell your doctor about them. The right diagnosis and treatment can help restore you to a life free of the discomforts of pelvic support problems.

The main causes of pelvic support defects are childbirth and aging. During childbirth, as the baby passes through the vagina, the fascia, ligaments, and muscles around the vagina stretch and may become weakened.

In later years, these tissues may become further thinned and weakened by the loss of the female hormone estrogen. This may cause the pelvic organs to bulge into and even out of the vagina.

Sometimes pelvic support problems occur in women who have never had children or who had no damage when they gave birth. In these women, the cause may be:
- △ Unusual weakening of the vaginal tissues after menopause (when menstrual periods end).
- △ Abnormal increases in abdominal pressure due to a chronic cough (often linked to smoking or lung disorders), heavy lifting, obesity, or constipation.
- △ A weakness of the tissues that is congenital (has been present since birth).

Symptoms

The symptoms of pelvic support problems depend on which organs are involved. These symptoms can range from minor discomfort to major problems that require surgery:
- △ Feeling of pelvic heaviness or fullness, or as though something is falling out of the vagina.
- △ Discomfort or aching pain in the pelvic area.
- △ Pulling or aching sensation in the lower abdomen, groin, or lower back.
- △ Leakage of urine.

All of these symptoms are apt to be more noticeable after you have been standing for a long time or at the end of the day. In very severe cases, the organs may protrude outside the vaginal opening, where they may be seen with a mirror or felt with the fingers. Sometimes it may be necessary to

push the organs back up into the vagina to completely empty the bladder or have a bowel movement.

If the organs stay outside of the vaginal opening, they may become irritated or infected or develop small sores or ulcers that bleed.

Types of pelvic support problems

Based on the organ or organs involved, the main types of pelvic support problems are described as:
- cystocele
- uterine prolapse
- enterocele
- rectocele
- vaginal vault prolapse

Although each problem is described separately, they most often occur in combination with each other.

■ Cystocele

When the base of the bladder descends from its normal position into the vagina, it is called cystocele. A large cystocele may tend to kink the opening of the bladder and interfere with the passing of urine.

If this occurs, you may have to strain or push the bladder up by reaching into the vagina in order to pass urine. If there is a very large cystocele and if the bladder loses some of its ability to contract, it may not completely empty. Urine may leak out when you cough, sneeze, lift objects, or even walk. Because there may be other reasons for loss of urine, your doctor can suggest methods to relieve the symptoms of a cystocele.

The junction of the bladder and the upper urethra is referred to as the bladder outlet or bladder neck. When the tissues that hold up the upper half of the urethra and the bladder neck are weakened, it is called a cystourethrocele.

Descent of the bladder neck often results in urine leakage. Urine is more likely to leak when there is an increase in abdominal pressure caused by walking, jumping, coughing, sneezing, laughing, lifting, or making sudden movements.

The amount of urine lost may be only a few drops, or it may be enough to require changing clothes or wearing pads. You should tell your doctor if you cannot control the leakage of urine.

■ Uterine prolapse

When the uterus drops or descends from its normal position, the condition is called uterine prolapse. The amount the uterus descends may vary. It may descend part of the way down the vagina and remain there, or it may protrude part or all of the way through the vaginal opening.

Women with more severe forms of this condition will often have a feeling of pelvic pressure or a pulling feeling in the groin or lower back. The cervix (the opening of the uterus) may protrude from the vagina, causing discomfort or interfering with intercourse. Uterine prolapse most often occurs when other pelvic organs are also displaced.

■ Enterocele

When a portion of the intestine bulges into the top of the vagina through the tissues at the bottom of the cul-de-sac, it is called an enterocele. An enterocele is felt by the doctor as a bulge into the top and upper back wall of the vagina. This is one of the causes of chronic low back pain.

■ Rectocele

When the rectum bulges into or out of the vagina, it is called a rectocele. A rectocele occurs lower on the back vaginal wall that an enterocele. It is caused by a weakness of the back vaginal wall. A fairly large rectocele may make it very hard to have a bowel movement, especially if you have constipation. Some women have to push the bulge back into the vagina in order to complete a bowel movement.

■ Vaginal vault prolapse

Sometimes after hysterectomy (removal of the uterus), the top, or vault, of the vagina loses its support and descends. This is called vaginal vault prolapse. The degree of the vaginal vault prolapse may vary. It may descend into the vagina and remain there, or it may extend part or all of the way through the vaginal opening. Most women who have vaginal vault prolapse also have an enterocele. Women who have complete vaginal vault prolapse can also have problems with the bladder. Sometimes the rectum protrudes outside of vaginal opening. If the vagina stays outside the body, it may develop ulcers and cause bleeding.

Diagnosis

The first step leading to treatment is proper diagnosis. Yet this is not always simple. The symptoms of pelvic support problems often mimic those of other conditions. Although a woman with these symptoms will usually realize that she has a problem, the exact cause of the problem must be found before the best treatment can be given.

In order to make an exact diagnosis, your doctor will have to obtain a detailed medical history and perform a thorough pelvic exam. He or she may have to examine you while you are lying down and again while you are standing up. Tests may also be done on your urine or bladder function.

If you have a problem with either passing or controlling urine, other tests may be needed:

▲ *Urethroscopy*: the inside of the urethra is viewed through a small, telescope-like instrument.

▲ *Cystoscopy*: the inside of the bladder is viewed through a small, telescope-like instrument.

▲ *Cystometry*: bladder capacity and control are measured.

▲ *Uroflowmetry*: urine flow is measured.

Treatment

Treatment of pelvic support problems may involve special exercises or devices to improve support, or a high-fiber diet or drugs to soften the stool and make bowel movements easier.

After menopause, the hormone estrogen may be given, either by itself or with another hormone called progesterone, to improve the strength of the tissues.

Many women with pelvic support problems do not require further treatment. Some bladder control problems respond best to drugs, while others may be treated by surgery.

Surgery is an elective procedure for which you give your informed consent. You are the best judge of whether symptoms of pelvic support problems are severe enough to warrant surgery. In patients with other medical problems, a special device may be used for support. While no form of treatment, even surgery, can be guaranteed to solve the problem, the chances for getting some degree of relief through a variety of methods are quite good.

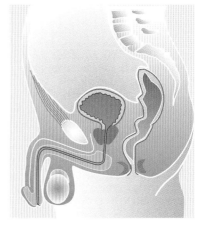

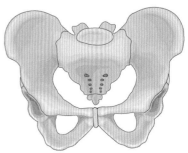

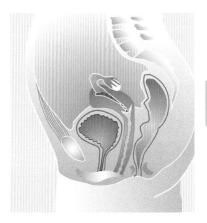

Side view of the male (top) and female (bottom) pelvis with genital organs. The pelvis is the lower (caudal) portion of the trunk of the body, bounded anteriorly and laterally by the hip bones and posteriorly by the sacrum and coccyx.

The frontal view of the bony skeleton of the pelvis is shown in the middle.

P

PEPTIC ULCER DISEASE

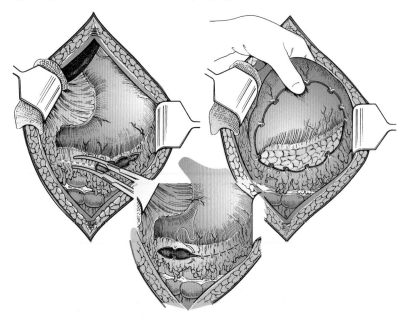

Description

A peptic ulcer is a circumscribed erosion in or loss of the mucous membrane lining of the gastro-intestinal tract. Peptic ulcers are chronic but may have acute exacerbations. They are most often solitary and occur at any level of the gastrointestinal tract exposed to the action of acid and pepsin. They are truly peptic. If acid and pepsin are diverted from an established ulcer, the ulcer will heal and not recur.

In decreasing order of incidence, they occur in the:
- duodenum;
- stomach;
- esophagus;

- stoma (artificial opening) of a stomach and small intestine;
- Meckel's diverticulum;
- jejunum.

However, the most significant sites of peptic ulcer disease are the duodenum and stomach. Peptic ulcers are caused by an increase in acid and pepsin, a decrease in the resistance of the mucosal lining, or a combination of the two.

In a high percentage of cases a bacterial growth of Helicobacter pylori is found. Furthermore the synthesis of prostaglandines (hormonelike fatty acids produced in small amounts in many body tissues) may be disturbed. Although they are often considered together, duodenal and gastric ulcers

have different symptoms and causes. However, both types may be induced by acids and pepsin stimulation.

Although there is a decline in the European countries in the overall incidence of peptic ulcer disease, there has been an increase in the percentage of patients over the age of 60 who have been hospitalized for both gastric and duodenal ulcer disease. Ulcers may recur even after surgical removal of the diseased tissue.

Both types have a low mortality but may cause morbidity. The disease does not occur in primitive tribes or lower primates until they live in conditions of "civilization." Peptic ulcer disease has serious health and economic consequences for society. It is a costly disease in terms of hospitalization, physician care, and medications as well as loss of productivity due to absenteeism.

Stomach ulcer

Stomach ulcers occur most often as single lesions along the lesser curvature and adjacent wall of the antrum up to within 4-5 cm of the sphincter of the pylorus (tubular portion of the stomach leading to the duodenum).

They may occur occasionally in the cardia (part of the stomach that connects with the esophagus), pyloric canal, and greater curvature of the body and fundus of the stomach. Increase in acidity is a less frequent observation in gastric ulcers than in duodenal ulcers. Gastric ulcer patients may have low or normal acid secretion.

However, there are areas of higher acidity in the stomach and duodenum. Acid seems more important in determining where, rather than when, a gastric ulcer will occur, so that lesser

Checking for a perforated posterior peptic ulcer by operative procedures. Dividing the greater omentum to open the lesser sac (left); inspecting the posterior wall of the stomach (right); repairing the omentum after closing the perforation (below).

P

curvature ulcers are frequently associated with diminished acid production.

Causes

Several theories have been proposed for the etiology of gastric ulcer disease. Among these are delayed emptying of the stomach and distention accompanied by increased gastric secretions.

Although this hypothesis is based on experimental and clinical observations, there are reasons to question its accuracy since some patients with gastric ulcers have normal gastric emptying times and low-acid secretion in the presence of high-gastrin level. As noted above, a certain type of bacterium (Helicobacter pylori) and prostaglandines may play a particular role in the cause of the ulcer.

Another theory holds that reflux of the contents of the duodenum, especially bile acids, is due to a dysfunction of the sphincter of the pylorus. Smoking, which is associated with an increased incidence of gastric ulcer, induces reflux. Bed rest improves ulcer healing and A reflux of bile salts may cause gastritis in the distal portion of the stomach and a break in the mucosal barrier. The damaged mucosa next to the acid-secreting mucosa is more susceptible to ulceration. Bile salts occur more frequently and in higher concentrations in the stomachs of gastric ulcer patients than in normal persons or patients with duodenal ulcers.

Gastric ulcers may result from an abnormality in the mucosa of the stomach. Normally, there is a relatively impermeable barrier called the stomach mucosal barrier that prevents the back diffusion of certain ions.

If the barrier is impaired and allows the back diffusion of hydrogen ions, bleeding and ulceration could occur. Other factors may be involved. A genetic factor is implied by the association of gastric ulcer in patients with blood type O and non-secretory status.

Smoking is associated with both stomach and duodenal ulcer. The use of aspirin on 4 or more days/weeks for at least 3 months is associated with a higher incidence of stomach but not

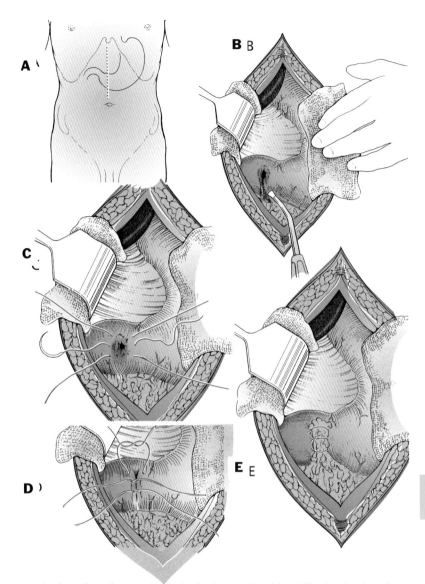

Repair of a perforated peptic ulcer in the duodenum. Site of the midline incision (A); identifying the perforation and aspirating fluid (B); inserting sutures (C); tying the sutures to close the perforation (D) and then again over a tag of the omentum (E).

duodenal ulcer.

Unknown environmental factors may cause ulcers, or the disease may be a heterogenous group of disorders that requires the interrelation of several factors in a predisposed individual.

Stomach ulcer disease is probably a multifactorial disease. Although acid and pepsin may not be the primary causative agents, they are still necessary for the occurrence of gastric ulcers.

Symptoms

Although the erosion of the stomach lining may occur without symptoms, the most common complaints are pain and bleeding. Stomach ulcer pain occurs 30-60 minutes after eating and lasts 60-90 minutes. The pain may be described as:
- "aching"
- "nagging"
- "cramp-like"
- "dull".

Its relationship to food intake results

Peptic ulcer   Questions & Answers

What is a peptic ulcer?

A peptic ulcer is a circumscribed erosion in or loss of the mucous membrane lining of the gastrointestinal tract. Peptic ulcers are chronic but may have acute exacerbations.

They are most often solitary and occur at any level of the gastrointestinal tract exposed to the action of acid and pepsin. They are truly peptic. If acid and pepsin are diverted from an established ulcer, the ulcer will heal and not recur.

Where do peptic ulcers occur in the body?

In decreasing order of incidence, they occur in the:

- duodenum;
- stomach;
- esophagus;
- stoma (artificial opening) of a stomach and small intestine;
- Meckel's diverticulum;
- jejunum.

However, the most significant sites of peptic ulcer disease are the duodenum and stomach.

What is the cause of peptic ulcers?

Peptic ulcers are caused by an increase in acid and pepsin, a decrease in the resistance of the mucosal lining, or a combination of the two.

In a high percentage of cases a bacterial growth of Helicobacter pylori is found. Furthermore the synthesis of prostaglandines (hormonelike fatty acids produced in small amounts in many body tissues) may be disturbed.

How often do peptic ulcers occur in the population?

Although there is a decline in the overall incidence of peptic ulcer disease, there has been an increase in the percentage of patients over the age of 60 who have been hospitalized for both gastric and duodenal ulcer disease.

Ulcers may recur even after surgical removal of the diseased tissue. Both types have a low mortality but may cause morbidity. The disease does not occur in primitive tribes or lower primates until they live in conditions of "civilization".

Peptic ulcer disease has serious health and economic consequences for society. It is a costly disease in terms of hospitalization, physician care, and medications as well as loss of productivity due to absenteeism.

Where to peptic ulcers occur in the stomach (stomach ulcer)?

Stomach ulcers occur most often as single lesions along the lesser curvature and adjacent wall of the antrum up to within 4-5 cm of the sphincter of the pylorus (tubular portion of the stomach leading to the duodenum).

They may occur occasionally in the cardia (part of the stomach that connects with the esophagus), pyloric canal, and greater curvature of the body and fundus of the stomach.Increase in acidity is a less frequent observation in gastric ulcers than in duodenal ulcers.

Gastric ulcer patients may have low or normal acid secretion. However, there are areas of higher acidity in the stomach and duodenum. Acid seems more important in determining where, rather than when, a gastric ulcer will occur, so that lesser curvature ulcers are frequently associated with diminished acid production.

from distention of inflamed areas and release of acid. The patient may associate the pain with eating and may stop eating, with resultant weight loss. Rhythm or chronicity associated with the pain is rare, and the pain covers a wide area in the upper middle part of the abdomen.

Pain radiating into the back indicates penetration, perforation, or obstruction. These three conditions constitute a medical emergency and referral to a hospital is indicated.

The following symptoms may also occur:

- ▲ nausea;
- ▲ bloating;
- ▲ anorexia;
- ▲ vomiting;
- ▲ weight loss.
- ▲ Diagnosis

A small percentage (depending on the diagnostic techniques ranging from five to seven per cent) of gastric ulcers are cancers of the stomach; therefore definitive diagnosis is needed for chronic or recurring symptoms. Bleeding, either acute or chronic, requires medical evaluation. Although the history of a patient is helpful, it is not as definitive for gastric ulcers as it is for duodenal ulcers.

Definitive diagnosis is made by:

- gastroscopy (endoscopy of the stomach);
- X-ray with radiopacque contrast media or computer scan methods;
- gastric analysis for acid and cells;
- testing for blood (occult or frank) in the faeces.

The mortality from gastric ulcers is low, but the morbidity is high. The most frequent and life threatening complications are bleeding and perforation. Gastric ulcers are less responsive to medical management than duodenal ulcers and require surgery more often.

Duodenal ulcer

Duodenal ulcers are lesions of the mucosal lining in the front wall of the first part of the duodenum just beyond the pyloric channel through which stomach contents enter the duodenum. Duodenal ulcers are caused by excessive acid and pepsin. The role of mucosal resistance has been incompletely evaluated. Several abnormalities may explain increased acid and pepsin delivery from the stomach to the duodenum.

The following factors may play a major role:

- ▲ an increased capacity to secrete due to a large parietal cell mass;
- ▲ an increased response to agents that normally stimulate secretion;
- ▲ an increased neural (vagal nerve) or hormonal drive to secrete;
- ▲ a defective inhibition of secretion;
- ▲ an increased gastric emptying rate.

Other factors may be interrelated. Familial or genetic influence is evidenced by the three-fold increase in the incidence of duodenal ulcer in first-degree or primary relatives of patients with duodenal ulcer.

Persons who smoke cigarettes are twice as likely to have duodenal ulceration. Emotional and psychological factors are believed to contribute to the disease but have never been documented.

An increased incidence of duodenal ulcers has been noted in patients with the following diseases:

- arthritis;
- chronic inflammation of the pancreas;
- chronic lung disease;
- increased function of the thyroid gland;
- cirrhosis of the liver.

It has been suggested that duodenal ulcer disease represents a mixture of disorders with different causes but a common pathologic expression which is increased acidity.

■ *Symptoms*

As in stomach ulcer, the primary symptoms of duodenal ulcer are pain and bleeding. However, key differences occur in the way the patient describes the symptoms.

Duodenal ulcer pain is rhythmical, periodic, and chronic. The rhythmical nature corresponds to the release of gastric acid. The pain usually begins 2-3 hours after meals and may continue until the next meal. It occurs when the stomach is empty and is relieved by food.

The sensation is described as:

- "gnawing"
- "burning"
- "pressing"
- "aching"
- resembling hunger pain.

The patient is often awakened at night by the pain. It is usually located in an area in the uppermiddle part of the abdomen. Typically the pain does not radiate. The pain is prone to exacerbation and remission with or without therapy. Exacerbations are most common in the spring and fall and may last for days or months.

If there is bleeding, stool colour and consistency may change. The stools become black and tarry because of partly digested blood (melaena). Other symptoms include:

- ▲ burning behind the breast bone;
- ▲ alteration in bowel habits;
- ▲ nausea;
- ▲ vomiting.

The patient's appetite is good; frequently, weight gain results from the increased food intake to allay pain.

The major complications of duodenal ulcer are bleeding, perforation, and obstruction.

The bleeding may cause anemia, iron deficiency, and low blood pressure. Iron deficiency anemia is characterized by the following symptoms:

- ▲ weakness;
- ▲ easy fatiguability;
- ▲ tachycardia (increased heart rate);
- ▲ dyspnea on exertion;
- ▲ inflammation of the tongue (glossitis);
- ▲ brittleness;
- ▲ deformity of nails;
- ▲ inflammation of the corners of the mouth;
- ▲ stomatitis (inflammation of the lining of the oral cavity).

Perforation and obstruction are indications for acute surgical intervention and are manifested by acute changes in symptoms. Perforation is accompanied by the following symptoms:

- ▲ sudden, severe, generalized abdominal pain or pain radiating to the back;
- ▲ prostration;
- ▲ abdominal rigidity;
- ▲ air or gas in the abdominal cavity.

Treatment

Therapy of gastric and duodenal ulcer is designed to neutralize or decrease acidity. If symptoms do not subside within a few days of such therapy, the diagnosis may be incorrect. Healing commonly requires from 4 to 8 weeks and may require a longer period, particularly for large and longstanding ulcers. Stomach ulcers will be monitored by regular X-ray or endoscopic examination, preferably the latter, until healing is complete.

Treatment is maintained until healing is confirmed, because otherwise the ulcer can be only presumed to be benign. If complete healing does not occur, the ulcer will be biopsied to rule out cancer. Duodenal ulcers heal in 4 to 6 weeks in about 80 per cent of persons, but demonstration of healing by endoscopy is less critical, since they are almost never malignant. Antacids give symptomatic relief, promote healing, and reduce recurrences.

A special group of medicines (histamine H receptor blocking agents; for instance, cimetidine (Tagamet) and ranitidine (Zantac) are preferred by most doctors. Both medicines have so far proved to be safe in both short- and long-term use. As a last resort the nervous supply (vagus nerve) may be decreased by cutting the small branches of this nerve leading to the stomach.

P

PERIODONTAL DISEASES

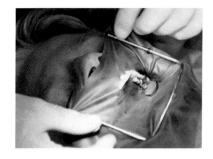

Description

Periodontal diseases inflame and destroy the structures surrounding and supporting the teeth, primarily the gums, the jawbones, and the outer layer of the tooth root.
The following tissues surround and support the tooth and are known collectively as the periodontium:
- gingiva
- periodontal ligament
- cementum
- alveolar process.

Gingiva

The gingiva is composed of keratinizing epithelium and connective tissue.

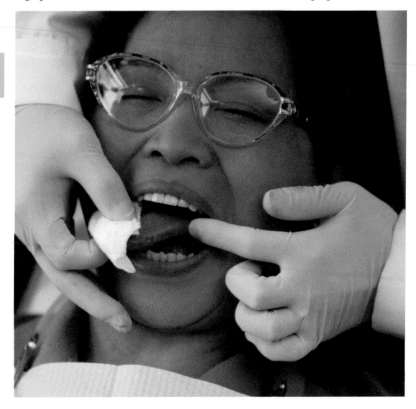

The following terminology is used when describing the gingiva:

▲ *Marginal (free) gingiva*
The portion of the gingiva surrounding the neck of the tooth, not directly attached to the tooth, and forming the soft tissue wall of the gingival sulcus. It extends from the free gingival margin to the free gingival groove.

▲ *Free gingival groove*
The shallow line or depression on the surface of the gingiva dividing the gingiva from the attached gingiva. The free gingival groove often, but not always, corresponds to the location of the bottom of the gingival sulcus.

▲ *Attached gingiva*
The portion of the gingiva that extends apically form the area of the free gingival groove to the mucogingival junction.

▲ *Keratinized gingiva*
Term used to describe the band of keratinized gingiva from the free gingival margin to the mucogingival junction.

▲ *Mucogingival junction*
The scalloped line dividing the attached gingiva from the alveolar mucosa.

▲ *Interdental groove*
The vertical groove, parallel to the long axes of adjacent teeth, found in the interdental area of the attached gingiva.

▲ *Interdental papilla*
The portion of the gingiva that fills the interproximal space between adjacent teeth.

▲ *Gingival sulcus*
The space bounded by the tooth and the free gingiva, and having the epithelial attachment as its base.

Cementum

Cementum, is the calcified structure that covers the anatomic roots of teeth. It consists of a calcified matrix containing collagenous fibers. The inorganic component is approximately 45 to 50 per cent.

▲ *Cementoid*
When first formed, cementum is uncalcified and is known as cemen-

Dentist taking a sample for bacterial examination.

P

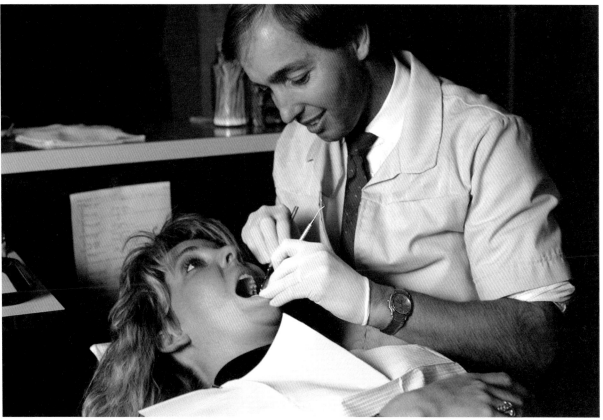

Treatment of gingivitis.

toid. As new layers are formed, the previously formed matrix is calcified and becomes mature cementum. Microscopically, cementum can be divided into two types, cellular and acellular. Functionally, however, there is no difference between the two.

The cellular cementum consists of lacunae that contain cells called cementocytes; the cells communicate with one another by means of canaliculi. The distribution of cellular and acellular cementum on the roots of teeth varies. Generally, cementum covering the coronal half of a root is acellular, whereas that covering the apical half is cellular. Cellular cementum is also more prevalent in the bifurcation and trifurcation areas and around the apices of teeth, and is the type of cementum initially formed during wound healing.

▲ *Functions*
The various functions of cementum can be summarized as follows:

▲ to anchor the tooth to the bony socket by means of the principal fibers of the periodontal ligament;
▲ to compensate, by its continued growth, for the loss of tooth structure through wear;
▲ to facilitate physiologic mesial drift of teeth, and
▲ to permit a continual rearrangement of the periodontal ligament.

Cementum is deposited throughout the life of the tooth. The presence of cementoid is considered a barrier to the apical migration of the epithelial attachment and to resorption of the root surface by the surrounding connective tissue.

Alveolar process
The alveolar process is that portion of the maxilla and mandible that forms and supports the sockets (alveoli) of the teeth.

On the basis of function and adaptation, the alveolar process can be divided into two parts:

■ *Alveolar bone proper*
This is a thin layer of bone that surrounds the root and gives attachment to the periodontal ligament. This bone is also known as the lamina dura or cribriform plate.

■ *Supporting alveolar bone*
This is the portion of the alveolar process that surrounds the alveolar bone proper and gives support to the sockets.

Gingivitis

Gingivitis is inflammation of the gums. It is an extremely common disease in which the gums become red and swollen and bleeds easily. Gingivitis causes little pain in its early stages and thus may not be noticed. However, gingivitis that is left untreated may progress to periodontitis, a more severe gum disease that can result in tooth loss.

Gingivitis may be caused by:

Periodontal disease Questions & Answers

What is the most common cause of periodontal disease?

The vast majority of diseases of the periodontal tissue results from bacterial infection. Although other factors may affect the periodontium in one way or another, the dominating causative agents of periodontal disease are colonized microorganisms and their products.

What is the significance of bacterial plaque for inflammatory processes of the gingiva and periodontium?

Bacterial plaque is directly responsible for the inflammatory diseases of the periodontium, such as gingivitis and periodontitis.

What kind of factors play a role in the development of periodontitis?

There are a number of systemic disorders that adversely affect the periodontium, but no systemic disorder is known to cause chronic destructive periodontitis in the absence of bacterial plaque.

Likewise, other local factors act in conjunction with bacterial plaque to produce chronic disease of the periodontium. Two factors which may initiate periodontal disease in the absence of bacterial plaque are malignancies and primary occlusal traumatism.

What are the major causes of periodontal disease?

The following aspects of the etiology of periodontal disease will be described:
- tooth accumulated materials
- bacterial plaque
- microorganisms of plaque
- other constituents of plaque
- mechanisms of action
- occurrence of disease
- systemic factors
- local contributing factors
- neoplasms

What is bacterial plaque?

Bacterial plaque is a material of densely packed, colonized and colonizing microorganisms, growing on and tenaciously attached to the tooth. Bacterial plaque is not removed with a forceful water spray, but it is readily removed by other mechanical means.

What is the pathological effect of bacterial plaque?

Although many and varied microorganisms normally reside in the oral cavity, their potential for causing damage to the teeth and the periodontium is not realized until they become attached to hard structures, such as teeth, restorations, and orthodontics or prosthetic appliances.

Once attached and undisturbed, the microorganisms multiply to form colonies of either the pure or mixed type, which are clinically recognizable on a wet tooth as either distinct round colonies or coalesced colonial masses. If the tooth is dried, the masses appear as a dull white film of varying thickness.

Unless they are present in massive amounts, colonies may be difficult to see without the most careful scrutiny in good light. Normally, white or transparent, they blend with the normal colour of the tooth but can be made readily visible by staining with disclosing materials.

- plaque formation
- certain drugs
- vitamin deficiency
- infections
- pregnancy
- menopause
- leukemia
- impacted tooth

Plague-induced gingivitis can be prevented with good oral hygiene - the daily use of a toothbrush and dental floss. Some mouthwashes also help control plaque. Medical conditions that might cause or worsen gingivitis should be treated or controlled. In case of infections antibiotics are also prescribed.

When a person has gingivitis due to an impacted tooth, a dentist may flush under the flap of gum to rinse out the debris and bacteria. If X-rays show that a lower tooth is not likely to emerge completely, a dentist may remove the upper tooth and prescribe antibiotics for a few days before removing the lower one. Sometimes a dentist removes the lower teeth immediately.

Periodontitis

Periodontitis is a severe form of gingivitis in which the inflammation of the gums extends to the supporting structures of the tooth. Once the inflammatory process involves the alveolar crest of teeth, the disease is called periodontitis. The periodontal fibers immediately apical to the sulcus are disrupted, and the junctional epithelium migrates along the root surface, resulting in a deeper sulcus (pocket).

Pocket formation

A pocket is a gingival sulcus pathologically deepened by periodontal disease. It is bordered by the tooth on one side, by ulcerated epithelium on the other, and has the junctional epithelium at its base.

Deepening of the sulcus can occur in three ways:
- By movement of the free gingival margin coronally, as observed in gingivitis.
- By movement of the junctional epithelium apically, with separation of the coronal portion from

the tooth.

▲ A combination of the above mentioned two mechanisms. Pockets may be classified as gingival pocket, suprabony pocket end infrabony pocket.

▲ Gingival pocket
Deepening of the gingival sulcus, mainly owing to an increase in the size of the gingiva, without any appreciable loss of the underlying tissues or apical migration of the junctional epithelium.

▲ Suprabony pocket
Deepening of the gingival sulcus, with destruction of the adjacent periodontal ligament and alveolar bone, associated with apical migration of the junctional epithelium. The bottom of the pocket and the junctional epithelium always remain coronal to the alveolar bone.

▲ Infrabony pocket
Deepening of the gingival sulcus to a level where the bottom of the pocket and the junctional epithelium are apical to the crest of the alveolar bone. In this type of pocket, the alveolar bone becomes a part of the pocket wall. One, two, or three osseous walls, or various combinations thereof, may remain, depending on the amount and pattern of bone loss.

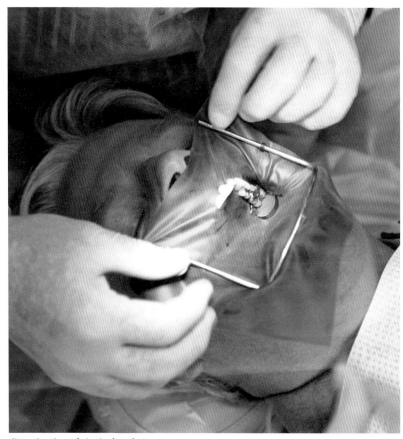

Examination of gingival pockets.

Spread of inflammation
Periodontitis usually develops as a sequel to persistent chronic gingivitis and has an identical etiology. Intendentally, inflammation and bacterial products spread from the gingiva to the alveolar process along the neurovascular bundle of the interdental canal at the crest of the septum.

Inflammation spreads along the course of the vascular channels because the loose connective tissue surrounding the neurovascular bundles offers less resistance than the dense fibers of the periodontal ligament.

The location where the inflammation enters the bone depends on the location of the vessels. In some instances, large vessels will exit at one side of the alveolar crest, permitting direct spread of inflammation into the marginal portion of the periodontal ligament.

After reaching the narrow spaces, the destructive process extends laterally into the periodontal ligament via the intra-alveolar openings. On the facial and lingual surfaces, the destructive process spreads along the supraperiosteal vessels and penetrates into the narrow spaces via the channels in the outer cortex.

Extension of the chronic inflammatory process into the alveolar bone is marked by infiltration of the marrow by leukocytes, new blood vessels, and proliferating fibroblasts.

Progressive extension is accompanied by destruction of the trabeculae and subsequent reduction in the height of the alveolar bone. This destruction is not a continuous process.

It is accompanied by osteoblastic activity and new bone formation even in the presence of inflammation. Likewise, there is a constant re-formation of the transseptal fibers as the attachment apparatus is destroyed.

Alveolar bone loss does not occur until the physiologic equilibrium of bone is disturbed to the point where resorption exceeds formation.

The general resistance factors of the individual play an important role in governing the rate at which bone loss progresses in untreated periodontal disease.

Symptoms
Pockets are usually asymptomatic, but patients occasionally complain of a "deep, gnawing pain," itchiness of the gums, sensitivity to heat and cold, a foul taste, bleeding gums, food sticking between the teeth, a toothache in the absence of caries, and increased spacing between their anterior teeth. It spite of a variety of signs and symptoms, or lack thereof, the only reliable method of detecting a pocket's existence is by probing the space between the gingiva and tooth surface.

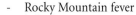

PNEUMONIA

Introduction

Pneumonia is an inflammation of the lungs caused primarily by bacteria, viruses, chemical irritants, vegetable dusts and allergic substances, but there are more than 50 different causes. The major causes of pneumonia are:

■ *Specific microbial causes*
- Influenza
- parainfluenza
- adenovirus
- respirovirus
- syncytial virus
- coxsackie viruses
- rhinoviruses
- echovirus
- reovirus
- cytomegalovirus
- Herpes simplex virus
- Mycoplasma pneumoniae
- pneumococcus
- staphylococcus
- hemolytic streptococcus
- Hemophilus influenzae
- Mycobacterium tuberculosis
- klebsiella
- Histoplasma capsulatum
- Coccidioides immitis
- viruses of certain childhood diseases such as measles

■ *Diseases accompanied by pneumonia*
- Tularaemia
- brucellosis
- rheumatic fever
- syphilis
- typhus
- Rocky Mountain fever
- infectious mononucleosis (glandular fever)
- trichinosis

■ *Pneumonias not caused by infections*
- Oil aspiration
- radiation
- chemicals
- allergy
- vegetable dusts
- silo-filler's disease

When the infection involves an entire lobe it is called lobar pneumonia; when it affects only parts of the lobe, it is called segmental or lobular pneumonia; and when it is confined to alveoli, it is referred to as bronchopneumonia.

Conditions that predispose a person to contract pneumonia include:
- the common cold;
- other acute respiratory infections caused by viruses;
- acute and chronic alcoholism;
- malnutrition;
- debility;
- exposure;
- coma;
- tumor of the bronchi;
- foreign matter in the airways;
- treatment with immunosuppressive drugs;
- hypostasis (stagnation of blood in a part due to inadequate circulation).

The two most common pneumonias are those caused by the pneumococcus bacterium and those caused by viruses.

■ *Pneumococcal pneumonia*
This is the most common pneumonia caused by bacteria, and many of its features are similar to those caused by other micro-organisms. The disease is generally sporadic but most frequent in winter. Healthy or convalescent car-

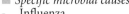

Macroscopic picture of lung tissue of a fatal viral infection.

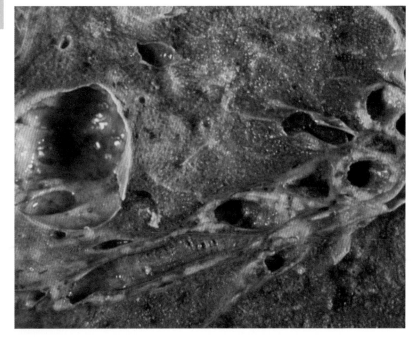

P

riers infect others but there is no practical way to distinguish these carriers, especially from those with chronic bronchitis, to eliminate the microorganisms.

The pneumococci reach the lungs via the airways. They lodge in the bronchioles and cause collapse of corresponding alveoli, where they proliferate and initiate an inflammatory process that begins with an outpouring of protein-rich fluid into the spaces of the air sacs (alveolar spaces). This fluid acts as a culture medium for the pneumococci and as a vehicle for their spread to other alveoli, segments and lobes of the lungs.

Signs and symptoms

The onset of signs and symptoms is sudden, with a shaking chill, sharp pain in the involved part of the chest, cough with early sputum production, fever and headache. Other symptoms may include nausea and vomiting and, in children, a convulsion ("fit"). Difficulty in breathing is frequent and respiration is rapid (25 to 40 breaths per minute) and painful due to the involvement of the pleura. An expiratory grunt is characteristic. Delirium may occur, especially in alcoholics when fever is high or cyanosis is marked. Often cyanotic and sweating profusely, the person is acutely ill.

The temperature rises rapidly to between 38°C and 40.5°C (100.4°-105°F); the pulse accelerates to between 100 and 130. Signs of consolidation may be lacking during the first few hours, but fine rales and suppressed breath sounds are heard by the doctor over the involved area. Frank consolidation, involving part of one or more lobes, is found later.

The cough is initially dry and hacking; however, if bronchitis preceded the pneumonia, coughing produces purulent sputum. Coughing usually occurs in extremely painful paroxysms, but later stages, the cough is more productive and usually painless.

The sputum, pinkish or blood-flecked at first, becomes rusty at the height of the illness, then yellow and foul-tasting as recovery advances.

Gastrointestinal symptoms - abdominal distention, jaundice, diarrhea - are

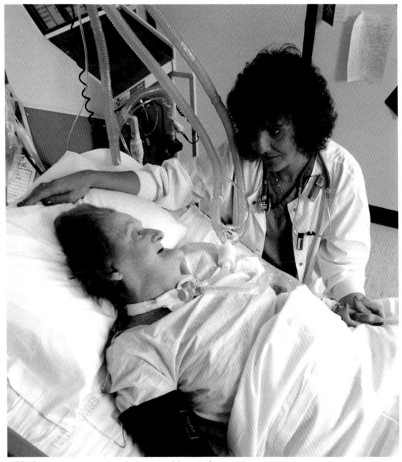

Elderly woman recovering from a viral lung infection.

often present. In pneumonia involving the middle or lower lobes of the right lung, tenderness and rigidity of the right side of the abdomen may mimic gall bladder disease, appendicitis or peritonitis.

Prognosis

Of those treated, 95 to 98 per cent of those between the ages of 2 and 50 survive; those treated during the first five days of illness being the most likely to recover.

Any of the following factors makes the outlook less favourable and convalescence more prolonged:

▲ age less than one year;
▲ age over 60 years;
▲ a positive blood culture (i.e. the bacteria have invaded the bloodstream);

▲ involvement of two or more lobes;
▲ more than 5000 white blood cells in the blood count (indicating widespread infection);
▲ underlying chronic disease;
▲ development of a pneumococci infection elsewhere, such as meningitis (inflammation of the membrane covering the brain and spinal cord) or endocarditis (inflammation of the membrane lining the heart).

Treatment

Pending the culturing of the pneumococci microorganisms, the doctor will tentatively base treatment on the person's medical history, physical examination and examination of the sputum, and it will consist of prescribing specific antibiotics. The response to

Pneumonia Questions & Answers

What are the cough characteristics in pneumonia?

The cough may be dry initially, but usually becomes productive with purulent, bloodstreaked or "rusty" sputum. These features are typically for pneumococcal pneumonia in a previously healthy person. In many instances, especially among patients at age extremes, the disease is more insidious with relatively fewer symptoms to suggest infection of the lower respiratory tract.

What are the common findings of pneumonia on physical examination?

Findings on physical examination are variable depending on the character of the process and the stage in which the patient is evaluated. The doctor may find typical lung signs of lobar pneumonia. A chest X-ray invariably shows a lung infiltrate, although findings may be minimal or undetectable during the first several hours.

How can the causing agent be demonstrated in pneumonia?

Pneumococci are clearly responsible for most cases of lobar pneumonia in which the chest X-ray shows dense consolidation confined to a single lobe with typical air bronchograms. The presence of the pneumococci in sputum can be demonstrated with various techniques in the laboratory of the doctor or hospital. Pneumococcal pneumonia will be suspected by the doctor in anyone with an acute febrile illness associated with chills, chest pain, and cough.

What are the common complications in pneumonia?

Serious, potentially lethal complications include overwhelming sepsis (spread of germs through the body), sometimes associated with adult respiratory distress syndrome and/or shock. Some patients develop so-called lung superinfections; during the usual course of treatment, temporary improvement is followed by deterioration with recurrence of fever and new lung infiltrates.

What is the prognosis of pneumonia in an adult patient?

Although the morbidity and mortality of pneumococcal pneumonia have changed substantially since the advent of antibiotics; these medicines have minimal impact on mortality during the first 5 days of illness. The overall mortality rate in developed countries is 5 per cent.

Factors that herald a prognosis include the following:
- age extremes, especially younger than 1 year and older than 60 years of age;
- involvement of more than 1 lobe of the lungs;
- presence of more than 5000 white blood cells per millilitre in the peripheral blood;
- presence of associated diseases (for instance, cirrhosis, heart failure, diabetes, uraemia, etc.);
- development of complications such as meningitis or valvular inflammation of the heart (endocarditis).

What is the best treatment for a common pneumonia?

Specific antibiotics are available for the various types of pneumonias. There are more than 80 different serotypes of pneumococci. Vaccines are available containing some 25 of the 80-plus antigens. These serotypes account for about 90 per cent of antigens that cause pneumococcal infections. Most children older than 2 years and adults show an antigenic response within 2 to 3 weeks after vaccination.

In case of pneumococcal pneumonia for whom is vaccination recommended?

Vaccination is recommended for children older than 2 years and adults who have an increased risk for pneumococcal disease or its complications.
Included are the following persons with:
- chronic heart disease;
- chronic lung diseases;
- dysfunction of the spleen;
- Hodgkin's disease;
- cirrhosis of the liver;
- alcoholism;
- kidney failure;
- organ transplant.

What is the antibiotic treatment schedule for pneumonia?

Treatment is with a specific antibiotic (usually a penicillin preparation). Mild ill patients who are treated relatively early in the course will usually defervesce during the first 24 to 48 hours; however, seriously ill patients and particularly those with the poor prognostic features noted above will often require more than 4 days to become without fever.

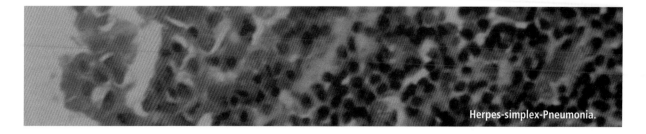

Herpes-simplex-Pneumonia.

the treatment is often prompt, but fever may persists for four days or longer in 50 per cent of patients.

Persisting fever without physical improvement demands careful re-examination of the patient. In uncomplicated illness, antibiotic therapy is continued until the person has been without fever for at least 48 hours. Supportive measures are also instituted immediately: complete bedrest, fluids and, if needed, oxygen and analgesics (painkillers) are given during the acute phase. Oxygen is given to patients with cyanosis, marked breathing difficulties, circulatory disturbances, feebleness or delirium.

Those who are treated during the first two days of illness and who respond rapidly may be allowed out of bed after they have been without fever for two to three days. Longer periods of partial bed rest may be required for those who survive a stormy course.

Pneumonia caused by viruses

Viral pneumonia may be caused by various agents (see above). The pneumonia usually results when a non-immune individual is exposed to infected persons shedding virus, and may account for about 75 per cent of all acute lung infections in some populations - for example, in schools and military recruits.

Most cases of viral pneumonia are mild, and lung involvement is often undetected. Severe and even fatal illness may result, however, especially with influenza A virus. Pneumonias due to varicella (chickenpox) or herpes simplex virus are associated with the disseminated form of these infections and may be extensive and severe. Symptoms vary widely, from those of the common cold to those of rapidly progressive respiratory failure. Constitutional symptoms may be pronounced, with severe headache, loss of appetite, fever and muscle pain; cough is common.

Identifying the microorganism responsible for sporadic viral pneumonia is difficult, but may be important in outbreaks confined to an institution or community.

The pneumonias complicating childhood infectious diseases - for instance, measles, herpes, chickenpox - may be identified tentatively by the

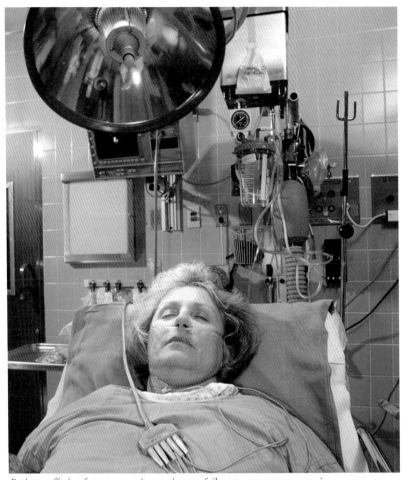

Patient suffering from progressive respiratory failure to a severe pneumonia.

structure and other characteristics of any rash.

Since isolation of viruses is still not feasible in many hospitals, the diagnosis of viral pneumonia is often based on clinical or epidemiological findings and the results of blood tests.

The prognosis varies widely with the specific virus, the extent of lung involvement, the patient's age and the presence or absence of underlying disease. Treatment involves the relief of symptoms.

Preventive vaccination with influenza is available for those at high risk of serious infection and may be given to persons over the age of 50, those with chronic heart or lung disease, and pregnant women. The drug amantadine, if given very early in the course of influenza A infection, may moderate the course of the disease.

Sputum with pneumococci from a patient suffering from a bacterial pneumonia.

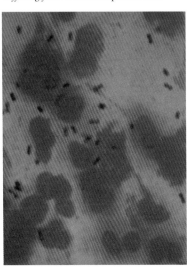

PREGNANCY

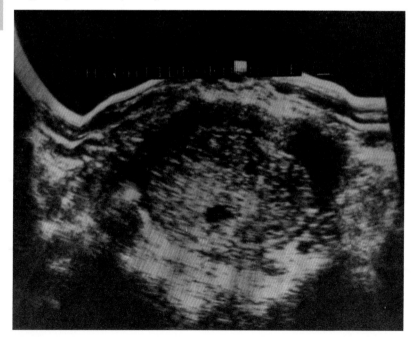

Introduction

Pregnancy is defined as the condition of having a developing embryo or fetus in the body. The average time of delivery is 280 days from the beginning of the last menstrual period, whereas the duration of pregnancy (age of the baby) is about 266 days (38 weeks). Pregnancy may extend to 300 days, or even more, in which case the baby tends to be heavier.

First trimester

You may have none, some or many of the following early signs of pregnancy. If you have had regular periods, you will probably notice that you have missed a period. However, some women do blood for the first two or three months even when they are pregnant, but bleeding is usually short and there is scant blood.

Also, about seven days or so after conception, the blastocyst, the tiny group of cells which becomes the embryo, attaches itself to the uterine wall, and you may have slight vaginal spotting, called implantation bleeding, while new blood vessels are being formed.

You may have to urinate more often because of increased hormonal changes; pituitary hormones affect the adrenals, glands which change the water balance in your body, so you retain more water. Also, your enlarging uterus presses against your bladder.

Your breasts will probably swell. They may tingle, throb or hurt. Your milk glands begin to develop. Because of an increased blood supply to your breasts, veins become more prominent. Your nipples and the area around them (areola) may darken and become broader.

Second trimester

At about the fourth month the fetus begins to take up much more space. Your waist becomes thicker, you clothes no longer fit you, your womb begins to swell below your waist and, around the fourth or fifth month, you can begin to feel light movements ("quickening"). The fetus has been moving for months, but it is only now that you can feel it. Often you will feel it first just before you fall asleep.

In some women the area around the nipple, the areola, becomes very dark due to hormonal changes. The line from the navel to the pubic region gets dark too, and sometimes pigment in the face becomes dark, making a kind of a mask.

Your uterus is changing too. It is growing. Its height increases and lines may appear, pink or reddish streaks. Your skin may become very dry; add oils to your bath and rub your skin with oil. By midpregnancy your breasts, stimulated by hormones, are functionally complete for nursing purposes. After about the nineteenth week a thin amber or yellow substance called colostrum may come out of your nipples; there is no milk yet.

As a result of pressure of pelvic organs, veins in your rectum (hemorrhoidal veins) may become dilated and sometimes painful. To prevent hemorrhoids, practice rectal Kegel exercises, which resemble the pelvic floor exer-

Ultrasonogram of a young embryo. Ultrasonography is the safest imaging procedure, to be performed at least once during a pregnancy to make sure the fetus is normally formed and to verify the expected date of delivery

P

cises except that you contract your rectal muscles instead.

Third trimester

Your uterus is becoming very large. It feels hard when you touch it. It is a strong muscular container. You can feel and see the movements of your fetus from the outside now, too, as it changes position, turns somersaults, hiccups.

Sometimes it puts pressure on your bladder, which makes you feel that you need to urinate when you don't, and which can hurt a little, or sometimes a lot, for very brief periods. Sometimes toward the end of pregnancy it puts pressure on the nerves at the top of your legs, which can be painful, too.

Your baby will be lying in a particular position, sometimes head down, back to your front, sometimes lying crossways. It moves around often. Your doctor can help you discover which position the baby is in.

It becomes increasingly uncomfortable for you to lie on our stomach. You may experience shortness of breath. There is pressure on your lungs from your uterus, and your diaphragm may be moved up as much as an 2-3 cm. Even so, because your thoracic (chest) cage widens, you breathe in more air when you are pregnant then when you are not.

Since your body becomes heavier, you will tend to walk differently for balance, often leaning back to counteract a heavier front.

This can cause backaches, for which there are exercises. Your pelvic joints are also much more separated. At about four to two weeks before birth, and sometimes as early as the seventh month, the baby's head settles into your pelvis. This is called "lightening" or "dropping." It takes pressure off your stomach.

Some women do feel much lighter. And if you have been having trouble breathing, pressure is now off your diaphragm. This "dropping" can cause constipation; your bowls are more obstructed than they were.

And for water retention, an average pregnant woman retains from 3 to 6 litres of liquid, half of this in the last ten weeks. Swollen ankles are common.

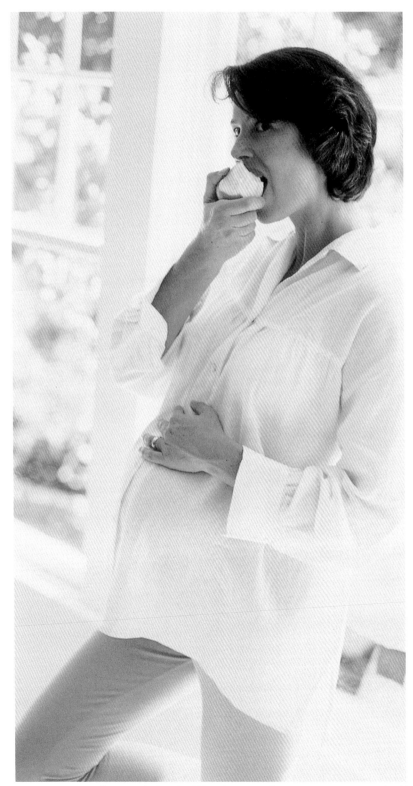

During pregnancy, the woman's diet should be adequate and nutritious. Most women should add about 250 calories to their daily diet to provide nourishment for the developing fetus.

P

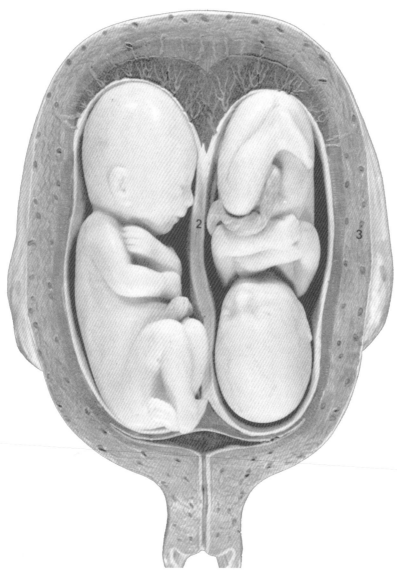

Pregnancy of twins; one baby in head presentation, the other one in breech presentation.

Exercises

Exercise is very important to you and your baby. If you stay active you will feel better. Outdoor exercises and recreation give you a chance to get sunshine and fresh air. Walking is particularly good because it strengthens some of the muscles you will use in labor.

If you are normally active in sports, continue to enjoy them. However, it is wise to stop when you get tired. Also, try team activities instead of individual games, and avoid strenuous workouts.

Do things with your friends and family - swim in a pool, dance, go on a picnic, and participate in light sports that pose no danger of falling or being bumped. If you are thinking of trying a new sport or exercise, or have been using a specific exercise routine, talk it over with your doctor or someone at the clinic.

Avoid lifting heavy objects and moving furniture while you are pregnant. Stretching will not harm you or your body, but do not reach for things from a chair or ladder because you might lose your balance and fall.

During the latter part of your pregnancy, you will probably begin to feel awkward because your balance is affected by your increasing size. At this point you may substitute walking for more active sports.

Rest

Rest is just as important as exercise during pregnancy. Be sure to get plenty of sleep at night. Most pregnant women need about 8 hours of sleep but your needs may be different. You may also need to rest during the day. If your work requires you to be on your feet most of the day, try to sit down, put your feet up, and close your eyes whenever it is convenient.

But if you spend most of your time sitting, get up and walk around for a few minutes every hour. When you are at home, take a nap during the day, especially if you have children who take naps.

Bathing

During pregnancy you will probably perspire more and have a slight vaginal discharge because your body is going through many hormonal

Pregnant lifestyle

Pregnancy is a perfectly natural state and should be a happy, healthy, and exciting period in your life.

But it does represent a major change, and you have to adapt your lifestyle to meet the needs of the baby developing inside you.

Your baby is completely dependent on you for everything, so your diet must include and supply what your baby needs to build a healthy body.

But remember, just as your baby gets its food from you,

▲ if you smoke, so does your baby;
▲ if you drink alcoholic beverages - so does your baby;
▲ if you use drugs or medicines - so does your baby.

All these things can harm your developing baby and may cause health and developmental problems later. If you do any of these potentially harmful things, this is a good time to "kick the habit."

Talk to your doctor or someone at the clinic; they will be able to advise and help you.

changes. Your usual daily bathing or showering will not only refresh and relax you, but also help prevent infection.

Special creams are available to soothe and soften dry, scaly skin should it occur. Never douche during pregnancy unless your doctor specifically tells you to.

It is always a good idea to put a rubber mat in the tub or shower to prevent slipping. Keep the water temperature warm but not hot, particularly in early and later pregnancy because hot water may make you feel dizzy or light-headed.

Tub baths may become more difficult near the end of pregnancy when your center of balance shifts. You may want to switch to showers or have someone help you in and out of the tub.

Breast care

Wearing a bra that provides firm support during your pregnancy may make your breasts more comfortable. About the third or fourth month, you may need to get a larger bra (such as a maternity bra) that fits well without pressing, binding, or rubbing against your nipples. If your breasts are large, you may be more comfortable wearing a bra at night as well as during the day.

About the middle of pregnancy, your nipples may drip a small amount of clear or yellowish fluid called colostrum. This is a sign that your body is preparing for breast feeding. Colostrum can dry into a crust around your nipples and should be washed off with only warm water since soap and alcohol dry out the skin and make your breasts sore. If colostrum leakage is a problem, wear a cotton or absorbent pad in your bra. To avoid irritation or infection, the pad should be replaced when wet.

Preparing to breast feed

If you plan to breast feed your baby, start to prepare your breasts during the seventh or eighth month. Your doctor or midwife may suggest some exercises every day.

They may include the following:
- Rubbing your nipples gently with a towel.
- Gently rolling each nipple between your thumb and finger

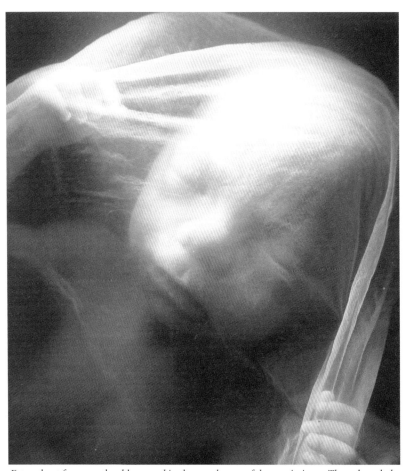

Fetus about four months old, covered in the membranes of the amniotic sac. The unborn baby is now about 6½ inches long and weighs 7 oz.

four or five times.
- Gently stretching each nipple to the side.
- Massaging your breasts.
- Exposing your breasts to sunlight and air.
- Letting your breasts rub against your clothing several times each day.

Care of teeth

Oral health is an important part of your total health and physical well-being. As early as possible in your pregnancy, see your dentist to be checked for tooth decay, gum disease, and other dental problems and get the necessary treatment. Because you require special care and attention at this time be sure to tell your dentist that you are pregnant - or suspect that you may be pregnant.

Discuss with your dentist the use of local X-rays, anesthetic agents, pain medications, and other drugs. Your dentist is trained to weigh the benefits and risks of your particular situation and recommend alternative procedures and treatments.

Brush and floss your teeth at least once a day. This disrupts plaque and bacteria that cause tooth decay and also will help you maintain healthy gums.

Oral hygiene practice and a well-balanced diet will help you maintain bright and healthy teeth. A well-balanced diet will also insure that your baby develops healthy second teeth.

Avoid sweets such as caramels, hard candies, sticky foods, and soft drinks. If you have some of these occasionally, eat or drink them at one time instead of several times throughout

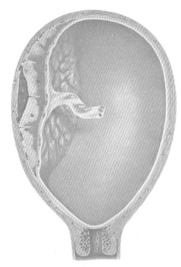

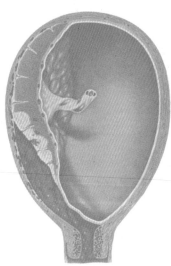

P

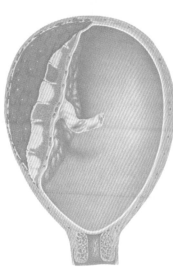

the day - and then brush your teeth or at least rinse with water. Sugar build-up in your mouth, even for a few hours, can contribute to tooth decay.

Clothing

During the fourth month of pregnancy you may notice that your clothes are tight and your bras are uncomfortable. Maternity clothes are not really necessary at this time, but loose clothing may be more comfortable. Some women feel much warmer during pregnancy and find lighter weight fabrics are more pleasant.

Avoid tight belts, bras, girdles, slacks, garters and knee socks. Clothes that cut circulation around the legs lead to varicose or enlarged veins.

A bra that fits provides good support to your breasts. If you plan to breast feed your baby, it may be more economical to buy a nursing bra to wear during pregnancy, too. Nursing bras are designed with flaps that unlock to allow easy access for breast feeding.

Your shoes should have a medium or low heel; and provide firm support. Wearing high heels may result in an accident or an aching back.

Sexual relations

For a healthy woman, there are few restrictions on sexual intercourse during pregnancy. However, it is perfectly normal for your feelings about sex to change during this time. You may go through temporary periods when you desire for sexual intercourse increases or decreases.

As the pregnancy progresses and your abdomen becomes large, intercourse may be uncomfortable and you and your partner may want to experiment with more comfortable positions.

Usually there is no problem with having intercourse into the ninth month, but it is best to discuss this with your doctor. There may be times when your doctor suggests that you do not have intercourse because it might interfere

Above: hematoma between placenta and uterine wall.
Middle: hematoma causing vaginal bleeding.
Below: large hematoma between placenta and uterine wall causing ablation of the placenta.

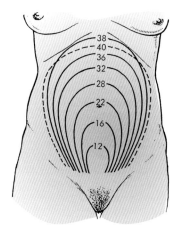

The uterus becomes abdominal by 12 weeks and increase in abdominal size is apparent by 16 weeks. The reduction in fundal height which occurs between 38 and 40 weeks is called "lightening", and is due to the descent of the foetus as the lower segment and cervix prepare for labour. It may not occur in women who have had a previous pregnancy; and the fundal height is an uncertain guide to maturity.

with the normal course of your pregnancy.

Intercourse is likely to be restricted in early pregnancy if you have a history of miscarriages, or later if you have had premature births.

See your doctor as soon as possible if intercourse is painful, if you have bleeding or infection, or if your water breaks prematurely. When you have any of these signs, discontinue intercourse.

Work

More women then ever are continuing work during pregnancy. It is best to discuss this matter with your doctor, however, because each woman should be evaluated individually. If your pregnancy is complicated by medical, obstetric, or other problems, you and your doctor must decide how long it is advisable for you to continue working.

In general, a normal, healthy woman who has no complications may work throughout pregnancy if her job presents no greater potential hazards than those she faces in normal daily life.

Special consideration should be given to occupational hazards such as heavy lifting, moving, other strenuous physical activities, or exposure to chemicals (gases, dusts, fumes), radiation, and infections.

Tell your nurse or doctor at your place of work as soon as you know you are pregnant. You may need to be reassigned temporarily to another type of work that does not pose any danger to your pregnancy.

It is even better to discuss the problem of occupational hazards when planning your baby. It is also important that you discuss any occupational hazards with the doctor or nurse who sees you for your prenatal care.

Travel

Traveling during your pregnancy is fine. Airplane, train, and bus travel are less tiring for long distances because you can get up and move around.

When you travel in a car, it is important to wear both a shoulder harness and a lap belt to protect you and the baby in case of an accident. Just fasten the belt as low as possible below the baby.

Sitting for long periods of time may cause leg cramps, discomfort, and tiredness, particularly late in the pregnancy. To keep from getting tired during a car trip, stop about every 2 hours to stretch, walk about, and go to the bathroom.

Late in your pregnancy, it is a good idea to avoid long trips. By staying close to home, your baby can be born where you planned and where your medical history is known. If you must travel at this time, ask your doctor to refer you to a doctor in the area you will be visiting and ask for a copy of your medical chart to take with you.

Smoking

Not smoking is one of the best gifts you can give your unborn child. Women who do not smoke are more likely to deliver a healthy baby of normal weight than women who do smoke.

Smoking cigarettes during pregnancy is directly associated with low birth weight, premature birth, miscarriage, and other complications. While there are no safe levels of smoking, the fewer cigarettes the better.

The risk of delivering a low birth weight baby may be reduced if a

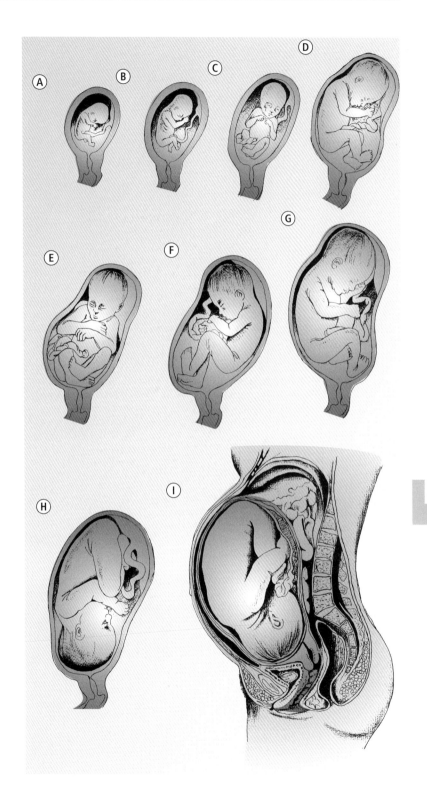

Development of embryonal and foetal stages during pregnancy. A. 8 weeks; B. 12 weeks; C. 16 weeks; D. 20 weeks; E. 24 weeks; F. 28 weeks; G. 32 weeks; H. 36 weeks; I. 40 weeks.

P

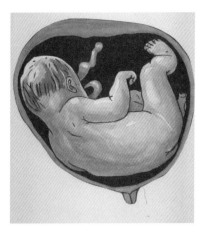
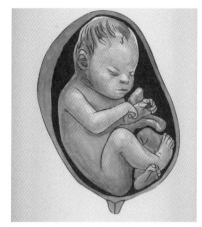
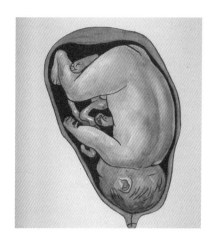

woman gives up smoking before the fourth month of pregnancy. Smoking during the time of breast feeding is also not advisable since the nicotine will be passed on to the baby through your breast milk. Babies born to mothers who smoked while pregnant and after delivery have a higher incidence of sudden infant death syndrome (SIDS, crib death).

Children whose mothers smoked during pregnancy are more susceptible to respiratory problems in early childhood and may be slightly behind in their age group in physical growth. If either parent continues to smoke after the baby is born, the child may have a greater risk of developing bronchitis or pneumonia.

Alcohol
Alcohol in any form can be harmful to a developing baby. All women of childbearing age should take the following precautions:
▲ do not drink alcoholic beverages when you are pregnant or are considering pregnancy. In the crucial early period of a baby's development - often before pregnancy is recognized - maternal consumption of alcohol increases the risk of abnormalities;
▲ be aware of the alcoholic content of food and drugs.

Researchers have found increased miscarriages and decreased birth weight associated with consumption of even 1 ounce or less of absolute (pure) alcohol per day.

This is the amount of alcohol found in 2 standard drinks. Women who drink 3 ounces (the amount in six standard drinks) or more of absolute alcohol per day are at very high risk of

Three normal presentations of the head of the foetus in labour. The occiput is the presenting part.

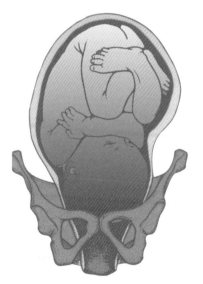
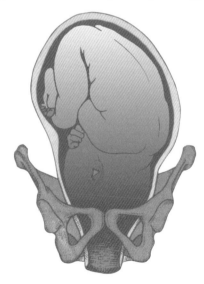
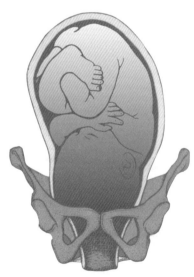

delivering a child with fetal alcohol syndrome (FAS).

You should also be aware that many cough medicines and nighttime cold medicines contain large amounts of alcohol. FAS can be entirely prevented if a pregnant woman does not take alcohol - in the form of alcoholic beverages or unprescribed medicine.

The alcohol in beverages such as wine, beer, and liquor is a rich source of calories, but these calories do not contribute to good nutrition. Alcohol can depress your appetite, causing you to replace nutritious food in your diet with empty calories.

Caution should be exercises even after your baby is born if you plan to breast feed. Alcohol passes to your baby through your breast milk in the same concentration as it is in your blood.

Medicines and drugs
You should take only those medicines prescribed by your doctor. This is particularly important during the first twelve weeks. *See the descriptions of the individual prescription and non-prescription drugs.*

Minor complaints

Heartburn
This is probably due to esophageal reflux of gastric acid. The enlarging uterus encourages some degree of hiatus hernia as pregnancy advances. Sleeping in a semi-recumbent position helps, so do alkalis, especially when they contain a local anesthetic which acts directly on the painful mucosa.

Leg cramps, backache
None of these complaints can be easily explained, but very probably have some connection with the postural changes of pregnancy - the "Pride of Pregnancy."

Alterations in the center of gravity cause a characteristic lordosis; and this along with the softening of ligaments caused by the steroid hormones may produce pressure on nerve roots (leading to nerve pain and cramps).

Treatment is directed mainly towards resting the muscles and preventing undue flexion of the vertebral joints

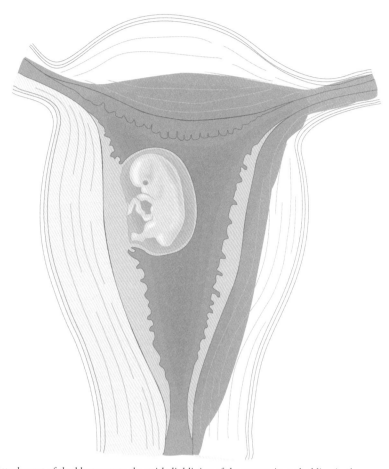

Attachment of the blastocyst to the epithelial lining of the uterus; its embedding in the compact layer. After some weeks the placenta is formed and the foetus becomes detached from the uterine wall.

by getting the patient to sleep with boards under her mattress.

Subjective complaints
This is due to steroid effects on smooth muscle, in part to obstruction by the gravid uterus at term. Attention to diet is the first step, but the patient is miserable if a bowel motion is not achieved every second or third day and laxatives are often required.

Morning sickness
The cause is not known, but is probably due to the effect of steroids on the liver and to reduced gastric motility. It is aggravated by cooking and fatigue.

The treatment in mild cases includes rest, light carbohydrate diet in the morning (biscuits and milk) and a variety of drugs including antihistamines (for their anti-emetic effects)

and antispasmodics such as belladonna derivatives.

Pressure in the pelvis
This gradually obstructs venous return and leads to hemorrhoids, varicose veins of legs, and varicosities of vulva and abdominal wall.

Treatment is symptomatic. The hemorrhoids can be helped by suppositories and only in rare cases is hemorrhoidectomy required. The legs can be clothed in special thigh stockings.

Vaginal discharge
The vaginal discharge becomes relatively copious in pregnancy because of the considerable increase in vascularity and the consequent transudation through the tissues. It is common, a frequent cause of complaint and difficult to eradicate.

PREMENSTRUAL SYNDROME (PMS)

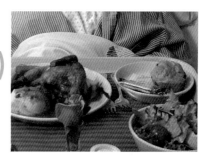

Introduction

Premenstrual syndrome (PMS) is the term used to describe a group of physical or behavioral changes that some women go through before their menstrual periods begin every month. Premenstrual syndrome can produce discomfort in different parts of the body; it can also cause unpleasant emotional feelings. For reasons that remain unclear, the physical discomforts or mood changes begin at various times near the end of the menstrual cycle and usually disappear after a woman has begun her menstrual period. They reappear at about the same time each month.

The degree of discomfort from premenstrual syndrome varies with each individual. Most women with premenstrual syndrome have symptoms that cause a mild or moderate degree of distress. In about 10 percent of women with premenstrual syndrome, symptoms may be severe.

Premenstrual syndrome can have a major impact on a woman's life.

▲ On the job or at home, a woman may not be able to function as well when symptoms occur.
▲ Problems caused by premenstrual syndrome may trigger marital and family conflicts.

▲ A woman may become less outgoing socially and avoid friends when symptoms occur.

Women who have premenstrual syndrome can be helped. Education is the most important step in understanding this condition. Certain treatments can be useful in some women. You should discuss any questions or concerns you might have about premenstrual syndrome with your doctor.

Symptoms and signs

A number of changes that cause various degrees of discomfort have been found in women with premenstrual syndrome:

■ *Physical changes*
· bloating
· weight gain
· breast soreness
· abdominal swelling
· headache
· clumsiness
· constipation
· swollen hands and feet
· fatigue

■ *Behavioral changes*
· depression
· irritability
· anxiety
· tension
· mood swings
· inability to concentrate
· change in sex drive

You do not have to have all of these problems to have premenstrual syndrome. Most women with premenstrual syndrome have only certain ones. Some women have more difficulty with changes that affect their bodies; others have more problems with emotional changes.

The severity of discomfort felt also

Sometimes changes in the types of foods you eat may help to relieve some premenstrual syndrome symptoms. Reduce caffeine - present in coffee, tea, cola and chocolate.

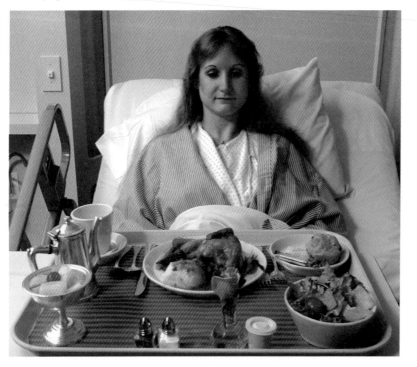

P

varies from woman to woman. Some months may be more stressful than others. Occasionally, premenstrual syndrome disappears temporarily for no reason.

Causes

No one knows for certain what causes premenstrual syndrome. It is probably related to the change in hormone levels that occurs in a woman's body before menstruation. Nor do doctors know why some women are more severely affected that others. Some well-publicized "simple answers" to premenstrual syndrome cannot be documented by scientific studies.

True, premenstrual syndrome occurs only when the ovaries are working to make both estrogen and progesterone - it has been detected only in women between puberty and menopause.

But premenstrual syndrome is probably not caused by hormone deficiencies or excesses. Hormone levels appear to be normal in women with premenstrual syndrome. Researchers are now studying the possibility that estrogen and progesterone may act in combination with chemicals made in the brain to cause some of the symptoms of premenstrual syndrome.

Diagnosis

The most important aspect of premenstrual syndrome is that it follows a pattern. Changes always occur during the second half of the menstrual cycle and are repeated each month. To be called premenstrual syndrome, symptoms must follow a certain pattern.

▲ Women with premenstrual syndrome may have discomfort during the last 3-14 days before their menstrual periods.

▲ They usually gain rapid relief of their symptoms once their menstrual periods start.

Treatment

No cure has yet been found for premenstrual syndrome. However, some of the individual symptoms can be

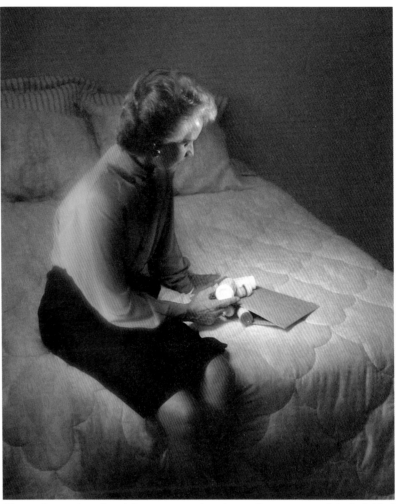

No cure has yet been found for premenstrual syndrome. However, some of the individual symptoms can be relieved with various medications.

relieved with various medications. Which treatment your doctor selects depends on the problems you are having and how severe they are. This is why it is important to describe physical and emotional changes carefully.

Diuretics, or "water pills," help the body eliminate excess fluid through the kidneys; your doctor may prescribe one of these drugs to reduce bloating if cutting down on foods high in salt does not help.

At present the most effective medication appears to be one type of mild diuretic. It is believed to work by interfering with the production of the hormones responsible for premenstrual syndrome as well as by getting rid of excess fluid.

Other treatments have been tried, such as vitamins, oral contraceptives (birth control pills), and natural progesterone suppositories (containing the hormone progesterone). However,l scientific studies have not proved these treatments to be effective for most women.

It is important to work closely with your doctor to find a treatment that works for you - you may have to try several different types of treatment to find relief.

Remember to keep charting your symptoms each month after you start any treatment. Your records will show whether it is having some effect. Let your doctor know if there is no change in your condition.

PSORIASIS

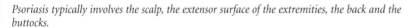

Introduction

Disorders and diseases of the skin are so varied and so common that dermatology is a specialty in the practice of medicine. The most remarkable fact about this field of medicine is how much there remains to be learned about it.

More than 95 per cent of all skin diseases and disorders are among the following ailments:

- acne;
- dermatitis;
- eczema;
- infections;
- psoriasis;
- tumors.

Psoriasis is a common chronic and recurrent disease characterized by dry, well-circumscribed, silvery, scaling papules and plaques of various sizes.

Psoriasis varies in severity from one to two lesions to a widespread skin disorder with disabling joint ailment and scaling of the skin.

About 2 to 4 per cent of the population are affected. Onset is usually between ages 10 and 40, but no age is exempt. A family history of psoriasis is common and usually reflects an autosomal dominant inheritance.

General health is not affected, except for the psychologic stigma of an unsightly skin disease, unless severe joint disease or intractable scaling of the skin develops.

Symptoms and signs

The onset is usually gradual. The typical course is one of chronic remissions and recurrences (or occasionally acute exacerbations) but vary in frequency and duration.

Factors precipitating eruptions include:

- ▲ local trauma, with lesions appearing at the trauma site;
- ▲ occasionally severe sunburn;
- ▲ irritation;
- ▲ topical medications;
- ▲ withdrawal of systemic corticosteroids.

Psoriasis characteristically involves the scalp, the extensor surface of the extremities (particularly at elbows and knees), the back, and the buttocks. The nails, eyebrows, axillas, navel, or anogenital region may also be affected.

The lesions are sharply demarcated (usually without itching phenomena), papules or plaques covered with overlapping, silvery or slightly opalescent, shiny scales.

The lesions heal without scarring, and hair growth is not altered. Papules sometimes extend and coalesce, producing large plaques in bizarre annular and gyrate patterns. Nail involvement may resemble a fungal infection, with stippling, pitting, fraying or separation on the distal margin, thickening, discoloration, and debris under the nail plate. There are a number of special appearances of psoriasis:

■ Psoriatic arthritis
A severe disorder of the joints often closely resembling rheumatoid arthritis. This condition is equally crippling, but the blood of the patient does not contain the rheumatoid factor.

■ Exfoliative psoriatic dermatitis
Severe skin disease which may be intractable and may lead to general debility; the entire skin is red and covered with fine scales.

Psoriasis typically involves the scalp, the extensor surface of the extremities, the back and the buttocks.

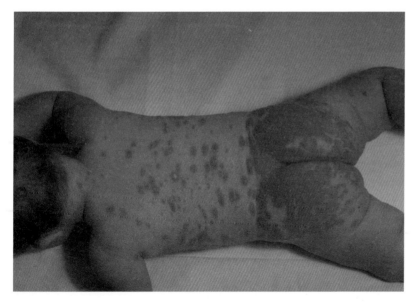

Light form of psoriasis involving the back and buttocks.

■ *Pustular psoriasis*
A condition characterized by sterile pustules that may be localized to the palms and soles or may be generalized; psoriatic lesions are not always present.

Diagnosis

Diagnosis by inspection is rarely difficult. In psoriasis of the scalp, as elsewhere, the well-defined, dry, heaped-up, lesions with large silvery scales are usually not hard to distinguish from the diffuse, greasy, yellowish scaling of seborrhoeic dermatitis. In psoriasis, removal of the superficial scale typically shows tiny bleeding points. Biopsy findings may be typical, but many other skin diseases may have psoriasis-like histologic features that make them difficult to distinguish.

Prognosis and treatment

The prognosis depends on the extent and severity of the initial involvement, and usually the earlier in life it begins, the greater the severity. Acute attacks usually clear up, but complete permanent remissions are rare. No therapeutic method assures a cure, but most cases can be well controlled. The simplest forms of treatment are:
- lubricants;
- keratolytics;
- topical corticosteroids.

These should be tried first for a limited number of lesions because effective remedies are not numerous. Exposure to sunlight is recommended, although occasionally sunburn makes the lesions worse. Strong medicines belonging to the group of antimetabolites should be used only in severe skin and joint involvement. Lubricating creams, hydrogenated vegetable (cooking) oils, or white petrolatum are applied alone or with the following medicines or agents:
- corticosteroids;
- salicylic acid;
- crude coal tar;
- dithranol or anthralin.

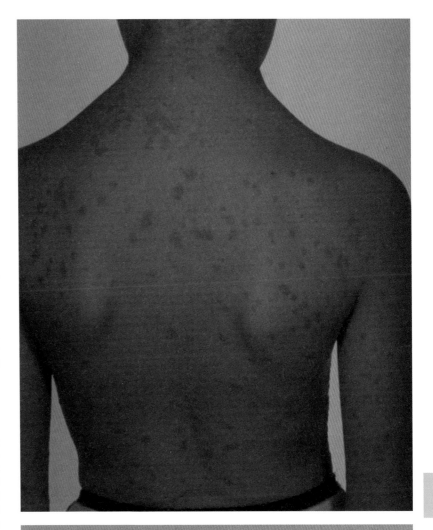

PUVA

▲ PUVA stands for the treatment of psoralen with ultraviolet A. Psoralen is any of the constituents of certain plants (for example, Psoralea corylifolia) that have the ability to produce dermatitis when an individual is first exposed to a psoralen and then to sunlight.

▲ PUVA is highly effective in treating ex-tensive psoriasis. Recently oral methoxalen - a derivative of psoralen - is used. The drug is followed, at a specific interval, by exposure to the skin to long-wave ultraviolet light. The dosage of both the medicine and the UV exposure must be tail-ored to each patient.

▲ Although the treatment is clean and may produce remissions for several months, repe-ated treatments with intense light may in-crease UV-induced skin cancer.

▲ The use of UV light to treat disease is called phototherapy. Psoriasis and atopic dermatitis are the disorders most commonly treated with phototherapy.

▲ Side effects of phototherapy include pain and reddening similar to sunburn with prolonged exposure to UV light.

▲ UV light exposure also increases the long-term risk of skin cancer, although the risk is small for brief courses of treatment.

Psoriasis Questions & Answers

What is psoriasis?
Psoriasis is a common chronic and recurrent disease characterized by dry, well-circumscribed, silvery, scaling papules and plaques of various sizes. Psoriasis varies in severity from one to two lesions to a widespread skin disorder with disabling joint ailment and scaling of the skin. About 2 to 4 per cent of the population are affected. Onset is usually between ages 10 and 40, but no age is exempt. A family history of psoriasis is common and usually reflects an autosomal dominant inheritance. General health is not affected, except for the psychologic stigma of an unsightly skin disease, unless severe joint disease or intractable scaling of the skin develops.

What are precipitating factors of psoriasis?
The onset is usually gradual. The typical course is one of chronic remissions and recurrences (or occasionally acute exacerbations) but vary in frequency and duration. Factors precipitating eruptions include:
- local trauma, with lesions appearing at the trauma site;
- occasionally severe sunburn;
- rritation;
- topical medications;
- withdrawal of systemic corticosteroids.

What are signs and symptoms of psoriasis?
Psoriasis characteristically involves the scalp, the extensor surface of the extremities (particularly at elbows and knees), the back, and the buttocks. The nails, eyebrows, axillas, navel, or anogenital region may also be affected. The lesions are sharply demarcated (usually without itching phenomena), papules or plaques covered with overlapping, silvery or slightly opalescent, shiny scales. The lesions heal without scarring, and hair growth is not altered. Papules sometimes extend and coalesce, producing large plaques in bizarre annular and gyrate patterns.

What is exfoliative psoriatic dermatitis?
This is a severe skin disease which may be intractable and may lead to general debility. The entire skin is red and covered with fine scales.

What is pustular psoriasis?
This is a condition characterized by sterile pustules that may be localized to the palms and soles or may be generalized; psoriatic lesions are not always present.

How is the diagnosis of psoriasis made?
Diagnosis by inspection is rarely difficult. In psoriasis of the scalp, as elsewhere, the well-defined, dry, heaped-up lesions with large silvery scales are usually not hard to distinguish from the diffuse, greasy, yellowish scaling of seborrhoeic dermatitis.

In psoriasis, removal of the superficial scale typically shows tiny bleeding points. Biopsy findings may be typical, but many other skin diseases may have psoriasis-like histologic features that make them difficult to distinguish.

Is somewthing known about the prognosis of psoriasis?
The prognosis of psoriasis depends on the extent and severity of the initial involvement, and usually the earlier in life it begins, the greater the severity. Acute attacks usually clear up, but complete permanent remissions are rare. No therapeutic method assures a cure, but most cases can be well controlled.

What is the best treatment of psoriasis?
The simplest forms of treatment are:
- lubricants;
- keratolytics;
- topical corticosteroids.
These should be tried first for a limited number of lesions because effective remedies are not numerous. Exposure to sunlight is recommended, although occasionally sunburn makes the lesions worse. Strong medicines belonging to the group of antimetabolites should be used only in severe skin and joint involvement.

What types of medications are used for psoriasis?
Lubricating creams, hydrogenated vegetable (cooking) oils, or white petrolatum are applied alone or with the following medicines or agents:
- corticosteroids;
- salicylic acid;
- crude coal tar;
- dithranol or anthralin.

Where stands PUVA for?
PUVA stands for the treatment of psoralen with ultraviolet A. Psoralen is any of the constituents of certain plants (for example, Psoralea corylifolia) that have the ability to produce dermatitis when an individual is first exposed to a psoralen and then to sunlight.

When is PUVA effective?
PUVA is highly effective in treating extensive psoriasis. Recently oral methoxalen - a derivative of psoralen - is used. The drug is followed, at a specific interval, by exposure to the skin to longwave ultraviolet light. The dosage of both the medicine and the UV exposure must be tailored to each patient. Although the treatment is clean and may produce remissions for several months, repeated treatments with intense light may increase UV-induced skin cancer.

Topical corticosteroids

Topical drugs (drugs applied to the skin) are used most commonly. Nearly everyone with psoriasis benefits from skin moisturizers (emollients). Other topical agents include corticosteroids, often used together with calcipotriene, a vitamin D derivative, or coal or pine tar.

Since topical corticosteroids have to be applied very carefully, a description is given of one of these preparations (aclometasone diproprionate), to provide patients with specific information about this tyupoe of drug.

Properties

This medicine contains aclometasone dipropionate, a corticosteroid, as active ingredient. Corticosteroids are used to help relieve redness, swelling, itching, inflammation, and discomfort of skin problems such as psoriasis. They exert this effect by interfering with natural body mechanisms that produce the rash, itching, or inflammation. They do not cure the underlying cause of the skin problem. This medication is applied to the skin.

Before using this medicine

Before you use this medicine check with your doctor, or pharmacist:

▲ if you ever had any unusual or allergic reaction to corticosteroids.

▲ if you are allergic to any substance, such as sulfites or other preservatives or dyes.

▲ if you are pregnant or intend to become pregnant while using this medicine. Studies have shown that corticosteroids applied to the skin in large amounts or over long periods of time can be the cause of birth defects.

▲ if you are breast-feeding an infant. Some corticosteroids pass into breast milk and may interfere with the infant's growth.

Treatment

Do not use this medicine more often or for a longer time than ordered. To do so may increase absorption through the skin and the chance of side effects. In addition, too much use, especially on areas with thinner skin (for example, face, armpits, groin), may result in thinning of the skin and stretch marks.

Before applying this medication, wash your hands. than, unless your doctor or pharmacist gives you different instructions, gently wash the area where the medication is to be applied. With a clean towel pat the area dry. Apply a small amount of the medication to the affected area in a thin layer. Do not bandage the area unless your doctor tells you to do so. If you miss a dose of this medication, apply the dose as soon as possible, unless it is almost time for the next application.

▲ Do not use this medicine for other skin problems without first checking with your doctor. You should not use a topical corticosteroid if you have a virus disease (such as herpes), fungal infection of the skin (such as athlete's foot), or tuberculosis of the skin.

Side effects

There are a number of side effects that usually do not require medical attention. Minor side effects are:

Acne
Burning sensations
Itching
Rash
Skin dryness

These possible side effects may go away during treatment; however, if they continue or are bothersome, check with your doctor, nurse, or pharmacist. Tell your doctor about any side effects that are persistent or particularly bothersome, such as:

Blistering
Increased hair growth
Irritation of the affected area
Loss of skin
Secondary infection of skin area
Thinning of the skin
Easy bruising

Interactions

None known as long as it is used according to the directions given to you by your doctor or pharmacist.

Storage

Cream, ointment, lotion, gel, spray, and aerosol should be stored at room temperature in tightly closed containers. This medication should never be frozen.

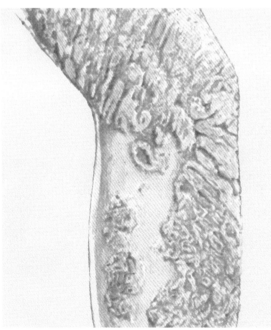

Severe form of psoriasis involving one of the extremities.

P

PSYCHOSES

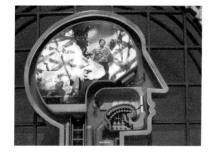

Description

Psychosis is a term formerly applied to any mental disorder, but now generally restricted to those disturbances of such magnitude that there is personality disintegration and loss of contact with reality. The disturbances are of psychogenic origin, or without clearly defined physical cause.

The psychoses include:
- organic psychoses
- schizophrenic disorders
- paranoid disorders
- manic-depression

These disorders present about 5 per cent of the overall psychiatric morbidity in family practice. Those mental disorders that occur in the elderly are comprised of the organic dementias and the functional disorders, of which the commonest is depression.

Schizophrenic illnesses uncommonly present for the first time after the age of 40 years and in three quarters of the cases that later exhibit the characteristic chronic syndrome, the illness begins between 15 and 25 years of age. Paranoid conditions, in which occur systematized delusions, most commonly of a persecutory character, but at times erotic, grandiose of hypochondriacal, tend to have a later age of onset.

A paranoid state which develops in middle age and which tends to become chronic (so-called involutional melancholia) is characterized by more or less systematic delusions, sometimes associated with hallucinations which in women are often related to the genitals and with delusional ideas.

The psychiatric interview

Several different levels of data are obtained simultaneously in the psychiatric interview. The data sources include the patient's verbal content (what he says), manner of speaking (how he says it), nonverbal communication (body language) and associated somatic clues, as well as the interviewer's own emotional responses.

Data at one level will often augment, modify or even contradict data at another level. Thus, the alert interviewer will note the patient who shifts position or fidgets with his watch while verbally denying that he is concerned about the item of history cur-

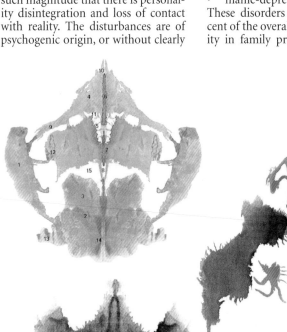

Rorschach inkblot test used to analyze certain components of human behavior. The test is nowadays rarely applied.

rently under discussion. Blushing, blanching, perspiration, increase in respiratory rate, and increase in tics or mannerism are all sensitive indicators of emotional arousal.

Often a subtle clue (a shift of gaze or slight change or expression) will suggest covert emotions, fantasies or impulses. Body language also may communicate more eloquently than words the pain of a deep depression, the terror of acute anxiety or the eroticism of seductive behavior.

The patient's or client's behavior is determined by the reality of the present situation, his past experiences, his personality and his outlook on life. The patient's or client's behavior is determined by the reality of the present situation, his past experiences, his personality and his outlook on life.

Commonly, he will initially have mixed feelings: while he usually acknowledges his need for help to share his concern with a potentially helpful professional, he may also be fearful of rejection, criticism or humiliation. Thus, his perceptions of and reactions to the interviewer contain both rational and irrational elements and his behavior may appear inconsistent, puzzling or inappropriate. In the table are listed the recording system of a history in the case of behavioral or psychotic disorders. The scheme is commonly used.

Alternatively, the developmental approach is used, starting at birth or with the family history so that the illness is described in the perspective of the patient's life history. The distinction between history and examination is even more blurred in psychiatry than in general medicine.

Most (and frequently all) of the mental status examination is carried out while the history is being obtained. A summary of the examination and recording of the mental state is given in the second table.

Organic psychoses

The organic psychoses are characterized by a basic syndrome consisting of impairment of orientation, memory, judgment, intellectual functions such as learning, calculation and comprehension, emotional lability and shal-

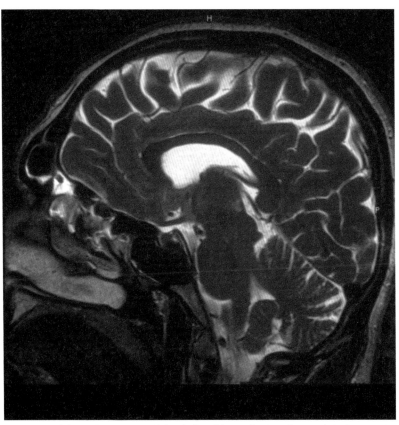

MRI-scan of the median section of the skull and brain showing characteristic degenerative changes in the cerebral cortex in Korsakow's syndrome.

lowness of affect.

Such a syndrome may be associated with other abnormal manifestations, for instance, depressive, manic or schizophrenic features; the exaggeration or emergence of personality traits, such as obsessional or attention-seeking features. There may be lowering of ethical standards and antisocial acts may be committed.

Paranoid symptoms in the elderly are occasionally seen as part of an organic process or a severe depressive picture but not infrequently they occur in isolation. The previous personalities of those in whom paranoid symptoms appear late in life are reportedly characterized by suspiciousness, querulousness and eccentricity.

Toxic-metabolic, inflammatory and structural brain disorders may produce symptoms simulating functional neurotic and psychotic syndromes, which may be the presenting or predominant feature of the disorder.

The psychotic or neurotic syndromes that occur wit brain involvement due to metabolic disease (for instance, deficiency of vitamin B12) or a secondary metabolic disorder (for instance, secondary to cancer of the pancreas) may be the earliest manifestations of the underlying disorder.

Any brain disorder may present as a psychotic syndrome, but drugs, brain tumors, temporal lobe epilepsy, multiple sclerosis, head injury, infarctions and degenerative disease are the commonest organic causes of psychosis.

The entire range of psychotic disorders can occur in the context of brain disease. Schizophrenic states due to excessive consumption of amphetamines, alcohol (alcoholic hallucinosis) or their toxic compounds are frequently misdiagnosed as primary schizophrenic illnesses.

Depressive states often follow influenza, typhoid, infectious hepatitis or childbirth or may be associated with

P

Psychosis - Examination of the mental state

- Appearance and behavior
  - dress
  - posture
  - facial expression
  - motor activity
  - impulsivity
  - mannerism
  - retardation

- Stream of talk
  - poverty of thought
  - rigidity of thought
  - pace and progression of speech
  - logical sequence of sentences
  - confusing and irrelevant remarks
  - presence of thought disorder
  - flight of ideas
  - obsessional qualification
  - distractibility

- Thought content
  - special preoccupations
  - obsessional ideas
  - misinterpretations
  - ideas of reference
  - ideas of influence
  - delusions
  - derogatory or grandiose ideas

- Perceptual abnormalities
  - auditory hallucinations
  - visual hallucinations
  - tactile hallucinations

- depersonalization
- derealization

- Affect
  - happiness
  - elation
  - sadness
  - depression
  - irritability
  - anger
  - suspicion
  - perplexity
  - fear or anxiety
  - blunting or incongruity of affect
  - lability of mood
  - reactivity of mood
  - appropriateness to context

- Cognitive functions
  - level of consciousness
  - memory and orientation
  - immediate recall
  - memory for recent events
  - memory for remote events
  - orientation in time
  - orientation in space
  - orientation in person
  - concentration in person
  - concentration
  - intelligence
  - psychometric testing
  - insight and judgment

medications such as antihypertensive drugs, notably reserpine. Sometimes gross euphoria may follow the administration of corticosteroids or ACTH.

Schizophrenic disorders

These psychotic conditions are defined as mental disorders with a tendency toward chronicity which impairs functioning and which is characterized by psychotic symptoms involving disturbances of thinking, feeling and behavior. *See Schizophrenia*

Paranoid disorders

These are states of heightened self-awareness with a ranked tendency to self-reference and projection of the patient's own ideas or others. In common usage "paranoid" implies persecutory ideas held by the client or patient.

Paranoid states range imperceptibly from a circumscribed delusional system with no loss of affect or associative processes, to the more complete disorganization seen in paranoid schizophrenia.

Signs and symptoms

The personality that spawns a paranoid illness reflects a need to shield sensitive portions of inner life, a hunger for recognition, and the fears and guilt feelings these conflicts and striving evoke. Sexual conflicts, often unconscious, may be operative and homosexual tendencies are often noted.

The paranoid patient characteristically has a tense and expectant affective state that stimulates his attention; he sees connections which do not exist and at times rationalizes his concepts into an extensive delusional system.

Brief paranoid states are often of a psychotic intensity. These reactive illnesses occur in persons whose personalities are characterized by the following elements:

- sensitivity
- insecurity
- inferiority
- suspiciousness

Isolation from social contact and physical problems (for instance, deafness) are often exacerbating factors, and alcoholism is commonly involved. In acute and chronic brain syndromes, the impaired comprehension and dulling of consciousness favour paranoid interpretations and delusions.

The paranoid psychosis is a disorder of a different nature and severity. Typically in these illnesses highly elaborated delusional systems gradually develop without hallucinations, disorganization of thinking, or other characteristic schizophrenic symptoms.

A few patients, however, eventually progress into frank schizophrenic psychosis. In this form of paranoid psychosis, core symptoms center on some minor or imagined physical defect.

The patient delusionally misinterprets scraps of conversation to confirm his beliefs that he or she is discriminated against because of this defect.

In other patients, a trivial or illusory asymmetry of the face and enlargement of the nose is the focus of a paranoid system. Such patients may trail from specialist to specialist incessantly demanding plastic surgery.

Real or imagined slights or injustices may lead to never-ending litigation, or religious fanaticism may insidiously progress to grandiose but encapsulated messianic beliefs. In one dangerous form of paranoid psychosis, delusional jealousy is the central theme.

Jealousy has a complex psychopathology, and morbid jealousy (the so-called Othello syndrome) occurs in a variety of condition, including paranoid states. A primary depression may underlie the illness.

The patient's anguish over delusions of his spouse's infidelity is readily converted to rage.

The patient may increasingly make accusations, spy upon or follow his spouse, examine undergarments for seminal stains, and misinterpret simple actions, such as the way a curtain is drawn, as a message of the lover.

He may demand confession constantly and asserts that forgiveness will ensue. Physical assault is a real danger. A persecutory delusional system may develop as a result of a close relationship with another person who already has a disorder with persecutory delusions.

This type of induction psychosis is a result of sharing the delusions of the dominant person. In rare instances more than 2 persons may be involved. The prognosis for what is called shared paranoid disorder is a function of the emotional strength of the person in whom the psychosis has been introduced.

Course and prognosis

The history may show that, as a child, the patient needed special appreciation, was moody, resented school, and parental discipline, could not form good play
adjustments and was suspicious.

While growing up, the rigidity and tendency to pride may have increased, as well as the patient's sensitivity to others' attitudes toward him of her. Before the psychosis becomes manifest, prodromal symptoms may occur. The patient may have reacted to numerous situations with wounded and bitter pride.

He analyses his moods and sensations, may become hypochondriacal, is reserved and withdrawn in disdain from discussing his problems. Gradually, the idea may be born that his failures have been due to the enmity of others, and he sees new and hidden significance in commonplace events, leading to the belief that people deliberately slight him and that his situation is endangered.

He experiences vague fears, becomes increasingly resentful and defends his suspicions vigorously. Hallucinations may or may not occur.

Patients with classic paranoia or reactions closely approximating it probably never recover; however, they do not necessarily deteriorate and may not require hospitalization.

If their conduct remains within bounds, society may view them as "cranks." However, some patients who at first appear to be suffering from circumscribed paranoid psychoses are later recognized to be schizophrenic.

Treatment

Whether the patient should be hospitalized is determined by his potential danger to himself and to others. If delusions are directed against specific persons, confinement probably is necessary; the greater the expressed hatred, the more imperative is hospitalization.

Establishing a relationship with the therapist is a vital step; psychotherapy will then alleviate distress and often modify behavior, even though essential delusional thinking is unaltered. Often the patient will follow reasonable suggestions and greatly modify his behavior.

The doctor may become the patient's one confidant and can help him by being tolerant and combining a philosophical detachment with sympathetic humility, discretion, understanding, warmth, and a sense of humour about his own possible inaptness as well as the patient's peccadilloes.

Phenothiazine drugs and other neuroleptic medicines are helpful and often minimize symptoms, though complete remission is uncommon, even after prolonged drug treatment.

Manic-depression

This psychosis is characterized by profound disturbance of affect, for instance, feelings and emotions. The illness usually appears unprovoked but may occasionally follow some stress. The psychosis has a strong tendency to recur and be self-limiting. *See Manic depreison*

Psychosis - Parameters of the history

1. Identifying characteristics
   - name, age, sex, race
   - marital status
   - occupation
   - source of referral

2. Presenting problems
   - in the form of a brief statement

3. History of present illness
   - current symptoms
   - behavioral changes
   - coincident life events
   - previous treatments
   - preset degree of disability

4. Personal history
   - birth and infancy
   - nature of delivery
   - ages passing milestones
   - relationships with siblings
   - relationships with peers
   - duration and details of schooling
   - achievements and adjustment
   - attitudes
   - work record
   - sexual maturation
   - sexual interest and practice

   - courtship, relationships
   - marriages, divorce

5. Previous medical history
   - physical disorders
   - psychological disorders

6. Personality prior to illness
   - social relationships at home
   - relationships at work
   - social toes in the community
   - social activities and interests
   - predominant moods
   - character traits
   - strengths and weaknesses
   - coping style
   - methods of handling challenge
   - methods of handling stress
   - temperament
   - religious and moral standards
   - ambitions and aspirations
   - drinking, drugs use, smoking

7. Family history
   - details of each parent
   - details of each sibling
   - familial diseases
   - dates and causes of death

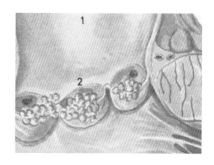

RHEUMATIC FEVER

Introduction

Rheumatic fever is defined as an acute inflammatory complication - without formation of pus - of streptococcal infections, characterized mainly by arthritis, chorea (involuntary, rapid and spastic jerks), or carditis (inflammation of heart tissues) appearing alone or in combination with residual heart disease as a possible sequel of the carditis. The skin and subcutaneous tissues also can be involved.

Both the incidence and the severity of this disease are declining and there is some evidence to suggest that the incidence of heart valve involvement is beginning to decline also.

Although much has been achieved in treatment and prevention, it seems likely that in this disease, like scarlet fever, there is a spontaneous trend inherent in the disease process which is not yet understood. There is now ample evidence implicating group A beta-hemolytic streptococcus as a major contributory factor of acute rheumatic fever.

Epidemiological evidence shows that the incidence of the disease follows that of sore throat caused by streptococcus, both seasonally, climatically, and socially. Both occur in temperate climates, in rather poor social circumstances and in minor epidemics in closed communities.

Serological evidence also indicates recent streptococcal infection which is usually in the upper respiratory tract, but may rarely be in wounds. Furthermore, treatment of streptococcal infections reduces the incidence of the disease.

Equally clearly, the streptococcus alone does not cause the disease directly. Although many are infected, few develop acute rheumatic fever, and their is a latent period between streptococcal infection and the onset

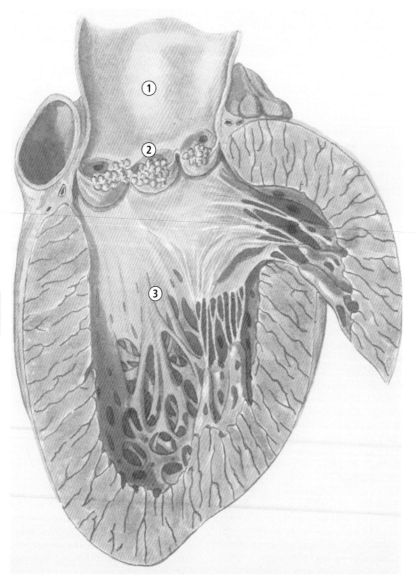

Degeneration of heart valves as a consequence of streptococcal infection.
1. Aorta
2. Degenerated aortic valves
3. Left ventricle

R

of the disease.

Elegant experimental work has shown that heart muscle, and some strains of streptococci share an antigenic determinant. Antibodies formed by the organisms might therefore also damage the heart, and indeed certain immunoglobulins have been demonstrated in the heart.

Signs and symptoms

The onset is acute and follows a streptococcal throat infection by 1 to 2 weeks. Males and females are equally affected and the first episode usually occurs between the ages of 5 and 15. Whereas in children the heart infection predominates, when adults are affected the joint ailment frequently overshadows the heart infection.

The joint disorder affects large joints such as the knees, wrists, ankles and elbows rather than the small joints of the hands, and is migratory, appearing in one joint and disappearing while it flares up in another.

The synovial membrane reveal an acute non-specific inflammation of white blood cells, but with little development of fibrosis and necrosis. The tissues around the joint may be more involved than the synovium. The arthritis is self-limiting and leaves no residual joint damage.

The inflammation of the heart involves the three layers of the heart wall: endocard, myocard, and epicard. An increase in heart rate (*tachycardia*) out of proportion to the fever, and enlargement of the heart suggest an inflammation of the muscular layer (*myocarditis*).

The inflammation of the inner lining of the heart (*endocarditis*) affects the valves in the left part of the heart (mitral and aortic valves) more than the valves in the right part (pulmonary and tricuspid valves). The first attacks of acute rheumatic fever, carditis is present in about 50 per cent of patients with arthritis. Since murmurs are the most frequent manifestation of carditis, careful examination by way of auscultation are required to avoid errors.

Heart decompensation in acutely ill children may remain undiagnosed, because its manifestations may be different from those expected in adults. Children's symptoms may be difficulty with breathing (dyspnoea) without rales, nausea and vomiting, an abdominal ache and a hacking nonproductive cough (due to lung congestion).

The lethargy, malaise, or fatigue often described to acute rheumatic fever can be caused by heart failure. In about 10 per cent of the patients the skin shows rounded pale-reddish spots (*erythema marginatum*) and subcutaneous nodules.

Course and prognosis

Except for the heart condition (carditis), all manifestations of acute rheumatic fever subside without residual effects. Joint pain and fever usually subside within 2 weeks, often more rapidly, and seldom last longer than a month.

Patients with carditis have overt auscultatory evidence of it when first encountered by a physician; if no worsening occurs during the next 2 to 3 weeks, new manifestations of carditis seldom occur thereafter.

Since murmurs often do not disappear and new heart phenomena are uncommon, inflammatory rather than heart manifestations are the best indexes of therapeutic response.

The evidence of acute inflammation usually subsides within 5 months in uncomplicated carditis. About 5 per cent of rheumatic patients have prolonged attacks (8 months or longer) with clinical and laboratory manifestations of inflammation appearing in spontaneously recurrent episodes unrelated to intervening streptococcal infection or to cessation of anti-inflammatory therapy.

Such recurrent attacks are more likely to be associated with carditis. Rheumatic fever does not seem to produce chronic "smoldering" heart inflammation. The long-term outcome depends on the severity of the initial heart inflammation.

Patients without carditis seldom develop damage to the heart valves and they are less likely to have rheumatic recurrences, and are unlikely to develop carditis during recurrences.

Those with severe carditis during the acute episode are usually left with residual heart disease that is often worsened by the rheumatic recurrences to which they are particularly susceptible. Murmurs eventually disappear in about half of the patients whose acute episodes were manifested by mild carditis without major heart enlargement or decompensation.

Treatment and prevention

In patients with arthritis only, therapy is directed toward relief of pain. In mild cases, codeine, other pain-relievers, or relatively small doses of aspirin are adequate. In more severe situations, a complete program with salicylates or similar medicines is necessary. Salicylates are given in an escalating pattern until effectiveness has been attained or toxicity supervenes. Salicylates will be abandoned in favour of a corticosteroid if a therapeutic effect has been produced by the 4th day. Preventive treatment of upper respiratory infections caused by streptococci reduces the incidence of acute rheumatic fever.

There is much to be said for administering an antibiotic to all patients with upper respiratory infections provided the patient is not sensitive to the drug. This, however, will not abolish the disease entirely since many streptococcal infections are symptomless.

It is common practice to prescribe 2 weeks of an oral antibiotic to patients with acute rheumatic fever although this course is rather like shutting the stable door when the horse has bolted. The acutely ill patient's choice of physical activities is usually as wise as arbitrary medical decisions. Patients generally limit themselves appropriately if symptomatic with arthritis, chorea, or heart failure.

In the absence of carditis, no restrictions are needed after the acute episode subsides. Advice about physical restrictions is most difficult for asymptomatic patients with carditis; strict bed rest has no proved value; and its enforcement by the physician may create undesirable psychologic reactions. Physical restrictions seem advisable only in patients with symptomatic heart failure to reduce or remove the symptoms.

655

RHEUMATOID ARTHRITIS

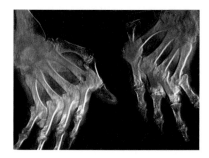

Definition and incidence

Rheumatoid arthritis is a systemic disease - one that affect the whole body. It is one of the most common of the rheumatic diseases which cause aches, pains, and stiffness in tissues within or around the joints.

Rheumatoid arthritis is a chronic inflammatory disease characterized by the presence of activated T lymphocytes, mnacrophages, and synoviocytes in the synovial membrane, converting the single-cell lining into an engorged inflammatory tissue called pannus.

Within the pannus, inflammation, proliferation, and humoural and cellular immune responses lead to release of metallo-protease enzymes and other mediators that degrade cartilage and connective tissue.

The inciting cause of rheumatoid arthritis, the role of T call activation, and the mechanism of synovial cell activation and proliferation are currently unknown. However, much recent evidence clearly indicates that the actions of certain pro-inflammatory cytokinines are responsible for many of the manifestations of the disease. Cytokinines are soluble proteins, secreted by cells of the immune system, that act as messengers to help regulate an immune response.

Rheumatoid arthritis is a chronic disease, meaning it may last throughout your lifetime. However, it can be managed through proper treatment programs. With proper treatment and possibly some changes in daily activities, most people with rheumatoid arthritis can lead a normal, productive life.

Features

Rheumatoid arthritis causes pain, stiffness, warmth, redness, and swelling - a process called inflammation - in the joints. The many symptoms of rheumatoid arthritis are

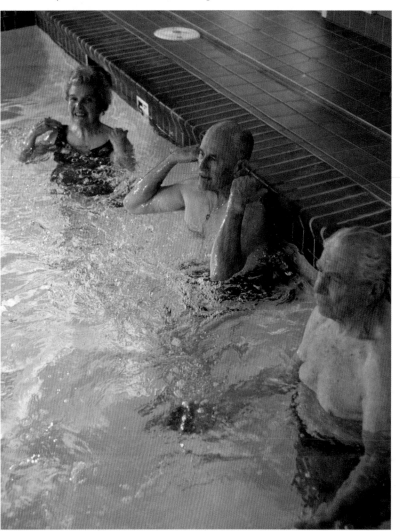

Along with drugs to reduce inflammation, a treatment plan for rheumatoid arthritis should include non-drug therapies, such as exercise, physical or occupational therapy, hydrotherapy. As the inflammation subsides, regular, active exercises can help, although a person should not exercises to the point of fatigue. For many people, exercise in water may be easier.

R

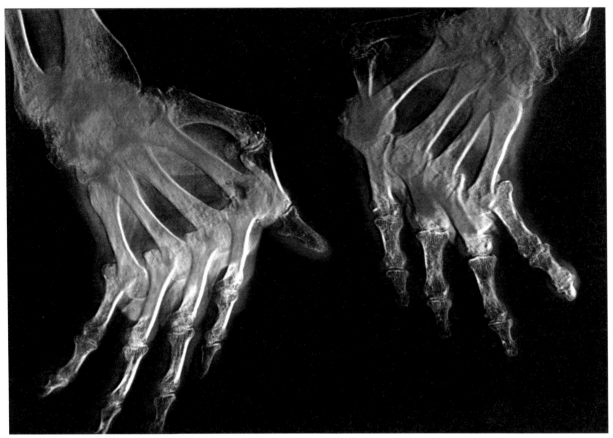

X-ray of hands showing rheumatoid arthritis.

caused by a general process called synovitis (an inflammation of the lining of the joint).

This causes the joint to appear swollen and feel painful and warm. Over time, this destructive inflammation may damage the entire joint. The disease affects two to three times more women than men. The disease usually begins in middle age (forties or fifties), but it can start at any age.

Signs and symptoms

The onset of rheumatoid arthritis is gradual, typically beginning with weakness, swelling and possibly pain in a few small joints, such as those of the hands or feet. Later, other joints may be affected.

The disease comes and goes unpredictably, in what is known as a "flare-and-remission" pattern. As it progresses, recurrent inflammation causes swelling and thickening of the membrane, called the synovia or synovium, that lines the joint.

Enzymes then attack and erode cartilage and other tissues, while spasms of surrounding muscles may pull the joint out of line. All this may be caused by the body's immune system being faulty and attacking the joints for no reason.

Joint pain

Rheumatoid arthritis starts as gradually developing joint and muscle stiffness. Although these symptoms usually develop over many weeks or months, they can also begin very suddenly. The pain usually occurs in the same joint on both sides of the body; that is, both hands, both feet, and so forth. Usually, you will notice joint pain in your hands and feet, first.

Rheumatoid arthritis can also affect joints in the wrists, elbows, shoulders, neck, knees, hips, and ankles. After a while, rheumatoid arthritis may cause joints to become bent or deformed. Fortunately, proper treatment can often prevent this process and can help correct it if it does occur.

Other general symptoms

In addition to joint and muscle pain, some people with rheumatoid arthritis may have a decreased appetite and lose weight, have a slight fever, and may be extremely fatigued.

Also, lumps called rheumatoid nodules may form under the skin in areas that receive pressure, such as the back of the elbows. They come and go during the course of the illness and usually don't cause problems. However, they sometimes become sore or infected.

Less commonly, rheumatoid arthritis may affect the heart or lungs, causing chest pain or difficulty breathing. It may also cause dryness and mild pain in the eyes.

Rheumatoid arthritis   Questions & Answers

What is rheumatoid arthritis?

Arthritis is an umbrella term that covers more than 100 diffe-rent diseases. It literally means "inflammation of a joint". This inflammation is what causes rheumatoid arthritis (RA). However, unlike osteoarthritis, RA is not localized to the joints. It can rarely affect other parts of the body such as the heart, skin, nerves, muscles and eyes.

Rheumatoid arthritis is one of the most severe forms of arthritis. It afflicts some 2.1 million Americans. It is a systemic disease and can be extremely painful and crippling. This chronic disease cannot be cured, but effective treatment is available.

What is the cause of RA?

The cause of RA is unknown. It is suspected, although unproven, that RA is caused by a viral infection. Genetics may also be a contributing factor. Women are afflicted two times more often than men.

What is inflammation?

When the body is injured, a normal inflammatory process begins. Cells in the blood rush to the injured area to eliminate toxic materials and speed healing. The outward signs are pain, swelling, heat and redness. In RA, the cells attack and destroy healthy tissue - starting with the membrane that surrounds the joint, extending to the cartilage that protects bone ends, and even affecting the underlying bone.

What are the symptoms?

The major symptoms of RA are joint pain, stiffness and muscle swelling. Other symptoms may include fatigue and joint deformity. In rare cases, damage to organs may result in shortness of breath or chest pain. Such symptoms may develop suddenly or over time.

Can RA be treated effectively?

Yes. Anti-inflammatory drugs are most commonly prescribed for early rheumatoid arthritis symptoms. However, now that more is known about RA, physicians recommend early treatment with more potent drugs such as hydroxychloroquine, methotrexate, newer biological treatments, or corticosteroids, which usually slow the disease down. Unless properly modified, these medications may have potentially serious side effects. Complete treatment of RA also requires learning how to protect affected joints by doing daily tasks in new ways and performing special exercises to strengthen muscles and maintain joint mobility. Because medication may not provide total symptom relief, hot or cold compresses and other physical therapy techniques also may be needed.

When is surgery considered?

Surgery may be considered when medical treatment does not work. If a joint becomes badly damaged, surgery may be required to remove the damaged tissue, stabilize the joint, or to replace it completely with an artificial joint.

Does the disease ever go away?

Rheumatoid arthritis sometimes gets worse - called a flare-up - or seems to subside or go away - called a remission - for unknown reasons. Both changes are usually temporary.

Causes of rheumatoid arthritis

The cause of rheumatoid arthritis is not yet known. For years, researchers have looked without success for an infection caused by a virus or bacterium as the cause of rheumatoid arthritis. It seems likely that a major disorder of the immune system plays a role. Researchers still suspect that something like a virus may trigger rheumatoid arthritis, but they do not think everyone who becomes infected with this "virus" will develop the illness. Scientists now believe that this unknown agent causes rheumatoid arthritis only in people who have a genetic, or inherited, tendency for the disease.

One clue supporting this idea is that most people with rheumatoid arthritis have a certain genetic marker called HLA-DR4. It is a common marker and occurs in about one-fourth of the United States population. Most people with the HLA-DR4 marker will not get rheumatoid arthritis, but may develop it more easily than those who don't have the marker.

Some people notice their rheumatoid arthritis begins or gets worse after a disturbing emotional event, such as a death in the family, divorce, or other emotional strain or shock. While such events don't cause rheumatoid arthritis, they may seem to trigger it or make it worse.

Diagnosis of rheumatoid arthritis

Because the symptoms of rheumatoid arthritis usually develop over a long period of time, it may take a while for your doctor to diagnose it.

The diagnosis of rheumatoid arthritis will not be based on one symptom or test alone, but on the overall pattern of the symptoms, your medical history, and the following tests:
- physical examination
- blood tests
- joint aspiration
- biopsy
- X-rays

R

Rheumatoid factor

This is an abnormal substance found in the blood of about 80 percent of adults with rheumatoid arthritis. It is also present in other diseases, so a positive factor does not always indicate rheumatoid arthritis. It is possible for people without the rheumatoid factor to have rheumatoid arthritis.

Erythrocyte sedimentation rate

This is a test which measures how fast red blood cells settle to the bottom of a thin tube. In people with chronic inflammation (including those with rheumatoid arthritis), the cells fall faster than normal. This test is a rough measurement of the activity of the disease.

Red blood cell count

This test is usually done during your first visit to the doctor. It shows if you have anemia, a condition which often occurs along with rheumatoid arthritis and causes extreme tiredness.

Joint aspiration

This is a test in which the doctor drains fluid from swollen joints and examines it to make sure the arthritis is not due to an infection or some other cause.

Biopsy

This is a test in which small bits of inflamed joint tissue or rheumatoid nodules are removed for examination with a microscope. This procedure may cause minor discomfort, but it is rarely used.

X-rays

X-rays may be used later in the disease to check the amount of damage in specific joints and to see if the stiffness is progressing.

Treatment

Rheumatoid arthritis can be severely crippling, as anyone knows who has seen the gnarled and twisted hands of a person who has the disease. To date, there is no cure for rheumatoid arthritis, but the disease can be controlled. And with continued treatment, the possibility of severe crippling is minimal.

Drugs used to treat rheumatoid arthritis

NSAIDs
- Aspirin
- Celecoxib
- Diclofenac
- Ibuprofen
- Naproxen
- Rofecoxib
- Valdecoxib, etc

Slow-acting compounds
- Cold compounds
- Hydroxychloroquine
- Penicillamine
- Sulfasalazine

Corticosteroid
- Prednisone, etc.

Immunosuppressive drugs
- Cyclophosphamide
- Cyclosporine
- Leflunomidee
- Methotrexate, etc

R

SCHIZOPHRENIA

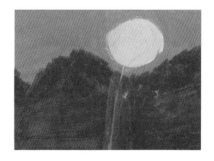

Description

Schizophrenia has a worldwide distribution. Using a relatively narrow concept of the disorder, studies of American, European and Asian populations have found the lifetime prevalence from 0.3 to 1.2 per cent. Even with the available forms of treatment, schizophrenic patients occupy about half of the hospital beds.

The high prevalence of schizophrenic disorders in lower socioeconomic classes has been mainly attributed to social disorganization and consequent stresses, but there is evidence that this association arises partly because some patients in a prepsychotic phase drift down the social scale.

Most cases of schizophrenia are now thought to be caused by a complex interaction between inherited and environmental factors. Approximately 10 per cent of relatives of schizophrenics will be recognized as schizophrenics. A genetic disposition is probably necessary if schizophrenia is to occur at all, but the overt manifestations of illness seem to be decided partly by stressful life experiences, such as faulty patterns of upbringing and disturbed relationships. Those who develop schizophrenia in middle age or later are often unmarried, widowed or deaf.

Although no specific type or premorbid personality is seen in all cases, many patients who develop schizophrenia show such traits as:
- sensitivity;
- shyness;
- unsociability;
- lack of affect;
- paranoid attitudes.

The term schizoid personality is used to describe persons with defective capacity to form social relationships; the term schizotypical personality is being introduced to describe those who, in addition to their deficiencies in social relations, show oddities of thinking, perception, communication and behavior which are not severe enough to meet the criteria of schizophrenia.

Signs and symptoms

Even in cases with acute onset and with an apparent relationship to stressful events in the environment, careful history taking often will reveal a prodromal period of weeks or months of increasing withdrawal and disorganization of the previous level of functioning. During the active phase, characteristic symptoms involve content of thought, language, perception, affect, collision, motor behavior, sense of self, and relationship to the external world. A residual phase often follows the active phase and may be similar to the prodromal phase, but at times with persistent

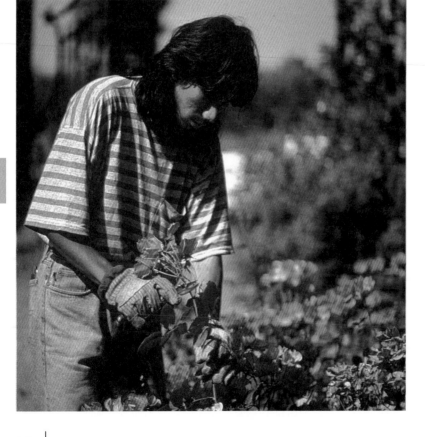

Community support activities are directed at teaching the skills needed to survive in the community.

S

delusional beliefs and with emotional blunting.

In order to distinguish schizophrenic disorders from short-term reversible illnesses, it is required that schizophrenia be diagnosed only when continuous signs have lasted for at least six months during the person's life, and that this period include an active phase of psychotic symptoms with or without a prodromal or residual phase. However, in many patients the deterioration is so gradual that it is difficult to trace back to a specific time when illness supervened in the schizoid personality.

In the early stages of schizophrenia, the patient may become increasingly uneasily aware that his psychological integrity is impaired. He may worry over his lack of concentration or fear that is going insane.

His personal identity may be threatened by doubts of his sexual gender. He may symbolize his wariness of illness in terms of an internal battle between good and evil or projects his feeling of internal dissolution onto the environment as fantasies of the annihilation of the world by some holocaust. Besides the group of specific symptoms there are also a number of nonspecific symptoms. Withdrawal from external reality and failure tom coordinate drive are frequent findings. There may be abnormality of psychomotor activity with rocking, pacing, peculiar motor response, or immobility.

The patient may often appear perplexed, eccentrically groomed or dressed, and disheveled.

Poverty of speech is common and ritualistic behavior associated with magical thinking often occurs. The patient may be depressed and exhibit anxiety, anger or a mixture of these. There may be ideas of reference and hypochondria concerns. Rarely, during a period of excitement, a patient may be found to be confused or disoriented, but usually there is significant disturbance in the sensorium.

Prognosis

Altered states of consciousness are rare in schizophrenic disorders. However, when this occurs and is

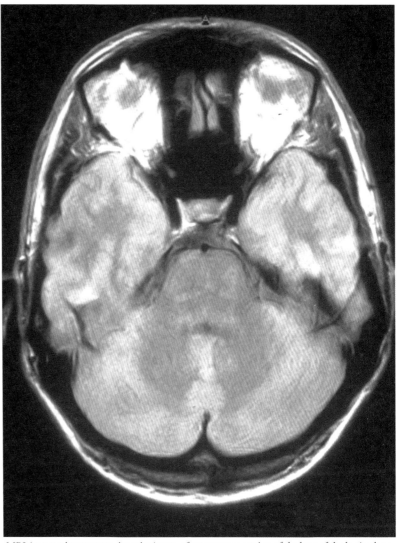

MRI (magnetic resonance imaging) scan of a transverse section of the base of the brain showing specific signs of degeneration of brain tissue.

accompanied by a clustering of schizophrenic symptoms, the symptoms may indicate an organic brain disorder caused by toxic (drugs, metabolic disturbances, infection) or other organic factors.

The organic delusional symptoms associated with amphetamines, cocaine and other drugs should be considered particularly. Paranoid disorders are usually distinguished from schizophrenic disorders by the absence of prominent hallucinations, incoherence or bizarre delusions.

Schizophrenia is not necessarily a chronic disorder.

About 30 per cent of patients recover completely and most of the remainder show some improvement. The florid symptoms can nearly always be controlled, but blunting of emotion and drive may remain intractable.

Although even minor defects may impair personal relationships and work efficiency, partial remission is compatible with a reasonable life adjustment. With treatment, an active psychosis commonly is controlled within 4 to 8 weeks, but residual defects of varying severity may persist

S

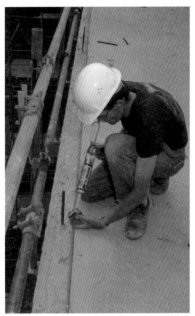
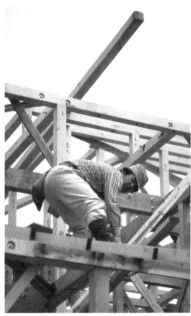

In taking psychoactive drugs, either for schizophrenia or any other psychological condition, one should take into account certain precautions:
▲ *Do not work around dangerous machinery.*
▲ *Do not climb ladders or work in dangerous places.*

Schizophrenia — Questions & Answers

What are the common symptoms of schizophrenia?

Schizophrenia is one of the most widespread and devastating of mental illnesses. While the word "schizophrenia" literally means "split mind." It is really an extensive deterioration of personality, a break with reality and a retreat into an unreal world. It is one type of psychosis.

People with advanced schizophrenia are easily recognized. They may see visions which appear totally real to them. They may have delusions of controlling others, including the world. They may withdraw, not speaking to others for weeks or months. They may be convinced of plots against them. They may daily repeat irrational acts.

The schizophrenic may be convinced he or she is some other person, such as Napoleon, Cleopatra, or God. In its early stages, when it may be more treatable, schizophrenia can be difficult to notice. People may seem to be more detached from their surroundings, or may throw themselves into some new activity in a bizarre way.

How can schizophrenia develop in a normal person; is anything known about the cause?

If left untreated, schizophrenia can advance to the point where the individual can no longer function in society. In schizophrenia, the disorganized type escapes reality through infantile behavior. Catatonics may sit motionless for hours or days, then go into wild frenzies. Paranoids may experience delusions of unbelievable grandeur.

Medical scientists still do not know for sure what causes schizophrenia. Some think that the disease is primarily psychological in nature and derives from problems in parent-child relationships. Others think that it is physical, a disorder of body chemistry. Others think it may be a combination of both.

Schizophrenic conditions are defined as mental disorders with a tendency toward chronicity which impairs functioning and which is characterized by psychotic symptoms involving disturbances of thinking, feeling and behavior.

Six specific criteria for the diagnosis of schizophrenic disorder include:
▲ certain psychotic symptoms, delusions, hallucinations, formal thought disorder;
▲ deterioration from a previous level of functioning;
▲ continuous signs of the illness for at least 6 months;
▲ a tendency towards onset before age 45;
▲ not due to affective disorders;
▲ not due to organic mental disorder or men-tal retardation.

for weeks or months before further improvement. Relapse is common unless adequate followup and medication intake is maintained. Acute exacerbations requiring therapeutic intervention often occur; residual impairment usually increases between episodes.

A favourable prognosis is associated with good premorbid personality with adequate social function, the presence of precipitating events, abrupt onset, onset late in life, a clinical picture that includes confusion or perplexity or a family history of affective disorder.

Treatment

The mainstays of treatment are:
- medicines;
- development of a therapeutic relationship with a skilled counsellor;
- social support;
- graded rehabilitation and retraining.

For the first illness or an acute relapse, hospitalization, even if it must be compulsory, is usually indicated for

Haldol

Properties

This medicine contains as active ingredient haloperidol, a psychoactive medicine that influences the activity of the brain. It is effective in reducing the violent aggressive manifestations of mental illnesses such as schizophrenia, mania, Alzheimer's dementia, and other disorders in which hallucinations are experienced.

The drug is prescribed for:

▲ Treatment for anxiety.
▲ Treatment for agitation and psychotic behavior.
▲ Treatment for Tourette's syndrome.
▲ Treatment for Huntington's chorea.

Before using this medicine

Before you use this medicine check with your doctor:

- if you ever had any unusual or allergic reaction to haloperidol.
- if you are pregnant or intend to become pregnant while using this medicine. Decide with your doctor if the drug benefits justify the risk to the unborn child.
- if you are breast-feeding an infant. The drug passes into the breast milk. Avoid the drug or discontinue nursing until you finish the medicine.
- if you have suffering from a depression.
- if you have Parkinson's disease.

Treatment

This medication is used to relieve or prevent the symptoms of your medical problem affecting your brain function.

▲ Tablet: swallow with liquid. If you can not swallow whole, crumble tablet and take with liquid or food.
▲ Drops: dilute dose in beverage before swallowing.
▲ Children: not recommended in children younger than 3 years. Side effects may be more common.
▲ Prolonged use: the patient may develop tardive dyskinesia. Talk to your doctor about the need for follow-up medical examinations or laboratory studies to check blood pressure, liver function.

Side effects

Along with the needed effects, a medicine may cause some unwanted effects. Side effects may include: High fever, Rapid pulse, Profuse sweating, Muscle rigidity, Confusion and irritability, Seizures, Jerky or involuntary movements, Slow-frequency tremor, Lack of facial expression, Inflexible movements, Pacing or restlessness

Overdose

Symptoms of overdose are: Weak, rapid pulse, Shallow, slow breathing, Tremor or muscle weakness, Very low blood pressure, Convulsions, Deep sleep ending in coma

▲ Call a doctor. Apply, if necessary, cardiac massage and mouth-to-mouth breathing.

Interactions

This medicine may interact with several other drugs. This medicine will add to the effects of alcohol, and CNS depressants. n Be sure to tell your doctor about any medications you are currently taking.

Driving or hazardous work

Do not drive until you learn how the medicine affects you. Do not work around dangerous machinery. Do not climb ladders or work in high places. Danger increases if you drink alcohol or take medicines affecting alertness and reflexes.

Storage

Store at room temperature in tightly closed, light-resistant containers. Keep out of the reach of children since overdose may be especially dangerous in children.

the following reasons:

▲ to stabilize the patient on a suitable regimen of medicines;
▲ to ensure the physical safety of the patient;
▲ to ensure the safety of other persons;
▲ to prevent damage to finances;
▲ to secure work prospects;
▲ to relieve the family.

Since schizophrenic patients are readily susceptible to institutionalism and since family ties are loosened by prolonged separation, hospitalization for more than a few months is harmful unless the severity of the illness makes it essential or it is part of an active rehabilitation program.

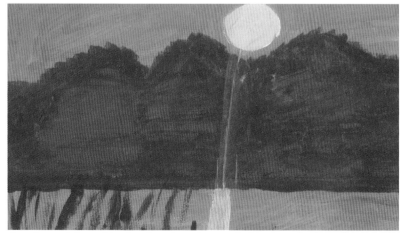

Drawing made by a schizophrenic patient who was asked to express her inner feelings.

SCIATICA

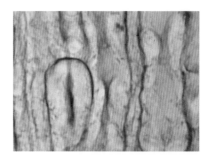

Description

Back pain or sciatica is a common disorder. What can go wrong in the back to produce backache, back trouble or a bad back? One or more of the bones in the spine may be injured or fractured. The site of the pain, its severity and how dangerous it is will depend on which bone is hurt.

Sciatic nerve
Course of the sciatic nerve in the pelvic region and the posterior part of the leg.

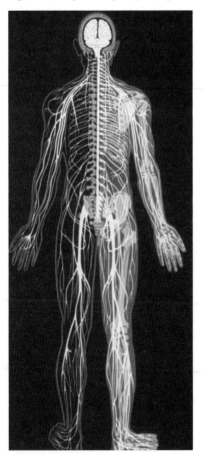

The back is vulnerable to most forms of arthritis, but the commonest is the kind caused over the years by wear and tear - osteoarthritis. Where you feel pain will depend on what part of the spine is involved.

Sciatic nerve

The components the sciatic nerve are derived from the spinal segments L4-S3. It is the largest nerve of the body and all roots of the sacral plexus contribute to it. In reality the sciatic nerve consists of two nerves within a common sheath: the common peroneal nerve and the tibial nerve.
The nerve leaves the pelvis through the infrapiriform part of the greater sciatic foramen. In the gluteal region the nerve courses laterally and then downward, leaving this area midway between the greater trochanter and the ischial tuberosity.
The sciatic nerve descends along the posterior surface of the thigh in a plane between the adductor magnus and hamstring muscles. At the lower half of the thigh at some distance above the popliteal fossa the main trunk divides into the common peroneal and tibial nerves.
In the thigh branches from the tibial portion of the sciatic nerve supply the following muscles;
- semitendinosus;
- semimembranosus;
- adductor magnus;
- biceps (long head).
The common peroneal portion of the sciatic nerve supplies the short head of the biceps. In close association with the sciatic nerve a number of small motor branches arise in the neighbourhood of the greater sciatic foramen to supply the external rotators of the thigh.

Lesions

Lesions to the sciatic nerve may usually result from a slipped disc. In general the common peroneal portion is affected more than the tibial portion. Various other conditions may injure the nerve:
- pelvic tumors;
- pelvic fractures;
- osteoarthritis;
- neuritis.
Paralysis of all the muscles makes much of the leg useless. A steppage gait is seen: the subject is unable to flex and extend at ankle and toe joints. Because of the hamstring paralysis, flexion at the knee joint is greatly impaired, but some flexion may be well performed by the sartorius muscles(innervated by the femoral nerve) and the gracilis muscle (innervated by the obturator nerve). The Achilles jerk and plantar reflex is also lost. Sensibility is lost on the outer side of the leg and most of the foot. Pain is present along the course of the nerve when the nerve is stretched by flexing the thigh and extending the knee.

Location of pain

The spinal column is surrounded by bands (ligaments) and muscles that protect it from injury and make sure its alignment does not go "out of whack."
When a bone is injured or diseased, these muscles go into spasm in order to protect it from excessive motion, and it's the spasm rather than the hurt bone that gives you most of the pain. Even a trivial bone disorder may trigger a crippling spasm, which accounts for the fact that many painful backs have normal X-rays. The most common variety of muscle spasm is not

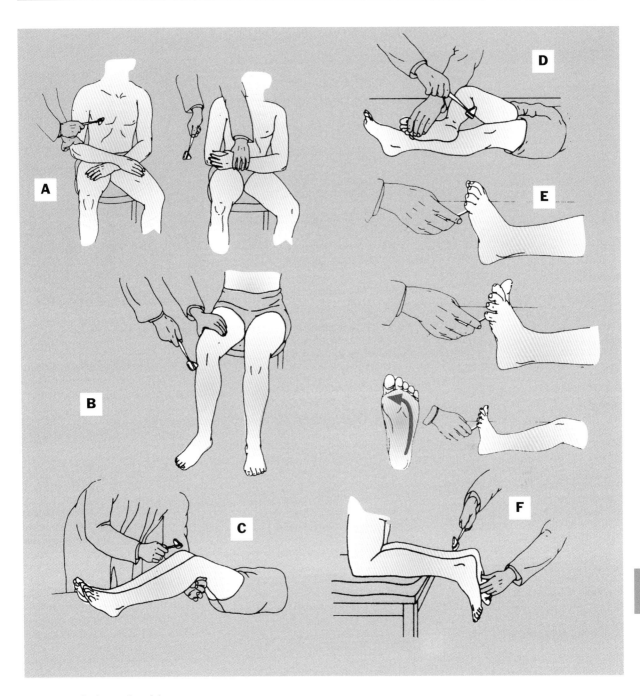

A. Biceps and triceps reflex of the arm.
Biceps reflex: contraction of the biceps muscle when its tendon is tapped. Triceps reflex: contraction of the belly of the triceps muscle, and slight extension of the arm when the tendon of the muscle is tapped directly, with the arm flexed and fully supported and relaxed.
C. Knee jerk: a kick reflex produced by sharply tapping the patellar ligament.
D and F. Achilles tendon reflex: plantar flexion of the foot elicited by a tap on the Achilles tendon, preferably while the patient kneels on a bed or chair, the feet hanging free over the edge.
E. Planter reflex: imitation of the sole contracts the toes. Babinski's reflex: dorsiflexion of the big toe on stimulation of the sole, occurring in lesions of the pyramidal tract.

S

Sciatica - Advice

Sleeping
- If you already have backache, you should never sleep on your stomach. For the sake of your back, lie on your side with the knees and hips bent or lie on your back with a pillow (or rolled blanket or similar object) under your knees to bend the knees and hips.
- It is best to sleep on a firm, flat mattress. Don't sleep on a soft, deep mattress or an old one with a depression in the middle.
- Your bed should not allow the middle of your body to sag as if it were in a hammock; it should support your hips firmly, with just enough softness for comfort.
- If your bed is too soft, you can get relief by putting a bed board (e.g. a sheet of plywood) under the mattress.
- When travelling, many hotels and motels will furnish bed boards on request or ask a hotel employee to move the mattress to the floor or simply spread blankets on the floor and sleep on them.

Standing
- If you must stand still for a long time, try to rest one foot higher than the other. If you are working on a ladder, put one foot on a rung higher than the other.
- If you are waiting at an airport or railway station, rest one foot on your suitcase. This standing position puts the least possible strain on your back.
- If you must be on your feet for a long time, try squatting; this will ease the strain on your back.

Fatigue
- It is best to avoid getting excessively tired during the day. Fatigue can exacerbate many lower back problems.
- Find a way to relax your back for five to ten minutes every day. If possible, lie flat on your back on a bed or floor. Elevate your legs on a pillow or cushion to exert a mild upward pull on your hips.

Bending
- When you bend over to get a closer look at something that is down on the ground, you should bend your knees as well as your back.
- If you must bend down to pick up something, avoid bending with your knees straight. It will be better for your back if you crouch down or rest on one knee only.
- When working with something on the ground, it is better to bend down on one knee rather than on both.

Lifting
- Bend your knees as well as your back when you bend over to pick up something.
- If you carry a heavy object for any distance, carry it close to your body with your elbows bent, not straight. Even with bent elbows it is dangerous to lift a heavy object higher than shoulder level.
- When carrying anything heavy, do not twist your body. If you must turn while heavily burdened, turn with your feet.
- Avoid lifting heavy objects that are in tight places.

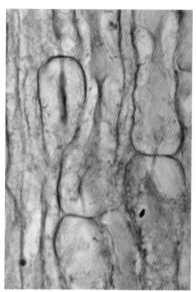

Microscopic picture of degeneration of the myelin sheath of the sciatic nerve.

the bones of the spine. These discs are normally of a gelatinous consistency. When they become dislocated or hardened, the bones they ordinarily separate ride on each other, and the nerves that go in and out of the spinal column are pressed.

The result is not only backache but numbness, tingling, pain and weakness of the arms and legs supplied by these nerves.

The arthritis process also thickens and deforms bones. When this happens, the holes through which nerves pass out of the bony spinal column become smaller and press on and irritate the nerves. This produces pain, not only in the diseased bone, but wherever the involved nerve happens to be going to, for example, an arm or leg. This explains the pain of sciatica, for example, which you feel in your buttock and down the back of the leg, even though the pressure is being exerted on the sciatic nerve in the low back.

Diagnosis

The diagnosis of backache is one thing; treatment is quite another. Diagnosis involves examination by looking, by touching, by assessment of muscle movement and, in order to

due to injury or disease but to nervous tension or bad posture.

Pain in the back can be transmitted to other parts of the body and mimic disease elsewhere. For example, a headache is much more likely to be due to spasm in the muscle at the back of the neck than to a brain tumor.

Back trouble is often due to disease and dislocation of the discs between

S

make sure that there are no underlying problems of the bones and spinal cord, by various X-ray methods. Moving from the neck downward, the doctor will check for mobility.

▲ How far can you bend forward to touch your toes?
▲ Does raising your legs cause pain in the back?

These and other movements reveal the presence and degree of any arthritis of the spine, the existence and severity of muscle spasm and whether or not there is a disc disease. Slipped discs are common in low back pain, producing pain in the sciatic area down the back of the leg. They can be detected by testing reflexes and sensation to see whether they are reduced or absent in the ankle and the knee.

Treatment

A few basic rules of treatment are generally accepted. If pain is due to bone injury, then rest and immobilization - as, for example, with a plaster cast - may be required. If you have a slipped disc, with pain and weakness of an arm or leg, before submitting to surgery try a good long period of bedrest, aspirin and moist heat.

As you improve, a program of planned progressive exercise may help, too. But remember, there is nothing worse than the wrong exercise, so make sure it is prescribed by a specialist in the field. Recently, injection of papain (a ferment obtained from the juice of the pawpaw) into slipped (herniated) discs to dissolve them has been tried, in many cases with good results. Many cases of chronic backache are due to physical inactivity, poor posture, obesity or bad mattresses that permit excessive curvature of the spine. Physically stressful jobs that require unnatural repetitive movements may also give rise to a sore back.

So, if you get recurrent aches in any part of your body, think about posture and the positions you assume during the day and at night. When you consult your doctor, be sure you tell him or her all about it, so that he/she can have a better understanding of the possible mechanisms that are giving you the symptoms.

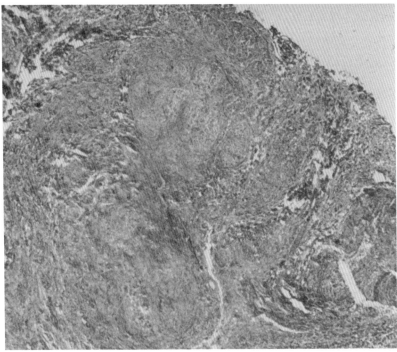

Microscopic picture of a neurinoma of the sciatic nerve causing severe attacks of pain.

Neurinoma of the sciatic nerve, probably due to repeated lesions.

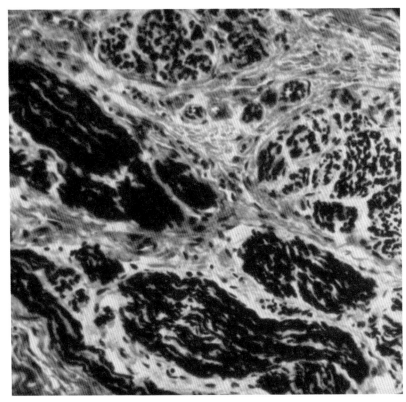

SEXUAL PROBLEMS

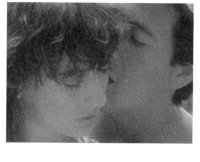

Introduction

Sexual problems may be classified as physiological, psychological, and social in origin. Any given problem may involve all three categories: a physiological problem, for example, will produce psychological effects, and these may result in some social maladjustment.

Sexuality is a normal part of the human experience. However, the types of sexual behavior, that are considered normal vary greatly within and among different cultures. Il fact, it may be impossible to define "normal" sexuality. There are wide variations not only in "normal" sexual behavior but also in the frequency of or need for sexual release.

Physiological problems

Physical problems of a specifically sexual nature are rather few. Only a small minority of people suffer from diseases of or deficient development of the genital organs or that part of the neurophysiology governing sexual response.

A large number of people, however, experience, at some point in life, sexual problems that are byproducts of other pathologies or injuries. Vaginal infections, for example, retroverted uterus, prostatitis, adrenal tumors, diabetes, senile changes of the vagina, and heart problems may cause disturbances of the sexual life.

In brief, anything that seriously interferes with normal bodily functioning generally causes some degree of sexu-

al trouble. Fortunately, the great majority of physiological sexual problems are solved through medication or surgery. Generally, only those problems involving damage to the nervous system defy therapy.

Psychological problems

Psychological problems constitute by far the largest category. They are not only the product of socially induced inhibitions, maladaptive attitudes, and ignorance but also of sexual myths held by society.

Premature ejaculation

Premature ejaculation is a common problem, especially for young males. Sometimes it is not the consequence of any psychological problem but the natural result of excessive tension in a male who has been sexually deprived. In such cases, more frequent coitus solves the problem.

A male suffers from premature ejaculation if he cannot delay ejaculation long enough to induce orgasm in a sexually normal female at least half a time. This generally means that vaginal penetration with some movement (although not continuous) must be maintained for more than one minute.

Various methods of preventing premature ejaculation have been tried. The most effective therapy is that advocated by Masters and Johnson in which the female brings the male nearly by orgasm and then prevents the male's orgasm by briefly compressing the penis between her fingers just below the head of the penis. The couple come to realize that premature ejaculation can thus be easily prevented, their anxiety disappears, and ultimately they can achieve normal coitus

Sexuality is a normal party of the human experience

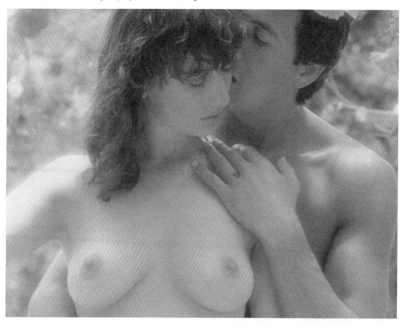

S

without resorting to this squeeze technique.

Erectile dysfunction

This is a medical condition characterized by the consistent inability to achieve and/or maintain an erection sufficient for satisfactory sexual activity.

Normally the male penis is soft and flaccid, but if sexually stimulated it becomes firm and erect. This is a reflex that cannot be consciously controlled by the man, and in fact if the man does try to consciously control an erection it is more likely to fail.

Stimulation of the penis, other sensitive areas of the body (e.g. nipple, small of back) and mental sexual imagery will result in a reflex in the nerves at the lower end of the spinal cord that sends a signal to muscle rings (valves) around the veins in the base of the penis that drain blood from the organ. These valves close, preventing blood from escaping from the penis while blood continues to be pumped into the organ through the arteries as normal. As a result it blows up in the same way as a sausage shaped balloon, the pressure of blood within the penis being the same as the maximum blood pressure elsewhere in the vascular system.

The penis has a long sponge filled sac (corpus cavernosum) along each side that fills with the blood under pressure to support the organ when erect. When ejaculation occurs or sexual stimulation ceases the valves around the veins open and allow the blood to drain out of the penis, and it becomes soft again. An inability to obtain an erection is called impotence or erectile dysfunction.

Vaginismus and dyspareunia

Vaginismus is a powerful spasm of the pelvic musculature constricting the vagina so that penetration is painful or impossible. It seems wholly due to anti-sexual conditioning or psychological trauma and serves as an

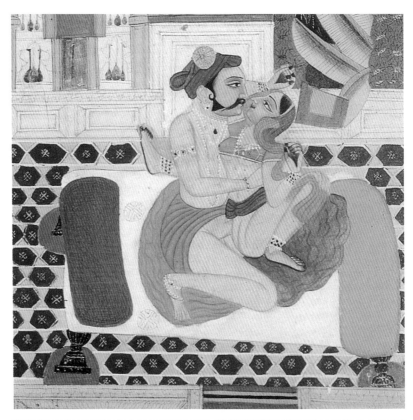

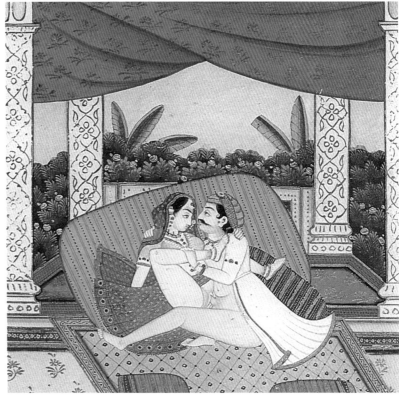

16th-century Indian drawings showing phases of love-making. The types of sexual behavior that are considered normal vary greatly within and among different cultures.

S

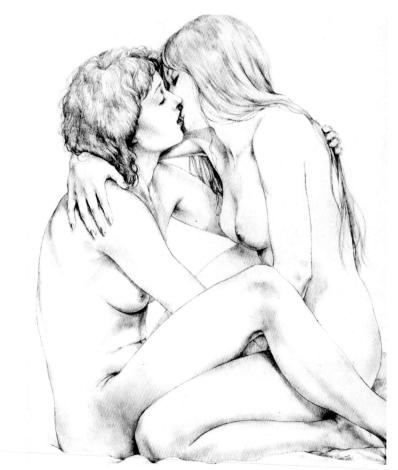

Homosexuals discover that they are attracted to people of the same sex, just as heterosexuals discover that they are attracted to people of the opposite sex. The attraction appears to be the end result of biological and environmental influences and is not a matter of choice.

Major sexuality disorders

Gender identity disorder
People who experience a significant discrepancy between their anatomy and their inner sense of self as masculine , feminine, mixed, or neutral often have a gender identity disorder. The extreme form of gender identity disorder is called transsexualism.

Paraphilias
Paraphilias are attractions that in extreme forms are socially unacceptable deviations from the traditionally held norms of sexual relationships and attractions. Examples are
- Fetishism
- Transvestic Fetishism
- Pedophilia
- Exhibitionism
- Voyeurism
- Sexual masochism and sadism

unconscious defense against coitus. It is treated by psychotherapy and by gradually dilating the vagina with increasingly large cylinders.

Dyspareunia, painful coitus, is generally physical rather that psychological. It is mentioned here because some inexperienced females fear they cannot accommodate a penis without being painfully stretched. This is a needless fear since the vagina is not only highly elastic but enlarges with sexual arousal, so that even a small female can, if aroused, easily receive en exceptionally large penis.

Disparity in sexual desire
Disparity in sexual desire constitutes the most common sexual problem. It is to some extent inescapable, since differences in the strength of the sexual impulse and the ability to respond are based on neurophysiological differences.

Much disparity, however, is the result of inhibition or of one person having been subjected to more sexual stimuli during the day than the other.

Another cause of disparity is a difference in viewpoint. Often a male will anticipate coitus as a palliative to compensate for the trials and tribulations of life, whereas many females are interested in sex only if the preceding hours have been reasonably problem-free and happy.

Even in cases of neurophysiological differences in sex drive, the less-motivated partner can be trained to a higher level of interest, since most humans operate well below their sexual capacities.

Anorgasmy
Lack of female orgasm, anorgasmy, is a very frequent problem. One should differentiate between females who become sexually aroused but do not reach orgasm and those who do not become aroused. Only the latter merit the label frigid.

It is common for females not to achieve orgasm during the first weeks or months of coital activity. It is almost as though many females must learn how to have orgasm, for after having had one, they respond with increasing frequency

Anorgasm is treated by removing inhibitions, teaching coital techniques, and by including orgasm through non-coital methods. The effective therapist should also impress upon the female that not reaching orgasm is no sign of failure or inadequacy on her part or her partner's and that sexual activity is very pleasurable to both, even, if orgasm does not ensue.

Sexual communication
Lastly, sexual problems are often perpatuated by the inability of the partners to communicate freely their feelings to one another. There is a curious and unfortunate reticence about

Erectile dysfunction   Questions & Answers

What is erectile dysfunction?

Erectile dysfunction is the consistent inability to achieve and/or maintain an erection sufficient for satisfactory sexual activity. That means not just an occasional problem, but one that has been occurring repeatedly for a period of time. It is a widespread condition.

What causes erectile dysfunction?

It was once believed that erectile dysfunction is all in your head, or just an inevitable result of getting older. Actually, the majority of erectile dysfunction cases are associated with physical conditions or events, including some that are age-related. The most common risk factors for erectile dysfunction include:

- Diabetes, high blood pressure, hardening of the arteries, or high cholesterol.
- Injury or illness, such as spinal cord injury, multiple sclerosis, depression, stroke, or surgery for the prostate gland or colon (bowel).
- Medications that may bring about erectile dysfunction as an unwanted side effect.
- Cigarette smoking or alcohol/drug abuse.
- Psychological conditions, such as anxiety and stress.

Can erectile dysfunction be treated?

Yes. Regardless of the cause, the vast majority of erectile dysfunction cases are treatable. Patients have a variety of treatment options from which to choose, including oral medication, hand-held vacuum pumps, self-administered injections, pellet suppositories and surgical implants.

Can anyone use these treatments?

It is important to remember that these treatments are not for everyone, but only for men diagnosed with erectile dysfunction. You and your doctor can determine the appropriate treatment for you.

How do I know if I have erectile dysfunction?

If you have erection problems, you probably already know it. But before your condition can be treated, you need to get a diagnosis from your doctor. There is no need to be embarrassed or ashamed when discussing erectile dysfunction with your doctor. He has probably diagnosed and treated erectile dysfunction many times but may not have discussed it with you out of respect for your privacy. Your doctor can provide you with understanding, support and best of all, information. To diagnose erectile dysfunction, doctors typically ask a few specific questions and give a routine physical examination. This should help your doctor arrive at a diagnosis.

informing one's partner as to what does or does not contribute to one's pleasure. The partner must function on a trial and error basis, ever on the alert for signs indicating the efficacy of his or her efforts.

This muteness is even more pronounced when it comes to an individual making suggestions to the partner. Many persons feel that a suggestion or request would be interpreted by the partner that he or she had been inapt or at least remiss. As with other problems, sexual problems can be overcome or ameliorated only if the individuals concerned communicate effectively.

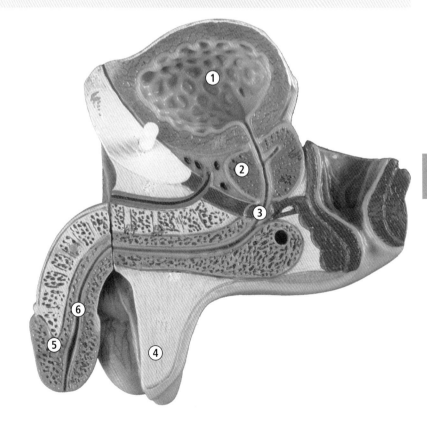

Side view of a model of the male reproductive organs.
1. Urinary bladder
2. Prostate gland
3. Urethra
4. Scrotum
5. Glans penis
6. Penis

S

SEXUALLY TRANSMITTED DISEASES (STD)

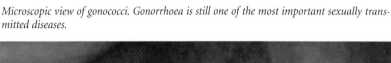

Introduction

About 85 per cent of cases of sexually transmitted diseases occur in persons aged between 15 and 20 years. In addition to syphilis and gonorrhea, the list of sexually transmitted diseases now includes:

- Human immunodeficiency virus (HIV) infection
- Chlamydia trachomatis infection
- Genital herpes virus infection
- Human papilloma virus (HPV) infection
- Chancroid
- Genital mycoplasma
- Cytomegalovirus infection
- Hepatitis B infection
- Certain types of vaginitis
- Certain enteric infections
- Certain ectoparasitic diseases

Chlamydial infection is the most common sexually transmitted disease.

Microscopic view of gonococci. Gonorrhoea is still one of the most important sexually transmitted diseases.

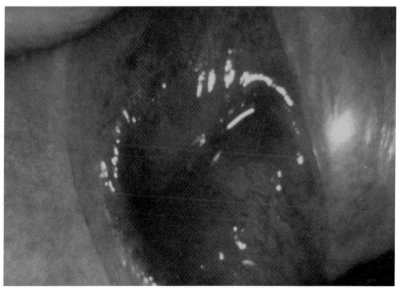

Although the incidence of gonorrhea and syphilis decreased in the early 1990s, these sexually transmitted diseases remain a persistent public health problem.

The consequences of sexually transmitted diseases are particularly troublesome for women and children. Apart from AIDS, the most serious complications of sexually transmitted diseases are:

- pelvic inflammatory disease
- an increased risk of cervical cancer
- ectopic pregnancy
- congenital infection
- congenital malformations
- delivery of premature infants
- delivery of low-birth-weight infants
- fetal death

Persons who are poor or medically under-served and racial and ethnic minorities also contract a disproportionate number of sexually transmitted diseases and the disabilities associated with them.

Individuals who are at increased risk for sexually transmitted diseases and HIV infection include:

- those who are or were recently sexually active, especially persons with multiple sexual partners
- those who use alcohol of illicit drugs
- gay or bisexual men who have sex with other men
- persons with a previous history of a documented sexually transmitted disease and their close contacts
- persons involed in the exchange of sex for drugs or money
- persons living in areas where the prevalence of human immunodeficiency virus infections and sexually transmitted diseases is high

Health authorities state that all adolescent and adult patients should be advised about risk factors for sexually transmitted diseases and HIV infection and counseled appropriately about effective measures to reduce risk of infection.

The recommendation is based on the proven efficacy of risk reduction, although the effectiveness of clinical counseling in the primary health care setting is uncertain. Counseling should be tailored to the individual risk factors, needs, and abilities of each patient.

Assessment of risk should be based on the local epidemiology of sexually transmitted diseases and HIV infection. Patients at risk of sexually transmitted diseases should receive information on their risk and be advised about measures to reduce their risk.

Effective measures include:

- abstaining from sex
- maintaining a mutually faithful monogamous sexual relationship

with a partner known to be uninfected
- regular use of latex condoms
- avoiding sexual contact with high-risk inividuals (e.g. injection drug users, commercial sex workers, and persons with numerous sex partners).

Women at risk of sexually transmitted diseases should be advised of options to reduce their risk in situations when their male partner does not use a condom, including the female condom. Warning should be provided that using alcohol and drugs can increase high-risk sexual behavior.

Basics of counseling
(1) Every patient's risk for sexually transmitted diseases should be determined. The physician should tailor counseling to the behaviors, circumstances, and specific needs of the person being served. Risk-reduction messages must be personalized and realistic. Counseling should be culturally appropriate, sensitive to issues of sexual identity, developmentally appropriate, and linguistically specific.
(2) All patients should be advised about the issue that any unprotected sexual behavior poses a risk for sexually transmitted diseases. A person who is infected can infect others during sexual intercourse, even if no symptoms are present.
(3) All sexually active patients should be instructed about the effective use and limitations of condoms, stressing that they are not foolproof, must be used properly, and may break during intercourse. The best preventive measure against transmission of HIV and other sexually transmitted diseases, after abstinence, is use of latex condoms (not "lambskin" or natural-membrane condoms).
Scientific research has demonstrated that latex condoms, when used consistently and correctly, are highly effective in stopping human immunodeficiency virus transmission.
(4) Myths about human immuno-deficiency virus transmission should be dispelled by informing patients that they cannot become

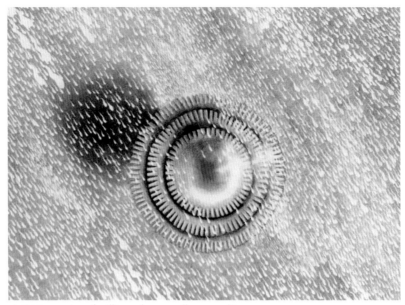

Artist impression of millions of sperm cells approaching an egg.

infected from mosquito bites; contact with toilet seats or other everyday objects, such as doorknobs, telephones, or drinking fountains; or manual contact with someone who is infected with human immunodeficiency virus of has AIDS, such as shaking hands, hugging, or a kiss on the cheek.
(5) Persons who continue to inject drugs should have periodic screening for human immuno-deficiency virus and hepatitis B. Hepatitis B vaccination should be considered for individuals lacking immunity who are negative for hepatitis B surface antigen. Measures to reduce the risk of infection caused by drug use should be discussed:
- use a new, sterile syringe for each injection
- never share or reuse injection equipment
- use clean (if possible, sterile) water to prepare drugs
- clean the injection site with alcohol before injection
- safely dispose of syringes after use

Examples of questions for taking clinical histories about sexual behavior

- ▲ Are you currently or were you recently in a sexual relationship?
- ▲ Do yu have sex with men, women, or both?
- ▲ How many men of women did you have sex with in the last week, last month, last year?
- ▲ Is each partner new, casual, or regular?
- ▲ Do you know if your partners have other sex partners?
- ▲ Have any of your partners been men who have sex with other men?
- ▲ Have any of your partners injected (shot) drugs?
- ▲ Have you had sex with someone that you know or suspect has human immuno-deficiency virus infection?
- ▲ Has anyone ever given you money, drugs, or other things of value in exchange for sex?

S

Sexually transmitted disease Questions & Answers

What are the most important STDs (Sexually Transmitted Diseases)?

Chlamydia, gonorrhoea, genital warts, herpes, hepatitis B and HIV infection are the most important STDs.

- Chlamydia is the most common and, just like gonorrhoea, can lead to infertility if left untreated.
- Genital warts and herpes are also very common and are particularly annoying because some people have regularly recurring bouts of them.
- Syphilis is a serious disease which is fortunately uncommon these days. Hepatitis B can have serious consequences if it is chronic.
- AIDS is an incurable, fatal disease caused by a virus (HIV). You can be infected without being ill. And you can then infect other people.

Other - less serious - STDs are trichomoniasis, pubic lice (crabs) and scabies.

How do you contract an STD?

You can contract an STD, including infection with HIV, from unsafe sex. Unsafe sex is:

- vaginal intercourse without a condom (penis enters vagina);
- intercourse without a condom (penis enters anus);
- to a certain extent oral sex (putting genitals in the mouth) without a condom.

Licking the vagina during menstruation or getting semen in the mouth can carry a risk of infection with HIV. HIV, hepatitis B, syphilis, chlamydia, herpes and gonorrhoea can also be

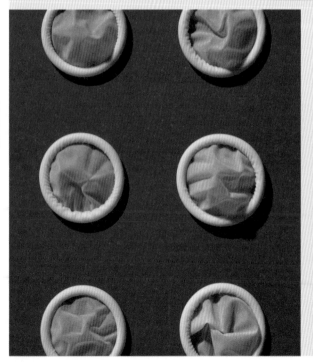

transmitted during pregnancy or birth if the mother is infected. HIV and hepatitis B can also be transmitted by sharing infected needles, during drug use or unhygienic tattooing.

Are there always symptoms of a sexually transmitted disease?

No, not always. It can take weeks, months and sometimes even years for symptoms to occur. Sometimes there are hardly any or no symptoms of they are so slight that they do not bother you. Women in particular often have no symptoms at all.

But without treatment you are and remain infectious and can unknowingly pass on the disease. People who are infected with the AIDS virus (HIV positive) are not necessarily aware of this. Often they can be symptom-free for years on end. And you cannot see they are infected. But they can transmit the AIDS virus.

What are the general complaints and symptoms of a sexually transmitted disease?

If complaints and symptoms do occur, these are mostly:

- Discharge or pus from penis, vagina or anus. In women there is increased discharge (as some discharge from the vagina is normal). The discharge can be watery, milky, yellowish or greenish and smell different.
- A burning feeling, irritation, pain during or after urinating or passing small amounts of urine frequently.
- Sores, warts or blisters on the penis, vagina, anus or mouth.
- Swollen glands in the groin.
- Pain in or near one or both testicles.
- Pain in the abdomen.
- Loss of blood after sex.

What are the consequences of not being treated for a STD (sexually transmitted disease)?

If you do not have a sexually transmitted disease treated there could be serious consequences. Some examples: it occurs more and more than women become infertile years after having contracted chlamydia and not having it treated. You are also more susceptible to infection with the AIDS virus if you have another STD.

What about pregnancy and an STD (sexually transmitted disease)?

If a woman contracts an STD before or during pregnancy, the baby can be infected during the pregnancy. The STD can also be passed on to the baby during birth. That is why pregnancy women are always tested for syphilis and hepatitis B. If these STDs are discovered early enough, then it is possible to prevent the baby becoming infected.

The test for AIDS virus is not automatically included in the antenatal. If you have run the risk of being infected with the AIDS virus, it is worth considering a test before becoming pregnant.

S

Sexually transmitted disease   Questions & Answers

What should you do if you (think you) have an STD (sexually transmitted disease)?

Most STDs are easy to treat, but they do not go away by themselves, even if the symptoms have disappeared. Treatment is always necessary. Do not try to be your own doctor. Even a doctor can only diagnose an STD after tests.

Some STD symptoms can be treated, but the symptoms will often recur (herpes, genital warts). You can go to your own doctor, the local health center or a family planning clinic.

Why a smear test and culture for an STD (sexually transmitted disease)?

The doctor takes a smear (this is not the same as a cervical smear). With a cotton bud (or a plastic spatula) some mucus and/or pus is taken from the spot where you might have been infected: penis, vagina, cervix (neck of the uterus), anus, sometimes the throat. Under the microscope it will then become visible if there is an STD. The material can also be sent to a laboratory. There they put the smear on a culture dish: the germ is cultivated.

What does treatment for a STD (sexually transmitted disease) consists of?

Each disease will have a different treatment. There are courses of tablets, one or more injections or ointments. The time it

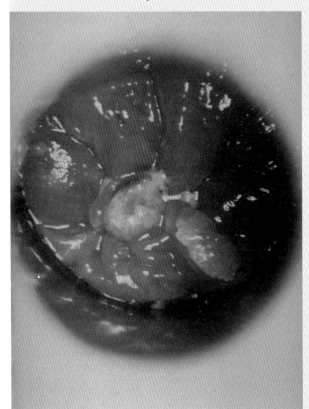

takes for an STD to be treated may vary. You should always take all the prescribed pills or tablets, even if the symptoms have disappeared.

Not finishing a course can be risky. For instance bacteria which have not yet been killed can then multiply again, and you will remain infected and capable of infecting others.It is better not to have sex during the time you are having treatment, so that the affected mucous membrane can heal. If you do have sex you can only do so with a condom or dental dam.

It is necessary to warn my partner if I have contact a STD (sexually transmitted disease)?

You can pass on the disease to everyone with whom you have sex from the moment you have been infected and during treatment. This is also the case when you have no or hardly any symptoms or when symptoms are so slight that they do not bother you.

That is why you should warn the people you have had sexual contact with. They could have the STD too, even if they have no symptoms. Advice them to visit a doctor and have a test. How far you have to go back in warning and tracing sexual partner(s) depends on the kind of STD and the stage of the infection. Discuss this with your doctor.

What is safer sex?

You can prevent contracting a sexually transmitted disease by always having safer sex. You then minimize the chance of catching a venereal disease.

Safer sex is:

- Only having sexual contact with one regular partner who never has sex with anyone else and not have a sexually transmitted disease.
- Caressing, French Kissing, kissing, cuddling, massage (mutual) masturbation.
- Using a condom for vaginal and anal intercourse.
- Using a condom or dental dam (a small sheet of thin rubber) for oral sex (licking the genitals) if you know or suspect that one of you has been infected.

How to use a condom?

Using a condom the right way minimizes the chance of a sexually transmitted disease. Stick to the following rules:

- Use a new condom every time you have intercourse (vaginal or anal).
- Avoid any contact between penis and vagina or anus before the condom has been put on.
- Do not put on the condom until the penis is completely erect. Hold on to the top of the condom with thumb and forefinger. Unroll the condom right down the penis.
- After you have come withdraw the penis from vagina or anus straightaway.
- Only use water-based lubricant which is specifically made for sex and not oil, vaseline or cream (these weaken the rubber).

S

SKIN CANCER

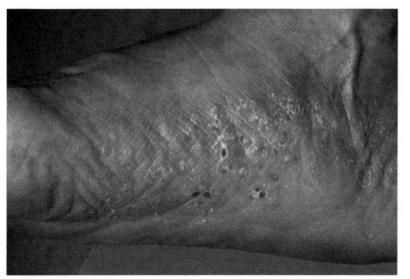

Description

The skin can also be involved in the development of malignant tumor or cancer as any other organ or tissue in the body. The two most common kinds of skin cancer are basal cell carcinoma and squamous cell carcinoma.

■ Basal cell carcinoma
Basal cell carcinoma accounts for more than 90 per cent of all skin cancers in the Western countries. It is a slow-growing cancer that seldom spreads to other parts of the body.

■ Squamous cell carcinoma
Squamous cell carcinoma also rarely spreads, but it does so more often than basal cell carcinoma.
However, it is important that skin cancers are found and treated in an early stage because they can invade and destroy nearby tissue. Basal cell

carcinoma and squamous cell carcinoma are sometimes called non-melanoma skin cancer, because another type of cancer that occurs in the skin is melanoma, which begins in the melanocytes.

■ Malignant melanoma
Melanomas are increasing in frequency. Malignant melanomas arise in areas of the skin, mucous membranes, the eye and central nervous system where pigment cells occur. They appear in different sizes, shapes, and colours (most commonly pigmented), and vary in propensity for invasion and metastasis.
Malignant melanoma is a highly malignant tumor that may spread so rapidly it is often fatal within months of its recognition, while in some forms the 5-year cure rate is nearly 100 per cent. Early suspicion by inspection and an adequate biopsy for histologi-

cal determination of tumor thickness are the only means of effective management and an optimum prognosis. Because the incidence of melanoma is increasing rapidly and early diagnosis and cure depend upon the patient's consulting a physician early, vigorous campaigns to alert the public are underway in most countries. Most malignant melanomas arise from melanocytes in normal skin; about 40 to 50 per cent develop from pigmented moles.
Danger signals that suggest malignant transformation of pigmented nevi include:
▲ changes in size;
▲ changes in colour, especially spread of pigmentation to surrounding normal skin and red, white, and blue colours;
▲ surface characteristics such as consistency and shape;
▲ surrounding skin alterations, especially with signs of inflammation.
Although melanomas are more common in pregnant than in nonpregnant women, pregnancy does not increase the likelihood that a mole will become a melanoma. Metastasis to the fetus is rare. Malignant melanomas are very rare in children, but can arise from very large pigmented moles (giant congenital nevi) that have been present from birth.

Cause and prevention

Skin cancer is the most common type of cancer in our country. According to present estimates 33-35 per cent of people living in this country who live to age 70 will have skin cancer at least once (most of them disappear spontaneously). Several risk factors increase the chance of getting skin cancer.

Old mycotic lesion showing the first sign of malignant degeneration.

S

Ultraviolet (UV) radiation from the sun is the main cause of skin cancer. Artificial sources of UV radiation, such as sunlamps and tanning booths, can also cause skin cancer.

Although anyone can get skin cancer, the risk is greatest for people who have fair skin and freckles easily - often those with red or blond hair and blue or light-coloured eyes. Worldwide, the highest rates of skin cancer are found in South Africa and Australia, areas that receive high amount of UV radiation.

In addition, skin cancer is related to lifetime exposure to UV radiation. Most skin cancers appear after age 50, but the sun's damaging effects begin at an early age. Therefore, protection should start in childhood to prevent skin cancer later in life.

Protective clothing, such as sun hats and long sleeves, can block out the sun's harmful rays. Also, lotions that contain sunscreens can protect the skin.

Sunscreens often contain PABA (para-aminobenzoic acid) and are rated in strength according to an SPF (Skin Protection Factor), which ranges from 2 to 15 or higher. The higher the number on the label, the greater the protection a sunscreen provides, meaning more of the sun's harmful rays will be blocked out.

Symptoms

The most common warning sign of skin cancer is a change on the skin, especially a new growth or a sore that does not heal. Skin cancer has many different appearances. For example, it may start as a small, smooth, shiny, pale, or waxy lump. The cancer may also appear as a firm red lump. Sometimes, the lump bleeds or develops a crust.

Skin cancer can also start as a flat, red spot that is rough, dry, or scaly. Pain is not a sign of skin cancer. Both basal and squamous cell cancers are found mainly on areas of the skin that are exposed to the sun - the head, face, neck, hands, and arms. However, skin cancer can occur anywhere.

Another condition that can affect the skin is actinic keratosis, which appears as rough, red or brown, scaly patches on the skin. Because actinic keratosis sometimes develops into squamous cell cancer, it is known as a precancerous condition. Like skin cancer, it usually appears on sun-exposed areas but can be found elsewhere. Changes in the skin are not sure signs of cancer; however, it is important to see a physician if any symptom lasts longer than two weeks.

Detection and diagnosis

The cure rate for skin cancer could be 100 per cent if all skin cancers were brought to a physician's attention before they had a chance to spread. Therefore, people should check themselves regularly for new growth or other changes in the skin.

Skin cancers are generally diagnosed and treated in the same way. When an area of skin does not look normal, the physician may remove all or part of the growth. This is called a biopsy. To check for cancer cells, the tissue is examined under a microscope by a pathologist or a dermatologist. A biopsy is the only sure way to tell if the problem is cancer.

Physicians generally divide skin cancer into two stages: local (affecting only the skin) or metastatic (spreading beyond the skin). In cases where the growth is very large or has been present for a long time, the physician will carefully check the lymph nodes in the area. In addition, the patient may need to have additional tests, such as special X-rays, to find out whether the cancer has spread to other parts of the body. Knowing the stage of a skin cancer helps the physician plan the best treatment.

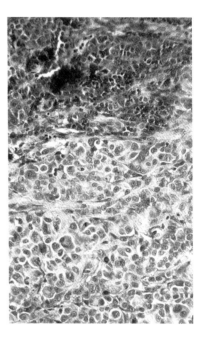

Microphotograph of a melanoma. These tumors can begin as a new, small, pigmented skin growth on normal skin, most often on sun-exposed areas, or it may develop from preexisting pigmented moles.

Treatment

Treatment for skin cancer may involve surgery, radiation therapy, or

Malignant melanoma - The facts

▲ Nearly all skin cancers are caused by the sun. There are two main types: malignant melanoma and non-melanoma.

▲ Malignant melanoma is the most dangerous form of skin cancer. It can spread rapidly, but if caught and treated early the chances of survival are good.
- over 16,000 new cases every year
- the number of new cases has more than doubled since 1990
- over 6,500 deaths every year
- about 60% more common in women than men
- affects young adults as well as older people

▲ Melanomas are most common among sun-sensitive people who spend most of the year indoors and then take a fortnight's holiday in the sun.

Skin cancer Questions & Answers

What is melanoma?

Melanoma is a kind of cancer that comes from the cells that give colour to the skin. These cells are called melanocytes. Some melanomas arise in normal skin and others arise in pigmented skin (moles).

Melanoma is a common type of cancer. If melanoma is not detected early, it can be fatal. Fortunately, melanoma is easy to detect. Almost all patients can be cured with minor surgery if melanoma is found early.

What causes melanoma or skin cancer?

Most experts agree than too much exposure to the sun is the main course of melanoma. Melanoma is also linked to moles. Some moles may turn into melanoma.

Who gets melanoma?

Anyone can get melanoma. People at increased risk of melanoma are those with fair hair, freckles, blond or red hair, and blue or grey eyes. If you have a large congenital nevus (sometimes called a congenital mole or birthmark) or many small moles, you may also have an increased risk. Melanoma can run in families, so tell your doctor if you have a relative who has had melanoma.

What is the difference between a melanoma and an ordinary mole?

Although it can be hard to tell the difference between a melanoma and a mole, there are some clues to look for. Normally, moles remain the same in size, shape and colour. A change in the appearance of a mole may be a sign of melanoma. If you notice that a mole has changed in any way - if it grows, bleeds, becomes scaly, changes colour, becomes itchy or painful - have your doctor look at it right away.

How can I remember the warning signs in case of melanoma of skin cancer?

The American Cancer Society recommends that people use the ABCD system to remember for warning signs of melanoma:

A = Asymmetry

Is the outline of the mole irregular or asymmetrical? If one half of the mole doesn't match the other half, it is asymmetrical. This can be a sign of melanoma.

B = Border

Are the edged, or border, of the mole uneven? Irregular edges may be a sign of melanoma.

C = Colour

Is the mole varied in colour? A melanoma is usually not uniform in colour. There may be shades of tan, brown and black present in a melanoma. Red, white and blue may also be seen.

D = Diameter

Is the diameter of the mole larger than normal (more than the size of a pencil eraser)? An increase in the size of a mole may be a sign of melanoma. See your doctor if you can answer yes to any of the questions above.

Can anything be done to prevent melanoma?

Yes. First, avoid prolonged exposure to strong sunlight and do not use tanning booths. Use a sunscreen lotion regularly when you are going to be in the sun. Wear clothes that cover you, such as broad-brimmed hat and shirts with long sleeves.

cryosurgery. Sometimes, a combination of these methods is used. The physician considers a number of factors to determine the best treatment for skin cancer, such as the location of the cancer, its size, and whether or not the cancer has spread beyond the skin. The physician's main objective is to destroy the cancer completely while causing as little as scarring as possible.

■ Surgery

Most skin cancers can be removed quickly and easily by surgery. Sometimes, the cancer is completely removed at the time of biopsy, and no further treatment is needed. To remove small skin cancers, physicians commonly use a special type of surgery called curettage. After a local anesthetic numbs the area, the cancer is scooped out with a curette, an instrument with a sharp, spoon-shaped end.

Then, the area is generally treated by electro-desiccation. An electric current from a special machine is used to control bleeding and kill any cancer cells around the edge of the wound. Mohn's technique is a special type of surgery used for skin cancer. It is especially helpful for treating skin cancer in cases where the shape and depth of the tumor are hard to determine. In addition, this method is used to treat cancers that have recurred. The cancer is shaved off one layer at a time until the entire tumor is removed. This method will be used by physicians who are specially trained in this type of surgery. Sometimes, when a large cancer is removed, a skin graft may be needed. For this procedure, the physician takes a piece of skin from another part of the body to replace the skin that was removed. Surgery to remove skin cancers, with or without skin grafts, may cause scars.

■ Cryosurgery

Extreme cold may be used to treat precancerous skin conditions, such as actinic keratosis, as well as skin cancers. In cryosurgery, liquid nitrogen is applied to the growth to freeze and kill the abnormal cells. After the area thaws, the dead tissue falls off. More than one freezing may be needed to remove the growth completely. Cryosurgery does not require anes-

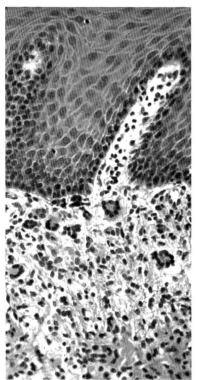

Microscopic picture of a xanthogranuloma, a disorder of lipid metabolism.

thesia, but patients may have pain after treatment. A white scar may form in the treated area.

■ Radiation therapy

Skin cancer responds well to radiation therapy, which uses high-energy rays to kill cancer cells. This treatment is used for cancers that occur in areas that are hard to treat with surgery. For example, radiation therapy might be used to treat skin cancers of the eyelid, the tip of the nose, and the ear. Several treatments may be needed to remove all of the cancer cells.

During radiation therapy, patients may notice skin reactions, such as rashes or redness, in the area being treated. Changes in skin colour and/or texture may develop, becoming more noticeable many years later.

■ Topical chemotherapy

This is the use of anticancer drugs in the form of a cream or lotion applied to the skin surface. Actinic keratosis can be treated effectively with a number of anticancer drugs. The lotion or cream may be applied daily for several weeks. Intense inflammation is common during treatment, but scars usually do not occur.

■ Follow-up therapy

Even though most patients with skin cancer are cured, this type of cancer is the one most likely to recur. That is why it is so important for patients to continue to examine themselves regularly, and to follow their physician's instructions on how to reduce their risk of developing skin cancer again.

■ New developments

Under study are: biological therapies, including interleukin-2 and interferon; therapeutic vaccines containing melanoma antigens, which are showing considerable promise.

Types of melanomas

Four major types of melanomas have been described. There is, however, little clinical significance as far as prognosis is concerned, since prognosis largely depends upon the histologically determined thickness of the melanoma.

Lentigo-maligna melanoma

This type of melanoma arises from lentigo maligna (Hutchinson's freckle) which appears on the face or other sun-exposed areas in elderly patients as an asymptomatic, large (1-2 inches), flat, tan or brown macula with darker brown or black spots scattered irre-gularly on its surface.
In this skin cancer both the normal and malignant melanocytes are not only confined to the epidermis, but also invade the der-mis.

Superficial spreading melanoma

Thus type accounts for about 65% of all melanomas. It is initially much smaller that the lentigo-maligna melanoma, is usual-ly asymptomatic, and occurs most commonly on the legs in women and on the trunk in men.
Consultation is sought because the pa-tient notes enlargement or irregular coloration of the lesion. It usually appears as a plague with raised, indurated edges, and often shows red, white, and blue spots or small, sometimes protuberant, blue-black nodules. Small indentation may be noted on the surface.

Nodular melanoma

This type comprises 10 to 15% of all melanomas. It may occur anywhere on the body and is seen in patients in their 20s to 60s. It is also asymptomatic, unless it ulcera-tes.
Consultation is usually sought because dark, protuberant papules or a pla-que rapidly enlarges, often with little radial growth. Colors vary from pearl to grey to black. Occasionally, a nodular mela-noma contains little if any pigment.

Acrolentiginous melanoma

This type is uncommon. It rises on palmar, plantar, and sublingual skin and has a cha-racteristic histological picture.

Warning signs of melanoma

▲ Enlarging pigmented (especially black or deep blue) spot or mole.

▲ Changes in colour of an existing mole, especially the spread of red, white, and blue pigmentation to surrounding skin.

▲ Changes in characteristics of skin over the pigmented spot, such as changes in consistency or shape.

▲ Signs of inflammation on skin surrounding an existing mole.

S

SKIN DISORDERS

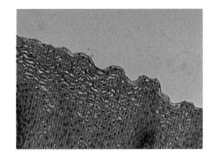

Introduction

Disorders and diseases of the skin are so varied and so common that dermatology is a specialty in the practice of medicine. The most remarkable fact about this field of medicine is how much there remains to be learned about it. For instance, that plague of adolescence, acne, is not completely understood even today. The same is true for psoriasis.

Although most microorganisms are parasites and thus pathogenic to man, there are numerous species that live on the skin at peace with us. Under certain conditions these microorganisms may become pathogenic and cause serious skin diseases.

Skin infection or dermatitis is not a specific illness but a general term for any inflammation of the skin. In the last decades it has been found that a great many such inflammations are allergic reactions.

The foreign proteins called allergens that cause these reactions are sometimes products of metabolism that appear after the intake of foods which the body is not accustomed to digesting. Among the most frequent offenders are such fruits as strawberries and certain proteins from such seafood as crabs and lobsters.

More than 95 per cent of all skin diseases and disorders are among the following ailments:

- acne
- eczema
- infections
- psoriasis
- tumors

Acne

Acne vulgaris is a chronic skin condition characterized mainly by comedones (whiteheads and blackheads) and papules (a small, firm raised skin lesion). In severe cases, inflammation, pustules (small, pus-containing elevations on the skin), cysts, and scaring may occur. Acne occurs most commonly on the face, back, and chest.

Although it does not pose a severe physical threat, acne should not be ignored since it may cause a great deal of emotional stress and anguish. The condition occurs most often in ado-

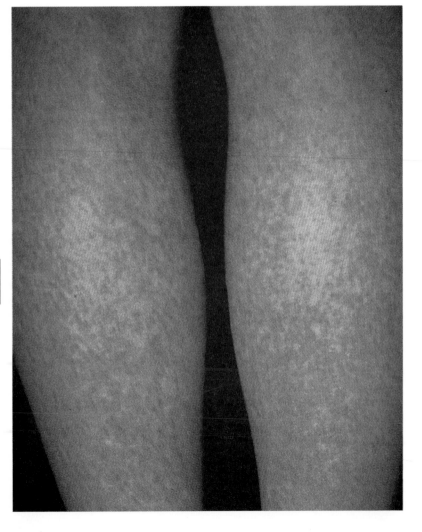

Exanthem; an acute but mild vital disease, with high fever for some 3 days, followed by a rash on the extremities and the trunk.

lescence, a period in which many physiologic, social, and psychological adjustments are made and when self-image and peer acceptance are extremely important. *See Acne*

Eczema

Eczema is a collective term for many inflammatory conditions of the skin. The term *dermatitis* is often used as a synonym for eczema, although in fact "dermatitis" means any inflammation of the skin.

All eczemas are forms of dermatitis, but dermatitis is not always eczema; for example, common sunburn is dermatitis but not eczema. An eczema causes a number of one physical changes to the skin.

Eczema can usually be controlled by a judicious combination of emollients and steroids applied to the skin, with the occasional use of antibiotics either taken by mouth or on the skin. Emollients are particularly useful for those with atopic eczema.

In the acute stage of eczema, all that may be useful to apply are soothing and cooling creams, ointments or liquids.

A fluorinated steroid cream or ointment becomes effective as soon as the acute stage has settled but should be substituted, after a few days, by a more diluted preparation. *See Eczema*

Infections

Skin (cutaneous) infections (dermatitis) may be caused by bacteria, fungi, viruses, or parasites. Many, but not all, bacterial and fungal infections are amenable to topical therapy. Careful assessment of the conditions must be made before appropriate treatment can be recommended.

The use of nonprescription topical antimicrobial products should be limited to superficial conditions that involve minimal areas, when no predisposing illnesses exist.

Self-administered topical products should be viewed as extensions of supportive treatment (proper cleaning, proper hygiene, and clean bandaging), and not as "miracle" treatments.

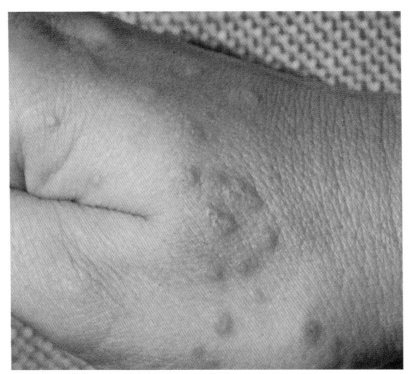

Small fluid-filled vesicles, probably due to an allergic reaction.

Surgical removal of a melanoma. Almost 100% of the earliest, most shallow melanomas are cured by surgery

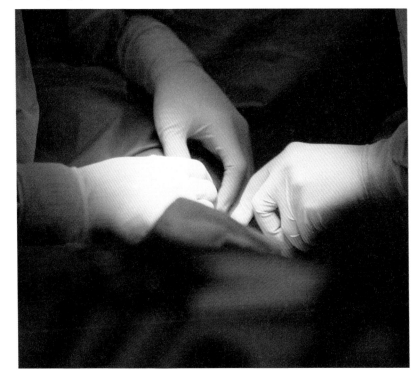

S

681

Skin infections — Questions & Answers

What causes skin infections?

Any damage to the surface of the skin offers an opportunity for bacteria, viruses or fungi to enter, allowing an infection to develop.

The skin surface can be broken either by a small cut, graze or scratch. Infection can sometimes enter through the site of insect bites. Other skin conditions such as eczema or psoriasis can also become infected, as can nappy rash.

Your general health will affect how your body responds to the infection and how well it fights it off. If you feel tired and run down or are under stress, or if you are not eating a balanced diet, you will be more prone to developing skin infections.

What treatments are available for skin infections?

Many minor skin infections can be treated with antiseptic washes, lotions and creams. Antiseptics kill organisms such as bacteria or prevent them growing and multiplying and, in doing so, prevent an infection spreading,

Use an antiseptic wash to clean the infected area. Then apply an antiseptic cream.

More stubborn bacterial infections may need treatment with antibiotic creams or tablets prescribed by your doctor.

Impetigo needs treatment with antibiotics. It is very infectious and spreads quickly among groups of children. Keep children with impetigo away from school until the infection has settled completely.

How can I help myself?

Apart from the treatment, personal hygiene and general cleanliness are all-important.

- Wash and bathe regularly. Change flannels, towels and bed linen at regular intervals.
- If a family member has a skin infection make sure they use separate flannels and towels.
- Take good care of any damaged area of skin to stop infection developing. Cover cuts and grazes and use an antibacterial cream or lotion to prevent infection.
- Do not pick or squeeze spots as this will damage the skin and spread infection.
- Keep hands and fingernails clear to reduce the chances of infection getting into a rash.

When should I see my doctor?

You will need to see your doctor if a skin infection has not cleared within a few days. Impetigo usually needs antibiotic treatment prescribed by your doctor, so if you think you or your child may have this, see your doctor.

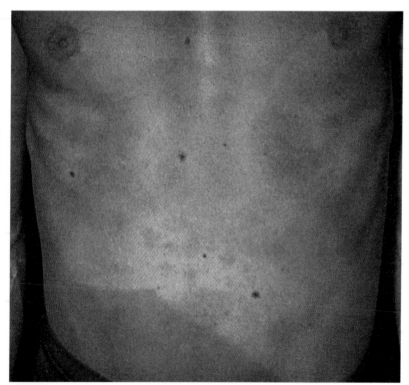

Dermatosis caused by exposure to sunlight.

Medical attention should be sought in all but the most superficial, uncomplicated skin infections, especially if it appears that systemic medication is needed. *See Dermatitis*

Psoriasis

Psoriasis is a common chronic and recurrent disease characterized by dry, well-circumscribed, silvery, scaling papules and plaques of various sizes. Psoriasis varies in severity from one to two lesions to a widespread skin disorder with disabling joint ailment and scaling of the skin.

About 2 to 4 per cent of the population are affected. Onset is usually between ages 10 and 40, but no age is exempt.

A family history of psoriasis is common and usually reflects an autosomal dominant inheritance.

General health is not affected, except for the psychologic stigma of an unsightly skin disease, unless severe joint disease or intractable scaling of the skin develops. *See Psoriasis*

S

Herpes simplex of the skin and shingles

▲ Herpes simplex is a viral infection of the skin and mucous membranes. The causative agent is a fairly large virus, Herpesvirus hominis.

▲ There are two strains:
  - herpesvirus Type-1 (herpes labialis or cold cores) is commonly found on the lips;
  - herpesvirus Type-2, which generally occurs as genital lesions and is sexually transmitted.

▲ Cold sores are a reactivation of latent virus which resides in the cranial nerve ganglion cells. When the general resistance is diminished for example by other infections.

▲ Shingles is a viral infection caused by the zoster-varicella virus, which is the same virus that causes chicken pox. The highly contagious, generalized, and usually benign chicken pox will develop in the nonimmune host, while the localized and painful zoster (shingles) will develop in the partially immune host.

▲ Shingles probably results from reactivation of latent virus, which resides in the dorsal root or cranial nerve ganglion cells. It is mainly a disease of adults who have unusually had chicken pox. After a few days of local pain, lesions appear suddenly and acutely along the course of a nerve or group of nerves on one side of the body.

▲ They appear as reddened, swollen round plaques ranging in size from bout 5 mm to areas larger than a hand; the spinal ganglia seem to be the primary site. The plaques may be painful after lesions form, and it is possible for them to appear as successive "showers" or crops over several days.

▲ The lesions develop into fairly large blisters that become crusty in 1-2 weeks. The regional lymph nodes generally are tender. The pain, particularly in the elderly, may persist for weeks or months. Sometimes the region of one eye is involved. The vesicles may damage the cornea and lead to disturbances of vision.

Tumors

The most common tumor encountered in day-to-day medical practice are tumors of the skin. Benign tumors are the most common types of benign epithelial growth and are primarily a cosmetic problem.

Clinically, they may sometimes be mistaken for malignant tumors. In all cases were the clinical diagnosis is in doubt, biopsy for histopathological examination will be performed.

Skin cancers such as basal cell and squamous cell carcinoma are among the most common malignancies and are usually curable.

Most of these tumors arise in sunexposed areas of skin. The incidence is highest in outdoor workers, sportsmen, and sunbathers, and is related to the amount of melanin pigment in the skin.

Light-skinned persons are more susceptible. Such tumors may also develop years after X-ray or radium burns or arsenic injection. *See Skin cancer*

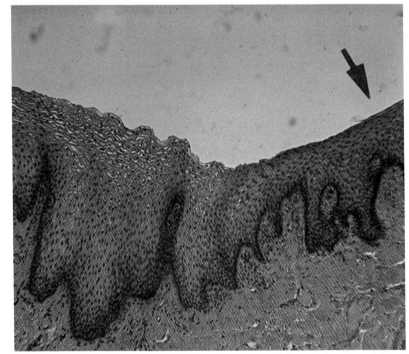

Microscopic section of the skin. Certain groups of squamous cells (arrow) show signs of altered keratosis.

S

SKULL DISORDERS

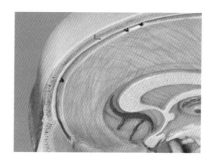

Description

The bony skeleton of the head, consisting of the cranium, made up of 8 bones that contain and protect the brain; and the facial skeleton, consisting of 14 bones.

The single occipital bone forms the back of the skull, while there is one parietal bone on each side, and the two frontal bones fuse soon after birth to form the forehead. The maxilla forms the upper jaw, while the zygoma arches out from the skull to support the cheek. Separate nasal bones form the base of the nose. The sphenoid bone has a very complex shape and supports the structures in the center of the skull behind the eye.

The eye socket is made of from parts of the sphenoid, frontal, zygoma and maxilla. The mastoid is a protrusion of the temporal bones, which form the lower sides of the skull and contain the ear canal. The sinuses are hollows in the front of the skull and around the eye sockets and nose.

There are about eighty five openings in the skull that vary from the large ones for the eyes and spine, to smaller ones for arteries and major nerves, and tiny ones for individual nerves and small veins.

Skull fracture

A break in a skull bone. Skull fractures can injury arteries and veins, which then bleed into spaces around the brain tissue. Fractures, especially at the base of the skull, can tear the meninges, the layers of tissue that line the brain. Cerebrospinal fluid, the fluid that circulates between the brain and the meninges, then can leak through the nose or ear. Bacteria occasionally enter the skull through such

fractures, causing infection and severe damage to the brain.

Most skull fractures don't require surgery unless bone fragments are pressing against the brain or the skull bones have been jolted out of alignment.

Head injuries

Skull and/or head injuries are most common in children under age 1 and adolescents over age 15. Boys are injured more often than girls. Major injuries are usually caused by motor vehicle and bicycles accidents. Minor head injuries are predominantly caused by falls in and around the home. Because any head injury is potentially serious, every child who has had a head injury should be evaluated carefully.

If the skull is fractures, a brain injury may be more severe. However, a brain injury commonly occurs without a skull fracture, and a skull fracture often occurs without a brain injury.

Fractures at the back or base of the skull usually indicate a forceful impact, because these parts of the skull are relatively thick. Such fractures often can not be seen on X-rays or computed tomography scans, but may be made visible on magnetic resonance imaging (MRI-scans).

Symptoms

A minor head injury may cause the following symptoms:
- vomiting;
- paleness;
- irritability;
- drowsiness;
- consciousness;
- immediate evidence of brain damage.

Symptoms of a severe head injury are:

- loss of consciousness;
- inability to move or feel part of the body;
- inability to recognise people or the environment;
- inability to speak or see;
- inability to maintain balance;
- clear fluid (cerebrospinal fluid) draining from the nose or mouth;
- severe headache.

If symptoms continue for more than 6 hours or worsen, a doctor should evaluate the child further to determine whether the injury is severe.

Fractures at the back or base of the skull are characterized by the following major symptoms:

▲ Cerebrospinal fluid (the clear fluid that surrounds the brain) draining form the nose or ears.

▲ Blood collecting behind the eardrum or bleeding from the ear if the eardrum is ruptured.

▲ Bruising behind the ear (Battle's sign) or around the eyes (racoon's sign).

▲ Blood collecting in the sinuses (can only be seen on X-rays or MRI-scans).

Prognosis

Head and/or skull injuries may bruise or tear brain tissue or blood vessels in or around the brain, causing bleeding and swelling inside the brain. The most common brain injury is diffuse (widespread) injury to brain cells. As a result, the patient may lose strength or sensation and becomes drowsy or unconscious. These symptoms suggest a severe brain injury, likely to result in permanent damage and the need for rehabilitation. As the swelling worsens, the pressure increases, so that even uninjured tissue can be compressed against the skull, causing permanent damage or death. Swelling with its dangerous results usually

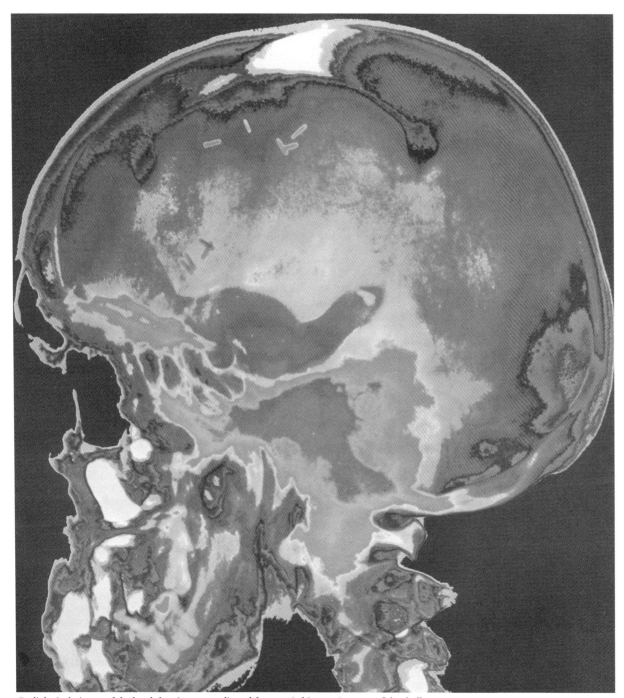

Radiological picture of the head showing a complicated fracture (white area) on top of the skull.

occurs in the first 18 to 72 hours after the injury.

Seizures

In depressed skull fractures, one or more fragments of bone press inward on the brain. The resulting bruising of the brain may cause seizures. Seizures may occur in about 5 per cent of children over age 5 years and in 10 per cent of those under age 5 during the first week after a serious head injury.

Seizures that start soon after the injury are less likely to result in a long-term seizure problem than those that start 7 or more days later.

S

SLEEP DISORDERS

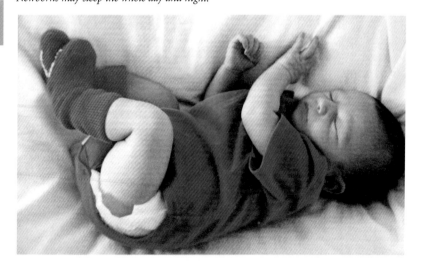

Introduction

Sleep is a normal, easily reversible, recurrent, and spontaneous state of decreased and less efficient responsiveness to external stimulation. The state contrasts with that of wakefulness, in which there is an enhanced potential for sensitivity and an efficient responsiveness to external stimuli.

Sleep disorders are divided into two major subgroups:

▲ dyssomnias; the predominant disturbance is in the amount, quality, or timing of sleep;
▲ parasomnias; the predominant disturbance is an abnormal event occurring during sleep.

Dyssomnias

The essential feature of this group of sleep disorders is a disturbance in the amount, quality, or timing of sleep.

The dyssomnias include three groups of disorders:

▲ insomnia disorders;
▲ hypersomnia disorders;
▲ sleep-wake schedule disorders.

Insomnia disorders

The essential feature of these disorders is a predominant complaint of difficulty in initiating or maintaining sleep, or of not feeling rested after sleep that is apparently adequate in amount (nonrestorative sleep).

The disturbance occurs at least three times a week for at least one month and is sufficiently severe to result in either a complaint of significant daytime fatigue or the observation by others of some symptom that is attributable to the sleep disturbance, e.g., irritability or impaired daytime functioning.

There are three insomnia disorders:

▲ insomnia related to another mental disorder (nonorganic);
▲ insomnia related to a known organic factor;
▲ primary insomnia.

There is great variability in the normal length of time it takes a person to fall asleep or in the amount of sleep normally required for a person to feel alert and rested. For the vast majority of people, sleep begins within 30 minutes of creating an environment that encourages sleep ("going to bed") and lasts from four to ten hours.

Typically, a young person with an insomnia disorder complains that it takes too long to fall asleep. An older person complains that he or she awakens too frequently, or is unable to stay asleep long enough to feel rested the next day. In some cases a person with insomnia complains only of nonrestorative sleep, despite apparently having no difficulty falling asleep or staying asleep.

In primary insomnia the essential feature is an insomnia disorder whose persistence is apparently not related to another mental disorder or to a known organic factor, such as a physical condition, or a medication. Characteristically, the person worries excessively during the day about not being able to fall and stay asleep; this may become a major preoccupation.

The person often makes intense efforts to fall asleep, but worries about these efforts' being unsuccessful, which increases tension of arousal; is able to fall asleep when he or she is not trying to sleep, for example, while watching television; and experiences a paradoxical improvement in sleep when away from his or her usual sleep environment.

Some people with primary insomnia report a lifelong pattern of poor sleep, often dating back to early childhood. Others develop the disorder later in life, often during a period of stressful life events.

Newborns may sleep the whole day and night.

Hypersomnia disorders

The essential feature of these disorders is either excessive daytime sleepiness or sleep attacks (not accounted for by an inadequate amount of sleep) or, more rarely, a prolonged transition to the fully awake state on awakening (sleep drunkenness).

The disturbance occurs nearly every day for at least one month, or episodically for longer periods of time, and is sufficiently severe or result in impaired occupational functioning or impairment in usual social activities or relationships with others.

Daytime sleepiness is defined as a tendency to fall asleep very easily (typically in five minutes or less), at almost any time during the day, even following a normal or prolonged amount of sleep at night.

Typically, in excessive daytime sleepiness the person falls asleep unintentionally at work, while driving, or at social gatherings. Thus, excessive fatigue, listlessness, or excessive bedrest are not synonymous with sleepiness.

Sleep attacks are discrete periods or sudden, irresistible sleep. In sleep drunkenness, the person requires much more time to become fully alert upon awakening than would be normal, and during this prolonged transition may be ataxic and disoriented. Usually the hypersomnia is present every day, as when related to sleep apnoea or narcolepsy. More rarely, the hypersomnia is episodic.

Sleep-wake schedule disorder

Even when people live in environments in which cues about the time of day have been removed, most biologic functions follow a rhythm with a period that lasts about 24 hours.

The essential feature of a sleep-wake schedule disorder is a mismatch between the normal sleep-wake schedule that is demanded by the person's environment and the person's circadian rhythm.

This results in a complaint of either insomnia (the person attempts to sleep, but is unable to do so) or hypersomnia (the person is unable to remain alert when wakefulness is expected).

However, if early in the development of such a sleep disorder the person is

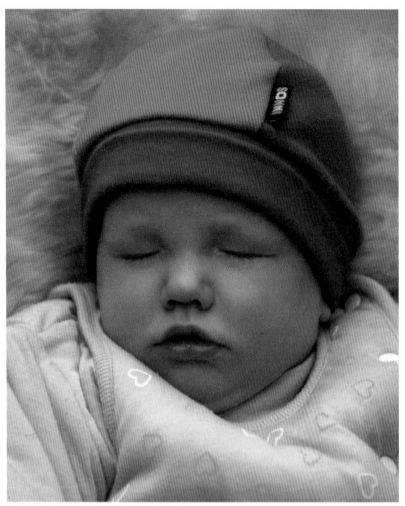

Children have a different sleep-wake schedule as adults.

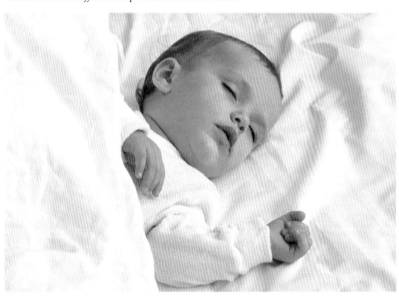

Sleep disorders   Questions & Answers

Is insomnia a common phenomenon?

Insomnia is interference in your normal sleep pattern to the extent that you do not get enough sleep to awake refreshed and to function well during the day. Insomnia may occur as a delay in getting to sleep, as awakening during the night but eventually returning to sleep, or as very early awakening before your sleep cycle is complete. Occasional insomnia should not worry you and usually disappears. But repeated insomnia merits attention. Nearly everyone occasionally has difficulty getting a good night's sleep. Few people actually stay awake all night, although many believe they do. Further, the occasional loss of a night's sleep is not really serious. It is far better to lose a night's sleep or to believe that you cannot go to sleep without a sleeping pill.

What causes insomnia?

Insomnia can be caused by psychological, physical or environmental problems. Most often, it is caused by anxiety or depression. When the problem causing the anxiety is solved or passes, transient insomnia usually disappears. When a major depression is the cause, psychotherapy and medicine treatment of the illness is necessary.

How can insomnia be treated?

First, it is important to determine the possible cause and obtain treatment, if necessary, to solve the underlying problem. Insomnia can be caused by physical factors such as:

- conditions causing pain, e.g., arthritis, ulcers, toothache, bruised muscles;
- prostate enlargement which lead to frequent wakening to urinate;
- leg cramps;
- excess consumption of caffeine or alcohol.

In most of these cases a causative treatment may be possible. In many other cases, insomnia can be helped by the following simple rules:

- do not overstimulate yourself with exciting TV shows or arguments before going to sleep;
- avoid caffeine, alcohol or cigarettes before going to bed;
- make sure your bedroom is at a comfortable temperature, with minimal light and noise;
- do not watch the clocks as the night hours pass. This only leads to anxiety that will, in itself, keep you awake;
- practice finding a comfortable position and lying perfectly still - resisting all temptation to move even a little to let your body quiet and relax for sleep.

Is narcolepsy a rare sleep disorder or a severe psychological problem?

Narcolepsy is a rare sleep disorder. Although its victims often complain of chronic drowsiness, narcolepsy is not related to insomnia. In contrast to people with insomnia, who can not fall asleep, people with narcolepsy fall asleep too often. Narcolepsy is characterized by recurrent sleep attacks - almost irresistible urges to sleep during the day. These attacks usually last 15 to 20 minutes.

However, if the person is lying down when the attack occurs, he may sleep for three hours or more. The frequency of sleep attacks varies widely from person to person - from a few to many in a single day. In addition, patients also may experience one or more of the following symptoms: cataplexy or sleep paralysis.

allowed to follow his or her own sleep-wake schedule, the insomnia or hypersomnia disappears. Transient sleep-wake mismatches commonly occur when people change time zones rapidly or occasionally stay up late for several days.

There are three types of sleep-wake schedule disorders:
- frequently changing type;
- advanced or delayed type;
- disorganized type.

In the advanced or delayed type, the essential feature is a disorder in which onset and offset of sleep are considerable advanced for the particular society. In some cases the person's sleep-wake schedule may occasionally appear to be normal only because medication or environmental demands interfere with sleep onset or offset.

In such a case, for example, the person may have a sleep-wake schedule that is delayed about four hours, so that without medication or environmental demands, he or she would go to sleep at about 3 AM and awaken at about 11 AM.

However, the person may actually have to awaken at 8 AM because of the need to be at work, or may go to sleep with a hypnotic medicine at 11 PM. Though these hours are the conventional societal times for onset and offset of sleep, in this instance the person's onset and offset of sleep that would occur without medication or environmental demands would reveal an underlying sleep-wake schedule disorder.

In the advanced type, most evening activity is preempted by an obligatory early bedtime, and the person may awaken for the day at 3 AM or earlier. In the delayed type, the person has great difficulty arising in time to fulfil his or her morning obligations.

The delayed type is frequently observed in younger people with few rigidly scheduled work or social commitments (e.g., students or unemployed). It is also frequent in "night people," i.e., those whose subjective arousal increases considerably at night, but who feel bad for a long time after the major sleep period has ended.

The advanced sleep pattern is often observed among older people.

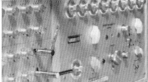
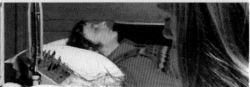

- The predominant complaint is of difficulty in initiating or maintaining sleep, or of nonrestorative sleep (sleep that is apparently adequate in amount, but leaves the person feeling unrested).

- The disturbance occurs at least three times a week for at least one month and is sufficiently severe to result in either a complaint of significant daytime fatigue or the observation by others of some symptom that is attributable to the sleep disturbance, e.g., irritability or impaired daytime functioning.

- Occurrence not exclusively during the course of sleep-wake schedule disorder or parasomnia.

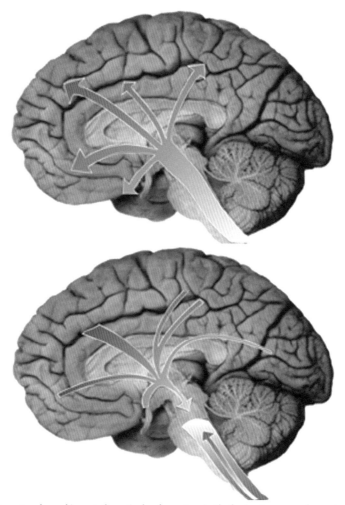

Brain networks making up the reticular formation in the brain stem may play a significant role in sleep-wake schedules.
Upper figure: The coordination of sensory stimuli reaching the brain stem is achieved by the reticular formation.
Bottom figure: Stimuli from various areas of the cerebral hemispheres converge in the reticular formation.

Because it also frequently results in early morning awakening, depression has to be differentiated from the advanced type of sleep by the presence of depressed mood or anhedonia and by other signs, such as loss of appetite and psychomotor disturbance.

In the disorganized type, the essential feature is a generally random or capricious pattern of sleep and wake times, in which there is no daily major sleep period. This type is seen in people who schedule their sleep hours haphazardly and snatch moments of sleep through the 24 hours. Some of these people may be elderly or bedridden and nap off and on throughout the day.

In the frequently changing type, the essential feature is a disorder apparently due to frequent changes in sleep and waking times. This is often associated with frequent airplane flights involving time-zone changes or with changing work schedules (shift work); sleep is then often divided into two or more periods (e.g., napping both before and after work).

On weekends or on days off, the person may temporarily attempt to revert to a normal sleep-wake schedule and thus undermine a long-term circadian adaptation to the new work schedule.

For reasons as yet unknown, people vary greatly in their ability to tolerate frequently changing sleep-wake schedules.

Some people work for years on rotating work shifts without experiencing any distress. In general, older people have more difficulty adjusting to frequent schedule changes.

"Night owls" seem to do better on shift work than those who typically rise early ("larks"). Some people attempt to force wakefulness during new work hours drinking excessive amounts of coffee. Less frequently, sleep is forced, through hypnotics, to fit the newly adopted sleep hours.

Parasomnias

The essential feature of this group of disorders is an abnormal event that occurs either during sleep or at the threshold between wakefulness and sleep; the predominant complaint focuses on this disturbance, not on its effect on sleeping or wakefulness.

For example, sleep apnoea and dream anxiety attacks both occur during

S

sleep; but the disturbance associated with sleep apnoea is classified as a dyssomnia because the person typically complains about excessive daytime sleepiness. Although rare, nocturnal seizure disorders may mimic the symptoms of a parasomnia, especially if the seizures do not occur at any particular time within the night.

Important subgroups are the following:

- dream anxiety disorder;
- sleep terror disorder;
- sleepwalking disorder.

Dream anxiety disorder

The essential feature is repeated awakenings from sleep with detailed recall of frightening dreams. These dreams are typically vivid and quite extended and usually include threats to survival security, or self-esteem.

Often there is a recurrence of the same or similar themes. The dream experience or the sleep disturbance resulting from the awakenings causes significant distress. Dream anxiety episodes often increase with mental stress, less often with physical fatigue, and, in a few cases, with changes in the sleep environment. This condition has also been called nightmare disorder.

Dream anxiety episodes occur during periods of REM sleep. Thus, although they may occur at almost any time during the night, they become more frequent toward the end of the night, when REM sleep is more abundant.

During a typical dream anxiety episode, there is remarkably little autonomic agitation. Large body movements are rarely observed during the episode because the REM-related loss of muscle tone inhibits body movement, but they are often present during the awakening.

Upon awakening from the frightening dream, the person rapidly becomes oriented and alert. Usually, a detailed account of the dream experience can be given, both immediately upon awakening and in the morning. Many people who suffer nightmares have difficulty returning to sleep after awakening from a nightmare.

Sleep terror disorder

The essential features of this disorder are repeated disorders of abrupt awakening from sleep, usually begin-

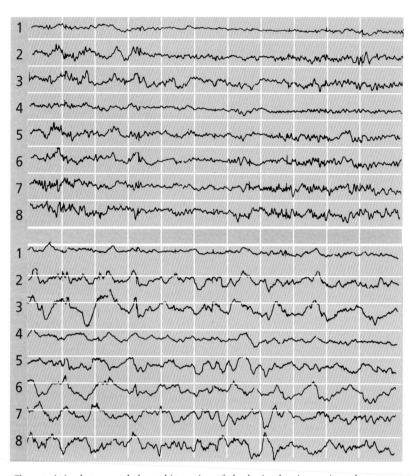

Characteristic electroencephalographic tracing of the brain showing various sleep stages; eight-channel recordings of the skull.
Above: first stage of sleep; below: second stage of sleep.
Sleep normally cycles through distinct stages five or six times during the night. Relatively little time is spent in deep sleep (stages 3 and 4). More time is spent in rapid eye movement (REM) stages as the night progresses, but this stage is interacted by brief returns to light sleep (stage 1). Brief awakenings may occur throughout the night.

ning with a panicky scream. The episode usually occurs during the first third of the major sleep period (the interval of NREM sleep that typically contains EEG delta activity, sleep stages 3 and 4) and lasts one to ten minutes. The condition has also been called pavor nocturnus.

During a typical episode, the person abruptly sits up in bed and has a frightened expression and signs of intense anxiety, dilated pupils, profuse perspiration, piloerection, rapid breathing, and a quick pulse. A person in this state is unresponsive to efforts of others to comfort him or her until the agitation and confusion subside.

The person may then recount having has a sense of terror and fragmentary dream images before arousal, but rarely a vivid and complete dream sequence. Morning amnesia for the entire period is a rule. Episodes are more likely to occur if the person is fatigued, or has experienced stress.

Before a severe period, the sleep EEG delta waves may be higher in amplitude than usual for the NREM phase of sleep, and breathing and heartbeat slower. There is no consistently associated psychopathology in children with this disorder. In contrast, adults with the disorder frequently have symptoms of other mental disorders,

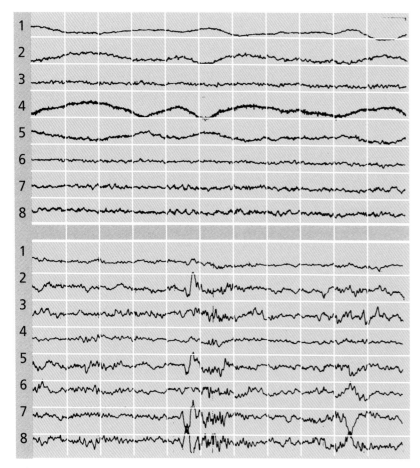

Characteristic electroencephalographic tracing of the brain showing various sleep stages; eight-channel recordings of the skull.
Above: third stage of sleep; below: fourth stage of sleep.
Sleep normally cycles through distinct stages five or six times during the night. Relatively little time is spent in deep sleep (stages 3 and 4). More time is spent in rapid eye movement (REM) stages as the night progresses, but this stage is interacted by brief returns to light sleep (stage 1). Brief awakenings may occur throughout the night.

such as a generalized anxiety disorder. Sleep terror disorder usually begins between the ages 4 and 12. When the disorder begins in adulthood, it usually begins in the 20s or 30s; onset after 40 is rare.

Sleepwalking disorder

The essential features of this disorder are repeated episodes of a sequence of complex behaviors that progress to leaving the bed and walking about, without the person's being conscious of the episode or later remembering it. The episode usually occurs during the first third of the major sleep period (the interval of nonrapid eye move-

ment sleep that typically contains EEG delta activity, sleep stages 3 and 4) and lasts from a few minutes to about a half-hour.

During a typical episode, the person sits up and initially performs preservative motor movements, such as picking at a blanket or sheet, then proceeds to semipurposeful motor acts, which, in addition to walking, may include dressing, opening doors, eating, and going to the bathroom. On some occasions the episode may terminate before the walking stage is reached.

During the episode the person has a blank, staring face, is relatively unre-

sponsive to the efforts of others to influence the sleepwalking or to communicate with him or her, and can be awakened only with great difficulty. During sleepwalking, coordination is poor; but the person may be able to see and walk around objects in his or her path. It is a myth that during sleepwalking the person is careful and safe; in fact, he or she can stumble or lose balance and be injured by taking hazardous routes such as through windows or down fire-escapes.

The walking behavior may terminate spontaneously, in which case the person awakens and is disoriented for several minutes. On the other hand, the person may return to bed without ever reaching consciousness, or may lie down in another place to continue sleeping, and be mystified the next morning at finding himself or herself there.

Upon awakening (either from the sleepwalking episode or the next morning), the person does not remember the route traversed and what happened during the episode. Fragmentary dream images may be recalled, but not complete dream sequences.

Frenzied behavior or aggression toward persons or objects during sleepwalking is frequent. Sleeptalking may accompany sleepwalking, but articulation is poor, and dialogue is rare.

The sleepwalking disorder usually begins between ages 6 and 12. Sleepwalking usually lasts several years in children and adolescents, whether it occurs infrequently or nightly. The great majority of children or adolescents with the disorder are asymptomatic by their 20s; when the disturbance begins in adulthood, it tends to be more chronic. Impairment is limited to avoidance of situations in which others might become aware of the disturbance, such as going to camp or visiting friends overnight. Accidental injury during the episodes is the major complication. Febrile illness as a child is a predisposing factor. It is estimated that 1-6 per cent of children have the disorder at some time. As many as 15 per cent of all children experience isolated episodes. Sleepwalking disorder is rarer in adults.

S

SMOKING

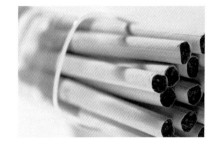

Introduction

There is no uncertainty among reputable scientists that cigarette smoking is eminently "dangerous to your health." A few questions about the details remain, but the main point had been proven: Cigarette smokers die younger that nonsmokers, and in large numbers.

The magnitude of the effect is hard for most people to grasp. In the United States, cigarette smoking is responsible every year for approximately 130,000 deaths from cancer, 170,000 deaths from heart disease, and 50,000 deaths from lung disease.

Health effects of smoking

Cigarettes attack the heart and lungs primarily. Smoking is responsible for one-third of all deaths from coronary disease and one-third of all cancer deaths - not only from lung cancer but from a variety of other tumors as well. Although men bore the brunt of illness from cigarettes for many decades, women, who have been increasing the amount they smoke for 30 or 40 years, are now shouldering an equivalent burden of disease.

Fifteen years ago, lung cancer caused only half as many deaths among women as breast cancer; not it slightly exceeds breast cancer as a killer of women. Cigarette smoking is also responsible for two-thirds of the heart attacks afflicting women under the age of 50. The baby of a cigarette-smoking woman is likely to have a low birth weight and possibly suffer other develop-mental failures.

In the first years of life, the child, if exposed to its parents' smoke, will have more bronchitis, tracheitis, bronchiolitis, colds, and other respiratory illnesses than a nonsmoker's baby. The children of smokers are also more likely to take up the habit.

And nonsmoking adult who breathe high levels of second-hand smoke are also injured by their exposure. At least 15 epidemiologic studies have asked whether "passive smokers" are more likely to develop lung cancer that people who live in a smoke-free environment. Thirteen of these studies have said yes. More recently, similar studies have bene looking at the rate of heart attacks in passive smokers - chiefly the wives of smoking men. These investigations indicate that being married to a current smoker triples the risk of having a heart attack.

Not incidentally, smoking endangers the lives not only of smokers but of nonsmokers by way of the fires that result from the habit. According to an estimate based on a 3-year survey of house fires in the city of Baltimore, cigarettes ignite house fires that kill almost 2,000 nonsmokers in the United States every year. This represents about 40 per cent of all deaths resulting from house fires.

Prepare yourself for quitting

The value of giving up cigarettes has been well publicized. People who quit smoking cigarettes get almost instant benefit to their heath (even though they may not feel better at first). In particular the risk of having a heart attack diminished rapidly within the first year. The following approach may be of value to you.

- Decide positively that you want to quit. Try to avoid negative thoughts about how difficult it might be.
- List all the reasons you want to quit. Every night before going to bed, repeat one of the reasons ten times.

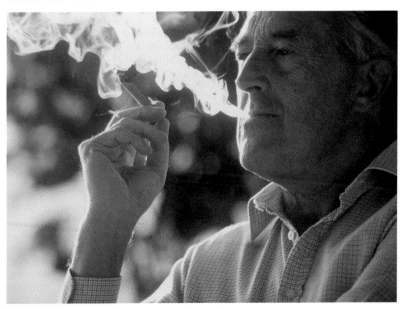

- Develop strong personal reasons in addition to your health and obligations to others. For example, think of all the time you waste taking cigarette breaks, rushing out to buy a pack, hunting for a light, etc.
- Begin to condition yourself physically: Start a modest exercise program; drink more fluids; get plenty of rest; and avoid fatigue.
- Set a target date for quitting - perhaps a special day such as your birthday, your 40th anniversary.
- If you smoke heavily at work, quit during your vacation so that you are already committed to quitting when you return. Make the data sacred, and don't let anything change it.
- Thus will make it easy for you to keep track of the day you became a nonsmoker and to celebrate that day every year.

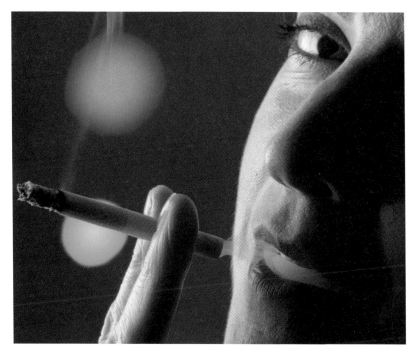

Knowing what to expect

- Have realistic expectations - quitting is not easy, but it is not impossible.
- Understand that withdrawal symptoms are temporary. They usually last only 1-2 weeks.
- Know that most relapses occur in the first week after quitting, when withdrawal symptoms are strongest and your body is still dependent on nicotine.
- Be aware that this will be your hardest time, and use all personal resources - willpower, family, friends, and the tips given here - to get you through this critical period successfully.
- Know that most other relapses occur in the first three months after quitting, when situational triggers - such as a particular stressful event - occur unexpectedly.
- These are the times when people reach for cigarettes automatically, because they associate smoking with relaxing.
- This is the kind of situation that is hard to prepare yourself for until it happens, so it is especially important to recognize it if it does happen. Remember that smoking is a habit, but a habit you can break.
- Realize that most successful ex-smokers quit for good only after several attempts You may be one of those who quit first try. But if you are not, do not give up. try again.
- Bet a friend you can quit on your target date. Put your cigarette money aside for every day, and forfeit it if you smoke.
- Ask your spouse or friend to quit with you. Tell your family and friends that you are quitting and when. They can be an important source of support, both before and after you quit.

Ways of quitting

There are many ways of quitting, the most important of which are:
- Switch brands
- Cut down the number of cigarettes you smoke
- Do not smoke automatically
- Make smoking inconvenient
- Make smoking unpleasant

■ *Switch brands*
- Switch to a brand you find distasteful.
- Change to a brand that is low in tar and nicotine a couple of weeks before your target date. This will help change your smoking behavior.
- However, do not smoke more cigarettes, inhale them more often or more deeply, or place your fingertips over the holes in the filters. All of these will increase your nicotine intake, and the idea is to get your body used to functioning without nicotine.

■ *Cut down the number of cigarettes you smoke*
- Smoke only half of each cigarette.
- Each day, postpone lighting your first cigarette 1 hour.
- Decide you will smoke only during odd or even hours of the day.
- Decide beforehand how many cigarettes you will smoke during the day. For each additional cigarette, give a dollar to your favourite charity.
- Change your eating habits to help you cut down. For example, drink milk, which many people consider incompatible with smoking. End meals or snacks with something that won't lead to a cigarette.
- Reach for a glass of juice instead of a cigarette for a "pick-me-up."

S

Smoking   Questions & Answers

How great are the risks of smoking?

Not all smokers will suffer from one or more of the smoking related diseases. But they are at much greater risk than nonsmokers. For example, emphysema is rarely seen in nonsmokers.

The following diseases or disease processes are related to smoking:
- coronary heart disease;
- cancer of lungs or bronchi;
- chronic bronchitis;
- lung emphysema;
- congestive heart failure;
- respiratory infections;
- decrease in lung function;
- atherosclerosis;
- peptic ulceration;
- cancer of the mouth, pharynx and larynx;
- tobacco amblyopia.

Death from a smoking related disease is more likely for a smoker than for a non-smoker. Ninety per cent of all death from lung cancer and chronic bronchitis are smokers.

What makes cigarettes harmful to the lungs and other organs of the body?

Tobacco smoke is made up of many compounds. These include nicotine (a powerful alkaloid), carbon monoxide, carcinogens and irritant substances; and traces of gases with unknown effects.
- Nicotine varies in its effect but acts on the catecholamine systems in the nervous system. Effects appear to vary according to the individual and the amount inhaled. In general, nicotine arouses or stimulates in small doses and depresses in large doses.
- Carbon monoxide has a high affinity for hemoglobin. Up to 15 per cent of hemoglobin can be converted to carboxyhemoglobin by carbon monoxide thus preventing it from carrying oxygen. This is particularly important in people who have heart disorders or asthma. Also especially harmful in pregnancy because it results in diminished oxygen supply to the uterus and fetus.
- Carcinogens are mainly found in the tar of condensate from smoke when cooled or filtered (in the lungs of the smoker). The tar has been shown to cause cancer in animals and man.
- Irritants are also found in the tar. They are generally responsible for the damage caused in the lungs, such as narrowing of bronchioles.

Is cough always a sign of lung disease?

Cough is a sudden explosive expiratory manoeuvre that tends to clear material from the airways. Cough is a familiar, but complex reflex. Differences exist among several sites from which cough stimuli can originate. Cough helps protect the lung against aspiration, and stimulation of the voice box will produce a choking type of cough without a preceding inspiration. Awareness of cough varies considerably; it can be distressing when it appears suddenly, particularly if it is associated with discomfort due to chest pain, dyspnea, or copious secretions.

However, if a cough develops slowly over decades (for instance, in a smoker with mild chronic bronchitis), the patient may hardly be aware of it, or may consider it normal. Cough can also be denied to avoid recommendations against cigarette smoking.

- Remember: Cutting down can help you quit, but it is not a substitute for quitting. If you are down to about seven cigarettes a day, it is time to set your target quit date and get ready to stick to it.

■ *Do not smoke automatically*
- Smoke only those cigarettes you really want. Catch yourself before you light up a cigarette out of pure habit.
- Do not empty your ashtrays. This will remind you of how many cigarettes you have smoked, and the sight and smell of stale butts will be very unpleasant.
- Make yourself aware of each cigarette by using the opposite hand or putting cigarettes in an unfamiliar location or a different pocket to break the automatic reach.
- If you light up many times during the day without even thinking about it, try to look in a mirror each time you put a match to your cigarette - you may decide you don't need it.

■ *Make smoking inconvenient*
- Stop buying cigarettes by the carton. Wait until one pack is empty before you buy another.
- Stop carrying cigarettes with you at home and at work. Make them difficult to get to.

■ *Make smoking unpleasant*
- Smoke only under circumstances that are not especially pleasurable for you. If you like to smoke with others, smoke alone. Turn your chair toward an empty corner and focus only on the cigarette you are smoking and its many negative effects.
- Collect all your cigarette butts in one large glass container as a visual reminder of the filth smoking represents.

Withdrawal symptoms

Within 12 hours after you have your last cigarette, your body will begin to heal itself. The levels of carbon monoxide and nicotine in your sys-

S

tem will decline rapidly, and your heart and lungs will begin to repair the damage caused by cigarette smoke. Within a few days, you will probably begin to notice some remarkable changes in your body. Your sense of smell and taste may improve.

You will breathe easier, and your smoker's hack will begin to disappear, although you may notice that you still cough for a whole. And you will be free from the mess, smell, inconvenience, expense, and dependence of cigarette smoking.

As your body begins to repair itself, instead of feeling better right away, you may feel worse for a while. It is important to understand that healing is a process - it begins immediately, but it continues over time. These "withdrawal pangs" are really symptoms of the recovery process.

Immediately after quitting, many ex-smokers experience "symptoms of recovery" such as temporary weight gain caused by fluid retention, irregularity, and dry, sore gums or tongue. You may feel edgy, hungry, more tires, an more short-tempered than usual, and have trouble sleeping and notice that you are coughing a lot.

These symptoms are the result of your body clearing itself of nicotine, a powerful addictive chemical. Most nicotine is gone from the body in 2-3 days. It is important to understand that the unpleasant after-effects of quitting are only temporary and signal the beginning of a healthier life. Now that you have quit, you have added a number of healthy productive days to each year of your life.

Most important, you have greatly improved your chances for a longer life. You have significantly reduced your risk of death from heart disease, stroke, chronic bronchitis, emphysema, and several kinds of cancer - not just lung cancer.

Microscopic view of a malignant growth in the lung. Cigarette smoking is the cause of about 90% of lung cancer cases in men and about 84% of cases in women. The greater the quantity and duration of smoking cigarettes, the greater the risk of developing lung cancer. About 10 to 12% of all smokers eventually develop lung cancer.

Smoking

Withdrawal symptoms and activities that might help

■ Dry mouth; sore throat, gums or tongue
Sip ice-cold water or fruit-juice, or chew gum.

■ Headaches
Take a warm bath or shower. Try relaxation or meditation techniques.

■ Trouble sleeping
Don't drink coffee, tea, or soda with caffeine after 6:00 PM. Again, try relaxation or meditation techniques.

■ Irregularity
Add roughage to your diet, such as raw fruit, vegetables, and whole-grain cereals. Drink 6-8 glasses of water a day.

■ Fatigue
Tale a nap. Try not to push yourself during this time. Do not expect too much of your body until it had had a change to begin to heal itself over a couple of weeks.

■ Hunger
Drink water or low-calorie liquids. Eat low-fat, low-calorie snacks.

■ Tenseness, irritability
Take a walk, soak in a hot bath, try relaxation or meditation techniques.

■ Couching
Sip warm herbal tea. Suck on cough drops or sugarless hard candy.

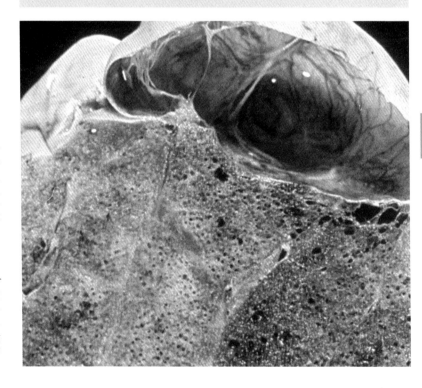

S

SPINAL CORD INJURIES

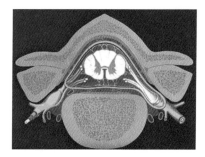

Description

That part of the central nervous system contained within the spinal column and extending from the skull to the level of the first or second lumbar vertebra; the nerve structures and nerve pathways within the vertebral canal, extending from the skull opening to the second lumbar vertebra.

Neurologist examining the X-rays of a patient with spinal cord injury.

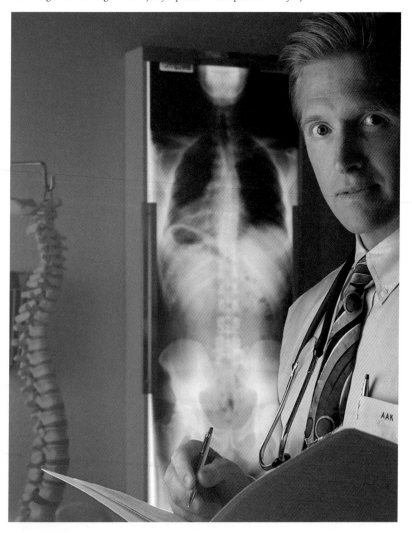

Injuries

The spinal cord may be injured directly by penetrating wounds, for example, stabs or gun-shot wounds, in which case it may be penetrated by a missile or by fragments of bone. When a fall or some other force fractures or dislocate the vertebral column, the vertebral bones that normally enclose and protect the cord can crush it, mechanically killing and damaging nerve fibers end neurons.

More frequently in civil life it may be penetrated indirectly as a result of injuries of the vertebral column, either fractures, dislocations, or fracture-dislocations. The commonest sites of spinal injury in civil life are the lower cervical region and the thoracolumbar junction. The upper cervical region suffers next in frequency. Though the spinal column may be injured as the result of a blow leading to fracture at the site of the impact, more frequently it is injured by transmitted violence. Forcible extension of the neck may cause fracture of the dens or contusion of the cervical cord, but most spinal injuries are the result of forcible flexion. A blow on the head which does not expend its violence in fracturing the skull may, by forcibly flexing the cervical spine, cause dislocation in the lower cervical region or herniation of an intervertebral disc.

Pathology

Concussion of the spinal cord is the term employed when the cord is injured by transmitted violence without fracture or dislocation of the vertebral column, for example, by the passage of a bullet near the spine without penetration of the dura.
The axis cylinders of the nerve cells

Effects of spinal injury

■ Level C1 to C5
Paralysis of muscles used for breathing and of all arm and leg muscles; usually fatal.

■ Level C5 to C6
Legs paralyzed; slight ability to flex arms.

■ Level C6 to C7
Paralysis of legs and part of wrists and hands; shoulder movement and elbow bending relatively preserved.

■ Level C8 to T1
Legs and trunk paralyzed; eyelids droop; arms relatively normal; hands paralyzed.

■ Level T2 to T4
Legs and trunk paralyzed; loss of feeling below the nipples.

■ Level T5 to T8
Legs and lower trunk paralyzed; loss of feeling below the rib cage.

■ Level T9 to T11
Legs paralyzed; loss of feeling below the umbilicus.

■ Level T12 to L1
Paralysis and loss of feeling below the groin.

■ Level L2 to S2
Different patterns of leg weakness and numbness.

are broken up but the myelin sheaths remain intact. Spinal contusion is defined as bruising of the cord without rupture of the pia mater, resulting from compression.
Microscopically, besides oedema and hemorrhages the contused cord exhibits swelling of the nerve fibers and disintegration of their myelin sheaths. In severe cases both completely disappear and the cord may be markedly softened. Ascending and descending degeneration of the long nerve tracts follows the focal lesion. Laceration of the cord implies an injury of greater severity than contu-

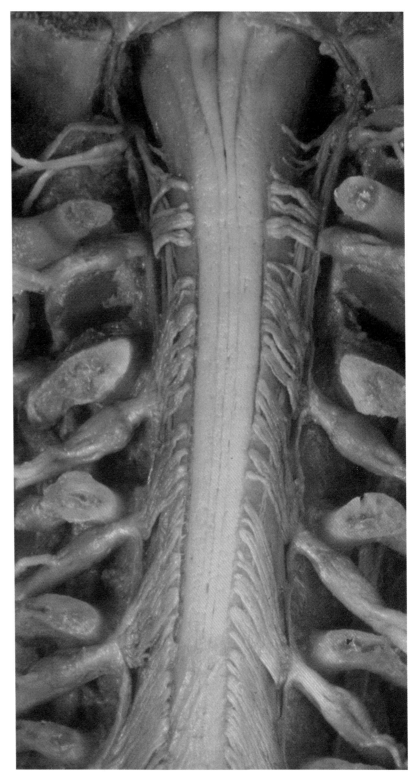

Dorsal view of the lower part of the medulla oblongata and the upper six segments of the cervical spinal cord. Injuries in this region causes paralysis of muscles used for breathing and of all arm and leg muscles. The injury is usually fatal.

S

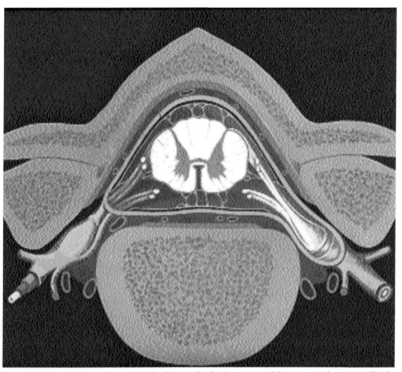

Cross section of the spinal cord inside the vertebral column. In addition to its function of body support and movement, as well as protection of the spinal cord, the vertebral column is built to withstand forces of compression many times the weight of the body.

sion, leading to rupture of the pia mater and in the most severe cases the cord is completely transected.

Signs and symptoms

The symptoms of spinal injury depend upon the severity and situation of the lesion.

Injury to the cord does not necessarily follow damage to the vertebral column; for example, dislocation of the cervical spine without injury to the cord is not rare.

An injury to the cord in the upper cervical region is usually rapidly, if not immediately, fatal, since it causes paralysis of the diaphragm and of the intercostal muscles. Complete interruption of the spinal cord leads immediately to flaccid paralysis with loss of all sensation and most reflex activity below the site of the lesion, and paralysis of the bladder and rectum.

Muscular paralysis and sensory loss are irrecoverable, but, as after from one to four weeks the stage of spinal shock passes off, reflex activity develops in the divided portion of the cord

Myelography (radiological examination of spinal cord and spinal canal) of a patient with spinal cord injury.

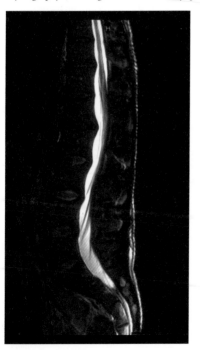
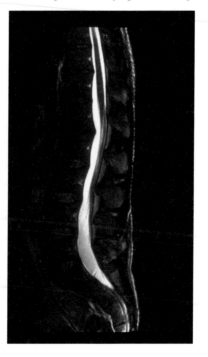
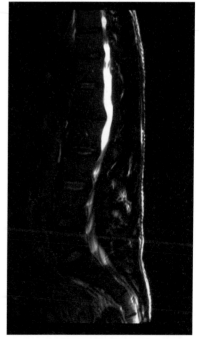

and the patient presents the picture of paraplegia-in-flexion.

Repair of damaged tissue

The end result of the injury is a complex state of disrepair. Axons that have been damaged become useless stumps, connected to nothing, and their several terminals disintegrate. Often many axons remain intact but are rendered useless by loss of their insulating myelin.

A fluid-like cavity or cyst, sits where neurones, other cells and axons used to be. And glial cells proliferate abnormally, creating clusters termed glial scars. Together the cyst and scars pose a formidable barrier to any cut axons that might somehow try to regrow and connect to cells that they once innervated.

A few axons may remain whole, myelinated and able to carry signals up or down the spine, but often their numbers are too small to convey useful directives to the brain or muscles.

If all these changes had to be fully reversed to help patients, the prospects for new treatments would be grim. Fortunately, it appears that salvaging normal activity in as little as 10 per cent of the standard axon complement would sometimes make walking possible for people who would otherwise lack that capacity.

The best therapy would not only reduce the extent of an injury but also repair damage. A key component of that repair would be stimulating the regeneration of damaged axons - that is, inducing their elongation and reconnection with appropriate target cells.

So far, few interventions in animals with well-established spinal cord injuries have achieved the magnitude of regrowth and synapse formation that would be needed to provide a hand grasp or the ability to stand and walk in human adults with long-term damage.

Because of the great complexities and difficulties involved in those aspects of cord repair, scientists cannot guess when reconstructive therapies might begin to become available. But researchers anticipate continued progress toward that end.

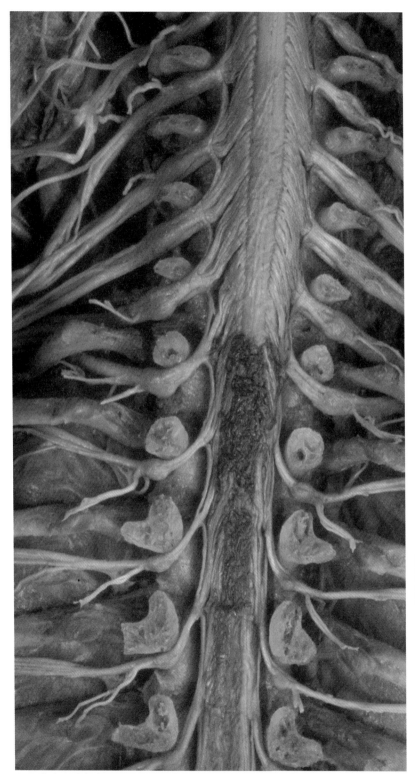

Dorsal view of the lower cervical and upper thoracic segments of the spinal cord. Injuries in this region causes paralysis of legs and part of wrists and hands; shoulder movements and elbow bending relatively preserved.

S

SPORTS INJURIES

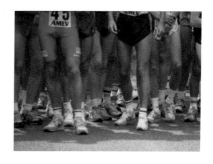

Introduction

Sports injuries are as common as a cold; more than 5 million occur every year in the UK and between 15 and 16 million in the United States. In is a common misconception that most amateur sports are free of injuries. In fact, its nature, variety of movements and the intensity of jumping expose the frequent participant to stress injuries.

Your muscles and joints are not accustomed to many of the movements in an aerobics routine. And with the amount of hopping, twisting and jumping necessary for a productive work-out, you will occasionally land badly. This has resulted in high injury rates among participants and instructors of aerobics.

The majority of these injuries are minor and require no treatment apart from rest. Most complaints are similar to those of runners - shin splints, runner's knee, metatarsal and arch pain, calf muscle stress and lower back pain. Many of these can be prevented by stretching, warming up and cooling down, and wearing shoes designed for aerobics. Barefoot exercisers run the gravest risk of injury.

Ankle injuries

The ankle's movements in sport are complex and involve a shift of weight in the balanced action between trunk, hip, knee, ankle and foot. The ankle must maintain a balance o fixed surfaces such as ice or water, and absorb impact on uneven surfaces.

In kicking the ankle develops intense momentum to transfer from the body to the foot the kinetic energy to propel the ball as in soccer. This synchronous movement requires a counterbalance thrust to the opposite ankle.

The relationship between ankle and knee is important but complex; for example, in place kicking, the instep and entire forefoot twist on a fixed knee. With rotatory instability of the knee the rotational forces are transmitted to the foot via the ankle, producing a chronic sprain of the ankle ligaments.

In dorsiflexion the ankle mortise widens due to the fact that the head of the talus is broader in front. Most commonly injuries to the ankle occur through forces applied to the mortise.

More than 10 million sports injuries are treated each year in the United States. Common sports injuries include: stress fractures of the foot, shin splints, tendinitis, runner's knee, hamstring injuries, tennis elbow, head injuries, foot injuries and myriad other sprains and pulled muscles

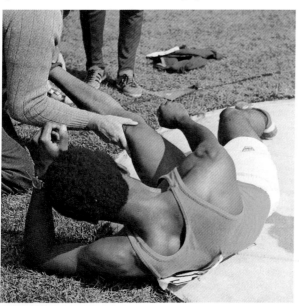

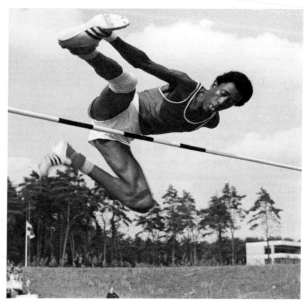

S

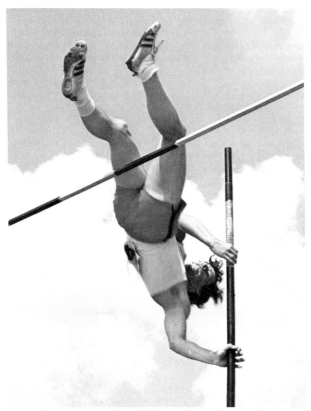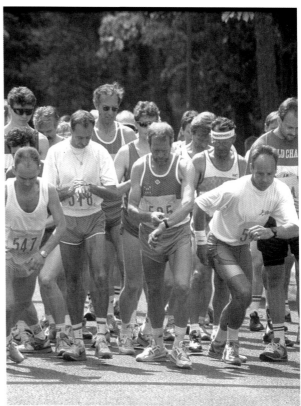

According to a survey, about half a sample population of runners reported a running injury in the previous year that was serious enough to make them reduce training, take medication or see a doctor.

Repeated stress causes capsular osteophytes.

Sprains

Acute capsular sprains of the ankle are probably the commonest single type of sports injury. The classic injury is one of inversion and internal rotation which results in sprain of the lateral ligament complex. In the acute injury with local pain and swelling the treatment is by strapping or plaster depending on the severity of the problem.

After 2-3 weeks the lesion resolves; more problematical is the less acute sprain which is often ignored because of the paucity of signs, the only gross physical sign being limitation of movement although careful inspection from behind shows filling of the sulcus on either side of the Achilles tendon due to backward bulging of the joint. This injury requires immobilization for it can be the precursor of a chronic sprained ankle.

Chronic sprained ankle

When a sprain has become chronic the local tender area in the capsule is demarcated and treated with ultrasound, manipulation under local or general anesthesia and local steroid injections. The ankle may have to be rested in plaster (below-knee) for 3-4 weeks, and a "raise and floaty" may have to be applied to the heel of the shoe (usually 5 mm).

Spikes or studs which give excessive grip predispose to ankle problems and correct release bindings should be used by skiers. Soccer players or football players who "dangle" their foot into a tackle should have this fault rectified.

Some doctors believe that ankle strapping may lead to local muscle wasting (atrophy) and the build-up of stresses which can lead to substantial injury. However, many professional football players or soccer players use ankle strapping especially after an ankle injury. Good muscle tone around the

ankle is very important.

In a ny ankle injury a series of X-rays must be taken to exclude margin fractures, osteochondritis dissecans, osteophytes (footballer's ankle) and a calcaneonavicular bar (with peroneal spasm); a stress film is examined for ligamentous rupture.

Ligament tears

In football, soccer and rugby the ankle is particularly vulnerable to sliding tackles or a clash of feet and the anterior fibers of the lateral ligament are torn with tenderness and swelling over the front aspect of the lateral ankle. When the opposing player's boot comes through in a tackle from behind the posterior and middle fibers of the lateral ligament may be damaged.

There is local pain and swelling on the lateral aspect of the ankle and severe bruising may be seen extending posteriorly to the Achilles region and on the dorsum and sole of the foot.

Sports injuries   Questions & Answers

Can a bursitis be cured with antibiotics or other medicines?

A bursitis is an acute or chronic inflammation of a bursa. Bursae are saclike cavities filled with synovial (joint) fluid and located at tissues where friction occurs, such as where tendons or muscles pass over bony prominences. Bursae facilitate normal movement and minimize friction between moving parts. Deep bursae may communicate with joints.

Most bursitis occurs in the shoulder, but other common forms exist:
- olecranon (elbow), also called miner's elbow;
- patella (housemaid's knee);
- calcaneus (Achilles);
- iliopectineal (iliopsoas);
- ischial (tailor's or weaver's bottom).

The cause of most bursitis is unknown. Acute bursitis is characterized by pain, localized tenderness, and limitation of motion. Swelling and redness are frequently present if the bursa is superficial. Chronic bursitis may follow previous attacks of bursitis or repeated trauma.

Is the inflammation of a tendon always caused by a microbe?

Inflammation of a tendon (tendinitis) is almost always accompanied by inflammation of the lining of the tendon sheath (tenosynovitis). The tendon sheath usually is the site of maximum inflammation, but the inflammatory response may involve the enclosed tendon.

Tendinitis and bursitis are terms which may be used interchangeable to describe the same process, since bursae are often located near tendons. The cause is unknown, but most instances occur in middle and older ages as the blood supply of the tendons attenuates and repetitive microtrauma may result in greater injury. Repeated or extreme trauma (short of rupture), strain, or excessive exercise is most frequently causative.

What is the common treatment for a tendinitis or tenosynovitis?

Symptomatic relief of the symptoms of a tendinitis is provided by immobilization (splint or cast) or rest of the part, application of heat or cold (whichever benefits the patient), pain relieving agents locally, and nonsteroidal anti-inflammatory agents systematically.

Injection into the tendon sheath of a depot corticosteroid indicated for soft-tissue injection, depending on site and severity, may be helpful. The injection is made blindly at the site of maximum tenderness if the specific inflammation side cannot be identified. Care will be taken not to inject the tendon, as it can weaken and rupture in active persons.

Reexamination of a less inflamed site 3 or 4 days later often discloses the specific lesion, and a second injection can be made with greater precision. Rest of the injected part is advisable to diminish risk of rupture of the tendon.

I am troubled with a so-called tennis-elbow but do not play tennis. What can be done about it?

A tennis elbow is defined as a strain of the lateral forearm muscles (extensors of the digits and wrist) or their tendinous attachments near their origin on the lateral condyle (bony extension) of the upper arm (humerus). The condition may be caused by repetitive strenuous supination of the wrist against resistance, as in manual screwdriving, or by violent extension of the wrist with the hand pronated, as in tennis.

Instability may be shown by stress firms, an arthrogram (special X-ray of the joint) or CT-scan may be used in acute tears to show the extent of ligamentous damage.

Treatment may be conservative or surgery. A walking cast may be applied for 3-4 weeks. Some doctors do not advocate repair of the lateral ligament unless instability is present in two planes and an arthrogram shows major damage. At surgery the joint is cleared of clotted blood and the shredded ligaments opposed with dexon. The foot is placed in slight valgus initially to take the strain off the suture line.

A plaster is worn for 3-4 weeks and mobilization exercises should be designed to regain full inversion before competition is resumed, especially football and soccer. Surgery is recommended in cases of chronic recurrent instability.

Footballer's ankle

This condition is not an osteoarthrosis of the ankle joint; examination of the joint surface at surgery reveals no damage to the hyaline cartilage. However, numerous small capsular tears cause marginal osteophytes which may impinge on the neck of the talus during kicking. This leads to discomfort on shooting and later a dull pain.

Tenderness is found over the anterior (and sometimes posterior) joint line and X-rays show the small spicules of bone. A somewhat similar condition involves fracture or degenerate changes in the back part of the talus and a small spur develops.

As far as treatment is concerned the following. In the early stages kicking should be reduced and short-wave diathermy given. Surgery is needed when the spicules have become prominent or fractured, and when loose bodies are present.

Fractures of the ankle

These may occur with or without dislocation or subluxation.

Usually the foot is anchored to the ground while the momentum of the body continues forwards. The most important forces are external rotation and either abduction or adduction of the ankle. The ankle is swollen and painful and the deformity is obvious. Conservative treatment and plaster immobilization for 6-12 weeks can be used when there is little or no place-ment or when there has been a very accurate reduction. The foot is placed at a right ankle to the leg and must be in na neutral position.

Surgery is required to ensure perfect reduction and to maintain it in unsta-ble fractures, to remove soft tissues which are intervening in the fracture and to repair the ligamentous dam-age.

It has been pointed out that the ankle mortise depends on the correct length of the fibula and the integrity of the anterior and posterior tibiofibular lig-aments. The fibula with its taut elastic attachment to the tibia takes absolute priority over the medial ankle.

Damage to the tibiofibular syndesmo-sis can be reduced from the level of the fracture. A fracture of the fibula at the level of the ankle or below this is never associated with a lesion of the syndesmosis. By contrast, a fracture of the fibula above this level is always associated with a lesion of either the anterior or the posterior tibiofibular ligament.

Besides injuries to the ankles and liga-ments where may be avulsion, shear osteochondral or chondral fractures of the talus, and these may produce loose fragments in the joints. Internal fixation of the lateral ankle is carried out with one or two screws or a small plate. Torn ligaments are repaired and stabilized with screws if necessary.

If the interosseous membrane has been torn, in addition to the repair, the syndesmosis is protected by fur-ther stabilization of the fibula. The medial ankle, back malleolus and del-toid ligament are repaired and stabi-lized using small screws or tension band wiring.

After the operation, the leg is elevated for 4-5 days and rests in a plaster splint with the leg at 90 degrees. After 48 hours dorsiflexion exercises are recommended. At 14 days partial weight-bearing is begun in a below-knee plaster of the original fixation was less than excellent; otherwise a removable splint can be used.

The placer is worn for 6-8 weeks. At the end of this period the screws or plate can be removed under local anesthesia. Sport begins at 4-5 months.

Boxing injuries

Boxing injury are defined in sports medicine as injuries acquired during boxing with fists. When a boxer decides to turn professional he under-goes an extensive medical examina-tion which is repeated annually by a doctor with knowledge of profession-al boxing and the danger entails there-in.

The doctor will not only ensure that the boxer is in excellent health, but he may also advice on matters of fitness, diet and training and report any prob-lems, physical symptoms or training difficulties which he discovers.

Should any ontoward features be noted during the examination, the specialists' reports are obtained and considered by a medical panel; only then is a recommendation for licens-ing made to the governing body.

Apart from the yearly examination, the boxer is also examined at lunchtime prior to his contest and has further checks both before and after the fight, regardless of the result or whether any injury has been sus-tained. The decision concerning a boxer's fitness always remains with the medical officer and his decision is final.

Two medical officers, both of whom should have a working knowledge of sports medicine and be able to treat such injuries as may arise, must be in attendance at a tournament; this per-mits one doctor to remain at the ring-side while the other is supervising medically in the dressing room.

The punch-drunk syndrome

This syndrome was quite common before World War II but is now fortu-nately rare, due to three different fac-tors:

- the great improvement in medical care and documentation, and especially the automatic suspen-sion of a boxer for a minimum of 21 days if he has lost any contest within a specific distance regard-less of why he has lost it;
- the fewer contests which each boxer undertakes;
- improved nutrition and knowl-edge of physical fitness which is available to professional athletes today.

The actual cause of the syndrome is still open to discussion; various theo-

Intercostal nerve block for rib fracture. Position of the patient (A); sites of infiltration with local anesthetic (B); "walking" the needle downwards until its top slips below the edge of the rib (C, D).

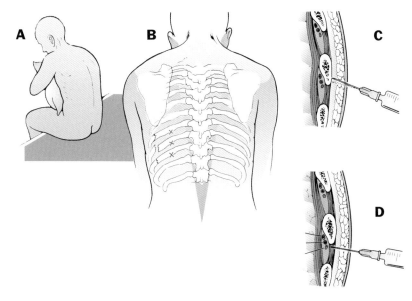

S

ries have been put forward but, until the exact etiology is discovered, we shall not be able to prevent the condition completely. The punch-drunk syndrome is not peculiar to boxing and has occurred in other contact sports, such as rugby, football, soccer and horse-riding. A great deal has been said recently about the wearing of headguards in both amateur and professional boxing and, although this may reduce the superficial trauma, experts are of the opinion that it would not prevent more serious and chronic lesions - on the contrary, headguards may actually increase the chances of these occurring.

Cuts around the eye
The commonest boxing injuries are cuts around the eyes resulting from either a punch or an accidental clash of heads. The immediate effect is to create the impression of gory mess which has undoubtedly captured the imagination of millions through the over-reaction of some sports commentators on TV.

However, they are easily dealt with after the contest is over. careful stitching by a competent doctor followed by six to eight weeks' rest from sparring or boxing allows ven the deepest cuts to heal properly.

The only danger from a cut around the eye is that the blood flowing profusely may impair the boxer's vision temporarily and therefore disturb his concentration and ability to avoid his opponent's punches.

Emergency treatment during the contest is carried out very efficiently by the boxer's trainer using 1:1000 aqueous adrenalin applied with a swab stick into the cut after cleansing with gauze; the wound is then covered with a thin film of vaseline.

All trainers and seconds musty have a working knowledge of how to treat cuts before being granted a license. The simple procedure described above is sufficient to stop the bleeding from the majority of cuts; it does not damage the tissues and enables the ring physician subsequently to suture without impairing healing.

In the past many compounds have been used to produce hemostasis, including ferric perchloride and trichloroacetic acid, but these set like concrete and caused severe tissue necrosis, although the initial result was satisfactory.

The doctor was then faced by all manner of problems and in many cases plastic surgery was required to excise the necrotic tissue before resuturing.

Eye injuries
Other eye injuries are not common. Temporary diplopia can result from bruising into the extra-ocular muscles, but, provided more serious problems have been excluded, this responds very well to a few days' rest. Retinal detachment, although again recently getting a great deal of press coverage, is not a common occurrence in boxing, in part due to the very stringent visual standards that have been attained.

Injuries to the ear
The cauliflower ear, which was the trademark of the professional boxer before World War II, is virtually unknown today although it has ben seen in judo and rugby players. Occasionally a boxer receives a direct blow to the ear and as a result sustains a traumatic perforation of the ear drum.

Provided he is allowed adequate time to recover with antibiotic prophylaxis, the perforation heals satisfactorily and would not preclude him from following his career. Deafness as a result of this type of injury is exceedingly rare.

Mouth injuries
Laceration of the lips and mouth are not common. So long as the boxer has adequate dental care and wears a well-fitting gum shield he is unlikely to suffer trauma to his mouth.

Musculoskeletal injuries
Fractures of the mandible are rare. fractures of the skull do not occur in professional boxing, partly because the ring is protected by a safety mat and the corners are well padded. Musculoskeletal injuries are unusual due to the superb fitness of the contestants. Bruising of the metacarpophalangeal and interphalangeal joints of the thumb and digits are usually due to incorrect punching which also results in the occasional fracture of the shaft of the metacarpal. Provided adequate orthopaedic treatment is at hand and rest afforded to allow complete resolution of the injury, no permanent deformity or disability will result.

Other injuries
Soft-tissue injuries, apart from lacerations, are quite common around the face and periorbital hematomas and occasionally quite large hematomas around the forehead can result in rather grotesque appearances, but a few days' treatment usually produces rapid resolution with no subsequent problems. Epistaxes (nose bleedings) are not unusual and are quite dramatic. They respond to treatment with 1:1000 aqueous adrenalin.

Apart from the impairment of breathing they are of no serious significance unless there is an underlying nasal fracture with may or may not require surgical treatment but would certainly necessitates a considerable lay-off from boxing.

Fractures of the ribs due to heavy body punches are quite unusual as the fitness program the boxer undertakes usually develops his intercostal muscles and sparring tends to toughen him up. A fractures rib would certainly necessitates a rest from boxing for three or four months.

Deaths in the ring
Despite the recent spate of ring deaths throughout the world serious injuries in the US are in fact rare due, in no small measure to the excellence of the referees who, before that receive their license, are instruct in the medical aspects of the sport.

Shoulder and arm problems

Rotator cuff disorder
Some people think that recurring shoulder pain is one of those little inconveniences that comes with the sport. Left untreated, however, the shoulder could eventually need reconstructive surgery. Rotator Cuff Impingement Syndrome (RCIS) is the most common affliction of athletes who participate in sports that require repetitive overhead arm movement. Such athletes include:

- swimming;
- baseball;
- tennis;
- softball;
- gymnastics;
- football;
- weightlifting;
- basketball.

The rotator cuff (ligaments, tendons, muscles, capsule and other soft tissue covering the shoulder joint) is vulnerable to injury because it is not strong. Athletes usually build up their chests and arms, and neglect the shoulder and back. As a result, the shoulder is not strengthened or stretched enough to accommodate the constant use.

Tennis elbow

Almost one-third of all tennis players - from novices to pros - end up with the classic overuse syndrome at one time or another. The first warning sign often is generalized soreness in the serving arm. Ignore it, and the pain intensifies, becomes more localized in the joint.

The cause of tennis elbow is usually faulty backhand technique - though weak arm muscles and improper equipment can also contribute to the condition. Your best defense is to train with a pro who can identify and correct the flaws in your stroke that put excessive stress on the elbow. It may also help to get a racket with a larger grip size of racket head, or switch to a two-handed backhand stroke.

If pain persists, see your doctor, who will probably insist that you take a court recess - until the muscle inflammation subsides - and then give you forearm-strengthening exercises, so that painful tennis elbow will be less likely to elbow its way into your game About half of the golf injuries involve the back and elbow. Researchers have found that women most frequently hurt their elbows, followed in order by backs, shoulders, hands and wrists, and knees.

There are few studies of golf injuries, particularly among recreational golfers. But compared to those professionals studied, it seems amateurs are at greater risk of elbow injury, while all players are subject to back woes. Most often pros' injuries resulted from overuse, whereas amateurs suffered from poor swing mechanics as

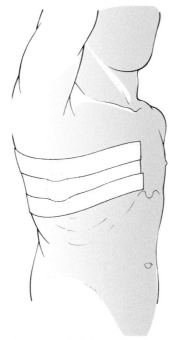 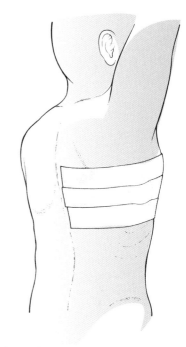

Fixing a small flail segment of the chest with a pad secured by adhesive tape. The tape extends from the midline anteriorly (A) to the midline posteriorly (B).

well as overuse, advanced age and weak physical condition.

The researchers recommended avoiding injury by:

- Learning and using proper swing technique.
- Regulating practice time to prevent overuse.
- Maintaining adequate physical conditioning.

Injuries from running

When you run, your feet strike the ground anywhere from 800 to 1,700 times a mile, at a force of about three to five times your body weight. A runner weighing 180 pounds may cumulatively absorb about 240 tons of force per mile. It is no wonder, then, that running injuries are so common. According to one survey, about half a sample population of runners reported a running injury in the previous year that was serious enough to make them reduce training, take medication or see a doctor. Most of the common runners' syndromes on the right are overuse, pr stress, injuries. Because they generally do not result in acute

sudden pain, stress injuries are insidious.

Typically, you first feel pain from such an injury as you get out of bed in the morning, when the muscles are short and inflexible after a period of inactivity. The discomfort subsides as the muscles stretch with use during the day. The pain returns and becomes most severe at the beginning of a work-out, diminishes during the run and then returns after the run.

Much of the time, these injuries are the result of running incorrectly, and you can prevent them by observing good form. In addition, it is important that you build your program gradually and that you take the time to warm up and cool down properly. Also wear a good pair of running shoes.

If you do sustain an injury, it may respond to home treatment. To reduce pain and swelling, you can apply ice to the affected area and take an analgesic such as aspirin. Limit your running or cease altogether during the recovery period. A chronic injury or any condition that results in severe pain should be treated by a doctor.

S

STOMACH CANCER

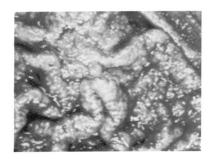

Desription

Tumors of the stomach may be benign or malignant. Benign tumors do not spread. They usually can be removed completely and are not likely to recur. But malignant tumors, or cancers of the stomach, invade neighbouring parts of the body. The incidence of stomach cancers shows enormous differences in worldwide distribution, which extremely high levels in Japan, Chile, and Iceland.

While its cause is unknown, stomach cancer is often associated with gastri-tis and intestinal metaplasia of the mucosa of the stomach. Such findings are not generally thought to result from gastric cancer rather than representing a common precursor state.

Gastric ulcer has been described as leading to cancer, but, if at all, it occurs in a very small proportion of patients, in most of whom an undetected cancer was probably present from the beginning.

Gastric polyps, also cited as precursors of cancer, are uncommon, but any polyp should be viewed with suspicion and removed.

Symptoms

In early stages, there are no specific symptoms. Patients and physicians alike tend to dismiss symptoms present for a year or more. Symptoms may suggest peptic ulcer, especially if a cancer involves the lesser curvature.

The first symptoms of stomach cancer are much like those of other digestive illnesses:

- ▲ persistent indigestion;
- ▲ a feeling of bloated discomfort after eating;
- ▲ slight nausea;
- ▲ loss of appetite;
- ▲ heartburn;
- ▲ sometimes mild stomach pain.

Later symptoms may be blood in the stool (either red of black in colour), vomiting, weight loss, and pain.

Diagnosis

To determine whether the symptoms are caused by stomach cancer or some other condition, samples of blood, stomach fluid, and stool are tested. The presence of anemia and lack of acid in the stomach are conditions often found in patients who have stomach cancer. Blood in the stool may be an indication of cancer in the gastrointestinal tract, including the stomach. An X-ray examination of the stomach also aids the physician in making a diagnosis. For this examination, you are asked to drink a liquid containing barium sulphate, a substance that makes parts of your body more visible in X-ray pictures.

Using an X-ray machine called a fluoroscope, the physician can observe the flow of barium sulphate into your stomach and see the outline of the stomach when it is filled. X-ray studies generally have been unreliable in find-

Laboratory analysis of gastric juice and biopsies taken with an endoscope (gastroscope).

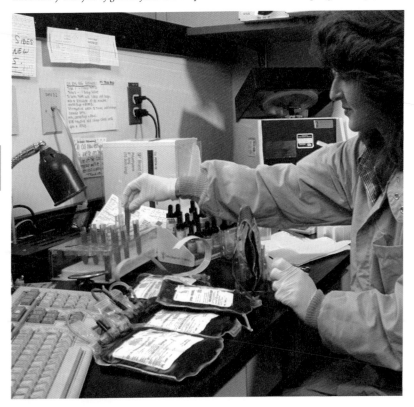

S

Barium X-rays are used to examine the inner part of the stomach. Special X-ray techniques allow for a three-D view of the stomach.

In addition to X-ray examination the doctor used endoscopy in which a flexible tube is used to visualize the inside of the digestive tract. It allows a doctor to view the stomach directly, to check for Helicobacter pylori, and to remove tissue samples for examination under a microscope.

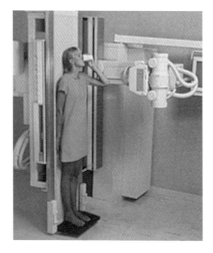
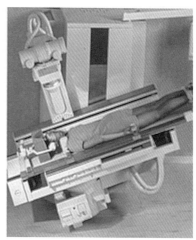

ing small, early lesions. However, by using double-contrast techniques that involve coating the mucosa of the stomach with barium and inflating the stomach to bring out mucosal details, radiologists report carcinomas as small as 1 cm in diameter.

In most cases the physician needs to examine the stomach with am instrument (gastroscope) passed through the mouth and esophagus. A sedative or an anesthetic may be given before this kind of examination so it is not to uncomfortable.

The instrument that may be used is a flexible tube (special type of endoscope called gastroscope) with a light and a series of mirrors that enable the physician to see and photograph the inside of the stomach.

If a growth is detected, a small sample of the tissue can be removed through the instrument. The sample can then be examined with a microscope to determine whether it is cancerous. The removal and microscopic examination of a tissue sample is called a biopsy.

Cytological studies of gastric washings are helpful in some patients; special techniques (for instance, spraying the surface of the tumor with a jet of water during endoscopy or using devices that abrase the surface of the tumor) may increase the yield of positive washings.

In experienced hands, use of a brush (to collect cells from the stomach surface) improves results.

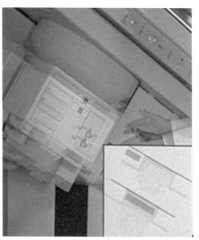
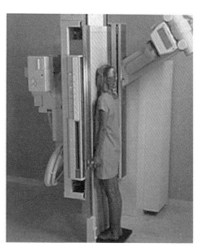

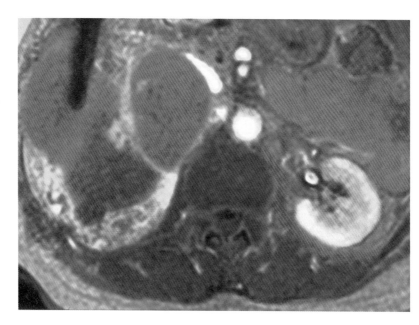

Cross section of the abdominal cavity, just below the diaphragm. This special radiological techniques shows the abdominal organs in different colors. To the left, the stomach; in the center, part of the spinal cord and to the right a cross section of the kidney.

S

Stomach cancer   Questions & Answers

Is stomach cancer a rare disease?

No. As far as the statistically stored data by the World Health Organization on cancer in the world is concerned, stomach cancer is judged to be the second most common cancer.

It remains the most frequent tumor in many parts of the world notably Japan and Iceland, where it accounts for roughly 30-33 percent of all new cancers. Incidence rates are also comparatively high in Europe and Latin America. However, the incidence of stomach cancer is declining at a rate if about two percent per year.

The reasons for this are not clearly understood, but it may be due to a decreasing reliance upon foodstuffs that have been stored or preserved in traditional ways (salting, pickling), and the greater availability of fresh and refrigerated food.

What are the characteristics of stomach cancer?

Cancer of the stomach, like other cancers, is a disease of the body's cells. Although cells of various organs differ in shape and function, all cells reproduce themselves by dividing.

Normal growth and repair of tissue take place in this orderly manner. When cell division is not orderly, abnormal growth takes place. Masses of tissue called tumors build up. Tumors of the stomach may be benign or malignant. Benign tumors do not spread.

They usually can be removed completely and are not likely to recur. But malignant tumors, or cancers of the stomach, invade neighbouring tissues and organs, and can spread to other parts of the body.

What are causative factors of stomach cancer?

While its cause is unknown, stomach cancer is often associated with gastritis and intestinal metaplasia of the mucosa of the stomach. Such findings are not generally thought to result from gastric cancer rather than representing a common precursor state.

What is the relationship of stomach cancer and peptic ulcer?

Peptic ulcer of the stomach has been described as leading to cancer, but, if at all, it occurs in a very small proportion of patients, in most of whom an undetected cancer was probably present from the beginning.

Stomach polyps, also cited as precursors of cancer, are uncommon, but any polyp will be viewed by the doctor with suspicion and removed.

What are the major symptoms of stomach cancer?

In early stages, there are no specific symptoms. Patients and doctors alike tend to dismiss symptoms present for a year or more. Symptoms may suggest peptic ulcer, especially if a cancer involves the lesser curvature. The first symptoms of stomach cancer are much like those of other digestive illnesses:

- persistent indigestion;
- a feeling of bloated discomfort after eating;
- slight nausea;
- loss of appetite;
- heartburn;
- sometimes mild stomach pain.

Later symptoms may be blood in the stool (either red or black in colour), vomiting, weight loss, and pain. See also p. 522.

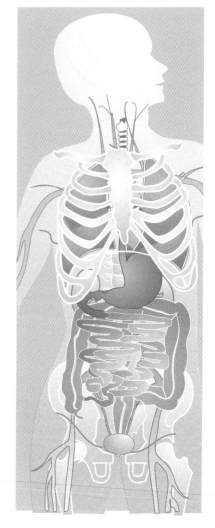

Localization of the stomach in the upper left part of the abdominal cavity.

Treatment

Treatment for stomach cancer is generally prompt removal of the tumor for surgery. This may require removing part or all of the stomach. Any post-operative difficulties in digestion can usually be prevented by eating several small meals a day rather than three large ones and by adhering to a low-sugar diet, high in protein and fat.

If the stomach cancer has started to spread, the surgeon may be able to stop it by removing the affected parts of neighbouring organs, such as the

S

Types of stomach cancer

Types of gastric carcinomas can be classified according to gross appearance:

- protruding (polypoid or fungating);

- penetrating; the tumor has a sharp, well-circumscribed border and may be ulcerated;

- spreading, either superficially along the mucosa or infiltrating within the wall;

- miscellaneous, showing characteristics of 2 of the other types; this is the largest group.

Protruding tumors have better prognosis than infiltrating tumors.

Stomach cancer Questions & Answers

How is the diagnosis of stomach cancer made?
To determine whether the symptoms are caused by stomach cancer or some other condition, samples of blood, stomach fluid, and stool are tested.
The presence of anemia and lack of acid in the stomach are conditions often found in patients who have stomach cancer. Blood in the stool may be an indication of cancer in the gastro-intestinal tract, including the stomach.
A sample of stomach lining can be obtained with a gastroscope. The sample can be examined with a microscope to determine whether it is cancerous. The removal and microscopic examination of a tissue sample is called a biopsy.

What is the value of cytological studies in the diagnosis of stomach cancer?
Cytological studies (microscopic investigation of cells) of stomach washings are helpful in some institutions. Special techniques (for instance, spraying the surface of the tumor with a jet of water during endoscopy or using devices that abrade the surface of the tumor) may increase the yield of positive washings. In experienced hands, use of a brush (to collect cells from the stomach surface), improves results.

What is the best treatment for stomach cancer?
Treatment for stomach cancer is generally prompt removal of the tumor by surgery. This may require removing part or all of the stomach. Any post-operative difficulties in digestion can usually be prevented by eating several small meals a day rather than three large ones and by adhering to a low-sugar diet, high in protein and fat.

If the stomach cancer has started to spread, the surgeon may be able to stop it by removing the affected parts of neighbouring organs, such as the spleen or pancreas. In recent years, advances in surgical techniques and medical care have made extensive surgery possible for persons previously considered too old or infirm for treatment.
Today, surgeons have the help of high sophisticated localizing techniques and the help of very competent teams of nurses, therapists, technicians, and other professionals to support patients throughout their post-operative period.
If all of the cancer present in the body cannot be removed by surgery, chemotherapy (treatment with anti-cancer medicines) may be given. Radiotherapy plays a limited role in the treatment of stomach cancer. The main reason is that radiation doses strong enough to destroy these cancer cells could seriously damage the surrounding healthy tissue.

What types of stomach cancer are known?
Types of stomach carcinomas can be classified according to gross appearance:
- protruding (polypoid or fungating);
- penetrating; the tumor has a sharp, well-circumscribed border and may be ulcerated;
- spreading, either superficially along the mucosa or infiltrating within the wall;
- miscellaneous, showing characteristics of 2 of the other types; this is the largest group.
Protruding tumors have better prognosis than infiltrating tumors.

spleen or pancreas. In recent years, advances in surgical techniques and medical care have made extensive surgery possible for persons previously considered too old or infirm for treatment.
Today, surgeons have the help of highly sophisticated localizing techniques and the help of very competent teams of nurses, therapists, technicians, and other professionals to support patients throughout their post-operative period.
If all of the cancer present in the body cannot be removed by surgery, chemotherapy (treatment with anti-cancer drugs) may be given. Anticancer drugs enter the bloodstream and circulate through the body to attack cancer in any location.
Because the drugs act on normal cells as well as cancerous ones, your physician must maintain a delicate balance of enough drugs to kill cancer cells without destroying too many healthy ones.
Radiation therapy plays a limited role in the treatment of stomach cancer. The main reason is that radiation doses strong enough to destroy these cancer cells could seriously damage the surrounding healthy tissue.

STOMACH DISEASES

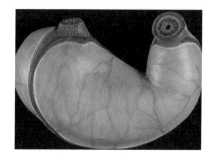

Introduction

Disorders of the stomach, or more generally of the alimentary canal or digestive system are fairly common. Almost everyone has had some degree of difficulty in this area at one time or another.

These disorders can be functional, because of the extensive nerve connections in the digestive system; fear, anger, and other nervous upsets may set off attacks of nausea, cramps, or diarrhea.

Organic diseases such as peptic ulcers and cancer can also affect these organs, as do contagious diseases, such as salmonellosis (eating food contaminated with Salmonella bacteria) and virus infections, as well as constipation, dyspepsia, allergies - and a list almost as long as the digestive tract itself.

Gastroesophageal reflux

Gastroesophageal reflux is the flow of gastric or duodenal contents across the gastroesophageal junction back into the esophagus. The effects depend on the mixture of stomach acid, pepsin, bile salts, and pancreatic enzymes refluxing into the esophageal mucosa.

Although gastroesophageal reflux may be without symptoms, the most common patient complaint is discomfort behind the breastbone, which radiates upward and is aggravated in the recumbent position.

Reflux esophagitis is also aggravated by the following conditions:

* obesity
* tight garments about the abdomen
* pregnancy

The patient may refer to these symptoms as "heartburn", "indigestion", or "sour stomach". The regurgitation of fluid while sleeping or bending over is conclusive evidence of gastroesophageal reflux.

Other less common symptoms include:

* painful swallowing
* difficult swallowing
* hemorrhage;
* lung complaints by choking on stomach contents

Although gastroesophageal reflux may exist simultaneously with a hiatus hernia (protrusion of part of the stomach through the diaphragm), the terms are not synonymous. Gastroesophageal reflux and hiatus hernia are two separate clinical entities, and one has no effect on the other.

In fact only about 5 per cent of patients with hiatal hernia complain of reflux symptoms. Hiatus hernia is a rather common disorder and in many cases produces no symptoms.

Location of the stomach in the left upper part of the abdominal cavity.
1. Stomach
2. Duodenum
3. Transverse colon
5. Small intestine
6. Peritoneum

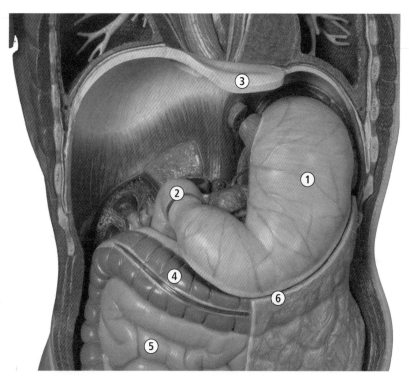

S

Cause and diagnosis

There is general agreement that dysfunction of the lower esophageal sphincter is the cause of reflux. Symptoms have been associated with unexplained, inappropriate, and transient relaxation of the lower esophageal sphincter. However, there is no explanation for the dysfunction of this sphincter. Other factors that may be associated with reflux are disordered peristalsis and delayed stomach emptying.

Gastroesophageal reflux is related to stomach volume. Overeating which increases stomach volume enhances reflux, and this is especially true at bedtime. A cycle of events occurs in which reflux causes inflammation and damage leading to esophagitis (inflammation of the lining of the esophagus). Esophagitis could result in defective peristalsis and incompetent lower esophageal sphincter.

An appropriate medical history as taken by the family doctor and prompt relief by acid neutralization usually indicate gastro-esophageal reflux. The doctor may feel that further diagnostic testing should be performed if disorders or diseases of the heart, gallbladder, stomach or duodenum are suspected.

Treatment

The treatment of gastroesophageal reflux is divided into three phases:

▲ phase I involves dietary and life style changes, measures to improve acid clearance and antacids;
▲ phase II utilizes specific medicines;
▲ phase III is antireflux surgery.

Although most therapy with medicines is aimed at improving the tone of the lower esophageal sphincter and/or neutralizing stomach acid, some very effective results can be obtained if the patient changes his or her life style. Smoking, and the ingestion of fatty foods, coffee, and chocolate, which can decrease lower esophageal sphincter tone, will be discouraged by the doctor.

The patient will be asked if he is taking any medicines known to decrease lower esophageal sphincter tone. These medicines include theophylline, diazepam, verapamil and

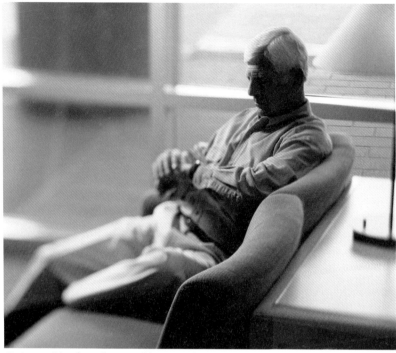

Patient waiting for endoscopy of the stomach.

anticholinergics. Individuals should eat slowly and not recline after meals. Carbonated beverages will also increase pressure in the stomach and should be avoided.

Perhaps the most effective treatment is to utilize gravity to diminish the gastro-esophageal pressure gradient by elevating the head of the bed with 15 cm blocks. Weight loss is also successful in decreasing symptoms.

Bethanechol and antacids have been used to increase competence of the lower esophageal sphincter. Alginic acid has been used to provide a physical barrier that will be neutral if refluxed, although there is controversy regarding the efficacy. Antireflux surgery is indicated only if other therapies fail.

Gastritis

Gastritis is defined as an inflammatory process of the stomach. It is characterized by pain or tenderness, nausea, vomiting and systemic electrolyte changes if vomiting persists. The mucosal lining of the stomach may be atrophic or hypertrophic.

On the basis of the clinical picture and the histological changes of the mucosal lining the following major types of gastritis can be distinguished:

· acute gastritis
· corrosive gastritis
· atrophic gastritis
· hypertrophic gastritis

See: *Gastritis*

Dyspepsia

This disorder may be defined as imperfect digestion; it is not a disease in itself, but symptomatic of other diseases or disorders. Dyspepsia is characterized by:

· vague abdominal discomfort
· heartburn
· nausea
· vomiting
· loss of appetite

The origin of the symptoms may be the stomach or the intestinal tract. Patients with such complaints are very common in the primary care setting and account for 30 to 50 per cent of the patients which are referred by the family doctor to the specialist in gastroenterology.

Stomach diseases   Questions & Answers

What is the structure of the stomach?

The stomach is a dilated, sac-like, distensible portion of the alimentary canal or digestive system below the esophagus and below the diaphragm. The organ is usually pear-shaped, divisible into a more expanded upper portion comprising about two-third of the volume and a narrower lower one-third that curves toward the right.

The junction of the two portions is referred to as gastric angle. At the upper end is the cardia, the aperture communicating with the esophagus. At the lower end is the pylorus, the aperture leading into the duodenum.

What are the borders and surfaces of the stomach?

The stomach has two borders and two surfaces. The right border forms the lesser curvature, which is concave and directly continuous with the right border of the esophagus.

The left border forms the greater curvature. It is convex and gives attachment to the greater omentum. This is a double layer of lining of the abdominal organs and wall - peritoneum attached to the stomach and connecting it with certain of the abdominal organs.

What is the fundus of the stomach?

The dilated portion of the stomach to the left and above the level of the cardia is the fundus. The fundus is continuous below with the body or corpus of the stomach. The third and narrower part of the stomach extends from the gastric angle to the pylorus and is designated as the pyloric portion.

This portion presents a variable dilation to the right of the gastric angle, the pyloric antrum. It is succeeded by a short constricted pyloric canal. When nearly empty, the stomach presents throughout a narrow, tubular form, except in the region of the fundus. This region, which contains the gas bubble, remains somewhat distended even when the remainder of the stomach is empty and contracted.

What happens when food is introduced into the stomach?

When food is introduced, it fills successively the various portions of the stomach, the body (corpus) and pyloric antrum being filled first and the pyloric canal usually last.

The J-shape is the most common form in the upright posture. In contrast to this type is the "cow-horn" stomach, a form that is rare in the upright, but common in the supine position. Here the greater curvature moves upward and the contents gather mainly in the fundus that becomes distended and displaced to the left.

What is the function of the glands of the stomach?

The glands of the mucosal layer secrete mucus, enzymes and hydrochloric acid. Three specific types of cells are found in the epithelium of the stomach glands:

- mucus secreting cells;
- chief cells that produce enzymes; particularly pepsinogen, which is activated in the presence of hydrochloric acid to the proteolytic enzyme pepsin;
- parietal cells that produce hydrochloric acid and intrinsic factor.

The mucosa has a total surface area of about 900 square meters and contains many billions of cells. The mucosal cells of the epithelium protect the stomach from the acid-pepsin complex by releasing an alkaline mucous secretion.

How is the stomach supplied by blood?

The stomach receives its blood supply from many branches. From the coeliac artery (a direct branch of the abdominal aorta) there is the left gastric artery. This vessel runs along the lesser curvature from left to right anastomosing with the right gastric branch of the liver artery.

Along the greater curvature run the right and left gastro-epiploic arteries, anastomosing at the middle of the border, the left being a branch of the splenic artery, the right a branch of the gastroduodenal artery. The blood from the stomach passes into the portal vein via the coronary vein and pyloric vein. There is a set of lymph nodes lying along the lesser curvature and the pyloric portion of the greater curvature, and others at the pyloric and cardiac ends.

How is the stomach supplied by nerves?

The nerves of the stomach are derived in part from the tenth cranial nerve (vagus nerve). The right vagus nerve descends on the back wall and the left on the front wall. The front trunk has four or more branches. They are distributed to the upper portion of the stomach along the lesser curvature and onto the front surface, passing toward the greater curvature.

The back trunk gives off about six branches. Most of these pass to the stomach from the lesser curvature independently. The distribution of the back trunk does not extend to the region of the pylorus. The fibers from the sympathetic part of the autonomic nervous system originate from the coeliac plexus (located around the root of the coeliac artery) and reach the stomach along the arterial branches.

What are the basic functions of the stomach?

The stomach receives the softened mass of food, the bolus, that has been masticated and mixed with saliva in the mouth and delivered by way of the pharynx (throat) and esophagus. The muscular wall of the stomach must complete the physical breakdown of large bits of food that the teeth failed to grind up.

The glands of the stomach produce hydrochloric acid and enzymes which are thoroughly mixed with the food converting the bolus in time into a semifluid mass called chyme. The enzymes can work in an acid medium. The chyme is then delivered to the small intestine, while solid particles are retained in the stomach until they too are converted to chyme.

Practically no absorption of food takes place in the stomach. Each anatomical area of the stomach has a different type of mucosa and contributes different secretions to the juice.

S

Although functional and nonspecific symptoms may in part derive from medical disease (for instance, peptic ulcer), the contributory psychological or cultural factors make the diagnosis difficult and medical treatment alone insufficient.

The term functional dyspepsia is defined as common discomfort, often described as "indigestion", gaseousness, dullness or pain, that is burning or gnawing in quality and localized to the upper abdomen or chest. The patient regards this condition as originating in the stomach or heart.

Signs and symptoms

Belching, abdominal distention and borborygmi (rambling noises caused by propulsion of gas through the intestines) are often described in addition to pain in the upper left part of the abdominal cavity or behind the breast bone.

Eating may worsen or relieve the pain. Other associated symptoms may include anorexia, nausea and change in bowel habits. Dysphoric states such as anxiety or depression may often be found.

These symptoms are not confined to a single organ or disease process and can have many causes. Dyspepsia may be reported in angina pectoris (in which the discomfort is worsened by exertion), gastro-esophageal reflux, diffuse esophageal spasm, peptic ulcer disease and inflammation of the mucosal lining of the gallbladder. Psychological causes include the following disorders:

- anxiety with or without swallowing of air (aerophagy);
- conversion disorder (specific emotional disorder);
- depressive syndrome;
- hypochondria (excessive concern about health; unrealistic interpretations of real or imagined symptoms).

A history of alternating constipation and diarrhea suggests a generalized motility disorder as the cause, such as the irritable bowel syndrome.

Treatment

Dyspepsia with no evidence of underlying bodily (somatic) disease usually calls first for reassurance and symptomatic management with observation

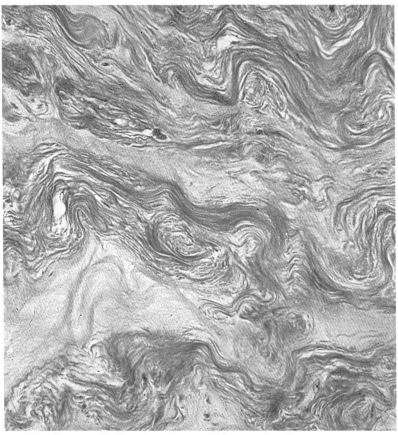

Histological micrograph of a malignant process of the stomach wall.

over time. Treatment of reflux symptoms or abdominal discomfort will be tried with antacids of specific medicines.

Changes in the clinical state may require more extensive evaluation if new problems arise or if symptoms persist and become disabling, but, for most patients with chronic nonspecific dyspepsia, continued observation by the family doctor is sufficient.

Stomach ulcer

Stomach ulcers belong to the group of digestive conditions called peptic ulcers. A peptic ulcer is a circumscribed erosion in or loss of the mucous membrane lining of the gastrointestinal tract. Peptic ulcers are chronic but may have acute exacerbations.

They are most often solitary and occur at any level of the gastrointestinal tract exposed to the action of acid and pepsin. T
hey are truly peptic. If acid and pepsin are diverted from an established ulcer, the ulcer will heal and not recur.

In decreasing order of incidence, they occur in the:
- duodenum
- stomach
- esophagus
- stoma of a stomach and small intestine
- Meckel's diverticulum
- jejunum

However, the most significant sites of peptic ulcer disease are the duodenum and stomach.

Peptic ulcers are caused by an increase in acid and pepsin, a decrease in the resistance of the mucosal lining, or a combination of the two.

In a high age of cases a bacterial growth of Helicobacter pylori is found.

See: *Peptic ulcer disease*

S

STRESS

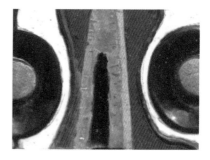

Description

In psychology and biology, stress is defined as any strain or interference that disturbs the functioning of an organism. Physical stresses such as cold, heat, or noise evoke biological reactions; and psychological stresses, such as frustration, deprivation, and conflict, evoke psychological defences. Many situations call forth both types of response. Disturbances of home-ostasis play an important role in the causation of stress.

People with chronic stress constantly feel worried or distressed; the workload may he too heavy.

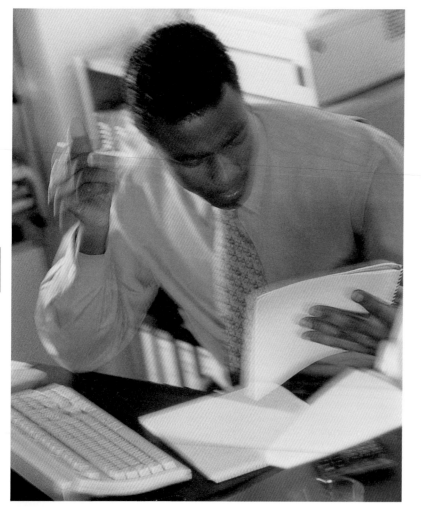

Homeostasis

Homeostasis, or the active maintenance of all the vital systems at the equilibrium levels conducive to optimum overall functioning, is common to all physiological concepts of stress. Each vital system may be considered to be a controlled system and every internal process that functions to maintain the homeostatic level of a particular system mat be called a controlling mechanism.

In the relatively simple case of human thermoregulation, the controlled system is body temperature, or more precisely brain temperature, and the controlling mechanisms include cardiac output, cutaneous blood flow, and sweating. A heat load, being an external stressor, will first activate the controlling mechanisms in the intact organisms, and if their response is sufficient, eventually the controlled system itself.

Throughout this process, the body can be said to be under stress - i.e., engaged in an effort to maintain thermal homeostasis however successfully. The physiological signs of increased cardiac output and increased cutaneous blood flow to provide greater heat loss by radiation, and sweating to provide heat loss by evaporation, are directly related to whole-body stress until those mechanisms are fully engaged or exhausted.

The final rise in body temperature is a more significant sign of stress as it indicates a pathological reaction, but it is obviously less sensitive. Physiological or psychological reactions that are not specifically related to thermoregulation but are instead correlates of stress in general would be of little interest if they did not occasionally lead to another reaction, e.g., impairment of the motivation or ability to perform a critical task in the heat, or in the long term or secondary system failure through general neuroendocrine activation. Correlates of adaptive stress reactions are certainly the least reliable and the most difficult to interpret among the signs of stress produced by physical agents. The psychosocial stressor is literally a creation of the human brain. That organ interprets perceived information in elation to information stored in the memory and an appraisal of its own capacity to overcome any threat the perceived information conveys.

The external psychosocial hazard is an event, of combination of events, that the brain interprets as a threat to its ability to maintain a comfortable state of equilibrium and/or a desired mode of behavior. These two factors may be viewed as constituting the controlled system.

Satisfactorily controlling mechanisms might be to act on the environment to eliminate the hazard, to reinterpret the hazard, to reduce its threat, or in some way to increase the capacity of the brain to challenge the threat more effectively. Such reactions can be categorized under the single title "coping". Unlike physiological adaptation to physical stressors, coping depends on having the freedom, experience, and ability to select the most effective form among a number of possible means. Many situational and individual factors limit coping.

Even when it is permitted within a given situation, the injudicious or merely unlucky selection of one particular means can intensify the threat and inhibit further attempt to cope.

Activation in the presence of a stressor

Cannon's famous "flight or fight" hypothesis pertains to man reacting to a threat as it does to the presence of a physical agent causing pain. Simply stated, the hypothesis is that the stressor activates all the physiological systems that have the function of sus-

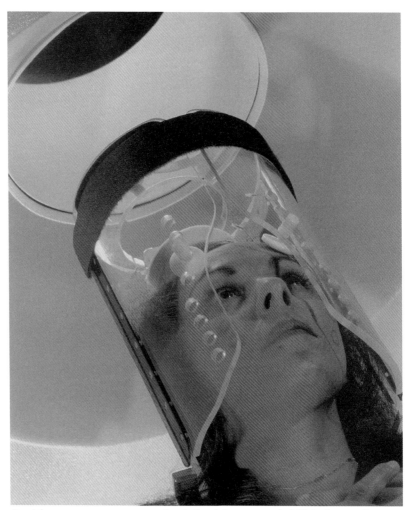

Special scan apparatus to measure electrical and electromagnetic fields in the central nervous system during experiments provoking stress situations.

Treatment strategies

- Remove the cause of the stress, which is much easier said than done in most cases.

- Rationalise stress by talking over the problem with a spouse, relatives, friends, doctor or priest. Writing down details of the problem makes it appear more manageable, particularly when all possible options are diagrammatically attached to it to give a rational view of the situation.

- Professional assistance may be given by a general practitioner, psychiatrist, psychologist, marriage guidance counsellor, child guidance officer or social worker.

- Medications that alter mood, sedate or relieve anxiety are used in a crisis, intermittently or for short periods of time. Some antidepressant drugs and treatments for psychiatric conditions are designed for long-term use, but most of the anxiety-relieving drugs can cause dependency if used regularly.

S

Methods for stress relief

Deep (abdominal) breathing

Deep breathing is one of the simplest yet most effective stress-management techniques there is. You can d it anywhere, any time, and it becomes even more effective with practice. By infusing the blood with extra oxygen, but also by causing the body to release endorphins, which are natural tranquillizing hormones, the effect may be longlasting.

To enjoy the benefits of deep breathing, however, you have to do it from the abdomen, not just the chest. This allows the lower lobes of the lungs (which accept oxygen best) to become more involved in the breathing process.

Here is how to do it:

- Slowly inhale through your nose, expanding your abdomen before allowing air to fill your chest.

- Slowly reverse the process as you exhale. Take a few minutes each day to practice this technique.

Massage

When faced with stress our bodies often tighten, causing pain. For some individuals, massage can help relieve this muscle tension and bring about a sense of relaxation. Shiatsu is a form of massage based on Chinese medicine that has been recorded since 200 BC.

In Shiatsu massage, pressure is applied to specific energetic pathways in the body, freeing up tension. There's one such area located on the wrist, for example, where blockage can reflect feelings of anxiety. A full Shiatsu treatment strategically performs similar prodigy all over the body, finding areas of tightness and working them out.

Yoga

Through combinations of movement, breathing awareness and relaxation techniques, yoga can reduce stress in three ways. It gives you time out to focus on yourself, which helps set the stage for stress reduction. It improves breathing, mus-

cle tone and posture, which can help you combat stress physically.

Yoga also can help you carry yourself in a way that can combat stress by giving you a greater sense of self-esteem. Shoulders relaxed, chest lifted, legs strong. Holding your body in this position, called mountain pose, gives a message to your mind about what's like to feel confident.

The good posture that yoga teaches can also combat low back pain, which can be a great source and cause of stress.

Body stretching

Stretching can help you feel more peaceful ad relaxed. Just as your mind affects your body, so can your body affects your mind. There are right and wrong ways to attempt this loosening up. First and foremost is to forget the creed of "no pain, no gain."

Pain defeats the purpose of stretching by causing muscles to tighten rather than relax. So never bounce when you stretch.

- Think about the area being stretched. Imagine the tension leaving them as you gently take them to their comfortable limit.

- Move slowly and fluidly.

- Exhale into the stretch; inhale on the release. Breathe deeply ad slowly and always through the nose. Never hold your breath during a stretch.

- Wear loose, comfortable clothing.

- Stretch with eyes close for better awareness of body responses.

- Wait several hours after eating before stretching. Physical movements diverts blood from the digestive system.

- Enjoy the process; do not worry about the end result.

taining maximum strength, speed of response, and endurance in the skeletal musculature. This included the following mechanisms:

- ▲ a rise in isometric muscle tension;
- ▲ a rise in cardiac output by means of increased myocardial strength and frequency of contraction;
- ▲ the contracture of arterioles in the cutaneous and mesenteric vascular beds;
- ▲ the neurohumoral mobilization of hepatic glucose and free fatty acids

and glycerol from the adipose tissue.

Though not known to Cannon, this general activation perpetuates the brain's own state of arousal medullary release of adrenaline which stimulates sites in the hypothalamus of the brain. Clearly this is a beneficial reaction in a short-lasting emergency when physical exertion is necessary to overcome the threat. But frequently repeated episodes of this sort, or prolonged activation of the autonomic nervous

system and various neuroendocrine systems, disturb homeostasis.

Stress and work

It is popular, in current psychosomatic medicine and biological psychiatry, to theorize that all sorts of diseases may be ascribed to the chronic effects of over-activation in people exposed to psychosocial hazards, particularly those encountered at work.

To prevent stress, observe mental health, such as for unusual irritability, anxiety, depressive symptoms.

The pathophysiological mechanisms of psychosomatic disease are exceedingly obscure, however, and though several possible mechanisms have been suggested none has been observed experimentally.

Many of the consequences to the systems of chronic over-activation, are mediated by an excessive production of adrenaline and noradrenaline. The hormones may also directly affect the organs, for instance,m the heart, causing arrhythmias, electrolyte imbalance, and even necrosis.

Chronic over-activation of the pituitary-suprarenal axis may produce local tissue damage, primarily as a result of the inhibition of cortisol and amino acid uptake by mucosal, skeletal muscle, skin, and lymphoid cells.

A loss of resistance in the gastrointestinal mucosa to acid and proteolytic enzymes, muscle wasting, and diminished antibody production which increases the susceptibility to infection, are some of the many possible results.

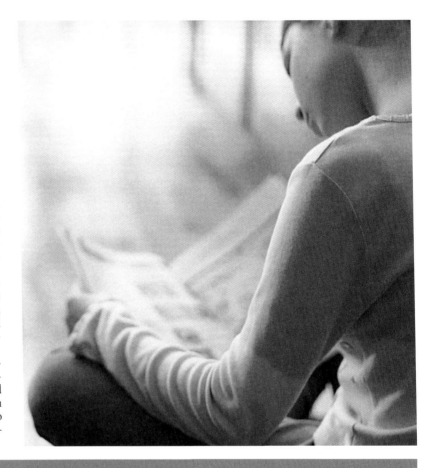

How to avoid stress

Eliminate stress points
Look for patterns in your daily life that trigger extra stress and get rid of them. Whenever you can, try to come up with plans in advance, so you'll avoid predictable crises.

Set priorities
Your priorities will not be the same every day. Some says you have to give more to your job; on others, you may put your kids first. The crucial point is that you consciously think about your needs, and do something to see that they are met.

Think of ways to say no
Use the time and energy to think of alternatives to a particular request. If you come up with an idea that appeals to you, go back and correct the situation.

Use your organizational skills
Simplify whatever you plan. Delegate if possible, ad try to create a supportive atmosphere. At home, ask for the cooperation of each member of the household rather that try to tackle everything yourself.

At work, negotiate for what you want. Instead of just talking about your problem, present a variety of possible solutions and invite others to make suggestions, too.

Establish routines and plan ahead
Try to anticipate stressful situation, such as a school holiday, so you can make arrangements.

Monitor yourself for signs of overload
All of us have early-warning signals of stress. When you see such symptoms, force yourself to stop and say, "I'm under stress. I need to do something about it." That might getting more sleep, or hiring a mother's helper for the weekend.

Be kinder and gentler to yourself
Relief may come just by talking to a friend. During your workday, take occasional breaks, whether it is 10 minutes to straighten up your desk or half an hour to eat lunch in the sun or meet a friend for coffee.

Try to get your partner to pitch in.
Make a list of everything that needs to be done. Then sit down with your partner and divide the various tasks.

S

STROKE

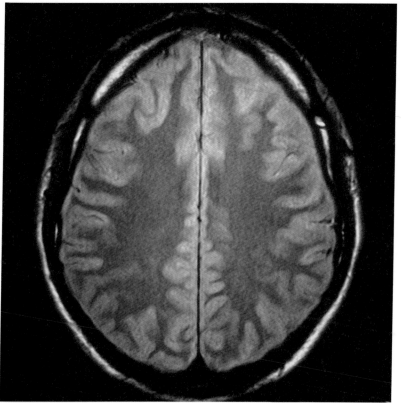

Description

A stroke, also called apoplexy and cerebrovascular accident (CVA), is the effect of either substantial reduction in blood flow to some part of the brain or intracranial bleeding. These effects may include transient or lasting paralysis on one or both sides of the body; difficulty in using words or in eating; or a loss in muscular coordination.

The term stroke is sometimes limited to the effects of a fall in blood flow to the brain, whereas the term apoplexy applies to the effects of intracranial bleeding. Both processes may result in cerebral infarctions - dead sections of brain tissue.

Causes of a stroke

Normally, an adequate blood flow to the brain is ensured by an efficient collateral system. The reduction in blood flow is often caused by formation of a blood clot (the process is called thrombosis) at the site of a fatty deposit (an atherosclerotic plaque) in the lining of a brain artery.

In these circumstances there may be, in advance of the full stroke (and in advance of the actual formation of an infarct), transient paralysis on one side of the face, for example, paralysis of an arm or a leg, or abnormal sensations on one side of the body. If the brainstem is the part of the brain affected, the effects may be on both sides of the body.

Treat of persons who have suffered strokes from thrombosis include measures to improve the blood supply to the brain and physical therapy and other measures directed toward rehabilitation.

Strokes may be caused by emboli, blood cloths or masses of other substance that have broken loose from their point of formation and have travelled through the bloodstream to a narrow point, where they lodge and obstruct the blood flow.

Emboli that cut off the blood supply to a section of the brain usually have formed in a diseased of malfunctioning heart. The outcome depends upon whether further emboli are formed and upon the seriousness of the heart disease if that is involved.

Treatment includes measures to restore the circulation of the blood and rehabilitation measures.

■ Intracranial bleeding
The intracranial bleeding that results in strokes mat be from a ruptured aneurysm (i.e., a ballooning out of an artery because of a weakened area of wall), from a ruptured angioma (a tangled knot of blood vessels containing abnormal interconnections between arteries and veins), or from rupture of blood vessels by abnormally high blood pressure.

Cross-section of the brain showing damage in one of the frontal areas due top a stroke.

Treatment is directed toward preservation of life, reducing the disability that has resulted from the stroke, and prevention of further strokes. Persons with some chance of survival may be operated upon to remove an aneurysm or correct any other source of bleeding or to relieve intracranial hypertension.

Symptoms, signs, and course

Two types of stroke can be distinguished: stroke in evolution and completed stroke.

s A *stroke in evolution* is defined as the clinical condition manifested by neurologic defects that increase over a 24- to 48-hour period, reflecting enlarging infarction, usually in the territory of the middle brain artery.

▲ A *completed stroke* is defined as the clinical condition manifested by neurologic deficits of varying severity, usually abrupt in onset and either fatal or showing variable improvement, resulting from infarction of brain tissue to atherosclerotic or hypertensive stenosis, thrombosis, or embolism.

In stroke in evolution, one-sided neurologic dysfunction (often beginning in one arm) increases painlessly and without headache or fever over several hours or a day or two to involve progressively more of the body on the same side. The progression is usually stepwise, interrupted by periods of stability, but may be continuous.

Acute completed stroke is by far the more common condition. Symptoms develop rapidly, and typically are maximal within a few more minutes. By convention, completed stroke also refers to the patient's condition, after either evolving or acute stroke, once symptoms have ceased to progress and are either stable or improving.

In either evolving or acute completed large strokes, deficits may worsen and consciousness may become clouded during the next few days because of swelling of the brain or, less often, from extension of the infarct.

Severe brain swelling can cause a potentially fatal shift in brain structures. However, early improvement in function is common unless severe

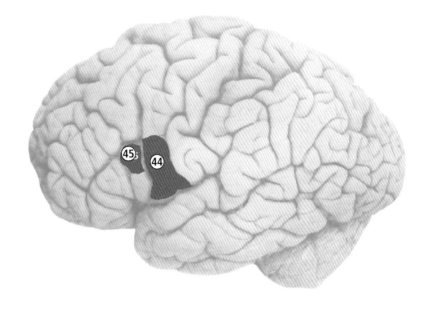

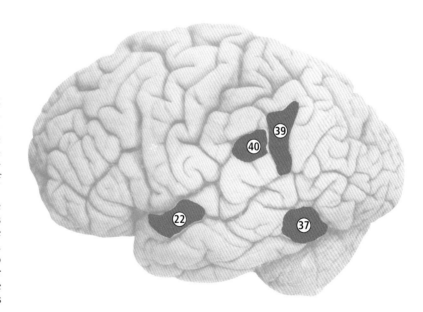

The various places in the brain where damage leads to speech disorders or other forms of aphasia. Motor aphasia occurs principally through damage to area 44 and 45. Damage to the other areas leads to sensory aphasia or a mixed form.

S

Stroke   Questions & Answers

What is a stroke?

A stroke is a form of cardiovascular disease. It affects the arteries or veins of the central nervous system and stops the flow of blood bringing oxygen and nutrients to the brain. A stroke occurs when one of these blood vessels either bursts or becomes clogged. Because of this rupture or blockage, part of the brain does not receive the flow of blood it needs. As a result, it starts to die.

Are there any warning signs of stroke?

The warning signs of stroke are:
- Sudden weakness or numbness of the face, arm and leg on one side of the body.
- Sudden dimness or loss of vision, particularly in one eye.
- Loss of speech, or trouble talking or understanding speech.
- Sudden, severe headaches with no apparent cause.
- Unexplained dizziness, unsteadiness or sudden falls, especially along with any of the previous symptoms.

What is a temporary stroke?

A transient ischemic attack or temporary stroke may occur days, weeks or even months before a major stroke.

A transient ischemic attack, also called TIA, results when a blood clot temporarily clogs an artery and part of the brain does not get the supply of blood it needs. The symptoms occur rapidly and last a relatively short time, usually from a few minutes to several hours. The usual symptoms are like those of a full-fledged stroke, except that the symptoms of a TIA are temporary, lasting 24 hours or less.

How can a stroke be prevented?

When a stroke occurs, severe losses in mental and bodily functions - even death - can result. That is why preventing a stroke is so important.

The best way to prevent a stroke is to reduce the factors that can cause one in the first place, such as hypertension, overweight, smoking, stress, etc.

What are the risk factors for stroke?

Some factors that increase the risk of stroke are genetically determined, others are simply a function of natural processes, but still others result from a person's lifestyle.

The factors resulting from heredity or natural processes cannot be changed, but those that are environmental can be modified with a doctor's help.

What are the risk factors that cannot be changed?

Five risk factors for stroke cannot be changed. These are:
- Age
- Sex
- Race
- Diabetes mellitus
- A prior stroke

The older the person gets, the greater the risk of stroke. Men are also more likely to have a stroke; blacks have a greater risk of stroke than whites. People with diabetes or who have had a prior stroke are also more likely to suffer stroke. It is possible that precise control of diabetes may reduce the risk of stroke in diabetic patients.

infarction has occurred. Further improvement is then gradual over days, weeks, or months.

Specific neurologic symptoms are determined by the site of the brain infarct. The involved artery can often be inferred from the symptom pattern, although the correlation is not exact. Occlusion of several arteries can cause a complex pattern of symptoms.

Diagnosis and prognosis

Stroke usually can be diagnosed clinically, especially in a patient over age 50 with high blood pressure, diabetes, or signs of atherosclerosis, or in any patient with a known source of emboli. Clinical diagnosis seldom is difficult. In the unusual case, differentiation from a rapidly growing or suddenly symptomatic tumor is aided by a negative skull X-ray or by a CTo or MRI-scan.

Determining the immediate cause of a stroke may be difficult for the general physician or specialist. Onset during sleep or on arising suggests infarction; onset during exertion, hemorrhage. headache, coma or stupor, marked high blood pressure, and convulsive seizures are more likely with bleeding (hemorrhage).

A stroke due to a large embolus tends to be an acute completed stroke, sudden in onset, with focal disorders that are maximal within a few minutes. Headache may precede it. Thrombosis is less frequent and is suggested by a slower onset, or a gradual progression of symptoms, as in evolving stroke.

As far as prognosis is concerned the following. During the early days of either evolving or completed stroke, neither progression nor ultimate outcome can be predicted. About 30 percent of patients die in the hospital; the mortality rate increases with age.

The eventual extent of neurologic recovery depends on the patient's age and general state of health as well as on the site and size of the infarction. Impaired consciousness, mental deterioration, aphasia, or severe brainstem signs all suggest a poor prognosis. Complete recovery is uncommon, but the sooner improvement begins, the better the prognosis.

S

About 50 percent of patients with moderate or severe hemiplegia, and most of those with lesser deficits, recover functionally by the time of discharge and are ultimately able to care for their basic needs, have a clear sensorium, and can walk adequately, although use of an affected limb mat be limited.

Any deficit remaining after 6 months is likely to be permanent, although some patients continue to improve slowly. Recurrence of brain infarction is common, and each recurrence is likely to add to the neurologic disability.

Treatment and rehabilitation

Immediate care of a comatose patient includes airway maintenance, adequate oxygenation, or intravenous fluids to maintain nutritional and fluid intake, attention to bladder and bowel function, and measures to prevent bed sore. Heart failure, rhythmic disorders of the heart, severe high blood pressure, and intercurrent respiratory infection will be treated by the specialist i the hospital.

Heparin may stabilize symptoms in evolving stroke, but anticoagulants are useless and probably dangerous) in acute completed stroke and are contraindicated in patients with high blood pressure because of increased possibility of bleeding (hemorrhage) into the brain or other organs.

Vascular surgery is not indicated as an emergency measure and is pointless after complete hemiplegic stroke or when atheromatous stenosis is widespread.

■ *Rehabilitation and aftercare*
Early and repeated appraisals of the patient's by physician, physical therapist, and nursing staff allow a remedial program to be designed. After someone survives a stroke, it is important to prevent further physical disability such as contractures and weakness from unnecessary bed rest and inactivity.

The next step in the care of the stroke patient is to teach him to perform necessary daily activities so that he may once again be independent. Most stroke patients can become independent in these activities with proper help and encouragement.

■ *General considerations*
If activities of daily living are started as soon as possible, the patient will maintain strength in his unaffected extremity and trunk muscles, will be more alert, and will have a more hopeful attitude. In addition, it may aid him in regaining some strength on his weak side.

Depending on the condition of the patient, it may be necessary to increase activities very gradually. However, some patients can progress at a rapid rate. In either case, frequent rest periods should be provided between activities so that the work is not too strenuous.

The attitude of the person working with the patient is extremely important. He must have a positive approach but not be too demanding. He must be firm and understanding, and must never be cross or impatient. By asking questions of the physician and watching the patient's progress, he will learn how much help to give, and when to give it, because it is important for the patient to succeed in his attempts to perform activities.

Unsuccessful attempts tend to be frustrating and to increase the patient's depression while success, even with help, is encouraging to him. It is important not to give too much assistance because when the helper performs the activity, the helper gets stronger; when the patient performs the activity, he gets stronger.

As soon as it is indicated by the doctor, the patient should begin activities such as rolling over in bed (using a side rail if necessary), changing his position in bed, lifting his hips on the bedpan, partially bathing himself, and feeding himself with his strong hand. If this is his left hand and he is left-handed, he should not encounter many difficulties except for not having his other hand to help. If his left hand is strong, ad he is right-handed, he will be very awkward at first but with encouragement, he should learn to feed himself with his left hand.

Those patients who do not regain use of the affected hand often do well with self-help devices, such as a curved rocker blade knife to cut their food.

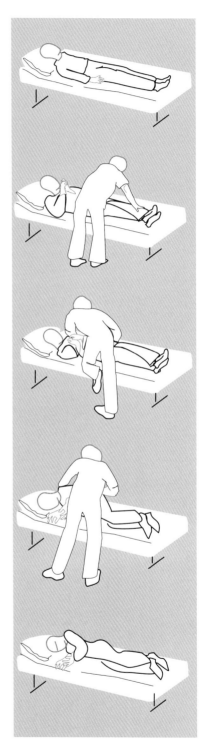

Physical therapy is an important part of the rehabilitation program of a stroke patient. Passive and active exercises are essential.

THYROID DISEASES

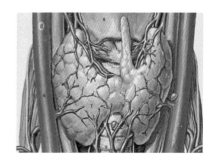

Description

The thyroid gland may be involved in a large number of pathological conditions such as decreased activity (hypothyroidism), increased activity (hyperthyroidism), autoimmune disease, cancers, etc.

Goitre

Goitre is defined as an enlarged thyroid gland. Thyroid enlargement may occur in association with a number of conditions such as:
- iodine deficiency;
- autoimmune thyroiditis;
- virus infection;
- congenital deficiency of any of the

enzymes concerned with the synthesis of thyroxine.

Since the iodisation of table salt there has been a significant decline in the incidence of goitre caused by deficiency of iodine. Hashimoto's disease is a common cause of goitre and may be associated with various functional conditions of the thyroid gland.

Thyroiditis caused by a virus produces a painful tender goitre which usually subsides spontaneously and which is accompanied by thyroid function tests typical of pathological increased activity of the gland. At puberty, especially in girls, and during pregnancy a small goitre may develop and later regress.

When the goitre is small most patients are quite unaware of its existence. As it enlarges it produces a visible palpable swelling and in that case of a viral infection there may be local tenderness. Marked enlargement of the gland may produce pressure symptoms with dyspnea or dysphagia.

In most patients with iodine-deficient goitre thyroxin production is adequate but with severe iodine lack and especially in children born of iodine-deficient mothers, decreased thyroid function may occur.

Such infants are called cretins and manifest growth and feeding problems and will become mentally subnormal, unless an early diagnosis is made and adequate treatment commenced.

Untreated cases show a number of characteristics:
- a typical appearance with pot-belly;
- constipation;
- a large tongue;
- thick skin;
- growth retardation.

In most cases the clinical feature will indicate the cause of goitre but the

Topography of the thyroid in the neck region.

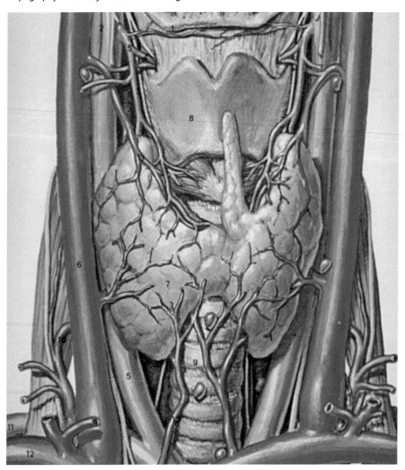

functional state of the thyroid gland is important. The treatment will depend on the underlying disease. Small iodine-deficient goitres will often decrease in size in response to physiological doses of thyroxine.

Larger long-standing goitres will probably be unaffected and if producing significant pressure, symptoms will require partial surgical removal of the gland. Thyroiditis caused by a virus infection usually subsides spontaneously and local pain and tenderness will respond to a regular painrelieving drug.

Hypothyroidism

This condition - also known as myoedema - is the characteristic reaction to thyroid hormone deficiency in the adult.

Primary hypothyroidism
The most common form, is probably an autoimmune disease, usually occurring as a sequel to Hashimoto's disease.

Secondary hypothyroidism
Occurs when there is a failure of the two controlling systems - the hypothalamus in the brain and/or pituitary gland - either due to deficient secretion of TRH from the hypothalamus or lack of secretion of TSH from the pituitary gland.

The symptoms and signs of primary hypothyroidism are generally in striking contrast to those of an increased activity of the thyroid gland and may be quite subtle and insidious in onset. The most characteristic symptoms and signs are the following:
- dull facial expression;
- puffiness in the face;
- swelling around the orbit;
- eyelids drip because of decreased adrenergic drive;
- hair is sparse, coarse and dry;
- skin is coarse, dry, scaly and thick.

The patients are forgetful and show other evidence of intellectual impairment with a gradual change in personality. There may be the occurrence of a frank psychosis; a condition sometimes called myoedema madness. There is bradycardia (slowing of the heart rate) due to a decrease in

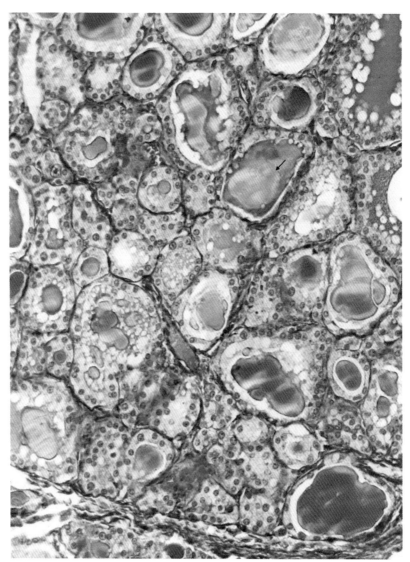

Microscopic structure of the thyroid gland. The gland is divided into lobules; each consisting of a number of structural units called the follicles. The follicles are irregularly-shaped, epithelial-lined vesicles that usually contain a homogeneous, acidophilic staining substance called colloid. The colloid is the stored secretion of the follicular cells. It consists primarily of a glycoprotein called thyroglobulin, which contains iodine and is the source of the thyroid hormones.

both thyroid hormone and adrenergic stimulation. The heart is enlarged due, in large measure, to accumulation of fluid in the pericardial sac.

Patients generally note constipation, which may be severe. Paraesthesia of the hands and feet are common. The reflexes may be very helpful diagnostically because of the brisk contraction and the slow relaxation time.

Hypothermia is commonly noted if the temperature is measured rectally. Anemia is often present. A variety of thyroid hormone preparations are available for replacement therapy.

Hyperthyroidism

This condition is characterized by an increased activity of the thyroid gland. This disorder is also known as:

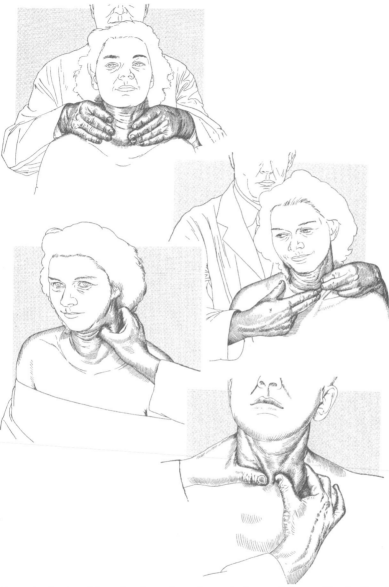

External palpation of the neck region to detect changes in the morphology and localization of the thyroid gland.

- tachycardia;
- insomnia;
- weakness;
- frequent bowel movements.

Eye signs in patients with hyperthyroidism include:
- stare;
- lid lag;
- lid retraction;
- mild degree of conjunctival injection;
- oedema-producing symptoms including orbital pain, lacrimation, irritation, and photophobia.

The diagnosis of hyperthyroidism is usually straightforward and depends on a careful clinical history and physical examination, a high index of suspicion and routine hormone determinations.

A number of approaches are utilized for the treatment of hyperthyroidism, for instance, the administration of iodine, radioactive iodine, certain antithyroid agents and surgery.

Surgery is indicated in a number of categories of patients;
▲ those below 21 years of age who should not receive radioiodine;
▲ in individuals who cannot tolerate other agents because of hypersensitivity or other problems;
▲ in patients with very large goitres;
▲ in some patients with toxic adenoma of the thyroid gland.

Surgery offers a good prospect for recovery. In experts hands, postoperative recurrences vary between 2 and 5 percent.

Hashimoto's disease

This autoimmune disease is thought to be the most common cause of primary hyperthyroidism. It is more prevalent (ratio 8:1) in women than men and most frequent between the ages of 30 and 50.

A family history of thyroid disorders is common and incidence is increased in patients with chromosomal disorders.

The patients complain of painless enlargement of the gland or fullness in the throat.

On examination the doctor finds a nontender goitre, smooth or nodular firm and more rubbery in consistency than the normal thyroid gland. The

- thyrotoxicosis;
- toxic diffuse goitre;
- Graves' disease;
- Basedow's disease;
- toxic nodular goitre.

Many symptoms and signs are associated with hyperthyroidism. The more common signs are the following:
- goitre;
- increased heart rate;
- widened pulse pressure;
- warm, fine, moist skin;

- tremor;
- eye signs;
- atrial fibrillation.

The most frequent symptoms are the following:
- nervousness and increased physical activity;
- hypersensitivity to heat;
- palpitations of the heart;
- fatigue;
- increased appetite;
- weight loss;

Congenital hypothyroidism

This condition results from abnormal functioning or development of the thyroid gland during fetal growth. An affected infant's family may occasionally have a history of thyroid disorders.

Symptoms of congenital hypothyroidism appear 6 to 12 weeks after birth. Facial features include a generally dull appearance with an underdeveloped nasal bridge, eyes that appear widely spaced, and a large, protruding tongue that prevents closing the lips. The neck appears short and thick, and the hands are broad and fat.

The skin is usually mottled (with a pattern of prominent veins) and cool to the touch. If the problem has been present for some time, the skin becomes dry and coarse, often developing a yellowish tinge reflecting an increase of an orange pigment, carotene, present in the blood. Perspiration is reduced. Nails and hair grow slowly and are coarse, dry, and brittle.

A child's heart rate and circulation are slowed; blood pressure is low. Appetite is usually reduced, and feeding of infants tends to be slow because of occasional difficulty in swallowing. Affected children, however, tend to be moderately overweight.

Because thyroid hormone is essential to the development of the central nervous system (brain, spinal cord, and their protective covering, the meninges), any deficiency during fetal development or early life causes slowed mental activity and responsiveness and, if untreated, may be associated with mental retardation.

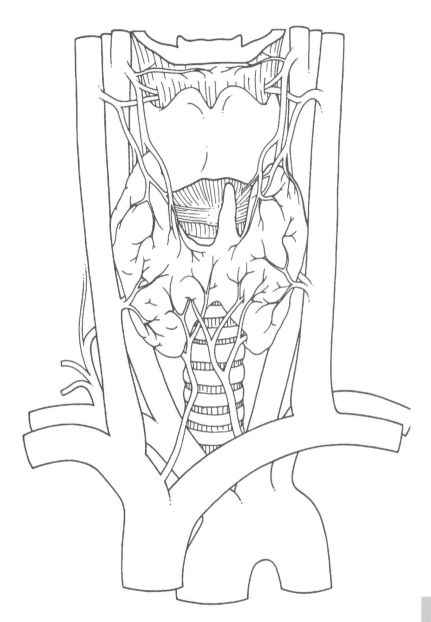

The thyroid gland lies in the anterior part of the neck, near the junction of the larynx with the trachea. Main arteries (carotid arteries) are located on both sides.

treatment of this disease requires life-long replacement with thyroid hormone to correct and prevent hypothyroidism.

Thyroid cancers

Usually, either the patient or the doctor notices an otherwise symptomless lump in the neck. Most thyroid nodules are benign and, as a rule, thyroid cancers are not highly malignant and generally compatible with normal life expectancy, if treated properly.

Near-total removal of the thyroid gland is the treatment of choice when operative intervention is required. The operation must be performed by a surgeon with proven expertise in thyroid surgery because of the risks inherent in such a procedure.

TOOTH DISORDERS

Common dental diseases

There are many diseases that affect the mouth, but the dental diseases constituting the main public health problem are dental caries (tooth decay) and periodontal disease. Both can be prevented or contained by removing the cause.

Caries

Caries, tooth decay, or dental decay, usually occurs within a few years of the teeth erupting.

It is thus primarily a disease of childhood and early adult life. It first affects the tooth enamel at localized sites; notably in the fissures in the tooth surfaces, around the contact points in adjacent, abutting teeth and near the gum margin.

If allowed to progress, a cavity forms and the dentine underlying the demineralized enamel becomes softened and infected with bacteria so that eventually the pulp is threatened.

Periodontal disease

Although periodontal disease can begin at any time after tooth eruption, it progresses slowly and, unlike caries, does not usually threaten the integrity of the dentition until early middle life or later.

Tooth decay

Tooth decay or caries is the gradual pathologic disintegration and dissolu-

X-rays of all teeth to check for cavities, peripheral abscesses, impacted teeth, and malocclusion.

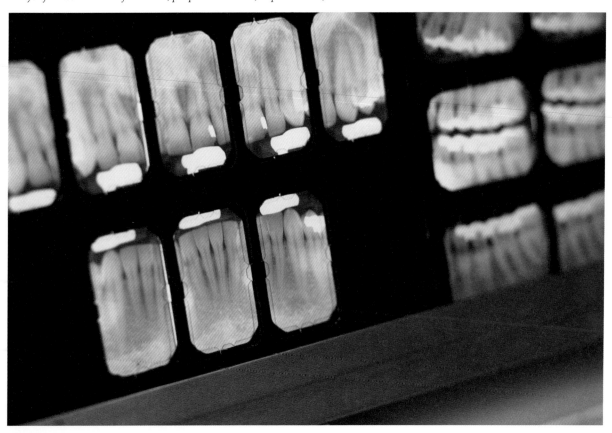

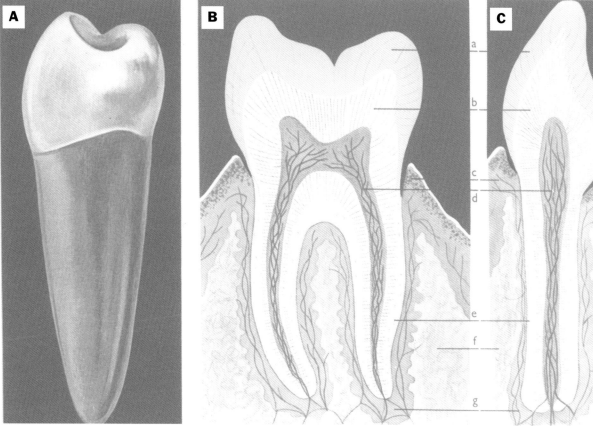

A. A tooth in which the crown and root can be differentiated.

B. Cross section of a tooth. The teeth and molars are held in place by sockets called alveoli (f) in the upper and lower jaws and consist, to a large extent, of matter that closely resembles bony tissue: dentine (b). The visible part, the crown, is covered by a smooth, very hard layer of glaze called the enamel (a). Under the surface of the gums (c), the crown merges into the root that rests in the socket. This root is attached to the root membrane (g) in the socket by bony tissue called cementum (e). The dental pulp (d) - connective tissue containing fine blood vessels and nerve branches - runs from the root to the innermost part of the tooth.

tion of tooth enamel and dentine, with eventual involvement of the pulp. Dental caries - is, except for the common cold, the most prevalent human disorder. The interaction of three factors results in dental cavities: a susceptible tooth surface, the proper microflora, and a suitable substrate for the microflora.

Dental cavities is mainly the result of eating sugar. Our teeth are naturally covered with a substance called plaque - a thin film of harmless bacteria and calcium salts - but when sugar is added, the bacteria Streptococcus mutans multiply and excrete acid. This dissolves the hard enamel, leading to decay.

Thus, sugar is the villain in dental cavities - nothing else we eat or drink has the same effect. How often we take sugar into our mouths is more important than the amount consumed. Having frequent between-meal snacks containing sugar is a good way of ensuring that sugar is present in the mouth for a longer time, and makes it much more likely that dental cavities will occur. Tooth decay begins on the external crown or exposed root surface of the tooth. Bacterial plaque, not food debris, causes dental cavities. Plaque is not flushed away by the action of oral musculature or saliva. The role of saliva in preventing dental cavities is in its buffering capacity and remineralization effect.

Acid action first demineralizes enamel with its high inorganic content; proteolysis of its organic matrix follows. When the carious process reaches the dentin or begins on the root surface, the tooth becomes sensitive to temperature or osmotic changes engendered by foods or by touch.

Dental cavities spreads rapidly because of the lower mineral content of dentin and cementum. As demineralization and necrosis of the dentin progress, microorganisms may invade the dentinal tubules.

Microbial products preceding the organisms in the dentinal tubules may cause inflammation of the dental pulp before destruction of the surrounding dentin is evident.

Symptoms and signs

A person is often unaware of the presence of caries until the decay is well

Tooth disorders   Questions & Answers

What are the causes of pathologic mobility of teeth?
Pathologic mobility has several principal causes:
▲ Gingival and periodontal inflammation.
▲ Parafunctional occlusal habits (bruxism, clenching, etc.).
▲ Occlusal prematurities.
▲ Loss of supporting bone.
▲ Traumatic torquing forces parallel to clasped teeth by removable partial dentures.
In addition, some transient mobility may follow periodontal therapy, endodontic therapy, and traumatic injuries.

Why is plaque control important?
Periodontal disease is a bacterial infection. Many local factors influence its initiation, but inadequate plaque control overshadows all others.
In study after study, the worldwide prevalence and severity of periodontal disease are associated with bacterial plaque, calculus, oral debris, and poor oral hygiene.
Neglect, then, is the principal cause of periodontal disease - neglect, on the part of the patient, to remove plaque; then, neglect to seek dental treatment; and last, neglect to remove plaque after periodontal therapy, thereby permitting the disease to recur.

What are the requirements of effective plaque control?
Effective plaque control requires that the patient have comprehension and motivation, manual dexterity, and reasonable access to all tooth surfaces.
Absence of one of these requisites will compromise treatment. The patient becomes involved in his treatment when he decides to accept all responsibility for daily control of plaque on a long-term basis.
His involvement is expressed by the action he takes to remove developing bacterial plaque every day. All of the various plaque control devices have their uses, depending on conditions present in the individual mouth. Generally speaking, any action is desirable if it is effective, safe, and practical.

How is effectiveness of plaque control achieved?
Effectiveness implies the cleansing of every surface of every tooth. Patients who brush frequently and manage to cleanse the occlusal and facial surfaces, from second bicuspid to second bicuspid, will benefit in these areas, but other surfaces may remain uncleaned, and their contiguous soft tissues will continue to be exposed to the destructive agents of bacterial plaque.
Many of these patients think their "tooth brushing" is effective and express surprise when their own ineffectiveness is demonstrated. They may simply not be aware of all the surfaces that need cleansing.

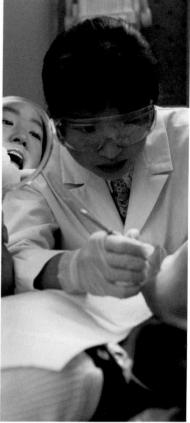

Dentist removing plaque. Plaque is a film-like substance composed of a mixture of bacteria, saliva, and dead cells that is continually being deposited on teeth, day and night. It occurs in everyone.

advanced. Common early symptoms are finding that it hurts to eat or drink hot and cold things, and discomfort after eating sugar-containing foods.
A darkened area between teeth or a hole (a cavity) may be noticed when the process has progressed sufficiently. Dental cavities is clinically diagnosed by the dentist when softened enamel or dentine is detected with a sharp instrument.
Radiographically, dental cavities appears as a radiolucent area, as do most resin filling materials and bases under metallic restorations.
Consequently, the dentist will couple the radiographic diagnosis with a visual examination.

Preventive measures
The most important thing is to reduce the amount of sugar you eat or drink and the frequency.
In addition, teeth are less susceptible to dental cavities if optimum amounts of fluoride are ingested while the teeth are developing (that is, up to the age of 11 or 13).
This can be achieved by drinking water that contains one part of fluoride to every million parts of water, or by taking fluoride drops or tablets. Fluoride combines with some of the crystals in the tooth structure to form a harder structure.
There is no clinical proof that drinking fluoridated water or taking fluoride supplements during pregnancy will significantly protect a child's teeth, but there is a little evidence that continuing to brush with a fluoride toothpaste may have some protective effect even on adult teeth.
If a child takes in too much fluoride before his or her first teeth erupt, while the enamel is forming, this may cause

permanent mottling of the enamel. During pregnancy, the placenta acts as a barrier against marked increases in fluoride concentration and thus protects the unborn baby's teeth against mottling.

Unfortunately, it has been found that brushing the teeth has no effect on dental cavities, except for the benefit that a fluoride toothpaste can give. Only by restricting the intake of sugar can you ensure having a set of teeth unmarked by fillings. It should be noted, however, that brushing is very important in avoiding gum disease.

Food particles and dental plaque should be removed from all accessible tooth surfaces at least once daily. Mechanical removal is the only effective method currently available. Proper use of a soft-bristled toothbrush removes plaque adequately from all areas except interproximal tooth surfaces and deep pits and fissures of the enamel.

Interproximal surfaces, highly susceptible to dental cavities, should be cleaned daily with dental floss or tape. Plaque-disclosing tablets or liquids composed of food colouring may be used to check the efficacy of plaque removal.

Since fluorides are relatively less effective for preventing pit and fissure caries, sealing enamel pits and fissures with a BIS-GMA-type resin is highly effective in preventing cavities and is performed increasingly by dentists. The sealed teeth should be checked annually and the sealant replaced when lost.

Treatment

Although dental cavities may be arrested, any tooth structure that has been destroyed cannot regenerate. Removal of all the affected parts of the tooth and proper replacement with a restorative material (a filling) is the best treatment.

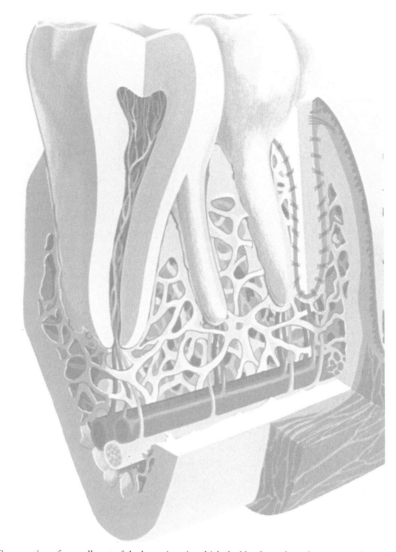

Cross section of a small part of the lower jaw, in which the blood supply and nerves are shown.

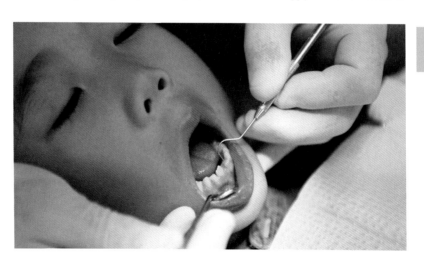

Dentist checking for cavities. Along with the common cold and gum disease, cavities are among the most common human afflictions. If cavities are not properly treated by a dentist, they continue to enlarge. Ultimately, an untreated cavity can lead to tooth loss.

TUBERCULOSIS

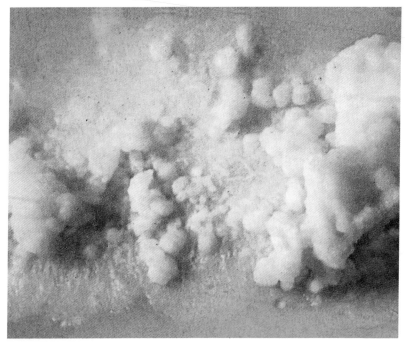

Description

Tuberculosis is a disease caused by several species of *Mycobacterium*, collectively called the tubercle bacillus. Tuberculosis in man is usually caused by the human and bovine varieties of the bacillus.

Humanity has probably recognized tuberculosis as a killer disease since the last Ice Age, if not before. Traces of tuberculosis lesions have been found in the lungs of 3000-year-old Egyptian mummies. In classic Greek times it was known as phthisis, from the verb phthinein, to waste away. Right up to the present century, it was commonly called consumption - for the same reason.

But it was in the 17th century that a Dutchman, Franciscus Sylvius of Leyden, first used the term "tubercle" to describe the knobby lesions found in the lungs of people who had died of the wasting disease. The name tuberculosis seems first to have been used in 1939, by Johann Schoenlein.

Although lung tuberculosis is a uncommon (though increasing) disease in our country it is still a major cause of morbidity and mortality in underdeveloped countries. There are about 12 million cases of active tuberculosis and 3 million deaths each year throughout the world.

Age, sex, heredity, and physical constitution seem to play a determining part in individual susceptibility and the severity of the infection. It is not clear whether a mild tuberculosis infection protects against reinfection.

Less than one-tenth of tuberculosis cases are not pulmonary; affected organs include:

- lymph nodes
- bones and joints
- serous surfaces
- genital organs
- kidneys and adrenal glands
- skin
- intestines

Generalization of tuberculosis infection, with dissemination through the bloodstream occasionally, occurs as a complication of nonpulmonary tuberculosis and is known as miliary tuberculosis.

Tuberculous meningitis (inflammation of the coverings of the brain and spinal cord), the most severe form of tuberculosis, is a frequent complication of miliary tuberculosis, occurring without grossly evident miliary tuberculosis.

Incidence

In Europe, the incidence of tuberculosis is increasing, mainly due to immigration of sufferers from developing countries. Between the 1950s and 1985, tuberculosis notifications decreased at a steady rate of 5 percent each year in the United States. However, between 1985 and 1995, tuberculosis notifications increased by 18 percent, resulting in an additional 39,000 unexpected causes of tuberculosis. The overall increase between 1995 and 2005 amounted to 13 percent. Over half of these cases were found among 25-44-year-olds.

Homelessness, drug abuse, deterioration of living conditions and of health care delivery to people, and immigra-

Culture of tuberculosis bacilli (Mycobacterium tuberculosis).

tion have also been implicated as factors contributing to the rapid increase of tuberculosis in the United States.

One of the major reasons for the increase in occurrence of tuberculosis may be the fact that we became complacent because we thought we had beaten tuberculosis. After the discovery of effective drugs between the 1960s and 1970s, the number of cases and deaths in the industrialized countries fell rapidly.

The sanatoria were closed down, public health measures for tuberculosis control were dismantled, and medical researchers working on the disease moved into other fields. Tuberculosis was presumed dead. Most health officials and scientists assumed that the developing world would subjugate the disease with equal ease using the new treatment programs.

These and other assumptions were wrong. Tuberculosis treatment turned out to be less straightforward than originally supposed. Tuberculosis drugs, nevertheless represent a heavy burden on developing countries. Poverty, economic recession, and malnutrition make populations more vulnerable to tuberculosis. Recent increases in human migration have rapidly mixed infected with uninfected communities.

To this already explosive mixture has been added the human immunodeficiency virus (HIV), a potent and dangerous ally of the TB bacilli, so that a person infected with both the TB bacillus and HIV is much more likely to develop active tuberculosis than someone infected with the tubercle bacillus alone.

Basic course of tuberculosis

Mycobacterium tuberculosis is the germ that carries tuberculosis. It is carried on droplets in the air and so can be spread by coughing or sneezing, entering the body through the airways.

If the immune system fails to stop the infection, the bacteria spread around the body and destroy tissues in the lungs, where they can multiply. Large numbers of bacteria are coughed out by the lungs into the outside world, infecting others.

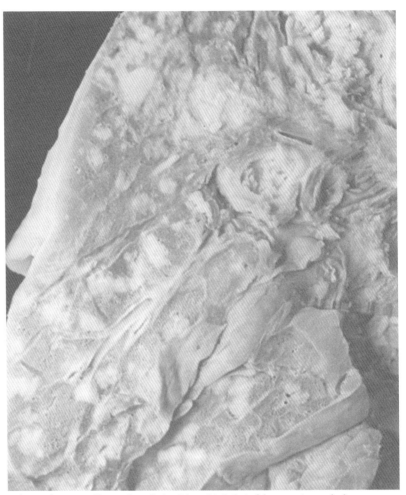

Advanced process of lung tuberculosis with multiple foci of degeneration and edema.

Tuberculosis medications

- A number of drugs can be used for the treatment of tuberculosis. Normally two or three are given simultaneously, and in the early stages of treatment they may be given by injection.

- Treatment is very slow, and the medication must be taken for months or years. Regular blood tests and X-rays are necessary while on treatment, and sometimes side effects may necessitate alterations in dosage or choice.

- Common medications in this group include:
  - ethambutol
  - isoniazid
  - pyrazinamide
  - rifampicin

- Because the side effects and precautions are so variable from drug to drug and patient to patient, it is not possible to list them in any meaningful way.

Tuberculosis   Questions & Answers

What is tuberculosis?
Tuberculosis (often called TB) is an infection caused by a germ called Mycobacterium tuberculosis. It most commonly affects the lungs, and is caught from other people. Once inhaled, the germ may be destroyed by the body's immune system and cause no problems, or they may cause an illness a few days to a few months later.

Does BCG give complete protection against tuberculosis?
Nearly all children will have had a vaccination against tuberculosis, called the BCG, either in the first few weeks after birth, or about the age of twelve. BCG vaccination does not give complete protection against tuberculosis, but does help the body's defenses to fight it off.

What are the symptoms of tuberculosis?
Tuberculosis can affect any part of the body, but most commonly affects the lungs and lymph glands. A cough is the commonest symptom sometimes accompanied by sputum (phlegm) which can be bloodstained.
There may also be chest pain, loss of appetite and weight, and a fever with sweating particularly at night. When tuberculosis affects the lymph glands, these may appear as lumps in the neck.

How is tuberculosis diagnosed?
Tuberculosis is usually diagnosed after a chest X-ray has been taken and a specimen of phlegm examined.

Can I affect other people?
If there are lots of TB germs in your phlegm, you may pass the disease on to other people. Doctors sometimes call this open tuberculosis or say that you are sputum positive. You can help prevent the spread of infection by covering your mouth and nose with a tissue when you cough, disposing of it carefully and then washing your hands.

How is tuberculosis treated?
Treatment for tuberculosis is with tablets which must be taken every single day for six to nine months. Many people have all their treatment at home but others may be admitted to hospital for the first week or so, particularly if they are very ill, at the time they are found to have tuberculosis or if they are thought to be highly infectious to other people.

Recent facts about tuberculosis

▲ Tuberculosis one thought to be under control, is fiercely on the rise in many places. Its increasing incidence affects people everywhere.
▲ Every year, three million people die from tuberculosis and eight million new people develop the disease. Tuberculosis is the world's foremost cause of death from a single infectious agent.
▲ One-third of the world's population is infected with tuberculosis.
▲ Tuberculosis is contagious. The disease is transmitted by bacilli spread into the air by a patient with active pulmonary tuberculosis. Coughing, sneezing, and even talking by a patient fills the air with droplets containing the tuberculosis germ.
▲ Once a person is infected, he or she risks developing active tuberculosis, and the risk persists throughout life.

With appropriate antibiotic therapy, persons with tuberculosis quickly become no longer infectious. One of the most urgent research needs, say scientists and health officials, is to cut down the time needed to securely diagnose tuberculosis in almost all cases so that treatment can begin earlier. This will speed the affected person's recovery and at the same time reduce the period in which they are - often without knowing it - spreading disease.

How easy is it to catch tuberculosis? The answer depends on the two-stage process that occurs with tuberculosis; first you have to be infected, and second, the infection has to progress to disease. Dealing first with injection, you are more likely to be infected if the person with tuberculosis with whom you are in contact (the index case) has cavities in the lungs.

These will be full of bacteria and when the person coughs, the bacteria are sprayed into the air. If you inhale a bacteria-laden droplet you may become infected. Clearly, the more time you spend with this index case, and the closer contact you have with him or her, the more likely you are to become infected.

Secondly, there is the process of the infection progressing to disease. This happens in about 10 percent of those infected, and it can happen at any time during the remainder of our lives. It is more likely to happen near the time the infection occurred - as time passes, it becomes less likely. However, if the immune system weakens, as happens with diabetes or cancer, or during treatment for kidney transplantation, or conditions of famine, malnutrition and AIDS, than tuberculosis can more easily develop.

Pulmonary tuberculosis

The tuberculosis bacillus is transmitted by inhalation or ingestion of droplets; it usually affects the lungs but may also affect other organs. The primary tuberculosis is beneath the pleura (subpleural) and the upper zones are most commonly affected. An average of 100 million tubercle bacilli are present in the lungs of a person with new, untreated tuberculosis. Tubercle bacilli deposited in an alveolus are surrounded by an exudate with neutrophils (type of white blood cell) which are later replaced by macrophages to form a tubercle. This is a lesion containing epithelium-like cells, Langhans giant cells, lymphocytes and a variable degree of fibrosis. The primary lesion may heal by fibrosis but viable dormant bacilli may remain for years. If active progression occurs, infection may spread by local extension, lymph channels and through the blood. Uncomplicated primary lung tuberculosis is often symptomless in older children or adults, but in younger children constitutional symptoms are usual.

■ Early symptoms include:
· fever
· loss of appetite
· fatigue
· vague chest pain

■ Later symptoms include:
· night sweats
· difficulty in breathing
· production of purulent sputum
· signs of severe lung involvement

Treatment

Treatment of tuberculosis includes bed rest and improved nutrition and hygiene, together with specific anti-tuberculosis drugs. Rifampicin, isoniazid, streptomycin-like antibiotics, and para-aminosalicylic acid used individually, or in combination, are effective chemotherapeutic agents. In a number of cases surgical procedures to remove part of the lug may also be necessary.

Tuberculosis is a terribly debilitating disease and, if untreated, kills around half of those affected. Fortunately, tuberculosis is still an available, curable disease. With proper management, more than 95 percent of patients are cured.

And treatment of tuberculosis costs less, in terms of the price for each year of life saved, than measles immunization. In stark contrast, the cost of ignoring tuberculosis could be catastrophic.

Multi-drug resistant tuberculosis
Resistant to treatment by a combination of drugs (multidrug treatment)

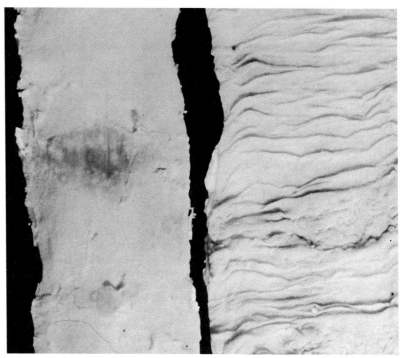

Advanced tuberculosis of the intestine.

has recently been recognized as a major problem in the United States. It has reached crisis proportions in New York City and in a few other cities, particularly among persons with HIV infection. There, an inadequate public health infrastructure and earlier lack of resources have impeded efforts to control the spread of these strains, which have been implicated in tuberculosis outbreaks in prisons, nursing homes and several hospitals.

Since these strains are resistant to isoniazid and rifampicin, the two most powerful and most commonly used anti-tuberculosis drugs, the disease is particularly difficult to treat and prevent, even in the absence of HIV infection. Associated mortality among persons with HIV infection has been in excess of 70%, and deaths have been reported among medical personnel and others working with tuberculosis patients.

Although this problem has been has been most extensively documented in New York City, it can certainly occur in other countries and other settings.

Facts about curing tuberculosis

▲ Tuberculosis has a cure, and treatment is inexpensive.
▲ Tuberculosis control is a very cost-effective health intervention Its cost-effectiveness is equivalent to that of the well-known childhood immunization programs.
▲ Successful treatment requires 6-8 months of consistent, uninterrupted medication.
▲ New, drug-resistant strains of tuberculosis are developing because patients are not completing their treatment.
▲ These drug-resistant strains are significantly more dangerous to the individual and the community because they are more difficult and more expensive to treat.
▲ The best way to prevent tuberculosis is to cure infectious cases in their early stages in order to prevent transmission to others.

UTERINE TUMORS

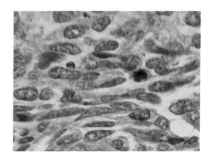

Description

The uterus (womb) is a hollow, pear-shaped organ located in a woman's lower abdomen between the bladder and the rectum. The narrow, lower portion of the uterus is the cervix; the broader, upper part is the corpus. Benign and malignant growth may develop in the cervix (see Cervical Disorders) or the corpus. This chapter deals with the latter tumors.

Benign tumors

Benign tumors are not cancer. They do not spread to other parts of the body and are seldom a threat to life. Several types of benign tumors occur in the corpus of the uterus. In some cases, these growths do not need to be treated. Sometimes, however, benign tumors must be removed by surgery. Once removed, these tumors are not likely to return.

Side view of the female pelvis. The uterus is located between the bladder and rectum.

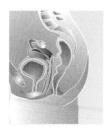

Fibroids

Fibroids are benign tumors in the wall of the uterus that are found most often in women over 35 years of age. While single fibroid tumors occur, multiple tumors are more common. Symptoms of fibroids depend on the size and location of the tumors and may include:

- irregular bleeding
- vaginal discharge
- frequent urination

When fibroids press against nearby organs and cause pain, surgery may be recommended. Often, however, fibroids do not cause symptoms and do not need to be treated, although they should be checked often. When a woman stops having menstrual periods (menopause), fibroids may become smaller and sometimes they disappear.

Endometriosis

Another benign condition of the uterus is endometriosis. In this condition, tissue that looks and acts like endometrial tissue begins to grow in unusual places, such as on the surface of the ovaries, on the outside of the uterus, and in other tissues in the abdomen. Endometriosis is most common in women in their thirties and forties. This condition causes painful menstrual periods and abnormal bleeding; sometimes, it can cause fertility. Some patients with endometriosis are treated with medication, and some are treated by surgery.

Hyperplasia

Hyperplasia is an increase in the number of normal cells lining the inside of the uterus. Although this condition is not cancer, it may develop into cancer in some women. The most common symptoms of hyperplasia are heavy menstrual periods and bleeding between periods.

Treatments depend on the extent of the condition (mild, moderate, or severe) and on the age of the patient. Young women usually are treated with female hormones, and the endometrial tissue is checked often. Hyperplasia in women near or after menopause may be treated with hormones if the condition is not severe. Surgery to remove the uterus is the usual treatment for severe cases.

Malignant tumors

Malignant tumors are cancer. They invade and destroy nearby healthy tissues and organs. Cancer cells also can metastasize, or spread, to other parts of the body and form new tumors. When cancer of the uterus spreads, it may travel through the bloodstream or lymphatic system.

Cancer cells can be carried along by blood or lymph, an almost colourless fluid discharged by tissues into the lymphatic system. Lymph nodes scattered along this system filter bacteria and abnormal substances such as cancer cells. For this reason, surgeons often remove pelvic lymph nodes to learn whether they contain cancer cells. Because uterine cancer can spread, it is important for the physician to find out as early as possible if a tumor is present and whether it is benign or malignant.

High risk women

Endometrial cancer most commonly occurs among women of menopausal age - that is, over 40 years of age. Certain menopausal women are at higher risk of endometrial cancer, including those

▲ who used estrogen for prolonged periods;

U

Above:
Microscopy of normal endometrium. The glands are tortuous with inspissated secretions within the lumen. The stroma shows a heavy granlocytic infiltrate (day 27 of menstrual cyclus).

Center:
The uterus has been opened anteriorly. The tubes and ovaries are still attached and appear normal. A large tumor mass with yellow tones fills the endometrial avity. Broad-based deep myometrial invasion is seen on the left.

Below:
Infection of the uterine wall (endometritis); two granulomas are present, and the one in de upper left has giant cells.

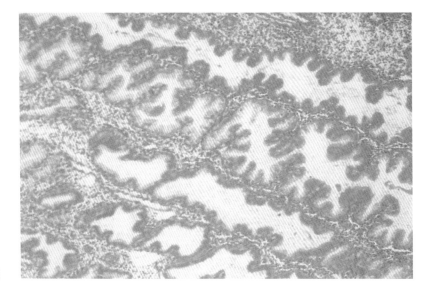

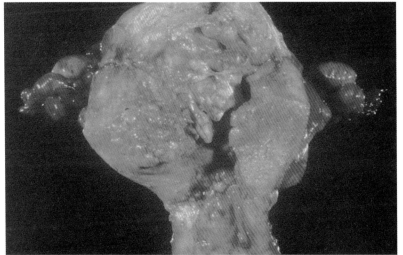

▲ who had irregular periods and failure of ovulation;
▲ who have hyperplasia (abnormal cells production) of the endometrium;
▲ who have had cancer of the breast, ovary or colon;
▲ women who are:
  • overweight
  • diabetic
  • hypertensive
  • infertile (never were able to have children)
  • nulliparous (never choose to have children)

Eestrogen use is contraindicated for all these at-risk women, and they should be thoroughly examined at least once a year by their physicians.

Incidence
The incidence of endometrial cancer among post-menopausal women who have not used estrogen during menopause is about one out of thousand each year. Research has shown that this rate is four to eight times higher among women who have used estrogen.
There is no evidence that a woman's risk increases with the amount of estrogen taken and the length of use, and decreases rapidly after she stops taking estrogen. Of course, a woman who has had a hysterectomy is not at risk because her uterus has been removed.

Symptoms
Abnormal bleeding after menopause is the most common symptom of can-

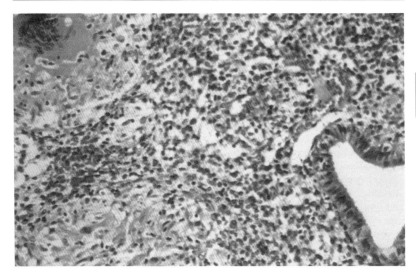

Uterine cancer   Questions & Answers

What are uterine fibroids?

Uterine fibroids are benign (not cancerous) growths in the uterus. They are the most common type of growth found in a women's pelvis. They occur in about 20-25 percent of all women. Fibroids are most common in women aged 30-40, but they can occur at any age. Fibroids occur more often in black women than in white women. They also seem to occur at a younger age in black women and to grow more quickly. Many women who have fibroids are not aware of them because the growths can remain small and not cause a problem. Although uterine fibroids are not cancer, they can cause problems due to their size, number, and location. Like any growth, fibroids should be checked by a doctor.

What are the main symptoms of fibroids?

Most fibroids, even large ones, produce no symptoms at all. When symptoms do occur, they often include the following:

- Changes in menstruation
  - more bleeding
  - longer or more frequent periods
  - menstrual pain or cramps
  - vaginal bleeding at times other than menstruation
  - anemia (from blood loss)
- Pain
  - in the abdomen or lower back
  - usually of a dull, heavy, aching nature
- Pressure
  - difficulty urinating
  - frequent urination
  - constipation
  - abdominal cramps
- Miscarriages and infertility

How are uterine fibroids diagnosed?

Most fibroids do not produce symptoms. During a routine pelvic examination, the first signs of fibroids can be detected. There are several tests that may show more information about fibroids:

- *Ultrasound.* This method uses sound waves to create a picture of the uterus or of the pelvic organs.
- *Hysteroscopy.* This method uses a slender instrument (the hysteroscope) to help the doctor see the inside of the uterus. It is inserted through the vagina and cervix. This permits the doctor to see some fibroids inside the uterine cavity.
- *Hysterosalpingography.* This is a special X-ray test. It may detect abnormal changes in the size and shape of the uterus and Fallopian tubes.
- *Laparoscopy.* With a slender instrument (laparoscope) the doctor can see the inside of the abdomen. It is inserted through a small cut just below or through the navel.

What is the best treatment for uterine fibroids?

Fibroids that do not cause symptoms, are small, or occur in a woman nearing menopause, often do not require treatment. In other cases, fibroids may be treated by removing them surgically. Drugs, such as gonadotropin-releasing hormone agonists, may be used to shrink fibroids temporarily and to control bleeding with myomectomy (removal of the fibroids leaving the uterus in place) or hysterectomy (removal of the uterus). The choice of treatment depends on factors such as your own wishes and medical advice about the size and location of fibroids.

The following signs and symptoms may signal the need for treatment: heavy or painful menstrual periods, bleeding between periods, rapid increase in growth of the fibroid, infertility, pelvic pain.

cer of the uterus. Bleeding may begin as a watery, blood-streaked discharge. Later, the discharge may contain more blood. Cancer of the uterus does not often occur before menopause, but it does occur around the time menopause begins.

The reappearance of bleeding should not be considered simply part of menopause; it should always be checked by a physician. Abnormal bleeding is not always a sign of cancer. It is important for a woman to see her physician, however, because that is the only way to find out what the problem is.

Any illness should be diagnosed and treated as soon as possible, but early diagnosis is especially important for cancer of the uterus.

Diagnosis

When symptoms suggest uterine cancer, the physician will ask a woman about her medical history and will conduct a thorough examination. In addition to checking general signs of health (temperature, pulse, blood pressure, and so on), the physician usually performs one of the following examinations.

Under study are tests for mutations in genes regulating DNA repair. These tests may help warn of endometrial cancer.

- *Pelvic examination*

The physician thoroughly examines the uterus, vagina, ovaries, bladder, and rectum. The physician feels these organs for any abnormality in their shape and size. A speculum is used to widen the opening of the vagina so that the physician can look at the upper portion of the vagina and the cervix.

- *Biopsy*

For a biopsy, the physician surgically removes a small amount of suspicious-looking uterine tissue, which is examined under a microscope by a pathologist.

- *D&C - Dilation and Curettage*

In a D&C, the physician dilates (widens) the cervix and inserts a curette (a small spoon-shaped instrument) to remove pieces of the inner lining of the uterus. A sample of uterine lining also can be removed by applying suction through a slender tube (called suction curettage). This tissue is examined for evidence of cancer.

■ *Pap test*

The Pap test is often used to detect cancer of the cervix. While it is sometimes done for cancer of the uterus, it is not a reliable test to exclude uterine cancer because it cannot always detect abnormal cells from the endometrium. If cancer cells are found, physicians use other tests to find out whether the disease has spread from the uterus to other parts of the body. These procedures include blood tests and a chest X-ray. For some patients special scan X-ray procedures are necessary or ultrasound investigations.

Treatment and prevention

Surgery, radiation therapy, hormone therapy, or chemotherapy may be used to treat uterine cancer.

Radiation therapy uses high-energy rays to kill cancer cells. Radiation may be given from a machine located outside the body (*external radiation therapy*), or radioactive material may be placed inside the body (*internal radiation therapy*).

In hormone therapy, female hormones are used to stop the growth of cancer cells. Chemotherapy is the use of drugs to treat cancer. Often, a combination of these methods is used. In some cases, the patient is referred to specialists in different kinds of cancer treatment.

In its earlier stages, cancer of the uterus is treated with surgery. The uterus and cervix are removed (hysterectomy), as well as the ovaries and Fallopian tubes (salpingo-oophorectomy). Some physicians recommend radiation therapy before surgery to shrink the cancer.

Others prefer to evaluate the patient carefully during surgery and recommend radiation therapy after surgery form patients whose tumors appear likely to recur. A combination of external and internal radiation therapy often is used. If the cancer has spread extensively or has recurred after treatment, the physician may

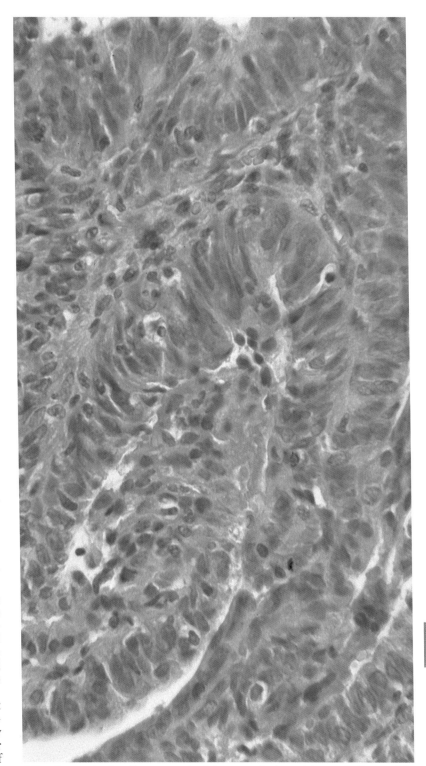

Microphotograph of malignant growth of the uterus (endometrial cancer). Cancer of the uterus begins in the lining of the uterus (endometrium) and is more precisely termed endometrial cancer. It is the most common gynecologic cancer and the fourth most common cancer among women.

Uterine cancer — Questions & Answers

What is endometrial cancer?

Endometrial carcinoma is cancer of the lining of the uterus (the endometrium). Growth and multiplication of malignant cells occur in the endometrium. The cancer usually develops in the womb's lining, but in rare cases in its muscular wall.

What is the incidence of endometrial cancer?

Cancer of the uterus is the 5th most common cancer affecting women, with around 4,800 new cases diagnosed each year in the UK.

Who is most at risk from endometrial cancer?

■ Age

The risk of endometrial cancer increases with age. Most cases occur in women after the menopause.

■ Estrogen replacement therapy

Having had hormone replacement therapy that did not contain progesterone may increase the risk of endometrial cancer.

■ Obesity

Being overweight can increase the risk of endometrial cancer. This may be because the more body fat you have generally the more estrogen you produce.

■ Family history

Some people inherit a greater than average risk of endometrial cancer. Members of their family may have been diagnosed with cancer of the bowel, breast, ovary or endometrium.

■ Childbearing and menopause

Women who have never been pregnant are more likely to develop endometrial cancer than women with children. Similarly, women who go through their menopause after the age of 52 may have an increased risk.

■ Personal history of other cancers

Women who have had breast or bowel cancer have a greater risk of developing endometrial cancer than women with no such history.

What are the immediate symptoms?

The symptoms of endometrial cancer include:

- Bleeding from the vagina after the menopause.
- Abnormal vaginal bleeding which could be "spotting" or very heavy, around the time of the menopause, or before.
- Vaginal discharge.
- Pain in the lower abdomen.
- An enlarged womb that feels swollen.
- Pain during intercourse.

If you recognise any of these symptoms, it is important to see your general physician as soon as possible.

How will my general physician know I have cancer of the womb?

■ Pelvic examination

Your general physician may perform a pelvic examination, to check the womb, vagina, ovaries and the bladder. If your doctor is at all concerned, you will be referred to the hospital form further tests.

■ Biopsy

You may have a biopsy which a small sample of tissue from the endometrium will be taken and analyzed for cancerous cells.

■ Ultrasound scan

You may also be given an ultrasound scan, using a small probe inserted into the vagina to measure the thickness of the endometrium. This is because increased thickness is often a sign of cancer.

recommend a female hormone (progesterone) or chemotherapy.

To reduce the risk of endometrial cancer, women should use estrogen only at the lowest effective dose and for the shortest possible length of time. Before and during estrogen therapy, the endometrium should be examined histologically at least on a yearly basis.

Early endometrial cancer has a 90 per cent cure rate. As with most medical problems, the earlier the diagnosis, the better the outcome. Therefore, all menopausal women should see their doctors at least once a year - especially of they were given estrogen for a prolonged period of time.

Side effects of treatment

The treatment used against uterine cancer must be very powerful. It is rarely possible to limit the effects of cancer treatments so that only cancer cells are destroyed.

Hysterectomy is major surgery. After the operation, the hospital stay usually lasts about one week. For several days after surgery, patients may have problems emptying their bladder and having normal bowel movements. The lower abdomen will be sore. Normal activities, including sexual intercourse, usually can be resumed in 4 to 8 weeks.

Women who have their uterus removed no longer have menstrual periods. When the ovaries are not removed, women do not have symptoms of menopause because their

Facts to remember

▲ Early endometrial cancer has a 90 per cent cure rate.

▲ Unusual vaginal bleeding can be done of the first signs of endometrial cancer.

▲ A woman who has vaginal bleeding after menopause should call her physician imme-dia-tely.

▲ Women who still have occasional periods should also remain alert for any unusual vaginal bleeding.

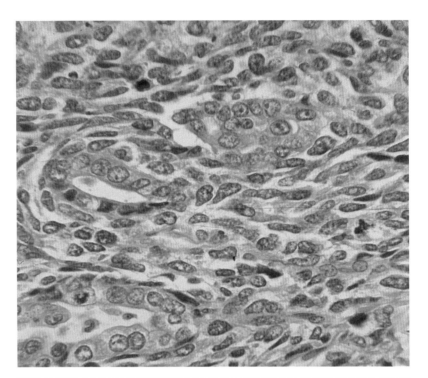

Microscopic picture (biopsy specimen) of malignant cells of the endometrium. If doctors suspect endometrial cancer or if Pap test results are abnormal, doctors perform an endometrial biopsy in their office. This test accurately detects endometrial cancer more than 90% of the time. If the diagnosis is still uncertain, doctors perform dilatation and curettage, in which tissue is scraped from the uterine lining.

ovaries still produce hormones. If the ovaries are removed or damaged by radiation therapy, menopause will occur. Hot flashes or other symptoms of menopause caused by treatment may be more severe than those from a natural menopause.

Sexual desire and the ability to have intercourse are not affected by hysterectomy. However, many women have an emotionally difficult time after a hysterectomy. They may have feelings of deep emotional loss because they are no longer able to become pregnant.

During radiation therapy, patients may notice a number of side effects, which usually disappear when treatment is completed. Patients may have skin reactions (redness or dryness) in the area being treated, and they may be unusually tired. Some have diarrhea and frequent uncomfortable urination.

Treatment can also cause dryness, itching, and burning in the vagina. Intercourse may be painful, and some women are advised not to have intercourse at this time. Most women can resume sexual activity within a few weeks after treatment ends. The side effects of chemotherapy depend on the drugs given and the individual responses of the patient.

Chemotherapy commonly affects hair cells, blood-forming cells, and cells lining the digestive tract. As a result, patients may have side effects such as:

- hair loss
- lowered blood counts
- nausea
- vomiting

Most side effects end after treatment is stopped.

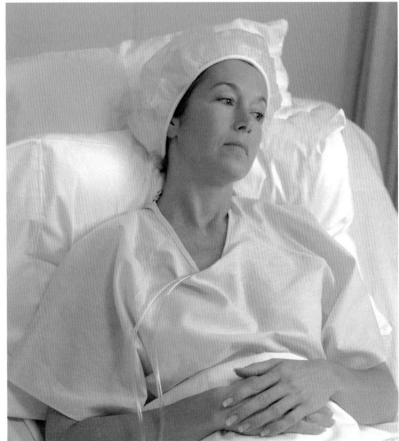

Woman hospitalized to undergo surgery for endometrial cancer.

VENOUS DISORDERS

Introduction

Vascular diseases of the extremities involve arteries and veins. Arteries are usually affected by atherosclerosis and veins are usually subject to thrombosis and dilatation (varicose veins). Since the peripheral vessels in the extremities are readily accessible to examination by the doctor, a correct clinical diagnosis can usually be made.

Special instrumentation and angiography (X-ray investigation of the blood vessels after introduction of a contrast medium) are rarely necessary to diagnose insufficiency of arteries, but are helpful to document the location and extent of disease if surgical correction is contemplated.

Noninvasive methods will confirm the diagnosis and are useful for the doctor to follow the patient being treated medically or after surgical interventions.

Venous disease of the legs is very prevalent. The most common condition is primary varicose veins, involving 10-15 per cent of the population over 20 years of age. It is prevalent in about 55 per cent of men and 75 per cent of women over 70 years of age.

In most American and European populations the prevalence rate for thrombophlebitis (inflammation affecting the superficial veins) and thrombosis (clotting in the deep veins) is about 2 per cent and up to 10 per cent in the over-60-year age group.

The cause of both conditions is similar: the development of a thrombus with inflammatory response of the venous wall. Deep vein thrombosis is of highest risk to the patient. It may result in the release of a thrombus (blood clot) and the development of possibly fatal pulmonary embolism (blockage of a blood vessel by a clot of blood).

Other complications of thrombosis are the chronic sequelae of deep vein obliteration, known as chronic venous insufficiency; i.e., edema of the leg, stasis, skin changes and venous ulcer ("open leg").

All diseases of the veins occur very frequently in the elderly. Although some, more often than others, develop in early adulthood, they do not give rise to complications until the patient is elderly.

Primary varicose veins

The diagnosis of primary varicose veins is simple. However, in the elderly in particular it must be determined absolutely, by clinical examination or by means of ultrasonography (use of high frequency sound waves), whether the varicosity is primary or secondary. The principal surgical procedures for the treatment of primary varicose veins are removal of the veins that are varicose and ligation of any insufficient perforating communicating veins. Surgery is not usually recom-

Deep and superficial veins of the abdominal region, pelvis and upper part of the lower extremities.

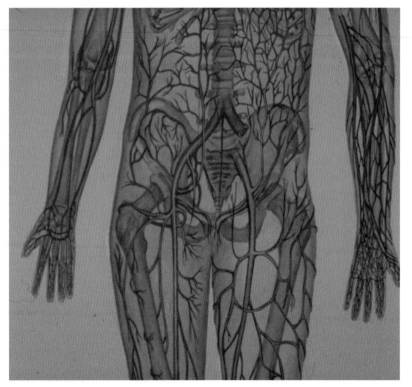

mended for patients over 65 years of age, because of the higher likelihood of complications.

Nevertheless, when an elderly patient has recurrent venous ulcers ligation of the insufficient perforating communicating veins is sometimes helpful. Sclerotherapy - injection of sclerosing solutions -, used fairly often for younger patients, is very rarely used for patients over 60 years of age.

Patients with large varicosities associated with marked reflux during elevation of intra-abdominal pressure, should wear an elastic bandage or an elastic stocking. All complications affecting the skin, particularly chronic or acute eczema, require careful attention and therapy. Patients need advice on life style.

They should avoid becoming overweight, be physically active, regularly exercise the lower limbs, put the legs up when lying or sitting, and avoid sitting or standing still for any length of time.

Phlebitis

The diagnosis of superficial phlebitis is simple, not requiring any type of instrumental diagnostic technique. The veins are swollen, red and painful.

Treatment can be given in an outpatient department. Hospital treatment is necessary only when the patient has extensive phlebitis involving the main trunks of the superficial veins up to their orifices.

Phlebitis is usually treated with a nonsteroidal anti-inflammatory medicine and the application of an elastic bandage. Immobilization and rest in bed are not necessary. Patients with massive phlebitis are advised to lie down frequently and to apply cold compresses to the diseased leg several times a day.

In some cases, an ointment containing a combination of butazolidine derivative and a heparinoid type medicine is applied over the diseased area. Broadspectrum antibiotics are administered for purulent phlebitis, which is characterized by massive local inflammatory reaction, and elevated temperature.

Thrombosis

While thrombosis in the veins of the legs after major surgery occurs in 20-25 per cent of patients over 40 years of age, it is even more common in elderly patients, occurring at a rate of 30-40 per cent after prostatectomy (sur-

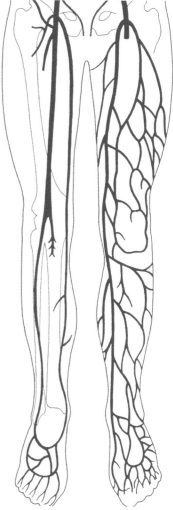

Initial phase of development of varicose veins in the leg. The precise cause of varicose veins is unknown, but the main problem is probably a weakness in the wall of the superficial veins. This weakness may be inherited. Over time, the weakness causes the veins to lose their elasticity.

gical removal of the prostate gland). Thrombosis occurs in about 40 per cent of patients immobilized in a hospital with stroke, and it is also common in older patients who, in addition to the primary disease, are in heart failure or have primary varicose veins.

Diagnosis
Deep vein thrombosis is difficult to diagnose because, in about 50 per cent of patients, it presents few, if any,

---

Summary table - Diseases of the veins

▲ Varicose veins are a common source of discomfort and ill health. Surgery and sclerotherapy, the principal therapeutic procedures for younger patients, recommended for patients over 60 years of age.

▲ Means of treating phlebitis include elastic bandages and nonsteroidal anti-inflammatory medicines.

▲ Deep vein thrombosis occurs frequently after surgery or after fracturing a hip, and may result in potentially fatal blood clots transported to the lungs.

▲ The treatment of deep vein thrombosis with thrombolytic and anticoagulant medicines requires caution.

▲ It is essential to take active steps to prevent deep vein thrombosis in all elderly patients at risk of developing thrombosis, particularly after surgery or serious injury.

▲ Preventive measures include exercising the lower limbs and other physical activities; walking as early as possible after surgery; and the administration of anticoagulant medicines.

Phlebitis   Questions & Answers

Where does a venous disease occur most often?

Venous disease of the legs is very prevalent. The most common condition is primary varicose veins, involving 10-15 per cent of the population over 20 years of age. It is prevalent in about 55 per cent of men and 75 per cent of women over 70 years of age.

The prevalence rate for thrombophlebitis (inflammation affecting the superficial veins) and thrombosis (clotting in the deep veins) is about 2 per cent and up to 10 per cent in the over-60-year age group.

How is phlebitis diagnosed?

The diagnosis of superficial phlebitis is simple, not requiring any type of instrumental diagnostic technique. The veins are swollen, red and painful. Treatment can be given in an outpatient department. Hospital treatment is necessary only when the patient has extensive phlebitis involving the main trunks of the superficial veins up to their orifices.

How is phlebitis treated?

Phlebitis is usually treated with a nonsteroidal anti-inflammatory medicine and the application of an elastic bandage. Immobilization and rest in bed are not necessary. Patients with massive phlebitis are advised to lie down frequently and to apply cold compresses to the diseased leg several times a day. In some cases, an ointment containing a combination of butazolidine derivative and a heparinoid type medicine is applied over the diseased area. Broadspectrum antibiotics are administered for purulent phlebitis, which is characterized by massive local inflammatory reaction, and elevated temperature.

What is the cause of thrombosis in the legs?

While thrombosis in the veins of the legs after major surgery occurs in 20-25 per cent of patients over 40 years of age, it is even more common in elderly patients, occurring at a rate of 30-40 per cent after prostatectomy (surgical removal of the prostate gland). Thrombosis occurs in about 40 per cent of patients immobilized in a hospital with stroke, and it is also common in older patients who, in addition to the primary disease, are in heart failure or have primary varicose veins.

How is deep vein thrombosis diagnosed?

Deep vein thrombosis is difficult to diagnose because, in about 50 per cent of patients, it presents few, if any, symptoms. All patients in the hospital, the older ones in particular, will be
examined clinically every day for signs of venous thrombosis.

Those in whom thrombosis is suspected will be submitted to additional diagnostic procedures, such as ultrasonography, or X-ray examination of the veins after injection of radioactive substances.

What is the clinical diagnosis of deep vein thrombosis?

The clinical diagnosis of deep vein thrombosis is more difficult in the elderly than in the young. Pitting edema may often be caused by another disease though asymmetry of the edema is an alerting sign.
Clinical signs of acute vein thrombosis are:
• oedema;
• tenderness;
• increased venous pressure;
• cyanosis;
• rise in temperature;

symptoms. All patients in the hospital, the older ones in particular, will be examined clinically every day for signs of venous thrombosis.

Those in whom thrombosis is suspected will be submitted to additional diagnostic procedures, such as ultrasonography, or X-ray examination of the veins after injection of radioactive substances. The clinical diagnosis of deep vein thrombosis is more difficult in the elderly than in the young. Pitting edema may often be caused by another disease though asymmetry of the edema is an alerting sign. Clinical signs of acute vein thrombosis are:
• edema
• tenderness
• increased venous pressure
• cyanosis
• rise in temperature
• increased collateral circulation

Ultrasonography is well suited to diagnosis in an outpatient department, and is reliable in particular for determining thrombosis of a large vein, such as the femoral or popliteal veins in the leg. Other instrumental procedures are usually carried out at centers or hospital departments specializing in venous diseases and angiology.

Therapy

All patients with acute deep vein thrombosis should be admitted to a hospital. Although the principles of treatment are much the same in the elderly as in younger patients, there are certain important differences.

Thrombolytic agents (agents that dissolve thrombi) will be prescribed with care for patients over 65 years of age because of the much greater risk of hemorrhagic complications, particularly brain hemorrhage.

Prevention

Adequate measures may significantly lower the occurrence of thrombosis after surgery or injury. Physical measures consist of lower limb exercises, pneumatic compression and electric stimulation of the muscles. Pharmacologic measures include heparin given in low doses, dextran, and antiplatelet agents.

Walking soon after surgery or injury is the most effective way to prevent deep vein thrombosis. Bedridden patients should exercise the feet - flexion up and down - for 1-2 minutes every hour. It has been proved that such exercises are beneficial also to patients with acute myocardial infarction.

Pneumatic boots are helpful in patients who are unconscious or unable to move their legs. Measures such as these can lower the incidence of thrombosis by as much as 60-65 per cent.

For a bedridden patient with heart failure or stroke standard treatment with an oral anticoagulant is the most effective preventive measure.

Deep vein thrombosis

This condition is defined as the formation of blood cloths in the deep veins. Three factors can contribute to deep vein thrombosis:
- injury to the vein's lining
- an increased tendency for blood to clot
- slowing of blood flow

Veins may be injured during surgery, by injecting of irritating substances, or by certain disorders of the vascular system. They may also be injured by a clot, making formation of a second clot more likely.

During prolonged bed rest, blood flow slows, because the calf muscles are not contracting and squeezing the blood toward the heart. For example, deep vein thrombosis may develop in people who have had a heart attack and lie in hospital beds for several days without sufficiently moving their legs or in people whose legs and lower body part are paralyzed.

Deep vein thrombosis can even occur in healthy people who sit for long periods, for example, during long drives or airplane flights.

Deep vein thrombosis may be difficult for doctors to detect, especially when pain and swelling are absent or very slight. When this disorder is suspected, color Doppler ultrasonography can confirm the diagnosis.

For deep vein thrombosis, treatment involves prevention of pulmonary embolism. Hospitalization may be necessary at first, but because of the advances in treatment, some people with deep vein thrombosis can be treated at home.

Varicose veins   Questions & Answers

What causes varicose veins?

They are the result of a malfunction of the valves, found at regular intervals in veins, which normally control the flow of blood back to the heart. The valves are supposed to prevent a backup of blood. When a series of valves degenerate, the weight of the blood in the vein tends to distend it.

Varicose veins are most often seen in people who are on their feet for long periods. An increase in internal pressure of the blood also can strain the valves. This may be caused by heavy filling, pregnancy, and abdominal tumors.

What are the symptoms of varicose veins?

In addition to - or instead of - the visual signs of varicose veins, there may be other symptoms including:

- feelings of heaviness;
- dull stabbing pain in the legs;
- leg cramps at night;
- itching around the ankles;
- tenderness along the vein;
- soreness along the vein.

If varicose veins are not treated, infections and leg ulcers may develop which can be very difficult to heal.

Can varicose veins be prevented?

There are no guarantees, because many cases seem to run in families. But some common sense measures can help prevent them.

- If your job requires to stand for long periods, be sure to take breaks to sit down and elevate your legs.
- On long trips, take breaks from sitting as well. Get up and stretch your legs at regular intervals.
- Get regular exercise to improve your circulation.
- If you are pregnant, discuss the use of support stockings with your physician.
- Never wear round garters or elastic girdles for long periods of time. They impair circulation.

How are varicose veins treated?

First, your doctor will recommend the life-style changes mentioned for prevention. Second, physicians now have a number of techniques to alleviate the swelling and help improve circulation. They may include medication, injections directly into the veins, surgery to remove the distended veins. Only your physician can make the decision about which treatment is best for you, depending on the degree of varicosity and your life-style.

WARTS

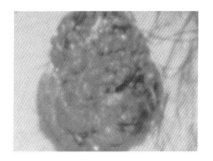

Introduction

Warts or verrucae are small skin growths caused by any of 60 related human papillomavirus types. Warts can develop at any age, but they are most common in children and least common in the elderly. Although

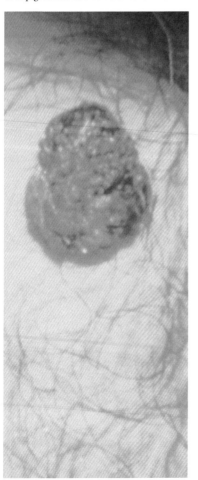

Macroscopic view of a wart; a solitary, verrucous pigmented lesion on the mons veneris.

W

warts on the skin are easily spread from one area of the body to another, most are not very contagious from one person to another. Genital warts, however, are contagious.

Characteristics

Warts are an extremely common affliction among people, old and young. Although sometimes associated with serious physical problems, warts are mostly a cosmetic annoyance that can cause embarrassment in the person who has them. Appearing on the face, hands, feet, knees, arms, genitals, and anus, warts are sometimes infectious and easily spread.

Types of warts

Warts are small, localized overgrowths of skin cells triggered by a family of viruses called papilloma. Appearing simply or in clusters, warts have various shapes and sizes depending on where they appear on the body and the degree of irritation the skin has sustained.

Warts are usually classified as follows:

▲ Common: a benign growth with a rough surface. These appear on the face, hands, scalp, knees, and arms.

▲ Plantar: these warts are also benign and appear on the soles of the feet. They are usually flat and can be extremely painful. Often, plantar warts appear in clusters and callous over.

▲ Periungual: these warts appear around nail beds and, like plantar warts, can be very painful if inappropriately placed.

▲ Venereal: these highly infectious warts appear on the genitals

and/or anus. They can become problematic if they tear or bleed during sex, especially those on the penis.

Though some doctors believe that certain types of venereal or genital warts can develop into cancer, several researchers dispute such notions, rightly pointing out that not all people with genital cancer have such warts. Genital warts can, however, infiltrate the urethra where they can grow rapidly, branching out like grape clusters and blocking the urine flow. This is a serious condition that should be attended to by a urologist at once.

Factors for development

Warts are a medical anomaly: they appear and disappear seemingly at random. Some warts remain in the same place for several years resistant to all treatments, while others shrivel up and vanish after no treatment at all.

Warts, however, appear to be highly suggestible. Virtually every grandparent has a "sure fire" wart cure and the cure rate appears to be directly linked to the person's faith that the cure will work.

In natural therapies, however, skin afflictions are typically indicative of poor elimination, especially by the liver. When the liver is not able to adequately filter toxins out of the blood, the body attempts to rid itself of them by directing them to the skin, another eliminative organ.

The immune system is also a factor in the appearance, constancy, and resolution of warts: if immunity is strong, warts are unlikely to appear. When, however, immunity is compromised by any of a number of factors (lack of sleep, drug or alcohol abuse, stress,

Warts Questions & Answers

What are genital warts?

Warts on the genitals and near the anus are very common and can be rather unpleasant. Sometimes they are very persistent. The warts are caused by a virus which is almost always transmitted through sexual contact. The warts are mainly found in moist places such as the skin of or near the genitals and between the buttocks.

The risk of infection is the greatest when the warts are clearly visible. A regular partner is usually also infected, even if warts have not (yet) formed. Warn anyone you have had sexual contact with in the past few months.

What are the major symptoms of genital warts in men and women?

The warts can appear from anything between a few weeks and eight months after infection with the virus. Women get them at the vaginal opening and in the vagina and/or on the cervix, while men get them on or near the penis. Both men and women get them on or near the anus.

Often it starts with a few small warts which grow and spread. They do not hurt, although they can itch. Women may find they get worse during menstruation or pregnancy. Sometimes it is difficult to detect them yourself. One someone has become infected with the virus they never get rid of it - as far is known until now.

The warts themselves can disappear. A well-known complication with regard to genital warts is that they can spread. This may look rather unpleasant. That is why it is important to start treatment early, even if it is for only one wart. The longer you wait and the more warts there are, the longer treatment will take.

What is the best treatment for genital warts?

The treatment is intensive. Your doctor may apply a solution to the warts. This can hurt. This solution should be washed off after about three hours. The warts often shrink and start disappearing after a while - but this can take some time. You cal also apply a solution to the warts yourself.

Sometimes the warts are removed by freezing, cauterization or surgery. This is usually done under anaesthesia. The warts may recur. You should check for this yourself and go for early repeat treatment.

What is a condylomata acuminata infection?

Condylomata acuminata are warts caused by a virus. Warts on the genitals and near the anus are very common and can be rather unpleasant. Sometimes they are very persistent. The warts are caused by a virus which is almost always transmitted through sexual contact.

The warts are mainly found in moist places such as the skin of or near the genitals and between the buttocks. The risk of infection is the greatest when the warts are clearly visible. A regular partner is usually also infected, even if warts have not (yet) formed. Warn anyone you have had sexual contact with in the past few months.

What are the major symptoms of an infection with condylomata acuminata in men and women?

The infection with condylomata acuminata or warts can appear from anything between a few weeks and eight months after infection with the virus. Women get them at the vaginal opening and in the vagina and/or on the cervix, while men get them on or near the penis. Both men and women get them on or near the anus.

Often it starts with a few small warts which grow and spread. They do not hurt, although they can itch. Women may find they get worse during menstruation or pregnancy. Sometimes it is difficult to detect them yourself. One someone has become infected with the virus they never get rid of it - as far is known until now.

The warts themselves can disappear. A well-known complication with regard to genital warts is that they can spread. This may look rather unpleasant. That is why it is important to start treatment early, even if it is for only one wart. The longer you wait and the more warts there are, the longer treatment will take.

What is the best treatment for an infection with condylomata acuminata?

The treatment is intensive. Your doctor may apply a solution to the warts. This can hurt. This solution should be washed off after about three hours. The warts often shrink and start disappearing after a while - but this can take some time. You cal also apply a solution to the warts yourself.

Sometimes the warts are removed by freezing, cauterization or surgery. This is usually done under anaesthesia. The warts may recur. You should check for this yourself and go for early repeat treatment.

---

smoking, poor nutrition, etc.), this opens the door for viral infections such as papilloma to occur.

Treatment

Treatment for warts depends on their location, type, and severity as well as how long they have been on the skin. Most common warts disappear without treatment within 2 years.

Daily application of a solution or plaster containing salicylic acid and lactic acids soften the infected skin, which can be peeled off to make the wart disappear faster. A doctor can freeze the wart using liquid nitrogen but may have to repeat the freezing process in 2 or 3 weeks to eliminate the wart completely.

Electrodesiccation (a treatment that uses an electric current) or laser surgery can destroy the wart, but each may cause scarring. Regardless of the treatment method, about a third of the time the wart comes back.

W

WOMEN'S DISEASES

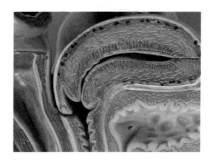

Major subjects on women's health issues have been described in the following chapters: Breast cancer, Cervix disorders, Genital herpes, Menopause, Menstrual disorders, Ovarian disorders, Pelvic disorders, Uterine tumors

Introduction

The female reproductive system consists of those structures within the female body that are designed to create and nourish new life. The system includes the ovaries, Fallopian tubes, uterus, cervix, and vagina.
Although the breasts, or mammary glands, are actually a type of sweat gland, their function (supporting new life) is closely related to that of the reproductive system.
Diseases of the female reproductive system are numerous and extremely common in clinical and pathologic practice, to the point at which they have been segregated into specialties unto themselves in gynecology and gynecologic pathology.
The following description presents the major entities that compose the bulk of the clinical problem, except for those disorders that have been described in oither chapters.

Endometriosis

Endometriosis is a condition in which tissue that looks and acts like endometrial tissue is found in places other than the lining of the uterus (endometrium). It occurs at menstruation when normal endometrial tissue backs up with menstrual blood through the Fallopian tubes and then implants and grows in other places such as:
• ovaries

• tubes
• outer surface of the uterus
• bowel
• other pelvic structures
Endometriosis may also develop on body tissues located anywhere in the abdomen; these tissues respond to the cycle of changes brought on by the female hormones just as the endometrium normally responds in the uterus. Thus, at the end of every cycle, when the hormones cause the uterus to shed its endometrial lining, endometrial tissue growing outside the uterus will break apart and bleed.
Unlike menstrual fluid from the uterus, which is discharged freely out of the body during menstruation, blood from the abnormal tissue has no place to go. Body tissues respond to this menstrual-type bleeding by
▲ surrounding it with inflammation (tissue that becomes red, swollen, and painful around the area);
▲ trying to absorb it back in the circulatory (blood) system.
The monthly inflammation subsides when the bleeding ends (at the same time normal menstrual bleeding ends), and scar tissue is produced around the area. This pattern occurs in the same cycle as the menstrual cycle: month after month, patches of endometriosis are triggered by the female hormones to menstruate blood; the blood is absorbed by the surrounding, inflamed area; and scar tissue forms. Endometriosis may also cause adhesions, abnormal tissue growth and binds organs together.
Sometimes a patch of endometriosis is surrounded by enough scar tissue to cut off its blood supply; such tissue can no longer respond completely to the hormones.
Other patches may rupture, or burst, during menstruation and spread their contents to other pelvic areas, causing

new spots of endometriosis to develop. Thus, the condition may become gradually worse with time, although symptoms may come and go.

Occurrence

Endometriosis can occur only after the menstrual flow begins; the disease has never been found in a young woman who has not yet begun to menstruate. After menopause, endometriosis is no longer active unless, for some reason, a woman's hormones become active again or she is given hormones for some other medical need. Endometriosis is most common among women in their 30s and 40s.
Little is known about why some women develop endometriosis and others do not. However, there is some evidence that the condition may be inherited.
A number of problems may be due to endometriosis, although they may also have other causes. If you have any of these symptoms, you should see your gynecologist:
▲ Increasing discomfort and pain during your menstrual period, called dysmenorrhea.
▲ A sharp, pain deep in the pelvis during intercourse. This may be a result of endometriosis that has lodged in the body space between the uterus and the rectum.
Cancer is found very rarely with endometriosis, occurring in less than 1 percent of women who have the condition. When it does occur, it is usually found in older, more advanced patches of endometriosis. However, the long-term outlook in these very rare situations is reasonably good.

Preventive factors

Because endometriosis is affected by hormone production, certain factors influence the progress of the disease:

▲ Since the hormones made by the placenta during pregnancy prevent proliferation, the progress of endometriosis is slowed or stopped during pregnancy.

▲ Oral contraceptives (birth control pills) are thought to protect against or halt the process of endometriosis in the same way that placental hormones do during pregnancy.

Women who have endometriosis tend to be less fertile (or able to become pregnant) than other women. Some women may find out that they have endometriosis after consulting a gynecologist for treatment of infertility. Once it is found, infertility caused by endometriosis can frequently be treated with good results.

Tests

Ordinarily, the doctor will look at your complete medical and menstrual background and perform a pelvic exam - an examination of the pelvic structures during which the doctor looks for signs of anything abnormal. The doctor may examine you between menstrual periods and then again during your menstrual periods in order to compare the change in certain findings from the pelvic exam at different times in the cycle. An accurate diagnosis can be obtained only by a procedure called laparoscopy. This is done under a local or general anesthetic, with a slender light-transmitting telescope that is inserted through a tiny cut made in the lower abdomen. This enables the doctor to view the pelvic organs and actually see 1f endometriosis is present.

Treatment

Different types of treatment may be needed for endometriosis:
· hormonal therapy
· conservative surgery
· major surgery

■ *Hormonal therapy*

During recent years, different types of hormone treatment have been developed. In such treatment, doses of hormones or drugs are given to temporarily change the patterns of the normal female hormones and thus slow the growth of endometriosis.

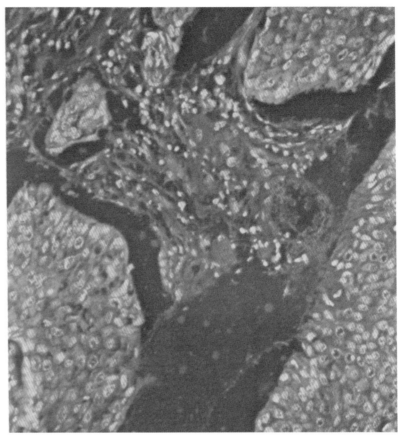

Malignant growth in the epithelial tissue of the vagina. The cancer is characterized by chaotic growth, differing sizes of cells and irregular mitosis (cell division). This malignant growth has been photographed by a special technique using a florescent microscope. The nuclei of the cells show up as yellow-green; RNA (nucleic acid) appears red. The presence of nucleic acid points to cell division.

One type of hormonal treatment mimics the hormones of pregnancy. Another causes your body to react in a way similar to menopause. Since hormonal therapy shuts off ovulation, women being treated for endometriosis will not get pregnant during such therapy, although some may become pregnant shortly after the therapy is stopped.

■ *Conservative surgery*

Surgery may be performed, during which spots of endometriosis are cut away from their abnormal locations. If you are concerned about infertility, you should be reassured that good ovarian tissue and normal tubal tissue are left intact as much as possible to aid the chances of achieving pregnancy after the operation. Such surgical treatment of infertile patients who have endometriosis is often, but not always, successful.

■ *Major surgery*

In cases of severe endometriosis it may be necessary to remove part or all of the reproductive organs to relieve symptoms and to stop the production of the female hormones that trigger further growth of endometriosis.

With surgical treatment of endometriosis, it is important that you understand the considerations of the gynecologist performing the surgery. Decisions concerning what type of surgical procedure is best for the individual woman can be made only during the surgery itself, when the gynecologist can actually see and evaluate the extent of the endometriosis.

W

747

Women's diseases Questions & Answers

What is endometriosis?

Endometriosis is a condition which occurs when endometrial tissue, the tissue that lines the uterus and is shed during menstruation, grows outside the uterus.

Once outside the uterus, endometrial tissue can develop into painful growths. Common sites for endometrial growths of endometriosis include the ovaries, the Fallopian tubes and the ligaments that support the uterus. Other possible sites for endometriosis include the bladder, bowel and vagina.

Endometriosis may also develop on body tissues located anywhere in the abdomen; these tissues respond to the cycle of changes brought on by the female hormones just as the endometrium normally responds in the uterus.

What causes endometriosis?

Endometriosis is one of the most puzzling conditions that affect women. The exact cause of the disease remains obscure. The most common theory is referred to as "retrograde menstruation."

According to this theory, a portion of the menstrual fluid flows backward into the Fallopian tubes, rather than into the vagina. Endometrial cells contained in the menstrual fluid may then attach themselves to various locations in the pelvic cavity.

Unlike menstrual fluid from the uterus, which is discharged freely out of the body during menstruation, blood from the abnormal tissue has no place to go. Body tissues respond to this menstrual-type bleeding by:

▲ Surrounding it with inflammation (tissue that becomes, red, swollen, and painful around the area).

▲ Trying to absorb it back into the circulatory system.

What is the consequence of the local inflammation in endometriosis?

The monthly inflammation subsides when the bleeding ends (at the same time normal menstrual bleeding ends), and scar tissue is produced around the area.

This pattern occurs in the same cycle as the menstrual cycle; month after month, patches of endometriosis are triggered by the female hormones to menstruate blood; the blood is absorbed by the surrounding, inflamed areas; and scar tissue forms. Endometriosis may also cause adhesions, abnormal tissue growth that binds organs together.

Sometimes a patch of endometriosis is surrounded by enough scar tissue to cut off its blood supply; such tissue can no longer respond completely to the hormones. This is called a burned-out plaque of endometriosis.

Who is most likely to develop endometriosis?

It is estimated that about 15 percent of all women develop some degree of endometriosis before reaching menopause. Although the disease more commonly occurs in childless women between the ages of 25 and 40, endometriosis can affect women, including those with children, at any time during the childbearing years. Endometriosis can occur only after the menstrual flow begins: the disease has never been found in a young woman who has not yet begun to menstruate.

After menopause, endometriosis is no longer active unless, for some reason, a woman's hormones become active again or she is given hormones for some other medical need.

Little is known about why some women develop endometriosis and others do not. However, there is some evidence that the condition may be inherited.

If surgery is needed, be sure that you talk with your doctor before the operation and that you understand fully what is involved.

Papillomavirus infection

Infection with human papillomavirus (HPV) is one of the most common sexually transmitted diseases. Genital warts, one of the diseases caused by the virus, has been around for centuries.

Today, though, more and more women are being diagnosed with human papillomavirus (HPV). There may be several reasons for this increase. Women today tend to have had more sexual partners, and they are less likely to rely on condoms for birth control.

Both of these habits increase the risk of infection. The fact that more women smoke today also may increase the problems that can arise with human papillomavirus (HPV) infection.

Finding out that you have been infected with human papillomavirus (HPV) may frighten you or upset you. Many women feel bad about themselves when they are diagnosed with genital warts. But human papillomavirus (HPV) infection is a very common problem.

Patience is the key to coping with genital warts. You may need to have repeat treatments for several weeks or months until all signs of the warts are gone. While this prolonged treatment may be a bother, it may be the best way of getting rid of all the growths. Even with successful treatment, the warts may come back later at any time.

If you have been infected, you may have a higher risk of some major health problems. But these problems can usually be treated. have a Pap test at least once a year, so that any new growths are caught early. Avoid smoking, which can increase problems related to human papillomavirus (HPV) infection. Working with your doctor, you can lessen the health risks of human papillomavirus (HPV) infection.

HPV, like all viruses, is a very small organism that needs to infect cells in

W

order to live. Once inside a cell, the virus directs the cell to make copies of itself and to infect other healthy cells. The cells infected with the virus eventually die. When this happen, they are shed from the body just as skin cells are shed. The virus is shed with the dead cells. When the virus is shed. it can be passed to another person, who can also become infected.

Once the virus has been passed on, it may be some time before the other person shows any signs of infection. These signs often appear several months after infection, but sometimes they may appear years later.

The virus can be passed from one person to another during sex. HPV is generally thought to be a sexually transmitted disease, although other, nonsexual forms of transmission may occur.

There are many types of HPV. Some types tend to infect cells in the genital of men and women, whole others tend to infect cells in other parts of the body. HPV can cause common warts, such as those that appear on fingers and hands. Sometimes these warts spread to the genital area, but this is rare. While unsightly, common warts to not pose any major health risks.

Types of HPV

The types of HPV that are found in the genital area cause condylomas, or genital warts. These growths may appear on the outside or inside of the genital area and can spread to nearby skin or to a sexual partner.

Genital warts are more likely to occur in women who have multiple sexual partners, or whose male partners have had multiple partners. Other vaginal infections often go along with genital warts.

While most HPV infections are not a serious threat to your health, some can increase the risk of getting cancer. This is why regular check-ups that include Pap tests are so important for women who have had genital warts. repeat treatments may be needed to make the warts go away.

Diagnosis

If you notice growths in the genital area, your doctor may perform tests to diagnose the problem. But HPV may be present without growths. This is because the virus can cause changes that cannot be seen by the naked eye. Sometimes human papillomavirus (HPV) infection can be indicated by a Pap test that is done as part of a regular check-up, even if no warts or other growth can be seen. For the Pap test, cells are wiped from the cervix and sent to a lab to be examined under a microscope.

If the results of a Pap test suggest that you may have human papillomavirus (HPV) infection, your doctor may check your cervix, vagina, and vulva. To do this, a magnifying instrument called a colposcope may be used to look at these areas. It is similar to binoculars on a stand. To help make the changes more visible, these areas may first be wiped with a vinegar solution. A speculum is placed in the vagina to separate the vaginal walls. The colposcope is then positioned outside your body so that the cervix, vagina, and vulva can be examined. Some doctors do not perform colposcopy in their offices, so you may be referred to another doctor or clinic for this exam.

An abnormal Pap test does not always mean that you have human papillomavirus (HPV) infection, or any other disorder. It does mean that you need to be examined. Your doctor may want merely to observe very early signs of infection. He or she may want you to have another Pap test in a few months.

If your doctor finds areas that look suspicious, he or she may perform a biopsy. In this procedure, a small sample of tissue is removed and sent to a lab to be checked for any signs of precancerous changes or cancer.

Doctors are now studying whether screening tests for human papillomavirus (HPV) infection other than the Pap test would be helpful for women with no symptoms.

Treatment

Although some signs of infection may go away on their own, treatment may be advised. There are many ways of treating the changes caused by the virus:

▲ Trichloroacetic acid (TCA) and bichloroacetic acid (BCA) are strong chemical sometimes painted on genital warts to destroy them. These drugs may cause some burning and must be used very carefully.

▲ Podophyllin is a drug that has been painted on genital warts to treat them. Because it can burn and should not be used during pregnancy, it is now used less often.

▲ Interferon is a new drug that can be used to treat genital warts. It may be injected into the warts themselves or into a muscle.

There is a new drug that you can apply to the warts at home. It is advailable by prescription and may cause burning and inflammation. Your doctor should show you how to apply it before you use it at home.

Several office procedures also are used to treat warts:

▲ *Cryotherapy* (cold cautery) destroys warts and other growths by freezing.

▲ *Laser treatment*, in which a high-intensity beam of light is used, may be used to destroy the growths.

▲ *Electrosurgery* uses an electric current to burn away the lesion or shave it with a tiny loop.

▲ *Excisional biopsy* (cutting away) may be needed to remove warts or other growths in some cases.

If you have many or large warts, they may need to be surgically removed in an operating room with anesthesia.

While these treatments can destroy the warts, which are caused by human papillomavirus (HPV) infection, the invisible virus can persist after treatment. The virus can produce new growths sometimes weeks or even months after the old ones have been destroyed.

In that case, you may need to return to your doctor for more treatment. You may feel frustrated or depressed when new warts appear, but over time, the warts usually go away either with treatment or on their own.

Because of the association of human papillomavirus (HPV) infection and abnormal growths, it is very important to have regular Pap tests. This way, if any changes occur that could suggest cancer, they can be treated promptly. Your doctor will advise you on how often you will need a Pap test.

W

Women's diseases   Questions & Answers

What are the symptoms of endometriosis?

The most common symptoms of endometriosis are pain before and during menstrual periods, pain during sexual intercourse, and heavy or irregular bleeding.

In more serious cases, scar tissue may form on the Fallopian tube and/or on the ovary, blocking the release of the egg and its passage through the tube toward the uterus. This, in turn, will inhibit a woman's ability to conceive.

However, some women with endometriosis may experience no symptoms. What is more, the amount of pain is not related to the extent of a patient's endometrial growths. Some women with numerous growths have no pain while others with minimal endometriosis experience severe pain.

How do female hormones affect endometrial growths?

During menstruation, endometrial growths can bleed, just like the uterine lining bleeds in response to the hormones of the menstrual cycle.

However, unlike the lining of the uterus, products of the endometrial growths have no way of leaving the body. This can result in irritation of the surrounding tissues. In reaction to this irritation, the body may surround this area with adhesions or scar tissue which can cause a woman severe pain.

In other words, as long as a woman's monthly menstrual cycle takes place, the endometrial tissue will be stimulated. This, in turn, can cause women to experience severe menstrual cramps, chronic pelvic pain or pressure, pain during sexual intercourse and/or bowel and bladder problems.

If a woman becomes pregnant or enters menopause, the endometrial growths shrink and much of the pain is eliminated.

How is a diagnosis of endometriosis made?

Ordinarily, the doctor will look at your complete medical and menstrual background and perform a pelvic examination - an examination of the pelvic structures during which the doctor looks for signs of anything abnormal.

If a physician suspects endometriosis, an accurate diagnosis of the disease can be made through a procedure called laparoscopy. During this minor surgical procedure, a slender light-transmitting microscope, the laparoscope, is inserted through a tiny incision made in the abdomen.

This procedure enables the physician to examine the condition of the abdominal organs and check the size and extent of the endometrial growths. This method also allows the physician to rule out other conditions with similar symptoms, such as ovarian cancer.

What kind of treatment is available for endometriosis?

Management of endometriosis is directed at suppressing a woman's levels of estrogen and progesterone, which stimulate the endometrial growths. Possible treatment options range from essentially no treatment in cases of minimal or even mild endometriosis to major surgery.

In general, patients have two broad choices; surgical treatment and drug therapy. For some women, a combination of the two may be required.

Endometriosis affects each woman differently. Ultimately the choice of treatment for endometriosis is up to each individual woman.

In choosing a treatment option for patients with endometriosis, physicians are concerned about:

▲ relieving pain and other symptoms;
▲ halting the progression of future lesions;
▲ restoring fertility to those patients who have lost the ability to become pregnant;
▲ preserving reproductive function for future childbearing.

HPV infection and pregnancy

Most of the time, human papillomavirus (HPV) infection and genital warts do not pose problems during pregnancy. Warts, which are caused by human papillomavirus (HPV) infection, can grow in number and size when a woman is pregnant, however. In very rare cases, the warts can grow so big that they narrow and sometimes even block the birth canal. If this occurs, a cesarean birth may be needed. In a cesarean birth, the baby is born through a surgical incision (cut) made in the mother's abdomen and uterus.

Most warts and vaginal infections caused by HPV can be treated during pregnancy. Pregnant women are most often treated with TCA, cryotherapy, or laser. Neither interferon nor podophyllin should be used during pregnancy.

Your doctor may prefer to wait until after you have your baby to treat you. He or she will watch your condition closely throughout your pregnancy.

Prevention

A good way to help prevent human papillomavirus (HPV) infection is to limit the number of your sexual partners. The more partners you have, the greater is your risk of picking up the virus. Intact condoms, used every time you have sex, may also help prevent the spread of HPV and other sexually transmitted diseases.

If your partner has genital warts, you should avoid having sex with him until after he has been treated. Otherwise, you run the risk of getting the infection from him.

If you have warts, avoid having sex until they are treated. Follow-up exams and Pap tests are important to prevent both the spread of the virus and its effects on your health.

Vaginitis

Vaginitis is an inflammation of the vagina; redness, swelling, and irritation of the vaginal tissues. It causes discharge, burning, itching, and odor. Infections of the vagina are most often the source of the problem, but other things that cause changes in the vagina can also result in vaginitis.

W

The cause of vaginitis must be detected before it can be treated, and this often takes time. Although it is usually not serious, vaginitis can be stubbornly persistent and very uncomfortable.

Symptoms of vaginitis are a very common problem among women. Vaginitis usually affects women of childbearing age, but it can also affect young girls and older women.

Some vaginal infections can be transmitted through sexual contact. These infections can affect male sexual partners of women who have the disease. Although men may show no symptoms, they can transmit such an infection. But it is not necessary to "catch" vaginitis - it can also occur without sexual contact.

Vaginitis does not pose major health problems, but it often does not go away on its own. Fortunately, medications can be very effective in treating and curing infections of the vagina. With proper treatment, according to your doctor's instructions, such infections are likely to disappear with no long-term effects. Other causes of vaginitis can also be eliminated once they are detected.

Vaginal acidity

The normal vagina harbors some microscopic organisms, as does the rest of the body. Some of these organisms break down substances in the vaginal secretions and produce an acidic environment in the vagina.

The natural acid environment of the vagina keeps the number of potentially harmful organisms in check. However, any number of things can alter the vaginal acidity:

- antibiotics prescribed for other diseases
- douching too often
- tampons irritating the vaginal walls
- tight slacks
- panties or panty hose without a cotton crotch
- extra weight
- diabetes
- pregnancy
- recent childbirth
- birth control pills

A change in the acidity of the vagina can allow these potentially harmful organisms living in the vagina to grow

Pain diary

An accurate description of your pain will help your doctor finds its cause. You may be asked to keep a pain diary so that more complete information can be obtained. In your pain diary, note when you feel pain:

- ▲ Time of day
- ▲ At certain times of your monthly cycle
- ▲ Before, during, or after
  - Eating
  - Urination
  - Bowel movement
  - Intercourse
  - Physical activity
  - Sleep

Describe the pain and note how long it lasts:
- ▲ Is it a sharp stab, or a dull ache?
- ▲ Does it come in phases, or is it steady?
- ▲ How long does it last?
- ▲ How intense is it?
- ▲ Does it always occur in the same place(s)?
- ▲ Is it mostly in one place, or over a general area?

rapidly. When this happens, they cause inflammation and abnormal discharge.

Not all types of vaginitis are caused by an upset in vaginal acidity, however. General resistance to infection can also be weakened by lack of sleep, poor diet, stress, or other illness. This lack of resistance can allow vaginal infections to thrive and cause inflammation. Some vaginal infections can be passed from one person to another during sexual intercourse.

Vaginal discharge

A certain amount of discharge from the vagina is normal. Normal vaginal discharge helps to cleanse the vagina and keep it healthy. Between periods some women notice a discharge that is clear or cloudy and whitish. This normal discharge does not smell, itch, or burn. It also does not require special care other than regular bathing.

Discharge caused by vaginitis is not normal. Identifying abnormal discharge is often a first step in identifying the problem. If you notice signs of abnormal discharge - or itching, burning, or odor - see your doctor at once.

Vaginal infections

Even though vaginitis is not a serious disease, the symptoms can be upsetting. Knowing the signs of vaginitis can lessen those fears and help a woman get to her doctor at the earliest stage of infection. The following are descriptions of three common types of vaginal infections that can cause vaginitis:

- candidiasis
- bacterial vaginosis
- trichomoniasis

■ Candidiasis

Candidiasis (al l fungus or yeast infection or moniliasis) is the most common type of vaginal infection that causes symptoms of irritation. It is often hard to get rid of, and recurrences are common.

Many women with this infection do not notice a discharge, but if it is present it is usually described as an odorless, "cheesy" discharge. The main symptom of this type of inflammation is intense itching, burning, and redness of the vaginal tissues.

Candidiasis is caused by a fungus, like yeast. Although it can affect any women, candidiasis is more frequent

W

Women's diseases Questions & Answers

What is the significance of the acidity of the vagina?

The normal vagina harbors some microscopic organisms, as does the rest of the body. Some of these organisms in the vagina break down substances in the vaginal secretions and produce an acidic environment. The natural acid environment of the vagina keeps the number of potentially harmful organisms in check. However, any number of things can alter the vaginal acidity such as antibiotics, tampons, diabetes, overweight, contraceptive devices etc.

What causes infection of the vaginal wall or vaginitis?

Vaginitis is an inflammation of the vagina: redness, swelling, and irritation of the vaginal tissues. It causes discharge, burning, itching, and odor.

Infections of the vagina are most often the source of the problem, but other things that cause changes in the vagina can also result in vaginitis.

Symptoms of vaginitis are a very common problem among women. Vaginitis usually affects women of childbearing age, but it can also affect young girls and older women.

Some vaginal infections can be transmitted through sexual contact. These infections can affect the male sexual partners of women who have the disease.

Although men may show no symptoms, they can transmit such an infection. But it is not necessary to "catch" vaginitis - it can also occur without sexual contact.

What can I do about vaginitis?

There are things you can do to help keep the vagina healthy. If you have recurrent vaginitis, keep in mind the following points:

▲ Avoid spreading bacteria from the rectum to the vagina. After a bowel movement, wipe from front to back, away from the vagina.
▲ Clean the vulva thoroughly and keep as dry as possible.
▲ Avoid irritating agents - harsh soaps or detergents, feminine hygiene sprays, perfumed toilet paper, perfumed tampons.
▲ Avoid using tampons alone throughout your entire menstrual period.
▲ Thoroughly clean diaphragms and spermicide applications.
▲ Avoid douching; practice good general hygiene.
▲ Avoid tight jeans, panties or panty hose without a cotton crotch, or other clothing than can trap moisture.

My doctor talked about the vulva; what did he mean by it?

The vulva is the outer part of the female genital area. To understand about the diseases that can affect the vulva, it is important to know about the anatomy of the external female genital area.

The mons veneris, or mons, lies directly over the joint of the pubic bones. Below the mons, the fleshy. hair-covered folds of tissue form the labia majora, or outer lips of the vulva.

Between the labia majora lie the labia minora, or inner lips. These are hairless and are sensitive to touch. In some women, the outer lips may be darker than the inner lips.

Within the labia minora is a space called the vestibulum. The vagina and urethra open into this space. At the top of the inner lips is the clitoris.

Just inside the vestibulum are the Bartholin glands, which you normally cannot feel. These glands produce some of the lubrication during sexual excitement. The area of thick muscular tissue between the anus and the vaginal opening is called the perineum.

among women who are pregnant, diabetic, or obese. These conditions can alter the body's metabolic balance and vaginal acidity and promote the growth of the fungus.

The use of antibiotics and birth control pills also make a woman more prone to this disorder. Antibiotics stimulate the growth of the fungus and eliminate certain protective bacteria. Birth control pills produce chemical changes in the vagina similar to those of pregnancy. In both cases, the fungus has a chance to overdevelop and cause inflammation.

If the physical exam and lab tests reveal that candidiasis is present, your doctor will prescribe medication to destroy the fungus causing the problem.

This may include vaginal suppositories or tablets or the application of a cream or gel into the vagina. The medication may be somewhat messy - you may need to wear a sanitary napkin during treatment. Your doctor will advise you in detail about what is involved.

In most cases, candidiasis will be cured with treatment. However, the infection resists treatment in some women - especially pregnant and diabetic women - and a cure may take some time.

Conditions that spur the growth of candidiasis will also have to be changed in order to get rid of the vaginal infection completely.

■ Bacterial vaginosis

Bacterial vaginosis (formerly called *Gardnerella vaginitis* or nonspecific vaginitis) is a complex condition that is not well understood at present.

The predominant symptom of bacterial vaginosis is an increase in vaginal discharge. Often the discharge has an unpleasant or "fishy" odor. Redness and itching are rare; however, since bacterial vaginosis can occur with other types of infections, other symptoms may be present. You should see your doctor to determine the exact cause of the problem.

The cause of this infection is thought to be an overgrowth of several different types of organisms. Some of these are *Gardnerella vaginalis*, *Mycoplasma species*, and a recently discovered organism called *Mobiluncus*.

Doctors usually recommend antibiotics taken by mouth for the treatment of bacterial vaginosis. A drug called metronidazole is an effective treatment. Sometimes drugs called ampicillin and amoxillin may be used. It is not clear whether the infection can be transmitted through sexual intercourse. For this reason, your doctor may advise that your partner be treated as well.

■ *Trichomoniasis*
Trichomoniasis is the third most common type of vaginal infection. This condition affects the urinary tract as well as the vagina. As with a *Gardnerella* infection, both women and men can be infected.

A woman may have an irritating discharge, frequently yellow-green in color. It may look frothy and have an offensive odor. The discharge can produce burning and itching, especially during urination. It also causes redness and swelling. Symptoms may be more severe just before and just after the menstrual period.

Trichomoniasis is caused by a protozoan - a one-celled organism much larger than a bacterium. This type of vaginitis is usually transmitted sexually.

Because trichomoniasis also affects the urinary tract, most doctors consider suppositories relatively ineffective in curing this condition. Metronidazole can cure almost all cases. A single large dose taken by mouth is usually effective. Sometimes smaller doses are taken over 7 days. Doctors often recommend treatment for both sexual partners to avoid reinfection.

Metronidazole is effective and has relatively few complications. However, undesirable side effects (nausea, vomiting, darkening of urine) can occur and should be promptly reported to the doctor.

In addition, anyone taking the drug should not drink alcohol during treatment - mixing this drug and alcohol can cause a violent reaction.

■ *Treatment for your sexual partner*
Trichomoniasis is often shared by sexual partners. Successful treatment depends on getting rid of the infection in both - even though the partner

Above: Macroscopic view of endometriosis of the peritoneum.
Middle: Microscopy of a vaginal smear. A Gram stain of vaginal discharge shows many polymorphicnuclear leukocytes. Gram-negative diplococci are seen in the cytoplasm of some of the leukocytes; this suggest the presence of an infection by Neisseria species.
Below: Macroscopy of the vulva showing signs of a herpes infection. This patient has early vesicular lesions of herpes simplex virus. The vesicles are small and surrounded by intense erythema.

may not show any symptoms. Unless both receive treatment at the same time, the infection can continue to occur.

Ideally, your partner should consult his doctor for examination and treatment. The important thing to remember is that he should be treated, even if he shows no signs of the infection.

For this reason, your doctor may prescribe metronidazole for both of you. If so, your partner should contact his personal doctor before taking the medication - he needs to be sure there are no reasons for him not to take metronidazole. You and your partner should both feel free to talk about any questions or concerns with your doctor.

Other causes of vaginitis
Vaginal inflammation is not always caused by infection. The vaginal area may have an adverse reaction to chemicals such as those used in feminine hygiene sprays or bubble baths. If injury to the vaginal walls occurs (for example, from improper tampon use), or if the outside organs are irritated by tight clothing or fabrics that do not "breathe," redness, swelling, and discharge can result.

Synthetic hormones (such as birth control pills) can also alter the hormonal balance of the vagina and cause symptoms of vaginitis.

After a woman reaches menopause, the vaginal tissues are no longer stimulated by the female estrogen from the ovaries. Tissue thins and becomes dry. The vagina is more prone to injury (from sexual intercourse, for example) and can more easily become irritated. Inflammation and discharge

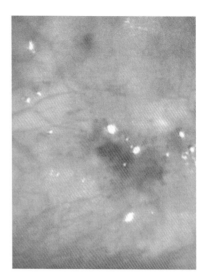

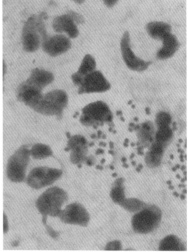

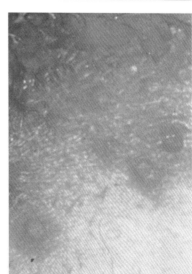

W

can develop. This is called atrophic vaginitis.

Vulvar diseases

The vulva, the outer part of the female genital area, can be the site of a variety of diseases. Many of the diseases are relatively minor. Others, such as cancer, though rare, can have more serious consequences if not treated early. To understand about the diseases that can affect the vulva, it is important to know about the anatomy of the external female genital area.

The mons veneris, or mons, lies directly over the joint of the pubic bones. Below the mons, the fleshy, hair-covered folds of tissue form the labia majora, or outer lips of the vulva. Between the labia majora lie the labia minora, or inner lips. These are hairless and are very sensitive to touch. In some women, the outer lips may be darker than the inner lips.

Within the labia minora is a space called the vestibule. The vagina and urethra (the short, narrow tube that conveys urine from the bladder out of the body) open into this space. You can see the small opening of the urethra just above the vaginal opening. At the top of the inner lips is the clitoris. This extremely sensitive organ is a source of sexual excitement in most women. The clitoris is partly covered by a fold of tissue called the hood.

Just inside the vestibule are the Bartholin glands, which you normally cannot feel. These glands produce some of the lubrication during sexual excitement. The area of thick muscular tissue between the anus and the vaginal opening is called perineum.

Vulvar self-examination

Because so many diseases that can affect the vulva have similar symptoms, it is important to be aware of any unusual changes in the vulvar area. One of the best ways to do this is to examine the vulvar area. This is especially important if you have ever had any disease that affects the vulva. Performing this exam will help you to be alert to any changes that could signal an infection or other problem. Any symptoms such as itching or discomfort should also be reported to

your doctor. If a problem does occur, your chances of catching it at an early stage - when treatment is most successful - are best if you have examined yourself regularly.

To find the cause of a particular vulvar disease, your doctor will ask questions about any symptoms you are having, and a number of tests may be performed. One of the most common and important of these tests is a biopsy, which is the removal of a small piece of tissue for examination under a microscope.

The following vulvar diseases have to be considered:
- contact dermatitis;
- vestibulitis;
- vulvodynia;
- vulvar dystrophies;
- Paget disease of the vulva;
- vulvar intra-epithelial neoplasia;
- invasive cancer;
- melanoma.

■ Contact dermatitis

Contact dermatitis is caused by chemical irritation of the skin of the vulva. This irritation may be caused by a variety of sources.
- Perfumed or dyed toilet tissue or underwear.
- Soaps, particularly those with strong deodorants.
- Talcum powder.
- Feminine hygiene sprays.
- Deodorant pads.
- Spermicidal foams, creams, and jellies.
- Rubber products such as those used in condoms.
- Poison ivy or similar plants.
- Insect bites or stings.

It is also possible to develop contact dermatitis by touching your vulva with irritants, such as nail polish or nail polish remover, that do not normally have contact with that part of your body. The chief symptoms of contact dermatitis are redness and itching. Your doctor may diagnose it after examining the vulvar area and asking you about the substances that come in contact with your vulva.

Treatment for contact dermatitis usually consists of getting rid of the source of the irritation and, if the dermatitis is severe, applying a steroid cream, such as hydrocortisone cream,

three times daily. You might also be told to apply cold compresses to relieve the itching.

To avoid getting contact dermatitis again, be sure to stay away from whatever substance caused it in the first place, as well as those listed here.

If you wear panty hose, be sure they have a cotton crotch, and wear white cotton underpants. Nylon and other synthetic fabrics do not "breathe" as well as cotton and may not allow enough air circulation to the vulvar area. It may also help to rinse out your underwear after it has been washed with detergent. Finally, always wash your hands before you touch your genital area to prevent the transfer of irritating substances.

■ Vestibulitis

Vestibulitis is an inflammation of the small glands around the vestibule. It is sometimes called "burning vulva," because one of the main symptoms is a burning sensation.

Other symptoms include pain, itching, and sometimes pain when urinating or during intercourse. The cause of vestibulitis is not definitely known, although infection or irritants may play a role.

After taking a medical history and performing a physical exam to detect possible causes your doctor may prescribe a cream or ointment to treat vestibulitis. Because it takes time for skin to heal, this treatment may continue for 4-6 weeks. If it does not work, further treatment with local injections or minor surgery may be needed.

■ Vulvodynia

Vulvodynia literally means "vulvar pain." Rather than a specific disease, it is a syndrome (a collection of signs and symptoms) that has no specific cause. The symptoms of vulvodynia include pain, especially during sexual intercourse; itching; and general discomfort.

It is usually diagnosed by ruling out other possible reasons for these symptoms. Many doctors feel that there may be a psychologic factor in chronic, persistent vulvar pain that has no known cause.

To find what is causing the symptoms of vulvodynia, your medical history

Above: Microscopic view of the skin of the vulva. This is a biopsy of a patient who had chronic dermatitis; a marked hyperkeratosis and acanthosis is present.
Middle: Macroscopic picture showing a large fungating verrucous carcinoma on the left vulva.
Below: The skin of the vulva shows chronic dermatitis, appears, dry, constricted, and whitish. The chronic changes distort the normal appearance of the vulva.

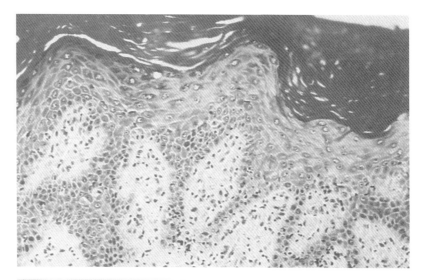

will first be taken. Secretions from your vagina will then be collected and examined under a microscope. this is done to find out whether you have a viral or bacterial infection that can be treated with specific drugs.

If no such cause is found, you may be given a cream or ointment that contains steroids or other hormones. or your doctor may advise measures to control pain, such as injections of steroid or nerve block. A nerve block is a procedure in which pain is blocked by injecting a long-acting local anesthetic or by surgically cutting the nerve.

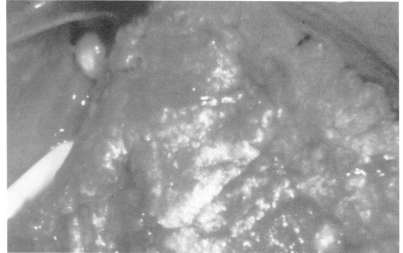

■ *Vulvar dystrophies*
In general, a dystrophy is a disease or condition in which tissue becomes wasted and shriveled. Vulvar dystrophies are usually chronic (long-lasting) and require long-term treatment. Some types of vulvar dystrophy can lead to cancer if they are not treated and watched carefully. For this reason, a biopsy may be performed if vulvar dystrophy is suspected.

Symptoms include white, hardened patches on the vulvar area. The vulvar skin may look like thin, wrinkled parchment. Treatment for vulvar dystrophy includes steroid creams or ointments (such as testosterone ointment).

These must be rubbed into the vulvar tissue, as simple application may not allow penetration. Your doctor may also advise a regimen of vulvar drying that may have to be continued indefinitely. The aim is to control, rather than cure, the disease. In some cases, surgery may be needed to remove the lesions.

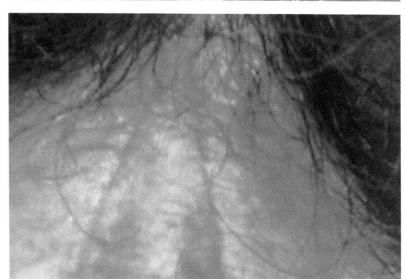

WORM INFESTATIONS

Description

Worms belong to the group of parasites, organisms that live in and feed off other organisms (the hosts). They are found worldwide and can cause infections in people of all ages. Parasitic infections are very common among children, who tend to put their unwashed fingers and hands in or near their mouths.

In the industrialized countries the most common parasitic infections are caused by adult worms and include pinworm, ascaris, whipworm, and hookworm infections. Less common worm infections include infestation by beef, pork, and fish tapeworms, and trichinosis.

The severity of any parasitic infection depends on the child's general health, the number of infective organisms inhabiting the child's body, the child's sensitivity to the parasite, and the presence of other parasites.

Although parasitic infections are huge problems in tropical and underdeveloped countries most cases in the United States and other industrialized countries clear up with proper treatment within a few days to a week. A child rarely suffers permanent complications.

Infestation

Worms generally enter the body through the mouth or skin. Worms that enter through the mouth are swallowed and can remain in the intestine or burrow through the intestinal wall and invade other organs.

Worms that enter through the skin bore directly through the skin or are introduced through the bites of infected insects (the vector). Some worms enter through the soles of the feet when a person walks barefoot or through the skin when a person swims or bathes in water where the parasites are present.

Diagnosis

A physician determines the presence of a worm by observing characteristic signs and symptoms and by isolating worms from stool, body fluids, ore body tissue. A history of travel outside the United States, especially to tropical countries, can also be an important clue.

Three fresh stool samples are usually required to confirm the presence of worms. Stool is also examined for white blood cells. Blood tests measure white-cell levels, and help determine whether worms, particularly those

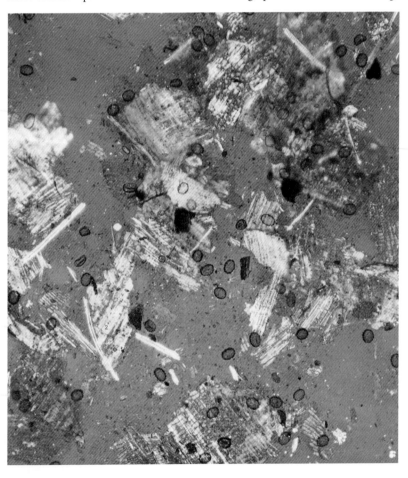

Microphotograph of eggs of roundworms and skin scales.

causing trichinosis, are present in the blood. If muscle pain is present, a muscle biopsy is performed to determine whether trichinosis is present.

Pinworm infestation may be confirmed by examining the child's buttocks and rectal area. Upon close observation, parents can often discover tiny threadlike worms. Deposits of eggs near the anus can be collected with cellophane tape. Once the eggs have been collected the tape should be folded over so only the smooth sides are exposed. A physician can attack the tape to a microscope slide and examine it for the presence of pinworm eggs.

If stool, fluid, or tissue examinations cannot detect the presence of worms, more involved tests such as liver X-rays may be performed.

Treatment

Worm infections do not always require treatment. For example, hookworm larvae causing cutaneous larval migrans usually die spontaneously within a week or two of infestation.

However, a child suffering from trichinosis must receive immediate treatment to prevent complications. Cases of amebiasis or pinworm, giardia, or tapeworm infestation must be treated promptly to prevent spread of infection to others.

In general, a physician must determine whether treatment of parasitic infections is needed. This is based on the severity of infestation, the type of treatment methods available, and whether severe side effects are likely to result from treatment.

If a physician decides that treatment is needed, an oral antiparasitic medication is usually prescribed. Duration of treatment depends on the parasite involved and the severity of infection. After treatment a patient's stool and blood are usually reexamined for evidence of remaining parasites.

An entire family is usually treated for pinworm infestation no matter how many members show symptoms. Treatment also includes taking extra care in the cleaning and trimming of nails and washing of hands.

In most cases treatment of mild worm

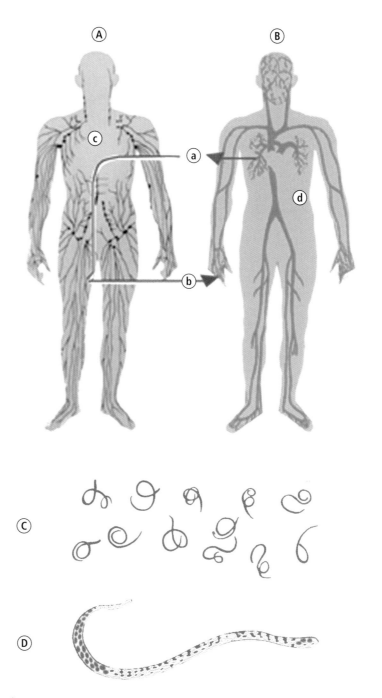

Infection with the parasitic worm Filaria bancrofti, causing elephantiasis. The adult worms live in the human lymphatic system (A). Larvae (C) released by female adults (D) are found in the blood (d) of infected patients (B). The infection is spread by many species of mosquitos (a) from one victim to another (b). The larvae penetrate the bite puncture and eventually reach the lymphatics, where they develop to adult stage, when (d) other people may become infected. Inflammation and fibrosis occur in the vicinity of adult worms, producing progressive lymphatic obstruction and great swelling of the affected area (elephantiasis).

A. Beef tapeworm infection; an intestinal infection caused by the tapeworm (cestode) Taenia saginata. The adult worm lives in the human intestine and may grow 15 to 30 feet in length. Egg-bearing sections of the worm (shown in the illustration) are passed into the stool and are eaten by cattle.

B. Pork tapeworm infection; an intestinal infection by an adult tapeworm: Taenia solium.

C. Dog tapeworm infection caused by Echinococcus granulosum. The worm may become several feet and may cause abdominal mass, pain, cough, coughing up blood.

Worms
Questions & Answers

What are common worms in children?

Worms are parasites that live in the gut. There are several different types, but threadworms most commonly affect children in the UK. Threadworms are thin, short white worms. They are easily passed on in schools or nurseries as the eggs can survive in sand, soil and clay. The eggs get into the body by being eaten with food or dirt.

What are the symptoms of a worm infestation?

Threadworms do not usually produce any symptoms while inside the gut. However, the females work their way out at night and leg eggs around the back passage which causes itching. Scratching results in the eggs getting under the fingernails. If the child then sucks his or her fingers, or handles food before eating it, new eggs enter the gut and the cycle is repeated. Even if your child has no symptoms, it is important to inspect the stools from time to time. Worms will not do your child any harm but they should be treated.

What treatments are available?

If you or your child has worms, it is important to treat the whole family and close contact such as nannies or grandparents. Several medicines are available from your pharmacy or on prescription. Some are only suitable for children over two. Some need to be repeated after two or three weeks.

How can I help my child?

During treatment, good hygiene is essential to ensure that any remaining eggs do not find their way back into the gut. Encourage children to wash their hands and scrub their nails before eating, after visiting the toilet and after playing with animals. A bath or shower first thing in the morning may help to wash away any eggs laid around the back passage overnight. Discourage children from sucking their fingers. Wash all vegetables and fruit well.

W

Threadworm
Questions & Answers

What is threadworm?
Threadworms are worms that can live and feed in the gut. They are not harmful but can cause irritation and are particularly common in children of school age. Threadworm eggs can survive in soil and sand and are caught when a child accidentally eats them on food or dirt.

What should I look out for?
Typical symptoms to look out for are:
- Itching and irritation around your child's back passage. Your child may complain of an itchy bottom or you may notice them scratching this area.
- Thin, short white worms that appear in your child's stools or around their anus. The worms are usually about a centimetre long and look like threads of cotton.
- Worms are usually easier to spot at night when they are more active.

What can I do to help my child?
Your pharmacist can advice you on appropriate medication. Threadworms are easily passed on, so the whole family should use the medication at the same time.
- Keep your child's fingernails short.
- Make sure they wash their hands regularly, especially before eating.

Should I talk to my general physician?
You should talk to a general physician if the child with threadworm is under 2 years old.

infections is successful within a few days to a week. Follow-up visits to a physician are always advised to determine whether treatment has been effective.

In some cases no treatment can completely eliminate parasites from a child's system. In such instances a parasitic infection may clear up by itself, although it may take months to several years.

Survey of common worm infestations

Pin- or threadworm
Pinworm infection (*enterobiasis*) is a disease caused by intestinal roundworms. Nearly 30 percent of all children worldwide are estimated to be infected with pinworm, regardless of their social or economic status.
■ *Treatment*
A single dose of mebendazole, albendazole or pyrantel pamoate, repeated after 2 weeks, effectively cures pinworm infection.

Hookworm
Hookworm infection (*ancylostomiasis*) is a disease of the intestines, resulting in anemia and occasionally skin rash, respiratory problems, or abdominal pain. The diagnosis is made by identifying hookworm eggs in a sample of stool.
■ *Treatment*
A doctor prescribes an oral drug, such as albendazole, mebendazole, or pyrantel pamoate. Because of possible adverse effects to the fetus, these drugs cannot be taken by pregnant women. Iron supplements are given to people with anemia.

Ascaris
Ascaris is a parasite resembling the earthworm. It is spread by contact with soil contaminated by human or animal excrement where adult worms have laid eggs. Most infested children do not have noticeable symptoms. However, a child may develop a cough, a slight fever, and symptoms of pneumonia during the migration of ascaris larvae through the lungs.
■ *Treatment*
The best strategies for preventing ascariasis include using adequate sanitation and avoiding uncooked foods.
To treat a person with ascariasis, a doctor prescribes mebendazole, albendazole, or pyrantel pamoate.

Tapeworm
Tapeworm infection is an intestinal disease caused by one of several species of tapeworms, including *Taenia saginata* (beef tapeworm), *Taenia solium* (pork tapeworm), and *Diphyllobothrium* latum (fish tapeworm).
■ *Treatment*
The first line of defense against tapeworms is careful evaluation of meat and fish by trained inspectors. A person with tapeworms is treated with a single oral dose of praziquantel. Sometimes corticosteroids are given, which help reduce inflammation.

Trichinosis
This is a worm infection caused by *Trichinella spiralis*, a worm found in contaminated animals, especially pigs. Unlike most other worm infections, trichinosis cannot be diagnosed by microscopic examination of the stool. Blood tests for antibodies to *Trichinella* are fairly reliable but only when performed 2 to 3 weeks after the start of the disease.
■ *Treatment*
Trichinosis is prevented by thoroughly cooking meats, especially pork. Oral doses of mebendazole or albendazole are effective against the parasite. Bed rest and analgesics help relieve muscle pain.

W

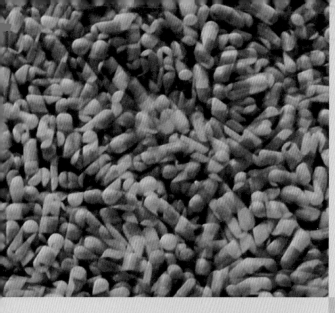
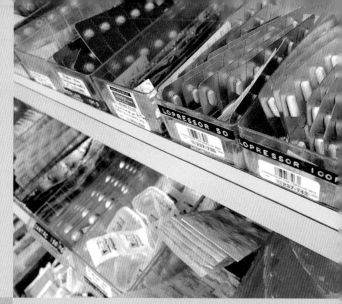
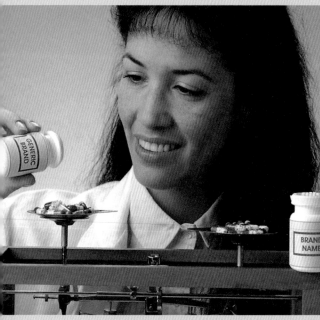
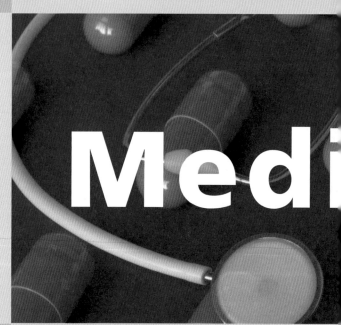

Medi

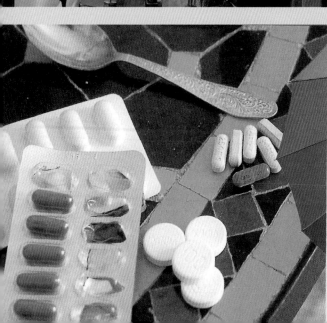
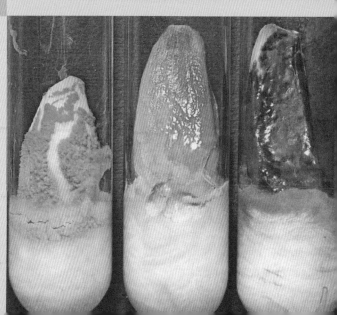

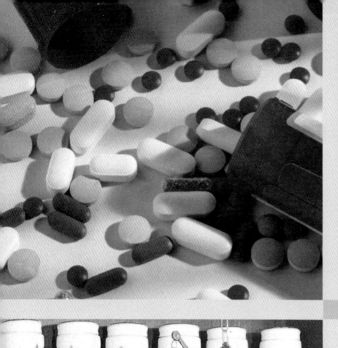
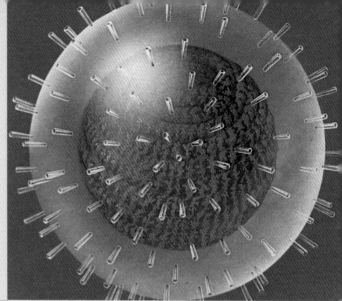
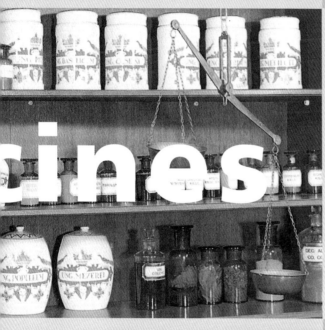
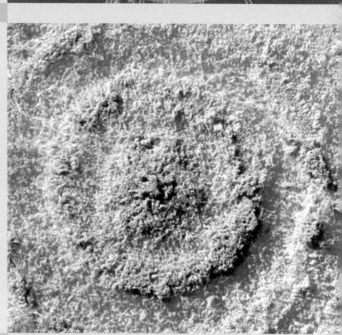
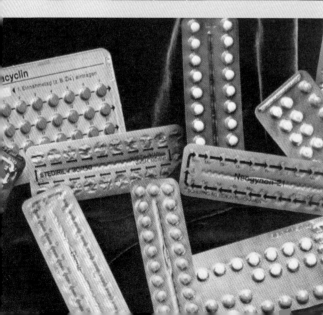
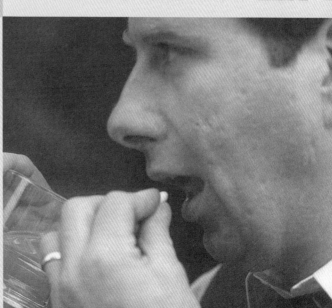

General Introduction

In this section of the encyclopaedia, the authors and editors have given a survey of the general characteristics of prescription and non-prescription medicines. For a substantial number of medicines, recommendations are made regarding indications, and descriptions of side effects and adverse reactions of drugs are offered.

Different people react to the same treatment, medication, test, or procedures in different ways. This section of the encyclopaedia does not attempt to answer all the questions about every situation that you may encounter in taking medicines.

Medicines play a major role in our lives, keeping us healthy and, for some people, prolonging life. A medicine or drug is a substance used as medicine in the treatment of disease, or a mood-altering substance, especially one that is addictive.

Medicines are chemical agents that affect the systems of the body. In general they are taken to treat or prevent disease, but certain drugs, such as the opium narcotics, amphetamines, barbiturates and hallucinogens, are taken for their psychological effects and are drugs of addiction or abuse.

Many medicines are the same as or similar to chemicals occurring naturally in the body and are used either to replace the natural substance (for instance, thyroid hormone) when deficient, or to induce effects that occur when these is an abnormal concentration of the substance, such as with steroids or oral contraceptives.

Other agents are known to interfere with a specific mechanism or to antagonize a normal process. Many other drugs are obtained from other biological systems; fungi, bacteria (antibiotics), plants (for example digitalis) and several others are chemical modifications of natural products.

In addition, there are a number of entirely synthetic drugs (for example barbiturates), some of which are based on active parts of naturally occurring drugs.

Basic mechanisms

A medicine is any drug or other agent used to treat or prevent disease or to treat injury. In devising medicines for treating common conditions, an especially desirable factor is that the medicine should be capable of being taken by mouth - that is, that it should be able to pass into the body unchanged in spite of being exposed to stomach acidity and the enzymes of the digestive system.

In many cases, this is possible but there are some important exceptions, such as insulin that has to be given by injection. This method may also be necessary if vomiting or a disease of the stomach or intestine prevent normal absorption. In most cases, the level of the drug in the blood or tissues determines its effectiveness.

Factors that can make a difference in the effectiveness of a drug include:
- the rate of distribution in the body
- the rate of breakdown
- interactions with other drugs

In addition, there is an individual variation in drug responsiveness that is also apparent with undesired side-effects. These arise because drugs acting on one system commonly act on others.

Side effects

Side effects may be of various kinds, either nonspecific, allergic or specific:
▲ non-specific side effects include nausea, vomiting, diarrhea, malaise or skin reactions;
▲ allergic side effects include urticaria (nettle rash), skin reactions and anaphylaxis (hypersensitivity leading to shock);
▲ specific side effects are related to the action of the medicine on the organ to be treated such as abnormal heart rhythm as a side effect of digitalis.

Mild side effects may be suppressed or simply accepted, but more serious ones must be watched for and the medicine stopped at the first sign of any adverse effect. Drugs may cross the placenta to reach the fetus during pregnancy, interfering with its development and perhaps causing deformity, as happened with thalidomide.

Actions of medicines

Medicines may be used for relief of symptoms - for example, analgesics (painkillers) and anti-emetics (drugs to reduce nausea and vomiting) - or to control a disease.

This can be accomplished by various mechanisms, such as:
▲ killing the infecting agents;
▲ by preventing specific infections;
▲ by restoring normal control over muscle activity (for example, drugs used in the treatment of Parkinson's disease);
▲ by restoring normal control over the mind (for example, antidepressants);
▲ by replacing a lost nutrient or other vital substance (for example, iron in anemia);
▲ by suppressing inflammatory responses (for example, by giving steroids);
▲ by improving the functioning of an organ (for example, digitalis in certain heart conditions);
▲ by protecting a diseased organ by altering the function of a normal one (for example, diuretics to reduce fluid retention in heart failure);
▲ by toxic actions on cancer cells.

New medicines

The search for new medicines or drugs is mainly in the hands of a few giant firms whose products and markets span the world. A large part of the industry is international in outlook, structure and organization, and its commitment to research is great.

This high rate of investment reflects the continuing demand for drugs in world markets and the heavy costs of development. For example, it has been calculated that, for every compound that is brought to therapeutic use, some 3000 or more substances have been made and tested. Today the search for new therapeutic agents can be regarded as a collaborative exercise between the pharmaceutical industry, drug authorities, health services and academic institutions.

Thus private enterprise and government, representing the public interest, are joined in a system of complex activities involving many technical languages and skills. In this system the motives are humanitarian, scientific and commercial.

Interactions

Drug interactions are defined as the alteration of the effects of one drug by the prior or concurrent administration of another and the usual result is an increase or decrease of the effects of one of the drugs.

Desired interactions are usually considered in the context of "combination therapy" (for example, in the treatment of raised blood pressure, asthma, certain infections and malignant tumors), in which two or more drugs are used to increase the therapeutic effects and/or reduce the toxicity of drugs. Unwanted interactions can cause side-effects or the ineffectiveness of the drugs.

Relatively few of the known or suggested drug interactions have been sufficiently analyzed to determine their clinical significance. If an interaction appears likely, a doctor will consider prescribing alternatives.

Drug interactions include the concurrent administration of drugs having the same (or opposing) pharmacological actions as well as alteration of the sensitivity or the responsiveness of the tissues to one drug or another. Many of these interactions can be predicted from a knowledge of the effects of each drug, and by monitoring patients, doctors will be able to detect deviations from expected effects and

dosages can be adjusted accordingly. Interactions that occur because of the way a drug passes through the body are more complicated and difficult to predict because the interacting drugs have unrelated actions. The interactions are mainly due to the processes of absorption, distribution, metabolism and excretion; the type of response expected from the drug is not changed, only the magnitude and duration.

The following general points concerning drug interactions warrant emphasis.

▲ The drugs for which interactions are most significant are those with potent effect and low safety margins, such as
  - digitalis preparations (used in the treatment of heart failure);
  - drugs for the treatment of hypertension (high blood pressure);
▲ drugs for the treatment of low blood sugar.
▲ It may be difficult to distinguish a drug interaction from symptoms of the illness or disease that can affect the body's response to a drug.

▲ Not all patients develop reactions, even when it is known that interactions may occur. Individual factors, such as dose and metabolism, determine whether the phenomenon occurs.
▲ When the effects of drugs are being closely monitored, an interaction usually requires a change of dosage or drug and does not result in significant problems for the patient.

Avoidance of drug interaction
To minimize the incidence and consequences of drug interactions, doctors should adhere to a number of general principles, and patients themselves should help doctors in detecting the symptoms of drug interaction.
▲ Doctors should know their patients' total drug intakes, including all agents prescribed by others and those that are purchased without a prescription. Patients should honestly tell their doctors about all chemicals and other agents they are using.
▲ Doctors should prescribe as few drugs in as low doses as possible for as short a time as needed to

How to use medicines

Important questions to ask your doctor or pharmacist.

- What is the name of this medicine or drug?

- What results can be expected from taking it?

- How long should I wait before reporting if this medicine does not help me?

- How does the substance work?

- What is the exact dose of the medicine or drug?

- What time(s) of the day should I take it?

- Can I drink alcoholic beverages while taking this medicine?

- Do I have to take special precautions with this medicine in combination with other prescription or non-prescription medicines I am taking?

- Do I have to take special precautions with this medicine if I am or want to become pregnant?

- Do I have ta take special precautions about driving and/or operating machinery while taking this medicine?

- Can I take this medicine without regard to whether it is meal time?

- Are there any special instructions I should have about how to use this medicine or drug?

- How long should I continue to take this medicine?

- Can I have a repeat prescription?

- Which side effects should I report?

- Do I have to take all this medicine, or can I stop when symptoms disappear?

- Can I sane any unused portion of this medicine for future use?

- How long can I keep this medicine?

- What should I do if I forget to take a dose of this medicine?

- If this medicine is available without a prescription would it be cheaper than the prescription medicine?

▲ Doctors should observe and monitor their patients for the drugs' effects, particularly after any alteration in therapy.

▲ Doctors should, with the aid of accurate information from their patients, consider drug interactions as possible causes of any unanticipated trouble. If unexpected responses do occur, blood levels of drugs being taken should be measured, if possible. Most importantly, the doses of drugs should be altered until the desired effect is obtained. If this fails, the drugs should be changed to alternatives that will not interact with others being taken.

Side effects

The term side effects, or "adverse drug reactions" embodies a wide variety of toxic drug reactions that occur in numerous types of treatment. Assessing the incidence and consequences of side effects is extremely difficult, as cause-and-effect relationships are often difficult or impossible to prove.

The ultimate proof, which may be unobtainable in cases of severe reactions, depends on disappearance of the effect on withdrawal of the suspected drug (although some severe reactions are irreversible) and reappearance on the administration of the drug.

It is also difficult to select a control population in a clinical setting to differentiate drug-related symptoms and signs from those that are non-drug-related; thus, there is a wide variation in the methods used to collect data on side effects of drugs.

Some studies of side effects rely on reactions reported voluntarily by doctors; others involve selected patient groups; information from patients may also be collected by direct questioning or by patients volunteering information.

There is also a potential for both under- and overestimating the incidence of side effects of drugs. Perhaps 2 to 3 per cent of admissions to hospital are due to drug reactions (excluding deliberate overdose or drug abuse), and among patients already in

achieve a desired effect, and should avoid unnecessary combinations.

▲ Doctors should know the effects, both wanted and unwanted, of all the drugs used (since the spectrum of drug interactions is usually contained within these effects) and know which doses produce which responses.

hospital, the incidence of mild to severe side effects may be as high as 8 to 10 per cent. These data are difficult to interpret in terms of cause-and-effect, mortality and physical damage. The incidence of drug-related deaths is unknown, but probably only a few deaths in medical units are drug-related, and these are often in patients with serious diseases that warrant such risks. The most commonly reported causes of drug-related deaths are:

▲ Gastrointestinal hemorrhage and peptic ulceration, caused by corticosteroids, aspirin and other anti-inflammatory drugs.

▲ Other hemorrhages, caused by anticoagulants (which reduce blood clotting) or cytostatic agents (anti-cancer drugs).

▲ Aplastic anemia, caused by chloramphenicol, phenylbutazone, gold salts or cytostatic agents.

▲ Damage to the liver, caused by paracetamol, chlorpromazine or isoniazid.

▲ Failure of the function of the kidney, caused by analgesics (painkillers).

▲ Infections, caused by corticosteroids or cytostatic drugs.

▲ Anaphylaxis, caused by penicillin or its derivatives or by antisera.

Although individuals vary considerably in their responsiveness to a particular drug effect, most toxic effects are related to the amount of drug taken. Previous contact with the drug is not necessary for the development of toxic reactions.

Side effects may be wanted under certain circumstances. For example, antihistamines given for hay fever may cause drowsiness as a side effect, but drowsiness may be a wanted effect when an antihistamine is given as a mild sleep remedy.

Side effects may also be the result of allergic reactions. These depend on whether the person has become sensitive as a result of prior contact with a drug that functions as an antigen or allergen. Allergic reactions are not related to the level of the dose; the symptoms and signs that develop are determined by the interactions of antigens and antibodies and are largely independent of the specific properties of the drug molecule. In a strict sense, allergic reactions are not com-

pletely unpredictable because a careful medical history and appropriate skin tests may make it possible to identify some of those at risk. This is not possible with all drugs, however, and with penicillin in particular.

Skin reactions

The great number of reactions of the skin to the administration of drugs warrants a separate discussion. The skin is the organ most commonly affected by severe, undesirable effects of drugs, and this can occur by a variety of different mechanisms: in rashes and the like, which follow the taking of drug, are often classed as allergic, but it must be said that the evidence for allergy is frequently scanty.

Allergic reactions
In order to be able, with absolute certainty, to classify such a drug reaction as "allergic" it is essential to demonstrate that antibodies or immune-competent cells directed against an antigen have been formed from the drug or one of its metabolites, and since drugs usually consist of fairly small molecules, the allergen that causes this reaction will as a rule be a compound formed by the drug and tissue protein.

In practice, the diagnosis of an allergic skin reaction to a drug is made only in those who have previously received the drug in question on one occasion and have tolerated it, but who, on renewed treatment, develop skin lesions with or without general symptoms such as high fever. Such people may develop an allergic reaction without having received exactly the same drug previously: for example, taking one sulphonamide drug can readily cause allergy to other sulphonamides in those sensitive to them.

Anaphylactic shock and nettle rash
These are caused by the formation of specific antibodies that become attached to tissue cells called mast cells. When an individual is again exposed to the drug, the allergen reacts with the specific antibodies, and histamines and other active substances are released from the mast cells and cause urticaria and, in some

cases, a fall in blood pressure, spasms of the muscles of the bronchi (airways), and edema (swelling) of the larynx.

In severe allergy, a person can die within minutes from allergic - or anaphylactic - shock. In moderate forms of allergy, urticaria alone may occur. Penicillin, aspirin, heparin (a drug that reduces blood clotting) and X-ray contrast media are fairly common examples of drugs that can cause these reactions.

Cytotoxic allergy
This mechanism takes place when antibodies develop against drug-protein coupling with certain cells, and the immune reaction results in cell damage. Such allergic blood disorders (thrombocytopaenias, leukopaenias and hemolytic anemias) are well known in general medicine.

Toxic-complex syndrome
This syndrome, also called Arthus reaction, is the result of the formation of antibodies that, on reaction with a drug-protein coupling, produce damage to blood vessels via complement, a constituent of blood serum. When antisera were in common use in the treatment of certain infections, they often produced these reactions. At present, penicillin is the commonest cause.

The sufferers develop pain in the joints, fever and blood disorders, and their skin becomes tender and urticaria often occurs.

765

Checklist for safer medicine use

- Make sure you tell the doctor everything that is wrong with you. The more information he/she has, the more effective will be your treatment.

- Make sure each doctor you see knows all the medicines you use regularly - that is, all prescription and non-prescription drugs or medicines, including herbal and homeopathic remedies.

- Carry important medical facts about yourself in your handbag or wallet. Information about drug allergies, chronic diseases or special requirements can be very useful

- Don't share your medicines with anyone. Your prescription was written for you and only you.

- Don't save unused medicine for future use unless you have consulted your doctor. Dispose of unused medicine by flushing it down the toilet.

- Tell your doctor about any medicine you take (even aspirin, allergy pills, cough and cold preparations, antacids, laxatives, vitamins, etc.) before you take any new medicine.

- Learn all you can about medicines you take before you take them. Information sources are your doctor, your nurse, your pharmacist, books in the public library, this computer database.

- Don't take medicines prescribed for some else - even if your symptoms are the same.

- Keep your prescription drugs to yourself. Your drugs may be harmful to someone else.

- Tell your doctor about any symptoms you believe are caused by a medicine that you take.

- Take only medicines that are necessary. Avoid taking non-prescription drugs while taking prescription drugs for a medical problem.

- Before your doctor prescribes for you, tell him about your previous experiences with any medicine - beneficial results, side effects, adverse reactions or allergies.

- Don't keep any medicines that change mood, alertness or judgment - such as sedatives, narcotics or tranquillizers - by your bedside. These cause many accidental deaths by overdose. You may unknowingly repeat a dose when you are half asleep or confused.

- Know the names of your medicines. These include the generic name, the brand name and the generic names of all ingredients in a medicine mixture. Your doctor, nurse or pharmacist can give you this information.

- Study the labels of all non-prescription medicines. If the information is incomplete or if you have questions, ask the pharmacist for more details.

- Obtain a standard measuring spoon from your pharmacy for liquid medicines. Kitchen teaspoons and tablespoons are not accurate enough.

- Store all medicines away from moisture and heat. Bathroom medicine cabinets are usually unsuitable.

- Follow diet instructions when you take medicines. Some work better on a full stomach, others on an empty stomach. Some drugs are more useful with special diets.

- Tell your doctor about any allergies you have. A previous allergy to a medicine may make it dangerous to prescribe again. People with other allergies, such as eczema, hay fever, asthma, bronchitis and food allergies, are more likely to be allergic to medicines.

- Prior to surgery, tell your doctor, anesthesiologist or dentist about any drugs you have taken in the past few weeks. Advise them of any cortisone drugs you have taken within two years.

- If you become pregnant while taking any medicine, including birth control pills, tell your doctor immediately.

- Avoid all drugs while you are pregnant, if possible. If you must take medicines during pregnancy, record names, amounts, dates and reasons.

- If you see more than one doctor, tell each one about medicines others have prescribed.

- Note the expiration date on each drug label. Discard outdated ones safely. If no expiration date appears and it has been at least one year since taking the medication, it may be best to discard it.

- Pay attention to the information in the charts about safety while driving, piloting or working in dangerous places.

Delayed allergy

Allergic contact eczema due to drugs applied directly to the skin is a common reaction. The same type of allergic reaction may be caused by taking the same drugs by mouth, injected into a vein, as a pessary, etc. Sulphonamides, chlorothiazide and numerous other drugs may produce this effect.

Addictive and abused drugs

The drugs that are addictive and/or often abused include very valuable substances that, taken in moderate doses that have been properly prescribed, relieve pain and produce sleep, but in large doses cause various physical and psychological effects, including stupor, coma and, commonly, convulsions. Among the habit-forming drugs are opium and its derivatives, cocaine, amphetamines and barbiturates.

One of the major issues regarding drug dependence refers to the question of why young people take such drugs. There appear to be three major reasons for doing so:

▲ To obtain something valued. For instance, to be accepted among their circle of friends (one of the main reasons for the epidemic quality of drug-taking), or to be awake, alert and lively, throughout weekend parties that may in themselves be a means of filling in time away from an unacceptable or unaccepting home.

▲ To remove discomfort or anxiety. For example, a boy who is shy and lonely finds that he can overcome his handicap with the help of alcohol or amphetamines. Another who is despondent or who has accepted social failure (especially with the opposite sex) may find temporary relief, a new identity, and at the same time may express, against himself, the resentment and aggression that frustration always produces (hence the seemingly self-destructive element of much drug-taking).

▲ To dispel boredom. All humans, especially the vigorous and intelligent young, have exploratory drives towards mastering things

and towards new and exciting, even dangerous, experiences; in their words they seek "kicks."

The problem is complicated by the varied effects of different drugs (not always the same in all people) and by the development of physical as well as psychological dependence. Thus, while drug-taking may be initiated in one way, it may be continued for quite different reasons.

One further general point concerns what is not known, and unfortunately the list is long. For example, we do not know the full extent of the problem - that is, how many are flirting with drugs, not just the factors that "hook" the few.

In particular, we do not know about treatment of severe cases; doctors are good at getting patients "off the hook" but very poor in keeping them off - all the more reason for trying to prevent addiction, and for the cooperation of lay people in the aftercare of former addicts.

Reflection on the above facts will suggest the principal ways of tackling the problem and where we, the general public, may help. Controlling sources of addictive drugs, law enforcement, the provision of treatment centers and research facilities are all of primary importance but are hardly our problems, except that, if responsible people repeatedly asked what was being done in these directions, there would be a powerful stimulus to getting something done, or getting something more done.

The most important thing for lay adults to be, if they are to help, is inquisitive, because if they are truly inquisitive either about the problem as a whole or about particular young persons, they will become concerned. They will not act on preconceived or emotional judgements but will try to find out, and that means that communication will be two-way and therefore potentially useful.

We know that it is no use talking at young people, or trying to scare them by depicting horrific consequences, but if there is a real exchange of facts, opinions and feelings between two parties, or within a

group, understanding and perhaps trust will have been gained on both sides and something practical may

Emergency action

If you think a child has swallowed a medicine or poison:

• **Get the child to the accident and emergency (casualty) department of the nearest hospital as soon as possible.**

• **Take the container of the medicine or poison with you so the doctor knows that the child has taken.**

• **Do not try and make the child sick. This may make the things worse.**

• **If the child is unconscious, lay him on his side to make breathing easier and to stop him inhaling vomit if he is sick.**

develop.

In this way, if young people admit to or are reported as misusing drugs, or if their erratic and variable behavior (their unhappiness and irritability, their exhaustion on Monday mornings, deterioration in their work, health and social relationships) suggests it, then we should begin thinking about the possible reasons as given here, and should make an opportunity to talk with them and to make plans with them.

A high priority in the discussion will be whom to call in, and of course parents must first be considered, as well as school principals, priests, doctors or social workers.

The majority of these cases, especially in the young, turn out to be based on familiar personal and family problems, directed into these new channels by unfortunate, but increasingly common, local conditions and opportunities. It is not quite such a new problem as may be supposed but it does need the active consideration and help of all responsible people, especially parents.

Many medicines, if taken by a woman when pregnant, may harm the unborn baby. Therefore, as a general rule it is best to avoid almost all medicines, including those that you purchase from your pharmacy or health food shop, if you think that you may be pregnant or are trying to conceive.

If you are taking any regular treatment, you should tell your doctor if you are trying to conceive or as soon as you know that you are pregnant. If you are on any medicines which the doctor thinks are essential, he or she will discuss the risks and benefits of continuing to take these medicines with you.

If you intend to self-medicate, do not simply take medicines that you have in the home and have used before in the belief that they will be all right. Always check with your doctor or pharmacist first, no matter how harmless you think the medicine is. There may be safer alternatives.

One rare exception is folic acid, a supplement that every woman planning a pregnancy should take. This has been shown to reduce the risk of spina bifida. If you are planning a pregnancy, you should take 1/2 mg of folic acid daily for at least a month before trying to conceive and continue taking it up until the 12th week of your pregnancy. Most women are unable to get sufficient folic acid from their diet, and therefore taking a supplement is the best way of ensuring that they get the right amount.

Ways to use medicines

There are many ways to take or use medicines, depending on their nature of characteristics, as well as on the nature of the illness. Medicines may be taken or used either
- by injection,
- topically (applied to the area where it is needed such as the skin, eye, ear, and nose).

Remember that one person's medicine can be another person's poison. The powerful ingredients in the medicine prescribed by the doctor to help you could harm someone else. So do not share your medicines with other people, especially children. You should never accept a medicine from a neighbour or relative, because they may have been prescribed for a different type of ailment.

Over half the cases of poisoning in children are caused by them swallowing medicines. Young children are naturally curious and do not understand danger. You cannot expect children to understand the difference between a brightly-coloured pill and a sweet. The reasons why pills can look like sweets are simple: there are only a few shapes and bright colours help people who take several medicines tell one type from another. Medicines come in many different forms. All of them can be dangerous to children. All bottles of tablets and capsules supplied from the pharmacy come with child-resistant tops. These tops make it harder for children to get at the medicine and some make a clicking noise to warn you that someone is trying to open the bottle. But they are not childproof: many children can open them. Even though those medicine bottles are safer you should still keep them out of children's reach.

Oral medicines

Tablets

Tablets contain the medicine's active component together with other ingredients in a compressed solid dosage form. With today's technology, many forms of tablets have been developed to cater to the needs of different kinds of people with different conditions.

▲ Sublingual tablet
When placed under the tongue, the medicine is absorbed rapidly into the blood by the blood vessels.

▲ Soluble effervescent tablet
This tablet dissolves in water to release the medicine. The liquid preparations is then drunk.

▲ Chewable tablet
This is chewed before swallowing, and is not to be swallowed whole. It is usually designed to coat the stomach lining. Most medicines in this form need to be broken down by physical action, i.e. chewing action.

▲ Enteric-coated tablet
This is to be swallowed whole. The special coating on this tablet form delays the release of the medicine until after it has passed the stomach. The medicine is then released in the intestine where the environment is less acidic. It s designed to release medicines in the intestine instead of the stomach to prevent from being destroyed by the stomach juices or irritate the lining of the stomach.
Since antacids make the stomach environment less acidic, do not take them with enteric-coated tablets, otherwise the medicine will be released in the stomach instead of the intestine.

▲ Slow-release tablet
Some conditions require a tablet that slowly releases the medicine over a prolonged period of time. The slow-release tablet works in this manner and since the time element is important, it should be taken according to the prescribed hour of dose.

Capsules

Capsules are solid dosage forms containing the drug substance enclosed in either a hard or soft, soluble container or shell made of gelatin.

▲ Hard gelatin capsule
This consists of two compartments, one slipped over the other, hence completely surrounding the medicine.

▲ Soft elastic capsule
This is a single soft gelatin shell that contains the medicine.

▲ Enteric capsule
Upon reaching the stomach, this capsule prevents the shell from breaking and releases the medicine only when it has reached the intestine.

▲ Slow-release capsule
Like the tablet, this capsule slowly releases the medicine over a prolonged time period. Since the time element is important, this should be taken according to the prescribed hour of dose.

Liquids

Liquid preparations are oral medicines combined with preservatives, flavours, colours, and other ingredients. These oral medicines are preferred when a patient is unable to swallow tablets or capsules. There are three important points to consider:

▲ Follow the Shake Well instruction on the label. This will mix the medicine evenly in the liquid base, this ensuring a correctly measured dose.

▲ Use only the measuring spoon to get the correct dose, unless otherwise directed by the doctor or pharmacist.

▲ Follow all the instructions written on the label, including those for storage. Some liquids undergo physical and chemical changes when not properly stored.

Injections

An injection may be done:
- intravenously (IV, into the vein);
- subcutaneously (under the skin).
Injections are often preferred or required when:

▲ the patient cannot take oral medicines due to unconsciousness, stomach irritations or obstructions in the oral cavity;

▲ rapid and localized action is needed, such as an injection in a joint in case of an inflammatory process.
The manner in which injections are administered depends on the nature of the ailment. Since injections are difficult to administer, they should be given only by qualified medical personnel, unless instructed to do so yourself (as with diabetics).

Suppositories and Pessaries

Suppository

A suppository is a medicated solid dosage form inserted into the rectum. It is used to treat hemorrhoids or loosen bowels during constipation.

▲ How to store suppositories
It is best to store suppositories in the refrigerator, but ensure that they are labelled and kept separately from the food. Chilling it for 30 minutes before insertion will prevent if from melting.

▲ How to insert a suppository
- Unwrap the suppository.
- Lie sideways, keeping your upper leg bent while the lower leg is resting on the floor.
- Wait for about 15 minutes.

Pessary

A pessary is a medicated solid dosage form inserted into the vagina or urethra. It is used to treat urinary tract infections. Consult your doctor on the safety of use during menstruation or pregnancy. Sexual intercourse should be avoided during the period of treatment.

▲ How to store pessaries
Store the pessaries in the refrigerator, properly labelled and kept separately from food. Chilling it for 30 minutes will prevent it from melting.

▲ How to insert a pessary
- Unwrap the pessary.
- Insert the pessary into the vagina, tapered end first, using a finger or an applicator.
- Wash your hands with soap and water.

Topical medicines

Topical medicines are drug preparations that are applied for local action usually on the skin, into the eyes, ear, and nose. Most of them can be bought without a prescription, but you must ask the pharmacist for the proper application or use.

Skin preparations

The most widely used topical medicines are those for the skin. They may come in the form of ointments, creams, lotions, or patches.

▲ What to consider when using skin preparations
- Follow closely the directions for use.
- Do not touch your mouth, eyes, or any part of your body immediately after applying skin preparations. A good soap-and-water wash should clean off the medicine from your fingers/hands.

▲ How to use creams, ointments and lotions
- Use soap and water to wash the infected area, as well as your hands.
- Replace the cover/cap of the cream/ointment/lotion. Do not allow the tip of the medicine container/tube to get into contact with the affected skin area, to avoid contamination.

▲ How to use transdermal patches
- Check the skin area on which the transdermal patch is to be applied for cuts, scratches, hair or other irritation.
- Apply the patch, making sure the whole skin area is covered.

Eye and ear preparations

The eyes and ears are some of the most sensitive body parts, and the most vulnerable to infections because their openings lend them to greater exposure. Eye and ear preparations are effective in treating local infections of the eye and the ear canals.

Eye and ear preparations may come in the form of drops or ointments. Since they are applied directly into the eye and ear canals sufficient medical advice should be sought as to their proper use and action.

▲ What to consider when using eye and ear preparations
- As with all medicines keep the preparations out of children's reach.
- Discard the preparation one month after use as they deteriorate rapidly.
- Do not overuse the preparations because the eyes and ears can only contain a limited amount of medication to fight the infection. Consult your doctor or pharmacist for the

proper use and dosing of the medications.

▲ How to use eye drops/ointments
- Use soap and water to wash hands.
- Tilt your head back and look up.
- Hold the dropper, instill the required number of drops into the lower eye pockets. For the ointment, gently squeeze the required amount of ointment into the lower eye pocket.
▲ Close the eyes gently for several seconds, blinking every now and then the spread the medication to the other parts of the eye.
▲ Replace the cap/cover of the medication and store it in a safe place.
▲ How to use ear drops
- Use soap and water to wash fingers/hands.
- Straighten the ear canal by pulling the ear lobe up or down, and then back.
- Stay in position for 2-3 minutes.
- Use soap and water to wash hands/fingers.

Nose preparations
They are drug preparations, in the form of drops or sprays, applied into the nasal cavity to treat local infections of the nose.
▲ What to consider when using nasal preparations
- Make sure that the inner walls of the nose are free from dirt, mucous and other foreign materials. A soft tissue of cloth may be used to clean the walls.
- These preparations are not to be taken into the mouth. Seek medical help in case of accidental ingestion.
▲ How to use nasal drops
- Wash your hands with soap and water.
- Insert the applicator into the nostrils, taking care not to allow contact with the inner walls of the nose.
- Stay in position for 2-3 minutes.
- Wash hands with soap and water.
▲ How to use nasal sprays
- Check the spray by actuating it into the air.
- Insert the nose-piece of the aerosol container into one nostril and close the other nostril by gently pressing a finger on it.
- Repeat the procedure with the other nostril.
- Replace the cap/cover of the canister and store in a safe place.

Inhaler

Many inhaled asthma medications are taken with a metered-dose inhaler. An inhaler can be used with a spacer, a device that holds the medication until you breathe it in. Inhalers and spacers must be used properly for the medication to be effective.
▲ How to use an asthma inhaler
- Breathe out deeply until no more air can be expelled from the lungs.
- Press the top of the canister down while inhaling deeply. It is essential to fire the aerosol as soon as you start breathing in so that your breath carries the particles of the drug as far down into the lungs as possible.
- Release pressure from the canister, remove inhaler from the mouth and breathe out gently.

Medicines A-Z

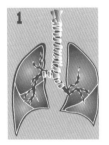 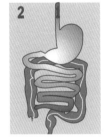 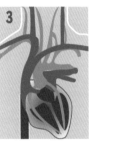 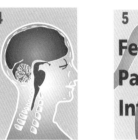

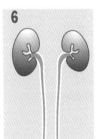 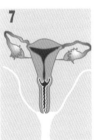 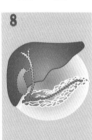 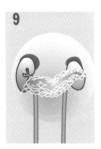 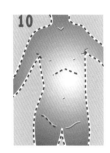

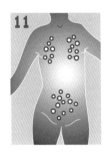 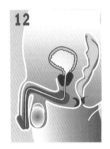 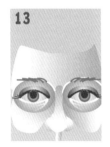 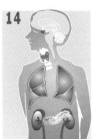 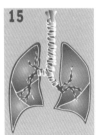

For a major group op medicines, drug profiles are designed to give you detailed information on the nations' most frequently prescribed medicines, plus widely used over-the-counter medications. To facilitate the classification of the drug, these descrioptions are accompanied by a small drawing indicating the major area of uses.

1. Disorders of the respiratory tract.
2. Digestive system.
3. Disease of heart and blood vessels.
4. Brain and nervous system.
5. Fever, pain and infection.
6. Kidneys and urinary tract disorders.
7. Female genital organs.
8. Liver, gallbladder, and pancreas.
9. Endocrine organs and diabetes.
10. Antibiotics.
11. Male genital; organs.
13. Disorders of sense organs.
14. Corticosteroids.
15. Musculoskeletal apparatus.

A

Abilify
A proprietary, prescription-only preparation of aripripazole. It is used for the psychotic symptoms in dementia.

Acarbose
An enzyme inhibitor that interferes with the conversion in the intestine of starch and sucrose in glucose and is used in diabetic treatment.

Accupro
A proprietary, prescription-only preparation of the ACE inhibitor quinapril. It can be used in the treatment of raised blood pressure.

Accuretic
A proprietary, prescription-only compound preparation of the quinapril and the thiazide diuretic drug. It can be used to treat raised blood pressure.

Acebutolol
A proprietary, prescription-only preparation of the beta-blocker type. It can be used in the treatment of raised blood pressure.

Acemetacin
A proprietary, prescription-only preparation of NSAID-type used to treat serious rheumatic complaints, arthritic and rheumatic pain and other musculoskeletal disorders.

Acetazolamide
A proprietary, prescription-only preparation of the carbonic anhydrase inhibitor type. It can be used as a glaucoma treatment.

Acetoxyl gelcupro
A proprietary, non-prescription preparation of the keratolytic and antimicrobial drug benzoyl peroxide, used for acne.

Acetylcysteine
A proprietary, prescription-only preparation which reduces the viscosity of sputum.

Alkaloids

Alkaloid is a chemical term applied to a group of compounds that are used as medicines. The majority of alkaloids were originally extracted from plants and are chemically heterocyclic, often complex, organic compounds with basic (alkali) properties and in medicine they are usually administered in the form of their salts.
Examples still in medical use include

- the belladonna alkaloids from *Atropa belladonna*: for instance, atropine sulphate and hyoscine hydrobromium;

- the alkaloids of opium from the poppy *Papaver somniferum*: for instance, codeine phosphate, morphine sulphate and papaverine;

- the ergot alkaloids: for instance, ergometrine maleate and ergotamine tartrate;

- the cinchone alkaloids: quinidine and quinine from the bark of the cinchona tree;

- the vinca alkaloids: for instance, vinblastine sulphate, vincristine sulphate and vindesine sulphate;

- ephedrine hydrochloride from ancient Chinese plants of the *Ephedra* species;

- nicotine from *Nicotina tabacum*;

- tubocurarine chloride, originally a South American arrow-poison from *Chondrodendrion tomentosum*;

- pilocarpine form a South American *Pilocarpus* shrub;

- ipecacuanha, which contains emetine and cephaline from ipecac (Brazilian root).

Acezide
A proprietary, prescription-only compound preparation of the ACE inhibitor quinapril and the thiazide diuretic. It can be used to treat raised blood pressure.

Achromycin
A proprietary, prescription-only preparation of the broad-spectrum antibacterial and antibiotic drug tetracycline. It can be used to treat a wide variety of infections.

Aciclovir
A proprietary, prescription-only preparation with antiviral properties used in the treatment of herpes infections and simular viral infections.

Acipimox
A proprietary, prescription-only preparation used as lipid-lowering drug in hyperlipidaemia (high blood levels of lipids).

Acitretin
A proprietary, prescription-only preparation vitamin A used in the treatment of psoriasis and other serious skin disorders.

Aclarubicin
A proprietary, prescription-only preparation with cytotoxic properties used in the treatment of various cancers.

Acnecide
A proprietary, non-prescription pre-

Acetoxyl gel

Properties
This medicine belongs to the family of topical (applied to the skin) anti-acne preparations, containing benzoyl peroxide as active ingredient. It is used in the treatment for acne and other skin conditions such as pressure sores. Acne is a condition of the skin that ranges in appearance from small raised bumps to pustules (large cysts and pimples). Acne is so common that more than 80 percent of the population will have some form of it at some time in their lives. This medication works by decreasing the cohesiveness of skin cells, causing the skin to peel, which is helpful in the treatment of mild acne and other skin conditions. The drug also slowly releases oxygen from the skin, which controls some skin bacteria. This drug is usually not effective in treating severe acne.

Before using this medicine
Before you use this medicine check with your doctor, or pharmacist:
- if you ever had any unusual or allergic reaction to tretinoin.
- if you are on a low-salt, low-sugar, or any other special diet, or if you are allergic to any substance, such as certain preservatives or dyes.
- if you are sunburned, or have an open skin wound.
- if you are pregnant, intending to become pregnant or breast-feeding an infant while using this medicine.

Treatment
This medication is used to relieve or prevent the symptoms of your medical problem. Take them as directed. Do not take more of them and do not take them more often than recommended on the label. To do so may increase the chance of absorption through the skin and the chance of side effects.
METHOD OF USE: Wash skin with non-medicated soap. Dry gently with towel. Rub medicine into affected areas. Keep away from eyes, nose, mouth. Apply one or more times daily. With a fair complexion, apply the drug only at bedtime. The time lapse before the drug works is 1 to 2 weeks. Use of the drug is not recommended for infants and children.

Side effects
The following side effects may occur:
- Painful skin
- Irritation

These side effects should disappear as your body adjusts to the medication. Tell your doctor about any side effects that are persistent or particularly bothersome.
You should discontinue the use of the drug when the following side effects occur:
- *Rash*
- *Blistering*
- *Swelling of skin area*
- *Excessive dryness of the skin*
- *Excessive peeling of the skin*

Foods with benzoic acid may cause the occurrence of a skin rash; as is also the case with cinnamon.

Interactions
This medicine may interact with several other skin medications. The combined use of this medicine with other anti-acne topical preparations may cause excessive skin irritation. The same holds true for the use of skin-peeling agents such as salicylic acid, sulphur, resorcinol; such as anti-acne topical preparations, medicated cosmetics, skin preparations with alcohol, and also with soaps or cleansers. The combined effect may cause severe skin irritation.

Storage
This medicine should be stored in a cool, dry place in a closed container. Store away from heat and direct light. Keep out of reach of children. Do not store in the bathroom medicine cabinet because the heat or moisture may cause the medicine to break down. Do not keep outdated medicine or medicine no longer needed. Flush the contents of the container down the toilet, unless otherwise directed.

---

paration of the keratolytic and antimicrobial drug benzoyl peroxide used for acne.

Acnegel
A proprietary, non-prescription preparation of the keratolytic and antimicrobial drug benzoyl peroxide used for acne.

Acnidazil
A proprietary, non-prescription preparation of the antifungal drug miconazole and benzoyl peroxide used to treat skin disorders.

Acnisal
A proprietary, non-prescription preparation of the keratolytic agent salicylic acid used for acne.

Acrivastine
A proprietary, prescription-only preparation of the antihistamine-type used for allergic conditions.

Acrosaxacin
An antibacterial and antibiotic drug used to treat gonorrhoea.

Actal Tablets
A proprietary, non-prescription preparation of the antacid alexitol sodium used for stomach conditions.

Act-HIB
A proprietary, prescription-only vaccine preparation for Hemophilus influenzae infection.

Actinac

Actinac
A proprietary, prescription-only compound preparation of the broad-spectrum antibiotic drug choramphenicol and the corticosteroid drug hydrocortisone.

Actonel
A proprietary, prescription-only preparation of risedronate. It is used to for the prevention and treatment of osteoporosis.

Actron
A proprietary, prescription-only preparation of the NSAID drug paracetamol, aspirin and the antacid sodium bicarbonate.

Acupan
A proprietary, prescription-only preparation of the NSAID drug nefopam used to treat pain conditions.

Acyclovir
A proprietary, prescription-only antiviral preparation for the treatment of viral diseases such as herpes infections.

Adalat
A proprietary, prescription-only preparation of the calcium-channel blocker nifedipine, used as an anti-angina treatment.

Adcortyl
A proprietary, prescription-only preparation of the corticosteroid and anti-inflammatory drug triamcinolone acetonide.

Adenosine
A proprietary, prescription-only drug used to correct heart irregularities.

Adifax
A proprietary, prescription-only preparation of the appetite-suppressant dexfenfluramine used for the treatment of obesity.

Adizem
A proprietary, prescription-only preparation of calcium-channel blocker diltiazem hydrochloride. It can be used to treat raised blood pressure and attacks of angina pectoris.

Advair
A proprietary, prescription-only preparation of fluticasone/salmeterol. It is an inhaler used in the treatment of asthmatic symptoms.

Aerobec
A proprietary, prescription-only preparation of the corticosteroid and anti-asthmatic drug beclomethasone diprionate used to prevent asthmatic attacks.

Aerocrom
A proprietary, prescription-only compound preparation of the anti-allergic drug sodium cromoglycate and the beta-receptor stimulant salbutamol used to prevent asthma symptoms.

Aerolin Autohaler
A proprietary, prescription-only preparation of the beta-receptor stimulant salbutamol used as a bronchodilator in reversible obstructive airways disease and asthma.

Afrazine
A proprietary, non-prescription preparation of the decongestant drug oxymetazoline hydrochloride. It can be used for the relief of nasal congestion.

Agarol
A proprietary, non-prescription compound preparation of the laxative phenolphthalein and the laxative liquid paraffin. It can be used to treat constipation.

Akineton
A proprietary, prescription-only preparation of the anticholinergic drug biperiden used in the treatment of parkinsonism.

Aknemin
A proprietary, prescription-only preparation of the antibacterial and antibiotic drug minocycline used to treat infections.

Albendazole
A proprietary, prescription-only anthelmintic preparation used for the treatment of Echinococcus infections.

Alclometasone
A proprietary, prescription-only preparation with corticosteroid properties. In can be used in the treatment of inflammatory skin disorders.

Alcobon
A proprietary, prescription-only preparation of the antifungal drug flucytosine used to treat systemic infections by yeasts.

Alcoderm
A proprietary, non-prescription preparation of liquid paraffin and emollient agents used for dry and itchy skin.

Aldactide
A proprietary, prescription-only compound preparation of the diuretic drugs spironolactone and hydroflumethazide, used for congestive heart failure treatment.

Aldactone
A proprietary, prescription-only preparation of diuretic drugs used to treat oedema and congestive heart failure.

Aldesleukin
A proprietary, prescription-only preparation of interleukin-2, an anti-cancer drug.

Aldomet
A proprietary, prescription-only preparation of the antisympathetic drug methyldopa, used to treat raised blood pressure.

Alexan
A proprietary, prescription-only preparation of the anticancer drug cytarabine. It can be used in the treatment of acute leukaemia.

Alexitol sodium
A proprietary, non-prescription preparation containing aluminium used as an antacid drug. In can be used in the treatment of hyperacidity, dyspepsia and indigestion.

Alfacalcidol
A proprietary, prescription-only preparation of calciferol. It can be used to treat calcium deficiency.

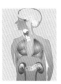

Adcortyl

Properties
This medicine belongs to the family of topical (applied to the skin) corticosteroids, containing an adrenocorticoid as active ingredient. It is used to relieve the symptoms of any itching, rash, or inflammation of the skin; it does not treat the underlying cause of the skin problem. It also relieves redness, swelling and itching caused by insect bites, poison ivy, poison oak, poison sumach, soaps, cosmetics, sunburn, and numerous skin rashes.
Topical adrenocorticosteroids are absorbed through the skin and may rarely affect growth in children. Before using this medicine in children you should discuss the use of it with your doctor.

Before using this medicine
Before you use this medicine check with your doctor, or pharmacist:
- if you ever had any unusual or allergic reaction to adrenocorticoids or corticosteroids in general.
- if you are on a low-salt, low-sugar, or any other special diet, or if you are allergic to any substance, such as certain preservatives or dyes.
- if you have diabetes, stomach ulcer, or infection at the treatment site.
- if you are pregnant, intending to become pregnant or breast-feeding an infant while using this medicine.
- if you have any of the following medical problems:
Diabetes mellitus (sugar diabetes)
Infection at the place of treatment
Ulceration at the place of treatment
Tuberculosis

Treatment
This medication is used to relieve or prevent the symptoms of your medical problem. Take them as directed. Do not take more of them and do not take them more often than recommended on the label.
To do so may increase the chance of absorption through the skin and the chance of side effects. In addition, too much use, especially on thin skin areas (for example, armpits, face, groin), may result in thinning of the skin and stretch marks.

Side effects
The following side effects may occur:
- Acne or oily skin
- Blistering
- Burning sensations
- Itching
- Dryness of the skin
- Secondary infection
- Thinning of skin
- Unusual hair growth
- Unusual loss of hair
These side effects should disappear as your body adjusts to the medication. Tell your doctor about any side effects that are persistent or particularly bothersome.
The above side effects are more likely to occur in children and elderly patients, who are usually more sensitive to the effects of this medicine.
When the gel, solution, lotion, or aerosol from this medicine is applied, a mild, temporary stinging may be expected.

Interactions
This medicine interacts with several other drugs such as antibiotics (causing a decreased antibiotic effect) and antifungals (causing a decreased antifungal effect).
Be sure to tell your doctor about any medications you are currently taking.

Storage
This medicine should be stored at room temperature in closed containers. Store away from heat and direct light. Keep out of reach of children, since overdose may be dangerous in children. Do not store in the bathroom medicine cabinet because the heat or moisture may cause the medicine to break down. Keep the medicine from freezing. Do not keep outdated medicine.

Alfentanil
A proprietary, prescription-only narcotic analgesic drug used for short surgical operations.

Alfyzosin
A proprietary, prescription-only alpha-adrenoreceptor blocker that is used to treat urinary retention.

Algesal
A proprietary, non-prescription preparation of diethylamide salicylate used to the skin for the relief of rheumatic conditions.

Algicon
A proprietary, non-prescription preparation containing various antacids used for the treatment of heartburn and gastric reflux.

Alginic acid
A proprietary, non-prescription preparation of alginate used to treat reflux esophagitis.

Algipan rub
A proprietary, non-prescription preparation of capsicum oleoresin, methyl nicotinate and glycol salicylate applied to the skin for the relief of muscle pain and stiffness.

Algipan spray
A proprietary, non-prescription preparation of capsicum oleoresin, methyl nicotinate and glycol salicylate applied to the skin for the relief of muscle pain and stiffness.

A

Alophen Pills

Properties

This medicine contains as active ingredients aloin and phenolphthalein, a stimulant laxative. Stimulant laxatives (also known as contact laxatives) are medicines taken by mouth to encourage bowel movements by acting on the intestinal wall. They increase the muscle contractions that move along the stool mass.

Before using this medicine

Before you use this medicine check with your doctor, or pharmacist:
-   if you ever had any unusual or allergic reaction to laxatives.
-   if you are on a low-salt, low-sugar, or any other special diet, or if you are allergic to any substance, such as sulfites or other preservatives or dyes.
-   if you are pregnant. Stimulant laxatives may cause unwanted effects in the expectant mother if improperly used. Some of the stimulant laxatives may cause contractions of the womb.
-   if you are breast-feeding an infant. Some stimulant laxatives may pass into the breast milk. Although the amount of laxative in the milk is generally thought to be too small to cause problems in the child, your doctor should be told that you plan to use such laxatives.
-   if you have any of the following medical problems:
    Appendicitis (or signs of)
    Colostomy
    Diabetes (sugar disease)
    Heart disease
    Hypertension
    Ileostomy
    Intestinal blockage
    Laxative habit
    Rectal bleeding

Treatment

For safe and effective use of bulk-forming laxatives.
Follow your doctor's orders if this laxative was prescribed.
Follow the manufacturer's package directions if you are treating yourself.
At least six to eight 8-ounce glasses of liquids should be taken each day.
Stimulant laxatives are usually taken on an empty stomach for rapid effect. Results are slowed if taken with food.
Laxatives should not be given to young children (up to 6 years of age) unless prescribed by their doctor. Since children cannot usually describe their symptoms very well, a doctor should check the child before giving this medicine.

Side effects

Along with the needed effects, a medicine may cause some unwanted effects.
Side effects that should be reported to your doctor: breathing difficulty; burning on urination; confusion; headache; irregular heartbeat; irritability; mood or mental changes; muscle cramps; skin rash; unusual tiredness.

Laxative habit

Laxatives are to be used to provide short-term relief only, unless otherwise directed by your doctor. Laxatives are overused by many people. Such a practice often leads to dependence on the laxative action to produce a bowel movement. In some cases, overuse of some laxatives has caused damage to the nerves, muscles, and tissues of the intestines and bowel.

Interactions

This medicine may interact with several other drugs, such as amiloride, antacids, other laxatives, potassium supplements, tetracycline antibiotics and triamterene.
Be sure to tell your doctor about any medications you are currently taking.

Storage

Store away from heat and direct light. Keep out of the reach of children. Do not store in the bathroom medicine cabinet because the heat or moisture may cause the medicine to break down.

Algitec

A proprietary, prescription-only preparation of cimetidine and alginic acid used as an ulcer-healing drug for benign peptic ulcers.

Alimix

A proprietary, prescription-only preparation of cisapride. It can be used to stimulate the stomach and intestine.

Alka-Seltzer

A proprietary, non-prescription preparation containing aspirin, citric acid and sodium bicarbonate used for general aches and pains.

Alkeran

A proprietary, prescription-only preparation of the anticancer drug melphalan. It can be used in the treatment of myelomatosis.

Allegra

A proprietary, prescription-only preparation of fexofenadine. It is used to for the symptomatic relief of rheumatic aches and pains.

Allegron

A proprietary, prescription-only preparation of the antidepressant drug nortriptyline used to treat depressive illness.

Allopurinol

A proprietary, prescription-only preparation used to treat excess uric acid in the blood in order to prevent attacks of gout.

Alphaderm

Properties
This medicine belongs to the family of topical (applied to the skin) corticosteroids, containing an adrenocorticoid as active ingredient. It is used to relieve the symptoms of any itching, rash, or inflammation of the skin; it does not treat the underlying cause of the skin problem. It also relieves redness, swelling and itching caused by insect bites, poison ivy, poison oak, poison sumach, soaps, cosmetics, sunburn, and numerous skin rashes.
Topical adrenocorticosteroids are absorbed through the skin and may rarely affect growth in children. Before using this medicine in children you should discuss the use of it with your doctor.

Before using this medicine
Before you use this medicine check with your doctor, or pharmacist:
- if you ever had any unusual or allergic reaction to adrenocorticoids or corticosteroids in general.
- if you are on a low-salt, low-sugar, or any other special diet, or if you are allergic to any substance, such as certain preservatives or dyes.
- if you have diabetes, stomach ulcer, or infection at the treatment site.
- if you are pregnant, intending to become pregnant or breast-feeding an infant while using this medicine.
- if you have any of the following medical problems:
  Diabetes mellitus (sugar diabetes)
  Infection at the place of treatment
  Ulceration at the place of treatment
  Tuberculosis

Treatment
This medication is used to relieve or prevent the symptoms of your medical problem. Take them as directed. Do not take more of them and do not take them more often than recommended on the label.
To do so may increase the chance of absorption through the skin and the chance of side effects. In addition, too much use, especially on thin skin areas (for example, armpits, face, groin), may result in thinning of the skin and stretch marks.

Side effects
The following side effects may occur:
- Acne or oily skin
- Blistering
- Burning sensations
- Itching
- Dryness of the skin
- Secondary infection
- Thinning of skin
- Unusual hair growth
- Unusual loss of hair

These side effects should disappear as your body adjusts to the medication. Tell your doctor about any side effects that are persistent or particularly bothersome.
The above side effects are more likely to occur in children and elderly patients, who are usually more sensitive to the effects of this medicine.
When the gel, solution, lotion, or aerosol from this medicine is applied, a mild, temporary stinging may be expected.

Interactions
This medicine interacts with several other drugs such as antibiotics (causing a decreased antibiotic effect) and antifungals (causing a decreased antifungal effect).
Be sure to tell your doctor about any medications you are currently taking.

Storage
This medicine should be stored at room temperature in closed containers. Store away from heat and direct light. Keep out of reach of children, since overdose may be dangerous in children. Do not store in the bathroom medicine cabinet because the heat or moisture may cause the medicine to break down. Keep the medicine from freezing. Do not keep outdated medicine.

Almodan
A proprietary, prescription-only preparation of the broad-spectrum antibacterial and antibiotic drug amoxycillin used to treat systemic bacterial infections.

Aloin
A proprietary, non-prescription laxative used to treat constipation.

Alophen Pills
A proprietary, non-prescription compound preparation of aloin and phenolphthalein used to treat constipation.

Aloxiprin
A proprietary, prescription-only preparation of the NSAID type used to treat pain symptoms.

Alpha VIII
A proprietary, prescription-only preparation of dried human factor VIII fraction, which acts as hemostatic drug to reduce or stop bleeding.

Alpha tocopheryl acetate
A form of vitamin E used to treat deficiency due to malabsorption.

Alphaderm
A proprietary, prescription-only compound preparation of hydrocortisone and urea used to treat inflammation of the skin.

Alphanine
A proprietary, prescription-only preparation of factor IX fraction of hu-

Alu-Cap

Properties
This medicine contains as active ingredient a neutralizing agent for excess stomach acid and is therefore called an antacid. Antacids are taken by mouth to relieve heartburn, sour stomach, or acid indigestion. Antacids alone or in combination with simethicone may be used to treat the symptoms of stomach or duodenal ulcers. This medication contains as active ingredient aluminum hydroxide.

Before using this medicine
Before you use this medicine check with your doctor, or pharmacist:
- if you ever had any unusual or allergic reaction to aluminum-, calcium-, magnesium-, sodium bicarbonate-, or simethicone containing medicines;
- if you are on a low-salt, low-sugar, or any other special diet, or if you are allergic to any substance, such as sulfites or other preservatives or dyes.
- if you are pregnant or intending to become pregnant while using this medicine. Although antacids have not been shown to cause problems in humans, the chance always exists.
- if you are breast-feeding an infant.
- if you have any of the following medical problems:
  Appendicitis (or signs of)
  Bone fractures
  Colitis or colostomy
  Constipation or diarrhea
  Heart disease
  High blood pressure
  Intestinal blockage
  Intestinal bleeding
  Kidney or liver disease
  Toxaemia of pregnancy
  Underactive parathyroids

Treatment
This medication is used to relieve or prevent the symptoms of your medical problem. Take them as directed. Do not take more of them and do not take them more often than recommended on the label, unless otherwise directed by your doctor. To do so may increase the chance of side effects.
When taking this medicine for a stomach or duodenal ulcer, take it exactly as ordered by your doctor to obtain maximum relief of your symptoms.
Antacids should not be given to young children (up to 6 years of age) unless prescribed by their doctor.

Side effects
Along with the needed effects, a medicine may cause some unwanted effects. Although the following side effects occur very rarely when this medicine is taken as recommended, they may be more likely to occur if:
- too much medicine is taken;
- it is taken in large doses;
- it is taken for a long period of time;
- it is taken by patients with kidney disease.
Check with your doctor as soon as possible if any of the following side effects or signs of overdose occur: constipation; cramping; difficult or painful urination; headache; loss of appetite; mood or mental changes; muscle pain or twitching; nausea or vomiting; stomach pain; unpleasant taste in mouth; unusual slow breathing; unusual tiredness or weakness.

Interactions
This medicine may interact with several other drugs such as adrenocorticosteroids, cellulose sodium phosphate, mecamylamine, and tetracyclines.
Be sure to tell your doctor about any medications you are currently taking.

Storage
Tablets, elixir, etc. should be stored at room temperature; store away from heat and direct light. Keep out of reach of children, since overdose may be very dangerous in children.

man blood used in treating patients with a deficiency of factor IX.

Alphavase
A proprietary, prescription-only preparation of prazosin. It can be used to treat raised blood pressure.

Alphosyl
A proprietary, non-prescription-only preparation of coal tar and allantoin. It can be used to treat eczema and psoriasis.

Alphosyl 2
A proprietary, non-prescription-only preparation of coal tar and allantoin used to treat dandruff, eczema and psoriasis.

Alphosyl HC
A proprietary, non-prescription-only preparation of coal tar, hydrocortisone and allantoin used to treat eczema and psoriasis.

Alprazolam
A proprietary, prescription-only preparation of the benzodiazepine type. It can be used to treat anxiety.

Alreumat
A proprietary, prescription-only preparation of ketoprofen used to relieve arthritic and rheumatic pain.

Altacite Plus
A proprietary, non-prescription preparation of hydrotalcite and dimethicone used for the relief of hyperacidity, flatulence, gastritis and dyspepsia.

Aluminium hydroxide

Properties
This medicine contains as active ingredient a neutralizing agent for excess stomach acid and is therefore called an antacid. Antacids are taken by mouth to relieve heartburn, sour stomach, or acid indigestion. Antacids alone or in combination with simethicone may be used to treat the symptoms of stomach or duodenal ulcers. This medication contains as active ingredient: aluminium carbonate.

Before using this medicine
Before you use this medicine check with your doctor, or pharmacist:
- if you ever had any unusual or allergic reaction to aluminum-, calcium-, magnesium-, sodium bicarbonate-, or simethicone containing medicines;
- if you are on a low-salt, low-sugar, or any other special diet, or if you are allergic to any substance, such as sulfites or other preservatives or dyes.
- if you are pregnant or intending to become pregnant while using this medicine. Although antacids have not been shown to cause problems in humans, the chance always exists.
- if you are breast-feeding an infant.
- if you have any of the following medical problems:
  Appendicitis (or signs of)
  Bone fractures
  Colitis or colostomy
  Constipation or diarrhea
  Heart disease
  High blood pressure
  Intestinal blockage
  Intestinal bleeding
  Kidney or liver disease
  Toxaemia of pregnancy
  Underactive parathyroids

µTreatment
This medication is used to relieve or prevent the symptoms of your medical problem. Take them as directed. Do not take more of them and do not take them more often than recommended on the label, unless otherwise directed by your doctor. To do so may increase the chance of side effects.
When taking this medicine for a stomach or duodenal ulcer, take it exactly as ordered by your doctor to obtain maximum relief of your symptoms.
Antacids should not be given to young children (up to 6 years of age) unless prescribed by their doctor.

Side effects
Along with the needed effects, a medicine may cause some unwanted effects. Although the following side effects occur very rarely when this medicine is taken as recommended, they may be more likely to occur if:
- too much medicine is taken;
- it is taken in large doses;
- it is taken for a long period of time;
- it is taken by patients with kidney disease.
Check with your doctor as soon as possible if any of the following side effects or signs of overdose occur: constipation; cramping; difficult or painful urination; headache; loss of appetite; mood or mental changes; muscle pain or twitching; nausea or vomiting; stomach pain; unpleasant taste in mouth; unusual slow breathing; unusual tiredness or weakness; dizziness.

Interactions
This medicine may interact with several other drugs such as adrenocorticosteroids, cellulose sodium phosphate, mecamylamine, and tetracyclines.
Be sure to tell your doctor about any medications you are currently taking.

Storage
Tablets, elixir, etc. should be stored at room temperature; store away from heat and direct light. Keep out of reach of children, since overdose may be very dangerous in children.

Altace
A proprietary, prescription-only preparation of ramipril. It is used for the reduction of the risk of heart attack and stroke.

Alteplase
A proprietary, prescription-only preparation used to break up blood clots in serious conditions such as myocardial infarction.

Alu-Cap
A proprietary, non-prescription preparation of the antacid aluminium hydroxide, for the relief of hyperacidity and dyspepsia.

Aludrox
A proprietary, non-prescription preparation of the antacid aluminium hydroxide, for the relief of hyperacidity and dyspepsia.

Aluminium acetate
A proprietary, non-prescription preparation with astringent properties. It is used primarily to clean sites of infection and inflammation.

Aluminium chloride
A proprietary, non-prescription preparation with astringent and antiperspirant properties. It can be used to treat hyperhidrosis (excessive sweating).

Alupent
A proprietary, prescription-only preparation of orciprenaline sulphate used as a bronchodilator in reversible obstructive airways disease.

Alverine citrate
A proprietary, prescription-only antispasmodic drug used to treat spasm in the gastrointestinal tract and dysmenorrhoea.

Amantadine
A proprietary, prescription-only antiparkinsonism drug. It can be used to treat the parkinsonian symptoms but has also some antiviral activity.

Ambaxin
A proprietary, prescription-only preparation of the broad-spectrum antibacterial and antibiotic drug bacampicillin used to treat systemic bacterial infections.

Ambien
A proprietary, prescription-only preparation of zodopem. It is indicated for the treatment of insomnia.

Ambisome
A proprietary, prescription-only preparation of the antifungal and antibiotic drug amphotericin, used for severe systemic, or deep-seated fungal infections.

Amethocaine
A proprietary, prescription-only local anesthetic drug used to treat localized pain and irritation and in ophthalmic treatments.

Amfipen
A proprietary, prescription-only preparation of the broad-spectrum antibacterial and antibiotic drug ampicillin, used to treat systemic bacterial infections.

Amikacin
A proprietary, prescription-only antibacterial and antibiotic drug used primarily against serious infections caused by Gram-negative bacteria.

Amikin
A proprietary, prescription-only preparation of the antibacterial and antibiotic drug amikacin, used to treat several serious bacterial infections.

Amil-Co
A proprietary, prescription-only compound preparation of the diuretic drugs amiloride and hydrochlorthiazide, used to treat oedema and hypertension.

Amilospare
A proprietary, prescription-only preparation of the diuretic drug amiloride used to treat oedema, congestive heart failure and hypertension.

Aminoglutethimide
A proprietary, prescription-only hormone antagonist. It can be used to treat breast cancer.

Aminoglycoside
A proprietary, prescription-only antibiotic and antibacterial drug. It can be used to treat severe bacterial infections.

Aminophylline
A proprietary, prescription-only bronchodilator used as an acute anti-asthmatic or a bronchitis treatment for severe acute attacks.

Aminosalicylate
A proprietary, prescription-only preparation of aminosalicylic acid used primarily to treat active Crohn's disease.

Amiodarone
A proprietary, prescription-only anti-arrhythmic drug used to treat certain severe irregularities of the heartbeat.

Amitriptyline
A proprietary, prescription-only preparation of the tricyclic group with quite marked sedative properties.

Amixo
A proprietary, prescription-only preparation of the broad-spectrum antibacterial and antibiotic drug amoxycillin used to treat systemic bacterial infections.

Amlodipine besylate
A proprietary, prescription-only preparation of the calcium-channel blocker type used to treat hypertension and angina.

Ammonium chloride
A proprietary, non-prescription expectorant. It can be used to treat cough.

Ammonium salicylate
A proprietary, prescription-only NSAID and antirheumatic drug used to treat rheumatic and other musculoskeletal disorders.

Amnivent
A proprietary, prescription-only preparation of aminophylline used as an anti-asthmatic and bronchitis treatment.

Amoram
A proprietary, prescription-only preparation of the broad-spectrum and antibacterial drug amoxycillin used to treat systemic bacterial infections.

Amorolfine
A proprietary, prescription-only antifungal drug used topically to treat fungal skin conditions.

Amoxapine
A proprietary, prescription-only antidepressant drug of the tricyclic group. It can be used to treat depressive illness.

Amoxicillin
A proprietary, prescription-only preparation of the broad-spectrum antibacterial and antibiotic drug amoxycilin used to treat systemic bacterial infections.

Amoxil
A proprietary, prescription-only preparation of the broad-spectrum antibacterial and antibiotic drug amoxycilin used to treat systemic bacterial infections.

Amoxycillin
A proprietary, prescription-only preparation of the broad-spectrum antibacterial and antibiotic drug amoxycilin used to treat systemic bacterial infections.

Amoxymed
A proprietary, prescription-only preparation of the broad-spectrum anti-

Amphotericin B

(Topical)

Properties
This medicine belongs to the family of topical (applied to the skin) antifungal preparations. It is used in the treatment of fungus infections on the skin and in the vagina. The medication fights infections such as ringworm of the scalp, athlete's foot, jockey itch, sun fungus, nail fungus and fungus infections of the vagina.
Fungal diseases may develop especially in people with disorders of immunity or diabetes and those on certain drugs (steroid, immunosuppressives, antibiotics). Thrush is common in the mouth and vagina but rarely causes systemic disease.
The drug kills fungi by damaging the fungal wall; it causes loss of essential elements to sustain fungus cell life.

Before using this medicine
Before you use this medicine check with your doctor, or pharmacist:
- if you ever had any unusual or allergic reaction to topical antifungal preparations.
- if you are on a low-salt, low-sugar, or any other special diet, or if you are allergic to any substance, such as certain preservatives or dyes.
- if you are sunburned, or have an open skin wound.
- if you are pregnant, intending to become pregnant or breast-feeding an infant while using this medicine.

Pregnant women should avoid using the vaginal cream during the first three months of pregnancy. They should use it during the next six months only if it is absolutely necessary.

Treatment
This medication is used to relieve or prevent the symptoms of your medical problem. Take them as directed. Do not take more of them and do not take them more often than recommended on the label. To do so may increase the chance of absorption through the skin and the chance

of side effects. If you forget to take a dose of this drug, take it as soon as you remember. If it is almost time for your next regularly scheduled application, skip the forgotten application and continue with your regular schedule.
CREAM, LOTION, OINTMENT, GEL: Bathe and dry area before use. Apply small amount and rub gently.
POWDER: Apply lightly to the skin.
VAGINAL CREAM & TABLETS: Insert into vagina with applicator as illustrated in instructions.
The treatment may require a period of 6 to 8 weeks for a complete cure. The usual schedule calls for an application twice a day, morning and evening, unless otherwise directed by your doctor or pharmacist. Be sure to complete the full course of treatment prescribed for you.

Side effects
The following side effects may occur:
- Itching
- Swelling of treated skin
- Redness of skin
- Vaginal burning and itching
- Irritation of vagina
- Swelling of labia
- Increased discharge

You should discontinue the use of the drug when these side effects occur. Call your doctor right away.

Interactions
This medicine may interact with several other medications applied to the skin or vagina. The combined effect may cause severe skin irritation or disorders of the labia or vagina.

Storage
This medicine should be stored cool, but do not freeze. Store away from heat and direct light. Keep out of reach of children. do not use on other members of the family without consulting your doctor. Do not store in the bathroom medicine cabinet because the heat or moisture may cause the medicine to break down. Do not keep outdated medicine or medicine no longer needed. Flush the contents down the toilet, unless otherwise directed.

bacterial and antibiotic drug amoxycilin used to treat systemic bacterial infections.

Amphocil
A proprietary, prescription-only preparation of the broad-spectrum antifungal and antibiotic drug amphotericin used to treat systemic and deep-seated fungal infections.

Amphotericin
A proprietary, prescription-only pre-

paration of the broad-spectrum antifungal and antibiotic drug amphotericin used to treat systemic and deep-seated fungal infections.

Ampicillin
A proprietary, prescription-only broad-spectrum antibacterial and antibiotic drug used to treat systemic bacterial infections.

Ampiclox
A proprietary, prescription-only pre-

paration of the broad-spectrum antibacterial and antibiotic drugs ampicillin and cloxacillin used to treat systemic bacterial infections.

Ampiclox neonatal
A proprietary, prescription-only preparation of the broad-spectrum antibacterial and antibiotic drugs ampicillin and cloxacillin used to treat systemic bacterial infections in the newborn.

Analgesics

An analgesic is a drug that relieves pain. There are many ways that drugs can be used to relieve pain. There are a number of major classes of analgesic medicines.

- The first class is the narcotic analgesics (for instance morphine sulphate), which have powerful actions on the central nervous system and alter the perception of pain. Because of the numerous possible side effects, the most important of which is drug dependence, this class is usually used under strict medical supervision. Other notable side effects include depression of respiration, nausea and vomiting, sometimes hypotension, constipation and inhibition of coughing.

- The second class is the non-narcotic analgesics, which are medicines that have no tendency to produce dependence, for example aspirin, but are by no means free of side effects. A very large number are referred to as non-steroidal anti-inflammatory drugs, abbreviated to NSAID. The latter term refers to the valuable anti-inflammatory action of some members of this class.

- Apart from the two main classes, there are other medicines that are sometimes referred to as analgesic because of their ability to relieve pain. For example, local anesthetics are referred to as local analgesics.

Amrit
A proprietary, prescription-only preparation of the broad-spectrum antibacterial and antibiotic drug amoxycilin used to treat systemic bacterial infections.

Amsacrine
A proprietary, prescription-only anticancer preparation which is used specifically in the treatment of acute myeloid leukaemia.

Amsidine
A proprietary, prescription-only preparation of the anticancer drug amsacrine. It can be used to treat acute myeloid leukaemia.

Amylobarbitone
A proprietary, prescription-only barbiturate preparation. It can be used as a hypnotic to treat severe and intractable insomnia.

Amytal
A proprietary, prescription-only barbiturate preparation amylobarbitone. It can be used as a hypnotic to treat severe and intractable insomnia.

Anacal
A proprietary, non-prescription preparation of heparinoids used for the symptomatic relief of hemorrhoids, perinatal eczema, itching and anal fissure.

Anadin Caplets
A proprietary, non-prescription compound preparation of aspirin and caffeine used for the treatment of mild to moderate pain and for symptomatic relief of feverish colds and flu.

Anadin Capsules
A proprietary, non-prescription compound preparation of aspirin and caffeine used for the treatment of mild to moderate pain and for symptomatic relief of feverish colds and flu.

Anadin Extra
A proprietary, non-prescription compound preparation of aspirin, paracetamol and caffeine used for the treatment of mild to moderate pain and for symptomatic relief of feverish colds and flu.

Anadin Extra Soluble Tablets
A proprietary, non-prescription compound preparation of aspirin, paracetamol and caffeine used for the treatment of mild to moderate pain and for symptomatic relief of feverish colds and flu.

Anadin Paracetamol
A proprietary, non-prescription preparation of paracetamol used for the treatment of headache, migraine, period pain and dental pain.

Anaflex
A proprietary, prescription-only preparation of the antifungal and antibacterial drug polynoxylin used topically to treat minor skin infections.

Anafranil
A proprietary, prescription-only preparation of clomipramine. It can used to relieve the symptoms of depressive illness.

Anapolon 50
A proprietary, prescription-only preparation of the steroid oxymetholone. It can be used to treat aplastic anemia.

Anbesol
A proprietary, non-prescription compound preparation of lignocaine and cetylpyridinum. It can be used for the temporary relief of pain caused by teething, mouth ulcers and denture irritation.

Anbesol Teething Gel
A proprietary, non-prescription compound preparation of lignocaine and cetylpyridinium used for the temporary relief of pain caused by teething, mouth ulcers and denture irritation.

Ancrod
A proprietary, prescription-only anticoagulant preparation used in the treatment of deep-vein thrombosis.

Andrews Answer A
A proprietary, non-prescription preparation of paracetamol and sodium bicarbonate used for headache with upset stomach and other general pain.

Anbesol

Properties
This medicine contains as active ingredient lignocaine. It belongs to a group of medicines known as topical local aesthetics. These drugs are used to relieve the pain, itching, and redness of minor skin disorders, including sunburn or other minor burns, insect bites or stings, poison ivy, poison oak, and minor cuts and scratches.
These drugs function by deadening the nerve endings in the skin. They do not cause drowsiness or disorders of consciousness as general aesthetics for surgery do.

Before using this medicine
Before you use this medicine check with your doctor, or pharmacist:
- if you ever had any unusual or allergic reaction to this medicine or to a local anesthetic, especially when applied to the skin.
- if you are allergic to any substance, such as para-aminobenzoic acid, parabens, paraphenylenediamine, sulfites or other preservatives or dyes.
- if you are pregnant or intending to become pregnant while using this medicine. Although local aesthetics have not been shown to cause problems in humans, the chance always exists.
- if you are breast-feeding an infant. Although this medicine has not been shown to cause problems in humans, it may pass into the breast milk in small amounts.
- if you have any of the following medical problems:
  Infection at or near the place of application
  Large sores
  Broken skin
  Severe injury at area of application

Treatment
This medication is used to relieve the pain, itching, and redness of minor skin disorders. For safe and effective use of this medicine follow your doctor's instructions. Unless otherwise stated by your doctor or pharmacist, do not use this medicine on large areas, especially if the skin is broken or scraped. Also, do not use it more often than directed on the package label, or for more than a few days at a time. To do so may increase the chance of absorption through the skin and the chance of unwanted effects. If you are using this medicine on your face, be very careful not to get it in your eyes. If you are using an aerosol or spray form of this medicine, spray it on your hand or an applicator before applying it to your face.

Side effects
Along with the needed effects, a medicine may cause some unwanted effects. These side effects may go away during treatment as your body adjusts to the medicine. Such minor side effects are: burning, stinging, or tenderness not present before treatment; skin rash, redness, itching or hives.
Signs of too much medicine being absorbed by the body are the following (! discontinue use of the drug and check with your doctor immediately):
- Blurred vision
- Double vision
- Dizziness
- Drowsiness
- Convulsions (seizures)
- Ringing in the ears
- Shivering or trembling
- Unusual anxiety
- Unusual increase in sweating
- Irregular heartbeat

Interactions
This medicine may interact with several other drugs such as antimyasthanics, long-acting eye drops or for glaucoma, sulfonamides.
Be sure to tell your doctor about any medications you are currently taking.

Storage
Store away from heat and direct light. Keep out of reach of children. Keep the medicine from freezing. Do not keep outdated medicine or medicine no longer needed.

Andrews Answer B
A proprietary, non-prescription preparation of calcium carbonate and magnesium carbonate used for the relief of upset stomach, heartburn, indigestion and trapped wind.

Androcur
A proprietary, prescription-only preparation of cyproterone acetate used to treat severe hypersexuality and sexual deviation in men.

Anectine
A proprietary, prescription-only preparation of suxamethonium chloride. It can be used to induce muscle paralysis during surgery.

Anestan Bronchial Tablets
A proprietary, non-prescription preparation of ephedrine and theophylline used as an anti-asthmatic drug for reversible bronchospasm.

Anexate
A proprietary, prescription-only preparation of flumazenil. It can be used to reverse the effects of benzodiazepines.

Angelettes
A preparation of aspirin used to help prevent the formation of thrombi.

Angilol
A proprietary, prescription-only pre-

paration of propranolol used in the treatment of hypertension, angina and heartrhythm irregularities.

Angiopine
A proprietary, prescription-only preparation of nifedipine used in the treatment of hypertension, angina and as a vasodilator in peripheral vascular disease.

Angiozem
A proprietary, prescription-only preparation of diltiazem. It can be used in the treatment of raised blood pressure and as an anti-angina drug.

Anhydrol Forte
A proprietary, non-prescription preparation of aluminium chloride, which can be used as an antiperspirant to treat hyperhidrosis.

Anistreplase
A proprietary, prescription-only fibrinolytic drug. It can be used to break up blood cloths.

Anodesyn
A proprietary, prescription-only preparation of benperidol. It can be used to treat and tranquillize psychotic patients.

Antabuse
A proprietary, prescription-only preparation of disulfiram. It can be used to assist in the treatment of alcoholism.

Antazoline
A proprietary, non-prescription antihistamine preparation. It can be used for the symptomatic relief of allergic symptoms.

Antepsin
A proprietary, prescription-only preparation of sucralfate used to treat gastric and duodenal ulcers.

Anthranol
A proprietary, non-prescription compound preparation of dithranol and salicylic acid used for subacute and chronic psoriasis.

Anturan
A proprietary, prescription-only pre-

paration of sulphinpyrazine. It can be used to treat and prevent gout.

Anugesic-HC
A proprietary, prescription-only compound preparation of hydrocortisone, zinc oxide, bismuth oxide, benzyl benzoate and pramoxine. It can be used to treat hemorrhoids and inflammation in the anal region.

Anusol
A proprietary, prescription-only compound preparation of zinc oxide and bismuth oxide. It can be used to treat hemorrhoids and inflammation in the anal region.

Anusol-HC
A proprietary, prescription-only compound preparation of hydrocortisone, zinc oxide, benzyl benzoate, bismuth subgallate and bismuth oxide. It can be used to treat hemorrhoids and inflammation in the anal region.

Apisate
A proprietary, prescription-only preparation of diethylproprion and vitamin supplements. It can be used as appetite suppressant.

Apomorphine hydrochloride
A proprietary, prescription-only preparation that has similar actions to bromocriptine used in the treatment of parkinsonism.

Aproclonidine
A proprietary, prescription-only preparation of clonidine used to control or prevent postoperative elevation of intraocular pressure after laser surgery.

Apresoline
A proprietary, prescription-only preparation of hydralazine used in long-term antihypertensive treatment and in hypertensive crisis.

Aprinox
A proprietary, prescription-only preparation with antifibrinolytic activity. It can be used to prevent life-threatening clot formation.

Apsifen
A proprietary, prescription-only pre-

paration of ibuprofen used to relieve pain, particularly of rheumatic disease and other musculoskeletal disorders.

Apsin
A proprietary, prescription-only preparation of the antibacterial and antibiotic drug phenoxymethylpenicillin, particularly effective in treating tonsillitis, infection of the middle ear and certain skin infections.

Apsolol
A proprietary, prescription-only preparation of oxprenolol used as an antihypertensive treatment for raised blood pressure, for angina and for rhythmic disorders of the heart.

Apstil
A proprietary, prescription-only preparation of stilboestrol used as an anticancer drug. It can be to treat prostate cancer.

Aquadrate
A proprietary, non-prescription-only preparation of urea. It can be used for dry, scaling, or itching skin.

Aramine
A proprietary, prescription-only preparation of metaraminol, most often used to raise blood pressure in a patient under general anesthesia.

Arbralene
A proprietary, prescription-only preparation of metoprolol used in the treatment of hypertension, angina, irregular heartbeat and to treat myocardial infection.

Aredia
A proprietary, prescription-only preparation of disodium pamidronate used to treat high calcium levels associated with malignant tumors.

Arelix
A proprietary, prescription-only preparation of piretanide. It can be used to treat raised blood pressure.

Arfonad
A proprietary, prescription-only preparation of trimetaphan camsylate

used as a hypotensive for controlled blood pressure during surgery.

Aricept

A proprietary, prescription-only preparation of donepezil. It is used for the symptomatic treatment of mild to moderate Alzheimer's disease.

Arimidex

A proprietary, prescription-only preparation of anastrozole. It is used for the adjuvant therapy of post-menopausal women with early breast cancer.

Arpicolin

A proprietary, prescription-only preparation of procyclidine. It can be used in the treatment of parkinsonism.

Arpimycin

A proprietary, prescription-only preparation of the antibacterial and antibiotic drug erythromycin, used to treat and prevent many forms of infection.

Arret

A proprietary, non-prescription preparation of loperamide.
It can be used for the relief of acute diarrhea and its associated pain and discomfort.

Artane

A proprietary, prescription-only preparation of benzhexol hydrochloride used in the treatment of parkinsonism and to control tremor and involuntary movement.

Arthrofen

A proprietary, prescription-only preparation of ibuprofen. It can be used to relieve pain, particularly that of rheumatic disease and other musculoskeletal disorders.

Arthrosin

A proprietary, prescription-only preparation of naproxen, used to relieve pain, particularly that of rheumatic disease and other musculoskeletal disorders.

Arthrotec

A proprietary, prescription-only pre-

Antibiotics

These medicines are, strictly speaking, natural products secreted by microorganisms into their environment where they inhibit the growth of competing microorganisms of different types.
But in common usage the term is often applied to any drug, natural or synthetic, that has selectively toxic action on bacteria or similar non-nucleated, single-celled microorganisms (including chlamydia, rickettsia and mycoplasma).
When administered by an appropriate route, such as topically (for instance the skin or eyes), orally, by injection, or by infusion, antibiotics kill microorganisms such as bacteria or inhibit their growth.
The selectively toxic action on invading microorganisms exploits differences between bacteria and their human host cells. Major target sites are the bacterial cell wall located outside the cell membrane and bacterial ribosome (the protein-synthesizing organelle within the cell), which in microorganisms is different in human cells.
Antibiotics of the penicillin and cephalosporin families attack the bacterial wall, whereas aminoglycoside and tetracycline antibiotics attack the ribosomes.
Unfortunately, because of the widespread use of antibiotics certain strains of common bacteria have developed resistance to antibiotics that were once effective against them.

paration of diclofenac and misoprostol, used to treat pain and inflammation in rheumatic disease.

Arthroxen

A proprietary, prescription-only preparation of naproxen, used to relieve pain, particularly that of rheumatic disease and other musculoskeletal disorders.

Artracin

A proprietary, prescription-only preparation of indomethacin, used to relieve pain and inflammation, particularly in rheumatism.

Arythmol

A proprietary, prescription-only preparation of propafenone hydrochloride, used to prevent and treat irregularities of the heartbeat.

Asacol

A proprietary, prescription-only preparation of mesalazine. It can be used to treat ulcerative colitis.

Ascabiol Emulsion

A proprietary, non-prescription preparation of benzyl benzoate for the treatment of lice infestation.

Asendis

A proprietary, non-prescription-only preparation of malic acid, benzoic acid and salicylic acid, used as a desloughing agent in the treatment of superficial ulcers, burns and bedsores.

Asilone

A proprietary, non-prescription compound preparation of aluminium hydroxide, dimethicome and magnesium oxide, used to treat dyspepsia, flatulence and associated abdominal distension, heartburn and to soothe the symptoms of peptic ulcers.

Asilone suspension

A proprietary, non-prescription compound preparation of aluminium hydroxide, dimethicone and magnesium oxide, used to treat dyspepsia, flatulence and associated abdominal distension, heartburn and to soothe the symptoms of peptic ulcers.

Asilone tablets

A proprietary, non-prescription compound preparation of aluminium hydroxide, dimethicone and magnesium oxide, used to treat dyspepsia, flatulence and associated abdominal distension, heartburn and to soothe the symptoms of peptic ulcers.

Askit powders
A proprietary, non-prescription compound preparation of aspirin, aloxiprin and caffeine used to treat mild to moderate pain and to relieve swelling.

Asmaven
A proprietary, prescription-only preparation of salbutamol used as a bronchodilator in reversible obstruction airways disease.

Aspav
A proprietary, prescription-only compound preparation of aspirin and indomethacin and some narcotic analgesic alkaloids used to relieve pain and inflammation, particularly in rheumatism.

Aspellin
A proprietary, non-prescription compound preparation of menthol, camphor, methyl salicylate, ethyl salicylate and ammonium salicylate. It can be used for symptomatic relief (applied to the skin) of underlying muscle or joint pain.

Aspirin
A proprietary, non-prescription preparation of acetylsalicylic acid. It can be used to relieve mild to moderate pain, particularly headache, toothache and period pain.

Aspro clear
A proprietary, non-prescription preparation of aspirin. It can be used to treat various aches and pains and fevers.

Aspro tablets
A proprietary, non-prescription preparation of aspirin. It can be used to treat various aches and pains and fevers.

Astemizole
A proprietary, prescription-only preparation of an antihistamine drug used for the symptomatic relief of allergic symptoms such as hay fever and urticaria.

AT 10
A proprietary, prescription-only preparation of dihydrotachysterol, a vitamin D analogue, used in the treatment of vitamin D deficiency.

Atarax
A proprietary, prescription-only preparation of hydroxyzine hydrochloride. It can be used for the relief of allergic symptoms.

Atenix
A proprietary, prescription-only preparation of atenolol, used as an antihypertensive treatment for raised blood pressure.

AtenixCo
A proprietary, prescription-only compound preparation of atenolol and chlorthalidone, used as an antihypertensive treatment for raised blood pressure.

Atenolol
A proprietary, prescription-only betablocker preparation. It can be used as an antihypertensive treatment for raised blood pressure.

Atensine
A proprietary, prescription-only preparation of the benzodiazepine drug diazepam, used as an anxiolytic drug to treat anxiety and as a hypnotic to relieve insomnia.

Ativan
A proprietary, prescription-only preparation of the benzodiazepine drug lorazepam used as an anxiolytic drug in the short-term treatment of anxiety and as a hypnotic to treat insomnia.

Atovaquone
A proprietary, prescription-only antiprotozoal drug. It can be used to treat pneumonia caused by Pneumocystis carinii.

Atracurium besylate
A proprietary, prescription-only preparation of a skeletal muscle relaxant drug. It can be used during surgery to induce muscle paralysis.

Atromid-S
A proprietary, prescription-only preparation of clofibrate. It can be used as a lipid-lowering drug in hyperlipidaemia.

Atropine sulphate
A powerful anticholinergic drug used as an antispasmodic preparation. It is commonly used during operations to dry up secretions and protect the heart.

Atrovent
A proprietary, prescription-only preparation of ipratropium bromide. It can be used to treat the symptoms of reversible airways obstructive disease.

Audicort
A proprietary, prescription-only compound preparation of trimacinolone and neomycine. It can be used to treat infections of the outer ear.

Augmentin
A proprietary, prescription-only compound preparation of amoxycillin and clavulanic acid. It can be used to treat a variety of infections.

Auranofin
A proprietary, prescription-only gold preparation used as an anti-inflammatory and antirheumatic treatment.

Aureocort
A proprietary, prescription-only compound preparation of triamcinolone and chlortetracycline used to treat severe inflammatory skin disorders.

Aureomycin
A proprietary, prescription-only preparation of the antibacterial and antibiotic drug chlortetracycline used to treat eye and skin infections.

Aureomycin topical
A proprietary, prescription-only preparation of the antibacterial and antibiotic drug chlortetracycline used to treat skin infections.

Avandia
A proprietary, prescription-only preparation of rosiglitazone. It is used in diabetes to improve blood sugar control.

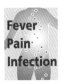

Fever
Pain
Infection

Aspirin

Properties
This medicine contains as active ingredient salicylic acid, used to relieve pain and reduce fever. Buffered salicylic acid is used only to relieve pain.

Before using this medicine
Before you use this medicine check with your doctor, or pharmacist:
- if you ever had any unusual or allergic reaction to salicylic acid or related compounds.
- if you are on a low-salt, low-sugar, or any other special diet, or if you are allergic to any substance, such as sulfites or other preservatives or dyes.
- if you are pregnant or intending to become pregnant while using this medicine. Studies on birth defects have not been done in humans.
- if you are breast-feeding an infant. Although this medicine has not been shown to cause problems in humans, it passes into the breast milk in small amounts.
- if you have any of the following medical problems:
  Virus infection of the liver
  Alcohol abuse
  Kidney disease
  Liver disease
- if you are now taking any of the following medicines:
  Anticoagulants
  Anticonvulsants
  Antihistamines
  Antineoplastics
  Barbiturates
  Contraceptives
  Corticosteroids
  Estrogens
  Sulphapreparations

Treatment
This medication is used to relieve pain and reduce fever. Unless otherwise directed by your doctor or pharmacist take this as directed.
Do not take more of them and do not take them more often than recommended on the label.
Children up to 12 years of age should not take this medicine more than 3 times a day or for more than 5 days in a row.

Side effects
Along with the needed effects, a medicine may cause some unwanted effects. Although the following side effects occur very rarely when this medicine is taken as recommended, they may be more likely to occur if:
- too much medicine is taken;
- it is taken in large doses;
- it is taken for a long period of time;
- it is taken by patients with kidney disease.
This drug is relatively free from side effects.
Check with your doctor immediately if any of the following side effects occur: yellowing of eyes or skin; bloody or cloudy urine; difficult or painful urination; skin rash, hives, or itching; sudden decrease in amount of urine; unexplained sore throat and fever; unusual bleeding or bruising; unusual tiredness or weakness.

Interactions
This medicine may interact with several other drugs such as adrenocorticosteroids, aspirin, caffeine-containing medications; theophylline, antibiotics, sulfonamides, etc.
Be sure to tell your doctor about any medications you are currently taking.

Storage
Tablets, elixir, suppository etc. should be stored at room temperature and away from direct light. Keep out of reach of children, since overdose may be very dangerous in children. Do not store in the bathroom medicine cabinet because the heat or moisture may cause the medicine to break down. Do not keep outdated medicine.

Aveeno cream
A proprietary, non-prescription preparation of colloidal oatmeal. It can be used for eczema, itching and other skin complaints.

Aveeno oiliated
A preparation of colloidal oatmeal. It can be used for eczema, itching and other skin complaints.

Aveeno regular
A proprietary, non-prescription preparation of colloidal oatmeal. It can be used for eczema, itching and other skin complaints.

Avloclor
A preparation of cloroquine. It can be used to prevent or suppress certain forms of malaria.

Avomine
A proprietary, non-prescription preparation of promethazine. It can be used as an antinauseant for nausea, motion sickness, vertigo and labyrinthine disorders.

Axid
A proprietary, prescription-only preparation of nizatidine. It can be used as an ulcer-healing drug for peptic ulcers, gastro-esophageal reflux, dyspepsia and associated conditions.

Axsain
A preparation of capsicum oleoresin applied to the skin for symptomatic relief of post-herpetic neuralgia.

Azactam
A proprietary, prescription-only pre-

Antihistamine

An antihistamine is a medicine that inhibits the effects of histamine in the body. Histamine is released naturally as the result of a patient coming into contact with a substance to which he or she is allergically sensitive and causes various symptoms such as hay fever, urticaria (itchy skin rash), itching (pruritus) or even asthma-like bronchoconstriction.

Many agents can act as triggers for histamine release, including inhalation of pollen, insect bites and stings, contact with some metal objects, food constituents, food dye additives, a number of medicine types and many environmental factors.

Consequently, antihistamines may be used for many purposes, but particularly for the symptomatic relief of allergy such as hay fever and urticaria and in the acute treatment of anaphylactic shock..

Many antihistamines also have anti-emetic properties and are therefore used to prevent vomiting associated with travel sickness, vertigo, or the effects of chemotherapy. All but some recently developed antihistamines produce drowsiness and this sedative action may be used to help induce sleep.

paration of the antibiotic drug aztreonam used to treat severe infections caused by Gram-negative bacteria.

Azamune

A proprietary, prescription-only preparation of azathioprine used to treat only serious cases of rheumatoid arthritis, acute gout and certain rheumatic diseases of the backbone.

Azapropazone

A non-narcotic, analgesic drug used to treat only serious cases of rheumatoid arthritis, acute gout and certain rheumatic diseases of the backbone.

Azatadine maleate

An antihistamine drug used for the symptomatic relief of allergic symptoms such as hay fever and urticaria.

Azathioprine

A powerful cytotoxic and immunosuppressant drug mainly used to reduce tissue rejection in transplant patients.

Azelaic acid

A drug with mild antibacterial and keratolytic properties. It can be used to treat skin conditions such as acne.

Azelastine hydrochloride

An antihistamine drug, which can be used for the symptomatic relief of allergic rhinitis.

Azithromycin

An antibacterial and antibiotic preparation. It can be used to treat infections.

Aztreonam

An antibacterial and antibiotic preparation. It can be used primarily to treat infections caused by Pseudomonas.

Aziocillin

An antibacterial and antibiotic preparation. It can be used primarily to treat infections caused by Gram-negative bacteria such as Pseudomonas aeruginosa.

B

Bacampicillin

A broad-spectrum antibacterial and antibiotic preparation. It can be used to treat a wide variety of infections.

Bacitracin zinc

An antibacterial and antibiotic drug used for the treatment of skin infections.

Baclofen

A skeletal muscle relaxant drug used for relaxing muscles that are in spasm, particularly when caused by an injury to or a disease of the central nervous system.

Baclospas

A proprietary, prescription-only preparation of the skeletal muscle relaxant drug baclofen used for relaxing muscles that are in spasm, particularly when caused by an injury to or a disease of the central nervous system.

Bactrim

A proprietary, prescription-only compound preparation of sulphamethoxazole and trimethoprim. It can be used to treat bacterial infections, especially infections of the urinary tract, prostatitis and bronchitis.

Bactroban

A proprietary, prescription-only preparation of the antibacterial and antibiotic drug mupirocin. It can be used to treat infections of the skin.

Bactroban Nasal

A proprietary, prescription-only preparation of the antibacterial and antibiotic drug mupirocin. It can be used to treat infections in and around the nostrils.

Balmosa Cream

A proprietary, non-prescription preparation of capsicum oleoresin, camphor, menthol and methyl salicylate. It can be applied to the skin for the symptomatic relief of muscular rheumatism, fibrosis and lumbago.

Baltar

A proprietary, non-prescription preparation of coal-tar used for conditions such as dandruff and psoriasis of the scalp.

Bambec

A proprietary, prescription-only preparation of bambuterol. It can be used as a bronchodilator in reversible obstructive airways disease and asthma.

Bambuterol

A proprietary, prescription-only preparation with beta-receptor properties. It can be used as a bronchodilator in reversible obstructive airways disease and asthma.

Baratol

A proprietary, prescription-only preparation of indoramin hydrochloride. It can be used in antihypertensive treatment, often in conjunction with other antihypertensive drugs.

Baxan

A proprietary, prescription-only preparation of the antibacterial and antibiotic drug cefadroxil. It can be used to treat many infections, especially those of the urinary tract.

Baycaron

A proprietary, prescription-only preparation of the diuretic drug mefruside. It can be used to treat raised blood pressure.

Becotide Rotacaps

A preparation of the corticosteroid beclomethasone. It can be used to prevent asthmatic attacks.

Bedranol

A proprietary, prescription-only preparation of the beta-blocker propranolol. It can be used as an antihypertensive treatment for raised blood pressure.

Beecham Pills

A proprietary, non-prescription preparation of aloin used to relieve constipation.

Beecham 75 mg Aspirin

A proprietary, non-prescription preparation of aspirin used to treat mild to moderate pain.

Beecham Hot Blackcurrant

A proprietary, non-prescription compound preparation of paracetamol, phenylephrine and vitamin C. It can be used for the symptomatic relief of mild to moderate pain, colds and flu, aches and pains.

Beecham Hot Lemon and Honey

A proprietary, non-prescription compound preparation of paracetamol, phenylephrine and vitamin C. It can be used for the symptomatic relief of mild to moderate pain, colds and flu, aches and pains.

Beecham Lemon Tablets

A proprietary, non-prescription compound preparation of aspirin and glycine. It can be used for the symptomatic relief of mild to moderate pain, colds and flu, aches and pains.

Beecham Powders

A proprietary, non-prescription compound preparation of aspirin and caffeine. It can be used for the symptomatic relief of mild to moderate pain, colds and flu, aches and pains.

Beecham Powders Capsules

A proprietary, non-prescription compound preparation of paracetamol, phenylephrine and caffeine. It can be used for the symptomatic relief of mild to moderate pain, colds and flu, aches and pains.

Bendogen

A proprietary, prescription-only preparation of bethanidine sulphate. It can be used to treat high blood pressure.

Bendrofluazide

A diuretic drug of the thiazide class. It can be used in antihypertensive treatment.

Bendroflumethiazide

A diuretic drug of the thiazide class. It can be used in antihypertensive treatment.

Benemid

A proprietary, prescription-only

Benzodiazepine

This type of medicine has a marked effect upon the central nervous system. The effect varies according to the level of dose, the frequency of dosage and which member of the group is used.

They have, to varying degrees, sedative, anxiolytic, hypnotic, anticonvulsant, anti-epileptic and skeletal muscle relaxant actions.

Benzodiazepines that are used as hypnotics have virtually replaced earlier drugs, such as the barbiturates and chloral hydrate, because they are just as effective but much safer in overdose.

There are now antagonists such as flumazenil, that can be used to reverse some of the central nervous system effects of benzodiazepines. However, it is now realized that dependence may result from prolonged use and that there may be a paradoxical increase in hostility and aggression in patients having long-term treatment.

There are a number of side effects, depending on use, dose and type, such as drowsiness and light-headedness the day after treatment, confusion and impaired gait (particularly in the elderly), dependence, amnesia, aggression, occasionally vertigo, headache, hypotension, salivation changes, rashes, visual disturbances, changes in libido, urinary retention, blood disorders, jaundice and gastrointestinal disorders.

Benoxyl 5/10/20

Properties
This medicine belongs to the family of topical (applied to the skin) anti-acne preparations, containing benzoyl peroxide as active ingredient. It is used in the treatment for acne and other skin conditions such as pressure sores. Acne is a condition of the skin that ranges in appearance from small raised bumps to pustules (large cysts and pimples). Acne is so common that more than 80 percent of the population will have some form of it at some time in their lives. This medication works by decreasing the cohesiveness of skin cells, causing the skin to peel, which is helpful in the treatment of mild acne and other skin conditions. The drug also slowly releases oxygen from the skin, which controls some skin bacteria. This drug is usually not effective in treating severe acne.

Before using this medicine
Before you use this medicine check with your doctor, or pharmacist:
- if you ever had any unusual or allergic reaction to tretinoin.
- if you are on a low-salt, low-sugar, or any other special diet, or if you are allergic to any substance, such as certain preservatives or dyes.
- if you are sunburned, or have an open skin wound.
- if you are pregnant, intending to become pregnant or breast-feeding an infant while using this medicine.

Treatment
This medication is used to relieve or prevent the symptoms of your medical problem. Take them as directed. Do not take more of them and do not take them more often than recommended on the label. To do so may increase the chance of absorption through the skin and the chance of side effects.
METHOD OF USE: Wash skin with non-medicated soap. Dry gently with towel. Rub medicine into affected areas. Keep away from eyes, nose, mouth. Apply one or more times daily. With a fair complexion, apply the drug only at bedtime. The time lapse before the drug works is 1 to 2 weeks. Use of the drug is not recommended for infants and children.

Side effects
The following side effects may occur:
- Painful skin
- Irritation

These side effects should disappear as your body adjusts to the medication. Tell your doctor about any side effects that are persistent or particularly bothersome.
You should discontinue the use of the drug when the following side effects occur:
- Rash
- Blistering
- Swelling of skin area
- Excessive dryness of the skin
- Excessive peeling of the skin

Foods with benzoic acid may cause the occurrence of a skin rash; as is also the case with cinnamon.

Interactions
This medicine may interact with several other skin medications. The combined use of this medicine with other anti-acne topical preparations may cause excessive skin irritation. The same holds true for the use of skin-peeling agents such as salicylic acid, sulphur, resorcinol; such as anti-acne topical preparations, medicated cosmetics, skin preparations with alcohol, and also with soaps or cleansers. The combined effect may cause severe skin irritation.

Storage
This medicine should be stored in a cool, dry place in a closed container. Store away from heat and direct light. Keep out of reach of children. Do not store in the bathroom medicine cabinet because the heat or moisture may cause the medicine to break down. Do not keep outdated medicine or medicine no longer needed. Flush the contents of the container down the toilet, unless otherwise directed.

preparation of probenecid used to prevent gout and to reduce the excretion of certain antibiotics by the kidney.

Bengué's Balsam
A proprietary, non-prescription preparation of menthol and methyl salicylate. It can be applied to the skin for symptomatic relief of underlying muscle or joint pain.

Benoral
A proprietary, non-prescription pre-

paration of benorylate. It can be used to treat mild to moderate pain, especially the pain of rheumatic disease.

Benorylate
A proprietary, non-prescription drug used to treat mild to moderate pain, especially the pain of rheumatic disease.

Benoxyl 5 Cream
A proprietary, non-prescription com-

pound preparation of miconazole and benzoyl peroxide used to treat acne.

Benoxyl 10 Lotion
A proprietary, non-prescription compound preparation of miconazole and benzoyl peroxide used to treat acne.

Benperidol
A powerful antipsychotic drug. It can be used to treat and tranquillize psychotics.

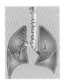

Benylin

Properties
This medicine contains pseudoephedrine as active ingredient; it is prescribed for symptomatic treatment of stuffy nose, upper respiratory congestion, or bronchospasms associated with asthma, asthmatic bronchitis or a similar condition.
The medication provides symptomatic relief of respiratory conditions, but does not treat the underlying disease.
The medicine decreases blood volume in nasal tissues, shrinking tissues and enlarging airways.

Before using this medicine
Before you use this medicine check with your doctor, or pharmacist:
- if you ever had any unusual or allergic reaction to any of the compounds of this medicine.
- if you are on a low-salt, low-sugar, or any other special diet, or if you are allergic to any substance, such as sulfites or other preservatives or dyes.
- if you are pregnant, intending to become pregnant or breast-feeding an infant while using this medicine.
- if you have any of the following medical problems:
  Overactive thyroid
  Diabetes
  Urination difficulty
  High blood pressure
  Depression

Treatment
This medication is used to relieve or prevent the symptoms of your medical problem. Take them as directed. Do not take more of them and do not take them more often than recommended on the label.
The medicine produces central nervous system stimulation, and it should not be taken by people with heart disease or high blood pressure.

Side effects
The following minor side effects may occur: dizziness; shakiness; weakness; paleness; agitation; insomnia.
These side effects should disappear as your body adjusts to the medication. Tell your doctor about any side effects that are persistent or particularly bothersome. It is especially important to tell your doctor about:
- Nausea or vomiting (severe)
- Irregular or slow heartbeat
- Painful or difficult urination
- Increased sweating
- Trembling
- Unusual fast, pounding, or irregular heartbeat
Discontinue use of the drug; call your doctor right away. Adverse reactions and side effects may be more frequent and severe in people over age 60 than in younger persons. Older adults with severe kidney problems may be more sensitive to the effects of this drug.
Signs of overdose include:
- *Nervousness*
- *Restlessness*
- *Headache*
- *Rapid or irregular heartbeat*
- *Nausea and vomiting*
- *Anxiety and/or confusion*
- *Delirium*
- *Hallucinations*

Interactions
This medicine interacts with several other drugs such as antihypertensives, beta-adrenergic blockers, calcium supplements, digitalis preparations.
Interaction with alcoholic beverages may produce drowsiness, sleepiness, and/or inability to concentrate.
Be sure to tell your doctor about any medications you are currently taking.

Storage
This medicine should be stored at room temperature in tightly closed containers. Store away from heat and direct light. Keep out of reach of children, since overdose may be very dangerous in children.

Benylin Chesty Coughs Non-Drowsy
A proprietary, non-prescription compound preparation of guaiphenesin and menthol. It can be used for the symptomatic relief of cough.

Benylin Chesty Coughs Original
A proprietary, non-prescription preparation of diphenhydramine. It can be used for the symptomatic relief of cough.

Benylin Children's Coughs Original
A proprietary, non-prescription preparation of diphenhydramine. It can be used for the symptomatic relief of cough and nasal congestion.

Benylin Children's Coughs Sugar Free/Colour Free
A proprietary, non-prescription compound preparation of diphenhydamine and menthol. It can be used for the symptomatic relief of cough and nasal congestion.

Benylin Day and Night
A proprietary, non-prescription compound preparation of paracetamol and phenylpropanolamine. It can be used for the symptomatic relief of colds and flu.

Benylin Dry Coughs Non-Drowsy
A proprietary, non-prescription pre-

Benzocaine

Properties

This medicine contains as active ingredient benzocaine. It belongs to a group of medicines known as topical local aesthetics. These drugs are used to relieve the pain, itching, and redness of minor skin disorders, including sunburn or other minor burns, insect bites or stings, poison ivy, poison oak, and minor cuts and scratches.

These drugs function by deadening the nerve endings in the skin. They do not cause drowsiness or disorders of consciousness as general aesthetics for surgery do.

Before using this medicine

Before you use this medicine check with your doctor, or pharmacist:
- if you ever had any unusual or allergic reaction to this medicine or to a local anesthetic, especially when applied to the skin.
- if you are allergic to any substance, such as para-aminobenzoic acid, parabens, paraphenylenediamine, sulfites or other preservatives or dyes.
- if you are pregnant or intending to become pregnant while using this medicine. Although local aesthetics have not been shown to cause problems in humans, the chance always exists.
- if you are breast-feeding an infant. Although this medicine has not been shown to cause problems in humans, it may pass into the breast milk in small amounts.
- if you have any of the following medical problems:
  Infection at or near the place of application
  Large sores
  Broken skin
  Severe injury at area of application

Treatment

This medication is used to relieve the pain, itching, and redness of minor skin disorders. For safe and effective use of this medicine follow your doctor's instructions. Unless otherwise stated by your doctor or pharmacist, do not use this medicine on large areas, especially if the skin is broken or scraped. Also, do not use it more often than directed on the package label, or for more than a few days at a time. To do so may increase the chance of absorption through the skin and the chance of unwanted effects. If you are using this medicine on your face, be very careful not to get it in your eyes. If you are using an aerosol or spray form of this medicine, spray it on your hand or an applicator before applying it to your face.

Side effects

Along with the needed effects, a medicine may cause some unwanted effects. These side effects may go away during treatment as your body adjusts to the medicine. Such minor side effects are: burning, stinging, or tenderness not present before treatment; skin rash, redness, itching or hives.

Signs of too much medicine being absorbed by the body are the following (! discontinue use of the drug and check with your doctor immediately):
- *Blurred vision*
- *Double vision*
- *Dizziness*
- *Drowsiness*
- *Convulsions (seizures)*
- *Ringing in the ears*
- *Shivering or trembling*
- *Unusual anxiety*
- *Unusual increase in sweating*
- *Irregular heartbeat*

Interactions

This medicine may interact with several other drugs such as antimyasthanics, long-acting eye drops or for glaucoma, sulfonamides.

Be sure to tell your doctor about any medications you are currently taking.

Storage

Store away from heat and direct light. Keep out of reach of children. Keep the medicine from freezing. Do not keep outdated medicine or medicine no longer needed.

---

paration of dextromethorphan. It can be used for the symptomatic relief of persistent, dry, irritating coughs.

Benylin with Codeine

A proprietary, non-prescription preparation of diphenhydramine and codeine. It can be used for the symptomatic relief of persistent, dry cough.

Benzagel

A proprietary, non-prescription preparation of miconazole and benzoyl peroxide used to treat acne.

Benzalkonium chloride

An antiseptic agent with keratolytic properties, used topically applied for skin disorders and wounds or ulcers.

Benzamycin

A proprietary, prescription-only preparation of the antibacterial and antibiotic drug erythromycin and benzoyl peroxide. It can be used to treat acne.

Benzhexol hydrochloride

An anticholinergic drug, which is used in the treatment of some types of parkinsonism.

Benzocaine

A local anesthetic drug used by topical application for the relief of pain in the skin surface or mucous membranes.

Benzoic acid
An antifungal and keratolytic preparation incorpotrated into non-proprietary and proprietary ointments and creams.

Benzoic acid ointment
A proprietary, non-prescription compound preparation of salicylic acid and benzoic acid. It can be used to treat patches of ringworm infection.

Benzoin tincture
A proprietary, non-prescription preparation of balsam resin and balsamic acid, used as a nasal decongestant for blocked nose in sinusitis and rhinitis.

Benzoyl peroxide
A keratolytic and antimicrobial drug used in combination with other drugs to treat conditions like acne.

Berkamil
A proprietary, prescription-only preparation of amiloride. It can be used to treat oedema, ascites, and congestive heart failure.

Berkaprine
A proprietary, prescription-only preparation of azathioprine. It can be used to treat tissue rejection in transplant patients and for a variety of autoimmune diseases.

Berkatens
A proprietary, prescription-only preparation of verapamil. It can be used to treat high blood pressure.

Berkmycen
A proprietary, prescription-only preparation of the antibacterial and antibiotic drug oxytetracycline used to treat a wide range of infections.

Berkolol
A proprietary, prescription-only preparation of propranolol. It can be used to treat raised blood pressure, angina and some irregularities of the heartbeat.

Berkozide
A proprietary, prescription-only preparation of bendrofluazide. It can be used in the treatment of oedema with congestive heart failure and high blood pressure.

Berotec
A proprietary, prescription-only preparation of fenoterol used as a bronchodilator in reversible obstructive airways disease.

Beta-Adalat
A proprietary, prescription-only preparation of nifedepine. It can be used to treat raised blood pressure.

Beta-Cardone
A proprietary, prescription-only preparation of sotalol hydrochloride. It can be used as an antihypertensive treatment for raised blood pressure and for angina and some irregularities of the heartbeat.

Betadine
A proprietary, non-prescription preparation of pividone-iodine. It can be used for the treatment of bacterial infections in the vagina and cervix.

Betadur CR
A proprietary, prescription-only preparation of propranolol. It can be used for the treatment of raised blood pressure, angina and some irregularities of the heartbeat.

Betagan
A proprietary, prescription-only preparation of levobunodol. It can be used for glaucoma treatment.

Betahistine hydrochloride
An antinauseant drug used to treat the vertigo, hearing loss and tinnitus associated with Ménière's disease.

Betaloc
A proprietary, prescription-only preparation of metoprolol. Ot can be used for the treatment of high blood pressure, angina pectoris and to regularize heartbeat.

Betaloc-SA
A proprietary, prescription-only preparation of metoprolol. It can be

Beta-blockers
These medicines inhibit some actions of the sympathetic nervous system by preventing the action of adrenaline and noradrenaline by blocking the beta-adrenoreceptors on which they act.

Correspondingly, drugs called alpha-blockers are medicines used to inhibit the remaining actions by occupying the other main class of adrenoreceptor, alpha-adrenoreceptors.

These two classes of receptors are responsible for the very widespread actions of adrenaline and noradrenaline in the body, both in normal physiology and in stress. For example, they speed the heart, constrict or dilate certain blood vessels (thereby increasing blood pressure) and suppress activity in the intestines. In general, they prepare the body for emergency action.

In disease, some of these actions may be inappropriate, exaggerated and detrimental to health, so beta-blockers may be used to restore a more healthy balance. Thus beta-blockers may be used as antihypertensives to lower blood pressure when it is abnormally raised in cardiovascular disease, as an anti-arrhythmic treatment to correct heartbeat irregularities; as an anti-angina treatment to prevent the pain of angina pectoris during exercise and to treat myocardial infarction associated with heart attacks.

Corticosteroids

These are steroid hormones secreted by the cortex (outer part) of the adrenal glands, or are synthetic substances that closely resemble the natural forms. There are two main types, glucocorticoids and mineralocorticoids. The latter assist in maintaining the salt- and waterbalance of the body.

Corticosteroids such as hydrocortisone (a glucocorticoid) and fludrocortisone (a mineralocorticoid) can be given to patients for replacement therapy where there is a deficiency, or in Addison's disease.

The glucocorticoids are potent anti-inflammatory and anti-allergic drugs and are frequently used to treat inflammatory and/or allergic reactions of the skin, airways and elsewhere.

Compound preparations are available that contain both an antibacterial or antifungal drug with an anti-inflammatory corticosteroid and can be used in conditions where an infection is also present.

However, these preparations must be used with caution because the corticosteroid component diminishes the patient's natural immune response to the infective agent. Absorption of a high dose of corticosteroid over a period of time may also cause undesirable, systemic side effects.

used for the treatment of high blood pressure, angina pectoris and to regularize heartbeat.

Betamethasone
A proprietary, prescription-only preparation of the corticosteroid class. It can be used in the treatment of many kinds of inflammation, particularly inflammation associated with skin conditions such as eczema and psoriasis and of the eyes, ears, or nose.

Betamethasone diproprionate
A proprietary, prescription-only preparation of the corticosteroid class. It can be used in the treatment of many kinds of inflammation, particularly inflammation associated with skin conditions such as eczema and psoriasis and of the eyes, ears, or nose.

Betamethasone sodium phosphate
A proprietary, prescription-only preparation of the corticosteroid. It can be class used in the treatment of many kinds of inflammation, particularly inflammation associated with skin conditions such as eczema and psoriasis and of the eyes, ears, or nose.

Betamethasone valerate
A proprietary, prescription-only preparation of the corticosteroid class. It can be used in the treatment of many kinds of inflammation, particularly inflammation associated with skin conditions such as eczema and psoriasis and of the eyes, ears, or nose.

Beta-Prograne
A proprietary, prescription-only preparation of propranolol used in the treatment of high blood pressure and angina and to regularize heartbeat.

Betaxolol hydrochloride
A beta-blocker preparation used to treat high blood pressure, angina and to regularize heartbeat.

Bethanechol chloride
A proprietary, prescription-only

parasympathicomimetic preparation. It can be used to stimulate motility in the intestines and to treat urinary retention.

Bethanidine sulphate
A proprietary, prescription-only preparation belonging to the antisympathetic class of drug. It prevents release of adrenaline from sympathetic nerves. It is used to treat high blood pressure.

Betim
A proprietary, prescription-only preparation of tomolol. It can be used to treat high blood pressure and angina and to regularize heartbeat.

Betnelan
A proprietary, prescription-only preparation of the corticosteroid betamethasone. It can be used to treat inflammation, especially in rheumatic or allergic conditions.

Betnesol
A proprietary, prescription-only preparation of the corticosteroid betamethasone. It can be used to treat local inflammation as well as more widespread rheumatic or allergic conditions.

Betnesol-N
A proprietary, prescription-only compound preparation of the corticosteroid betamethasone and the antibiotic neomycin. It can be used to treat eye, ear and nose conditions.

Betnovate
A proprietary, prescription-only preparation of the corticosteroid betamethasone. It can be used to treat severe, non-infective inflammation of the skin, rectum and scalp.

Betnovate-C
A proprietary, prescription-only compound preparation of the corticosteroid betamethasone and clioquinol. It can be used to treat severe, non-infective inflammation of the skin such as eczema.

Betnovate-RD
A proprietary, prescription-only preparation of the corticosteroid be-

Betamethasone
(Topical)

Properties
This medicine belongs to the family of topical (applied to the skin) corticosteroids, containing an adrenocorticoid as active ingredient. It is used to relieve the symptoms of any itching, rash, or inflammation of the skin; it does not treat the underlying cause of the skin problem. It also relieves redness, swelling and itching caused by insect bites, poison ivy, poison oak, poison sumach, soaps, cosmetics, sunburn, and numerous skin rashes.
Topical adrenocorticosteroids are absorbed through the skin and may rarely affect growth in children. Before using this medicine in children you should discuss the use of it with your doctor.

Before using this medicine
Before you use this medicine check with your doctor, or pharmacist:
- if you ever had any unusual or allergic reaction to adrenocorticoids or corticosteroids in general.
- if you are on a low-salt, low-sugar, or any other special diet, or if you are allergic to any substance, such as certain preservatives or dyes.
- if you have diabetes, stomach ulcer, or infection at the treatment site.
- if you are pregnant, intending to become pregnant or breast-feeding an infant while using this medicine.
- if you have any of the following medical problems:
  Diabetes mellitus (sugar diabetes)
  Infection at the place of treatment
  Ulceration at the place of treatment
  Tuberculosis

Treatment
This medication is used to relieve or prevent the symptoms of your medical problem. Take them as directed. Do not take more of them and do not take them more often than recommended on the label.
To do so may increase the chance of absorption through the skin and the chance of side effects. In addition, too much use, especially on thin skin areas (for example, armpits, face, groin), may result in thinning of the skin and stretch marks.

Side effects
The following side effects may occur:
- Acne or oily skin
- Blistering
- Burning sensations
- Itching
- Dryness of the skin
- Secondary infection
- Thinning of skin
- Unusual hair growth
- Unusual loss of hair
These side effects should disappear as your body adjusts to the medication. Tell your doctor about any side effects that are persistent or particularly bothersome.
The above side effects are more likely to occur in children and elderly patients, who are usually more sensitive to the effects of this medicine.
When the gel, solution, lotion, or aerosol from this medicine is applied, a mild, temporary stinging may be expected.

Interactions
This medicine interacts with several other drugs such as antibiotics (causing a decreased antibiotic effect) and antifungals (causing a decreased antifungal effect).
Be sure to tell your doctor about any medications you are currently taking.

Storage
This medicine should be stored at room temperature in closed containers. Store away from heat and direct light. Keep out of reach of children, since overdose may be dangerous in children. Do not store in the bathroom medicine cabinet because the heat or moisture may cause the medicine to break down. Keep the medicine from freezing. Do not keep outdated medicine.

tamethasone. It can be used to treat severe, non-infective inflammation of the skin and scalp.

Betoptic
A proprietary, prescription-only preparation of betaxolol hydrochloride used for glaucoma treatment.

Bezafibrate
A proprietary, prescription-only preparation of the lipid-lowering class. It can be used to reduce the levels of various lipids in the bloodstream.

Bezalip
A proprietary, prescription-only preparation of the lipid-lowering drug bezafibrate, used to reduce the levels of various lipids in the bloodstream.

Bezalip Mono
A proprietary, prescription-only preparation of the lipid-lowering drug bezafibrate, used to reduce the levels of various lipids in the bloodstream.

Bicillin
A proprietary, prescription-only preparation of the antibacterial and antibiotic drug penicillin. In can be used to treat conditions such as syphilis and gonorrhoea.

BiCNU
A proprietary, prescription-only preparation of the cytotoxic (anticancer) drug carmustive. It can be used in the treatment of certain myelomas, lymphomas and brain tumors.

Bisacodyl

Properties
This medicine contains as active ingredient bisacodyl, a stimulant laxative. Stimulant laxatives (also known as contact laxatives) are medicines taken by mouth to encourage bowel movements by acting on the intestinal wall. They increase the muscle contractions that move along the stool mass.

Before using this medicine
Before you use this medicine check with your doctor, or pharmacist:
- if you ever had any unusual or allergic reaction to laxatives.
- if you are on a low-salt, low-sugar, or any other special diet, or if you are allergic to any substance, such as sulfites or other preservatives or dyes.
- if you are pregnant. Stimulant laxatives may cause unwanted effects in the expectant mother if improperly used. Some of the stimulant laxatives may cause contractions of the womb.
- if you are breast-feeding an infant. Some stimulant laxatives may pass into the breast milk. Although the amount of laxative in the milk is generally thought to be too small to cause problems in the child, your doctor should be told that you plan to use such laxatives.
- if you have any of the following medical problems:
  Appendicitis (or signs of)
  Colostomy
  Diabetes (sugar disease)
  Heart disease
  Hypertension
  Ileostomy
  Intestinal blockage
  Laxative habit
  Rectal bleeding

Treatment
For safe and effective use of bulk-forming laxatives:
Follow your doctor's orders if this laxative was prescribed.
Follow the manufacturer's package directions if you are treating yourself.
At least six to eight 8-ounce glasses of liquids should be taken each day.
Stimulant laxatives are usually taken on an empty stomach for rapid effect. Results are slowed if taken with food.
Laxatives should not be given to young children (up to 6 years of age) unless prescribed by their doctor. Since children cannot usually describe their symptoms very well, a doctor should check the child before giving this medicine.

Side effects
Along with the needed effects, a medicine may cause some unwanted effects.
Side effects that should be reported to your doctor: breathing difficulty; burning on urination; confusion; headache; irregular heartbeat; irritability; mood or mental changes; muscle cramps; skin rash; unusual tiredness.

Laxative habit
Laxatives are to be used to provide short-term relief only, unless otherwise directed by your doctor. Laxatives are overused by many people. Such a practice often leads to dependence on the laxative action to produce a bowel movement. In some cases, overuse of some laxatives has caused damage to the nerves, muscles, and tissues of the intestines and bowel.

Interactions
This medicine may interact with several other drugs, such as amiloride, antacids, other laxatives, potassium supplements, tetracycline antibiotics and triamterene.
Be sure to tell your doctor about any medications you are currently taking.

Storage
Store away from heat and direct light. Keep out of the reach of children. Do not store in the bathroom medicine cabinet because the heat or moisture may cause the medicine to break down.

Biguanide
A hypoglycaemic drug used in diabetic treatment for Type II diabetes.

BiNovum
A compound hormonal preparation. It can be used as an oral contraceptive and for some menstrual problems.

Bioplex
A proprietary, prescription-only preparation of carbenoxolone sodium. It can be used to treat mouth ulcers.

Bioral Gel
A proprietary, prescription-only preparation of carbenoxolone sodium. It can be used to treat mouth ulcers.

Biorphen
A proprietary, prescription-only preparation of orphenadrine hydrochloride. It can be used to relieve some of the symptoms of parkinsonism.

Biperiden
An anticholinergic preparation used in the treatment of some types of parkinsonism.

Biphasic insulin
A form of purified insulin, which is prepared from bovine insulin crystals, used in diabetic treatment.

Biphasic isophane insulin
A form of purified insulin, which is prepared from porcine insulin or human insulin complex. It can be used in diabetic treatment.

Bisodol

Properties

This medicine contains as active ingredient a neutralizing agent for excess stomach acid and is therefore called an antacid. Antacids are taken by mouth to relieve heartburn, sour stomach, or acid indigestion. Antacids alone or in combination with simethicone may be used to treat the symptoms of stomach or duodenal ulcers. This medication contains as active ingredients calcium carbonate and magnesia.

Before using this medicine

Before you use this medicine check with your doctor, or pharmacist:
- if you ever had any unusual or allergic reaction to aluminum-, calcium-, magnesium-, sodium bicarbonate-, or simethicone containing medicines;
- if you are on a low-salt, low-sugar, or any other special diet, or if you are allergic to any substance, such as sulfites or other preservatives or dyes.
- if you are pregnant or intending to become pregnant while using this medicine. Although antacids have not been shown to cause problems in humans, the chance always exists.
- if you are breast-feeding an infant.
- if you have any of the following medical problems:
  Appendicitis (or signs of)
  Bone fractures
  Colitis or colostomy
  Constipation or diarrhea
  Heart disease
  High blood pressure
  Intestinal blockage
  Intestinal bleeding
  Kidney or liver disease
  Toxaemia of pregnancy
  Underactive parathyroids

Treatment

This medication is used to relieve or prevent the symptoms of your medical problem. Take them as directed. Do not take more of them and do not take them more often than recommended on the label, unless otherwise directed by your doctor. To do so may increase the chance of side effects.

When taking this medicine for a stomach or duodenal ulcer, take it exactly as ordered by your doctor to obtain maximum relief of your symptoms.

Antacids should not be given to young children (up to 6 years of age) unless prescribed by their doctor.

Side effects

Along with the needed effects, a medicine may cause some unwanted effects. Although the following side effects occur very rarely when this medicine is taken as recommended, they may be more likely to occur if:
- too much medicine is taken;
- it is taken in large doses;
- it is taken for a long period of time;
- it is taken by patients with kidney disease.

Check with your doctor as soon as possible if any of the following side effects or signs of overdose occur: bone pain; constipation, feeling of discomfort; loss of appetite; mood or mental changes; muscle weakness; swelling of wrists or ankles; unusual loss of weight.

Interactions

This medicine may interact with several other drugs such as adrenocorticosteroids, cellulose sodium phosphate, mecamylamine, methenamine, and tetracyclines.

Be sure to tell your doctor about any medications you are currently taking.

Storage

Tablets, elixir, etc. should be stored at room temperature; store away from heat and direct light. Keep out of reach of children, since overdose may be very dangerous in children. Do not keep outdated medicine or medicine no longer needed.

Bisacodyl

A stimulant laxative used to promote defecation and relieve constipation.

Bismag Tablets

A proprietary, non-prescription compound preparation of sodium bicarbonate, calcium carbonate and mixed magnesium carbonates. It can be used for the symptomatic relief of hyperacidity, indigestion, dyspepsia and flatulence.

Bismuth oxide

A mild astringent agent, which is used in the treatment of hemorrhoids.

Bismuth subnitrate

A mild astringent agent, which is used in the treatment of hemorrhoids.

Bisodol Antacid Powder

A proprietary, non-prescription compound preparation of sodium bicarbonate and magnesium bicarbonate. It can be used for the relief of indigestion, heartburn, dyspepsia, acidity and flatulence.

Bisodol Antacid Tablets

A proprietary, non-prescription compound preparation of sodium bicarbonate and magnesium bicarbonate. It can be used for the relief of indigestion, heartburn, dyspepsia, acidity and flatulence.

Bisodol Extra Tablets

A proprietary, non-prescription com-

Bisodol Heartburn

pound preparation of sodium bicarbonate, magnesium bicarbonate, and simethicone. It can be used for the relief of indigestion, heartburn, dyspepsia, acidity and flatulence.

Bisodol Heartburn

A proprietary, non-prescription compound preparation of sodium bicarbonate, magaldrate and alginic acid. It can be used for the relief of indigestion, heartburn, dyspepsia, acidity and flatulence.

Bisoprolol fumarate

A proprietary, prescription-only preparation of the beta-blocker class. It can be used to treat high blood pressure and angina and to regularize heartbeat.

Blemix

A proprietary, prescription-only preparation of the antibacterial and antibiotic drug minocycline. It can be used to treat a wide range of infections.

Bleomycin

A proprietary, prescription-only preparation of the anticancer drug class used to treat certain types of cancer.

Blisteze

A proprietary, non-prescription preparation of phenol. It can be used for cold sores and chapped cracked lips.

Blocadren

A proprietary, prescription-only preparation of the beta-blocker timolol. It can be used to treat high blood pressure and angina and to regularize heartbeat.

BN Linement

A proprietary, non-prescription preparation of turpentine oil, ammonia and ammonium chloride. It can be applied to the skin for the symptomatic relief of pain associated with rheumatism, neuralgia, fibrosis and sprains.

Bocasan

A proprietary, non-prescription preparation of the antiseptic agent sodium perborate. It can be used to cleanse and disinfect the mouth.

Bolvidon

A proprietary, prescription-only preparation of mianserin. It can be used to treat depressive illness, especially where sedation is required.

Bonefos

A proprietary, prescription-only preparation of sodium chlodronate. It can be used to treat high calcium levels associated with malignant tumors.

Boniva

A proprietary, prescription-only preparation of bandronate. It is used for the prevention of postmenopausal osteoporosis.

Bonomint

A proprietary, non-prescription preparation of the laxative phenolphthalein. It can be used in the treatment of constipation.

Boots Covering Cream

A proprietary, non-prescription preparation used to mask scars and other skin disfigurements.

Boots Travel Calm Tablets

A proprietary, non-prescription preparation of hyoscine hydrobromide used as antinauseant in the treatment of motion sickness.

Botoxro

A proprietary, prescription-only preparation of botulinum A toxin-hemaglutin complex. It can be used for treating blepharospasm.

Bradosol Plus

A proprietary, non-prescription compound preparation of domiphen bromide and lignocaine. It can be used for the symptomatic relief of a painful sore throat.

Bradosol Sugar-Free Lozenges

A proprietary, non-prescription compound preparation of benzalkonium chloride. It can be used for the symptomatic relief of a painful sore throat.

Brasivol

A proprietary, non-prescription preparation of particles of aluminium oxide, that can be used to cleanse skin with acne.

Brelomax

A proprietary, prescription-only preparation of tulobuterol used as a bronchodilator in reversible obstructive airways disease and as an anti-asthmatic treatment in severe acute asthma.

Bretylate

A proprietary, prescription-only preparation of bretylium tosylate used to treat abnormal heart rhythms.

Bretylate tosylate

A proprietary, prescription-only preparation of the antisympathetic class of drug. It can be used to treat abnormal heart rhythms.

Brevibloc

A proprietary, prescription-only preparation of the beta-blocker esmolol hydrochloride. It can be used to treat high blood pressure, angina and to regularize heartbeat.

Brevinor

A proprietary, prescription-only compound hormonal preparation. It can be used as an oral contraceptive and also for certain menstrual problems.

Bricanyl

A proprietary, prescription-only preparation of pertutaline sulphate. It can be used as a bronchodilator in reversible obstructive airways disease and to treat acute asthma.

Brietal Sodium

A proprietary, prescription-only preparation of methoxitone sodium. It can be used for the induction and maintenance of anesthesia.

Britaject

A proprietary, prescription-only preparation of apomorphine hydrochloride. It can be used to treat symptoms of parkinsonism.

Britiazim

A proprietary, prescription-only pre-

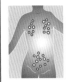

Brompheniramine

Properties
This medicine contains brompheniramine as active ingredient; it is used to treat or prevent symptoms of allergy. This medication belongs to a group known as antihistamines. Antihistamines block the action of histamine, a chemical that is released by the body during an allergic reaction. Some of the antihistamines are also used to prevent motion sickness, nausea, vomiting, and dizziness.

Before using this medicine
Before you use this medicine check with your doctor, or pharmacist:
- if you ever had any unusual or allergic reaction to antihistamines.
- if you are on a low-salt, low-sugar, or any other special diet, or if you are allergic to any substance, such as sulfites or other preservatives or dyes.
- if you are pregnant or intending to become pregnant while using this medicine.
- if you are breast-feeding an infant. Small amounts of antihistamines pass into the breast milk. Use is not recommended since the chances are greater for most antihistamines to cause side effects, such as unusual excitement or irritability in the infant.
- if you have any of the following medical problems:
  Asthma attack
  Enlarged prostate
  Glaucoma
  Urinary tract blockage
  Difficult urination

Treatment
This medication is used to relieve or prevent the symptoms of your medical problem. Take them as directed. Do not take more of them and do not take them more often than recommended on the label, unless otherwise directed by your doctor. To do so may increase the chance of side effects.

Side effects
The following minor side effects may occur:
- Blurred vision
- Confusion
- Constipation
- Diarrhea
- Difficult or painful urination
- Dizziness
- Dry mouth, throat, or nose
- Headache
- Irritability
- Loss of appetite
- Nausea or stomach upset
- Ringing or buzzing in the ears
- Unusual increase in sweating..

These side effects should disappear as your body adjusts to the medication.
Tell your doctor about any side effects that are persistent or particularly bothersome. It is especially important to tell your doctor about a change in menstruation, clumsiness, feeling faint, flushing of the face, hallucinations, rash, palpitations, seizures, shortness of breath, fever, sleeping disorders, sore throat, tightness in the chest, unusual bleeding or bruising, or unusual tiredness or weakness.

Interactions
This medicine interacts with several other drugs such as central nervous system depressants and it can decrease the activity of oral anticoagulants.
Be sure to tell your doctor about any medications you are currently taking.

Storage
Tablets, elixir, etc. should be stored at room temperature in tightly closed containers. Store away from heat and direct light. Keep out of reach of children, since overdose may be very dangerous in children. Do not keep outdated medicine or medicine no longer needed. Flush the contents of the container down the toilet, unless otherwise directed.

---

paration of diltiazem hydrochloride. It can be used to treat high blood pressure, angina and to prevent angina attacks.

BritLofex
A proprietary, prescription-only preparation of lofexidine hydrochloride. It can be used to alleviate symptoms of opioid withdrawal.

Brocadopa
A proprietary, prescription-only preparation of levodopa used to treat parkinsonism.

Broflex
A proprietary, prescription-only preparation of benzhexol hydrochloride. It can be used in the treatment of parkinsonism.

Brolene Eye Drops
A preparation of the antibacteriaL drug propamidine isethionate. It can be used to treat infections of the eyelids.

Brolene Eye Ointments
A proprietary, prescription-only preparation of the antibacteriaL drug dibromopropamidine isothionate. It can be used to treat infections of the eyelids.

Brol-eze Eye Drops
A proprietary, non-prescription preparation of the anti-allergic drug sodium cromoglycate. It can be used to treat allergic conjunctivitis.

Fever
Pain
Infection

Brufen

Properties
This medicine contains as active ingredient ibuprofen. It belongs to the group of medicines called non-steroidal anti-inflammatory drugs (NSAIDs). These drugs are taken by mouth to relieve some symptoms caused by arthritis or rheumatism, such as inflammation, swelling, stiffness, and joint pain. However, these medicines do not cure arthritis and will help you only as long as you continue to take them. Some of these medicines are also used to relieve other kinds of pain or to treat other painful conditions, such as gout attacks, bursitis, tendinitis, sprains, strains, menstrual cramps. The drug reduces the tissue concentration of prostaglandins (hormonal substances which produce inflammation and pain).

Before using this medicine
Before you use this medicine check with your doctor, or pharmacist:
- if you ever had any unusual or allergic reaction, such as skin rash, hives, or itching or breathing problems, to any of the anti-inflammatory analgesics.
- if you are on a low-salt, low-sugar, or any other special diet, or if you are allergic to any substance, such as sulfites or other preservatives or dyes.
- if you are pregnant or intending to become pregnant while using this medicine. Studies on birth defects have not been done in humans. However, if taken regularly during the last months of pregnancy, there is a chance that these medicines may cause unwanted effects on the heart or blood flow in the fetus or newborn infant.
- if you are breast-feeding an infant. Although this medicine has not been shown to cause problems in humans, it passes into the breast milk in small amounts.
- if you have any of the following medical problems:
  Asthma
  Bleeding problems
  Colitis
  Stomach ulcer
  Heart disease
  Kidney or liver disease

Treatment
This medication is used to relieve pain or other symptoms caused by arthritis. For safe and effective use of this medicine, do not take more of it, do not take it more often, and do not take it for a longer period of time than ordered by your physician or directed by the package label.
If you are taking this medication on a regular schedule and you miss a dose, take the missed dose as soon as possible, unless it is almost time for your next dose. In that case do not take the missed dose at all.
To lessen stomach upset, anti-inflammatory analgesics may be taken with food or antacids.

Side effects
Along with the needed effects, a medicine may cause some unwanted effects. These side effects may go away during treatment as your body adjusts to the medicine. Such minor side effects are: dizziness; nausea; pain; headache; drowsiness; swollen feet, face or leg; constipation or diarrhea; vomiting; dry mouth.
Check with your doctor immediately if any of the following side effects occur:
- *Muscle cramps*
- *Numbness or tingling*
- *Mouth ulcers*
- *Convulsions or confusion*
- *Rash, hives, or itch*
- *Tightness in chest*

Interactions
This medicine may interact with several other drugs.
Be sure to tell your doctor about any medications you are currently taking.

Storage
The medicine should be stored at room temperature in a tightly closed, light-resistant container. Store away from heat and direct light. Keep out of reach of children.

Bromazepam
A proprietary, prescription-only preparation of benzodiazepine class, which is used as an anxiolytic in the short-term treatment of anxiety.

Bromocriptine
A proprietary, prescription-only preparation of an ergot alkaloid used primarily to treat parkinsonism.

Brompheniramine maleate
An antihistamine drug used to treat the symptoms of allergic conditions such as hay fever and urticaria.

Bronalin Dry Cough Elixir
A proprietary, non-prescription compound preparation of dextromethorphan hydrobromide, pseudoephedrine and alcohol. It can be used for the symptomatic relief of dry, ticklish coughs and colds.

Bronchodil
A proprietary, prescription-only preparation of reproterol. It can be used as a bronchodilator in reversible obstructive airways disease and as an anti-asthmatic drug.

Brooklax
A proprietary, non-prescription preparation of phenolphthalein used to relieve constipation.

Brufen

A proprietary, prescription-only preparation of ibuprofen. It can be used to relieve pain, particularly the pain of rheumatic disease and other musculoskeletal disorders.

Brufen Retard

A proprietary, prescription-only preparation of ibuprofen. It can be used to relieve pain, particularly the pain of rheumatic disease and other musculoskeletal disorders.

Brulidine

A proprietary, non-prescription preparation of dibromopropanidine isothiolate. It can be used to treat minor burns and abrasions.

Brush Off Cold Sopre Lotion

A proprietary, only-prescription preparation of povidone-iodine. It can be used for the treatment of cold sores.

Buccastem

A proprietary, prescription-only preparation of prochlorperazine. It can be used to relieve symptoms of nausea caused by vertigo and loss of balance.

Buclizine hydrochloride

A proprietary, prescription-only antihistamine drug used in the treatment of migraine.

Budesonide

A proprietary, prescription-only preparation of the corticosteroid class. It can be used to prevent attacks of asthma, rhinitis and severe inflammatory skin disorders.

Bupivacaine

A local anesthetic drug commonly used for spinal anesthesia.

Buprenorphine

An opioid that is long-acting and used to treat moderate to severe pain.

Burinex

A proprietary, prescription-only preparation of the diuretic bumetamide. It can be used to treat oedema, particularly lung oedema.

Burinex K

A proprietary, prescription-only compound preparation of the diuretic bumetamide and potassium chloride. It can be used to treat oedema, particularly lung oedema and congestive heart failure.

Buscopan

A proprietary, prescription-only preparation of hyoscine butylbromide. It can be used as an antispasmodic drug.

Buserelin

An analogue of the hypothalamic hormone gonadorelin. It reduces secretion of gonadotrophin by the pituitary gland, which results in reduced secretion of sex hormones by the ovaries and testes.

Buspar

A proprietary, prescription-only preparation of the anxiolytic drug busipirone hydrochloride. It can be used in the short-term treatment of anxiety.

Buspirone hydrochloride

A proprietary, prescription-only preparation of the anxiolytic class. It can be used in the short-term treatment of anxiety.

Busulphan

A cytotoxic drug that is used as an anticancer treatment, particularly for chronic myeloid leukaemia.

Butacote

A proprietary, prescription-only preparation of phenylbutazone. It is used solely in the treatment of ankylosing spondylitis.

Butobarbitone

A proprietary, prescription-only preparation of the barbiturate class. It can be used to treat severe and intractable insomnia.

C

Cabergoline

A proprietary, prescription-only preparation with similar properties as bromocryptine. It can be used to treat parkinsonism and some hormonal disorders.

Caduet

A proprietary, prescription-only preparation of amlodipine. It is used for the treatment of high blood pressure and high cholesterol.

Cafergot

A proprietary, prescription-only preparation of ergotamine tartrate and caffeine. It can be used as an antimigraine treatment.

Calabren

A proprietary, prescription-only preparation of glibenclamide. It can be used in treatment of non-insulin dependent diabetes.

Caladryl Cream

A proprietary, non-prescription preparation of diphenhydramine hydrochloride, camphor and zinc oxide. It can be used for the relief of skin irritation associated with urticaria, herpes and minor skin afflictions.

Caladryl Lotion

A proprietary, non-prescription preparation of diphenhydramine hydrochloride, camphor and zinc oxide. It can be used for the relief of skin irritation associated with urticaria, herpes and minor skin afflictions.

Calamine

A proprietary, non-prescription preparation of zinc carbonate. It can be used to cool and soothe itching skin.

Calamine and coal tar ointment

A proprietary, non-prescription compound preparation of zinc carbonate and coal tar. It is used to treat chronic eczema and psoriasis.

C

Cephalosporins

These are broad-spectrum anti-bacterial and antibiotic drugs that act against both Gram-positive and Gram-negative bacteria. Their chemical structure bears a strong resemblance to that of the penicillins as they both contain a beta-lactam ring, hence their classification as beta-lactam antibiotics.

As a group, the cephalosporins are generally active against streptococci, staphylococci and a number of Gram-negative bacteria, including many coliforms.

Some of the latest, third-generation, cephalosporins (for instance ceftizoxime and cefodizime) act as antibacterials against certain Gram-negative bacteria (for instance Hemophilus influenzae) and pseudomonal infections (for instance Pseudomonas aeruginosa).

Many cephalosporins are actively excreted by the kidney and therefore reach considerably higher concentrations in the urine than in the blood. For this reason, they may be used to treat infections of the urinary tract during their own excretion.

The cephalosporins currently used are relatively non-toxic, and only occasional blood-clotting problems, superinfections and hypersensitivity reactions occur (only 10 per cent of patients allergic to penicillin show sensitivity to cephalosporins).

Calamine cream
A proprietary, non-prescription compound preparation of zinc carbonate zinc oxide, liquid paraffin and other constituents. It is used to cool and soothe itching skin.

Calamine lotion
A proprietary, non-prescription compound preparation of zinc carbonate zinc oxide, liquid paraffin and other constituents. It is used to cool and soothe itching skin.

Calcijex
A proprietary, prescription-only preparation of calcitrol, a vitamin D analogue, that can be used in vitamin D deficiency.

Calcilat
A proprietary, prescription-only preparation of nifedipine. It is used to treat angina, angina attacks and high blood pressure.

Calciparine
A proprietary, prescription-only preparation of heparin. It is used to treat various forms of thrombosis.

Calcipotriol
A proprietary preparation used to treat chronic of milder forms of psoriasis.

Calcisorb
A proprietary, non-prescription preparation of sodium cellulose phosphate, used to help reduce high calcium levels in the bloodstream.

Calcitare
A proprietary, prescription-only preparation of the thyroid hormone calcitonin. It can be used to lower blood levels of calcium.

Calcitonin
A thyroid hormone produced and secreted by the thyroid gland. Its function is to lower the levels of calcium and phosphate in the blood.

Calcitrol
A synthesized form of vitamin D that is used in the treatment of vitamin D deficiency.

Calcium carbonate
A chemical compound used therapeutically as an antacid. It is used to relieve hyperacidity, dyspepsia, heartburn and symptoms of peptic ulcer.

Calcium-500
A proprietary, non-prescription preparation of calcium carbonate. It can be used as a mineral supplement for calcium in cases of deficiency.

Calcium-Sandoz
A proprietary, non-prescription preparation of calcium carbonate. It can be used as a mineral supplement for calcium in cases of deficiency.

Calfig California Syrup of Figs
A proprietary, non-prescription preparation of the laxative senna. It can be used for the relief of constipation.

Calmurid
A proprietary, non-prescription compound preparation of lactic acid and urea. It can be used for dry, scaly, or hard skin.

Calmurid HC
A proprietary, prescription-only compound preparation of hydrocortisone, lactic acid and urea. It can be used for mild inflammation of the skin.

Calpol Infant Suspension
A proprietary, non-prescription preparation of paracetamol. It can be used to treat mild to moderate pain and to reduce fever.

Calpol Infant Suspension Sugar-Free
A proprietary, non-prescription preparation of paracetamol. It can be used to treat mild to moderate pain and to reduce fever.

Calpol Six Plus
A proprietary, non-prescription preparation of paracetamol. It can be used to treat mild to moderate pain and to reduce fever.

Calsynar
A proprietary, prescription-only preparation of the thyroid hormone calcitonin. It can be used to lower blood levels of calcium.

Calcium carbonate

Properties
This medicine contains as active ingredient a neutralizing agent for excess stomach acid and is therefore called an antacid. Antacids are taken by mouth to relieve heartburn, sour stomach, or acid indigestion. Antacids alone or in combination with simethicone may be used to treat the symptoms of stomach or duodenal ulcers. This medication contains as active ingredient: calcium carbonate.

Before using this medicine
Before you use this medicine check with your doctor, or pharmacist:
- if you ever had any unusual or allergic reaction to aluminum-, calcium-, magnesium-, sodium bicarbonate-, or simethicone containing medicines;
- if you are on a low-salt, low-sugar, or any other special diet, or if you are allergic to any substance, such as sulfites or other preservatives or dyes.
- if you are pregnant or intending to become pregnant while using this medicine. Although antacids have not been shown to cause problems in humans, the chance always exists.
- if you are breast-feeding an infant.
- if you have any of the following medical problems:
  Appendicitis (or signs of)
  Bone fractures
  Colitis or colostomy
  Constipation or diarrhea
  Heart disease
  High blood pressure
  Intestinal blockage
  Intestinal bleeding
  Kidney or liver disease
  Toxaemia of pregnancy
  Underactive parathyroids

Treatment
This medication is used to relieve or prevent the symptoms of your medical problem. Take them as directed. Do not take more of them and do not take them more often than recommended on the label, unless otherwise directed by your doctor. To do so may increase the chance of side effects.
When taking this medicine for a stomach or duodenal ulcer, take it exactly as ordered by your doctor to obtain maximum relief of your symptoms.
Antacids should not be given to young children (up to 6 years of age) unless prescribed by their doctor.

Side effects
Along with the needed effects, a medicine may cause some unwanted effects. Although the following side effects occur very rarely when this medicine is taken as recommended, they may be more likely to occur if:
- too much medicine is taken;
- it is taken in large doses;
- it is taken for a long period of time;
- it is taken by patients with kidney disease.
Check with your doctor as soon as possible if any of the following side effects or signs of overdose occur: bone pain; constipation, feeling of discomfort; loss of appetite; mood or mental changes; muscle weakness; swelling of wrists or ankles; unusual loss of weight.

Interactions
This medicine may interact with several other drugs such as adrenocorticosteroids, cellulose sodium phosphate, mecamylamine, methenamine, and tetracyclines.
Be sure to tell your doctor about any medications you are currently taking.

Storage
Tablets, elixir, etc. should be stored at room temperature; store away from heat and direct light. Keep out of reach of children, since overdose may be very dangerous in children. Do not keep outdated medicine or medicine no longer needed.

CAM
A proprietary, prescription-only preparation of ephedrine hydrochloride. It can be used as bronchodilator in reversible obstructive airways disease and asthma.

Camcolit 400
A proprietary, prescription-only preparation of lithium. It can be used to prevent and treat mania and manic-depressive bouts.

Camphor
An aromatic substance with mild counter-irritant properties.

Camsilon
A proprietary, prescription-only preparation of edrophonium chloride. It is used in the diagnosis of myasthenia gravis.

Canesten
A proprietary, prescription-only preparation of the antifungal drug clotri-

mazol. It can be used to treat fungal infections, particularly vaginal candidiasis and skin infections.

Canesten 1 VT
A proprietary, prescription-only preparation of the antifungal drug clotrimazol. It can be used to treat fungal infections, particularly vaginal candidiasis.

Canesten 1 %
A proprietary, prescription-only preparation of the antifungal drug clotri-

mazol. It can be used to treat fungal infections, particularly vaginal candidiasis and skin infections.

Canesten 10% VC

A proprietary, prescription-only preparation of the antifungal drug clotrimazol. It can be used to treat fungal infections, particularly vaginal candidiasis.

Canesten-HC

A proprietary, prescription-only compound preparation of the antifungal drug clotrimazol and the corticosteroid hydrocortisone. It can be used to treat fungal infections, particularly those associated with inflammation.

Cantil

A proprietary, prescription-only preparation of mepenzolate. It can be used as an antispasmodic for the symptomatic relief of smooth muscle spasm.

Capasal

A proprietary, non-prescription compound preparation of coal tar and salicylic acid. It can be used for conditions such as dandruff and psoriasis.

Capastat

A proprietary, prescription-only preparation of the antibacterial and antibiotic drug capreomycin. It can be used to treat tuberculosis.

Capitol

A proprietary, prescription-only preparation of the antiseptic agent benzalkonium chloride. It can be used to treat dandruff and other scalp conditions.

Caplenal

A proprietary, prescription-only preparation of allopurinol. It can be used to treat excess uric acid to prevent kidney stones and attacks of gout.

Capoten

A proprietary, prescription-only preparation of captopril. It can be used to treat high blood pressure and heart failure.

Capozide

A proprietary, prescription-only preparation of captopril. It can be used

to treat high blood pressure and heart failure.

Capreomycin

A proprietary, prescription-only preparation of an antibacterial and antibiotic drug used specifically in the treatment of tuberculosis.

Caprin

A proprietary, non-prescription preparation of aspirin. It can be used to treat headache and rheumatic conditions.

Capsaicin

The active principle of capsicum. When rubbed in topically to the skin it causes a feeling of warmth that offsets the pain from underlying tissues.

Capsicum oleoresin

The active principle of capsicum. When rubbed in topically to the skin it causes a feeling of warmth that offsets the pain from underlying tissues.

Captopril

A proprietary, prescription-only drug with powerful vasodilator properties. It can be used to treat high blood pressure and heart failure.

Carace

A proprietary, prescription-only preparation of lisinopril. It can be used to treat high blood pressure and heart failure.

Carace Plus

A proprietary, prescription-only compound preparation of lisinopril and hydrochlorthiazide. It can be used to treat high blood pressure.

Carbachol

A parasympathicomimetic drug used in glaucoma treatment.

Carbalax

A proprietary, non-prescription preparation of the laxative sodium acid phosphate. It can be used to relieve constipation.

Carbamazepine

A proprietary, prescription-only preparation with anticonvulsant and anti-epileptic properties. It is used in

the preventive treatment of most forms of epilepsy.

Carbaryl

A proprietary, non-prescription-only pediculicidal preparation used in the treatment of head lice and crab lice.

Carbenicillin

A proprietary, prescription-only antibacterial and antibiotic preparation of the penicillin family. It is used to treat serious infections caused by sensitive Gram-negative organisms.

Carbenoxolone sodium

A synthetic derivative of glycyrrhinic acid. It can be used as an ulcer-healing drug for benign gastric ulcers.

Carbidopa

A proprietary, prescription-only preparation. It can be used in the treatment of parkinsonism.

Carbimazole

A proprietary, prescription-only hormone antagonist of the thyroid gland. It is used to treat an excess in the blood of thyroid hormones.

Carbocisteine

A proprietary, prescription-only mucolytic preparation. It can be used in patients with disorders of the upper respiratory tract, such as chronic asthma.

Carbo-Cort

A proprietary, prescription-only compound preparation of hydrocortisone and coal tar. It can be used by topical application to treat eczema and psoriasis.

Carbo-Dome

A proprietary, prescription-only preparation of coal tar. It can be used by topical application to treat eczema and psoriasis.

Carbomer

A proprietary, prescription-only synthetic agent that can be used in artificial tears where there is dryness of the eye.

Carbomix

A proprietary, non-prescription preparation of charcoal. It can be used to

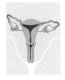

Canesten (Vaginal, topical)

Properties
This medicine belongs to the family of topical (applied to the skin) antifungal preparations. It is used in the treatment of fungus infections on the skin and in the vagina. The medication fights infections such as ringworm of the scalp, athlete's foot, jockey itch, sun fungus, nail fungus and fungus infections of the vagina.

Fungal diseases may develop especially in people with disorders of immunity or diabetes and those on certain drugs (steroid, immunosuppressives, antibiotics). Thrush is common in the mouth and vagina but rarely causes systemic disease.

The drug kills fungi by damaging the fungal wall; it causes loss of essential elements to sustain fungus cell life.

Before using this medicine
Before you use this medicine check with your doctor, or pharmacist:
- if you ever had any unusual or allergic reaction to topical antifungal preparations.
- if you are on a low-salt, low-sugar, or any other special diet, or if you are allergic to any substance, such as certain preservatives or dyes.
- if you are sunburned, or have an open skin wound.
- if you are pregnant, intending to become pregnant or breast-feeding an infant while using this medicine.

Pregnant women should avoid using the vaginal cream during the first three months of pregnancy. They should use it during the next six months only if it is absolutely necessary.

Treatment
This medication is used to relieve or prevent the symptoms of your medical problem. Take them as directed. Do not take more of them and do not take them more often than recommended on the label. To do so may increase the chance of absorption through the skin and the chance of side effects. If you forget to take a dose of this drug, take it as soon as you remember. If it is almost time for your next regularly scheduled application, skip the forgotten application and continue with your regular schedule.

CREAM, LOTION, OINTMENT, GEL: Bathe and dry area before use. Apply small amount and rub gently.
POWDER: Apply lightly to the skin.
VAGINAL CREAM & TABLETS: Insert into vagina with applicator as illustrated in instructions.

The treatment may require a period of 6 to 8 weeks for a complete cure. The usual schedule calls for an application twice a day, morning and evening, unless otherwise directed by your doctor or pharmacist. Be sure to complete the full course of treatment prescribed for you.

Side effects
The following side effects may occur:
- Itching
- Swelling of treated skin
- Redness of skin
- Vaginal burning and itching
- Irritation of vagina
- Swelling of labia
- Increased discharge

You should discontinue the use of the drug when these side effects occur. Call your doctor right away.

Interactions
This medicine may interact with several other medications applied to the skin or vagina. The combined effect may cause severe skin irritation or disorders of the labia or vagina.

Storage
This medicine should be stored cool, but do not freeze. Store away from heat and direct light. Keep out of reach of children. do not use on other members of the family without consulting your doctor. Do not store in the bathroom medicine cabinet because the heat or moisture may cause the medicine to break down. Do not keep outdated medicine or medicine no longer needed. Flush the contents down the toilet, unless otherwise directed.

---

treat patients suffering from poisoning or a drug overdose.

Carboplatin
A proprietary, prescription-only preparation of cisplatin. It can be used as an anticancer treatment specifically for cancer of the ovary.

Carboprost
A proprietary, prescription-only analogue of prostaglandin used to treat hemorrhage following childbirth.

Cardene
A preparation of nicardipine hydrochloride. It can be used to treat high blood pressure and angina.

Cardene SR
A proprietary, prescription-only preparation of nicardipine hydrochloride. It can be used to treat high blood pressure and angina.

Cardilate MR
A proprietary, prescription-only pre-

paration of nifedipine used in the treatment of high blood pressure and angina.

Cardinol
A preparation of propranolol. It can be used to treat high blood pressure and angina and regularize heartbeat.

Cardura
A proprietary, prescription-only preparation of doxazosin. It can be used to treat high blood pressure.

Carisoma
A proprietary, prescription-only preparation of carisoprolol. It can be used to treat muscle spasm caused by injury to or a disease of the central nervous system.

Carmustine
A proprietary, prescription-only preparation of cytostatic drug class used as an anticancer drug.

Carteolol
A proprietary, prescription-only preparation of the beta-blocker type used for chronic simple glaucoma.

Carvedilol
A proprietary, prescription-only preparation of the beta-blocker type used to treat high blood pressure.

Carylderm
A proprietary, non-prescription preparation of carbaryl used to treat infestations of lice in the scalp and pubic hair.

Catapres
A proprietary, prescription-only preparation of clonidine hydrochloride used in the treatment of high blood pressure.

Caved-S
A proprietary, non-prescription compound preparation of aluminium hydroxide, magnesium carbonate, sodium bicarbonate, bismuth subnitrate and liquorice. It can be used to treat peptic ulcers.

Caverject
A proprietary, prescription-only preparation of alprostadil used for men to manage penile erectile dysfunction.

Cedax
A proprietary, prescription-only preparation of the antibacterial and antibiotic drug ceftibuten. It can be used to treat acute bacterial infections of the urinary and respiratory tracts.

Cedocard
A proprietary, prescription-only preparation of isosorbide nitrate. It can be used to treat angina pectoris and heart failure.

Cedocard-Retard
A proprietary, prescription-only preparation of isosorbide nitrate. It can be used to prevent angina pectoris.

Cefaclor
A proprietary, non-prescription antibacterial and antibiotic preparation, primarily used to treat infections of the respiratory and urinary tracts.

Cefadroxil
A proprietary, prescription-only antibacterial and antibiotic broad-spectrum preparation primarily used to treat infections of the urinary tract.

Cefodizime
A proprietary, prescription-only antibacterial and antibiotic broad-spectrum preparation primarily used to treat infections of the urinary tract and lower respiratory tract.

Cefotaxime
A proprietary, prescription-only antibacterial and antibiotic drug. It can be used to treat many infections.

Cefpodoxine
A proprietary, prescription-only antibacterial and antibiotic drug. It can be used to treat a wide range of infections of the respiratory tract.

Cefuroxime
A proprietary, prescription-only antibacterial and antibiotic drug. It can be used to treat a wide range of infections of the urinary, respiratory and genital tracts.

Celebrex
A proprietary, prescription-only preparation of celecoxib. It is used to for the symptomatic relief of symptoms osteoarthritis and adult rheumatoid arthritis.

Celectol
A proprietary, prescription-only preparation of methylcellulose, used to treat a number of gastrointestinal disorders.

Celiprolol
A proprietary, prescription-only preparation of the beta-blocker type. It can be used to treat high blood pressure.

Cephalexin
A proprietary, prescription-only antibacterial and antibiotic preparation. It can be used to treat a wide range of infections, particularly of the urinary tract.

Cephazolin
A proprietary, prescription-only antibacterial and antibiotic preparation. It can be used to treat a wide range of infections, particularly of the skin, soft tissues, and urinary, genital and respiratory tracts.

Cephradine
A proprietary, prescription-only antibacterial and antibiotic preparation. It can be used to treat a wide range of infections, particularly of the skin, soft tissues, and urinary, genital and respiratory tracts.

Cerumol
A proprietary, non-prescription compound preparation of chlorbutol and arachis oil, used to remove earwax.

Cetavlex
A proprietary, non-prescription compound preparation of chlorbutol and arachis oil. It can be used to treat cuts and abrasions.

Cetrimide
An antiseptic and disinfectant agent, used therapeutically for cleansing the skin and scalp, burns and wounds.

Chenofalk
A proprietary, prescription-only preparation of chenodeoxycholic acid, used to dissolve gallstones.

Chloractil
A proprietary, prescription-only preparation of chlorpromazine hydrochloride, used in patients undergoing behavioral disturbances, or who are psychotic.

Chloramphenicol
A proprietary, prescription-only antibacterial and antibiotic broad-spectrum preparation. It can be used to treat many forms of infection.

Fever
Pain
Infection

Celebrex

What is Celebrex?
Celebrex is a proprietary, prescription preparation (generic name Celecoxib) believed to fight pain and inflammation by inhibiting the effect of a natural enzyme called COX-2.

Why is this drug prescribed?
This drug is prescribed for acute pain, menstrual cramps, and the pain and inflammation of osteoarthritis and rheumatoid arthritis.

What are important facts about this drug?
Although this drug is easy on the stomach, it still poses some degree of risk, especially if you have had a stomach ulcer or gastrointestinal bleeding in the past.

How should I take this medication?
For best results, take this drug regularly, exactly as prescribed. You can take it with or without food.
If you miss a dose, take it as soon as possible. If it is almost time for your next dose, skip the one you missed and go back to your regular schedule. Do not take 2 doses at the same time.

What side effects may occur?
Side effects cannot be anticipated. If any develop or change in intensity, inform your doctor as soon as possible. Only your doctor can determine if it is safe for you to continue taking this medicine.
▲ More common side effects
  - Abdominal pain
  - diarrhea
  - headache
  - indigestion
  - nausea
  - respiratory infection
  - sinus inflammation
▲ Less common side effects
  - Back pain
  - dizziness
  - insomnia
  - rash
  - swelling
▲ Rare side effects
  - Allergic reactions
  - anxiety
  - blood disorders
  - chest pain
  - depression
  - severe diarrhea
  - skin reaction due to sunlight

Why should this drug not be prescribed?
Do not take this medicine if you are allergic to sulphonamide drugs such as sulphadiazine, sulphisoxazole. Also avoid this medicine if you have ever suffered an asthma attach, face and throat swelling, or skin eruptions after taking aspirin or other NSAIDs. If you find that you are allergic to this medicine, you will not be able to use is.

Are there any special warnings about this drug?
▲ Remember to tell your doctor about any stomach ulcers or bleeding if you have had in the past. Also alert your doctor if you develop any digestive problems, swelling, or rash.
▲ If you have asthma, use this drug with caution. It could trigger an attack, especially if you are sensitive to aspirin.
▲ If you are taking a steroid medication for your arthritis, do not discontinue it abruptly when you begin with this medicine. It is not a substitute for steroids. This medicine has been known to cause kidney or liver problems, particularly in people with an existing problem. If you have such a disorder, take this medicine with caution. If you develop symptoms of liver poisoning, stop taking this medicine and see your doctor immediately. Warning signs include: nausea, fatigue, itching, itching, yellowish skin, pain in the right side of the abdomen, flu-like symptoms
▲ This drug sometimes causes water retention, which can aggravate swelling, high blood pressure, and heart failure. Use this drug with caution if you have any of these conditions.
▲ The safety and effectiveness of this drug have not been tested in children under 18 years.

Can I take this drug during pregnancy and/or breastfeeding?
This drug can harm a developing baby if taken during the third trimester, and its safety earlier in pregnancy has not been confirmed. Take it during pregnancy only if you and your doctor feel the risk is justified.
It is possible that this medicine makes its way into breast milk, and it could cause serious reactions in a nursing infant. If this drug is essential to your health, your doctor may advice you to discontinue breastfeeding.

What is the recommended dosage?
▲ Osteoarthritis
  The recommended daily dose is 200 milligrams, taken as a single dose or in 100-milligramme doses twice a day.
▲ Rheumatoid arthritis
  The recommended daily dose is 100 to 200 milligrammes twice a day.
▲ Acute pain and menstrual cramps
  The recommended daily dose is 400 milligrammes, followed by an additional 200 milligrammes if needed on the first day. On subsequent days. the recommended dosage is 200 milligrammes twice a day

Chlordiazepoxide
A proprietary, prescription-only preparation of the benzodiazepine class. It can be used as an anxiolytic in the short-term treatment of anxiety.

Chlormycetin
A proprietary, prescription-only preparation of the antibacterial and antibiotic drug chloramphenicol. It can be used to treat potentially dangerous bacterial infections, such as typhoid fever.

Chlormycetin hydrocortisone
A compound preparation of the antibacterial and antibiotic drug chloramphenicol and the corticosteroid drug hydrocortisone. It can be used to treat eye infections with inflammation.

Chloroquine
A proprietary, prescription-only preparation used to treat and to prevent malaria. The drug is also used as an antirheumatic to slow the progress of rheumatic disease.

Chlorothiazide
A proprietary, non-prescription diuretic preparation, used to treat high blood pressure and oedema.

Chlorphenamine maleate
A proprietary, prescription-only antihistamine preparation. It is used to treat the symptoms of allergic conditions such as hay fever and urticaria.

Chlorpheniramine maleate
A proprietary, prescription-only antihistamine preparation. It is used to treat the symptoms of allergic conditions such as hay fever and urticaria.

Chlorpromazine hydrochloride
A proprietary, prescription-only preparation of the phenothiazine group. It is used as an antipsychotic drug and has marked sedative effects.

Chlorpropamide
A proprietary, non-prescription hypoglycaemic preparation used in the treatment of type-II diabetes.

Chlortetracycline
A proprietary, prescription-only broad-spectrum antibacterial and antibiotic preparation, used to treat many forms of infection, especially of the eye and skin.

Chlorthalidone
A proprietary, prescription-only diuretic preparation, used to treat oedema and high blood pressure.

Cholestyramine
A resin that binds bile acids in the gut and is used as a lipid-lowering drug to reduce levels of lipids in the bloodstream.

Choline salicylate
A proprietary, non-prescription preparation with mild, local pain-relieving properties.

Chorionic gonadotrophin
Hormone secreted by the placenta and so is obtained form the urine of pregnant women. It can be used as an infertility treatment.

Cicatrin
A proprietary, non-prescription preparation of the antibacterial and antibiotic drug neomycin. It can be used to treat skin infections.

Cidomycin
A proprietary, prescription-only preparation of the antibacterial and antibiotic drug gentamycin. It can be used to treat many forms of infection.

Cidomycin Topical
A proprietary, prescription-only preparation of the antibacterial and antibiotic drug gentamycin for topical application. It can be used to treat many forms of infection.

Cilastin
A proprietary, prescription-only enzyme inhibitor which breaks down imipenem and so prolongs and enhances the antibiotic's effects.

Cilazepil
A proprietary, non-prescription powerful vasodilator, used in the treatment of high blood pressure.

Ciloxan
A proprietary, prescription-only preparation of the antibacterial and antibiotic drug ciprofloxacin. It can be used to treat a variety of infections.

Cimetidine
A proprietary, prescription-only ulcer-healing drug. It is used to assist in the treatment of benign peptic ulcers, to relieve heartburn in cases of reflux esophagitis and a variety of conditions where reduction of acidity is beneficial.

Cinchocaine
A proprietary, non-prescription local anesthetic used to relieve pain, particularly in dental surgery.

Cineole
A proprietary, non-prescription preparation of terpene plant oils and resins. It can be used as a nasal decongestant.

Cinnarizine
A proprietary, prescription-only preparation with antihistamine properties, mainly used as an antinauseant.

Cinobac
A proprietary, prescription-only preparation of the antibacterial and antibiotic drug cinoxacin. It can be used to treat various infections.

Cinoxacin
A proprietary, prescription-only preparation of the antibacterial and antibiotic drug cinoxacin. It can be used to treat various infections.

Ciprofibrate
A proprietary, prescription-only lipid-lowering drug. It can be used to reduce lipid levels in the bloodstream.

Ciprofloxacin
A proprietary, prescription-only antibacterial and antibiotic preparation. It can be used to treat infections in patients who are allergic to penicillin.

Ciproxin
A proprietary, prescription-only antibacterial and antibiotic preparation. It can be used to treat infections in patients who are allergic to penicillin.

Cisapride
A proprietary, prescription-only preparation with motility stimulant properties. It can be used to treat esophageal reflux, dyspepsia and some other conditions.

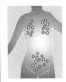

Chlorpheniramine

Properties

This medicine contains chlorpheniramine as active ingredient; it is used to treat or prevent symptoms of allergy. This medication belongs to a group known as antihistamines. Antihistamines block the action of histamine, a chemical that is released by the body during an allergic reaction. Some of the antihistamines are also used to prevent motion sickness, nausea, vomiting, and dizziness.

Before using this medicine

Before you use this medicine check with your doctor, or pharmacist:
- if you ever had any unusual or allergic reaction to antihistamines.
- if you are on a low-salt, low-sugar, or any other special diet, or if you are allergic to any substance, such as sulfites or other preservatives or dyes.
- if you are pregnant or intending to become pregnant while using this medicine.
- if you are breast-feeding an infant. Small amounts of antihistamines pass into the breast milk. Use is not recommended since the chances are greater for most antihistamines to cause side effects, such as unusual excitement or irritability in the infant.
- if you have any of the following medical problems:
  Asthma attack
  Enlarged prostate
  Glaucoma
  Urinary tract blockage
  Difficult urination

Treatment

This medication is used to relieve or prevent the symptoms of your medical problem. Take them as directed. Do not take more of them and do not take them more often than recommended on the label, unless otherwise directed by your doctor. To do so may increase the chance of side effects.

Side effects

The following minor side effects may occur:
- Blurred vision
- Confusion
- Constipation
- Diarrhea
- Difficult or painful urination
- Dizziness
- Dry mouth, throat, or nose
- Headache
- Irritability
- Loss of appetite
- Nausea or stomach upset
- Ringing or buzzing in the ears
- Unusual increase in sweating.

These side effects should disappear as your body adjusts to the medication.

Tell your doctor about any side effects that are persistent or particularly bothersome. It is especially important to tell your doctor about a change in menstruation, clumsiness, feeling faint, flushing of the face, hallucinations, rash, palpitations, seizures, shortness of breath, fever, sleeping disorders, sore throat, tightness in the chest, unusual bleeding or bruising, or unusual tiredness or weakness.

Interactions

This medicine interacts with several other drugs such as central nervous system depressants and it can decrease the activity of oral anticoagulants.

Be sure to tell your doctor about any medications you are currently taking.

Storage

Tablets, elixir, etc. should be stored at room temperature in tightly closed containers. Store away from heat and direct light. Keep out of reach of children, since overdose may be very dangerous in children. Do not keep outdated medicine or medicine no longer needed. Flush the contents of the container down the toilet, unless otherwise directed.

Cisplatin

A proprietary, prescription-only cytotoxic preparation, used to treat certain forms of cancer.

Citanest

A proprietary, prescription-only preparation of the local anesthetic drug prilocaine. It can be used for various types of anesthesia.

Citanest with Octapressin

A proprietary, prescription-only compound preparation of the local anesthetic drug prilocaine and felypressin. It can be used in dental surgery.

Claforan

A preparation of the antibacterial and antibiotic drug cefotaxine. It can be used a wide variety of infections.

Clarinex

A proprietary, prescription-only preparation of desloratadine. It is used to for the symptomatic treatment of allergic rhinitis.

Clarithromycin

A proprietary, non-prescription preparation of the antibacterial and antibiotic drug erythromycin. It is usually given to patient who are allergic to penicillin.

C

Claritin
A proprietary, prescription-only preparation of loratadine/pseudoephedrine. It is used for allergic conditions such as runny nose, sneezing, watery eyes.

Clavulanic acid
A proprietary, prescription-only antibiotic preparation that is only weakly antibacterial, but which prevents bacterial resistance.

Clearine Eye Drops
A proprietary, non-prescription preparation of naphazoline hydrochloride. It can be used redness in the eyes due to minor infections.

Clemastine
A proprietary, prescription-only antihistamine preparation, used for the symptomatic relief of allergic symptoms.

Cexane
A proprietary, prescription-only preparation of enoxaparin. It can be used for long-duration prevention of venous thrombo-embolism.

Climagest
A proprietary, prescription-only compound preparation of oestradiol and norethisterone, used to treat menopausal problems.

Climaval
A proprietary, prescription-only preparation of oestradiol, used to treat menopausal problems.

Clindamycin
A proprietary, prescription-only antibacterial and antibiotic drug, used to treat infections of bones and joints, peritonitis and to assist in the prevention of endocarditis.

Clinicide
A proprietary, non-prescription preparation of carbaryl, used to treat infestation of the scalp and pubic hair by lice.

Clinitar
A proprietary, non-prescription preparation of coal tar. It can be used by topical application to treat eczema and psoriasis.

Clinoril
A proprietary, prescription-only preparation of sulindac, used to treat rheumatic conditions and other musculoskeletal disorders.

Clioquinol
A proprietary, prescription-only antimicrobial preparation used to treat Candida fungal infections of the skin.

Clobazam
A proprietary, non-prescription benzodiazepine preparation used in the short-term treatment of anxiety.

Clobetazol propionate
A proprietary, prescription-only corticosteroid preparation used in the treatment of skin conditions such as eczema and psoriasis.

Clobetazol butyrate
A proprietary, prescription-only corticosteroid preparation used in the treatment of skin conditions such as eczema and certain types of dermatitis.

Clofazimine
A proprietary, prescription preparation used in the treatment of leprosy.

Clofibrate
A proprietary, prescription-only lipid-lowering preparation used to reduce the levels of lipids in the bloodstream.

Clomid
A proprietary, prescription-only preparation of clomiphene citrate, used in the treatment of infertility.

Clomiphene
A proprietary, prescription-only preparation of clomiphene citrate, used in the treatment of infertility.

Clomipramine hydrochloride
A proprietary, prescription-only antidepressant preparation used to treat depressive illness.

Clonazepam
A proprietary, prescription-only benzodiazepine preparation used for all forms of epilepsy.

Clonidine hydrochloride
A proprietary, prescription-only anti-sympathetic preparation, used in the treatment of high blood pressure.

Clopamide
A proprietary, prescription-only antidiuretic preparation used in the treatment of high blood pressure.

Clopixol
A proprietary, prescription-only preparation of zuclopenthixol used for the treatment of schizophrenia and other psychoses.

Clopixol Acuphase
A proprietary, prescription-only preparation of zuclopenthixol used for the short-term treatment of schizophrenia and other psychoses.

Clopixol Concentrate
A proprietary, prescription-only preparation of zuclopenthixol used for the long-term treatment of schizophrenia and other psychoses.

Clorazepate dipotassium
A proprietary, prescription-only benzodiazepine preparation, used for the short-term treatment of anxiety.

Clotrimazole
A proprietary, prescription-only antibacterial and antifungal preparation, used for the treatment of fungal infections of the skin.

Cloaxillin
A proprietary, prescription-only antibacterial and antibiotic preparation of the penicillin family, used for the treatment of a variety of infections.

Clozapine
A proprietary, prescription-only antipsychotic preparation, used for the treatment of schizophrenia.

Clozaril
A proprietary, prescription-only preparation of clozapine. It can be used for the treatment of schizophrenia.

Coal tar
A black, viscous liquid obtained by distillation of coal, used on the skin for the treatment of inflammation and itching.

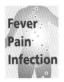

Clinoril

Properties
This medicine contains as active ingredient sulindac. It belongs to the group of medicines called non-steroidal anti-inflammatory drugs (NSAIDs). These drugs are taken by mouth to relieve some symptoms caused by arthritis or rheumatism, such as inflammation, swelling, stiffness, and joint pain. However, these medicines do not cure arthritis and will help you only as long as you continue to take them. Some of these medicines are also used to relieve other kinds of pain or to treat other painful conditions, such as gout attacks, bursitis, tendinitis, sprains, strains, menstrual cramps. The drug reduces the tissue concentration of prostaglandins (hormonal substances which produce inflammation and pain).

Before using this medicine
Before you use this medicine check with your doctor, or pharmacist:
- if you ever had any unusual or allergic reaction, such as skin rash, hives, or itching or breathing problems, to any of the anti-inflammatory analgesics.
- if you are on a low-salt, low-sugar, or any other special diet, or if you are allergic to any substance, such as sulfites or other preservatives or dyes.
- if you are pregnant or intending to become pregnant while using this medicine. Studies on birth defects have not been done in humans. However, if taken regularly during the last months of pregnancy, there is a chance that these medicines may cause unwanted effects on the heart or blood flow in the fetus or newborn infant.
- if you are breast-feeding an infant. Although this medicine has not been shown to cause problems in humans, it passes into the breast milk in small amounts.
- if you have any of the following medical problems: Asthma, Bleeding problems, Colitis or other intestinal problems Stomach ulcer, or other stomach problems Heart disease Kidney or liver disease

Treatment
This medication is used to relieve pain or other symptoms caused by arthritis. For safe and effective use of this medicine, do not take more of it, do not take it more often, and do not take it for a longer period of time than ordered by your physician or directed by the package label.
If you are taking this medication on a regular schedule and you miss a dose, take the missed dose as soon as possible, unless it is almost time for your next dose. In that case do not take the missed dose at all.
To lessen stomach upset, anti-inflammatory analgesics may be taken with food or antacids.

Side effects
Along with the needed effects, a medicine may cause some unwanted effects. These side effects may go away during treatment as your body adjusts to the medicine. Such minor side effects are: dizziness; nausea; pain; headache; drowsiness; swollen feet, face or leg; constipation or diarrhea; vomiting; dry mouth.
Check with your doctor immediately if any of the following side effects occur:
- *Muscle cramps*
- *Numbness or tingling*
- *Mouth ulcers*
- *Convulsions or confusion*
- *Rash, hives, or itch*
- *Tightness in chest*

Interactions
This medicine may interact with several other drugs.
Be sure to tell your doctor about any medications you are currently taking.

Storage
The medicine should be stored at room temperature in a tightly closed, light-resistant container. Store away from heat and direct light. Keep out of reach of children.

Coal tar and salicylic acid
Coal tar is a black, viscous liquid obtained by distillation of coal. With salicylic acid it is used for the treatment of chronic eczema and psoriasis.

Co-amilofruse 5/40
A proprietary, prescription-only compound preparation of amiloride hydrochloride and frusemide, used for the treatment of high blood pressure and congestive heart failure.

Co-amilofruse 10/80
A proprietary, prescription-only compound preparation of amiloride hydrochloride and frusemide, used for the treatment of high blood pressure and congestive heart failure.

Co-amilozide 2.5/25
A preparation of amiloride hydrochloride and hydrochlorothiazide, used for the treatment of high blood pressure and congestive heart failure.

Co-amilozide 5/50
A proprietary, prescription-only preparation of amiloride hydrochloride and hydrochlorothiazide, used for the treatment of high blood pressure and congestive heart failure.

Co-amoxclav
A proprietary, prescription-only preparation of amoxycillin and clavulanic acid, used for the treatment of various types of infection.

Cobadex

A proprietary, prescription-only compound preparation of hydrocortisone and dimethicone, used for the treatment of inflammatory skin conditions.

C

Cobalin-H

A proprietary, prescription-only preparation of hydroxocobalamin, used to correct deficiency of vitamin B_{12}.

Co-beneldopa

A proprietary, prescription-only compound preparation of levodopa and benserazide, used for the treatment of parkinsonism.

Co-Betaloc

A proprietary, prescription-only compound preparation of metoprolol and chlorothiazide, used for the treatment of raised blood pressure.

Co-Betaloc SA

A proprietary, prescription-only compound preparation of metoprolol and chlorothiazide, used for the treatment of raised blood pressure.

Co-Careldopa

A proprietary, prescription-only compound preparation of levodopa and carbidopa, used for the treatment of parkinsonism.

Cocois

A proprietary, non-prescription preparation of salicylic acid, coal tar and sulphur, used for the treatment of eczema and psoriasis.

Co-codamol

A proprietary, prescription-only compound preparation of codeine phosphate and paracetamol, used for the treatment of mild to moderate pain.

Co-codaprin

A proprietary, prescription-only compound preparation of codeine phosphate and aspirin, used for the treatment of pain conditions.

Codafen Continus

A proprietary, prescription-only preparation of codeine phosphate and ibuprofen, used for the treatment of pain of musculoskeletal disorders.

Codalax

A proprietary, prescription-only preparation of danthron, used for the treatment of constipation.

Codalax Forte

A proprietary, prescription-only preparation of danthron. It can be used for the treatment of constipation.

Coda-Med

A proprietary, non-prescription preparation of codeine phosphate, paracetamol and caffeine, used for the symptomatic relief of pain.

Codanin Tablets

A proprietary, non-prescription preparation of codeine phosphate and paracetamol, used for the symptomatic relief of pain.

Co-danthramer 25/200

A proprietary, prescription-only compound preparation of danthron and poloxamer, used for the treatment of constipation.

Co-danthramer 75/1000

A proprietary, prescription-only compound preparation of danthron and poloxamer, used for the treatment of constipation.

Co-danthusate 50/60

A proprietary, prescription-only compound preparation of danthron and docusate sodium, used for the treatment of constipation.

Codeine phosphate

An opioid narcotic analgesic that has pain-relieving properties and is also an antitussive.

Co-dergocrine mesylate

A proprietary, prescription-only compound preparation of dihydroergocornine mesylate and alpha- and beta-dihydroergocornine mesylate, used for the treatment of certain brain dysfunctions.

Codis 500

A proprietary, prescription-only com-pound preparation of codeine phosphate and aspirin, used for the relieve of mild to moderate pain.

Co-dydramol

A proprietary, prescription-only compound preparation of paracetamol and dihydrocodeine, used for the treatment of mild to moderate pain.

Co-fluampicil

A proprietary, prescription-only compound preparation of ampicillin and fluxloxacillin, used for the treatment of a variety of infections.

Co-flumactone 25/25

A proprietary, prescription-only compound preparation of spironolactone and hydroflumethiazide, used for the treatment of oedema, high blood pressure and congestive heart failure.

Cogentin

A proprietary, prescription-only preparation of benztropine mesylate. It can be used for treatment of parkinsonism.

Cojene Tablets

A proprietary, non-prescription compound preparation of aspirin, codeine phosphate and caffeine, used for the treatment of fever and cold and rheumatic pain.

Colchicine

A proprietary, prescription-only preparation derived from Colchicum autumnale. It can be used for the treatment of gout.

Cold Relief Capsules

A proprietary, non-prescription compound preparation of paracetamol and caffeine, used for the relief of cold and flu symptoms.

Coldrex Powders

A proprietary, non-prescription compound preparation of paracetamol, phenylefrine and vitamin C, used for the relief of cold and flu symptoms.

Coldrex Tablets

A proprietary, non-prescription compound preparation of paracetamol, phenylefrine, caffeine and vitamin C, used for the relief of cold and flu symptoms.

C

Colestid
A proprietary, prescription-only lipid-lowering preparation, used for the reduction of high levels of lipids in the bloodstream.

Colestipol hydrochloride
A resin that binds bile acids and lowers LDL-cholesterol. It can be used as lipid-lowering drug.

Colifoam
A proprietary, prescription-only preparation of the corticosteroid hydrocortisone, used for the treatment of colitis and proctitis.

Colistin
A proprietary, prescription-only antibacterial and antibiotic preparation of the polymixin family, used in the treatment of a variety of infections.

Colofac
A proprietary, prescription-only preparation of mebeverine hydrochloride, used in the treatment of gastrointestinal spasms.

Colomycin
A proprietary, prescription-only preparation of the antibacterial and antibiotic drug colestin, used by topical application for the treatment of skin infections, burns and wounds.

Colpermin
A proprietary, non-prescription preparation of peppermint oil, used to relieve of the discomfort of abdominal colic and distention.

Combantrin
A proprietary, prescription-only preparation of pyrantel, used for the treatment of infestations by pinworm, threadworm and hookworm.

Comixco
A proprietary, prescription-only compound preparation of sulphamethoxazole and trimethoprim, used to treat bacterial infections.

Comox
A proprietary, prescription-only compound preparation of sulphamethoxazole and trimethoprim, used to treat bacterial infections.

Concordin
A proprietary, prescription-only compound preparation of protriptyline hydrochloride, used for the treatment of depressive illness.

Condolyne
A proprietary, prescription-only compound preparation of podophyllum, used for the removal of penile warts.

Conjugated estrogens
Naturally obtained estrogens, which are used in hormone replacement therapy.

Conotrane
A proprietary, non-prescription compound preparation of benzalkonium chloride and dimethicone, used for the relief of nappy rash and skin sores.

Conova 30
A proprietary, prescription-only compound preparation of female sex hormones, used as oral contraceptive and also for certain menstrual problems.

Contac 400
A proprietary, non-prescription compound preparation of phenylpropanolamine and chlorpheniramine maleate, used for symptomatic relief of nasal oversecretion.

Contac Coughcaps
A proprietary, non-prescription preparation of dextromethorphan, used for the treatment of unproductive coughs.

Contraflam
A proprietary, prescription-only preparation of nefenamic acid, used for the treatment of pain in rheumatoid arthritis.

Convulex
A proprietary, prescription-only preparation of valproic acid, used for the treatment of all forms of epilepsy.

Co-phenotrope
A proprietary, prescription-only compound preparation of diphenoxalate hydrochloride and atropine sulphate, used for the treatment of chronic diarrhea.

Copholco
A proprietary, non-prescription compound preparation of pholcodine, terpin, cineole and menthol. It is used for the symptomatic treatment of ticklish cough.

Copholcoids Cough Pastilles
A proprietary, non-prescription compound preparation of pholcodine, terpin, cineole and menthol. It is used for the symptomatic treatment of ticklish cough.

Co-praxamol
A proprietary, prescription-only compound preparation of dextroproxyphene hydrochloride and paracetamol, used for the relief of moderate to mild pain.

Coracten
A proprietary, prescription-only preparation of nifedipine, used for the treatment of raised blood pressure.

Cordarone X
A proprietary, prescription-only preparation of amiodarone hydrochloride, used for the treatment of heartbeat irregularities.

Cordilox
A proprietary, prescription-only preparation of verapamil. It can be used for the treatment of raised blood pressure.

Coreg
A proprietary, prescription-only preparation of carvedilol. It is used for the prevention of another heart attack or stroke.

Corgard
A proprietary, prescription-only compound preparation of nadolol, used for the treatment of raised blood pressure, angina pectoris and to regularize heartbeat.

Corgaretic 40
A proprietary, prescription-only compound preparation of nadolol and bendrofluazide, used for the treatment of raised blood pressure.

Corgaretic 80
A proprietary, prescription-only com-

pound preparation of nadolol and bendrofluazide, used for the treatment of raised blood pressure.

Corlan
A proprietary, non-prescription preparation of the corticosteroid hydrocortisone, used for the treatment of ulcers and sores in the mouth.

Coro-nitro Spray
A proprietary, prescription-only preparation of glyceryl trinitrate, used for the treatment and prevention of angina pectoris and heart failure.

Correctol
A proprietary, non-prescription preparation of chlorhexidine, used for the treatment of inflammation and infection of the mouth.

Corticotrophin
A hormone produced and secreted by the pituitary gland in order to control the secretion and production of other hormones in the adrenal glands. It is used for various deficiency syndromes.

Cortisone acetate
A proprietary, prescription-only corticosteroid drug used to make up for deficiency.

Cortistab
A preparation of the corticosteroid cortisone acetate, used to make up for hormonal deficiency.

Cortisyl
A proprietary, prescription-only preparation of the corticosteroid cortisone acetate, used to make up for hormonal deficiency.

Corwin
A proprietary, prescription-only preparation of amoterol, used for the treatment of moderate heart failure.

Cosalgesic
A proprietary, prescription-only preparation of dextropropoxyphene hydrochloride, used for the treatment of many types of pain.

Cosmogen Lyovac
A proprietary, prescription-only pre-

paration of the cytotoxic drug dactinomycin, used for the treatment of certain forms of cancer.

Cosuric
A proprietary, prescription-only preparation of allopurinol, used for the treatment of attacks of gout and the prevention of renal stones.

Co-tenidone
A proprietary, prescription-only compound preparation of atenolol and chlorthalidone, used for the treatment of raised blood pressure.

Co-triamterzide 50/25
A proprietary, prescription-only compound preparation of triamterine and hydrochlorthiazide, used for the treatment of oedema and raised blood pressure.

Co-trimoxazole
A proprietary, prescription-only compound preparation of sulphamethoxazole and trimethoprin, used for the treatment and prevention of urinary tract infections.

Coversyl
A proprietary, prescription-only preparation of perindopril, used for the treatment of raised blood pressure and heart failure.

Covonia Bronchial Balsam
A compound preparation of dextramethorphan hydrobromide, menthol and guaiphenesin. It is used for the symptomatic relief of non-productive coughs.

Covonia for Children
A proprietary, non-prescription preparation of dextramethorphan hydrobromide. It is used for the symptomatic relief of non-productive coughs, including those associated with the common cold.

Cremalgin Balm
A proprietary, non-prescription compound preparation of capsicum oleoresin, methyl nicotinate and glycol salicylate, used in topical application for symptomatic relief of underlying joint and muscle pain.

Creono
A proprietary, non-prescription preparation of pancreatin, used for the treatment of deficiency of digestive juices.

Cristantaspase
A proprietary, prescription-only preparation of asparginase. It can be used for the treatment of acute lymphoblastic leukaemia.

Crotamiton
A proprietary, non-prescription drug used to relieve itching of the skin.

Crystal violet
A dye with astringent and oxidizing properties that is used as an antiseptic agent.

Crystapen
A proprietary, prescription-only preparation of the antibacterial and antibiotic drug benzylpenicillin, used for the treatment of infections of the skin, middle ear, the respiratory tract and certain severe systemic infections.

Cultivate
A proprietary, prescription-only preparation of fluticasone proprionate, used for the treatment of inflammatory skin disorders.

Cupanol Over 6 Paracetamol Oral Suspension
A proprietary, non-prescription preparation of paracetamol, used for the treatment of mild to moderate pain, toothache, headache and feverish conditions.

Cupanol Under 6 Paracetamol Oral Suspension
A proprietary, non-prescription preparation of paracetamol, used for the treatment of mild to moderate pain such as teething and feverish conditions.

Cuplex
A proprietary, non-prescription compound preparation of salicylic acid, lactic acid and copper acetate. It is used to remove warts and hard skin.

Cuprofen
A proprietary, non-prescription

Cortistab

Properties
This medicine belongs to the family of topical (applied to the skin) corticosteroids, containing an adrenocorticoid as active ingredient. It is used to relieve the symptoms of any itching, rash, or inflammation of the skin; it does not treat the underlying cause of the skin problem. It also relieves redness, swelling and itching caused by insect bites, poison ivy, poison oak, poison sumach, soaps, cosmetics, sunburn, and numerous skin rashes.
Topical adrenocorticosteroids are absorbed through the skin and may rarely affect growth in children. Before using this medicine in children you should discuss the use of it with your doctor.

Before using this medicine
Before you use this medicine check with your doctor, or pharmacist:
- if you ever had any unusual or allergic reaction to adrenocorticoids or corticosteroids in general.
- if you are on a low-salt, low-sugar, or any other special diet, or if you are allergic to any substance, such as certain preservatives or dyes.
- if you have diabetes, stomach ulcer, or infection at the treatment site.
- if you are pregnant, intending to become pregnant or breast-feeding an infant while using this medicine.
- if you have any of the following medical problems:
Diabetes mellitus (sugar diabetes)
Infection at the place of treatment
Ulceration at the place of treatment
Tuberculosis

Treatment
This medication is used to relieve or prevent the symptoms of your medical problem. Take them as directed. Do not take more of them and do not take them more often than recommended on the label.
To do so may increase the chance of absorption through the skin and the chance of side effects. In addition, too much use, especially on thin skin areas (for example, armpits, face, groin), may result in thinning of the skin and stretch marks.

Side effects
The following side effects may occur:
- Acne or oily skin
- Blistering
- Burning sensations
- Itching
- Dryness of the skin
- Secondary infection
- Thinning of skin
- Unusual hair growth
- Unusual loss of hair
These side effects should disappear as your body adjusts to the medication. Tell your doctor about any side effects that are persistent or particularly bothersome.
The above side effects are more likely to occur in children and elderly patients, who are usually more sensitive to the effects of this medicine.
When the gel, solution, lotion, or aerosol from this medicine is applied, a mild, temporary stinging may be expected.

Interactions
This medicine interacts with several other drugs such as antibiotics (causing a decreased antibiotic effect) and antifungals (causing a decreased antifungal effect).
Be sure to tell your doctor about any medications you are currently taking.

Storage
This medicine should be stored at room temperature in closed containers. Store away from heat and direct light. Keep out of reach of children, since overdose may be dangerous in children. Do not store in the bathroom medicine cabinet because the heat or moisture may cause the medicine to break down. Keep the medicine from freezing. Do not keep outdated medicine.

---

preparation of ibuprofen, used for the relief of headache, period pain, muscular pain, dental pain, feverishness and cold and flu symptoms.

CX Antiseptic Dusting Powder
A proprietary, non-prescription preparation of chlorhexidine, used for the topical application for disinfection and antisepsis.

Cyanocabalamin
A form of vitamin B_{12}, used for the treatment of deficiency syndromes and certain forms of anemia.

Cyclimorph
A proprietary, prescription-only compound preparation of morphine tartrate and cyclizine tartrate. It can be used for the treatment of moderate to severe pain.

Cyclodox
A proprietary, prescription-only preparation the antibacterial and antibiotic drug doxycycline. It can be used to treat a wide variety of infections.

Cyclopenthiazide
A proprietary, prescription-only diuretic preparation of the thiazide class. It is used for the treatment of oedema.

Cyclopentolate hydrochloride
A proprietary, prescription-only anticholinergic drug, which can be used to dilate the pupil and paralyse the fo-

C

cusing of the eye for ophthalmic examination.

Cyclophosphamide
A proprietary, prescription-only cytotoxic preparation. It can be used for the treatment of certain forms of cancer.

Cyclo-Progynova
A proprietary, prescription-only compound preparation of female sex hormones. It can be used in hormone replacement therapy.

Cycloserine
A proprietary, prescription-only preparation of the antibacterial drug cycloserine. It can be used for the treatment of tuberculosis.

Cyclosporin
A proprietary, prescription-only immunosuppressant drug. It can be used to limit tissue rejection.

Cyklokapron
A proprietary, prescription-only preparation of tranexamic acid. It can be used to stop bleeding.

Cymevene
A proprietary, prescription-only preparation of ganciclovir, used to treat life-threatening and sight-threatening viral infections.

Cyproheptadine hydrochloride
A proprietary, non-prescription antihistamine preparation, used for the symptomatic relief of allergic symptoms.

Cyprostat
A proprietary, prescription-only preparation of cyprosterone, used as an anticancer drug for cancer of the prostate gland.

Cyprosterone acetate
A proprietary, prescription-only preparation, used as an anticancer drug for cancer of the prostate gland.

Cystrin
A proprietary, prescription-only preparation of oxybutynin hydrochloride, used in the treatment of urinary frequency and incontinence.

Cytarabine
A proprietary, prescription-only cytotoxic drug. It can be used for the treatment of acute leukaemia.

Cytosar
A proprietary, prescription-only preparation of cytarabine. It can be used for the treatment of acute leukaemia.

Cytotec
A proprietary, prescription-only preparation of misoprostol. It can be used to treat gastric and duodenal ulcers.

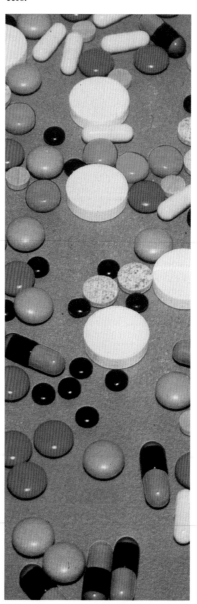

D

Dacarbazine
A proprietary, prescription-only cytotoxic drug, used to treat the skin cancer melanoma,

Dactinomycin
A proprietary, prescription-only cytotoxic drug. It is used to treat cancer in children.

Daktacort
A proprietary, prescription-only preparation of the corticosteroid hydrocortisone and miconazole. It is used to treat fungal skin infection with inflammation.

Daktarin
A proprietary, prescription-only preparation of the antifungal drug miconazole. It is used to treat fungal infections.

Daktarin Cream
A proprietary, non-prescription preparation of the antifungal drug miconazole. It is used to treat fungal infections of the skin.

Daktarin Oral Gel
A proprietary, non-prescription preparation of the antifungal drug miconazole. It is used to treat fungal infections of the mouth.

Daktarin Powder
A preparation of the antifungal drug miconazole. It is used to treat infections of the skin.

Daktarin Spray Powder
A proprietary, non-prescription preparation of the antifungal drug miconazole. It is used to treat infections of the mouth.

Dalacin
A proprietary, prescription-only preparation of antibacterial and antibiotic drug clindamycin. It is used to treat vaginal infections.

Dalacin C
A proprietary, prescription-only pre-

Danthron

Properties
This medicine contains as active ingredient danthron, a stimulant laxative. Stimulant laxatives (also known as contact laxatives) are medicines taken by mouth to encourage bowel movements by acting on the intestinal wall. They increase the muscle contractions that move along the stool mass.

Before using this medicine
Before you use this medicine check with your doctor, or pharmacist:
- if you ever had any unusual or allergic reaction to laxatives.
- if you are on a low-salt, low-sugar, or any other special diet, or if you are allergic to any substance, such as sulfites or other preservatives or dyes.
- if you are pregnant. Stimulant laxatives may cause unwanted effects in the expectant mother if improperly used. Some of the stimulant laxatives may cause contractions of the womb.
- if you are breast-feeding an infant. Some stimulant laxatives may pass into the breast milk. Although the amount of laxative in the milk is generally thought to be too small to cause problems in the child, your doctor should be told that you plan to use such laxatives.
- if you have any of the following medical problems:
  Appendicitis (or signs of)
  Colostomy
  Diabetes (sugar disease)
  Heart disease
  Hypertension
  Ileostomy
  Intestinal blockage
  Laxative habit
  Rectal bleeding

Treatment
For safe and effective use of bulk-forming laxatives:
Follow your doctor's orders if this laxative was prescribed.
Follow the manufacturer's package directions if you are treating yourself.
At least six to eight 8-ounce glasses of liquids should be taken each day.
Stimulant laxatives are usually taken on an empty stomach for rapid effect. Results are slowed if taken with food.
Laxatives should not be given to young children (up to 6 years of age) unless prescribed by their doctor. Since children cannot usually describe their symptoms very well, a doctor should check the child before giving this medicine.

Side effects
Along with the needed effects, a medicine may cause some unwanted effects.
Side effects that should be reported to your doctor: breathing difficulty; burning on urination; confusion; headache; irregular heartbeat; irritability; mood or mental changes; muscle cramps; skin rash; unusual tiredness.

Laxative habit
Laxatives are to be used to provide short-term relief only, unless otherwise directed by your doctor. Laxatives are overused by many people. Such a practice often leads to dependence on the laxative action to produce a bowel movement. In some cases, overuse of some laxatives has caused damage to the nerves, muscles, and tissues of the intestines and bowel.

Interactions
This medicine may interact with several other drugs, such as amiloride, antacids, other laxatives, potassium supplements, tetracycline antibiotics and triamterene.
Be sure to tell your doctor about any medications you are currently taking.

Storage
Store away from heat and direct light. Keep out of the reach of children. Do not store in the bathroom medicine cabinet because the heat or moisture may cause the medicine to break down.

paration of antibacterial and antibiotic drug clindamycin. It is used to treat infections of the bones and joints and peritonitis.

Dalacin T
A proprietary, prescription-only preparation of antibacterial and antibiotic drug clindamycin. It is used to treat acne.

Dalmane
A proprietary, prescription-only pre-

paration of the benzodiazepine drug flurazepam. It is used to treat insomnia.

Dalsaparoid sodium
A proprietary, prescription-only preparation of a heparin-like drug. It can be used to prevent venous thromboembolism.

Dalteparin
A proprietary, prescription-only preparation of a heparin-like drug. It can

be used to prevent venous thromboembolism.

Danazol
A proprietary, prescription-only hormonal preparation. It is used to treat endometriosis.

Daneral SA
A proprietary, prescription-only preparation of the antihistamine drug pheniramine. It can be used to treat the symptoms of allergic disorders.

Danol

A proprietary, prescription-only hormonal preparation of danazol. It is used to treat inflammation of the endometrium, gynaecomastia and menstrual disorders.

Danthron

A proprietary, non-prescription laxative preparation. It is used to treat constipation.

Dantrium

A proprietary, prescription-only preparation of dantrolene sodium. It is used to treat severe spasticity in skeletal muscles.

Dantrolene sodium

A proprietary, prescription-only drug. It is used to treat severe spasticity in skeletal muscles.

Dantron

A proprietary, non-prescription laxative preparation. It is used to treat constipation.

Daonil

A proprietary, prescription-only preparation of glibenclamide, used in the treatment of diabetes Type II.

Dapsone

A proprietary, prescription-only antibacterial drug, used in the treatment of lepra.

Daranide

A proprietary, prescription-only preparation of the diuretic drug dichlorphenamide. It is used to treat glaucoma.

Daraprim

A proprietary, prescription-only preparation of the antimalarial drug pyrimethamine. It is used to treat or prevent malaria.

Day Nurse Capsules/ Liquid

A proprietary, non-prescription compound preparation of paracetamol, phenylpropanolamine and dextromethorphan. It is used for the relief of cold and flu symptoms.

Debrisoquine

A proprietary, prescription-only adrenergic neuron blocker. It is used to treat severe high blood pressure.

Decadron

A proprietary, prescription-only preparation of the corticosteroid dexamethasone. It is used to treat allergic and inflammatory conditions in shock.

Decadron Shock-Pak

A proprietary, prescription-only preparation of the corticosteroid dexamethasone. It is used to treat allergic and inflammatory conditions in shock.

Deca-Durabolin

A proprietary, prescription-only preparation of the corticosteroid nandralone. It is used to treat osteoporosis in postmenopausal women.

Decazate

A proprietary, prescription-only preparation of flufenazine deconate. It is used in the long-term maintenance of the tranquillization of psychotic patients.

Declinax

A proprietary, prescription-only preparation of debrisoquine. It is used to treat severe high blood pressure.

Decortisyl

A proprietary, prescription-only preparation of the corticosteroid prenisolone. It is used to treat a variety of inflammatory and allergic disorders.

Delfen

A proprietary, non-prescription spermicidal contraceptive for use in combination with barrier methods of contraception.

Deltacortril Enteric

A proprietary, prescription-only preparation of the corticosteroid prenisolone. It is used to treat allergic and rheumatoid conditions.

Deltastab

A proprietary, prescription-only preparation of the corticosteroid prenisolone. It is used to treat allergic and rheumatoid conditions.

Delvas

A proprietary, prescription-only compound preparation of the diuretic drugs amiloride and hydrochlorothiazide. It is used to treat oedema, congestive heart failure, and raised blood pressure.

Demeclocycline

A proprietary, prescription-only antibacterial and antibiotic tetracycline drug. It is used to treat a wide variety of infections.

Demix

A proprietary, prescription-only antibacterial and antibiotic preparation of doxycycline. It is used to treat infections of many kinds.

De-Nol

A proprietary, non-prescription preparation of tropotassium dicitratobismuthate. It is used as an ulcer-healing drug for benign peptic ulcers.

Dentomycin

A proprietary, prescription-only preparation of the antiprotozoal drug metronidazole. It is used for the treatment of local infections in dental surgery.

Depixol

A preparation of the antipsychotic drug flupenthixol. It is used to treat psychotic disorders including schizophrenia.

Depo-Medrone

A proprietary, prescription-only preparation of corticosteroid methylprednisolone. It is used to relieve allergic and inflammatory disorders.

Deponit

A proprietary, prescription-only preparation of glyceryl trinitrate. It is used to treat and prevent angina pectoris.

Depo-Provera

A proprietary, prescription-only preparation of medroxyprogesterone. It is used as an anticancer drug and as a hormonal supplement.

Depostat

A proprietary, prescription-only hor-

Dermovate

Properties
This medicine belongs to the family of topical (applied to the skin) corticosteroids, containing an adrenocorticoid as active ingredient. It is used to relieve the symptoms of any itching, rash, or inflammation of the skin; it does not treat the underlying cause of the skin problem. It also relieves redness, swelling and itching caused by insect bites, poison ivy, poison oak, poison sumach, soaps, cosmetics, sunburn, and numerous skin rashes.
Topical adrenocorticosteroids are absorbed through the skin and may rarely affect growth in children. Before using this medicine in children you should discuss the use of it with your doctor.

Before using this medicine
Before you use this medicine check with your doctor, or pharmacist:
- if you ever had any unusual or allergic reaction to adrenocorticoids or corticosteroids in general.
- if you are on a low-salt, low-sugar, or any other special diet, or if you are allergic to any substance, such as certain preservatives or dyes.
- if you have diabetes, stomach ulcer, or infection at the treatment site.
- if you are pregnant, intending to become pregnant or breast-feeding an infant while using this medicine.
- if you have any of the following medical problems:
Diabetes mellitus (sugar diabetes)
Infection at the place of treatment
Ulceration at the place of treatment
Tuberculosis

Treatment
This medication is used to relieve or prevent the symptoms of your medical problem. Take them as directed. Do not take more of them and do not take them more often than recommended on the label.
To do so may increase the chance of absorption through the skin and the chance of side effects. In addition, too much use, especially on thin skin areas (for example, armpits, face, groin), may result in thinning of the skin and stretch marks.

Side effects
The following side effects may occur:
- Acne or oily skin
- Blistering
- Burning sensations
- Itching
- Dryness of the skin
- Secondary infection
- Thinning of skin
- Unusual hair growth
- Unusual loss of hair
These side effects should disappear as your body adjusts to the medication. Tell your doctor about any side effects that are persistent or particularly bothersome.
The above side effects are more likely to occur in children and elderly patients, who are usually more sensitive to the effects of this medicine.
When the gel, solution, lotion, or aerosol from this medicine is applied, a mild, temporary stinging may be expected.

Interactions
This medicine interacts with several other drugs such as antibiotics (causing a decreased antibiotic effect) and antifungals (causing a decreased antifungal effect).
Be sure to tell your doctor about any medications you are currently taking.

Storage
This medicine should be stored at room temperature in closed containers. Store away from heat and direct light. Keep out of reach of children, since overdose may be dangerous in children. Do not store in the bathroom medicine cabinet because the heat or moisture may cause the medicine to break down. Keep the medicine from freezing. Do not keep outdated medicine.

---

monal preparation of gestronol hexonate. It is used to treat cancer of the endometrium and benign enlargement of the prostate gland.

Dequacaine Lozenges
A proprietary, non-prescription compound preparation of dequalinium chloride and benzocaine. It is used to relieve the discomfort of severe sore throat.

Dequadin Lozenge
A proprietary, non-prescription pre-

paration of dequalinium chloride. It is used to treat common infections of the mouth and throat.

Dequalinium chloride
A proprietary, non-prescription drug used to treat common infections of the mouth and throat.

Derbac-C
A proprietary, non-prescription preparation of carbaryl. It is used to treat infestations of the scalp and pubic hair by lice.

Derbac-M
A proprietary, non-prescription preparation of malathion. It is used to treat infestations of the scalp and pubic hair by lice.

Dermalex
A proprietary, non-prescription preparation of the antiseptic agent hexachlorophane. It is used to treat urinary rash.

Dermovate
A proprietary, prescription-only pre-

D

Desoxymetasone (Topical)

Properties
This medicine belongs to the family of topical (applied to the skin) corticosteroids, containing an adrenocorticoid as active ingredient. It is used to relieve the symptoms of any itching, rash, or inflammation of the skin; it does not treat the underlying cause of the skin problem. It also relieves redness, swelling and itching caused by insect bites, poison ivy, poison oak, poison sumach, soaps, cosmetics, sunburn, and numerous skin rashes.
Topical adrenocorticosteroids are absorbed through the skin and may rarely affect growth in children. Before using this medicine in children you should discuss the use of it with your doctor.

Before using this medicine
Before you use this medicine check with your doctor, or pharmacist:
- if you ever had any unusual or allergic reaction to adrenocorticoids or corticosteroids in general.
- if you are on a low-salt, low-sugar, or any other special diet, or if you are allergic to any substance, such as certain preservatives or dyes.
- if you have diabetes, stomach ulcer, or infection at the treatment site.
- if you are pregnant, intending to become pregnant or breast-feeding an infant while using this medicine.
- if you have any of the following medical problems:
  Diabetes mellitus (sugar diabetes)
  Infection at the place of treatment
  Ulceration at the place of treatment
  Tuberculosis

Treatment
This medication is used to relieve or prevent the symptoms of your medical problem. Take them as directed. Do not take more of them and do not take them more often than recommended on the label.
To do so may increase the chance of absorption through the skin and the chance of side effects. In addition, too much use, especially on thin skin areas (for example, armpits, face, groin), may result in thinning of the skin and stretch marks.

Side effects
The following side effects may occur:
- Acne or oily skin
- Blistering
- Burning sensations
- Itching
- Dryness of the skin
- Secondary infection
- Thinning of skin
- Unusual hair growth
- Unusual loss of hair

These side effects should disappear as your body adjusts to the medication. Tell your doctor about any side effects that are persistent or particularly bothersome.
The above side effects are more likely to occur in children and elderly patients, who are usually more sensitive to the effects of this medicine.
When the gel, solution, lotion, or aerosol from this medicine is applied, a mild, temporary stinging may be expected.

Interactions
This medicine interacts with several other drugs such as antibiotics (causing a decreased antibiotic effect) and antifungals (causing a decreased antifungal effect).
Be sure to tell your doctor about any medications you are currently taking.

Storage
This medicine should be stored at room temperature in closed containers. Store away from heat and direct light. Keep out of reach of children, since overdose may be dangerous in children. Do not store in the bathroom medicine cabinet because the heat or moisture may cause the medicine to break down. Keep the medicine from freezing. Do not keep outdated medicine.

paration of the corticosteroid clobetasol proprionate. It is used to treat severe inflammatory skin disorders.

Dermovate-NN
A proprietary, prescription-only compound preparation of the corticosteroid clobetasol proprionate, neomysin sulphate and nystatin. It is used to treat severe inflammatory skin disorders.

Deseril
A proprietary, prescription-only preparation of methylsergide. It is used to treat and prevent severe, recurrent migraine.

Desferal
A proprietary, prescription-only preparation of the chelating agent desferrioxamine mesylate. It is used as an antidote to treat iron poisoning.

Desferrioxamine mesylate
A proprietary, prescription-only chelating agent, used as an antidote to treat iron poisoning.

Desflurane
A proprietary, prescription-only general anesthetic drug. It is used for the introduction and maintenance of anesthesia.

Desipramine hydrochloride
A proprietary, prescription-only antidepressant drug. It is used to treat depressive illness.

Desmopressin
A proprietary, prescription-only analogue of the antidiuretic hormone va-

sopressin. It is used to treat and test diabetes insipidus.

Desmospray

A proprietary, prescription-only preparation of desmopressin, an analogue of the antidiuretic hormone vasopressin. It is used to treat and test diabetes insipidus.

Desmotabs

A proprietary, prescription-only preparation of desmopressin, an analogue of the antidiuretic hormone vasopressin. It is used to treat and test diabetes insipidus.

Desogestrel

A proprietary, prescription-only hormonal preparation, used as part of a contraceptive.

Desoximetasone

A proprietary, prescription-only corticosteroid. It is used to treat severe, acute inflammation of the skin and chronic skin disorders.

Desoxymethasone

A proprietary, prescription-only corticosteroid. It is used to treat severe, acute inflammation of the skin and chronic skin disorders.

Destolit

A proprietary, prescription-only preparation of ursodeoxycholic acid. It is used to dissolve gallstones.

Deteclo

A proprietary, prescription-only compound preparation of the antibacterial and antibiotic drugs chlortetracycline and demeclocycline. It is used to treat many kinds of infection.

Dexamethasone

A proprietary, prescription-only preparation of the corticosteroid dexamethasone. It is used in the suppression of allergic and inflammatory conditions and in the treatment of shock. (see page 650)

Dexamphetamine

A proprietary, prescription-only preparation of amphetamine. It is used to treat narcolepsy and ADHD.

Decongestants

These are drugs administered to relieve or reduce the symptoms of congestion of the airways and/or nose. Nasal decongestants are generally applied in the form of nose-drops or as a nasal spray, which avoids the tendency of such medicines to have side effects, such as raising the blood pressure, though some are administered orally.

Most decongestants are sympathomimetic drugs, which work by constricting blood vessels in the mucous membranes of the airways and nasal cavity, so reducing the membranes' thickness, improving drainage and possibly decreasing mucous and fluid secretions.

However, rhinitis (nasal congestion), especially when caused by an allergy (for instance hay fever), is usually dealt with by using antihistamines, which inhibit the detrimental and congestive effects of histamine released by an allergic response, or by drugs which inhibit the allergic response itself and so effectively reduce inflammation.

Decongestant drugs are often included in compound preparations that are used to treat colds and which may contain a number of other constituents.
However, most people are unaware of this, but it is important to realize that the vasoconstriction, speeding of the heart and hypertension often caused by these drugs are detrimental and potentially dangerous in a number of cardiovascular disorders.

Dexa-Rhinaspray

A proprietary, prescription-only compound preparation of the corticosteroid dexamethasone, neomycin and tramazoline. It is used to treat allergic rhinitis.

Dexedrine

A proprietary, prescription-only preparation of dexamphetamine. It is used to treat narcolepsy and ADHD.

Dexfenfluramine

A proprietary, prescription-only appetite suppressant, used to treat obesity.

Dextromethorphan hydrobromide

A proprietary, prescription-only drug, used to relieve dry or painful coughs.

Dextromoramide

A proprietary, prescription-only synthetic derivative of morphine. It is used to treat severe and intractable pain, particularly in the final stages of terminal illness.

Dextropropoxyphene hydrochloride

A proprietary, prescription-only opioid drug. It is used to relieve severe pain.

DF 118

A proprietary, prescription-only preparation of the narcotic analgesic drug dihydrocodeine tartrate. It is used to treat acute and chronic severe pain.

DF 118 Forte

A proprietary, prescription-only preparation of the narcotic analgesic drug dihydrocodeine tartrate. It is used to treat acute and chronic severe pain.

DHC Continus

A proprietary, prescription-only preparation of the narcotic analgesic drug dihydrocodeine tartrate. It is used to treat acute and chronic severe pain.

Diabetamide

A proprietary, prescription-only

Dexamethasone
(Topical)

Properties
This medicine belongs to the family of topical (applied to the skin) corticosteroids, containing an adrenocorticoid as active ingredient. It is used to relieve the symptoms of any itching, rash, or inflammation of the skin; it does not treat the underlying cause of the skin problem. It also relieves redness, swelling and itching caused by insect bites, poison ivy, poison oak, poison sumach, soaps, cosmetics, sunburn, and numerous skin rashes.
Topical adrenocorticosteroids are absorbed through the skin and may rarely affect growth in children. Before using this medicine in children you should discuss the use of it with your doctor.

Before using this medicine
Before you use this medicine check with your doctor, or pharmacist:
- if you ever had any unusual or allergic reaction to adrenocorticoids or corticosteroids in general.
- if you are on a low-salt, low-sugar, or any other special diet, or if you are allergic to any substance, such as certain preservatives or dyes.
- if you have diabetes, stomach ulcer, or infection at the treatment site.
- if you are pregnant, intending to become pregnant or breast-feeding an infant while using this medicine.
- if you have any of the following medical problems:
  Diabetes mellitus (sugar diabetes)
  Infection at the place of treatment
  Ulceration at the place of treatment
  Tuberculosis

Treatment
This medication is used to relieve or prevent the symptoms of your medical problem. Take them as directed. Do not take more of them and do not take them more often than recommended on the label.
To do so may increase the chance of absorption through the skin and the chance of side effects. In addition, too much use, especially on thin skin areas (for example, armpits, face, groin), may result in thinning of the skin and stretch marks.

Side effects
The following side effects may occur:
- Acne or oily skin
- Blistering
- Burning sensations
- Itching
- Dryness of the skin
- Secondary infection
- Thinning of skin
- Unusual hair growth
- Unusual loss of hair

These side effects should disappear as your body adjusts to the medication. Tell your doctor about any side effects that are persistent or particularly bothersome.
The above side effects are more likely to occur in children and elderly patients, who are usually more sensitive to the effects of this medicine.
When the gel, solution, lotion, or aerosol from this medicine is applied, a mild, temporary stinging may be expected.

Interactions
This medicine interacts with several other drugs such as antibiotics (causing a decreased antibiotic effect) and antifungals (causing a decreased antifungal effect).
Be sure to tell your doctor about any medications you are currently taking.

Storage
This medicine should be stored at room temperature in closed containers. Store away from heat and direct light. Keep out of reach of children, since overdose may be dangerous in children. Do not store in the bathroom medicine cabinet because the heat or moisture may cause the medicine to break down. Keep the medicine from freezing. Do not keep outdated medicine.

---

preparation of glibenclamide. It is used in diabetic treatment of Type II diabetes.

Diabenese
A preparation of chlorpropamide. It is used in diabetic treatment of Type II diabetes.

Diagesil
A proprietary, prescription-only preparation of diamorphine hydrochloride. It is used to relieve intractable pain.

Dialar
A preparation of benzodiazepine drug diazepam. It is used to treat anxiety and insomnia.

Diamorphine hydrochloride
A proprietary, prescription-only narcotic analgesic drug. It is used to treat severe, intractable pain.

Diamox
A proprietary, prescription-only preparation of azetazolamide. It is used to treat glaucoma.

Dianette
A proprietary, prescription-only compound hormonal preparation of ethinyloestradiol and cyproterone. It is used for contraception.

Diaphine
A proprietary, prescription-only preparation of diamorphine hydrochloride. It is used to relieve intractable pain.

Diarphen
A proprietary, prescription-only com-

pound preparation of diphenoxylate hydrochloride and atropine sulphate. It is used to treat chronic diarrhea.

Diarrest
A proprietary, prescription-only preparation of codeine salts. It is used to supplement or replace minerals.

Diazemuls
A proprietary, prescription-only preparation of the benzodiazepine drug diazepam. It is used to treat anxiety and insomnia.

Diazepam
A proprietary, prescription-only benzodiazepine drug. It is used to treat anxiety, epilepsy and insomnia.

Diazepam Rectubes
A proprietary, prescription-only benzodiazepine drug. It is used to treat anxiety, epilepsy and insomnia.

Diazoxide
A proprietary, prescription-only drug. It is used to treat raised blood pressure and as oral antidiabetic drug.

Dibenyline
A preparation of phenoxybenzamine hydrochloride. It is used to treat raised blood pressure and shock symptoms.

Dibromopropamidine isethionate
A proprietary, prescription-only antibacterial drug. It is used to treat infections of the eyelids.

Dichlorphenamide
A proprietary, prescription-only drug used as a glaucoma treatment.

Diclofenac
A proprietary, prescription-only non-narcotic analgesic and antirheumatic drug. It is used to treat pain and inflammation in rheumatic disease and other musculoskeletal disorders.

Diclomax Retard
A proprietary, prescription-only preparation of diclofenac. It is used to treat pain and inflammation in rheumatic disease and other musculoskeletal disorders.

Diuretics

These medicines are used to reduce fluid in the body by increasing the excretion of water and mineral salts by the kidney, so increasing urine production. They have a wide range of uses, because oedema (accumulation of fluid in the tissues) in sites such as the lungs, ankles and eyeball is symptomatic of a number of disorders.

Reducing oedema is, in itself, of benefit in some of these disorders, and diuretic drugs may be used in acute lung oedema, congestive heart failure, some liver and kidney disorders, glaucoma and in certain electrolyte disturbances.

Their most common use is in antihypertensive treatment, where their action of reducing oedema is of value in relieving the load on the heart, which then gives way to a beneficial reduction in blood pressure.

In relation to their specific actions and uses, the diuretics are divided into a number of distinct classes.

- Osmotic diuretics (for instance mannitol) are inert compound secreted into the kidney proximal tubules and are not resorbed and therefore carry water and salts with them into the urine.

- Loop diuretics (for instance frusemide) have a very vigorous action on the ascending tubules of the loop of Henle (inhibiting resorption of sodium and water) and are used for short periods, especially in heart failure.

- Thiazide and thiazide-like diuretics (for instance chlorothiazide) are the most commonly used and have a moderate action in inhibiting sodium reabsorption at the distal tubule of the kidney, allowing their prolonged use as antihypertensives.

- Potassium-sparing diuretics (for instance amiloride hydrochloride) have a weak action on the distal tubule of the kidney and cause retention of potassium.

- Aldosterone antagonists (for instance spironolactone) work by blocking the action of the normal mineralocorticoid hormone aldosterone and this makes them suitable for treating oedema associated with aldosteronism, liver failure and certain heart conditions.

- Carbonic anhydrase inhibitors (for instance acetazolamide) are useful in reducing fluid in the anterior chamber of the eye which causes glaucoma.

Diclozip
A preparation of diclofenac. It is used to treat pain and inflammation in rheumatic disease and other musculoskeletal disorders.

Dicobalt edeate
An antidote used in acute cyanide poisoning.

Diconal
A proprietary, prescription-only preparation of dipipanone. It is used to treat moderate to severe pain.

Dicyclomine hydrochloride
A proprietary, prescription-only anticholinergic drug that can be used as an antispasmodic for the sympto-

Diflunisal

Properties
This medicine contains as active ingredient diflunisal. It belongs to the group of medicines called non-steroidal anti-inflammatory drugs (NSAIDs). These drugs are taken by mouth to relieve some symptoms caused by arthritis or rheumatism, such as inflammation, swelling, stiffness, and joint pain. However, these medicines do not cure arthritis and will help you only as long as you continue to take them. Some of these medicines are also used to relieve other kinds of pain or to treat other painful conditions, such as gout attacks, bursitis, tendinitis, sprains, strains, menstrual cramps. The drug reduces the tissue concentration of prostaglandins (hormonal substances which produce inflammation and pain).

Before using this medicine
Before you use this medicine check with your doctor, or pharmacist:
- if you ever had any unusual or allergic reaction, such as skin rash, hives, or itching or breathing problems, to any of the anti-inflammatory analgesics.
- if you are on a low-salt, low-sugar, or any other special diet, or if you are allergic to any substance, such as sulfites or other preservatives or dyes.
- if you are pregnant or intending to become pregnant while using this medicine. Studies on birth defects have not been done in humans. However, if taken regularly during the last months of pregnancy, there is a chance that these medicines may cause unwanted effects on the heart or blood flow in the fetus or newborn infant.
- if you are breast-feeding an infant. Although this medicine has not been shown to cause problems in humans, it passes into the breast milk in small amounts.
- if you have any of the following medical problems: Asthma

Bleeding problems
Colitis
Stomach ulcer
Heart disease
Kidney or liver disease

Treatment
This medication is used to relieve pain or other symptoms caused by arthritis. For safe and effective use of this medicine, do not take more of it, do not take it more often, and do not take it for a longer period of time than ordered by your physician or directed by the package label.
If you are taking this medication on a regular schedule and you miss a dose, take the missed dose as soon as possible, unless it is almost time for your next dose. In that case do not take the missed dose at all.
To lessen stomach upset, anti-inflammatory analgesics may be taken with food or antacids.

Side effects
Along with the needed effects, a medicine may cause some unwanted effects. These side effects may go away during treatment as your body adjusts to the medicine. Such minor side effects are: dizziness; nausea; pain; headache; drowsiness; swollen feet, face or leg; constipation or diarrhea; vomiting; dry mouth.
Check with your doctor immediately if any of the following side effects occur:
- *Muscle cramps*
- *Numbness or tingling*
- *Mouth ulcers*
- *Convulsions or confusion*
- *Rash, hives, or itch*
- *Tightness in chest*

Interactions
This medicine may interact with several other drugs.
Be sure to tell your doctor about any medications you are currently taking.

Storage
The medicine should be stored at room temperature in a tightly closed, light-resistant container. Store away from heat and direct light. Keep out of reach of children.

matic relief of muscle spasm in the gastrointestinal tract.

Dicyverine hydrochloride
A proprietary, prescription-only anticholinergic drug that can be used as an antispasmodic for the symptomatic relief of muscle spasm in the gastrointestinal tract.

Didanosine
A proprietary, prescription-only an-

tiviral drug that can be used in the treatment of AIDS.

Didronal PMO
A compound preparation of disodium etidronate and calcium carbonate. It is used to treat Paget's disease of the bone and high calcium levels associated with malignant tumors.

Didronel
A proprietary, prescription-only com-

pound preparation of disodium etidronate and calcium carbonate. It is used to treat Paget's disease of the bone and high calcium levels associated with malignant tumors.

Didronel IV
A compound preparation of disodium etidronate and calcium carbonate. It is used to treat Paget's disease of the bone and high calcium levels associated with malignant tumors.

Dienoestrol

A proprietary, prescription-only synthetic estrogen used as part of hormone replacement therapy.

Diethylamine salicylate

A proprietary, non-prescription drug applied to the skin for symptomatic relief of underlying muscle or joint pain.

Diethyl ether

An inhalant general anesthetic drug.

Diethylpropion hydrochloride

A proprietary, prescription-only preparation related to amphetamine and used as appetite suppressant for the treatment of obesity.

Difflam

A proprietary, non-prescription preparation of benzydamine hydrochloride. It is used for symptomatic relief of pain on the skin, mouth ulcers and other sores.

Diflucan

A proprietary, prescription-only preparation of the antifungal drug fluconazole. It is used to treat candidiasis of the vagina, mouth and other tissue areas.

Diflucortone valerate

A proprietary, prescription-only corticosteroid drug. It is used to treat severe, acute inflammatory skin disorders.

Diflunisal

A proprietary, prescription-only preparation of aspirin. It is used to treat pain and rheumatic disorders.

Digibind

A proprietary, prescription-only drug used as antidote to overdosage by the digoxin and digitoxin.

Digitoxin

A proprietary, prescription-only drug derived from the leaves of Digitalis foxgloves. It is used as heart stimulant, because it increases the force of contraction of the heart muscle.

Digoxin

A proprietary, prescription-only drug derived from the leaves of Digitalis foxgloves. It is used as heart stimulant, because it increases the force of contraction of the heart muscle.

Dihydrocodeine tartrate

A proprietary, prescription-only narcotic analgesic drug with similar actions as codeine phosphate.

Dihydrotachysterol

A synthetic form of vitamin D that is used to make up body deficiencies of this vitamin.

Dijex

A compound preparation of aluminium hydroxide and magnesium hydroxide. It is used to relieve acid indigestion and dyspepsia.

Dijex Tablets

A proprietary, non-prescription compound preparation of aluminium hydroxide and magnesium hydroxide. It is used to relieve acid indigestion and dyspepsia.

Diloxanide furoate

A proprietary, prescription-only antiprotozoal and amoebicidal drug. It can be used to treat chronic infection of the intestine to amoebae.

Diltiazem hydrochloride

A proprietary, prescription-only calcium-channel drug. It is used to treat raised blood pressure and to prevent attacks of angina pectoris.

Diltizem SR

A proprietary, prescription-only calcium-channel drug. It is used to treat raised blood pressure and to prevent attacks of angina pectoris.

Diltizem XL

A proprietary, prescription-only calcium-channel drug. It is used to treat raised blood pressure and to prevent attacks of angina pectoris.

Dimenhydrinate

A proprietary, non-prescription antinauseant drug. It is used to treat motion sickness.

Dimercaprol

A chelating agent used as antidote to poisoning with antimony, arsenic, bismuth, gold, mercury, thallium and lead.

Dimethicone

A water-repellent silicone used as antifoaming agent to reduce flatulence.

Dimotane Expectorant

A proprietary, non-prescription compound preparation of guaiphenesin, brompheniramine maleate and pseudoephedrine. It is used for the symptomatic relief of upper respiratory tract disorders.

Dimotane with Codeine

A proprietary, non-prescription compound preparation of codeine phosphate, brompheniramine maleate and pseudoephedrine. It is used for the symptomatic relief of upper respiratory tract disorders.

Dimotane with Codeine Paediatric

A proprietary, non-prescription compound preparation of codeine phosphate, brompheniramine maleate and pseudoephedrine. It is used for the symptomatic relief of upper respiratory tract disorders.

Dimotapp Elixir

A proprietary, non-prescription compound preparation of phenylpropanolamine, phenylephrine and brompheniramine maleate. It is used for the symptomatic relief of upper respiratory tract disorders.

Dimotapp Elixir Paediatric

A proprietary, non-prescription compound preparation of phenylpropanolamine, phenylephrine and brompheniramine maleate. It is used for the symptomatic relief of upper respiratory tract disorders.

Dimotapp LA Tablets

A proprietary, non-prescription compound preparation of phenylpropanolamine, phenylephrine and brompheniramine maleate. It is used for the symptomatic relief of upper respiratory tract disorders.

Dindevan

A proprietary, prescription-only pre-

Diovol

Properties
This medicine contains as active ingredient a neutralizing agent for excess stomach acid and is therefore called an antacid. Antacids are taken by mouth to relieve heartburn, sour stomach, or acid indigestion. Antacids alone or in combination with simethicone may be used to treat the symptoms of stomach or duodenal ulcers. This medication contains as active ingredients alumina, magnesia, and simethicone.

Before using this medicine
Before you use this medicine check with your doctor, or pharmacist:
- if you ever had any unusual or allergic reaction to aluminum-, calcium-, magnesium-, sodium bicarbonate-, or simethicone containing medicines;
- if you are on a low-salt, low-sugar, or any other special diet, or if you are allergic to any substance, such as sulfites or other preservatives or dyes.
- if you are pregnant or intending to become pregnant while using this medicine. Although antacids have not been shown to cause problems in humans, the chance always exists.
- if you are breast-feeding an infant.
- if you have any of the following medical problems:
  Appendicitis (or signs of)
  Bone fractures
  Colitis or colostomy
  Constipation or diarrhea
  Heart disease
  High blood pressure
  Intestinal blockage
  Kidney or liver disease
  Toxaemia of pregnancy
  Underactive parathyroids

Treatment
This medication is used to relieve or prevent the symptoms of your medical problem. Take them as directed. Do not take more of them and do not take them more often than recommended on the label, unless otherwise directed by your doctor. To do so may increase the chance of side effects.
When taking this medicine for a stomach or duodenal ulcer, take it exactly as ordered by your doctor to obtain maximum relief of your symptoms.
Antacids should not be given to young children (up to 6 years of age) unless prescribed by their doctor.

Side effects
Along with the needed effects, a medicine may cause some unwanted effects. Although the following side effects occur very rarely when this medicine is taken as recommended, they may be more likely to occur if:
- too much medicine is taken;
- it is taken in large doses;
- it is taken for a long period of time;
- it is taken by patients with kidney disease.
Check with your doctor as soon as possible if any of the following side effects or signs of overdose occur: constipation; cramping; difficult or painful urination; headache; loss of appetite; mood or mental changes; muscle pain or twitching; nausea or vomiting; stomach pain; unpleasant taste in mouth; unusual slow breathing; unusual tiredness or weakness.

Interactions
This medicine may interact with several other drugs such as adrenocorticosteroids, cellulose sodium phosphate, mecamylamine, and tetracyclines.
Be sure to tell your doctor about any medications you are currently taking.

Storage
Tablets, elixir, etc. should be stored at room temperature; store away from heat and direct light. Keep out of reach of children, since overdose may be very dangerous in children.

---

paration of phenindione. It is used to treat and prevent thrombosis.

Dinoprost
A proprietary, prescription-only prostaglandin preparation. It is used almost solely to induce termination of pregnancy.

Dinoprostone
A proprietary, prescription-only prostaglandin preparation. It is used almost solely to induce termination of pregnancy.

Diocalm
A proprietary, non-prescription compound preparation of morphine hydrochloride, attapulgite and magnesium aluminium silicate. It is used to treat diarrhea and associated pain and discomfort.

Diocalm Replenisher
A proprietary, non-prescription compound preparation of sodium chloride, sodium citrate, potassium chloride and glucose. It is used as an electrolyte replacement.

Diocalm Ultra
A proprietary, non-prescription preparation of loperamide. It is used to treat diarrhea and associated pain and discomfort.

Diocaps
A proprietary, non-prescription preparation of loperamide. It is used to treat diarrhea and associated pain and discomfort.

Dioctyl
A proprietary, non-prescription com-

pound preparation of ducosate sodium and several other ingredients. It is used to relieve constipation.

Dioctyl Ear Drops

A proprietary, non-prescription compound preparation of ducosate sodium and several other ingredients. It is used for the dissolution and removal of earwax.

Dioderm

A proprietary, prescription-only preparation of the corticosteroid hydrocortisone. It is used to treat mild, inflammatory skin disorders.

Diovol

A proprietary, non-prescription compound preparation of aluminium hydroxide, magnesium hydroxide and dimethicone. It is used for the symptomatic relief of dyspepsia, hyperacidity, hiatus hernia, flatulence and peptic ulcers.

Dipentum

A proprietary, prescription-only preparation of olsalazine sodium. It is used to treat ulcerative colitis.

Diphenhydramine hydrochlorid

A proprietary, prescription-only drug used for the symptomatic relief of allergic symptoms.

Diphenoxylate hydrochloride

A proprietary, prescription-only drug that is used to treat severe diarrhea.

Diphenylpyraline hydrochloride

A proprietary, prescription-only antihistamine preparation, used for the symptomatic relief of allergic symptoms.

Dipipanone

A proprietary, prescription-only powerful narcotic analgesic drug. It is used to treat acute, moderate and severe pain.

Dipivefrine hydrochloride

A proprietary, prescription-only derivative of adrenaline. It is used to treat glaucoma.

Diprivan

A proprietary, prescription-only pre-

paration of propofol. It is used for induction and maintenance of anesthesia.

Diprobase

A proprietary, non-prescription preparation of liquid paraffin that is used as emollient for dry skin.

Diprobath

A proprietary, non-prescription preparation of liquid paraffin that is used as emollient for dry skin.

Diprosalic

A proprietary, prescription-only compound preparation of the corticosteroid betamethasone and salicylic acid. It is used to treat severe inflammatory skin disorders.

Diprosalic XL

A proprietary, prescription-only preparation of the corticosteroid betamethasone. It is used to treat severe inflammatory skin disorders.

Dipyridamole

A proprietary, prescription-only antiplatelet drug. It is used to prevent thrombosis.

Dirythmin SA

A proprietary, prescription-only preparation of disopyramide. It is used to treat irregularities of the heartbeat.

Disipal

A proprietary, prescription-only preparation of orphenadrine. It is used to treat symptoms of parkinsonism.

Disodium etidronate

A proprietary, prescription-only drug used to treat disorders of bone metabolism due to hormone disorders.

Disodium pamidronate

A proprietary, prescription-only drug used to treat disorders of bone metabolism due to hormone disorders.

Disopyramide

A proprietary, prescription-only drug used to treat irregularities of the heartbeat.

Disprin

A proprietary, non-prescription preparation of aspirin. It is used to treat mild to moderate pain and to relieve flu end cold symptoms.

Disprin CV

A proprietary, non-prescription antiplatelet aggregation drug aspirin.It is used to prevent cardiovascular diseases, including heart attack.

Disprin Direct

A proprietary, non-prescription preparation of aspirin. It is used to treat mild to moderate pain, to relieve flu and cold symptoms.

Disprin Extra

A proprietary, non-prescription preparation of aspirin. It is used to treat mild to moderate pain, to relieve flu and cold symptoms.

Disprol

A proprietary, non-prescription preparation of paracetamol. It is used to treat mild to moderate pain, to relieve flu and cold symptoms, feverishness and rheumatic aches and pains.

Disprol Infant

A proprietary, non-prescription preparation of paracetamol. It is used to treat mild to moderate pain, to relieve flu and cold symptoms and feverishness.

Disprol Junior

A proprietary, non-prescription preparation of paracetamol. It is used to treat mild to moderate pain, to relieve flu and cold symptoms and feverishness.

Distaclor

A proprietary, prescription-only preparation of antibacterial and antibiotic drug cefaclor. It is used to treat a wide range of bacterial infections.

Distaclor MR

A proprietary, prescription-only preparation of antibacterial and antibiotic drug cefaclor. It is used to treat a wide range of bacterial infections, particularly of the urinary tract.

Distalgesic

A proprietary, prescription-only compound preparation of dextropropoxyphene and paracetamol. It is used to treat pain anywhere in the body.

Distamine

A proprietary, prescription-only preparation of penicillamine. It is used as an antidote to copper or lead poisoning.

Distigmine bromide

A proprietary, prescription-only anticholinergic drug. It is used to treat urinary retention and paralytic ileus.

Disulfiram

An enzyme inhibitor which blocks a stage in the break down of alcohol. It is used to treat alcoholism.

Dithranol

A proprietary, non-prescription drug used to treat chronic and milder forms of psoriasis.

Dithranol Ointment

A proprietary, non-prescription drug used to treat chronic and milder forms of psoriasis.

Dithranol Triacetate

A proprietary, non-prescription drug used to treat chronic and milder forms of psoriasis.

Dithrocream

A proprietary, non-prescription preparation of dithranol, used to treat chronic and milder forms of psoriasis.

Dithrocream S

A proprietary, non-prescription compound preparation of dithranol and salicylic acid, used to treat chronic and milder forms of psoriasis.

Ditropan

A proprietary, prescription-only preparation of oxybutynin. It is used for the symptomatic treatment of overactive bladder.

Diumide-K Continus

A proprietary, prescription-only compound preparation of frusemide and potassium chloride. It is used to treat oedema.

Diurexan

A proprietary, prescription-only preparation of diuretic drug xipamide. It is used to treat oedema and raised blood pressure.

Dixarit

A proprietary, prescription-only preparation of clonidine hydrochloride. It is used reduce the frequency of migraine attacks.

Doan's Backache Pills

A proprietary, non-prescription preparation of paracetamol and sodium salicylate. It is used for the symptomatic relief of rheumatic aches and pains.

Dobutamine hydrochloride

A proprietary, prescription-only cardiac stimulant drug. It is used to treat serious heart disorders.

Dobutrex

A proprietary, prescription-only preparation of the cardiac stimulant drug dobutamine hydrochloride, used to treat serious heart disorders.

Docusate sodium

A proprietary, non-prescription laxative drug that is used to treat constipation.

Do-Do Expectorant Linctus

A preparation of guaiphenesin. It can be used for the relief of productive and non-productive cough associated with irritation due to infection of the upper airways.

Do-Do Tablets

A proprietary, non-prescription compound preparation of ephedrine hydrochloride and theophylline. It can be used for the relief of productive and non-productive cough, wheezing and breathlessness.

Dolmatil

A proprietary, prescription-only preparation of the antipsychotic drug sulpiride. It can be used to treat schizophrenia and other psychotic conditions.

Dolobid

A proprietary, prescription-only preparation of diflunisal. It can be used to treat moderate to mild pain, the pain of rheumatic disease and other musculoskeletal disorders.

Doloxene

A proprietary, prescription-only preparation of dextropropoxyphene hydrochloride. It can be used to treat mild to moderate pain anywhere in the body.

Doloxene Compound

A proprietary, prescription-only compound preparation of dextropropoxyphene hydrochloride, caffeine and aspirin. It can be used to treat mild to moderate pain anywhere in the body.

Domical

A proprietary, prescription-only preparation of amitriptyline. It can be used to treat depressive illness and bed-wetting by children.

Domiphen bromide

A proprietary, non-prescription antiseptic agent used in throat lozenges.

Domperidone

A proprietary, prescription-only antiemetic and antinauseant drug used particularly for the relief of nausea and vomiting in patients undergoing treatment for cancer.

Dopacard

A proprietary, prescription-only preparation of cardiac stimulant dopexamine. It can be used to treat certain heart diseases.

Dopamet

A proprietary, prescription-only preparation of methyldopa. It can be used to treat raised blood pressure.

Dopamine hydrochloride

A proprietary, prescription-only preparation of the naturally occurring neurotransmitter dopamine. It can be used to treat cardiac shock following a heart attack.

Dopexamine hydrochloride

A proprietary, prescription-only car-

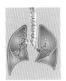

Dolobid

Properties
This medicine contains as active ingredient diflunisal. It belongs to the group of medicines called non-steroidal anti-inflammatory drugs (NSAIDs). These drugs are taken by mouth to relieve some symptoms caused by arthritis or rheumatism, such as inflammation, swelling, stiffness, and joint pain. However, these medicines do not cure arthritis and will help you only as long as you continue to take them. Some of these medicines are also used to relieve other kinds of pain or to treat other painful conditions, such as gout attacks, bursitis, tendinitis, sprains, strains, menstrual cramps. The drug reduces the tissue concentration of prostaglandins (hormonal substances which produce inflammation and pain).

Before using this medicine
Before you use this medicine check with your doctor, or pharmacist:
- if you ever had any unusual or allergic reaction, such as skin rash, hives, or itching or breathing problems, to any of the anti-inflammatory analgesics.
- if you are on a low-salt, low-sugar, or any other special diet, or if you are allergic to any substance, such as sulfites or other preservatives or dyes.
- if you are pregnant or intending to become pregnant while using this medicine. Studies on birth defects have not been done in humans. However, if taken regularly during the last months of pregnancy, there is a chance that these medicines may cause unwanted effects on the heart or blood flow in the fetus or newborn infant.
- if you are breast-feeding an infant. Although this medicine has not been shown to cause problems in humans, it passes into the breast milk in small amounts.
- if you have any of the following medical problems:
Asthma

Bleeding problems
Colitis
Stomach ulcer
Heart disease
Kidney or liver disease

Treatment
This medication is used to relieve pain or other symptoms caused by arthritis. For safe and effective use of this medicine, do not take more of it, do not take it more often, and do not take it for a longer period of time than ordered by your physician or directed by the package label.
If you are taking this medication on a regular schedule and you miss a dose, take the missed dose as soon as possible, unless it is almost time for your next dose. In that case do not take the missed dose at all.
To lessen stomach upset, anti-inflammatory analgesics may be taken with food or antacids.

Side effects
Along with the needed effects, a medicine may cause some unwanted effects. These side effects may go away during treatment as your body adjusts to the medicine. Such minor side effects are: dizziness; nausea; pain; headache; drowsiness; swollen feet, face or leg; constipation or diarrhea; vomiting; dry mouth.
Check with your doctor immediately if any of the following side effects occur:
- *Muscle cramps*
- *Numbness or tingling*
- *Mouth ulcers*
- *Convulsions or confusion*
- *Rash, hives, or itch*
- *Tightness in chest*

Interactions
This medicine may interact with several other drugs.
Be sure to tell your doctor about any medications you are currently taking.

Storage
The medicine should be stored at room temperature in a tightly closed, light-resistant container. Store away from heat and direct light. Keep out of reach of children.

---

diac stimulant, used to treat certain heart disorders.

Dopram
A preparation of doxapram hydrochloride. It can be used to relieve severe respiratory difficulties in patients with chronic obstructive airways disease.

Doralese
A proprietary, prescription-only pre-

paration of indoramin. It can be used to treat urinary retention en benign prostatic hyperplasia.

Dormonoct
A proprietary, prescription-only preparation of the benzodiazepine drug flurazepam. It can be used to treat insomnia.

Dostinex
A proprietary, prescription-only pre-

paration of cabergoline. It can be used to treat the symptoms of parkinsonism.

Dothapax
A proprietary, prescription-only preparation of dothiepin hydrochloride. It can be used to treat depressive illness.

Dothiepin hydrochloride
A proprietary, prescription-only drug

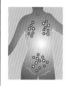

Doxylamine

Properties
This medicine contains doxylamine as active ingredient; it is used to treat or prevent symptoms of allergy. This medication belongs to a group known as antihistamines. Antihistamines block the action of histamine, a chemical that is released by the body during an allergic reaction. Some of the antihistamines are also used to prevent motion sickness, nausea, vomiting, and dizziness.

Before using this medicine
Before you use this medicine check with your doctor, or pharmacist:
- if you ever had any unusual or allergic reaction to antihistamines.
- if you are on a low-salt, low-sugar, or any other special diet, or if you are allergic to any substance, such as sulfites or other preservatives or dyes.
- if you are pregnant or intending to become pregnant while using this medicine.
- if you are breast-feeding an infant. Small amounts of antihistamines pass into the breast milk. Use is not recommended since the chances are greater for most antihistamines to cause side effects, such as unusual excitement or irritability in the infant.
- if you have any of the following medical problems:
  Asthma attack
  Enlarged prostate
  Glaucoma
  Urinary tract blockage
  Difficult urination

Treatment
This medication is used to relieve or prevent the symptoms of your medical problem. Take them as directed. Do not take more of them and do not take them more often than recommended on the label, unless otherwise directed by your doctor. To do so may increase the chance of side effects.

Side effects
The following minor side effects may occur:
- Blurred vision
- Confusion
- Constipation
- Diarrhea
- Difficult or painful urination
- Dizziness
- Dry mouth, throat, or nose
- Headache
- Irritability
- Loss of appetite
- Nausea or stomach upset
- Ringing or buzzing in the ears
- Unusual increase in sweating.

These side effects should disappear as your body adjusts to the medication.
Tell your doctor about any side effects that are persistent or particularly bothersome. It is especially important to tell your doctor about a change in menstruation, clumsiness, feeling faint, flushing of the face, hallucinations, rash, palpitations, seizures, shortness of breath, fever, sleeping disorders, sore throat, tightness in the chest, unusual bleeding or bruising, or unusual tiredness or weakness.

Interactions
This medicine interacts with several other drugs such as central nervous system depressants and it can decrease the activity of oral anticoagulants.
Be sure to tell your doctor about any medications you are currently taking.

Storage
Tablets, elixir, etc. should be stored at room temperature in tightly closed containers. Store away from heat and direct light. Keep out of reach of children, since overdose may be very dangerous in children. Do not keep outdated medicine or medicine no longer needed. Flush the contents of the container down the toilet, unless otherwise irected.

---

that can be used to treat depressive illness.

Double Check
A proprietary, non-prescription spermicidal contraceptive, which is used in combination with barrier methods of contraception.

Dovonex
A proprietary, prescription-only preparation of calcipotriol. It can be used to treat psoriasis.

Doxapram hydrochloride
A respiratory stimulant drug. It can be used to relieve severe respiratory difficulties in chronic obstructive airways disease.

Doxazosin
A proprietary, prescription-only alpha-blocker drug. It can be used to treat raised blood pressure.

Doxepin
A proprietary, prescription-only tricyclic antidepressant drug. It can be used to treat depressive illness.

Doxorubicin hydrochloride
A proprietary, prescription-only cytotoxic drug, which is used as an anti-cancer treatment.

Doxycycline
A proprietary, prescription-only antibacterial and antibiotic drug of the tetracycline class. It can be used to treat a wide variety of infection.

Dulco-lax

Properties
This medicine contains as active ingredient bisacodyl, a stimulant laxative. Stimulant laxatives (also known as contact laxatives) are medicines taken by mouth to encourage bowel movements by acting on the intestinal wall. They increase the muscle contractions that move along the stool mass.

Before using this medicine
Before you use this medicine check with your doctor, or pharmacist:
-   if you ever had any unusual or allergic reaction to laxatives.
-   if you are on a low-salt, low-sugar, or any other special diet, or if you are allergic to any substance, such as sulfites or other preservatives or dyes.
-   if you are pregnant. Stimulant laxatives may cause unwanted effects in the expectant mother if improperly used. Some of the stimulant laxatives may cause contractions of the womb.
-   if you are breast-feeding an infant. Some stimulant laxatives may pass into the breast milk. Although the amount of laxative in the milk is generally thought to be too small to cause problems in the child, your doctor should be told that you plan to use such laxatives.
-   if you have any of the following medical problems:
    Appendicitis (or signs of)
    Colostomy
    Diabetes (sugar disease)
    Heart disease
    Hypertension
    Ileostomy
    Intestinal blockage
    Laxative habit
    Rectal bleeding

Treatment
For safe and effective use of bulk-forming laxatives:
Follow your doctor's orders if this laxative was prescribed.
Follow the manufacturer's package directions if you are treating yourself.
At least six to eight 8-ounce glasses of liquids should be taken each day.
Stimulant laxatives are usually taken on an empty stomach for rapid effect. Results are slowed if taken with food.
Laxatives should not be given to young children (up to 6 years of age) unless prescribed by their doctor. Since children cannot usually describe their symptoms very well, a doctor should check the child before giving this medicine.

Side effects
Along with the needed effects, a medicine may cause some unwanted effects.
Side effects that should be reported to your doctor: breathing difficulty; burning on urination; confusion; headache; irregular heartbeat; irritability; mood or mental changes; muscle cramps; skin rash; unusual tiredness.

Laxative habit
Laxatives are to be used to provide short-term relief only, unless otherwise directed by your doctor. Laxatives are overused by many people. Such a practice often leads to dependence on the laxative action to produce a bowel movement. In some cases, overuse of some laxatives has caused damage to the nerves, muscles, and tissues of the intestines and bowel.

Interactions
This medicine may interact with several other drugs, such as amiloride, antacids, other laxatives, potassium supplements, tetracycline antibiotics and triamterene.
Be sure to tell your doctor about any medications you are currently taking.

Storage
Store away from heat and direct light. Keep out of the reach of children. Do not store in the bathroom medicine cabinet because the heat or moisture may cause the medicine to break down.

Doxylar
A proprietary, prescription-only anti-bacterial and antibiotic drug of the tetracycline class. It can be used to treat a wide variety of infection.

Doxic
A proprietary, prescription-only preparation of haloperidol. It can be used to treat psychotic disorders.

Dramamine
A proprietary, non-prescription preparation of the antihistamine drug dimenhydrinate. It can be used to treat nausea and vomiting.

Drogenil
A proprietary, prescription-only preparation of flutamide. It can be used to treat certain types of cancer.

Droleptan
A proprietary, prescription-only preparation of droperidol. It can be used to treat psychotic conditions.

Droperidol
A proprietary, prescription-only antipsychotic drug. It can be used to treat psychotic conditions.

Dryptal
A proprietary, prescription-only preparation of the diuretic drug fursemide. It can be used to treat oedema.

Dulco-lax Suppositories
A proprietary, non-prescription

preparation of the laxative bisacodyl. It can be used to treat constipation.

Dulco-lax Suppositories for Children
A proprietary, non-prescription preparation of the laxative bisacodyl. It can be used to treat constipation.

Dulco-lax Tablets
A proprietary, non-prescription preparation of the laxative bisacodyl. It can be used to treat constipation.

Duofilm
A proprietary, non-prescription preparation of salicylic acid. It can be used to remove warts and hard skin.

Duovent
A proprietary, prescription-only compound preparation of fenoterol and ipratropium bromide. It can be used to treat asthma and chronic bronchitis.

Duphalac
A proprietary, non-prescription preparation of lactulose. It can be used to treat constipation.

Duphaston
A proprietary, prescription-only preparation of dydrogesterone. It can be used to treat many conditions of hormonal deficiency in women.

Duracreme
A proprietary, non-prescription spermicidal contraceptive that is used in combination with barrier methods of contraception.

Durogesic
A proprietary, prescription-only preparation of fentanyl. It can be used to treat moderate to severe pain.

Duromine
A proprietary, prescription-only preparation of phentermine. It can be used to treat obesity.

Dyazide
A proprietary, prescription-only compound preparation of the diuretic drugs hydrochlorothiazide and triamterene. It can be used to treat oedema and raised blood pressure.

Dydrogesterone
A proprietary, prescription-only analogue of the hormone progesterone, used to treat many disorders of hormonal deficiency in women.

Dynese
A proprietary, non-prescription preparation of magaldrate. It can be used for the symptomatic relief of dyspepsia.

Dysman 250
A proprietary, prescription-only preparation of mefenamic acid. It can be used to treat pain and inflammation in rheumatic disorders.

Dysman 500
A proprietary, prescription-only preparation of mefenamic acid. It can be used to treat pain and inflammation in rheumatic disorders.

Dyspamet
A proprietary, prescription-only preparation of cimetidine. It can be used to treat dyspepsia, gastro-esophageal reflux and peptic ulcers.

Dysport
A proprietary, prescription-only preparation of botulinum A toxin-hemagglutin complex. It can be used to treat blepharospasm.

Dytac
A proprietary, prescription-only preparation of diuretic drug triamterene. It can be used to treat oedema.

Dytide
A proprietary, prescription-only preparation of diuretic drug triamterene. It can be used to treat oedema.

E

E45 Cream
A proprietary, non-prescription compound preparation of liquid paraffin, white soft paraffin and wool fat. It can be used as an emollient for dry skin and minor abrasions and burns.

Ebufac
A proprietary, prescription-only preparation of ibuprofen. It can be used to relieve pain, particularly the pain of rheumatic disease and other musculoskeletal disorders.

Econacort
A proprietary, prescription-only compound preparation of hydrocortisone and econazole nitrate. It can be used to treat fungal infections.

Econacort
A proprietary, prescription-only antifungal drug, used to treat fungal infections of the skin, nails, or mucous membranes, such as vaginal candidiasis.

Ecostatin
A proprietary, prescription-only antifungal drug, used to treat fungal infections of the skin and mucous membranes, especially of the vagina and vulva.

Edecrin
A proprietary, prescription-only preparation of the diuretic drug ethacrynic acid. It can be used to treat oedema in patients with heart failure.

Edrophonium chloride
A proprietary, prescription-only preparation of acetylcholine. It can be in the diagnosis of myasthenia gravis.

Efalith
A proprietary, prescription-only compound preparation of lithium succinate and zinc sulphate. It can be used to treat seborrhoeic dermatitis.

Efamast
A proprietary, prescription-only preparation of gamolenic acid. It can be used for the relief of breast pain.

Efcortelan

A proprietary, prescription-only preparation of the corticosteroid hydrocortisone. It can be used to treat mild inflammatory skin disorders.

Efcortesol

A proprietary, prescription-only preparation of the corticosteroid hydrocortisone. It can be used to treat inflammation caused by allergy and to treat shock.

Effercitrate

A proprietary, non-prescription-only preparation of potassium citrate. It can be used to relieve the mild discomfort of urinary tract infection.

Effexor

A proprietary, prescription-only preparation of venlafaxine. It can be used to treat depressive illness.

Efudix

A proprietary, prescription-only preparation of fluorouracil. It can be used to treat malignant skin lesions.

Elantan

A proprietary, prescription-only preparation of isosorbide mononitrate. It can be used to treat and prevent angina pectoris and for heart failure.

Elantan LA

A proprietary, prescription-only preparation of isosorbide mononitrate. It can be used to treat and prevent angina pectoris and for heart failure.

Elavil

A proprietary, prescription-only preparation of amitriptyline hydrochloride. It can be used to treat depressive illness.

Eldepryl

A proprietary, prescription-only preparation of selegilline. It can be used to treat symptoms of parkinsonism.

Eldisine

A proprietary, prescription-only preparation of the anticancer drug vindicine sulphate. It can be used to treat acute leukaemia, lymphomas and some solid tumors.

Eltroxin

A proprietary, prescription-only preparation of thyroxine sodium. It can be used to make up for hormonal deficiency of the thyroid gland.

Eludril Mouthwash

A proprietary, non-prescription preparation of chlorhexidine. It can be used to treat and prevent gingivitis and minor throat problems.

Eludril Spray

A proprietary, non-prescription preparation of chlorhexidine. It can be used to treat and prevent gingivitis and minor throat problems.

Elyzol

A proprietary, non-prescription preparation of metrodinazole. It can be used to treat local infections in dental surgery.

Emblon

A proprietary, prescription-only preparation of tamoxifen. It can be used to treat cancers that depend on the presence of estrogen in women.

Emcor

A preparation of the beta-blocker bisoprolol fumarate. It can be used to treat raised blood pressure and angina pectoris.

Emeside

A proprietary, prescription-only preparation of ethosuximide. It can be used to treat absence (petit mal), myoclonic and some other types of seizure.

Emflex

A proprietary, prescription-only preparation of acemetacin. It can be used to treat the pain of rheumatic and other musculoskeletal disorders.

Eminase

A proprietary, prescription-only preparation of amistreplase. It can be used to treat myocardial infarction.

Emia

A proprietary, prescription-only com-

Enzyme inhibitors

These medicines work by inhibiting enzymes, which are proteins that play an essential part in the metabolism by acting as catalysts in specific, necessary biochemical reactions. Certain medicines have been developed that act only on certain enzymes and so can be used to manipulate the biochemistry of the body.

Monoamine-oxidase inhibitors, or MAOIs (for instance isocarboxazid) are one of the three major classes of antidepressant drugs. They work by inhibiting en enzyme in the brain that metabolizes monoamines (including noradrenaline and serotonin), which results in a change of mood. However, this same enzyme detoxifies other amines, so if certain foods are eaten or medicines taken that contain amines, then dangerous side effects could occur.

ACE inhibitors (angiotensine-converting enzyme inhibitors), such as captopril and ramipril, are medicines that are used in the treatment of raised blood pressure and in heart failure. They work by inhibiting the conversion of the natural circulating hormone angiotensin.

Further examples of enzyme inhibitor drugs include the carbonic anhydrase inhibitor drugs (which are used for their diuretic actions and in glaucoma treatment) and the phosphodiesterase inhibitors (for congestive heart failure treatment).

pound preparation of lignocaine and prilocaine hydrochloride. It can be used for surface anesthesia.

Emmolate

A proprietary, non-prescription preparation of liquid paraffin. It has an emollient action.

Emulsiderm

A proprietary, non-prescription compound preparation of the antiseptic agent benzalkonium chloride and paraffin, used for skin disorders.

Enalapril maleate

A proprietary, prescription-only ACE inhibitor drug. It can be used to treat raised blood pressure, heart failure treatment and to prevent ischemia.

Enbrel

A proprietary, prescription-only preparation of etanercept. It is used for the symptomatic relief rheumatoid arthritis.

Enfluranea

A proprietary, prescription-only inhalant anesthetic drug, used for general anesthesia.

Eno

A proprietary, non-prescription compound preparation of calcium carbonate, citric acid and calcium carbonate. It can be used to treat indigestion, flatulence and nausea.

Enoxaparin

A preparation of heparin. It can be used for prevention of thrombo-embolism.

Enoximone

A proprietary, prescription-only preparation of a phosphodiesterase inhibitor. It can be used to treat congestive heart failure.

Entamizole

A proprietary, prescription-only preparation of diloxamide furoate. It can be used to treat chronic intestinal infection of Entamoeba histolytica.

Epanutin

A proprietary, prescription-only preparation of phenytoin. It can be used

to treat and prevent most forms of seizure and also the pain of trigeminal neuralgia.

Ephedrine hydrochloride

A proprietary, prescription-only alkaloid with sympathicomimetic action. It can be used as bronchodilator and vasoconstrictor.

Epifoam

A proprietary, prescription-only compound preparation of the corticosteroid hydrocortisone and pramoxine hydrochloride. It can be used to treat inflammation and pain in the perineal region.

Epilim

A proprietary, prescription-only preparation of sodium valproate. It can be used to treat all forms of epilepsy.

Epilim Chrono

A proprietary, prescription-only preparation of sodium valproate. It can be used to treat all forms of epilepsy.

Epilim Intravenous

A preparation of sodium valproate. It can be used to treat all forms of epilepsy.

Epimaz

A proprietary, prescription-only preparation of carbamazepine. It can be used to treat all forms of epilepsy and trigeminal neuralgia.

Epipen

A proprietary, prescription-only preparation of the natural hormone adrenaline. It can be used in the emergency treatment of acute and severe bronchoconstriction.

Epirubicin hydrochloride

A proprietary, prescription-only cytotoxic drug. It can be used to treat severe breast and kidney tumors.

Epoetin

A proprietary, prescription-only preparation of human erythropoietin. It can be used in chronic renal failure.

Epogam

A proprietary, prescription-only preparation of gamolenic acid. It can be used to treat atopic eczema.

Epoprostenol

A proprietary, prescription-only preparation of a prostaglandin. It can be used as vasodilator and anticoagulant drug.

Eppy

A proprietary, prescription-only preparation of adrenaline. It can be used to treat glaucoma.

Eprex

A proprietary, prescription-only preparation of epoetin alpha. It can be used in the treatment of anemia.

Equagesic

A proprietary, prescription-only compound preparation of meprobamate, aspirin and ethoheptazine citrate. It can be used to treat rheumatic pain and the symptoms of other musculoskeletal disorders.

Equanil

A proprietary, prescription-only preparation of meprobamate. It can be used to treat anxiety.

Eradacin

A proprietary, prescription-only preparation of acrosoxacin. It can be used to treat a range of infections.

Ergocalciferol

A proprietary, non-prescription natural form of calciferol. It can be used to make up deficiencies.

Ergometrine maleate

A proprietary, prescription-only alkaloid. It can be used to speed up the third stage of labour.

Ergotamine tartrate

A proprietary, prescription-only alkaloid. It can be used to treat attacks of migraine.

Erwinase

A proprietary, prescription-only preparation of cristantaspase. It can be used to treat acute lymphoblastic leukaemia.

Epifoam

Properties

This medicine belongs to the family of topical (applied to the skin) corticosteroids, containing an adrenocorticoid as active ingredient. It is used to relieve the symptoms of any itching, rash, or inflammation of the skin; it does not treat the underlying cause of the skin problem. It also relieves redness, swelling and itching caused by insect bites, poison ivy, poison oak, poison sumach, soaps, cosmetics, sunburn, and numerous skin rashes.

Topical adrenocorticosteroids are absorbed through the skin and may rarely affect growth in children. Before using this medicine in children you should discuss the use of it with your doctor.

Before using this medicine

Before you use this medicine check with your doctor, or pharmacist:

- if you ever had any unusual or allergic reaction to adrenocorticoids or corticosteroids in general.
- if you are on a low-salt, low-sugar, or any other special diet, or if you are allergic to any substance, such as certain preservatives or dyes.
- if you have diabetes, stomach ulcer, or infection at the treatment site.
- if you are pregnant, intending to become pregnant or breast-feeding an infant while using this medicine.
- if you have any of the following medical problems:
  Diabetes mellitus (sugar diabetes)
  Infection at the place of treatment
  Ulceration at the place of treatment
  Tuberculosis

Treatment

This medication is used to relieve or prevent the symptoms of your medical problem. Take them as directed. Do not take more of them and do not take them more often than recommended on the label.

To do so may increase the chance of absorption through the skin and the chance of side effects. In addition, too much use, especially on thin skin areas (for example, armpits, face, groin), may result in thinning of the skin and stretch marks.

Side effects

The following side effects may occur:

- Acne or oily skin
- Blistering
- Burning sensations
- Itching
- Dryness of the skin
- Secondary infection
- Thinning of skin
- Unusual hair growth
- Unusual loss of hair

These side effects should disappear as your body adjusts to the medication. Tell your doctor about any side effects that are persistent or particularly bothersome.

The above side effects are more likely to occur in children and elderly patients, who are usually more sensitive to the effects of this medicine.

When the gel, solution, lotion, or aerosol from this medicine is applied, a mild, temporary stinging may be expected.

Interactions

This medicine interacts with several other drugs such as antibiotics (causing a decreased antibiotic effect) and antifungals (causing a decreased antifungal effect).

Be sure to tell your doctor about any medications you are currently taking.

Storage

This medicine should be stored at room temperature in closed containers. Store away from heat and direct light. Keep out of reach of children, since overdose may be dangerous in children. Do not store in the bathroom medicine cabinet because the heat or moisture may cause the medicine to break down. Keep the medicine from freezing. Do not keep outdated medicine.

Erycen

A proprietary, prescription-only preparation of the antibacterial and antibiotic drug erythromycin. It can be used to treat and prevent many forms of infection.

Erymax

A proprietary, prescription-only preparation of the antibacterial and antibiotic drug erythromycin. It can be used to treat and prevent many forms of infection.

Erymcin

A proprietary, prescription-only preparation of the antibacterial and antibiotic drug erythromycin. It can be used to treat and prevent many forms of infection.

Erythromid

A proprietary, prescription-only preparation of the antibacterial and antibiotic drug erythromycin. It can be used to treat and prevent many forms of infection.

Erythromycin

A proprietary, prescription-only antibacterial and antibiotic drug. It can be used to treat and prevent many forms of infection.

Erythroped

A proprietary, prescription-only preparation of the antibacterial and antibiotic drug erythromycin. It can be used to treat and prevent many forms of infection.

Erythroped A

A proprietary, prescription-only preparation of the antibacterial and antibiotic drug erythromycin. It can be used to treat and prevent many forms of infection.

Eskazole

A proprietary, prescription-only antibiotic drug albendazole. It can be used to treat and prevent Echinococcus infection.

Eskornade Capsules

A proprietary, non-prescription compound preparation of phenylpropanolamine hydrochloride and diphenylpyraline. It can be used for the symptomatic relief of congestive symptoms of colds, allergy and flu.

Eskornade Syrup

A proprietary, non-prescription compound preparation of phenylpropanolamine hydrochloride and diphenylpyraline. It can be used for the symptomatic relief of congestive symptoms of colds, allergy and flu.

Esmeron

A proprietary, prescription-only preparation of rocuronium bromide. It can be used to induce muscle paralysis in surgery.

Esmolol hydrochloride

A proprietary, prescription-only beta-blocker drug. It can be used to treat raised blood pressure and irregularities of the heartbeat.

Estracombi

A proprietary, prescription-only compound preparation of the female sex hormones oestradiol and norethisterone. It can be used to treat menopausal problems.

Estracyr

A proprietary, prescription-only preparation of the cytotoxic drug estramustine phosphate. It can be used to treat cancer of the prostate gland.

Estraderm TTS

A proprietary, prescription-only preparation oestradiol. It can be used in hormone replacement therapy.

Estramustine phosphate

A proprietary, prescription-only cytotoxic drug. It can be used to treat prostate cancer.

Estrapak 50

A proprietary, prescription-only compound preparation of the female sex hormones oestradiol and norethisterone. It can be used to treat menopausal problems.

Estring

A proprietary, prescription-only preparation oestradiol. It can be used in postmenopausal disorders such as urogenital complaints.

Etacrinic acid

A proprietary, prescription-only diuretic drug. It can be used to treat oedema in patients with chronic heart failure of kidney disorders.

Etacrynic acid

A proprietary, prescription-only diuretic drug. It can be used to treat oedema in patients with chronic heart failure of kidney disorders.

Etamsylate

A proprietary, prescription-only antifibrinolytic drug. It can be used to treat bleeding in premature infants.

Ethambutol hydrochloride

A proprietary, prescription-only antibacterial drug. It can be used to treat various types of infection.

Ethamsylate

A proprietary, prescription-only antifibrinolytic drug. It can be used to treat bleeding in premature infants.

Ethanolamine Oleate

A proprietary, prescription-only drug. It can be used to treat varicose veins (sclerotherapy).

Ethinyloestradiol

A proprietary, prescription-only female sex hormone. It can be used to treat gynaecological disorders and prostate gland cancer.

Ethmozine

A proprietary, prescription-only preparation of moracizine hydrochloride. It can be used to treat irregularities of the heartbeat.

Ethosuximide

A proprietary, prescription-only anticonvulsant drug. It can be used to treat absence, myoclonic and some other types of seizure.

Ethynodiol diacetate

A proprietary, prescription-only female sex hormone used as a constituent of oral contraceptive drugs.

Etodalac

A proprietary, prescription-only drug. It can be used primarily to treat the pain and inflammation of rheumatoid arthritis and osteoarthritis.

Etomidate

A general anesthetic drug, which is used for the initial induction of anesthesia.

Etoposide

A proprietary, prescription-only cytotoxic drug. It can be used to treat small cell lung cancer, lymphomas and cancer of the testes.

Eucardic

A proprietary, prescription-only preparation of the beta-blocker carvediol. It can be used to treat raised blood pressure.

Eudemine Injection

A proprietary, prescription-only preparation of diazoxide. It can be used to treat raised blood pressure and hypertensive crisis.

Eudemine Tablets

A proprietary, prescription-only preparation of diazoxide. It can be used to treat raised blood pressure and hypertensive crisis.

Euglucon

A proprietary, prescription-only preparation of glibenclamide. It can be used in the treatment of Type II diabetes.

Eugynon

A proprietary, prescription-only hormonal compound preparation of

Ex-Lax

Properties
This medicine contains as active ingredient phenolph-thalein, a stimulant laxative. Stimulant laxatives (also known as contact laxatives) are medicines taken by mouth to encourage bowel movements by acting on the intestinal wall. They increase the muscle contractions that move along the stool mass.

Before using this medicine
Before you use this medicine check with your doctor, or pharmacist:
-   if you ever had any unusual or allergic reaction to lax-atives.
-   if you are on a low-salt, low-sugar, or any other special diet, or if you are allergic to any substance, such as sulfites or other preservatives or dyes.
-   if you are pregnant. Stimulant laxatives may cause un-wanted effects in the expectant mother if improperly used. Some of the stimulant laxatives may cause con-tractions of the womb.
-   if you are breast-feeding an infant. Some stimulant laxatives may pass into the breast milk. Although the amount of laxative in the milk is generally thought to be too small to cause problems in the child, your doc-tor should be told that you plan to use such laxatives.
-   if you have any of the following medical problems:
    Appendicitis (or signs of)
    Colostomy
    Diabetes (sugar disease)
    Heart disease
    Hypertension
    Ileostomy
    Intestinal blockage
    Laxative habit
    Rectal bleeding

Treatment
For safe and effective use of bulk-forming laxatives:
Follow your doctor's orders if this laxative was prescribed.
Follow the manufacturer's package directions if you are treating yourself.
At least six to eight 8-ounce glasses of liquids should be taken each day.
Stimulant laxatives are usually taken on an empty stomach for rapid effect. Results are slowed if taken with food.
Laxatives should not be given to young children (up to 6 years of age) unless prescribed by their doctor. Since children cannot usually describe their symptoms very well, a doctor should check the child before giving this medicine.

Side effects
Along with the needed effects, a medicine may cause some unwanted effects.
Side effects that should be reported to your doctor: breathing diffi-culty; burning on urination; confusion; headache; irregular heart-beat; irritability; mood or mental changes; muscle cramps; skin rash; unusual tiredness.

Laxative habit
Laxatives are to be used to provide short-term relief only, unless otherwise directed by your doctor. Laxatives are overused by many people. Such a practice often leads to dependence on the laxative action to produce a bowel movement. In some cases, overuse of some laxatives has caused damage to the nerves, muscles, and tissues of the intestines and bowel.

Interactions
This medicine may interact with several other drugs, such as amiloride, antacids, other laxatives, potassium supple-ments, tetracycline antibiotics and triamterene.
Be sure to tell your doctor about any medications you are currently taking.

Storage
Store away from heat and direct light. Keep out of the reach of children. Do not store in the bathroom medicine cabinet because the heat or moisture may cause the medi-cine to break down.

---

oestradiol and levonergestrel. It can be used as oral contraceptive and to treat menstrual problems.

Eumovate
A proprietary, prescription-only preparation of the corticosteroid clo-betasone butyrate. It can be used to treat eczema and various forms of dermatitis.

Eumovate-N
A proprietary, prescription-only com-pound preparation of the corticos-teroid clobetasone butyrate and neomycin. It can be used to treat in-flammation of the eye.

Eurax
A proprietary, non-prescription preparation of crotaminon. It can be used to treat itching in scabies.

Eurax-Hydrocortisone
A proprietary, prescription-only com-pound preparation of crotaminon

and the corticosteroid hydrocorti-sone. It can be used to treat itching in scabies.

Evorel
A proprietary, prescription-only pre-paration of oestradiol. It can be used in hormone replacement ther-apy.

Evorel Pak
A proprietary, prescription-only com-pound preparation of oestradiol and

norethisterone. It can be used in hormone replacement therapy.

Exelderm
A proprietary, prescription-only preparation of the antifungal drug sulconazole nitrate. It can be used to treat fungal skin infections.

Exirel
A proprietary, prescription-only preparation of pirbuterol. It can be used as a bronchodilator in severe acute asthma and chronic bronchitis.

Ex-Lax Chocolate
A proprietary, non-prescription preparation of the laxative phenolphthaleine. It can be used to treat constipation.

Ex-Lax Pills
A proprietary, non-prescription preparation of the laxative phenolphthaleine. It can be used to treat constipation.

Exocin
A proprietary, prescription-only preparation of antibacterial and antibiotic drug ofloxacin. It can be used to treat bacterial infections of the eye.

Expelix
A proprietary, non-prescription preparation of piperazine. It can be used to treat infestation by threadworms or roundworms.

Expulin Cough Linctus
A proprietary, non-prescription compound preparation of chlorpheniramine and pholcodeine. It can be used for the symptomatic relief of cough.

Expulin Dry Cough Linctus
A proprietary, non-prescription preparation of pholcodeine. It can be used for the symptomatic relief of dry cough.

Exterol
A proprietary, non-prescription preparation of the antiseptic agent hydrogen peroxide. It can be used to dissolve and wash out earwax.

F

Fabrol
A proprietary, prescription-only preparation of the mucolytic drug acetylcysteine. It can be used to reduce viscosity of sputum and so facilitate expectoration.

Famciclovir
A proprietary, prescription-only antiviral drug that is similar to aciclovir. It can be used to treat infection caused by herpes zoster.

Famel Expectorant
A preparation of guaiphenesin. It can be used for the symptomatic relief of coughs, bronchial congestion and catarrh.

Famel Honey and Lemon Pastilles
A proprietary, non-prescription preparation of guaiphenesin. It can be used for the symptomatic relief of coughs, bronchial congestion and catarrh.

Famel Linctus
A proprietary, non-prescription preparation of pholcodeine. It can be used for the symptomatic relief of dry and irritating coughs.

Famel Original
A proprietary, non-prescription preparation of codeine phosphate. It can be used for the symptomatic relief of dry troublesome coughs.

Famotidine
A proprietary, prescription-only ulcer-healing drug. It can be used to treat benign peptic ulcers, to relieve heartburn and a variety of gastric conditions.

Famvir
A proprietary, prescription-only compound preparation of pyrimethamine and sulfadoxine. It can be used to treat malaria.

Fartulal
A proprietary, prescription-only preparation of the female sex hormone medroxyprogesterone acetate. It can be used to treat cancer of the breast or uterine endometrium.

Fasigyn
A proprietary, prescription-only preparation of the antibacterial and antiprotozoal drug tinidazole, used to treat anaerobic infections.

Faverin
A proprietary, prescription-only preparation of fluvoxamine. It can be used to treat depressive illness.

Fectrim
A proprietary, prescription-only compound preparation of sulphamethoxazole and trimethoprim. It can be used to treat a variety of bacterial infections.

Fefol
A proprietary, non-prescription preparation of ferrous sulphate and folic acid. It can be used as an iron and folic acid supplement during pregnancy.

Feldene
A proprietary, prescription-only preparation of or piroxicam. It can be used to treat acute gout, arthritic and rheumatic pain and other musculoskeletal disorders.

Feldene Gel
A proprietary, prescription-only preparation of or piroxicam. It can be applied to the skin for symptomatic relief of underlying muscle or joint pain.

Felodipine
A proprietary, prescription-only calcium-channel blocker drug. It can be used to treat raised blood pressure.

Felypressin
A proprietary, prescription-only analogue of vasopressin. It can be used as a vasoconstrictor.

Femeron
A proprietary, non-prescription preparation of miconazole. It can be used to treat external vaginal itching due to Candida infection.

**Fever
Pain
Infection**

Feldene

Properties
This medicine contains as active ingredient piroxicam. It belongs to the group of medicines called non-steroidal anti-inflammatory drugs (NSAIDs). These drugs are taken by mouth to relieve some symptoms caused by arthritis or rheumatism, such as inflammation, swelling, stiffness, and joint pain. However, these medicines do not cure arthritis and will help you only as long as you continue to take them. Some of these medicines are also used to relieve other kinds of pain or to treat other painful conditions, such as gout attacks, bursitis, tendinitis, sprains, strains, menstrual cramps. The drug reduces the tissue concentration of prostaglandins.

Before using this medicine
Before you use this medicine check with your doctor, or pharmacist:
- if you ever had any unusual or allergic reaction, such as skin rash, hives, or itching or breathing problems, to any of the anti-inflammatory analgesics.
- if you are on a low-salt, low-sugar, or any other special diet, or if you are allergic to any substance, such as sulfites or other preservatives or dyes.
- if you are pregnant or intending to become pregnant while using this medicine. Studies on birth defects have not been done in humans. However, if taken regularly during the last months of pregnancy, there is a chance that these medicines may cause unwanted effects on the heart or blood flow in the fetus or newborn infant.
- if you are breast-feeding an infant. Although this medicine has not been shown to cause problems in humans, it passes into the breast milk in small amounts.
- if you have any of the following medical problems:
  Asthma
  Bleeding problems
  Colitis, or other intestinal problems
  Stomach ulcer,
  Heart disease,
  High blood pressure
  Kidney or liver disease

Treatment
This medication is used to relieve pain or other symptoms caused by arthritis. For safe and effective use of this medicine, do not take more of it, do not take it more often, and do not take it for a longer period of time than ordered by your physician or directed by the package label.
If you are taking this medication on a regular schedule and you miss a dose, take the missed dose as soon as possible, unless it is almost time for your next dose. In that case do not take the missed dose at all.
To lessen stomach upset, anti-inflammatory analgesics may be taken with food or antacids.

Side effects
Along with the needed effects, a medicine may cause some unwanted effects. These side effects may go away during treatment as your body adjusts to the medicine. Such minor side effects are: dizziness; nausea; pain; headache; drowsiness; swollen feet, face or leg; constipation or diarrhea; vomiting; dry mouth.
Check with your doctor immediately if any of the following side effects occur:
- *Muscle cramps*
- *Numbness or tingling*
- *Mouth ulcers*
- *Convulsions or confusion*
- *Rash, hives, or itch*
- *Tightness in chest*

Interactions
This medicine may interact with several other drugs.
Be sure to tell your doctor about any medications you are currently taking.

Storage
The medicine should be stored at room temperature in a tightly closed, light-resistant container. Store away from heat and direct light. Keep out of reach of children.

Femigraine
A proprietary, non-prescription compound preparation of cyclizine hydrochloride and aspirin. It can be used to treat acute migraine attacks and associated nausea.

Feminax
A compound preparation of codeine phosphate and hyoscine hydrobromide. It can be used for the relief of period pain.

Femodene
A proprietary, prescription-only compound preparation of an estrogen and a progestogen. It can be used as oral contraceptive drug.

Femodene ED
A proprietary, prescription-only compound preparation of an estrogen and a progestogen. It can be used as oral contraceptive drug.

Femulen
A proprietary, prescription-only preparation of a progestogen. It can be used as oral contraceptive drug.

Fenbid
A preparation of ibuprofen. It can be used to treat all kinds of pain, especially pain from rheumatic disorders.

Fenbufen
A proprietary, prescription-only

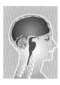

Fenoprofen

Bleeding problems
Colitis
Stomach ulcer
Heart disease
Kidney or liver disease

Properties

This medicine contains as active ingredient fenoprofen. It belongs to the group of medicines called non-steroidal anti-inflammatory drugs (NSAIDs). These drugs are taken by mouth to relieve some symptoms caused by arthritis or rheumatism, such as inflammation, swelling, stiffness, and joint pain. However, these medicines do not cure arthritis and will help you only as long as you continue to take them. Some of these medicines are also used to relieve other kinds of pain or to treat other painful conditions, such as gout attacks, bursitis, tendinitis, sprains, strains, menstrual cramps. The drug reduces the tissue concentration of prostaglandins (hormonal substances which produce inflammation and pain).

Before using this medicine

Before you use this medicine check with your doctor, or pharmacist:

- if you ever had any unusual or allergic reaction, such as skin rash, hives, or itching or breathing problems, to any of the anti-inflammatory analgesics.
- if you are on a low-salt, low-sugar, or any other special diet, or if you are allergic to any substance, such as sulfites or other preservatives or dyes.
- if you are pregnant or intending to become pregnant while using this medicine. Studies on birth defects have not been done in humans. However, if taken regularly during the last months of pregnancy, there is a chance that these medicines may cause unwanted effects on the heart or blood flow in the fetus or newborn infant.
- if you are breast-feeding an infant. Although this medicine has not been shown to cause problems in humans, it passes into the breast milk in small amounts.
- if you have any of the following medical problems: Asthma

Treatment

This medication is used to relieve pain or other symptoms caused by arthritis. For safe and effective use of this medicine, do not take more of it, do not take it more often, and do not take it for a longer period of time than ordered by your physician or directed by the package label.

If you are taking this medication on a regular schedule and you miss a dose, take the missed dose as soon as possible, unless it is almost time for your next dose. In that case do not take the missed dose at all.

To lessen stomach upset, anti-inflammatory analgesics may be taken with food or antacids.

Side effects

Along with the needed effects, a medicine may cause some unwanted effects. These side effects may go away during treatment as your body adjusts to the medicine. Such minor side effects are: dizziness; nausea; pain; headache; drowsiness; swollen feet, face or leg; constipation or diarrhea; vomiting; dry mouth.

Check with your doctor immediately if any of the following side effects occur:

- *Muscle cramps*
- *Numbness or tingling*
- *Mouth ulcers*
- *Convulsions or confusion*
- *Rash, hives, or itch*
- *Tightness in chest*

Interactions

This medicine may interact with several other drugs.

Be sure to tell your doctor about any medications you are currently taking.

Storage

The medicine should be stored at room temperature in a tightly closed, light-resistant container. Store away from heat and direct light. Keep out of reach of children.

---

pain-relieving drug. It can be used to treat all kinds of pain, especially pain from rheumatic disorders.

Fenbuzip

A proprietary, prescription-only pain-relieving drug. It can be used to treat all kinds of pain, especially pain from rheumatic disorders.

Fenfluramine hydrochloride

A proprietary, prescription-only ap-

petite suppressant. It can be used to treat obesity.

Fenofibrate

A proprietary, prescription-only lipid-lowering drug. It can be used to reduce high lipid levels in the bloodstream.

Fenoprofen

A proprietary, prescription-only antirheumatic drug. It can be used to re-

lieve pain and inflammation of rheumatic and other musculoskeletal disorders.

Fenopron 300/600

A proprietary, prescription-only preparation of the antirheumatic drug fenoprofen. It can be used to relieve pain and inflammation of rheumatic and other musculoskeletal disorders.

Ferospan

Properties
This medicine contains iron as active ingredient and is therefore called an iron supplement. Iron shortage may occur in iron-deficiency anemia. In this condition the body does not have enough iron to produce the amount of normal red blood cells needed to keep you in good health. Your doctor can determine if you have an iron deficiency, what is causing the deficiency, and if an iron supplement is necessary. The iron supplement works by being incorporated into red blood cells, where it can help carry oxygen throughout the body.

Before using this medicine
Before you use this medicine check with your doctor, or pharmacist:
- if you ever had any unusual or allergic reaction to iron medicine.
- if you are pregnant or intending to become pregnant while using this medicine. During the first 3 months of pregnancy, a proper diet usually provides enough iron; however, during the last 6 months, in order to meet the increased needs of the developing baby, an iron supplement may be recommended by your doctor.
- if you are breast-feeding an infant. Iron normally is present in breast milk in small amounts. Nursing mothers are advised to check with their doctor or pharmacist before taking iron supplements.
- if you have any of the following medical problems:
Alcoholism
Blood disease (other than iron)
deficiency anemia)
Infection
Intestinal disorders
Liver disease
Pancreatitis
Peptic ulcer
Stomach upset
Ulcerative colitis
When iron combines with certain foods it loses much of its value. The following foods should be avoided or taken in very small amounts within 1 hour before or 2 hours after the iron supplement: cheese and cottage cheese; eggs; ice cream; milk; tea or coffee; whole-grain breads and cereals.

Treatment
This medication is used to treat anemias due to iron deficiency. The iron supplement is best taken on an empty stomach, with water or fruit juice, about 1 hour before or 2 hours after a meal.
For safe and effective use of this iron supplement:
Follow your doctor's instructions if this medicine was prescribed.
Follow the manufacturer's package directions if you are treating yourself.

Side effects
Along with the needed effects, a medicine may cause some unwanted effects. Possible side effects include:
- Abdominal pain
- Stomach upset and irritation
- Nausea
- Diarrhea
- Constipation

Interactions
This medicine may interact with several other drugs such as oral Tetracycline and antacids. In these cases avoid taking iron supplements until your other medical condition clears up.
Be sure to tell your doctor about any medications you are currently taking.

Storage
Capsules, tablets, elixir, etc. should be stored at room temperature; store away from heat and direct light. Keep out of reach of children, since overdose may be very dangerous in children. As few as 3 or 4 adult iron tablets can cause serious poisoning in small children. Do not store in the bathroom medicine cabinet because the heat or moisture may cause the medicine to break down.

Fenoterol hydrobromide
A proprietary, prescription-only beta-receptor stimulant drug. It can be used to treat asthmatic attacks and for the alleviation of symptoms of chronic bronchitis and emphysema.

Fenox Nasal Drops
A proprietary, non-prescription preparation of phenylephrine hydrochloride. It can be used for the symptomatic relief of nasal congestion associated with colds, catarrh and sinusitis.

Fenox Nasal Spray
A preparation of phenylephrine hydrochloride. It can be used for the symptomatic relief of nasal congestion associated with colds, catarrh and sinusitis.

Fentanyl
A proprietary, prescription-only opioid narcotic drug. It can be used to treat moderate to severe pain.

Fentazin
A proprietary, prescription-only preparation of perphenazine. It can be used to treat schizophrenia and other psychoses.

Ferospan
A proprietary, non-prescription preparation of ferrous sulphate. It can be

Ferrous fumarate

Properties

This medicine contains iron as active ingredient and is therefore called an iron supplement. Iron shortage may occur in iron-deficiency anemia. In this condition the body does not have enough iron to produce the amount of normal red blood cells needed to keep you in good health. Your doctor can determine if you have an iron deficiency, what is causing the deficiency, and if an iron supplement is necessary. The iron supplement works by being incorporated into red blood cells, where it can help carry oxygen throughout the body.

Before using this medicine

Before you use this medicine check with your doctor, or pharmacist:
- if you ever had any unusual or allergic reaction to iron medicine.
- if you are pregnant or intending to become pregnant while using this medicine. During the first 3 months of pregnancy, a proper diet usually provides enough iron; however, during the last 6 months, in order to meet the increased needs of the developing baby, an iron supplement may be recommended by your doctor.
- if you are breast-feeding an infant. Iron normally is present in breast milk in small amounts. Nursing mothers are advised to check with their doctor or pharmacist before taking iron supplements.
- if you have any of the following medical problems:
  Alcoholism
  Blood disease (other than iron)
  deficiency anemia)
  Infection
  Intestinal disorders
  Liver disease
  Pancreatitis
  Peptic ulcer
  Duodenal ulcer
  Stomach upset

  Ulcerative colitis

When iron combines with certain foods it loses much of its value. The following foods should be avoided or taken in very small amounts within 1 hour before or 2 hours after the iron supplement: cheese and cottage cheese; eggs; ice cream; milk; tea or coffee; whole-grain breads and cereals.

Treatment

This medication is used to treat anemias due to iron deficiency. The iron supplement is best taken on an empty stomach, with water or fruit juice, about 1 hour before or 2 hours after a meal.

For safe and effective use of this iron supplement:

Follow your doctor's instructions if this medicine was prescribed.

Follow the manufacturer's package directions if you are treating yourself.

Side effects

Along with the needed effects, a medicine may cause some unwanted effects. Possible side effects include:
- Abdominal pain
- Stomach upset and irritation
- Nausea
- Diarrhea
- Constipation

Interactions

This medicine may interact with several other drugs such as oral Tetracycline and antacids. In these cases avoid taking iron supplements until your other medical condition clears up.

Be sure to tell your doctor about any medications you are currently taking.

Storage

Capsules, tablets, elixir, etc. should be stored at room temperature; store away from heat and direct light. Keep out of reach of children, since overdose may be very dangerous in children.

As few as 3 or 4 adult iron tablets can cause serious poisoning in small children. Do not store in the bathroom medicine cabinet because the heat or moisture may cause the medicine to break down.

used to treat certain types of anemia.

Ferfolic SV

A proprietary, prescription compound preparation of ferrous gluconate, folic acid and ascorbic acid. It can be used as an iron and folic acid supplement during pregnancy.

Fergon

A proprietary, non-prescription preparation of ferrous gluconate. It can be used to treat certain types of anemia.

Ferric ammonium citrate

A proprietary, non-prescription preparation of iron salt. It can be used to treat certain types of anemia.

Ferrocap-F 350

A proprietary, prescription-only compound preparation of ferrous fumarate and folic acid. It can be used as an iron and folic acid supplement during pregnancy.

Ferrocontin Continus

A proprietary, non-prescription preparation of ferrous glycine sulphate.

It can be used as an iron supplement.

Ferrocontin Continus
A proprietary, non-prescription compound preparation of ferrous glycine sulphate and folic acid. It can be used as an iron and folic acid supplement during pregnancy.

Ferrograd
A preparation of ferrous sulphate. It can be used to treat certain types of anemia.

Ferrograd Folic
A proprietary, non-prescription compound preparation of ferrous sulphate and folic acid. It can be used as an iron and folic acid supplement during pregnancy.

Ferrous fumarate
A proprietary, non-prescription preparation of iron salts. It can be used to treat certain types of anemia.

Ferrous gluconate
A proprietary, non-prescription preparation of iron salts. It can be used to treat certain types of anemia.

Ferrous sulphate
A proprietary, non-prescription preparation of iron salts. It can be used to treat certain types of anemia.

Ferrous sulphate oral solution, paediatric
A proprietary, non-prescription preparation of ferrous sulphate. It can be used to treat certain types of anemia.

Fertiral
A proprietary, prescription-only preparation of gonadorelin. It can be used to treat women for infertility.

Filair Forte
A proprietary, prescription-only preparation of the corticosteroid beclomethasone diproprionate. It can be used to treat and prevent asthmatic attacks.

Finasteride
A proprietary, prescription-only anti-androgen. It can be used to treat benign prostatic hyperplasia.

Fisherman's Friend
A proprietary, non-prescription lozenge of menthol, liquorice and aniseed oil. It can be used to treat cold symptoms.

Flagyl
A proprietary, prescription-only preparation of metronidazole. It can be used to treat many types of anaerobic infection.

Flagyl Compak
A proprietary, prescription-only preparation of metronidazole. It can be used to treat many types of anaerobic infection.

Flamatrol
A proprietary, prescription-only preparation of piroxican. It can be used to treat rheumatic and arthritic pain.

Flamazine
A proprietary, prescription-only preparation of sulphadiazine. It can be used to treat wounds, burns, ulcers and bedsores.

Flamrase
A proprietary, prescription-only preparation of diclofenac sodium. It can be used to treat pain and inflammation, particularly arthritic and rheumatic pain.

Flavixate hydrochloride
A proprietary, prescription-only anticholinergic drug. It can be used to treat urinary frequency and incontinence.

Flaxedil
A proprietary, prescription-only preparation of gallamine triethiodide. It can be used to induce muscle paralysis during surgery.

Flecainide acetate
A proprietary, prescription-only anti-arrhythmic drug. It can be used to treat irregularities of the heartbeat.

Fleet Ready-to-Use Enema
A proprietary, non-prescription compound preparation of sodium phosphate and sodium acid phosphate. It can be used to treat constipation.

Flemoxin Solutab
A proprietary, prescription-only preparation of the antibacterial and antibiotic drug amoxycillin. It can be used to treat a wide variety of infection.

Fletchers' Arachis Oil Retention Enema
A proprietary, non-prescription preparation of arachis oil. It can be used to treat constipation.

Fletchers' Enemette
A proprietary, non-prescription preparation of docusate sodium and glycerol. It can be used to treat constipation.

Fletchers' Phosphate Enema
A proprietary, non-prescription preparation of sodium phosphate and sodium acid phosphate. It can be used to treat constipation.

Flexin
A proprietary, prescription-only preparation of indomethacin. It can be used to treat the pain and inflammation of rheumatic and other acute, severe musculoskeletal disorders.

Flexin-25 Continus
A proprietary, prescription-only preparation of indomethacin. It can be used to treat the pain and inflammation of rheumatic and other acute, severe musculoskeletal disorders.

Flexin-L5 Continus
A proprietary, prescription-only preparation of indomethacin. It can be used to treat the pain and inflammation of rheumatic and other acute, severe musculoskeletal disorders.

Flixonase
A proprietary, prescription-only preparation of the corticosteroid fluticasone. It can be used to treat nasal allergy.

Flolan
A proprietary, prescription-only preparation of epoprostenol. It can be used to prevent formation of blood clots.

Florinef

Properties
This medicine belongs to the family of topical (applied to the skin) corticosteroids, containing an adrenocorticoid as active ingredient. It is used to relieve the symptoms of any itching, rash, or inflammation of the skin; it does not treat the underlying cause of the skin problem. It also relieves redness, swelling and itching caused by insect bites, poison ivy, poison oak, poison sumach, soaps, cosmetics, sunburn, and numerous skin rashes.
Topical adrenocorticosteroids are absorbed through the skin and may rarely affect growth in children. Before using this medicine in children you should discuss the use of it with your doctor.

Before using this medicine
Before you use this medicine check with your doctor, or pharmacist:
- if you ever had any unusual or allergic reaction to adrenocorticoids or corticosteroids in general.
- if you are on a low-salt, low-sugar, or any other special diet, or if you are allergic to any substance, such as certain preservatives or dyes.
- if you have diabetes, stomach ulcer, or infection at the treatment site.
- if you are pregnant, intending to become pregnant or breast-feeding an infant while using this medicine.
- if you have any of the following medical problems:
  Diabetes mellitus (sugar diabetes)
  Infection at the place of treatment
  Ulceration at the place of treatment
  Tuberculosis

Treatment
This medication is used to relieve or prevent the symptoms of your medical problem. Take them as directed. Do not take more of them and do not take them more often than recommended on the label.
To do so may increase the chance of absorption through the skin and the chance of side effects. In addition, too much use, especially on thin skin areas (for example, armpits, face, groin), may result in thinning of the skin and stretch marks.

Side effects
The following side effects may occur:
- Acne or oily skin
- Blistering
- Burning sensations
- Itching
- Dryness of the skin
- Secondary infection
- Thinning of skin
- Unusual hair growth
- Unusual loss of hair

These side effects should disappear as your body adjusts to the medication. Tell your doctor about any side effects that are persistent or particularly bothersome.
The above side effects are more likely to occur in children and elderly patients, who are usually more sensitive to the effects of this medicine.
When the gel, solution, lotion, or aerosol from this medicine is applied, a mild, temporary stinging may be expected.

Interactions
This medicine interacts with several other drugs such as antibiotics (causing a decreased antibiotic effect) and antifungals (causing a decreased antifungal effect).
Be sure to tell your doctor about any medications you are currently taking.

Storage
This medicine should be stored at room temperature in closed containers. Store away from heat and direct light. Keep out of reach of children, since overdose may be dangerous in children. Do not store in the bathroom medicine cabinet because the heat or moisture may cause the medicine to break down. Keep the medicine from freezing. Do not keep outdated medicine.

Flonase
A proprietary, prescription-only preparation of fluticasone. It is used as nasal spray for runny nose, nasal congestion, itchy nose, and sneezing.

Florinef
A proprietary, prescription-only preparation of the corticosteroid fludrocortisone acetate. It can be used to treat adrenal gland insufficiency.

Floxapen
A proprietary, prescription-only preparation of the antibacterial and antibiotic drug flucloxacillin. It can be used to treat bacterial infections, particularly staphylococcal infections.

Flu-Amp
A proprietary, prescription-only compound preparation of the antibiotics flucloxacillin and ampicillin. It can be used to treat severe infections where the causative agent has not been identified.

Fluxanol
A proprietary, prescription-only preparation of flupenthixol. It can be used to treat depressive illness.

Fluclomix
A preparation of the antibacterial and antibiotic drug flucloxacillin. It can be used to treat bacterial infections, particularly staphylococcal infections.

Flucloxacillin
A proprietary, prescription-only anti-

bacterial and antibiotic drug. It can be used to treat bacterial infections, particularly those resistant to penicillin.

Fluconazole
A proprietary, prescription-only antifungal drug. It can be used to treat fungal infections..

Flucytosine
A proprietary, prescription-only antifungal drug. It can be used to treat fungal infections such as systemic candidiasis.

Fludara
A proprietary, prescription-only cytotoxic drug. It can be used to treat acute leukaemia.

Fludrocortisone acetate
A proprietary, prescription-only corticosteroid drug. It can be used to treat deficiencies of hormones from the adrenal gland.

Flumazanil
A proprietary, prescription-only benzodiazepine antagonist. It can be used to reverse the sedative affects of benzodiazepine preparations.

Flunisolide
A proprietary, prescription-only anti-allergic and corticosteroid drug. It can be used to treat nasal allergy and hay fever.

Flunitrazepam
A proprietary, prescription-only benzodiazepine drug. It can be used to treat insomnia.

Fluocinolone acetonide
A proprietary, prescription-only preparation of corticosteroid drug. It can be used to treat inflammatory skin disorders.

Fluocinonide
A proprietary, prescription-only preparation of corticosteroid drug. It can be used to treat inflammatory skin disorders.

Fluocortolone
A proprietary, prescription-only preparation of corticosteroid drug. It can be used to treat inflammatory skin disorders.

Fluocortolone
A proprietary, prescription-only preparation of corticosteroid drug. It can be used to treat inflammatory eye disorders.

Fluorouracil
A proprietary, prescription-only cytotoxic drug. It can be used to treat solid tumors (for example of the colon and breast).

Fluoro-uracil
A proprietary, prescription-only cytotoxic drug. It can be used to treat solid tumors (for example of the colon and breast).

Fluothane
An anesthetic inhalant used for the induction and maintenance of anesthesia during surgery.

Fluoxetine
A proprietary, prescription-only antidepressant drug. It can be used to treat depressive illness.

Flupenthixol
A proprietary, prescription-only phenothiazine derivative. It can be used to treat schizophrenia and other psychoses.

Flupenthixol deconate
A proprietary, prescription-only phenothiazine derivative. It can be used to treat schizophrenia and other psychoses.

Flupentixol
A proprietary, prescription-only phenothiazine derivative. It can be used to treat schizophrenia and other psychoses.

Flupentixol decanoate
A phenothiazine derivative. It can be used to treat schizophrenia and other psychoses.

Fluphenazine decanoate
A proprietary, prescription-only phenothiazine derivative. It can be used to treat schizophrenia and other psychoses.

Fluphenazine hydrochloride
A proprietary, prescription-only phenothiazine derivative. It can be used to treat schizophrenia and other psychoses.

Flurandrenolone
A proprietary, prescription-only corticosteroid drug. It can be used to treat inflammatory skin disorders such as eczema.

Flurazepam
A proprietary, prescription-only benzodiazepine drug. It can be used to treat insomnia and anxiety.

Flurbiprofen
A proprietary, prescription-only analgesic and antirheumatic drug. It can be used to treat pain and inflammation in musculoskeletal disorders and rheumatism.

Flurex Cold Capsules with Cough Suppressant
A proprietary, non-prescription-only preparation of phenylephrine hydrochloride, paracetamol and dextromethorphan hydrobromnide. It can be used for the relief of nasal congestion during colds and flu.

Flurex Flu Capsules with Cough Suppressant
A proprietary, non-prescription-only preparation of phenylephrine hydrochloride, paracetamol and dextromethorphan hydrobromnide. It can be used for the relief of nasal congestion during colds and flu.

Flurex Tablets
A proprietary, non-prescription-only preparation of phenylephrine hydrochloride, paracetamol and dextromethorphan hydrobromnide. It can be used for the relief of nasal congestion during colds and flu.

Fluspirilene
A proprietary, prescription-only antipsychotic drug. It can be used to treat schizophrenia.

Flutamide
A proprietary, prescription-only anti-androgen drug. It can be used to treat prostate cancer.

Fluticasone
(Topical)

Properties
This medicine belongs to the family of topical (applied to the skin) corticosteroids, containing an adrenocorticoid as active ingredient. It is used to relieve the symptoms of any itching, rash, or inflammation of the skin; it does not treat the underlying cause of the skin problem. It also relieves redness, swelling and itching caused by insect bites, poison ivy, poison oak, poison sumach, soaps, cosmetics, sunburn, and numerous skin rashes.
Topical adrenocorticosteroids are absorbed through the skin and may rarely affect growth in children. Before using this medicine in children you should discuss the use of it with your doctor.

Before using this medicine
Before you use this medicine check with your doctor, or pharmacist:
- if you ever had any unusual or allergic reaction to adrenocorticoids or corticosteroids in general.
- if you are on a low-salt, low-sugar, or any other special diet, or if you are allergic to any substance, such as certain preservatives or dyes.
- if you have diabetes, stomach ulcer, or infection at the treatment site.
- if you are pregnant, intending to become pregnant or breast-feeding an infant while using this medicine.
- if you have any of the following medical problems:
  Diabetes mellitus (sugar diabetes)
  Infection at the place of treatment
  Ulceration at the place of treatment
  Tuberculosis

Treatment
This medication is used to relieve or prevent the symptoms of your medical problem. Take them as directed. Do not take more of them and do not take them more often than recommended on the label.
To do so may increase the chance of absorption through the skin and the chance of side effects. In addition, too much use, especially on thin skin areas (for example, armpits, face, groin), may result in thinning of the skin and stretch marks.

Side effects
The following side effects may occur:
- Acne or oily skin
- Blistering
- Burning sensations
- Itching
- Dryness of the skin
- Secondary infection
- Thinning of skin
- Unusual hair growth
- Unusual loss of hair

These side effects should disappear as your body adjusts to the medication. Tell your doctor about any side effects that are persistent or particularly bothersome.
The above side effects are more likely to occur in children and elderly patients, who are usually more sensitive to the effects of this medicine.
When the gel, solution, lotion, or aerosol from this medicine is applied, a mild, temporary stinging may be expected.

Interactions
This medicine interacts with several other drugs such as antibiotics (causing a decreased antibiotic effect) and antifungals (causing a decreased antifungal effect).
Be sure to tell your doctor about any medications you are currently taking.

Storage
This medicine should be stored at room temperature in closed containers. Store away from heat and direct light. Keep out of reach of children, since overdose may be dangerous in children. Do not store in the bathroom medicine cabinet because the heat or moisture may cause the medicine to break down. Keep the medicine from freezing. Do not keep outdated medicine.

Fluticasone propionate
A proprietary, prescription-only corticosteroid drug. It can be used to treat inflammatory skin disorders.

Fluvastatin
A proprietary, prescription-only lipid-lowering drug. It can be used to reduce the levels of various lipids in the bloodstream.

Fluvoxamine maleate
A proprietary, prescription-only antidepressant drug. It can be used to treat depressive illness.

FML
A proprietary, prescription-only preparation of fluorometholone. It can be used to treat inflammatory eye conditions.

Folex-350
A preparation of ferrous fumarate and folic acid. It can be used as an iron and folic acid supplement.

Folic acid
A vitamin of the B complex. Its consumption is particularly necessary during pregnancy to prevent congenital disorders.

Folinic acid
A derivative of folic acid; a vitamin of the B complex. Its consumption is particularly necessary during pregnancy to prevent congenital disorders.

Fever Pain Infection

Froben

Properties
This medicine contains as active ingredient ibuprofen. It belongs to the group of medicines called non-steroidal anti-inflammatory drugs (NSAIDs). These drugs are taken by mouth to relieve some symptoms caused by arthritis or rheumatism, such as inflammation, swelling, stiffness, and joint pain. However, these medicines do not cure arthritis and will help you only as long as you continue to take them. Some of these medicines are also used to relieve other kinds of pain or to treat other painful conditions, such as gout attacks, bursitis, tendinitis, sprains, strains, menstrual cramps. The drug reduces the tissue concentration of prostaglandins (hormonal substances which produce inflammation and pain).

Before using this medicine
Before you use this medicine check with your doctor, or pharmacist:
- if you ever had any unusual or allergic reaction, such as skin rash, hives, or itching or breathing problems, to any of the anti-inflammatory analgesics.
- if you are on a low-salt, low-sugar, or any other special diet, or if you are allergic to any substance, such as sulfites or other preservatives or dyes.
- if you are pregnant or intending to become pregnant while using this medicine. Studies on birth defects have not been done in humans. However, if taken regularly during the last months of pregnancy, there is a chance that these medicines may cause unwanted effects on the heart or blood flow in the fetus or newborn infant.
- if you are breast-feeding an infant. Although this medicine has not been shown to cause problems in humans, it passes into the breast milk in small amounts.
- if you have any of the following medical problems: Asthma

Bleeding problems
Colitis
Stomach ulcer
Heart disease
Kidney or liver disease

Treatment
This medication is used to relieve pain or other symptoms caused by arthritis. For safe and effective use of this medicine, do not take more of it, do not take it more often, and do not take it for a longer period of time than ordered by your physician or directed by the package label.
If you are taking this medication on a regular schedule and you miss a dose, take the missed dose as soon as possible, unless it is almost time for your next dose. In that case do not take the missed dose at all.
To lessen stomach upset, anti-inflammatory analgesics may be taken with food or antacids.

Side effects
Along with the needed effects, a medicine may cause some unwanted effects. These side effects may go away during treatment as your body adjusts to the medicine. Such minor side effects are: dizziness; nausea; pain; headache; drowsiness; swollen feet, face or leg; constipation or diarrhea; vomiting; dry mouth.
Check with your doctor immediately if any of the following side effects occur:
- *Muscle cramps*
- *Numbness or tingling*
- *Mouth ulcers*
- *Convulsions or confusion*
- *Rash, hives, or itch*
- *Tightness in chest*

Interactions
This medicine may interact with several other drugs.
Be sure to tell your doctor about any medications you are currently taking.

Storage
The medicine should be stored at room temperature in a tightly closed, light-resistant container. Store away from heat and direct light. Keep out of reach of children.

Fomac
A preparation of mebeverine hydrochloride. It can be used to treat gastrointestinal spasm.

Formestane
A proprietary, prescription-only cytotoxic drug. It can be used to treat advanced breast cancer.

Fortagesic
A proprietary, prescription-only com-

pound preparation of pentazocine and paracetamol. It can be used to relieve pain anywhere in the body.

Fortral
A proprietary, prescription-only compound preparation of pentazocine and paracetamol. It can be used to relieve pain anywhere in the body.

Fortum
A proprietary, prescription-only pre-

paration of the antibacterial and antibiotic drug ceftazidine. It can be used to treat infections of the respiratory tract.

Foscarnet sodium
A proprietary, prescription-only antiviral drug. It can be used to treat cytomegaloviral retinitis.

Foscavir
A proprietary, prescription-only pre-

paration of the antiviral drug foscarnet sodium. It can be used to treat viral infections.

Fosfestrol tetrasodium
A proprietary, prescription-only drug that is converted in the body to stilbestrol. It can be used in men as an anticancer treatment for cancer of the prostate gland.

Fosinopril
A proprietary, prescription-only ACE inhibitor drug. It can be used to treat raised blood pressure.

Fragmin
A proprietary, prescription-only preparation of the anticoagulant drug dalteparin. It can be used to prevent venous thrombo-embolism.

Framycetin sulphate
A proprietary, prescription-only antibacterial and antibiotic drug. It can be used to treat a wide variety of infections.

Franol
A proprietary, prescription-only compound preparation of theophylline and ephedrine hydrochloride. It can be used to treat asthma and chronic bronchitis.

Franol Plus
A proprietary, prescription-only compound preparation of theophylline and ephedrine hydrochloride. It can be used to treat asthma and chronic bronchitis.

Franolyn for Chesty Coughs
A proprietary, non-prescription compound preparation of theophylline, guaiphensin and ephedrine hydrochloride. It can be used to treat asthma and chronic bronchitis.

Franolyn for Dry Coughs
A proprietary, non-prescription preparation of dextromethorphan hydrobromide. It can be used for the symptomatic relief of dry, irritating cough.

Frisium
A proprietary, prescription-only preparation of the benzodiazepine drug clobazam. It can be used to treat anxiety.

Froben
A proprietary, prescription-only preparation of flurbiprofen. It can be used to treat arthritis and rheumatic pain. (see page 675)

Froop
A proprietary, prescription-only preparation of the diuretic drug fursemide. It can be used to treat oedema.

Fru-Co
A proprietary, prescription-only compound preparation of the diuretic drugs fursemide and amiloride hydrochloride. It can be used to treat oedema.

Frumil
A proprietary, prescription-only compound preparation of the diuretic drugs fursemide and amiloride hydrochloride. It can be used to treat oedema.

Fursemide
A proprietary, prescription-only diuretic drug. It can be used to treat oedema due to heart or kidney disorders.

Fucebet
A proprietary, prescription-only compound preparation of betamethasone and fusidic acid. It can be used to treat skin disorders, such as psoriasis and eczema.

Fucidin
A proprietary, prescription-only preparation of the antibacterial and antibiotic drug fusidic acid. It can be used to treat staphylococcal infections.

Fucidin H
A proprietary, prescription-only compound preparation of betamethasone and fusidic acid. It can be used to treat skin inflammation.

Fulcin
A proprietary, prescription-only preparation of the antifungal and antibiotic drug griseofulvin. It can be used to treat fungal infections of the scalp, skin and nails.

Fungillin
A proprietary, prescription-only preparation of the antifungal and antibiotic drug amphotericin. It can be used to treat fungal infections, especially candidiasis.

Furadantin
A proprietary, prescription-only preparation of the antibacterial drug nitreofurantoin It can be used to treat infections of the urinary tract.

Furamide
A proprietary, prescription-only preparation of the antiprotozoal and amoebicidal drug diloxamide furoate. It can be used to treat chronic intestinal infection by Entamoeba histolytica.

Fusafungine
A proprietary, prescription-only anti-inflammatory and antibiotic drug. It can be used to treat infection and inflammation of the nose and throat.

Fusidic acid
A proprietary, prescription-only preparation of antibacterial and antibiotic drug. It can be used to treat staphylococcal infections.

Fybogel
A proprietary, non-prescription preparation of the laxative ispaghula husk. It can be used to treat a number of gastrointestinal disorders.

Fybogel Mebeverine
A proprietary, non-prescription compound preparation of the laxative ispaghula husk and mebeverine hydrochloride. It can be used to treat a number of gastrointestinal disorders characterized by spasms.

Fynnon Calcium Aspirin
A proprietary, non-prescription preparation of aspirin and calcium carbonate. It can be used to treat rheumatic pain, stiffness and swelling of joints.

G

Gabapentin
A proprietary, prescription-only anti-epileptic and anticonvulsant drug, used to assist in the control of seizures.

Galake
A proprietary, non-prescription compound preparation of diohydrocodeine tartrate and paracetamol. It can be used to relieve pain and to reduce high body temperature.

Galcodine
A proprietary, prescription-only preparation of codeine phosphate. It can be used to relieve a dry, painful cough.

Galcodine Paediatric
A proprietary, prescription-only preparation of codeine phosphate. It can be used to relieve a dry, painful cough.

Galenamet
A proprietary, prescription-only preparation of cimetidine. It can be used as an ulcer-healing drug for benign peptic ulcer.

Galeamox
A preparation of the antibacterial and antibiotic drug amoxycillin. It can be used to treat systemic bacterial infections.

Galenphol Linctus
A proprietary, non-prescription preparation of pholcodeine. It can be used to treat a dry, painful cough.

Galenphol Linctus Strong
A proprietary, non-prescription preparation of pholcodeine. It can be used to treat a dry, painful cough.

Galenphol Paediatric Linctus
A proprietary, non-prescription preparation of pholcodeine. It can be used to treat a dry, painful cough.

Galfer
A proprietary, non-prescription pre-paration of ferrous fumarate. It can be used to treat some forms of anemia.

Galfer FA
A proprietary, non-prescription compound preparation of ferrous fumarate and folic acid. It can be used as an iron and folic acid supplement during pregnancy.

Galfloxin
A proprietary, prescription-only preparation of the antibacterial and antibiotic drug flucloxacillin. It can be used to treat bacterial infections, especially staphylococcal infections.

Gallamine triethiodide
A proprietary, prescription-only skeletal muscle relaxant. It can be used to induce muscle paralysis during surgery.

Galpseud
A proprietary, non-prescription preparation of pseudoephedrine hydrochloride. It can be used as a nasal decongestant.

Galpseud Plus
A proprietary, non-prescription compound preparation of pseudoephedrine hydrochloride and chlorpheniramine maleate. It can be used as a nasal decongestant and for the relief of cold symptoms.

Gamanil
A proprietary, prescription-only preparation of lofepramine. It can be used to treat depressive illness.

Gammabulin
A preparation of human normal immunoglobulin. It can be used to confer immediate passive immunity against infection by viruses.

Ganciclovir
A proprietary, prescription-only antiviral drug. It can be used to treat cytomegalovirus infections.

Ganda
A proprietary, prescription-only compound preparation of guanethidine monosulphate and adrenaline. It can be used to treat glaucoma.

Garamycin
A proprietary, prescription-only preparation of antibacterial and antibiotic drug gentamycin. It can be used to treat many forms of eye and ear infections.

Gardenal Sodium
A proprietary, prescription-only preparation of phenobarbitone. It can be used to treat most forms of epilepsy.

Gastrobid Continus
A proprietary, prescription-only preparation of metoclopramide hydrochloride. It can be used to treat nausea and vomiting.

Gastrocote
A proprietary, prescription-only compound preparation of aluminium hydroxide, sodium bicarbonate and magnesium trisilicate. It can be used for the symptomatic relief of heartburn, reflux esophagitis and hernia hiatus.

Gastroflux
A proprietary, prescription-only preparation of metoclopramide hydrochloride. It can be used to treat nausea and vomiting.

Gastromax
A proprietary, prescription-only preparation of metoclopramide hydrochloride. It can be used to treat nausea and vomiting.

Gastron
A proprietary, non-prescription-only preparation of aluminium hydroxide, sodium bicarbonate, alginic acid and magnesium trisilicate. It can be used for the relief of dyspepsia.

Gastrozepin
A proprietary, prescription-only preparation of pirenzepine. It can be used to treat gastric and duodenal ulcers.

Gaviscon 250
A proprietary, non-prescription-only preparation of aluminium hydroxide, sodium bicarbonate, alginic acid and magnesium trisilicate. It can be used for the relief of dyspepsia.

G

Gaviscon

Properties
This medicine contains as active ingredient a neutralizing agent for excess stomach acid and is therefore called an antacid. Antacids are taken by mouth to relieve heartburn, sour stomach, or acid indigestion. Antacids alone or in combination with simethicone may be used to treat the symptoms of stomach or duodenal ulcers. This medication contains as active ingredients alumina, magnesium carbonate, magnesium trisilicate.

Before using this medicine
Before you use this medicine check with your doctor, or pharmacist:
- if you ever had any unusual or allergic reaction to aluminum-, calcium-, magnesium-, sodium bicarbonate-, or simethicone containing medicines;
- if you are on a low-salt, low-sugar, or any other special diet, or if you are allergic to any substance, such as sulfites or other preservatives or dyes.
- if you are pregnant or intending to become pregnant while using this medicine. Although antacids have not been shown to cause problems in humans, the chance always exists.
- if you are breast-feeding an infant.
- if you have any of the following medical problems:
  Appendicitis (or signs of)
  Bone fractures
  Colitis or colostomy
  Constipation or diarrhea
  Heart disease
  High blood pressure
  Intestinal blockage or bleeding
  Kidney or liver disease
  Toxaemia of pregnancy
  Underactive parathyroids

Treatment
This medication is used to relieve or prevent the symptoms of your medical problem. Take them as directed. Do not take more of them and do not take them more often than recommended on the label, unless otherwise directed by your doctor. To do so may increase the chance of side effects.
When taking this medicine for a stomach or duodenal ulcer, take it exactly as ordered by your doctor to obtain maximum relief of your symptoms.
Antacids should not be given to young children (up to 6 years of age) unless prescribed by their doctor.

Side effects
Along with the needed effects, a medicine may cause some unwanted effects. Although the following side effects occur very rarely when this medicine is taken as recommended, they may be more likely to occur if:
- too much medicine is taken;
- it is taken in large doses;
- it is taken for a long period of time;
- it is taken by patients with kidney disease.
Check with your doctor as soon as possible if any of the following side effects or signs of overdose occur: constipation; cramping; difficult or painful urination; headache; loss of appetite; mood or mental changes; muscle pain or twitching; nausea or vomiting; stomach pain; unpleasant taste in mouth; unusual slow breathing; unusual tiredness or weakness.

Interactions
This medicine may interact with several other drugs such as adrenocorticosteroids, cellulose sodium phosphate, mecamylamine, and tetracyclines.
Be sure to tell your doctor about any medications you are currently taking.

Storage
Tablets, elixir, etc. should be stored at room temperature; store away from heat and direct light. Keep out of reach of children, since overdose may be very dangerous in children.

Gaviscon Liquid
A proprietary, non-prescription-only preparation of aluminium hydroxide, sodium bicarbonate, alginic acid and magnesium trisilicate. It can be used for the symptomatic relief of dyspepsia and heartburn.

Geangin
A proprietary, prescription-only preparation of verapamil. It can be used to treat raised blood pressure and angina pectoris.

Gee's Linctus
A proprietary, non-prescription-only compound preparation of tolu syrup, camphorated tincture of opium and anhydrous morphine. It can be used to treat coughs.

Gelcosal
A compound preparation of salicylic acid and coal tar. It can be used to treat psoriasis and dermatitis.

Gemeprost
A proprietary, prescription-only prostaglandin preparation. It can be used during the induction of labour.

Gemfibrozil
A proprietary, prescription-only lipid-lowering drug. It can be used to reduce lipid levels in the bloodstream.

Genisol
A proprietary, prescription-only compound preparation of coal tar and sodium sulphosuccinate. It can be used to treat skin conditions such as dandruff and psoriasis.

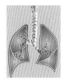

Gee's Linctus

Properties

This medicine contains guaifenesin as active ingredient; it is used to treat severe cough symptoms. This medication is taken by mouth to relieve coughs due to colds or influenza. Guaifenesin works by loosening the mucus or phlegm in the lungs. It increases production of watery fluids to thin mucus so it can be coughed out or absorbed. *Regular use for 5 to 7 days is necessary for maximum benefit.*

Before using this medicine

This medicine is not to be used for the chronic cough that occurs with smoking, asthma, or emphysema or when there is an unusually large amount of mucus or phlegm with the cough. Before you use this medicine, check with your doctor or pharmacist:
- if you ever had any unusual or allergic reaction to any of the compounds of this medicine.
- if you are on a low-salt, low-sugar, or any other special diet, or if you are allergic to any substance, such as sulfites or other preservatives or dyes.
- if you are pregnant, intending to become pregnant or breast-feeding an infant while using this medicine.

Do not take this drug with other medicine without consulting your doctor or pharmacist.

Treatment

This medication is used to relieve or prevent the symptoms of your medical problem. Take them as directed. Do not take more of them and do not take them more often than recommended on the label. To help loosen mucus or phlegm in the lungs, drink a glass of water after each dose of this medicine, unless otherwise directed by your doctor. If you must take this medicine regularly and you miss a dose, take it as soon as possible. However, if it is almost time for your next dose, skip the missed dose and go back to your regular dosing schedule. Do not double doses.

Side effects

Along with its needed effects, a medicine may cause some unwanted effects. Although not all of these side effects appear very often, when they do occur they may require medical attention. The following minor side effects may occur:
- Diarrhea
- Drowsiness
- Nausea
- Skin rash
- Stomach pain
- Vomiting

Symptoms of overdose include the following:
- Drowsiness
- Mild weakness
- Nausea and vomiting

An overdose is unlikely to threaten life. If a person takes much larger doses than prescribed, call a doctor, poison control center or hospital emergency room for instructions. The side effects should disappear as your body adjusts to the medication. Tell your doctor about any side effects that are persistent or particularly bothersome. Adverse reactions and side effects may be more frequent and severe in people over 60 years than in younger persons.

Driving, piloting or hazardous work should be avoided if you feel drowsy.

Interactions

This medicine interacts with several other drugs such as anticoagulants. There exists a possible risk of bleeding.

Storage

This medicine should be stored at room temperature in tightly closed containers. Store away from heat and direct light. Keep out of reach of children, since overdose may be dangerous in children. Do not store in the bathroom medicine cabinet because the heat or moisture may cause the medicine to break down. Do not refrigerate the syrup form of this medicine. Do not keep outdated medicine or medicine no longer needed.

Genotropin

A proprietary, prescription-only preparation of somatropin. It can be used to treat growth hormone deficiency.

Gentamycin

A proprietary, prescription-only antibacterial and antibiotic drug. It can be used to treat serious infections caused by Gram-negative bacteria.

Gentisone HC

A proprietary, prescription-only combined preparation of gentamycin and hydrocortisone. It can be used to treat bacterial infections of the middle ear.

Germoline Cream

A proprietary, non-prescription compound preparation of chlorhexidine and phenol. It can be used for cleaning all types of lesions.

Germoline Ointment

A compound preparation of zinc oxide, phenol, octaphonium and methyl salicylate. It can be used for cleaning minor skin disorders.

Germoloids

A proprietary, non-prescription compound preparation of lignocaine hydrochloride and zinc oxide. It can be used for the symptomatic relief of pain and itching of hemorrhoids.

G

Gestodene
A proprietary, prescription-only progestogen preparation. It can be used as a constituent of an oral contraceptive drug.

Gestone
A proprietary, prescription-only preparation of progesterone. It can be used to treat hormonal deficiency disorders.

Gestronol hexanoate
A synthetic form of progestogen used as an anticancer treatment for cancer of the endometrium.

Glandosane
A proprietary, non-prescription preparation of carmellose sodium, sorbitol, potassium chloride, sodium chloride and other salts. It can be used as a form of artificial saliva.

Glauicol
A proprietary, prescription-only preparation of tomolol maleate. It can be used to treat glaucoma.

Glibenclamide
A proprietary, prescription-only drug used in the treatment of diabetes Type II.

Glibenese
A proprietary, prescription-only drug. It can be used to treat diabetes Type II.

Glipzide
A proprietary, prescription-only drug. It can be used to treat diabetes Type II.

Glucobay
A proprietary, prescription-only preparation of acarbose, used to treat diabetes Type II.

Glucophage
A proprietary, prescription-only preparation of metformin hydrochloride, used to treat diabetes Type II.

Glucovance
A proprietary, prescription-only preparation of glyburide/metformin. It is used in diabetics to lower blood sugar levels.

Glurenorm
A proprietary, prescription-only preparation of gliquidone, used to treat diabetes Type II.

Glutarol
A proprietary, non-prescription preparation of glutaraldehyde. It can be used to treat warts and to remove hard, dead skin.

Glyceryl trinitrate
A proprietary, prescription-only vasodilator drug. It can be used to treat and prevent angina pectoris.

Glycol salicylate
A proprietary, non-prescription drug used on topical application to relieve inflammatory pain in joints and muscles.

Glypressin
A proprietary, prescription-only preparation of vasopressin. It can be used to treat bleeding from varices.

Glytrin Spray
A proprietary, non-prescription-only preparation of glyceryl trinitrate. It can be used to treat and prevent attacks of angina pectoris.

Goddard's Embrocation
A proprietary, non-prescription preparation of turpentine oil, ammonia and acetic acid. It can be applied to the skin for symptomatic relief of underlying muscle or joint pain.

Golden Eye Drops
A proprietary, non-prescription-only preparation of propamidine isethionate. It can be used to treat infections of the eyelids or conjunctiva.

Golden Eye Ointment
A proprietary, non-prescription-only preparation of dibromopropamidine isethionate. It can be used to treat infections of the eyelids or conjunctiva.

Gonadotrophin LH
A proprietary, prescription-only preparation of human chorionic gonadotrophin. It can be used to treat undescended testicles and delayed puberty.

Gopten
A proprietary, prescription-only preparation of trandolapril. It can be used to treat raised blood pressure.

Goserelin
An analogue of human gonadorelin, used as an anticancer drug for cancer of the prostate gland.

Gramicidin
A proprietary, prescription-only antibacterial and antibiotic drug. It can be used to treat eye and ear conditions.

Graneodin
A proprietary, prescription-only preparation of the antibacterial and antibiotic drug neomycin sulphate. It can be used to treat numerous bacterial infections.

Granisetron
A proprietary, prescription-only antiemetic and antinauseant drug, used to give relief from nausea and vomiting.

Gregoderm
A proprietary, prescription-only compound preparation of hydrocortisone, polymyxin B and neomycin sulphate. It can be used to treat inflammation of the skin.

Griseofulvin
A proprietary, prescription-only antifungal and antibiotic drug. It can be used to treat large-scale skin infections.

Grisovin
A proprietary, prescription-only preparation of the antifungal and antibiotic drug griseofulvin. It can be used to treat infections of the scalp, skin and nails.

Guaiphenesin
A proprietary, non-prescription expectorant. It can be used to relieve the symptoms of colds.

Guanethidine monosulphate
A adrenergic neurone blocker. It can be used to treat raised blood pressure.

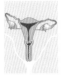

Gyno-Daktarin

Properties
This medicine belongs to the family of topical (applied to the skin) antifungal preparations. It is used in the treatment of fungus infections on the skin and in the vagina. The medication fights infections such as ringworm of the scalp, athlete's foot, jockey itch, sun fungus, nail fungus and fungus infections of the vagina.

Fungal diseases may develop especially in people with disorders of immunity or diabetes and those on certain drugs (steroid, immunosuppressives, antibiotics). Thrush is common in the mouth and vagina but rarely causes systemic disease.

The drug kills fungi by damaging the fungal wall; it causes loss of essential elements to sustain fungus cell life.

Before using this medicine
Before you use this medicine check with your doctor, or pharmacist:
- if you ever had any unusual or allergic reaction to topical antifungal preparations.
- if you are on a low-salt, low-sugar, or any other special diet, or if you are allergic to any substance, such as certain preservatives or dyes.
- if you are sunburned, or have an open skin wound.
- if you are pregnant, intending to become pregnant or breast-feeding an infant while using this medicine.

Pregnant women should avoid using the vaginal cream during the first three months of pregnancy. They should use it during the next six months only if it is absolutely necessary.

Treatment
This medication is used to relieve or prevent the symptoms of your medical problem. Take them as directed. Do not take more of them and do not take them more often than recommended on the label. To do so may increase the chance of absorption through the skin and the chance of side effects. If you forget to take a dose of this drug, take it as soon as you remember. If it is almost time for your next regularly scheduled application, skip the forgotten application and continue with your regular schedule.

CREAM, LOTION, OINTMENT, GEL: Bathe and dry area before use. Apply small amount and rub gently.

POWDER: Apply lightly to the skin.

VAGINAL CREAM & TABLETS: Insert into vagina with applicator as illustrated in instructions.

The treatment may require a period of 6 to 8 weeks for a complete cure. The usual schedule calls for an application twice a day, morning and evening, unless otherwise directed by your doctor or pharmacist. Be sure to complete the full course of treatment prescribed for you.

Side effects
The following side effects may occur:
- Itching
- Swelling of treated skin
- Redness of skin
- Vaginal burning and itching
- Irritation of vagina
- Swelling of labia
- Increased discharge

You should discontinue the use of the drug when these side effects occur. Call your doctor right away.

Interactions
This medicine may interact with several other medications applied to the skin or vagina. The combined effect may cause severe skin irritation or disorders of the labia or vagina.

Storage
This medicine should be stored cool, but Do not freeze. Store away from heat and direct light. Keep out of reach of children. Do not use on other members of the family without consulting your doctor. Do not store in the bathroom medicine cabinet because the heat or moisture may cause the medicine to break down. Do not keep outdated medicine or medicine no longer needed. Flush the contents down the toilet, unless otherwise directed.

Guarem
A preparation of guar gum. It is used as a form of diabetic treatment.

Guar gum
A form of diabetic treatment in as much that if it is taken in sufficient quantities it reduces the rise in blood glucose which occurs after meals.

Guarina
A proprietary, non-prescription preparation of guar gum. It is used as a form of diabetic treatment.

Gyno-Daktarin
A proprietary, prescription-only preparation of the antifungal drug miconazide. It can be used to treat fungal infections of the vagina or vulva.

Gynol II
A proprietary, non-prescription spermicidal contraceptive used in combination with barrier methods of contraception.

Gyno-Pevaryl
A proprietary, prescription-only preparation of the antifungal drug econazole nitrate. It can be used to treat fungal infections of the vagina, vulva or penis.

H

Haelan
A proprietary, prescription-only preparation of the corticosteroid flurandrenolone. It is used to treat inflammatory skin disorders such as eczema.

Haelan XL
A proprietary, prescription-only compound preparation of the corticosteroid flurandrenolone and clioquinol. It is used to treat inflammatory skin disorders such as eczema.

Halciderm Topical
A proprietary, prescription-only preparation of the corticosteroid halcinonide. It is used to treat skin disorders such as eczema and psoriasis.

Haldol
A preparation of the antipsychotic drug haloperidol. It is used to treat psychotic disorders and to tranquillize patients undergoing behavioral disturbance.

Haldol Decanoate
A proprietary, prescription-only preparation of the antipsychotic drug haloperidol. It is used to treat psychotic disorders and to tranquillize patients undergoing behavioral disturbance.

Halfan
A proprietary, prescription-only preparation of halofantrine. It is used to treat and prevent malaria.

Half-Betadur CR
A proprietary, prescription-only preparation of the beta-blocker propranolol hydrochloride. It can be used to treat raised blood pressure.

Half-Beta-Prograne
A proprietary, prescription-only preparation of the beta-blocker drug propranolol. It is used to treat raised blood pressure.

Half-Inderal LA
A proprietary, prescription-only preparation of the beta-blocker drug propranolol. It is used to treat raised blood pressure.

Half Securon SR
A proprietary, prescription-only preparation of verapamil hydrochloride. It can be treat raised blood pressure and to prevent angina attacks.

Half Sinemet CR
A proprietary, prescription-only compound preparation of levodopa and carbidopa. It is used to treat symptoms of parkinsonism.

Halofantrine hydrochloride
A proprietary, prescription-only antimalarian drug. It is used to treat infections by Plasmodium falciparum.

Haloperidol
A proprietary, prescription-only antipsychotic drug. It is used to treat psychotic disorders including schizophrenia.

Halothane
A proprietary, prescription-only anesthetic drug. It is used for the induction and maintenance of anesthesia during surgery.

Hamarin
A proprietary, prescription-only preparation of allopurinol. It is used to treat attacks of gout and to prevent renal stones.

Harmogen
A proprietary, prescription-only preparation of the estrogen piperazone estrone sulphate. It is used in hormone replacement therapy.

Hay-Crom
A proprietary, prescription-only preparation of cromoglycate. It is used to treat allergic conjunctivitis.

Haymine
A proprietary, non-prescription compound preparation of chlorpheniramine and ephedrine hydrochloride. It is used for the symptomatic relief of allergic symptoms.

Healonid
A proprietary, prescription-only preparation of sodium hyaluronate. It is used during surgical procedures of the eye.

Hedex Extra Tablets
A proprietary, non-prescription compound preparation of paracetamol and caffeine. It is used fore the pain of headache, neuralgia, period pain and to relieve cold symptoms.

Hedex Tablets
A proprietary, non-prescription preparation of paracetamol. It is used fore the pain of headache, neuralgia, period pain and to relieve cold symptoms.

Hemabate
A proprietary, prescription-only preparation of carboprost. It is used to treat hemorrhage following childbirth.

Hemionevrin
A preparation of chlormethiazole. It is used to treat insomnia, epilepsy and eclampsia.

Hemocane
A proprietary, non-prescription preparation of lignocaine, zinc oxide, bismuth oxide and benzoic acid. It is used for the symptomatic relief of the pain and itching of hemorrhoids.

Heparin
A natural anticoagulant in the body, which is produced mainly by the liver. It is used to treat thrombosis and similar conditions.

Heparinoid
A version of the heparin, the natural anticoagulant in the body, which is produced mainly by the liver. It is used to treat thrombosis and similar conditions.

Herpid
A proprietary, prescription-only preparation of the antiviral drug idoxuridine. It can be used to treat infections of the skin by herpes simplex or herpes zoster.

Hewletts Cream
A proprietary, non-prescription preparation of zinc oxide. It can be used to treat minor abrasions and burns.

Halcinderm
(Topical)

Properties

This medicine belongs to the family of topical (applied to the skin) corticosteroids, containing an adrenocorticoid as active ingredient. It is used to relieve the symptoms of any itching, rash, or inflammation of the skin; it does not treat the underlying cause of the skin problem. It also relieves redness, swelling and itching caused by insect bites, poison ivy, poison oak, poison sumach, soaps, cosmetics, sunburn, and numerous skin rashes.

Topical adrenocorticosteroids are absorbed through the skin and may rarely affect growth in children. Before using this medicine in children you should discuss the use of it with your doctor.

Before using this medicine

Before you use this medicine check with your doctor, or pharmacist:

- if you ever had any unusual or allergic reaction to adrenocorticoids or corticosteroids in general.
- if you are on a low-salt, low-sugar, or any other special diet, or if you are allergic to any substance, such as certain preservatives or dyes.
- if you have diabetes, stomach ulcer, or infection at the treatment site.
- if you are pregnant, intending to become pregnant or breast-feeding an infant while using this medicine.
- if you have any of the following medical problems:
  Diabetes mellitus (sugar diabetes)
  Infection at the place of treatment
  Ulceration at the place of treatment
  Tuberculosis

Treatment

This medication is used to relieve or prevent the symptoms of your medical problem. Take them as directed. Do not take more of them and do not take them more often than recommended on the label.

To do so may increase the chance of absorption through the skin and the chance of side effects. In addition, too much use, especially on thin skin areas (for example, armpits, face, groin), may result in thinning of the skin and stretch marks.

Side effects

The following side effects may occur:

- Acne or oily skin
- Blistering
- Burning sensations
- Itching
- Dryness of the skin
- Secondary infection
- Thinning of skin
- Unusual hair growth
- Unusual loss of hair

These side effects should disappear as your body adjusts to the medication. Tell your doctor about any side effects that are persistent or particularly bothersome.

The above side effects are more likely to occur in children and elderly patients, who are usually more sensitive to the effects of this medicine.

When the gel, solution, lotion, or aerosol from this medicine is applied, a mild, temporary stinging may be expected.

Interactions

This medicine interacts with several other drugs such as antibiotics (causing a decreased antibiotic effect) and antifungals (causing a decreased antifungal effect).

Be sure to tell your doctor about any medications you are currently taking.

Storage

This medicine should be stored at room temperature in closed containers. Store away from heat and direct light. Keep out of reach of children, since overdose may be dangerous in children. Do not store in the bathroom medicine cabinet because the heat or moisture may cause the medicine to break down. Keep the medicine from freezing. Do not keep outdated medicine.

Hexachlorophane

A proprietary, non-prescription antiseptic agent. It is used to treat prevent infections.

Hexachlorophene

A proprietary, non-prescription antiseptic agent. It is used to treat prevent infections.

Hexamine hippurate

A proprietary, prescription-only antibacterial drug. It is used to prevent infections during urinogenital surgery.

Hexetidine

A proprietary, non-prescription antiseptic preparation. It is used for routine oral hygiene.

Hexopal

A proprietary, non-prescription-only preparation of inositol nicotinate. It is used to help improve blood circulation of the hands.

Hibisol

A proprietary, preparation of the antiseptic agent chlorhexidine. It is used to treat minor wounds and burns.

Hibitane

A proprietary, non-prescription preparation of the antiseptic agent chlorhexidine. It is used to treat minor wounds and burns.

Hioxyl

A proprietary, non-prescription pre-

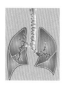

Hismanal

Properties
This medicine contains astemiazole as active ingredient; it is prescribed for symptomatic treatment of stuffy nose, upper respiratory congestion, or bronchospasms associated with asthma, asthmatic bronchitis or a similar condition.

The medication provides symptomatic relief of respiratory conditions, but does not treat the underlying disease. The medicine decreases blood volume in nasal tissues, shrinking tissues and enlarging airways.

Before using this medicine
Before you use this medicine check with your doctor, or pharmacist:
- if you ever had any unusual or allergic reaction to any of the compounds of this medicine.
- if you are on a low-salt, low-sugar, or any other special diet, or if you are allergic to any substance, such as sulfites or other preservatives or dyes.
- if you are pregnant, intending to become pregnant or breast-feeding an infant while using this medicine.
- if you have any of the following medical problems:
  Overactive thyroid
  Diabetes
  Urination difficulty
  Heart condition
  High blood pressure

Treatment
This medication is used to relieve or prevent the symptoms of your medical problem. Take them as directed. Do not take more of them and do not take them more often than recommended on the label.

The medicine produces central nervous system stimulation, and it should not be taken by people with heart disease or high blood pressure.

Side effects
The following minor side effects may occur: dizziness; shakiness; weakness; paleness; agitation; insomnia.

These side effects should disappear as your body adjusts to the medication. Tell your doctor about any side effects that are persistent or particularly bothersome. It is especially important to tell your doctor about;
- Nausea or vomiting (severe)
- Irregular or slow heartbeat
- Painful or difficult urination
- Increased sweating
- Trembling
- Unusual fast, pounding, or irregular heartbeat

Discontinue use of the drug; call your doctor right away. Adverse reactions and side effects may be more frequent and severe in people over age 60 than in younger persons. Older adults with severe kidney problems may be more sensitive to the effects of this drug. Signs of overdose include:
- *Nervousness*
- *Restlessness*
- *Headache*
- *Rapid or irregular heartbeat*
- *Nausea and vomiting*
- *Anxiety and/or confusion*
- *Delirium*
- *Hallucinations*

Interactions
This medicine interacts with several other drugs such as antihypertensives, beta-adrenergic blockers, calcium supplements, digitalis preparations. Interaction with alcoholic beverages may produce drowsiness, sleepiness, and/or inability to concentrate.

Be sure to tell your doctor about any medications you are currently taking.

Storage
This medicine should be stored at room temperature in tightly closed containers. Store away from heat and direct light. Keep out of reach of children, since overdose may be very dangerous in children.

---

paration of the antiseptic agent chlorhexidine. It is used to treat minor wounds, bedsores and burns.

Hiprex
A proprietary, non-prescription preparation of the antibacterial drug hexamine hippurate. It is used to treat infections of the urinary and gastrointestinal tract.

Hirudoid
A preparation of heparinoids. It is used to improve circulation in conditions such as bruising and hematoma.

Hismanal
A preparation of astemizole. It is used to treat allergic disorders such as hay fever and urticaria.

Hivid
A proprietary, prescription-only preparation of zalcitabine. It is used in the treatment of AIDS.

Honvan
A proprietary, prescription-only preparation of fosferol tetrasodium. It is used in men for the treatment of prostate cancer.

Hormonin
A proprietary, prescription-only compound preparation of the hormones oestradiol and oestriol. It is used in hormone replacement therapy for menopausal disorders.

HRF
A proprietary, prescription-only preparation of gonadorelin. It is used as a diagnostic aid in the functioning of the pituitary body.

Human Actraphane 30/70
A proprietary, prescription-only preparation of human insulin. It is used to treat diabetes.

Human Actrapid
A proprietary, prescription-only preparation of synthesized insulin. It is used to treat diabetes.

Human Initard 50/50
A proprietary, prescription-only preparation of insulin. It is used to treat diabetes.

Human Insulatard
A proprietary, prescription-only preparation of human insulin. It is used to treat diabetes.

Human Mixtard 30/70
A proprietary, prescription-only preparation of human insulin. It is used to treat diabetes.

Human Protaphane
A proprietary, prescription-only preparation of human insulin. It is used to treat diabetes.

Human Protaphane
A proprietary, prescription-only preparation of human insulin zinc suspension. It is used to treat diabetes.

Human Velosulin
A proprietary, prescription-only preparation of human insulin. It is used to treat diabetes.

Humatrope
A proprietary, prescription-only preparation of somatropin. It is used to treat hormonal deficiency.

Humegon
A proprietary, prescription-only preparation of human menopausal gonadotrophin. It is used to treat infertility in women.

Humiderm
A proprietary, prescription-only preparation of pyrolidone. It is used as an emollient to treat dry skin.

Hormones

These are substances produced and secreted by glands. In the case of endocrine hormones they are carried by the bloodstream to the organs on which they have their effect. Hormones can be divided into several families.

- The adrenal hormones are secreted by the adrenal glands, of which there are two distinct types: adrenal cortical hormones (for instance corticosteroids) and adrenal medullary hormones (for instance adrenaline and noradrenaline).

- The thyroid hormones and the parathyroid hormones come from the thyroid and parathyroid glands at the base of the neck (for instance calcitonin, triiodothyronine).

- The glucose-regulatory hormones are produced by the pancreas (for instance glucagon and insulin).

- The sex hormones come mainly from the ovaries and testes (for instance testosterone, estrogens, progestogens).

- The pituitary gland, situated at the base of the skull, is an important producer of several vital hormones. There are two distinct classes of pituitary hormones: the posterior pituitary hormones oxytocin and vasopressin, and the anterior pituitary hormones, which include corticotrophin and somatotropin.

Humelin I
A proprietary, prescription-only preparation of human isophane insulin. It is used in diabetic treatment to treat and maintain diabetic patients.

Humelin Lente
A preparation of human insulin zinc suspension. It is used in diabetic treatment to treat and maintain diabetic patients.

Humelin M1
A proprietary, prescription-only preparation of human isophane insulin. It is used in diabetic treatment to treat and maintain diabetic patients.

Humelin M2
A proprietary, prescription-only preparation of human isophane insulin 80/20. It is used in diabetic treatment to treat and maintain diabetic patients.

Humelin M3
A proprietary, prescription-only preparation of human isophane insulin 70/30. It is used in diabetic treatment to treat and maintain diabetic patients.

Humelin M3
A proprietary, prescription-only preparation of human isophane insulin 40/60. It is used in diabetic treatment to treat and maintain diabetic patients.

Humelin S
A proprietary, prescription-only preparation of synthesized neural soluble insulin. It is used in diabetic treatment to treat and maintain diabetic patients.

Humelin Zn
A proprietary, prescription-only preparation of human insulin zinc suspension. It is used in diabetic treatment to treat and maintain diabetic patients.

Hyalase

A proprietary, prescription-only preparation of hyaluronidase. It is used to increase the permeability of soft tissues.

Hydergine

A proprietary, prescription-only preparation of co-dergocrine mesylate. It is used as vasodilator.

Hydralazine hydrochloride

A proprietary, prescription-only vasodilator drug. It is used to treat acute and chronic cardiovascular disorders.

Hydrea

A proprietary, prescription-only preparation of the cytotoxic drug hydroxyurea. It is used to treat myeloid leukaemia.

Hydrenox

A proprietary, prescription-only preparation of the diuretic drug hydroflumethiazide. It is used to treat oedema.

Hydrocal

A proprietary, prescription-only compound preparation of hydrocortisone and calamine. It is used to treat inflammatory skin disorders.

Hydrochlorothiazide

A proprietary, prescription-only diuretic drug. It is used to treat oedema associated with congestive heart failure.

Hydrocortisone

A proprietary, prescription-only corticosteroid drug. It is used to treat any kind of inflammation.

Hydrocortisone acetate

A proprietary, prescription-only corticosteroid drug. It is used to treat any kind of inflammation.

Hydrocortisone butyrate

A proprietary, prescription-only corticosteroid drug. It is used to treat any kind of inflammation.

Hydrocortisone sodium succinate

A proprietary, prescription-only corticosteroid drug. It is used to treat any kind of inflammation.

Hydrocortisyl

A proprietary, prescription-only preparation of the corticosteroid drug hydrocortisone. It is used to treat any kind of inflammation of the skin.

Hydrocortone

A proprietary, prescription-only preparation of the corticosteroid drug hydrocortisone. It is used to treat any kind of inflammation and to make up hormonal deficiency.

Hydroflumethiazide

A proprietary, prescription-only diuretic drug. It is used to treat oedema associated with congestive heart failure.

Hydrogen peroxide

A general antiseptic drug, used for a wide range of purposes.

Hydromet

A proprietary, prescription-only compound preparation of hydrochlorothiazide and methyldopa. It is used to treat raised blood pressure.

Hydromol

A proprietary, non-prescription preparation of liquid paraffin and arachis oil. It is used to treat dry skin.

Hydrosaluric

A proprietary, prescription-only preparation of hydrochlorothiazide. It is used to treat oedema and raised blood pressure.

Hydroxycobalamin

A form of vitamin B12, used in deficiency disorders.

Hydroxychloroquine sulphate

A proprietary, prescription-only anti-inflammatory and antirheumatic drug. It is used to treat rheumatoid arthritis.

Hydroxyprogesterone caproate

A progestogen. It is used to treat recurrent abortion (habitual abortion).

Hydroxyprogesterone hexanoate

A proprietary, prescription-only progestogen. It is used to treat recurrent abortion (habitual abortion).

Hydroxyurea

A proprietary, prescription-only cytotoxic drug. It is used to treat chronic myeloid leukaemia.

Hydroxyzine hydrochloride

A proprietary, prescription-only antihistamine drug with anxiolytic properties. It is used to treat allergic conditions.

Hygroton

A preparation of the diuretic drug chlothalidone. It is used to treat oedema and raised blood pressure.

Hyoscine butylbromide

A proprietary, prescription-only anticholinergic drug. It is used for the relief of smooth muscle spasm.

Hyoscine hydrobromide

A proprietary, prescription-only belladonna alkaloid drug.It is used to induce sedation.

Hunomidate

A proprietary, prescription-only preparation of etomidate. It is used to treat insomnia.

Hypnovel

A proprietary, prescription-only preparation of modazolam. It is used to treat anxiety and insomnia.

Hypovase

A proprietary, prescription-only preparation of prazosin. It is used to treat raised blood pressure and in congestive heart failure.

Hypovase Benign Prostatic Hypertrophy

A proprietary, prescription-only preparation of prazosin. It is used to treat urinary retention in benign prostatic hypertrophy.

Hypurin Isophane

A proprietary, non-prescription-only preparation of isophane insulin. It is used to treat diabetes.

Hypurin Lente

A proprietary, non-prescription-only preparation of insulin zinc suspension. It is used to treat diabetes.

Hydrocortisone
(Topical)

Properties

This medicine belongs to the family of topical (applied to the skin) corticosteroids, containing an adrenocorticoid as active ingredient. It is used to relieve the symptoms of any itching, rash, or inflammation of the skin; it does not treat the underlying cause of the skin problem. It also relieves redness, swelling and itching caused by insect bites, poison ivy, poison oak, poison sumach, soaps, cosmetics, sunburn, and numerous skin rashes.

Topical adrenocorticosteroids are absorbed through the skin and may rarely affect growth in children. Before using this medicine in children you should discuss the use of it with your doctor.

Before using this medicine

Before you use this medicine check with your doctor, or pharmacist:
- if you ever had any unusual or allergic reaction to adrenocorticoids or corticosteroids in general.
- if you are on a low-salt, low-sugar, or any other special diet, or if you are allergic to any substance, such as certain preservatives or dyes.
- if you have diabetes, stomach ulcer, or infection at the treatment site.
- if you are pregnant, intending to become pregnant or breast-feeding an infant while using this medicine.
- if you have any of the following medical problems:
  Diabetes mellitus (sugar diabetes)
  Infection at the place of treatment
  Ulceration at the place of treatment
  Tuberculosis

Treatment

This medication is used to relieve or prevent the symptoms of your medical problem. Take them as directed. Do not take more of them and do not take them more often than recommended on the label.

To do so may increase the chance of absorption through the skin and the chance of side effects. In addition, too much use, especially on thin skin areas (for example, armpits, face, groin), may result in thinning of the skin and stretch marks.

Side effects

The following side effects may occur:
- Acne or oily skin
- Blistering
- Burning sensations
- Itching
- Dryness of the skin
- Secondary infection
- Thinning of skin
- Unusual hair growth
- Unusual loss of hair

These side effects should disappear as your body adjusts to the medication. Tell your doctor about any side effects that are persistent or particularly bothersome. The above side effects are more likely to occur in children and elderly patients, who are usually more sensitive to the effects of this medicine.

When the gel, solution, lotion, or aerosol from this medicine is applied, a mild, temporary stinging may be expected.

Interactions

This medicine interacts with several other drugs such as antibiotics (causing a decreased antibiotic effect) and antifungals (causing a decreased antifungal effect).

Be sure to tell your doctor about any medications you are currently taking.

Storage

This medicine should be stored at room temperature in closed containers. Store away from heat and direct light. Keep out of reach of children, since overdose may be dangerous in children.

▲ Do not store in the bathroom medicine cabinet because the heat or moisture may cause the medicine to break down.

▲ Keep the medicine from freezing. Do not keep outdated medicine.

Hypurin Neutral
A preparation of protamine zinc insulin. It is used to treat diabetes.

Hytrin
A proprietary, prescription-only preparation of terazosin hydrochloride. It is used to treat high blood pressure.

Hytrin BPH
A proprietary, prescription-only preparation of terazosin hydrochloride. It is used to treat urinary retention.

I

Ibugel
A proprietary, prescription-only preparation of the analgesic and antirheumatic drug ibuprofen. It is used as topical medicine to treat rheumatic and musculoskeletal pain and inflammation.

Ibular
A proprietary, prescription-only preparation of the analgesic and antirheumatic drug ibuprofen. It is used to treat rheumatic and musculoskeletal pain and inflammation.

Ibuleve Gel
A proprietary, prescription-only preparation of the analgesic and antirheumatic drug ibuprofen. It is used as topical drug to treat rheumatic and musculoskeletal pain and sports injuries.

Ibuleve Sports Gel
A proprietary, prescription-only preparation of the analgesic and antirheumatic drug ibuprofen. It is used as topical drug to treat rheumatic and musculoskeletal pain and sports injuries.

Ibumed
A proprietary, prescription-only preparation of the analgesic and antirheumatic drug ibuprofen. It is used to treat rheumatic and musculoskeletal pain and inflammation.

Ibuprofen
A proprietary, prescription-only analgesic and antirheumatic drug. It is used to treat rheumatic and musculoskeletal pain and inflammation.

Ibuspray
A proprietary, prescription-only preparation of the analgesic and antirheumatic drug ibuprofen. It is used as topical drug to treat rheumatic and musculoskeletal pain and inflammation.

Ichthammol
A proprietary, non- prescription preparation of bituminous oil. It is used for the topical treatment of ulcers and inflammation of the skin.

Idarubicin hydrochloride
A proprietary, prescription-only preparation cytotoxic drug. It can be used to treat acute leukaemia and breast cancer.

Idoxene
A proprietary, prescription-only preparation of the antiviral drug idoxuridine. It is used to treat local viral infection, particularly herpes simplex eye infections.

Idoxuridine
A proprietary, prescription-only antiviral drug. It is used to treat local viral infection, particularly herpes simplex eye infections.

Iduridin
A proprietary, prescription-only preparation of the antiviral drug idoxuridine. It is used to treat local viral infection, particularly herpes simplex eye infections.

Ifisfamide
A proprietary, prescription-only cytotoxic drug. It is used to treat some systemic cancers.

Ikorel
A preparation of microrandil. It is used to treat and prevent attacks of angina pectoris.

Ilosone
A proprietary, prescription-only preparation of the antibacterial and antibiotic drug erythromycin. It is used to treat and prevent many forms of infection.

Ilube
A proprietary, prescription-only preparation of acetylcysteine. It is used to treat some disorders of the lacrimal system.

Imbrilon
A proprietary, prescription-only preparation of indomethacin. It is used to treat the pain and inflammation of rheumatic disease and other musculoskeletal disorders.

Imigran
A proprietary, prescription-only preparation of sumatriptan. It is used to treat acute migraine attacks and cluster headache.

Imipramine hydrochloride
A proprietary, prescription-only antidepressant drug. It is used to treat depressive illness.

Imitrex
A proprietary, prescription-only preparation of sumatriptan. It is used for the treatment of symptoms of migraine.

Immukin
A proprietary, prescription-only preparation of interferon. It is used to treat serious infections in patients with chronic granulomatous disease.

Immunoprin
A proprietary, prescription-only preparation of azathioprine. It is used to treat a variety of autoimmune diseases and also tissue rejection in transplant patients.

Imodium Capsules
A proprietary, non-prescription preparation of loperamide. It is used for the symptomatic relief of acute diarrhea.

Imtack Spray
A proprietary, non-prescription preparation of isorbide dinitrate. It is used to treat and prevent angina pectoris.

Imunovir
A proprietary, prescription-only preparation of the antiviral drug inosine pranobex. It is used to treat herpes simplex infections.

Imuran
A proprietary, prescription-only preparation of azothioprine. It is used to treat a variety of autoimmune diseases and to treat tissue rejection in transplant patients.

Indapamide
A proprietary, prescription-only diuretic drug. It is used to treat raised blood pressure.

Fever
Pain
Infection

Ibuprofen

Properties
This medicine contains as active ingredient ibuprofen. It belongs to the group of medicines called non-steroidal anti-inflammatory drugs (NSAIDs). These drugs are taken by mouth to relieve some symptoms caused by arthritis or rheumatism, such as inflammation, swelling, stiffness, and joint pain. However, these medicines do not cure arthritis and will help you only as long as you continue to take them. Some of these medicines are also used to relieve other kinds of pain or to treat other painful conditions, such as gout attacks, bursitis, tendinitis, sprains, strains, menstrual cramps. The drug reduces the tissue concentration of prostaglandins (hormonal substances which produce inflammation and pain).

Before using this medicine
Before you use this medicine check with your doctor, or pharmacist:
- if you ever had any unusual or allergic reaction, such as skin rash, hives, or itching or breathing problems, to any of the anti-inflammatory analgesics.
- if you are on a low-salt, low-sugar, or any other special diet, or if you are allergic to any substance, such as sulfites or other preservatives or dyes.
- if you are pregnant or intending to become pregnant while using this medicine. Studies on birth defects have not been done in humans. However, if taken regularly during the last months of pregnancy, there is a chance that these medicines may cause unwanted effects on the heart or blood flow in the fetus or newborn infant.
- if you are breast-feeding an infant. Although this medicine has not been shown to cause problems in humans, it passes into the breast milk in small amounts.
- if you have any of the following medical problems:
  Asthma

Bleeding problems
Colitis
Stomach ulcer
Heart disease
Kidney or liver disease

Treatment
This medication is used to relieve pain or other symptoms caused by arthritis. For safe and effective use of this medicine, do not take more of it, do not take it more often, and do not take it for a longer period of time than ordered by your physician or directed by the package label.
If you are taking this medication on a regular schedule and you miss a dose, take the missed dose as soon as possible, unless it is almost time for your next dose. In that case do not take the missed dose at all.
To lessen stomach upset, anti-inflammatory analgesics may be taken with food or antacids.

Side effects
Along with the needed effects, a medicine may cause some unwanted effects. These side effects may go away during treatment as your body adjusts to the medicine. Such minor side effects are: dizziness; nausea; pain; headache; drowsiness; swollen feet, face or leg; constipation or diarrhea; vomiting; dry mouth.
Check with your doctor immediately if any of the following side effects occur:
- *Muscle cramps*
- *Numbness or tingling*
- *Mouth ulcers*
- *Convulsions or confusion*
- *Rash, hives, or itch*
- *Tightness in chest*

Interactions
This medicine may interact with several other drugs.
Be sure to tell your doctor about any medications you are currently taking.

Storage
The medicine should be stored at room temperature in a tightly closed, light-resistant container. Store away from heat and direct light. Keep out of reach of children.

Indaxa 25
A proprietary, prescription-only preparation of the diuretic drug indapamide. It is used to treat raised blood pressure.

Inderal
A preparation of the beta-blocker propranolol hydrochloride. It is used to treat raised blood pressure and to prevent and treat attacks of angina pectoris.

Inderal-LA
A proprietary, prescription-only preparation of the beta-blocker propranolol hydrochloride. It is used to treat raised blood pressure and to prevent and treat attacks of angina pectoris.

Inderetic
A proprietary, prescription-only preparation of the beta-blocker propranolol hydrochloride. It is used to treat raised blood pressure and to prevent and treat attacks of angina pectoris.

Inderex
A compound preparation of the beta-blocker propranolol hydrochloride and bendrofluaxide. It is used to treat raised blood pressure.

Indocid
A proprietary, prescription-only pre-

paration of the analgesic and antirheumatic drug indomethacin. It is used to treat the pain of rheumatic disease and other musculoskeletal disorders.

Indocid PDA
A proprietary, prescription-only preparation of indomethacin. It is used in some emergency situations of premature infants.

Indolar SR
A preparation of the analgesic and antirheumatic drug indomethacin. It is used to treat the pain of rheumatic disease and other musculoskeletal disorders.

Indomax
A proprietary, prescription-only preparation of the analgesic and antirheumatic drug indomethacin. It is used to treat the pain of rheumatic disease and other musculoskeletal disorders.

Indometacin
A proprietary, prescription-only analgesic and antirheumatic drug. It is used to treat the pain of rheumatic disease and other musculoskeletal disorders.

Indomethacin
A proprietary, prescription-only analgesic and antirheumatic drug. It is used to treat the pain of rheumatic disease and other musculoskeletal disorders.

Indomod
A proprietary, prescription-only preparation of the analgesic and antirheumatic drug indomethacin. It is used to treat the pain of rheumatic disease and other musculoskeletal disorders.

Indoramin
A proprietary, prescription-only adrenoreceptor drug. It is used to treat raised blood pressure.

Infacol
A proprietary, non-prescription preparation of dimethicone. It is used to relieve infant colic and griping pain.

Infant Gaviscon Liquid
A proprietary, non-prescription compound preparation of alginic acid, mannitol and silica. It is used for gastric reflux and regurgitation.

Initard 50/50
A proprietary, non-prescription preparation of biphasic, isophane insulin. It is used to treat and maintain diabetic patients.

Innohep
A proprietary, prescription-only preparation of tinzaparin. It is used to prevent venous thrombo-embolism.

Innovace
A proprietary, prescription-only preparation of enalapril maleate. It is used to treat high blood pressure and heart failure.

Innozide
A proprietary, prescription-only compound preparation of enalapril maleate and hydrochlorothiazide. It is used to treat raised blood pressure.

Inosine pranobex
A proprietary, prescription-only antiviral drug. It is used to treat herpes simplex infections.

Inositol nicotinate
A proprietary, prescription-only vasodilator drug. It is used to help improve blood circulation.

Inoven
A preparation of ibuprofen. It is used for the relief of headache, period pain, muscular pain, dental pain and feverishness.

Instillagel
A proprietary, non-prescription compound preparation of chlorhexidine and lignocaine. It is used to treat painful inflammation of the urethra.

Insulatard
A proprietary, prescription-only preparation of isophane insulin. It is used in diabetic therapy to treat and maintain diabetic patients.

Insulin
A protein hormone produced and se-

Insulin

Insulin is a protein hormone produced and secreted by the islets of Langerhans within the pancreas. It has the effect of reducing the level of glucose (blood sugar) in the bloodstream and is part of a balancing mechanism with the opposing hormone glucagon (which increases blood sugars).

Its deficiency (in the disorder called diabetes mellitus) results in high levels of blood sugar, which can rapidly lead to severe symptoms and potentially coma and death.

Patients suffering from diabetes can be divided into two groups, which largely determines the nature of their treatment. Those who have Type 1 diabetes (insulin-dependent diabetes) are generally maintained for life on one or other of the insulin preparations. Those who develop type 2 diabetes (non-insulin dependent diabetes) can usually be managed by treatment with oral hypoglycaemic drugs or by diet alone and less commonly require insulin injections.

Modern genetic engineering has enabled the production of quantities of the human form of insulin, which is now replacing the former insulins extracted from cows (bovine insulin).

There are marked differences in absorption time - which dictates both the rate of onset and duration of action - between insulin preparations. There are short-acting, intermediate-acting and long-acting preparations.

creted by the islets of Langerhans within the pancreas. It is used, in numerous preparation, in diabetic therapy to treat and maintain diabetic patients.

Insulin Zinc Suspension
A proprietary, prescription-only preparation of insulin zinc suspension. It is used in diabetic therapy to treat and maintain diabetic patients.

Intal
A proprietary, prescription-only preparation of sodium cromoglycate. It is used to treat and prevent asthmatic attacks.

Interferon
A protein produced in tiny quantities by cells infected by a virus. It is used to assist in the treatment of certain cancers.

Intralgin
A proprietary, non-prescription compound preparation of benzocaine and salicylamide. It can be applied to the skin for symptomatic relief of underlying muscle or joint pain.

Intraval Sodium
A proprietary, prescription-only preparation of thiopertone sodium. It can be used as general anesthetic drug.

Intron
A preparation of interferon. It is used to assist in the treatment of certain cancers.

Intropin
A proprietary, prescription-only preparation of dopamine hydrochloride. It is used to treat cardiogenic shock following a heart attack.

Ionamin
A proprietary, prescription-only preparation of phentermine. It is used to treat obesity.

Ionil T
A proprietary, non-prescription compound preparation of benzalkonium chloride and salicylic acid. It is used to treat dandruff and other scalp conditions.

Ipecac
A proprietary, non-prescription extract of the ipecac plant. It can be used to clear the stomach in certain cases of non-corrosive poisoning.

Ipecacuanha
A proprietary, non-prescription extract of the ipecac plant. It can be used to clear the stomach in certain cases of non-corrosive poisoning.

Ipecacuanha and Morphine
A proprietary, non-prescription extract of the ipecac plant combined with minute amounts of morphine. It can be used as an antitussive

Ipral
A proprietary, prescription-only preparation of the antibacterial and antibiotic drug trimethoprim. It can be used to treat infections of the upper respiratory tract.

Ipratropium bromide
A proprietary, prescription-only bronchodilator drug. It is used to treat chronic bronchitis.

Isclofen
A proprietary, prescription-only preparation of diclofenac sodium. It can be used to treat the pain and inflammation of arthritis and rheumatism.

Isisfen
A proprietary, prescription-only preparation of ibuprofen. It can be used to treat the pain and inflammation of arthritis and rheumatism.

Isisfen
A proprietary, prescription-only preparation of ibuprofen. It is used to relieve the pain of rheumatism and other musculoskeletal disorders.

Ismelin
A proprietary, prescription-only preparation of guanethidine monosulphate. It is used to treat raised blood pressure.

Ismo
A preparation of isosorbide mononitrate. It is used to treat and prevent attacks of angina pectoris.

Ismo Retard
A proprietary, non-prescription preparation of isosorbide mononitrate. It is used to treat and prevent attacks of angina pectoris.

Isocarboxazid
A proprietary, prescription-only antidepressant drug. It is used to treat depressive illness.

Isoconazole
A proprietary, prescription-only antifungal drug. It is used to treat fungal infections of the vagina.

Isoflurane
A proprietary, prescription-only general anesthetic drug. It is used for the induction and maintenance of general anesthesia.

Isogel
A proprietary, non-prescription preparation of ispagula husk. It is used to treat constipation

Isoket
A proprietary, prescription-only preparation of vasodilator drug isosorbide dinitrate. It is used in heart failure treatment.

Isoket Retard
A proprietary, prescription-only preparation of vasodilator drug isosorbide dinitrate. It is used in heart failure treatment.

Isometheptene mucate
A proprietary, prescription-only sympathicomimetic drug. It is used to treat acute migraine attacks.

Isomide CR
A proprietary, prescription-only preparation of disopyramide. It is used to regularize the heartbeat.

Isoniazid
A proprietary, prescription-only antibacterial drug. It is used to prevent the contraction of tuberculosis.

Isophane insulin
A proprietary, prescription-only purified form of bovine insulin. It is used to treat diabetes.

Isoprenaline
A proprietary, prescription-only synthetic sympathicomimetic substance similar to adrenaline. It is used to treat certain heart conditions.

Isopto Alkaline
A proprietary, non-prescription preparation of hypromellose. It is used to treat dryness of the eyes.

Isopto Atropine
A proprietary, prescription-only preparation of atropine sulphate. It is used to dilate the pupil for ophthalmologic procedures.

Isopto Carbachol
A proprietary, prescription-only preparation of carbachol. It is used to treat glaucoma.

Isopto Carpine
A proprietary, prescription-only preparation of pilocarpine. It can be used in glaucoma treatment.

Isopto Frin
A proprietary, non-prescription preparation of phenylephrine hydrochloride. It is used to treat tear deficiency.

Isopto Plain
A proprietary, non-prescription preparation of hypromellose. It is used to treat dryness of the eyes.

Isordil
A proprietary, prescription-only preparation of isorbide dinitrate. It can be used to treat and prevent attacks of angina pectoris.

Isordil Tembids
A proprietary, prescription-only preparation of isorbide dinitrate. It can be used to treat and prevent attacks of angina pectoris.

Isordide dinitrate
A proprietary, prescription-only vasodilator drug. It can be used to treat and prevent attacks of angina pectoris.

Isordide mononitrate
A proprietary, prescription-only vasodilator drug. It can be used to treat and prevent attacks of angina pectoris and heart failure conditions.

Isotrate
A proprietary, prescription-only preparation of the vasodilator drug isosorbide mononitrate. It can be used to treat and prevent attacks of angina pectoris and heart failure conditions.

Isotretinoin
A proprietary, non-prescription derivative of retinol. It is used to treat severe acne.

Isotrex
A proprietary, non-prescription preparation of isotretinoin, a derivative of retinol. It is used to treat severe acne.

Ispaghula husk
A proprietary, non-prescription bulking agent laxative. It can be used constipation treatment.

Isradipine
A proprietary, prescription-only calcium-channel blocker agent. It is used to treat raised blood pressure.

Istin
A proprietary, prescription-only preparation of the calcium-channel blocker agent amlodipoine. It is used to treat raised blood pressure.

Itraconazole
A proprietary, prescription-only broadspectrum antifungal drug. It can be used to treat resistant forms of candidiasis.

Ivermectin
A proprietary, prescription-only anthelminthic drug. It can be used to treat onchocerciasis disease.

J

Jackson's All Fours
A proprietary, non-prescription preparation of guaiphenesin. It can be used for the symptomatic relief of coughs.

Jackson's All Fours
A proprietary, non-prescription preparation of sodium salicylate. It can be used for the symptomatic relief of flu, sore throat, feverish colds and muscle pain.

J Collis Browne's Mixture
A proprietary, non-prescription compound preparation of anhydrous morphine and peppermint. It is used for the symptomatic relief of occasional diarrhea.

J Collis Browne's Tablets
A proprietary, non-prescription compound preparation of anhydrous morphine, kaolin and calcium carbonate. It is used for the symptomatic relief of occasional diarrhea.

Japps Health Salts
A proprietary, non-prescription compound preparation of bicarbonate and sodium potassium tartrate. It is used to treat heartburn and indigestion.

Jexin
A proprietary, prescription-only preparation of tubocurarine chloride. It is used to induce muscle paralysis during surgery.

Joy-Rides
A proprietary, non-prescription preparation of hyoscine hydrobromide. It is used to treat nausea and motion sickness.

Junifen
A proprietary, prescription-only preparation of ibuprofen. It is used to relieve pain such as earache, sore throats, minor aches and sprains.

K

Kabiglobulin
A proprietary, prescription-only preparation of human normal immunoglobulin. It is used in immunization to confer immediate passive immunity to infection by viruses.

Kabikinase
A proprietary, prescription-only preparation of streptokinase. It is used to treat thrombosis and embolism.

Kalspare
A proprietary, prescription-only preparation of the diuretic drug chlorthalidone. It is used to treat raised blood pressure.

Kalten
A proprietary, prescription-only compound preparation of atenolol and hydrochlorothiazide. It is used to treat raised blood pressure.

Kamillosan
A proprietary, non-prescription preparation of arachis oil and liquid paraffin. It is used to treat and sooth nappy rash.

Kanamycin
A proprietary, prescription-only antibiotic and antibacterial drug. It is used to treat serious infections caused by Gram-negative bacteria.

Kannasyn
A proprietary, prescription-only preparation of the antibiotic and antibacterial drug kanamycin. It is used to treat serious infections caused by Gram-negative bacteria.

Kaodene
A proprietary, non-prescription preparation of kaolin and codeine phosphate. It is used to treat diarrhea.

Kaolin
A proprietary, non-prescription preparation of white clay. It is used to treat diarrhea.

Kaolin and Morphine Mixture
A proprietary, non-prescription preparation of kaolin and morphine. It is used to treat diarrhea.

Kaopectate
A proprietary, non-prescription preparation of kaolin (white clay). It is used to treat diarrhea.

Karvol Decongestant Capsules
A proprietary, non-prescription compound preparation of menthol, chlorbutol and thymol. It is used for the symptomatic relief of colds.

Kefadim
A proprietary, prescription-only preparation of the antibacterial and antibiotic drug ceftazidine. It is used to treat many infections.

Kefadol
A proprietary, prescription-only preparation of the antibacterial and antibiotic drug cephamandole. It is used to treat many infections.

Keflex
A proprietary, prescription-only preparation of the antibacterial and antibiotic drug cephalexin. It is used to treat many infections.

Kefzol
A proprietary, prescription-only preparation of the antibacterial and antibiotic drug cephazolin. It is used to treat many infections.

Kelfizine
A proprietary, prescription-only preparation of the sulpha-drug sulfametopyrazine. It is used to treat chronic bronchitis and infections of the urinary tract.

Kelocyanor
A proprietary, prescription-only preparation of dicobalt edeate. It is used as an antidote to acute cyanide poisoning.

Kemadrin
A proprietary, prescription-only preparation of procyclidine hydrochloride. It is used to treat the symptoms of parkinsonism.

Kemicetine
A proprietary, prescription-only preparation of the antibacterial and antibiotic drug chloramphenicol. It is used to treat life-threatening infections.

Kenalog
A proprietary, prescription-only preparation of the corticosteroid drug triamcinolone acetonide. It is used to treat inflammation and allergic conditions.

Kenalog Intracapsular
A proprietary, prescription-only preparation of the corticosteroid drug triamcinolone acetonide. It is used to treat inflammation of the joints and soft tissues.

Kenalog Intramuscular
A proprietary, prescription-only preparation of the corticosteroid drug triamcinolone acetonide. It is used to treat inflammation of the joints and soft tissues.

Keri
A proprietary, non-prescription compound preparation of liquid paraffin and lanolin oil. It is used as an emollient to soften dry skin.

Kerlone
A proprietary, prescription-only preparation of the beta-blocker drug betaxolol hydrochloride. It is used to treat raised blood pressure and to prevent and treat attacks of angina pectoris.

Ketalar
A proprietary, prescription-only preparation of the general anesthetic drug ketamine. It is used for the induction and maintenance of general anesthesia.

Ketamine
A proprietary, prescription-only general anesthetic. It is used for the induction and maintenance of general anesthesia.

Ketoconazole
A proprietary, prescription-only antifungal drug. It is used to treat deep-seated, serious fungal infections.

Ketoprofen

A proprietary, prescription-only analgesic and antirheumatic drug. It can be used to treat rheumatic and muscular pain caused by inflammation, acute gout and period pain.

Ketoprofen CR

A proprietary, prescription-only analgesic and antirheumatic drug. It can be used to treat rheumatic and muscular pain caused by inflammation, acute gout and period pain.

Ketorolac Trometamol

A proprietary, prescription-only preparation of ketoprofen. It is used to relieve pain of arthritis and rheumatism.

Ketotifen

A proprietary, prescription-only preparation of sodium cromoglycate. It is used to treat and prevent attacks of asthma.

Ketovail

A proprietary, prescription-only preparation of ketoprofen. It is used to relieve pain of arthritis and rheumatism.

Kinidin Durules

A proprietary, prescription-only preparation of quinidine. It is used to treat and prevent irregularities of the heartbeat.

Klaricid

A proprietary, prescription-only preparation of the antibacterial and antibiotic drug clarithromycin. It is used to treat and prevent many forms of infection.

Klean-Prep

A proprietary, non-prescription compound preparation of macrogol with sodium and potassium salts. It is used as a bowel-cleansing solution.

KLN Suspension

A proprietary, non-prescription-only preparation of kaolin, peppermint oil and sodium citrate. It is used to treat diarrhea in children.

Kogenate

A proprietary, prescription-only preparation of dried human factor VIII. It is used to reduce or stop bleeding.

Kolanticon Gel

A proprietary, non-prescription preparation of aluminium hydroxide, magnesium oxide and dicyclomine hydrochloride. It is used to treat gastrointestinal spasm, hyperacidity, flatulence and the symptoms of peptic ulcer.

Konakion

A proprietary, prescription-only preparation of vitamin K1. It is used to treat deficiency of vitamin K.

Kwells Junior

A proprietary, non-prescription preparation of hyoscine hydrobromide. It is used to treat nausea and motion sickness.

Kwells Tablets

A proprietary, non-prescription preparation of hyoscine hydrobromide. It is used to treat nausea and motion sickness.

Kytril

A proprietary, prescription-only preparation of granisetron. It is used to give relief from nausea and vomiting.

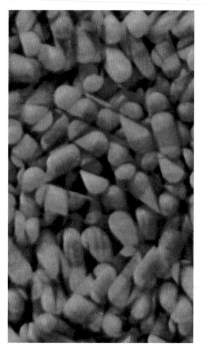

L

Labetalol

A proprietary, prescription-only beta-blocker drug. It can be used to treat raised blood pressure.

Labophylline

A proprietary, prescription-only preparation of theophylline. It can be used to treat asthma and chronic bronchitis.

Labosept Pastilles

A proprietary, non-prescription preparation of the antiseptic agent dequalinium chloride. It can be used to treat sore throats.

Lacidipine

A proprietary, prescription-only calcium-channel blocker drug. It can be used to treat raised blood pressure.

Lacri-Lube

A proprietary, non-prescription preparation of liquid paraffin and white soft paraffin. It can be used as an eye lubricant.

Lacticare

A proprietary, non-prescription compound preparation of sodium pyrrolidine carboxylate and lactic acid. It can be used as en emollient for dry skin conditions.

Lactilol

A proprietary, non-prescription osmotic laxative. It can be used to treat constipation.

Lactugal

A proprietary, non-prescription preparation of lactulose. It can be used to treat constipation.

Lactulose

A proprietary, non-prescription laxative preparation. It can be used to treat constipation.

Ladropen

A proprietary, prescription-only preparation of the antibacterial and antibiotic drug flucloxacillin. It can be used to treat staphylococcal infections.

Lamictal
A proprietary, prescription-only preparation of lamotrigine. It can be used to treat seizures.

Lamistil
A proprietary, prescription-only preparation of the antifungal drug terbinafine. It can be used to treat fungal infections of the nails and ringworm.

Lamotrigine
A proprietary, prescription-only anticonvulsant drug. It can be used to treat various types of seizures.

Lamprene
A proprietary, prescription-only preparation of the antibacterial and antibiotic drug clofazimine. It can be used to treat leprosy.

Lanolin
A non-proprietary constituent of wool fat and is incorporated in several emollient preparations.

Lanoxin
A proprietary, prescription-only preparation of digoxin. It can be used to treat heart failure conditions and to regularize heartbeat.

Lanoxin-PG
A proprietary, prescription-only preparation of digoxin. It can be used to treat heart failure conditions and to regularize heartbeat.

Lanzoprazole
A proprietary, prescription-only ulcer-healing drug. It can be used to treat gastric and duodenal ulcers.

Lanvis
A proprietary, prescription-only preparation of the cytotoxic drug thioguanine. It can be used to treat leukaemia.

Laractone
A proprietary, prescription-only preparation of the diuretic drug spironolactone. It can be used to treat oedema.

Laxatives

These medicines promote defecation and so relieve constipation. They can be divided into several different types of natural and synthetic types.

- The *faecal softener laxatives*, for instance, liquid paraffin, soften the faeces for easier evacuation.

- The *bulking agent laxatives* increase the overall volume of the faeces, which then stimulates bowel movement. Bulking agents are normally some form of fiber, for instance bran, ispaghula, methylcellulose and stergulia.

- The stimulant laxatives act on the intestinal muscles to increase motility.
  Many traditional remedies for constipation are stimulants, such as cascara, castor oil, figs elixir and senna. However, there are modern variants with less of a stimulant action and which also have other properties, for instance:
  - Bisacodyl;
  - Danthron;
  - Docussate sodium.

- Finally, the osmotic laxatives, which are chemical salts that work by retaining water in the intestine so increasing overall liquidity, for instance:
  - lactulose;
  - magnesium hydroxide;
  - magnesium sulphate.

Larafen CR
A proprietary, prescription-only preparation of ketoprofen. It can be used to relieve pain, particularly rheumatic and arthritic pain and to treat other musculoskeletal disorders.

Laraflex
A proprietary, prescription-only preparation of naproxen. It can be used to relieve pain, particularly rheumatic and arthritic pain and to treat other musculoskeletal disorders.

Larapam
A proprietary, prescription-only preparation of piroxicam. It can be used to relieve pain, particularly rheumatic and arthritic pain and to treat other musculoskeletal disorders.

Laratrim
A proprietary, prescription-only preparation of the antibacterial and antibiotic drug trimethoprim. It can be used to treat bacterial infections, particularly infections of the urinary tract.

Largactil
A proprietary, prescription-only preparation of the antipsychotic drug chlorpromazine hydrochloride. It can be used to treat patients with behavioral disturbances.

Lariam
A proprietary, prescription-only preparation of mefloquine. It can be used to treat and prevent malaria.

Larodopa
A proprietary, prescription-only preparation of larodopa. It can be used to treat symptoms of parkinsonism.

Lasikal
A proprietary, prescription-only compound preparation of frusemide and

potassium chloride. It can be used to treat oedema.

Lasilaktone

A proprietary, prescription-only preparation of spironolactone and frusemide. It can be used to treat resistant oedema.

Lasix

A proprietary, prescription-only preparation of the diuretic drug frusemide. It can be used to treat oedema, associated with lung or heart conditions.

Lasix+K

A proprietary, prescription-only compound preparation of the diuretic drug frusemide and potassium chloride. It can be used to treat oedema, associated with lung or heart conditions.

Lasix Paediatric Liquid

A proprietary, prescription-only compound preparation of the diuretic drug frusemide and potassium chloride. It can be used to treat oedema.

Lasma

A proprietary, prescription-only preparation of theophylline. It can be used to treat and prevent asthma and chronic bronchitis.

Lasonil

A proprietary, non-prescription compound preparation of heparinoids and hyaluronidase. It can be used to improve circulation in the skin.

Lasoride

A proprietary, prescription-only preparation of the diuretic drugs frusemide and amiloride hydrochloride. It can be used to treat oedema.

Laxoberol

A proprietary, non-prescription preparation of the laxative drug picosulphate. It can be used to treat constipation.

Laxose

A proprietary, non-prescription preparation of the laxative drug lactulose. It can be used to treat constipation.

Ledercort

A proprietary, prescription-only preparation of the corticosteroid drug triamcinolone. It can be used to treat severe infections and allergic conditions of the skin.

Lederfen

A proprietary, prescription-only preparation of fenbufen. It can be used to treat rheumatic and arthritic pain.

Ledermycin

A proprietary, prescription-only preparation of the antibacterial and antibiotic drug demeclocycline hydrochloride. It can be used to treat a wide range of infections.

Lederspan

A proprietary, prescription-only preparation of the corticosteroid drug triamcinolone. It can be used to treat severe infections of the joints and the soft tissues.

Lemsip

A proprietary, non-prescription compound preparation of paracetamol, phenylephrine, sodium citrate and vitamin C. It can be used for the relief of cold and flu symptoms.

Lenium

A proprietary, non-prescription preparation of selenium. It can be used to treat dandruff.

Lentard MC

A proprietary, prescription-only preparation of insulin zinc suspension. It can be used to treat diabetes.

Lentaron

A proprietary, prescription-only preparation of formestane. It can be used to treat advanced stages of breast cancer.

Lentizol

A proprietary, prescription-only preparation of the antidepressant drug amitriptyline hydrochloride. It can be used to treat depressive illness.

Lescol

A proprietary, prescription-only preparation of chlorambucil. It can

be used to treat various forms of cancer and rheumatoid arthritis.

Leuprorelin acetate

A proprietary, prescription-only analogue of gonadorelin. It can be used to treat endometriosis and is also used as anticancer drug.

Levamisole

A proprietary, prescription-only anthelminthic drug. It can be used to treat roundworm infections.

Levobunolol hydrochloride

A proprietary, prescription-only beta-blocker drug. It can be used to treat chronic simple glaucoma.

Levodopa

A neurotransmitter present in the central and peripheral nervous system. It can be used to treat the symptoms of parkinsonism.

Levonorgestrel

A proprietary, prescription-only progestogen. It can be used to as oral contraceptive and in hormone replacement treatment.

Levophed

A proprietary, prescription-only preparation of noradrenaline. It can be used in emergencies to raise the blood pressure.

Lexotan

A proprietary, prescription-only preparation of the benzodiazepine drug bromazepam. It can be used to treat anxiety syndromes.

Lexpec

A proprietary, prescription-only preparation of folic acid. It can be used as a vitamin supplement, for example, during pregnancy.

Lexpec with Iron

A proprietary, prescription-only combined preparation of folic acid and an iron salt. It can be used as a vitamin supplement, for example, during pregnancy.

Lexpec with Iron-M

A proprietary, prescription-only combined preparation of folic acid and

Lignocaine

Properties
This medicine contains as active ingredient lidocaine. It belongs to a group of medicines known as topical local anesthetics. These drugs are used to relieve the pain, itching, and redness of minor skin disorders, including sunburn or other minor burns, insect bites or stings, poison ivy, poison oak, and minor cuts and scratches.
These drugs function by deadening the nerve endings in the skin. They do not cause drowsiness or disorders of consciousness as general anesthetics for surgery do.

Before using this medicine
Before you use this medicine check with your doctor, or pharmacist:
-   if you ever had any unusual or allergic reaction to this medicine or to a local anesthetic, especially when applied to the skin.
-   if you are allergic to any substance, such as para-aminobenzoic acid, parabens, paraphenylenediamine, sulfites or other preservatives or dyes.
-   if you are pregnant or intending to become pregnant while using this medicine. Although local anesthetics have not been shown to cause problems in humans, the chance always exists.
-   if you are breast-feeding an infant. Although this medicine has not been shown to cause problems in humans, it may pass into the breast milk in small amounts.
-   if you have any of the following medical problems:
    Infection at or near the place of
    application
    Large sores
    Broken skin
    Severe injury at area of application

Treatment
This medication is used to relieve the pain, itching, and redness of minor skin disorders. For safe and effective use of this medicine follow your doctor's instructions. Unless otherwise stated by your doctor or pharmacist, do not use this medicine on large areas, especially if the skin is broken or scraped. Also, do not use it more often than directed on the package label, or for more than a few days at a time. To do so may increase the chance of absorption through the skin and the chance of unwanted effects. If you are using this medicine on your face, be very careful not to get it in your eyes. If you are using an aerosol or spray form of this medicine, spray it on your hand or an applicator before applying it to your face.

Side effects
Along with the needed effects, a medicine may cause some unwanted effects. These side effects may go away during treatment as your body adjusts to the medicine. Such minor side effects are: burning, stinging, tenderness not present before treatment; skin rash, redness, itching or hives.
Signs of too much medicine being absorbed by the body are the following (! discontinue use of the drug and check with your doctor immediately):
-   *Blurred vision*
-   *Double vision*
-   *Dizziness*
-   *Drowsiness*
-   *Convulsions (seizures)*
-   *Ringing in the ears*
-   *Shivering or trembling*
-   *Unusual excitement*
-   *Unusual increase in sweating*
-   *Unusually irregular heartbeat*

Interactions
This medicine may interact with several other drugs such as antimyasthanics, long-acting eye drops or for glaucoma, sulfonamides.
Be sure to tell your doctor about any medications you are currently taking.

Storage
Store away from heat and direct light. Keep out of reach of children. Keep the medicine from freezing. Do not keep outdated medicine or medicine no longer needed.

ferric ammonium citrate. It can be used as a vitamin supplement, for example, during pregnancy.

Libanil
A proprietary, prescription-only preparation of glibenclamide. It can be used to treat Type II diabetes.

Librium
A proprietary, prescription-only preparation of the benzodiazepine drug chlordiazepoxide. It can be used in the treatment of anxiety and acute alcohol withdrawal symptoms.

Librofen
A proprietary, prescription-only preparation of ibuprofen. It can be used for the relief of period pain and also for headache, muscular pain and feverishness.

Lidifen
A proprietary, prescription-only preparation of ibuprofen. It can be used for the relief of rheumatic pain, period pain and also for headache, muscular pain and feverishness.

Lignocaine
A proprietary, prescription-only preparation of the local anesthetic drug lignocaine hydrochloride. It can be

used to treat irregularities of the heartbeat.

Lignocaine hydrochloride

A proprietary, prescription-only anesthetic drug. It can be used to treat irregularities of the heartbeat.

Li-Liquid

A proprietary, prescription-only preparation of the antipsychotic drug lithium. It can be used to prevent and treat mania, manic-depressive bouts and recurrent depression.

Limclair

A preparation of trisodium edeate. It can be used to treat the symptoms of hypercalcaemia.

Lindane

A proprietary, non-prescription pediculicidal drug. It can be used to treat infestation by itch-mites (scabies).

Lingraine

A proprietary, prescription-only preparation of ergotamine tartrate. It can be used to treat acute attacks of migraine.

Lioresal

A proprietary, prescription-only preparation of baclofen. It can be used to treat muscle spasm caused by injury or disease of the central nervous system.

Liothyronine sodium

A proprietary, prescription-only form of the natural thyroid hormone iodothyronine. It can be used to make up a hormonal deficiency.

Lipantil

A proprietary, prescription-only preparation of fenofibrate. It can be used to reduce lipid levels in the bloodstream.

Lipostat

A proprietary, prescription-only preparation of pravastatin. It can be used to reduce lipid levels in the bloodstream.

Liquid paraffin

A non-prescription laxative drug. It can be used to treat constipation.

Liquorice

A non-prescription preparation of polyvinyl alcohol. It can be used to treat dryness of the eyes.

Lisinopril

A proprietary, prescription-only ACE inhibitor. It can be used to treat raised blood pressure.

Liskonium

A proprietary, prescription-only preparation of lithium. It can be used to treat mania, manic-depressive bouts and recurrent depression.

Lithium

A prescription-only preparation antipsychotic drug. It can be used to treat mania, manic-depressive bouts and recurrent depression.

Livial

A preparation of tibolone. It can be used to treat hormone replacement therapy.

Lloyd's Cream

A proprietary, non-prescription preparation of diethylamine salicylate. It can be used to the skin to treat for symptomatic relief of underlying muscle or joint pain.

Lobak

A proprietary, prescription-only compound preparation of chlormezanone and paracetamol. It can be used for the relief of muscle pain.

Locabiotal

A proprietary, prescription-only preparation of the antibacterial and antibiotic drug fusafungine. It can be used to treat infection and inflammation in the nose and throat.

Loceryl

A proprietary, prescription-only preparation of the antifungal drug amorolfine. It can be used to treat fungal skin infections.

Locoid

A proprietary, prescription-only preparation of the corticosteroid drug hydrocortisone. It can be used to treat serious inflammatory skin conditions, such as eczema and psoriasis.

Locoid C

A proprietary, prescription-only compound preparation of the corticosteroid drug hydrocortisone and chloroquinaldol. It can be used to treat serious inflammatory skin conditions, such as eczema and psoriasis.

Lococorten-Vioform

A proprietary, prescription-only compound preparation of the corticosteroid drug flumethasone and clioquinol. It can be used to treat mild inflammatory conditions of the middle ear.

Lodine

A proprietary, prescription-only preparation of etodolac. It can be used to treat the pain of osteoarthritis and rheumatoid arthritis.

Loestrin 20

A proprietary, prescription-only compound preparation of an estrogen and progestogen. It can be used as oral contraceptive and to treat some menstrual problems.

Loestrin 30

A proprietary, prescription-only compound preparation of an estrogen and progestogen. It can be used as oral contraceptive and to treat some menstrual problems.

Lofepramine

A proprietary, prescription-only antidepressant drug. It can be used to treat depressive illness.

Lofexidine hydrochloride

A proprietary, prescription-only drug that is used to alleviate opioid withdrawal symptoms.

Logynon

A proprietary, prescription-only compound preparation of an estrogen and progestogen. It can be used as oral contraceptive and to treat some menstrual problems.

Logynon ED

A proprietary, prescription-only compound preparation of an estrogen and progestogen. It can be used as oral contraceptive and to treat some menstrual problems.

Lomotil
A proprietary, prescription-only compound preparation of atropine sulphate and diphenoxylate hydrochloride. It can be used to treat chronic diarrhea.

Lomustine
A proprietary, prescription-only cytotoxic drug that is used to treat Hodgkin's disease.

Loniten
A preparation of minoxidil. It can be used to treat severe acute hypertension.

Loperamide hydrochloride
A proprietary, prescription-only antidiarrheal drug. It can be used to treat diarrhea.

Lopid
A proprietary, prescription-only preparation of gemfibrozil. It can be used to reduce high levels of lipids in the bloodstream.

Lopidine
A proprietary, prescription-only preparation of apraclonidine. It can be used to treat intraocular pressure.

Loprazolam
A proprietary, prescription-only benzodiazepine drug. It can be used to treat insomnia.

Lopresor
A proprietary, prescription-only preparation of the beta-blocker drug metoprolol tartrate. It can be used to treat raised blood pressure and to prevent and treat attacks of angina pectoris.

Lopresor SR
A proprietary, prescription-only preparation of the beta-blocker drug metoprolol tartrate. It can be used to treat raised blood pressure and to prevent and treat attacks of angina pectoris.

Loratadine
A proprietary, prescription-only antihistamine drug. It can be used for the symptomatic relief of allergic symptoms.

Lorazepam
A proprietary, prescription-only benzodiazepine drug. It can be used to treat insomnia and epilepsy.

Loron
A proprietary, prescription-only preparation of sodium chlodronate. It can be used to treat high calcium levels in the bloodstream.

Losec
A proprietary, prescription-only preparation of omeprazole. It can be used as an ulcer-healing drug.

Lotriderm
A proprietary, prescription-only compound preparation of betamethasone and clotrimazole. It can be used to treat fungal infections.

Loxapac
A proprietary, prescription-only preparation of the antipsychotic drug loxapine. It can be used to treat acute and chronic psychoses.

Luborant
A proprietary, non-prescription compound preparation of carmellose sodium, sorbitol, potassium chloride and other salts. It can be used to treat dry mouth.

Lubrifilm
A proprietary, non-prescription compound preparation of liquid paraffin, yellow soft paraffin and wool fat. It can be used as an eye lubricant.

Ludiomil
A proprietary, prescription-only preparation of maprotiline. It can be used to treat depressive illness.

Lunesta
A proprietary, prescription-only preparation of eszopiclone. It is used for the treatment of insomnia.

Lurselle
A proprietary, prescription-only preparation of probucol. It can be used to reduce high levels of lipids in the bloodstream.

Lustral
A proprietary, prescription-only preparation of sertraline. It can be used to treat depressive illness.

Lymecycline
A proprietary, prescription-only antibacterial and antibiotic drug. It can be used to treat infections of many kinds.

Lypressin
A proprietary, prescription-only analogue of vasopressin. It can be used to treat diabetes insipidus.

Lysuride maleate
A proprietary, prescription-only preparation of ergo-alkaloids. It can be used to treat symptoms of parkinsonism.

Lipid-lowering drugs

These medicines are used in clinical conditions of hyperlipidaemia, when the blood plasma contains very high levels of the lipids cholesterol and/or triglycerides (natural fats of the body).

Current medical opinion suggests that if diet, or drugs, can be used to lower levels of LDL-cholesterol (low-density lipoprotein) while raising HDL-cholesterol (high-density lipoprotein), then there may be a regression of the progress of coronary atherosclerosis (a diseased state of the arteries of the heart when plaques of lipid material narrow blood vessels, which contributes to angina pectoris attacks and the formation of abnormal clots that can go on to cause heart attacks and stroke).

Currently, lipid-lowering drugs are generally only used when there is a family history of hyperlipidaemia, or clinical signs indicating the need for intervention. In most individuals, an appropriate low-fat diet can adequately do what is required.

M

Maalox Plus Suspension

A proprietary, non-prescription compound preparation of magnesium hydroxide, aluminium hydroxide and dimethicone. It can be used for the symptomatic relief of dyspepsia, heartburn and flatulence.

Maalox Plus Tablets

A proprietary, non-prescription compound preparation of magnesium hydroxide and aluminium hydroxide. It can be used for the symptomatic relief of dyspepsia, heartburn and flatulence.

Maalox TC Suspension

A proprietary, non-prescription compound preparation of magnesium hydroxide and aluminium hydroxide. It can be used for the symptomatic relief of dyspepsia, heartburn and flatulence.

Maclean Indigestion Tablets

A proprietary, non-prescription compound preparation of magnesium carbonate, aluminium hydroxide and calcium carbonate. It can be used for the symptomatic relief of dyspepsia, nausea, heartburn and flatulence.

Macrobid

A proprietary, prescription-only preparation of the antibacterial drug nitrofurantoin. It can be used to treat infections of the urinary tract.

Macrodantin

A proprietary, prescription-only preparation of the antibacterial drug nitrofurantoin. It can be used to treat infections of the urinary tract.

Madopar

A proprietary, prescription-only compound preparation of levodopa and benserazide hydrochloride. It can be used to treat the symptoms of parkinsonism.

Magaldrate

A proprietary, non-prescription compound preparation of aluminium hydroxide and magnesium hydroxide. It can be used to treat severe dyspepsia.

Magnapen

A proprietary, prescription-only compound preparation of ampicillin and flucloxacillin. It can be used to treat severe infection.

Magnatol

A proprietary, non-prescription preparation of potassium bicarbonate, magnesium carbonate and alexitol sodium. It can be used for the symptomatic relief of heartburn.

Magnesium carbonate

An antacid that also has laxative properties. It is used for the relief of hyperacidity, dyspepsia, heartburn and peptic ulcer.

Magnesium chloride

The chemical form of magnesium that is most commonly used to make up a magnesium deficiency.

Magnesium hydroxide

An antacid that also has laxative properties. It is used for the relief of hyperacidity, dyspepsia, heartburn and peptic ulcer.

Magnesium sulphate

An osmotic laxative drug. It is used for the relief of constipation.

Magnesium trisilicate

An antacid with a long duration of action. It is used for the relief of hyperacidity, dyspepsia, heartburn and peptic ulcer.

Malix

A proprietary, prescription-only preparation of glibenclamide. It can be used to treat Type II diabetes.

Maloprim

A proprietary, prescription-only compound preparation of antibacterial and antibiotic drug dapsone and pyrimethamine. It can be used to prevent malaria.

Manerix

A proprietary, prescription-only preparation of moclobemide. It can be used to treat major depressive illness.

Manevax

A proprietary, prescription-only compound preparation of ipaghula husk and senna. It can be used to treat a number of gastrointestinal disorders.

Mannitol

A proprietary, prescription-only osmotic diuretic drug. It can be used to treat oedema.

Maprotiline hydrochloride

A proprietary, prescription-only preparation of antidepressive drug. It can be used to treat depressive illness.

Marcain

A proprietary, prescription-only preparation of the local anesthetic drug bupivacaine hydrochloride. It can be used in long-term treatment.

Marcain with Adrenaline

A proprietary, prescription-only preparation of the local anesthetic drug bupivacaine hydrochloride and the vasoconstrictor drug adrenaline. It can be used in long-term treatment.

Marevan

A proprietary, prescription-only preparation of warfarin sodium. It can be used to prevent blood clot formation.

Marplan

A proprietary, prescription-only preparation of the antidepressant drug isocarboxazid. It can be used to treat depressive illness.

Marvelon

A proprietary, prescription-only hormonal preparation of estrogen and progestogen. It can be used as oral contraceptive and for certain menstrual disorders.

Masnoderm

A proprietary, prescription-only preparation of the antifungal; drug clotrimazole. It can be used to treat fungal skin infections.

Massé Breast Cream

A proprietary, non-prescription compound preparation of arachis oil, wool fat, glycerol and glyceryl mono-

Maalox

Properties
This medicine contains as active ingredient a neutralizing agent for excess stomach acid and is therefore called an antacid. Antacids are taken by mouth to relieve heartburn, sour stomach, or acid indigestion. Antacids alone or in combination with simethicone may be used to treat the symptoms of stomach or duodenal ulcers. This medication contains as active ingredients alumina and magnesia.

Before using this medicine
Before you use this medicine check with your doctor, or pharmacist:
- if you ever had any unusual or allergic reaction to aluminum-, calcium-, magnesium-, sodium bicarbonate-, or simethicone containing medicines;
- if you are on a low-salt, low-sugar, or any other special diet, or if you are allergic to any substance, such as sulfites or other preservatives or dyes.
- if you are pregnant or intending to become pregnant while using this medicine. Although antacids have not been shown to cause problems in humans, the chance always exists.
- if you are breast-feeding an infant.
- if you have any of the following medical problems:
  Appendicitis (or signs of)
  Bone fractures
  Colitis or colostomy
  Constipation or diarrhea
  Heart disease
  High blood pressure
  Intestinal blockage
  Kidney or liver disease
  Toxaemia of pregnancy
  Underactive parathyroids

Treatment
This medication is used to relieve or prevent the symptoms of your medical problem. Take them as directed. Do not take more of them and do not take them more often than recommended on the label, unless otherwise directed by your doctor. To do so may increase the chance of side effects.
When taking this medicine for a stomach or duodenal ulcer, take it exactly as ordered by your doctor to obtain maximum relief of your symptoms.
Antacids should not be given to young children (up to 6 years of age) unless prescribed by their doctor.

Side effects
Along with the needed effects, a medicine may cause some unwanted effects. Although the following side effects occur very rarely when this medicine is taken as recommended, they may be more likely to occur if:
- too much medicine is taken;
- it is taken in large doses;
- it is taken for a long period of time;
- it is taken by patients with kidney disease.
Check with your doctor as soon as possible if any of the following side effects or signs of overdose occur: constipation; cramping; difficult or painful urination; headache; loss of appetite; mood or mental changes; muscle pain or twitching; nausea or vomiting; stomach pain; unpleasant taste in mouth; unusual slow breathing; unusual tiredness or weakness.

Interactions
This medicine may interact with several other drugs such as adrenocorticosteroids, cellulose sodium phosphate, mecamylamine, and tetracyclines.
Be sure to tell your doctor about any medications you are currently taking.

Storage
Tablets, elixir, etc. should be stored at room temperature; store away from heat and direct light. Keep out of reach of children, since overdose may be very dangerous in children.

---

sterate. It can be used as emollient for sore nipples.

Matrex
A proprietary, prescription-only preparation of the cytotoxic drug methotrexate. It can be used to treat lymphoblastic leukaemia, lymphomas and rheumatoid arthritis.

Maxepa
A proprietary, prescription-only preparation of omega-3 marine triglycerides. It can be used to reduce high lipid levels in the bloodstream.

Maximum Strength Aspro Clear
A proprietary, non-prescription preparation of aspirin. It can be used to relieve pain, including headache, neuralgia, period and dental pain.

Maxitrol
A proprietary, prescription-only compound preparation of the corticosteroid dexamethasone, polymyxin B and neomycin sulphate. It can be used to treat inflammation of the eye.

Maxivent
A proprietary, prescription-only pre-paration of salbutamol. It can be used to treat asthmatic attacks and to alleviate symptoms of chronic bronchitis.

MCR-50
A proprietary, prescription-only preparation of isosorbide mononitrate. It can be used to treat and prevent attacks of angina pectoris and in heart failure treatment.

Mebendazole
A proprietary, prescription-only anthelminthic drug. It can be used to

treat infections by roundworm, threadworm, whipworm and hookworm.

Mebeverine hydrochloride

A proprietary, prescription-only antispasmodic drug. It can be used to treat muscle spasm in the gastrointestinal tract.

Meclozine hydrochloride

A proprietary, prescription-only antihistamine drug. It can be used to treat or prevent motion sickness.

Mectizan

A proprietary, prescription-only preparation of ivermectin. It can be used to treat onchocerciasis.

Mediclair 5/10 Acne Cream

A proprietary, non-prescription preparation of the keratolytic and antimicrobial drug benzoyl peroxide. It can be used to treat acne.

Mediclair Acne Lotion

A proprietary, non-prescription preparation of the keratolytic and antimicrobial drug benzoyl peroxide. It can be used to treat acne.

Medicoal

A proprietary, non-prescription preparation of activated charcoal. It can be used to treat patients suffering from poisoning or a drug overdose.

Medihaler-Epi

A proprietary, prescription-only preparation of the sympathicomimetic drug adrenaline acid tartrate. It can be used to treat acute and severe allergic reactions.

Medihaler-Ergotamine

A proprietary, prescription-only preparation of the vasoconstrictor drug ergotamine tartrate. It can be used to treat attacks of migraine.

Medihaler-Iso

A proprietary, prescription-only preparation of the beta-receptor stimulant isoprenaline. It can be used to treat severe acute asthma.

Medilave

A proprietary, non-prescription compound preparation of cetylpyridinium chloride and benzocaine. It can be used to relieve pain of sores and ulcers in the mouth.

Medised

A proprietary, non-prescription compound preparation of paracetamol and promethazine hydrochloride. It can be used to treat pain and feverish conditions.

Medrone

A proprietary, prescription-only preparation of the corticosteroid methylprednisolone. It can be used to treat allergic disorders, shock and cerebral oedema.

Medroxyprogesterone acetate

An female sex hormone, a synthetic progestogen. It can be used as constituent of oral contraceptive drugs and as hormonal supplement.

Mefenamic acid

A proprietary, prescription-only analgesic and antirheumatic drug. It can be used to treat mild to moderate pain and inflammation in rheumatoid arthritis.

Mefloquine

A proprietary, prescription-only antimalarian drug. It can be used to treat and prevent malaria infection.

Mefoxin

A proprietary, prescription-only preparation of the antibacterial and antibiotic drug cefoxitin. It can be used to treat many types of bacterial infection.

Mefruside

A proprietary, prescription-only diuretic drug. It can be used to treat raised blood pressure and oedema.

Megace

A proprietary, prescription-only progestogen drug. It can be used to treat estrogen-linked cancers.

Meggezones

A proprietary, non-prescription preparation of menthol. It can be used for the symptomatic relief of sore throat, coughs, colds, catarrh and congestion.

Melleril

A proprietary, prescription-only preparation of thioridazine. It can be used to treat and tranquillize patients with psychotic disorders.

Melphalan

A proprietary, prescription-only cytotoxic drug. It can be used to treat cancer of the bone marrow.

Meltus Dry Couch Elixir

A proprietary, non-prescription compound preparation of pseudephedrine hydrochloride and dextromethorphan hydrobromide. It can be used for the symptomatic relief of dry, painful, tickly cough and catarrh.

Meltus Junior Dry Couch Elixir

A proprietary, non-prescription compound preparation of pseudephedrine hydrochloride and dextromethorphan hydrobromide. It can be used for the symptomatic relief of dry, painful, tickly cough and catarrh.

Menadiol sodium phosphate

A synthetic form of vitamin K. It is used in deficiency syndromes.

Menotropin

A proprietary, prescription-only hormone preparation. It can be used in deficiency syndromes.

Mentholatum Deep Heat Rub

A proprietary, non-prescription compound preparation of turpentine oil, eucalyptus oil, menthol and methyl salicylate. It can be applied to the skin for symptomatic relief of underlying muscle of joint pain.

Menzol

A proprietary, prescription-only preparation of norethisterone. It can be used to treat uterine bleeding, abnormal heavy menstruation, premenstrual tension and other menstrual problems.

Mepacrine hydrochloride

A proprietary, prescription-only antiprotozoal drug. It can be used to treat intestinal protozoan infection by Giardia lamblia.

M

Metamucil

Properties
This medicine contains as active ingredient psyllium, a bulk-forming laxative. Bulk-forming laxatives are medicines taken by mouth to encourage bowel movements to relieve constipation and to prevent straining. This type of laxative is not digested but absorbs liquid in the intestines and swells to form a soft, bulky stool. The bowel is than stimulated normally by the presence of the bulky mass.

Before using this medicine
Before you use this medicine check with your doctor, or pharmacist:
- if you ever had any unusual or allergic reaction to laxatives.
- if you are on a low-salt, low-sugar, or any other special diet, or if you are allergic to any substance, such as sulfites or other preservatives or dyes.
- if you are pregnant or intending to become pregnant while using this medicine. Some bulk-forming laxatives contain a large amount of sodium or sugars, which may have possible unwanted effects such as increasing blood pressure or causing water to be held in the tissues.
- if you have any of the following medical problems:
  Appendicitis (or signs of)
  Diabetes (sugar disease)
  Heart disease
  Hypertension
  Intestinal blockage
  Laxative habit
  Rectal bleeding
  Swallowing difficulty

Treatment
For safe and effective use of bulk-forming laxatives:
Follow your doctor's orders if this laxative was prescribed.
Follow the manufacturer's package directions if you are treating yourself.
Do not try to swallow in the dry form. Take with liquid.
Each dose should be taken in or with a full glass of water or more of cold water or fruit juice.
At least six to eight 8-ounce glasses of liquids should be taken each day.

Side effects
Along with the needed effects, a medicine may cause some unwanted effects.
Side effects that should be reported to your doctor:
- *Asthma*
- *Intestinal blockage*
- *Itching*
- *Skin rash*
- *Swallowing difficulty*

Laxatives should not be given to young children (up to 6 years of age) unless prescribed by their doctor. Since children cannot usually describe their symptoms very well, a doctor should check the child before giving this medicine.

Laxative habit
Laxatives are to be used to provide short-term relief only, unless otherwise directed by your doctor. Laxatives are overused by many people. Such a practice often leads to dependence on the laxative action to produce a bowel movement. In some cases, overuse of some laxatives has caused damage to the nerves, muscles, and tissues of the intestines and bowel.

Interactions
This medicine may interact with several other drugs, such as anticoagulants, aspirin or other salicylates, digitalis preparations, potassium supplements, antibiotics and triamterene.
Be sure to tell your doctor about any medications you are currently taking.

Storage
Store away from heat and direct light. Keep out of the reach of children. Do not store in the bathroom medicine cabinet because the heat or moisture may cause the medicine to break down.

Mepenzolate bromide
A proprietary, prescription-only preparation of the beta-blocker drug metropolol tartrate. It can be used to treat raised blood pressure and angina pectoris.

Meprobamate
A proprietary, prescription-only anxiolytic drug. It can be used to treat anxiety.

Meptazinol
A proprietary, prescription-only narcotic analgesic drug. It can be used to treat moderate to severe pain.

Meptid
A preparation of the narcotic analgesic drug meptazinol. It can be used to treat moderate to severe pain.

Merbentyl
A proprietary, prescription-only preparation of diclomine hydrochloride. It can be used to treat smooth muscle spasm in the gastrointestinal tract.

Merbentyl 20
A proprietary, prescription-only preparation of diclomine hydrochloride. It can be used to treat smooth muscle spasm in the gastrointestinal tract.

Mercaptopurine

A proprietary, prescription-only cytotoxic drug. It can be used to treat acute leukaemia.

Mercilon

A proprietary, prescription-only compound of female sex hormones. It can be used to treat menstrual problems and as oral contraceptive drug.

Merocaine Lozenges

A proprietary, non-prescription compound preparation of cetylpyridinium and benzocaine. It can be used to treat pain and discomfort of a sore throat and superficial minor mouth infections.

Mercets Gargle

A proprietary, non-prescription preparation of the antiseptic agent cetylpyridinium. It can be used to treat pain and discomfort of a sore throat and superficial minor mouth infections.

Mercets Mouthwash

A proprietary, non-prescription preparation of the antiseptic agent cetylpyridinium. It can be used to treat pain and discomfort of a sore throat and superficial minor mouth infections.

Merothol Lozenges

A proprietary, non-prescription compound preparation of the antiseptic agent cetylpyridinium, cineole and menthol. It can be used to treat pain and discomfort of a sore throat and nasal congestion.

Merovit Lozenges

A proprietary, non-prescription compound preparation of the antiseptic agent cetylpyridinium and vitamin C. It can be used to treat pain and discomfort of a sore throat.

Mersalyl

A proprietary, prescription-only diuretic drug. It can be used to treat oedema and high blood pressure.

Mesalazine

A proprietary, prescription-only aminosalicylate drug. It can be used to treat ulcerative colitis.

Mesna

A proprietary, prescription-only cytotoxic drug. It can be used as an adjunct in the treatment of certain forms of cancer.

Mesterolone

A proprietary, prescription-only androgen drug. It can be used to treat hormonal deficiency.

Mestinon

A proprietary, prescription-only preparation of pyridostigmine. It can be used to treat myasthenia gravis.

Mestranol

A proprietary, prescription-only synthetic estrogen. It can be used as an oral contraceptive drug and in hormone replacement therapy.

Metalpha

A proprietary, prescription-only preparation of methyldopa. It can be used to treat high blood pressure.

Metamucil

A proprietary, non-prescription preparation of ispaghula husk. It can be used to treat constipation. (see page 703)

Metanium

A proprietary, non-prescription preparation of titanium dioxide. It can be used as a barrier cream for nappy rash.

Metaraminol

A vasoconstrictor drug. It can be used to treat active hypotension.

Metenix 5

A proprietary, prescription-only preparation of the diuretic drug metolazone. It can be used to treat oedema and raised blood pressure.

Meterfolic

A proprietary, non-prescription compound preparation of ferrous fumarate and folic acid. It can be used as supplement during pregnancy.

Metformin hydrochloride

A proprietary, prescription-only preparation of giguanide. It can be used to treat diabetes.

Methadone hydrochloride

A proprietary, prescription-only narcotic analgesic drug. It can be used to treat severe pain. It is also used as a substitute for addictive opioids in detoxification therapy.

Methicillin

A proprietary, prescription-only antibacterial and antibiotic drug. It can be used to treat a wide variety of infection.

Methionine

An antidote to poisoning caused by an overdose of paracetamol.

Methionine Tablets

An antidote to poisoning caused by an overdose of paracetamol.

Methocarbamol

A skeletal muscle relaxant drug. It can be used to treat muscle spasm.

Methohexitone sodium

A proprietary, prescription-only barbiturate drug. It can be used for induction and maintenance of anesthesia during short operations.

Methotrexate

A proprietary, prescription-only cytotoxic drug. It can be used to treat lymphoblastic leukaemia, other lymphomas and some solid tumors.

Methotrimeprazine

A preparation of phenothiazine. It can be used to treat psychotic disorders.

Methoxamine hydrochloride

A proprietary, prescription-only vasoconstrictor drug. It can be used to raise lowered blood pressure.

Methylcellulose

A proprietary, non-prescription-only bulking agent laxative. It can be used to treat constipation.

Methyl cysteine hydrochloride

A proprietary, prescription-only mucolytic drug. It can be used as an expectorant.

Methyldopa

A proprietary, prescription-only anti-

Methylcellulose

Properties
This medicine contains as active ingredient methylcellulose, a bulk-forming laxative. This medicine is taken by mouth to encourage bowel movements to relieve constipation and to prevent straining. This type of laxative is not digested but absorbs liquid in the intestines and swells to form a soft, bulky stool. The bowel is than stimulated normally by the presence of the bulky mass.

Before using this medicine
Before you use this medicine check with your doctor, or pharmacist:
- if you ever had any unusual or allergic reaction to laxatives.
- if you are on a low-salt, low-sugar, or any other special diet, or if you are allergic to any substance, such as sulfites or other preservatives or dyes.
- if you are pregnant or intending to become pregnant while using this medicine. Some bulk-forming laxatives contain a large amount of sodium or sugars, which may have possible unwanted effects such as increasing blood pressure or causing water to be held in the tissues.
- if you have any of the following medical problems:
  Appendicitis (or signs of)
  Diabetes (sugar disease)
  Heart disease
  Hypertension
  Intestinal blockage
  Laxative habit
  Rectal bleeding
  Swallowing difficulty

Treatment
For safe and effective use of bulk-forming laxatives:
Follow your doctor's orders if this laxative was prescribed.
Follow the manufacturer's package directions if you are treating
yourself.
Do not try to swallow in the dry form. Take with liquid.
Each dose should be taken in or with a full glass of water or more of cold water or fruit juice.
At least six to eight 8-ounce glasses of liquids should be taken each day.

Side effects
Along with the needed effects, a medicine may cause some unwanted effects.
Side effects that should be reported to your doctor:
- *Asthma*
- *Intestinal blockage*
- *Itching*
- *Skin rash*
- *Swallowing difficulty*
Laxatives should not be given to young children (up to 6 years of age) unless prescribed by their doctor. Since children cannot usually describe their symptoms very well, a doctor should check the child before giving this medicine.

Laxative habit
Laxatives are to be used to provide short-term relief only, unless otherwise directed by your doctor. Laxatives are overused by many people. Such a practice often leads to dependence on the laxative action to produce a bowel movement. In some cases, overuse of some laxatives has caused damage to the nerves, muscles, and tissues of the intestines and bowel.

Interactions
This medicine may interact with several other drugs, such as anticoagulants, aspirin or other salicylates, digitalis preparations, potassium supplements, antibiotics and triamterene.
Be sure to tell your doctor about any medications you are currently taking.

Storage
Store away from heat and direct light. Keep out of the reach of children. Do not store in the bathroom medicine cabinet because the heat or moisture may cause the medicine to break down.

M

---

sympathetic drug. It can be used to treat raised drug pressure.

Methyldopate hydrochloride
A preparation of the sympathetic drug methyldopa. It can be used to treat raised drug pressure.

Methyl nicotinate
A proprietary, prescription-only drug. It can be used to treat mild to moderate pain.

Methylphenobarbitone
A proprietary, prescription-only barbiturate drug. It can be used to treat all forms of epilepsy.

Methylprednisolone
A proprietary, prescription-only corticosteroid drug. It can be used to treat allergic reactions, cerebral oedema, shock and rheumatic disease.

Methyl salicylate
A proprietary, prescription-only salicylate derivative. It can be used to treat local pain.

Methysergide
A proprietary, prescription-only antimigraine drug. It can be used to treat severe recurrent migraine.

Metipranolol
A proprietary, prescription-only beta-

Miconazole
(Topical)

Properties
This medicine belongs to the family of topical (applied to the skin) antifungal preparations. It is used in the treatment of fungus infections on the skin and in the vagina. The medication fights infections such as ringworm of the scalp, athlete's foot, jockey itch, sun fungus, nail fungus and fungus infections of the vagina. Fungal diseases may develop especially in people with disorders of immunity or diabetes and those on certain drugs (steroid, immunosuppressives, antibiotics). Thrush is common in the mouth and vagina but rarely causes systemic disease.
The drug kills fungi by damaging the fungal wall; it causes loss of essential elements to sustain fungus cell life.

Before using this medicine
Before you use this medicine check with your doctor, or pharmacist:
- if you ever had any unusual or allergic reaction to topical antifungal preparations.
- if you are on a low-salt, low-sugar, or any other special diet, or if you are allergic to any substance, such as certain preservatives or dyes.
- if you are sunburned, or have an open skin wound.
- if you are pregnant, intending to become pregnant or breast-feeding an infant while using this medicine.
Pregnant women should avoid using the vaginal cream during the first three months of pregnancy. They should use it during the next six months only if it is absolutely necessary.

Treatment
This medication is used to relieve or prevent the symptoms of your medical problem. Take them as directed. Do not take more of them and do not take them more often than recommended on the label. To do so may increase the chance of absorption through the skin and the chance of side effects. If you forget to take a dose of this drug, take it as soon as you remember. If it is almost time for your next regularly scheduled application, skip the forgotten application and continue with your regular schedule.
CREAM, LOTION, OINTMENT, GEL: Bathe and dry area before use. Apply small amount and rub gently.
POWDER: Apply lightly to the skin.
VAGINAL CREAM & TABLETS: Insert into vagina with applicator as illustrated in instructions.
The treatment may require a period of 6 to 8 weeks for a complete cure. The usual schedule calls for an application twice a day, morning and evening, unless otherwise directed by your doctor or pharmacist. Be sure to complete the full course of treatment prescribed for you.

Side effects
The following side effects may occur:
- Itching
- Swelling of treated skin
- Redness of skin
- Vaginal burning and itching
- Irritation of vagina
- Swelling of labia
- Increased discharge
You should discontinue the use of the drug when these side effects occur. Call your doctor right away.

Interactions
This medicine may interact with several other medications applied to the skin or vagina. The combined effect may cause severe skin irritation or disorders of the labia or vagina.

Storage
This medicine should be stored cool, but Do not freeze. Store away from heat and direct light. Keep out of reach of children. Do not use on other members of the family without consulting your doctor. Do not store in the bathroom medicine cabinet because the heat or moisture may cause the medicine to break down. Do not keep outdated medicine or medicine no longer needed. Flush the contents down the toilet, unless otherwise directed.

blocker drug. It can be used to treat chronic simple glaucoma.

Metirosine
A proprietary, prescription-only antisympathetic drug. It can be used in the preoperative treatment of phaeochromocytoma.

Metoclopramide hydrochloride
A proprietary, prescription-only antiemetic and antinauseant drug. It can be used to prevent vomiting caused by gastrointestinal disorders.

Metolazone
A proprietary, prescription-only diuretic drug. It can be used to treat oedema and raised blood pressure.

Metopirone
A proprietary, prescription-only preparation of metyrapone. It can be used to treat Cushing's syndrome.

Metoprolol tartrate
A proprietary, prescription-only beta-blocker drug. It can be used to treat raised blood pressure.

Metosyn
A proprietary, prescription-only preparation of flucononide. It can be used to treat severe, acute inflammatory skin disorders.

Metriphonate
A proprietary, prescription-only organophosphorus compound. It can be used to treat infection with Schistosoma hematobium.

Metrodin High Purity
A proprietary, prescription-only pre-

paration of urofollitrophin. It can be used to treat women suffering from specific hormonal deficiencies.

Metrogel
A proprietary, prescription-only preparation of metrodinazole. It can be used to treat acute acne rosacea outbreaks.

Metronidazole
A proprietary, prescription-only antimicrobial drug. It can be used to treat acute acne rosacea outbreaks.

Metrotop
A proprietary, prescription-only preparation of metrodinazole. It can be used to treat fungating, malodorous tumors.

Metyrapone
A proprietary, prescription-only enzyme inhibitor. It can be used to treat Cushing's syndrome.

Mexiletine hydrochloride
A proprietary, prescription-only cardiac drug. It can be used to regularize heartbeat.

Mexitil
A proprietary, prescription-only preparation of the cardiac drug mexiletine hydrochloride. It can be used to regularize heartbeat.

Mexitil PL
A proprietary, prescription-only preparation of the cardiac drug mexiletine hydrochloride. It can be used to regularize heartbeat.

Miacalcic
A proprietary, prescription-only preparation of calcitonin. It can be used to lower blood levels of calcium.

Mianserin hydrochloride
A proprietary, prescription-only antidepressant drug. It can be used to treat depressive illness.

Micolette Micro-enema
A proprietary, non-prescription preparation of sodium citrate, sodium alkylsulphoacetate, sorbic acid and glycerol. It can be used to treat constipation.

Miconazole
A proprietary, prescription-only antifungal drug. It can be used to treat fungal infections of the skin and intestines.

Micralax Micro-enema
A proprietary, non-prescription preparation of sodium citrate, sodium alkylsulphoacetate, sorbic acid and glycerol. It can be used to treat constipation.

Microgynon 30
A proprietary, prescription-only preparation of an estrogen and progestogen. It can be used as oral contraceptive drug and to treat certain menstrual problems.

Micronor
A proprietary, prescription-only preparation of progestogen. It can be used as a contraceptive drug.

Micronor HRT
A proprietary, prescription-only preparation of progestogen. It can be used in hormone replacement therapy.

Microval
A proprietary, prescription-only preparation of progestogen. It can be used as oral contraceptive drug.

Mictral
A proprietary, prescription-only preparation of the diuretic drug amiloride. It can be used to treat oedema and raised blood pressure.

Midazolam
A proprietary, prescription-only benzodiazepine drug. It can be used to treat anxiety and insomnia.

Midrid
A proprietary, non-prescription compound preparation of isometheptene and paracetamol. It can be used to treat acute migraine attacks.

Mifegyne
A proprietary, prescription-only preparation of mifepristone. It can be used for the termination of pregnancy at up to 63 days of gestation.

NSAID

NSAID is an abbreviation for non-steroidal anti-inflammatory drug, which is used to describe a large group of medicines, of which aspirin is an original member. Although they are all acidic components of different chemical structure, they have several important actions in common.

They can be used
- **as anti-inflammatory drugs, to the extent that some may be sued as antirheumatic treatments;**
- **as non-narcotic analgesics, particularly when the pain is associated with inflammation;**
- **as antipyretic drugs, with the added advantage that they lower body temperature only when it is raised in fever;**
- **additionally, some NSAIDs may be used as antiplatelet drugs, because they can be used to beneficially reduce platelet aggregation.**

All these actions are thought to be due to the ability of NSAIDs to change the synthesis and metabolism of the natural local hormones the prostaglandins. In practice, the side effects of NSAIDs are so extensive that the use of individual members depends on the ability of individual patients to tolerate their side effects.

Some with the least side effects are regarded as safe enough for non-prescription, over-the-counter sale, such as aspirin and ibuprofen.

M

Milk of Magnesia
Liquid

Properties
This medicine contains as active ingredient a neutralizing agent for excess stomach acid and is therefore called an antacid. Antacids are taken by mouth to relieve heartburn, sour stomach, or acid indigestion. Antacids alone or in combination with simethicone may be used to treat the symptoms of stomach or duodenal ulcers. This medication contains as active ingredient: milk of magnesia.

Before using this medicine
Before you use this medicine check with your doctor, or pharmacist:
- if you ever had any unusual or allergic reaction to aluminum-, calcium-, magnesium-, sodium bicarbonate-, or simethicone containing medicines;
- if you are on a low-salt, low-sugar, or any other special diet, or if you are allergic to any substance, such as sulfites or other preservatives or dyes.
- if you are pregnant or intending to become pregnant while using this medicine. Although antacids have not been shown to cause problems in humans, the chance always exists.
- if you are breast-feeding an infant.
- if you have any of the following medical problems:
  Appendicitis (or signs of)
  Bone fractures
  Colitis
  Colostomy
  Constipation
  Diarrhea
  Heart disease
  High blood pressure
  Intestinal blockage
  Intestinal bleeding
  Kidney disease
  Liver disease
  Toxaemia of pregnancy
  Underactive parathyroids

Treatment
This medication is used to relieve or prevent the symptoms of your medical problem. Take them as directed. Do not take more of them and do not take them more often than recommended on the label, unless otherwise directed by your doctor. To do so may increase the chance of side effects.

When taking this medicine for a stomach or duodenal ulcer, take it exactly as ordered by your doctor to obtain maximum relief of your symptoms.
Antacids should not be given to young children (up to 6 years of age) unless prescribed by their doctor.

Side effects
Along with the needed effects, a medicine may cause some unwanted effects. Although the following side effects occur very rarely when this medicine is taken as recommended, they may be more likely to occur if:
- too much medicine is taken;
- it is taken in large doses;
- it is taken for a long period of time;
- it is taken by patients with kidney disease.

Check with your doctor as soon as possible if any of the following side effects or signs of overdose occur: constipation; cramping; difficult or painful urination; headache; loss of appetite; mood or mental changes; muscle pain or twitching; nausea or vomiting; stomach pain; unpleasant taste in mouth; unusual slow breathing; unusual tiredness or weakness; dizziness,

Interactions
This medicine may interact with several other drugs such as adrenocorticosteroids, cellulose sodium phosphate, mecamylamine, and tetracyclines.

Be sure to tell your doctor about any medications you are currently taking.

Storage
Tablets, elixir, etc. should be stored at room temperature; store away from heat and direct light. Keep out of reach of children, since overdose may be very dangerous in children.

Migepristone
A proprietary, prescription-only hormonal preparation. It can be used for the termination of pregnancy at up to 63 days of gcstation.

Migraleve
A compound preparation of buclizine hydrochloride, paracetamol and codeine sulphate. It can be used to treat acute migraine attacks.

Micravess
A proprietary, prescription-only compound preparation of metoclopramide and aspirin. It can be used to treat to treat migraine.

Micravess XL
A proprietary, prescription-only compound preparation of ergotamine tartrate and caffeine. It can be used to treat to treat migraine.

Mildison
A preparation of the corticosteroid drug hydrocortisone. It can be used to treat mild inflammatory skin conditions.

Milk of Magnesia Liquid
A proprietary, non-prescription preparation of magnesium hydroxide. It can be used for the relief of stomach discomfort, indigestion, hyperacidity, heartburn and flatulence.

M

Milk of Magnesia Tablets

A proprietary, non-prescription preparation of magnesium hydroxide. It can be used for the relief of stomach discomfort, indigestion, hyperacidity, heartburn and flatulence.

Milrinone

A proprietary, prescription-only phosphodiesterase inhibitor. It can be used to treat acute heart failure.

Minihep

A proprietary, prescription-only preparation of heparin. It can be used to treat various forms of thrombosis.

Minihep Calcium

A proprietary, prescription-only preparation of heparin. It can be used to treat various forms of thrombosis.

Min-I-Jet Adrenaline

A proprietary, prescription-only preparation of adrenaline. It can be used to treat acute and severe bronchial asthma attacks.

Min-I-Jet Aminophylline

A proprietary, prescription-only preparation of aminophylline. It can be used to treat acute and severe bronchial asthma attacks.

Min-I-Jet Bretylate Tosylate

A proprietary, prescription-only preparation of bretylate tosylate. It can be used to treat ventricular arrhythmias.

Min-I-Jet Frusemide

A proprietary, prescription-only preparation of frusemide. It can be used to treat oedema.

Min-I-Jet Isoprenaline

A proprietary, prescription-only preparation of isoprenaline hydrochloride. It can be used to treat acute heart block and bradycardia.

Min-I-Jet Lignocaine

A proprietary, prescription-only preparation of lignocaine hydrochloride. It can be used to treat irregularities of the heartbeat.

Min-I-Jet Mannitol

A proprietary, prescription-only preparation of mannitol. It can be used to treat oedema.

Min-I-Jet Morphine Sulphate

A proprietary, prescription-only preparation of morphine sulphate. It can be used to treat severe pain.

Min-I-Jet Naloxone

A proprietary, prescription-only preparation of naloxone hydrochloride. It can be used to treat overdosage with opioids.

Min-I-Jet Sodium Bicarbonate

A proprietary, prescription-only preparation of sodium bicarbonate. It can be used to treat metabolic acidosis.

Minims Amethocaine

A proprietary, prescription-only preparation of amethocaine. It can be used by topical application for ophthalmic procedures.

Minims Artificial Tears

A proprietary, prescription-only preparation of hydroxyethylcellulose. It can be used by topical application for dryness of the eyes.

Minims Atropine Sulphate

A proprietary, prescription-only preparation of atropine sulphate. It can be used by topical application for dilatation of the pupil.

Minims Benoxinate

A proprietary, prescription-only preparation of benoxinate hydrochloride. It can be used by topical application for ophthalmic procedures.

Minims Chloramphenicol

A proprietary, prescription-only preparation of chloramphenicol. It can be used by topical application bacterial infection of the eye.

Minims Cyclopentolate

A proprietary, prescription-only preparation of cyclopentolate. It can be used by topical application for dilatation of the pupil.

Minims Fluorescein Sodium

A preparation of fluorescein sodium. It can be used by topical application for diagnostic ophthalmologic procedures.

Minims Gentamycin

A proprietary, prescription-only preparation of gentamycin. It can be used by topical application for infection of the eyes.

Minims Homatropine

A proprietary, prescription-only preparation of homatropine. It can be used by topical application to dilate the pupils.

Minims Metipranolol

A proprietary, prescription-only preparation of metipranolol. It can be used by topical application for glaucoma treatment.

Minims Neomycin Sulphate

A proprietary, prescription-only preparation of neomycin sulphate. It can be used by topical application for bacterial infections in the eye.

Minims Phenylephrine

A proprietary, prescription-only preparation of phenylephrine. It can be used by topical application for ophthalmic procedures.

Minims Pilocarpine Nitrate

A proprietary, prescription-only preparation of pilocarpine nitrate. It can be used by topical application to treat glaucoma.

Minims Prednisolone

A proprietary, prescription-only preparation of prednisolone. It can be used by topical application for conditions in and around the eye.

Minims Rose Bengal

A proprietary, prescription-only preparation of the dye Rose Bengal. It can be used by topical application for ophthalmic procedures.

Minims Sodium Chloride

A proprietary, prescription-only preparation of sodium chloride. It can be used by topical application for irrigation of the eye.

Minims Tropicamide

A proprietary, prescription-only pre-

M

paration of tropicamide. It can be used by topical application for ophthalmic procedures.

Minitran
A proprietary, non-prescription preparation of glyceryl trinitrate. It can be used to treat and prevent angina pectoris.

Minocin
A proprietary, prescription-only preparation of antibacterial and antibiotic drug minocycline. It can be used to treat a wide variety of infection.

Minocin MR
A preparation of antibacterial and antibiotic drug minocycline. It can be used to treat a wide variety of infection.

Minocycline
A proprietary, prescription-only antibacterial and antibiotic drug. It can be used to treat a wide variety of infection.

Minodiab
A proprietary, prescription-only preparation of glipizide. It can be used to treat diabetes.

Minoxidil
A proprietary, prescription-only vasodilator drug. It can be used to treat male-pattern baldness.

Mintec
A proprietary, non-prescription preparation of peppermint oil. It can be used to relieve the discomfort of abdominal colic and distension.

Mintezol
A proprietary, prescription-only preparation of thiabendazole. It can be used to treat intestinal infestations.

Mirulet
A proprietary, prescription-only compound preparation of an estrogen and a progestogen. It can be used to treat menstrual problems and as an oral contraceptive.

Miochol
A proprietary, prescription-only pre-

paration of acetylcholine. It can be used to contract the pupils.

Misoprostol
A proprietary, prescription-only synthetic analogue of a prostaglandin. It can be used as an ulcer-healing drug.

Mithracin
A proprietary, prescription-only preparation of plicamycin. It can be used to treat excess levels of calcium in the bloodstream.

Mitomycin
A proprietary, prescription-only cytotoxic drug. It can be used to treat various types of cancer.

Mitomycin C Kyowa
A proprietary, prescription-only cytotoxic drug. It can be used to treat various types of cancer.

Mitoxana
A proprietary, prescription-only preparation of the cytotoxic drug ifosamide. It can be used to treat various types of cancer.

Mitoxantrone
A proprietary, prescription-only cytotoxic drug. It can be used to treat several types of cancer.

Mitozantrone
A proprietary, prescription-only cytotoxic drug. It can be used to treat several types of cancer.

Mivacron
A proprietary, prescription-only preparation of mivacurium. It can be used to induce muscle paralysis during surgery.

Mivacurium chloride
A proprietary, prescription-only drug. It can be used to induce muscle paralysis during surgery.

Mixtard 30/70
A proprietary, prescription-only preparation of biphasic isophane insulin. It can be used to treat diabetes.

Mobiflex
A proprietary, prescription-only preparation of tenoxicam. It can be used

to treat the pain and inflammation of rheumatism.

Mobilan
A proprietary, prescription-only preparation of indomethacin. It can be used to treat the pain and inflammation of rheumatism.

Meclobemide
A proprietary, prescription-only antidepressant drug. It can be used to treat major depressive illness.

Modalim
A proprietary, prescription-only preparation of ciprofibrate. It can be used to reduced high levels of lipids in the bloodstream.

Modecate
A proprietary, prescription-only preparation of fluphenazine. It can be used to treat psychotic patients including schizophrenia.

Moditen
A proprietary, prescription-only preparation of fluphenazine. It can be used to treat psychotic patients including schizophrenia.

Modrasone
A proprietary, prescription-only preparation of the corticosteroid drug alclometasone diprorionate. It can be used to treat inflammatory skin conditions such as eczema.

Modrenal
A proprietary, prescription-only preparation of trilostane. It can be used to treat conditions that result from the excessive secretion of corticosteroids.

Moducren
A proprietary, prescription-only compound preparation of the betablocker timolol maleate and hydrochlorothiazide. It can be used to treat raised blood pressure and to treat oedema.

Moduret-25
A proprietary, prescription-only compound preparation of the diuretic drugs hydrochlorothiazide and amiloride hydrochloride. It can be

used to treat oedema and raised blood pressure.

Moduretic

A proprietary, prescription-only compound preparation of the diuretic drugs hydrochlorothiazide and amiloride hydrochloride. It can be used to treat oedema and raised blood pressure.

Mogadon

A proprietary, prescription-only preparation of the benzodiazepine drug nitrazepam. It can be used to treat insomnia.

Molcer

A proprietary, non-prescription preparation of docussate sodium. It can be used for the dissolution and removal of earwax.

Molipaxin

A proprietary, prescription-only preparation of the antidepressant drug trazodone hydrochloride. It can be used to treat depressive illness.

Monit

A proprietary, prescription-only preparation of isorbide mononitrate. It can be used to treat and prevent angina pectoris.

Monit SR

A proprietary, prescription-only preparation of isorbide mononitrate. It can be used to treat and prevent angina pectoris.

Mono-Cedocard

A proprietary, prescription-only preparation of isorbide mononitrate. It can be used to treat and prevent angina pectoris.

Mono-Cedocard Retard-50

A proprietary, prescription-only preparation of isorbide mononitrate. It can be used to treat and prevent angina pectoris.

Monoclate-P

A proprietary, prescription-only preparation of dried human factor VIII fraction. It can be used to reduce or stop bleeding.

Monocor

A proprietary, prescription-only preparation of the beta-blocker bisoprolol fumarate. It can be used to treat raised blood pressure and to prevent and treat angina pectoris.

Mononine

A proprietary, prescription-only preparation of factor IX fraction prepared from human blood plasma. It can be used to treat deficiency of this factor.

Monoparin

A proprietary, prescription-only preparation of heparin. It can be used to treat various forms of thrombosis.

Monoparin Calcium

A proprietary, prescription-only preparation of heparin calcium. It can be used to treat various forms of thrombosis.

Monotrim

A proprietary, prescription-only preparation of the antibacterial and antibiotic drug trimethoprim. It can be used to treat infections of the upper respiratory tract.

Monovent

A proprietary, prescription-only preparation of terbutaline sulphate. It can be used as bronchodilator to treat reversible airways disorders.

Monozide 10

A proprietary, prescription-only compound preparation of bisoprolol and hydrochlorothiazide. It can be used to treat raised blood pressure.

Monphytol

A proprietary, non-prescription preparation of antiseptic agents. It can be used to treat skin infections.

Monuril

A proprietary, prescription-only preparation of antibacterial and antibiotic drug fosfomycin. It can be used to treat infections of the urinary tract.

Moorland Tablets

A proprietary, non-prescription compound preparation of calcium carbonate, aluminium hydroxide, magnesium carbonate, magnesium trisilicate and bismuth aluminate. It can be used to treat indigestion, heartburn and flatulence.

Moracizine hydrochloride

A proprietary, prescription-only cardiac drug. It can be used to treat irregularities of the heartbeat.

Morhulin Ointment

A proprietary, non-prescription preparation of zinc oxide and cod-liver oil. It can be used as an emollient for minor wounds, pressure sores and skin ulcers.

Morphine hydrochloride

A powerful opioid narcotic analgesic drug. It can be used to treat severe pain and to relieve the associated stress and anxiety.

Morphine sulphate

A powerful opioid narcotic analgesic drug. It can be used to treat severe pain and to relieve the associated stress and anxiety.

Motens

A proprietary, prescription-only preparation of diclofenac sodium. It can be used to treat the pain and inflammation of arthritis and rheumatism.

Motilium

A proprietary, prescription-only preparation of domperidone. It can be used to treat drug-induced nausea and vomiting.

Motipress

A proprietary, prescription-only compound preparation of fluphenazine hydrochloride and nortriptyline hydrochloride. It can be used to treat depressive illness with anxiety.

Motival

A proprietary, prescription-only compound preparation of fluphenazine hydrochloride and nortriptyline hydrochloride. It can be used to treat depressive illness with anxiety.

Motrin

A proprietary, prescription-only

M

M

Motrin

Fever
Pain
Infection

Properties

This medicine contains as active ingredient ibuprofen. It belongs to the group of medicines called non-steroidal anti-inflammatory drugs (NSAIDs). These drugs are taken by mouth to relieve some symptoms caused by arthritis or rheumatism, such as inflammation, swelling, stiffness, and joint pain. However, these medicines do not cure arthritis and will help you only as long as you continue to take them. Some of these medicines are also used to relieve other kinds of pain or to treat other painful conditions, such as gout attacks, bursitis, tendinitis, sprains, strains, menstrual cramps. The drug reduces the tissue concentration of prostaglandins (hormonal substances which produce inflammation and pain).

Before using this medicine

Before you use this medicine check with your doctor, or pharmacist:
- if you ever had any unusual or allergic reaction, such as skin rash, hives, or itching or breathing problems, to any of the anti-inflammatory analgesics.
- if you are on a low-salt, low-sugar, or any other special diet, or if you are allergic to any substance, such as sulfites or other preservatives or dyes.
- if you are pregnant or intending to become pregnant while using this medicine. Studies on birth defects have not been done in humans. However, if taken regularly during the last months of pregnancy, there is a chance that these medicines may cause unwanted effects on the heart or blood flow in the fetus or newborn infant.
- if you are breast-feeding an infant. Although this medicine has not been shown to cause problems in humans, it passes into the breast milk in small amounts.
- if you have any of the following medical problems:
  Asthma

Bleeding problems
Colitis
Stomach ulcer
Heart disease
Kidney or liver disease

Treatment

This medication is used to relieve pain or other symptoms caused by arthritis. For safe and effective use of this medicine, do not take more of it, do not take it more often, and do not take it for a longer period of time than ordered by your physician or directed by the package label.

If you are taking this medication on a regular schedule and you miss a dose, take the missed dose as soon as possible, unless it is almost time for your next dose. In that case do not take the missed dose at all.

To lessen stomach upset, anti-inflammatory analgesics may be taken with food or antacids.

Side effects

Along with the needed effects, a medicine may cause some unwanted effects. These side effects may go away during treatment as your body adjusts to the medicine. Such minor side effects are: dizziness; nausea; pain; headache; drowsiness; swollen feet, face or leg; constipation or diarrhea; vomiting; dry mouth.

Check with your doctor immediately if any of the following side effects occur:
- *Muscle cramps*
- *Numbness or tingling*
- *Mouth ulcers*
- *Convulsions or confusion*
- *Rash, hives, or itch*
- *Tightness in chest*

Interactions

This medicine may interact with several other drugs.
Be sure to tell your doctor about any medications you are currently taking.

Storage

The medicine should be stored at room temperature in a tightly closed, light-resistant container. Store away from heat and direct light. Keep out of reach of children.

---

preparation of ibuprofen. It can be used to relieve pain and inflammation of rheumatic disease.

Movelat Cream

A proprietary, non-prescription preparation of salicylic acid and mono-polysaccharide polysulphate. It can be applied to the skin for symptomatic relief of underlying muscle or joint pain.

MST Contin

A proprietary, prescription-only preparation of morphine sulphate. It can be used to treat severe pain.

Mucaine

A proprietary, prescription-only compound preparation of aluminium hydroxide, magnesium hydroxide and oxethazaine It can be used to relieve reflux esophagitis and hiatus hernia.

Mucodyne

A proprietary, prescription-only preparation of carbocisteine. It can be used to relieve viscosity of sputum and thus facilitate expectoration.

Mucogel Suspension

A proprietary, non-prescription compound preparation of aluminium hydroxide and magnesium hydroxide. It can be used to relieve indigestion, dyspepsia and heartburn.

Mu-Cron Tablets
A proprietary, non-prescription compound preparation of paracetamol and phenylpropanolamine hydrochloride. It can be used for the symptomatic relief of sinus pain and nasal congestion.

Multiparin
A proprietary, prescription-only preparation of heparin. It can be used to treat various forms of thrombosis.

Mupirocin
A proprietary, prescription-only antibacterial and antibiotic drug. It can be used to treat bacterial skin infection.

Muripsin
A proprietary, non-prescription preparation of glutamic acid hydrochloride. It can be used to treat hypochlohydria and achlorhydria.

Mustine hydrochloride
A proprietary, prescription-only cytotoxic drug. It can be used to treat Hodgkin's disease.

Myambutol
A proprietary, prescription-only preparation of the antibacterial drug ethambutol hydrochloride. It can be used to treat tuberculosis.

Mycardol
A proprietary, prescription-only preparation of pentaerythitrol tetranitrate. It can be used to treat and prevent angina pectoris.

Mycifradin
A proprietary, prescription-only preparation of the antibacterial and antibiotic drug neomycin sulphate. It can be used to treat certain intestinal infections.

Mycil Athlete's Foot Ointment
A proprietary, non-prescription preparation of tolnaftate. It can be used to treat fungal skin infections.

Mycil Athlete's Foot Spray
A proprietary, non-prescription preparation of tolnaftate. It can be used to treat fungal skin infections.

Mycobutin
A proprietary, prescription-only preparation of the antibacterial and antibiotic drug rifabutin. It can be used to treat and prevent tuberculosis.

Mycota Cream
A proprietary, non-prescription compound preparation of undecenoate and undecenoic acid. It can be used to treat fungal skin infections.

Mycota Powder/ Spray
A proprietary, non-prescription compound preparation of undecenoate and undecenoic acid. It can be used to treat fungal skin infections.

Mydriacyl
A proprietary, prescription-only preparation of tropicamide. It can be used to dilate the pupils.

Mydrilate
A proprietary, prescription-only preparation of cyclopentolate hydrochloride. It can be used to dilate the pupils.

Myleran
A proprietary, prescription-only preparation of the cytotoxic drug busulphan. It can be used to treat chronic myeloid leukaemia.

Myocrisin
A proprietary, prescription-only preparation of aurothiomalate. It can be used to treat rheumatoid arthritis and juvenile arthritis.

Myotonine
A proprietary, prescription-only preparation of bethanechol chloride. It can be used to stimulate motility in the intestines.

Mysoline
A proprietary, prescription-only preparation of primidone. It can be used to treat all forms of epilepsy.

Mysteclin
A proprietary, prescription-only compound preparation of the antibacterial and antibiotic drugs tetracycline and nystatin. It can be used to treat a variety of infections.

N

Nabilone
A synthetic drug derived from cannabis. It is used to treat vomiting and nausea.

Nabumetone
A proprietary, prescription-only non-narcotic analgesic and antirheumatic drug. It is used to relieve pain and inflammation, particularly in osteoarthritis and rheumatoid arthritis.

Nacton
A proprietary, prescription-only preparation of poldine methylsulphate. It is used for the symptomatic relief of smooth muscle spasm.

Nadolol
A proprietary, prescription-only beta-blocker drug. It is used to treat raised blood pressure.

Nafarelin
A proprietary, prescription-only analogue of gonadorelin. It is used to treat endometriosis and in in vitro fertilization.

Naftidrofuryl oxalate
A proprietary, prescription-only vasodilator drug. It is used to treat peripheral vascular disease.

Nalcrom
A proprietary, prescription-only preparation of cromoglycate. It is used to treat certain allergic conditions.

Nalidixic acid
A proprietary, prescription-only antibacterial and antibiotic drug. It can be used to treat a variety of infection.

Nalorex
A proprietary, prescription-only preparation of naltrexone hydrochloride. It is used in detoxification therapy.

Naloxone hydrochloride
A proprietary, prescription-only opioid antagonist drug. It is used as an

antidote to an overdose of narcotic analgesics.

Naltrexone hydrochloride
A opioid antagonist of narcotic analgesic drugs. It is used in detoxification therapy.

Nandrolone
A anabolic steroid. It is used to treat osteoporosis and aplastic anemia.

Naphazoline hydrochloride
A proprietary, prescription-only vasoconstrictor drug. It is used for the symptomatic relief of conjunctivitis.

Napratec
A proprietary, prescription-only compound preparation of naproxen and misoprostol. It is used to treat the pain and inflammation of rheumatoid arthritis and osteoarthritis.

Naprosyn
A preparation of naproxen. It is used to treat the pain and inflammation of rheumatoid arthritis and osteoarthritis.

Naproxen
A antirheumatic drug. It is used to treat the pain and inflammation of rheumatoid arthritis and osteoarthritis.

Nardil
A proprietary, prescription-only preparation of phenelzine. It is used to treat depressive illness.

Narphen
A proprietary, prescription-only preparation of phenazocine. It is used to relieve severe pain.

Nasacort
A proprietary, prescription-only preparation of mometasone. It is applied intranasally to treat congestion and other seasonal nasal allergy symptoms.

Nasanex
A proprietary, prescription-only preparation of clonidine. It is used to for the symptomatic relief of rheumatic aches and pains.

Naseptin
A proprietary, prescription-only compound preparation of the antibacterial and antibiotic drug neomycin sulphate and chlorhexidine. It is used to treat staphylococcal infections in and around the nostrils.

Natrilix
A proprietary, prescription-only preparation of indapamide. It can be used to treat raised blood pressure.

Natulan
A proprietary, prescription-only preparation of the cytotoxic drug procarbazine. It can be used in the treatment of lymphatic cancer.

Navidrex
A proprietary, prescription-only preparation of cyclopenthiazide. It is used to treat oedema.

Navispare
A proprietary, prescription-only compound preparation of the diuretic drugs amiloride hydrochloride and cyclopenthiazide. It is used to treat raised blood pressure.

Navoban
A proprietary, prescription-only preparation of tropisetron. It is used to treat nausea and vomiting.

Nebcin
A proprietary, prescription-only preparation of the antibacterial and antibiotic drug tobramycin. It is used to treat serious bacterial infections.

Nedocromil sodium
A proprietary, prescription-only anti-asthmatic drug. It is used to prevent recurrent attacks of asthma.

Negram
A preparation of the antibacterial and antibiotic drug nalidixic acid. It is used to treat infections of the urinary tract.

Neocon
A proprietary, prescription-only compound preparation of an estrogen and progestogen. It is used to treat menstrual problems and as an oral drug for contraception.

Neo-Cortef
A proprietary, prescription-only compound preparation of the corticosteroid drug hydrocortisone and neomycin sulphate. It is used to treat bacterial infections of the outer ear and eye.

Neogest
A proprietary, prescription-only preparation of progestogen. It is used as an oral contraceptive.

Neo-Medrone
A proprietary, prescription-only preparation of the corticosteroid methylprednisolone and neomycin sulphate. It is used to treat inflammatory skin conditions.

Neo-Mercazole
A proprietary, prescription-only preparation of carbimazole. It is used to treat the effects of an excess of thyroid hormones in the bloodstream.

Neomycin sulphate
A proprietary, prescription-only preparation antibacterial and antibiotic drug. It is used to treat superficial skin infections and inflammation of the eye and ear.

Neo-NaClex
A proprietary, prescription-only preparation of the diuretic drug bendrofluazide. It is used to treat heart failure disorders.

Neo-NaClex-K
A compound reparation of the diuretic drug bendrofluazide and potassium chloride. It is used to treat heart failure disorders, oedema and raised blood pressure.

Neosporin
A preparation of neomycin sulphate. It is used to treat superficial skin infections and inflammation of the eye and ear.

Neostigmine
A proprietary, prescription-only anticholinesterase drug. It is used to treat urinary retention and paralytic ileus.

Neotigason
A proprietary, prescription-only preparation of acitretin. It is used to treat severe psoriasis and other skin disorders.

Naprosyn

Properties

This medicine contains as active ingredient naproxen. It belongs to the group of medicines called non-steroidal anti-inflammatory drugs (NSAIDs). These drugs are taken by mouth to relieve some symptoms caused by arthritis or rheumatism, such as inflammation, swelling, stiffness, and joint pain. However, these medicines do not cure arthritis and will help you only as long as you continue to take them. Some of these medicines are also used to relieve other kinds of pain or to treat other painful conditions, such as gout attacks, bursitis, tendinitis, sprains, strains, menstrual cramps. The drug reduces the tissue concentration of prostaglandins (hormonal substances which produce inflammation and pain).

Before using this medicine

Before you use this medicine check with your doctor, or pharmacist:

- if you ever had any unusual or allergic reaction, such as skin rash, hives, or itching or breathing problems, to any of the anti-inflammatory analgesics.
- if you are on a low-salt, low-sugar, or any other special diet, or if you are allergic to any substance, such as sulfites or other preservatives or dyes.
- if you are pregnant or intending to become pregnant while using this medicine. Studies on birth defects have not been done in humans. However, if taken regularly during the last months of pregnancy, there is a chance that these medicines may cause unwanted effects on the heart or blood flow in the fetus or newborn infant.
- if you are breast-feeding an infant. Although this medicine has not been shown to cause problems in humans, it passes into the breast milk in small amounts.
- if you have any of the following medical problems: Asthma

Bleeding problems
Colitis
Stomach ulcer
Heart disease
Kidney or liver disease

Treatment

This medication is used to relieve pain or other symptoms caused by arthritis. For safe and effective use of this medicine, do not take more of it, do not take it more often, and do not take it for a longer period of time than ordered by your physician or directed by the package label.

If you are taking this medication on a regular schedule and you miss a dose, take the missed dose as soon as possible, unless it is almost time for your next dose. In that case do not take the missed dose at all.

To lessen stomach upset, anti-inflammatory analgesics may be taken with food or antacids.

Side effects

Along with the needed effects, a medicine may cause some unwanted effects. These side effects may go away during treatment as your body adjusts to the medicine. Such minor side effects are: dizziness; nausea; pain; headache; drowsiness; swollen feet, face or leg; constipation or diarrhea; vomiting; dry mouth.

Check with your doctor immediately if any of the following side effects occur:

- *Muscle cramps*
- *Numbness or tingling*
- *Mouth ulcers*
- *Convulsions or confusion*
- *Rash, hives, or itch*
- *Tightness in chest*

Interactions

This medicine may interact with several other drugs.

Be sure to tell your doctor about any medications you are currently taking.

Storage

The medicine should be stored at room temperature in a tightly closed, light-resistant container. Store away from heat and direct light. Keep out of reach of children.

Nephril

A proprietary, prescription-only preparation of the diuretic drug polythiazide. It is used to treat oedema.

Nericur

A proprietary, non-prescription compound preparation of the antifungal drug micronazole and benzoyl peroxide. It is used to treat acne

Nerisone

A proprietary, prescription-only preparation of the corticosteroid difluocortolone valerate. It can be used to treat severe, acute inflammatory skin disorders.

Netillin

A proprietary, prescription-only preparation of the antibacterial and antibiotic drug netilmicin. It is used to treat a range of serious bacterial infections.

Netilmicin

A proprietary, prescription-only antibacterial and antibiotic drug. It is used to treat a range of serious bacterial infections.

Neulasta

A proprietary, prescription-only preparation of pegfilgrastim. It is used for the stimulation of growth of neutrophils.

Neurontin

A proprietary, prescription-only preparation of gabapentin. It is used to assist in the control of seizures.

Nexium

A proprietary, prescription-only preparation of esomeprazole. It is used to for the symptomatic relief of acid reflux and heartburn.

Nicardipine hydrochloride

A proprietary, prescription-only calcium-channel blocker. It is used to treat and prevent angina pectoris end raised blood pressure.

Niclosamide

A proprietary, prescription-only synthetic anthelminthic drug. It is used to treat infestation by tapeworms.

Nicobrevin

A proprietary, non-prescription compound preparation of methyl valerate, quinine and camphor. It is used to alleviate the withdrawal symptoms experienced when giving up smoking.

Niconil

A proprietary, non-prescription preparation of nicotine. It is used to alleviate the withdrawal symptoms experienced when giving up smoking.

Nicorette

A proprietary, non-prescription preparation of nicotine. It is used to alleviate the withdrawal symptoms experienced when giving up smoking.

Nicorette Patch

A proprietary, non-prescription preparation of nicotine. It is used to alleviate the withdrawal symptoms experienced when giving up smoking.

Nicorette Plus

A proprietary, non-prescription preparation of nicotine. It is used to alleviate the withdrawal symptoms experienced when giving up smoking.

Nicotinell TTS

A proprietary, non-prescription preparation of nicotine. It is used to alleviate the withdrawal symptoms experienced when giving up smoking.

Nicotinic acid

A B-complex vitamin. Dietary deficiency results in the disease pellagra. Nicotinic acid is commonly used as a vasodilator.

Nicotinyl alcohol

A proprietary, prescription-only vasodilator drug. It is used to improve blood circulation.

Nicoumalone

A proprietary, prescription-only synthetic anticoagulant drug. It can be used to prevent the formation of cloths in heart disease.

Nifedipine

A proprietary, prescription-only calcium channel blocker drug. It is used as a vasodilator in peripheral vascular disease.

Night Cold Comfort Capsules

A proprietary, non-prescription compound preparation of pseudo-ephedrine hydrochloride, paracetamol, pholcodeine and diphenhydramine hydrochloride. It is used to relieve nasal congestion during colds and flu, aches, cough and fever.

Night Nurse Capsules

A proprietary, non-prescription compound preparation of pseudo-ephedrine hydrochloride, paracetamol, pholcodeine and promethazine hydrochloride. It is used for the symptomatic relief of colds and flu, aches, cough and fever.

Night Nurse Liquid

A proprietary, non-prescription compound preparation of pseudo-ephedrine hydrochloride, paracetamol, pholcodeine and promethazine hydrochloride. It is used for the symptomatic relief of colds and flu, aches, cough and fever.

Nimodipine

A proprietary, prescription-only calcium-channel blocker drug. It is used to treat and prevent ischemic damage following subarchnoidal hemorrhage.

Nimotop

A proprietary, prescription-only preparation of the calcium-channel blocker drug nimodipine. It is used to treat and prevent ischemic damage following subarachnoidal hemorrhage.

Nipride

A proprietary, prescription-only preparation of nitroprusside. It is used to treat acute high blood pressure.

Nirolex

A proprietary, non-prescription compound preparation of guaiphenesin, ephedrine hydrochloride, glycerin and menthol. It is used for the symptomatic relief of chesty coughs.

Nirolex X

A proprietary, non-prescription preparation of guaiphenesin. It is used for the symptomatic relief of dry and chesty coughs.

Nirolex Lozenges

A proprietary, non-prescription preparation of dextromethorphan hydrobromide. It is used for the symptomatic relief of dry and chesty coughs.

Nitoman

A proprietary, prescription-only preparation of tetrabenazine. It is used to assist a patient to regain voluntary control of movement.

Nitrazepam

A proprietary, prescription-only benzodiazepine drug. It is used to treat insomnia.

Nitrocine

A proprietary, prescription-only preparation of glycerol trinitrate. It is used to treat and prevent angina pectoris.

Nitrocontin Continus

A proprietary, prescription-only preparation of glycerol trinitrate. It is used to treat and prevent angina pectoris.

Nitrodur

A proprietary, prescription-only preparation of glycerol trinitrate. It is used to treat and prevent angina pectoris.

Nitrofurantoin

A proprietary, prescription-only antibacterial drug. It is used to treat infections of the urinary tract.

Nizoral
(Topical)

Properties

This medicine belongs to the family of topical (applied to the skin) antifungal preparations. It is used in the treatment of fungus infections on the skin and in the vagina. The medication fights infections such as ringworm of the scalp, athlete's foot, jockey itch, sun fungus, nail fungus and fungus infections of the vagina.

Fungal diseases may develop especially in people with disorders of immunity or diabetes and those on certain drugs (steroid, immunosuppressives, antibiotics). Thrush is common in the mouth and vagina but rarely causes systemic disease.

The drug kills fungi by damaging the fungal wall; it causes loss of essential elements to sustain fungus cell life.

Before using this medicine

Before you use this medicine check with your doctor, or pharmacist:

- if you ever had any unusual or allergic reaction to topical antifungal preparations.
- if you are on a low-salt, low-sugar, or any other special diet, or if you are allergic to any substance, such as certain preservatives or dyes.
- if you are sunburned, or have an open skin wound.
- if you are pregnant, intending to become pregnant or breast-feeding an infant while using this medicine.

Pregnant women should avoid using the vaginal cream during the first three months of pregnancy. They should use it during the next six months only if it is absolutely necessary.

Treatment

This medication is used to relieve or prevent the symptoms of your medical problem. Take them as directed. Do not take more of them and do not take them more often than recommended on the label. To do so may increase the chance of absorption through the skin and the chance of side effects. If you forget to take a dose of this drug, take it as soon as you remember. If it is almost time for your next regularly scheduled application, skip the forgotten application and continue with your regular schedule.

CREAM, LOTION, OINTMENT, GEL: Bathe and dry area before use. Apply small amount and rub gently.

POWDER: Apply lightly to the skin.

VAGINAL CREAM & TABLETS: Insert into vagina with applicator as illustrated in instructions.

The treatment may require a period of 6 to 8 weeks for a complete cure. The usual schedule calls for an application twice a day, morning and evening, unless otherwise directed by your doctor or pharmacist. Be sure to complete the full course of treatment prescribed for you.

Side effects

The following side effects may occur:

- Itching
- Swelling of treated skin
- Redness of skin
- Vaginal burning and itching
- Irritation of vagina
- Swelling of labia
- Increased discharge

You should discontinue the use of the drug when these side effects occur. Call your doctor right away.

Interactions

This medicine may interact with several other medications applied to the skin or vagina. The combined effect may cause severe skin irritation or disorders of the labia or vagina.

Storage

This medicine should be stored cool, but Do not freeze. Store away from heat and direct light. Keep out of reach of children. Do not use on other members of the family without consulting your doctor. Do not store in the bathroom medicine cabinet because the heat or moisture may cause the medicine to break down. Do not keep outdated medicine or medicine no longer needed. Flush the contents down the toilet, unless otherwise directed.

N

Nitrolingual Spray

A proprietary, prescription-only preparation of glycerol trinitrate. It is used to treat and prevent angina pectoris.

Nitronal

A preparation of glycerol trinitrate. It is used to treat and prevent angina pectoris.

Nivaquine

A proprietary, prescription-only preparation of chloroquine. It is used to prevent or suppress certain forms of malaria.

Nivemycin

A proprietary, prescription-only preparation of the antibacterial and antibiotic drug neomycin sulphate. It is used to reduce bacterial levels in the intestines before surgery.

Nitazidine

A proprietary, prescription-only ulcer-healing drug. It is used to assist in the treatment of benign peptic ulcer, to relieve heartburn and dyspepsia.

Nizoral

A proprietary, prescription-only preparation of the antifungal drug ketoconazole. It is used to treat serious systemic and skin-surface fungal infections.

Noctec

A proprietary, prescription-only

preparation of chloral hydrate. It is used to treat insomnia.

Noltam

A proprietary, prescription-only preparation of tamoxifen. It is used to treat estrogen-dependent cancers.

Nolvadex

A proprietary, prescription-only preparation of tamoxifen. It is used to treat estrogen-dependent cancers.

Nonoxinol

A spermicidal drug that is used to assist barrier methods of contraception.

Nootropil

A proprietary, prescription-only preparation of piracetam. It can be used to treat cortical myoclonus.

Norditropin

A proprietary, prescription-only preparation of somatropin. It is used to treat hormonal deficiency.

Nordox

A proprietary, prescription-only preparation of the antibacterial and antibiotic drug doxycycline. It is used to treat a range of infections.

Norethisterone

A proprietary, prescription-only progestogen drug. It is used to in hormone replacement therapy.

Norflex

A proprietary, prescription-only preparation of orphenadrine citrate. It is used to treat skeletal muscle spasm.

Norfloxacin

A proprietary, prescription-only antibacterial and antibiotic drug. It is used to treat a wide variety of infections.

Norgalex Micro-enema

A proprietary, non-prescription preparation of docussate sodium. It is used to treat constipation.

Norgeston

A proprietary, prescription-only progestogen drug. It is used to as an oral contraceptive.

Norgestrel

A proprietary, prescription-only progestogen drug. It is used to as an oral contraceptive.

Noriday

A proprietary, prescription-only progestogen drug. It is used to as an oral contraceptive.

Norimin

A proprietary, prescription-only compound preparation of an estrogen and a progestogen. It is used to treat certain menstrual disorders and as an oral contraceptive.

Norinyl-1

A proprietary, prescription-only compound preparation of an estrogen and a progestogen. It is used to treat certain menstrual disorders and as an oral contraceptive.

Normacol

A proprietary, non-prescription preparation of sterculia. It is used to treat constipation.

Normacol Plus

A proprietary, non-prescription compound preparation of sterculia and frangula bark. It is used to treat constipation.

Normax

A proprietary, prescription-only preparation of co-danthramer. It is used to treat constipation.

Normegon

A proprietary, prescription-only preparation of human gonadotrophins. It can be used to treat infertility in women.

Norplant

A proprietary, prescription-only preparation of a prostogen drug. It is used as an oral contraceptive.

Nortriptyline hydrochloride

A proprietary, prescription-only antidepressant drug. It is used to treat depressive illness.

Norval

A proprietary, prescription-only preparation of mianserin hydrochlo-ride. It is used to treat depressive illness.

Novantone

A proprietary, prescription-only preparation of nitrozantrone. It is used to treat certain types of cancer.

Nozinan

A proprietary, prescription-only preparation of methotrimeprazine. It is used to tranquillize patients with psychotic disorders.

Nubain

A proprietary, prescription-only preparation of nalbuphine hydrochloride. It is used to treat moderate to severe pain.

Nuelin

A proprietary, prescription-only preparation of theophylline. It is used to treat and prevent asthmatic attacks.

Nulacin Tablets

A proprietary, non-prescription compound preparation of calcium carbonate, magnesium carbonate, magnesium oxide and magnesium tricilicate. It can be used for the relief of indigestion, heartburn, acid indigestion and hiatus hernia.

Nurofen

A proprietary, prescription-only preparation of ibuprofen. It is used to relieve pain and inflammation in rheumatic disorders.

Nurse Sykes Powders

A proprietary, non-prescription preparation of aspirin, paracetamol and caffeine. It is used to relieve the symptoms colds and flu, mild to moderate pain and aches.

Nutrizym 10/22/GR

A proprietary, non-prescription preparation of the digestive enzyme pancreatin. It is used to treat deficiencies of digestive juices.

Nuvelle

A proprietary, prescription-only compound preparation of an estrogen and a progestogen drug. It is used in hormonal replacement therapy.

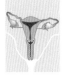 Nystatin

Properties

This medicine belongs to the family of topical (applied to the skin) antifungal preparations. It is used in the treatment of fungus infections on the skin and in the vagina. The medication fights infections such as ringworm of the scalp, athlete's foot, jockey itch, sun fungus, nail fungus and fungus infections of the vagina.

Fungal diseases may develop especially in people with disorders of immunity or diabetes and those on certain drugs (steroid, immunosuppressives, antibiotics). Thrush is common in the mouth and vagina but rarely causes systemic disease.

The drug kills fungi by damaging the fungal wall; it causes loss of essential elements to sustain fungus cell life.

Before using this medicine

Before you use this medicine check with your doctor, or pharmacist:

- if you ever had any unusual or allergic reaction to topical antifungal preparations.
- if you are on a low-salt, low-sugar, or any other special diet, or if you are allergic to any substance, such as certain preservatives or dyes.
- if you are sunburned, or have an open skin wound.
- if you are pregnant, intending to become pregnant or breast-feeding an infant while using this medicine.

Pregnant women should avoid using the vaginal cream during the first three months of pregnancy. They should use it during the next six months only if it is absolutely necessary.

Treatment

This medication is used to relieve or prevent the symptoms of your medical problem. Take them as directed. Do not take more of them and do not take them more often than recommended on the label. To do so may increase the chance of absorption through the skin and the chance of side effects. If you forget to take a dose of this drug, take it as soon as you remember. If it is almost time for your next regularly scheduled application, skip the forgotten application and continue with your regular schedule.

CREAM, LOTION, OINTMENT, GEL: Bathe and dry area before use. Apply small amount and rub gently.

POWDER: Apply lightly to the skin.

VAGINAL CREAM & TABLETS: Insert into vagina with applicator as illustrated in instructions.

The treatment may require a period of 6 to 8 weeks for a complete cure. The usual schedule calls for an application twice a day, morning and evening, unless otherwise directed by your doctor or pharmacist. Be sure to complete the full course of treatment prescribed for you.

Side effects

The following side effects may occur:

- Itching
- Swelling of treated skin
- Redness of skin
- Vaginal burning and itching
- Irritation of vagina
- Swelling of labia
- Increased discharge

You should discontinue the use of the drug when these side effects occur. Call your doctor right away.

Interactions

This medicine may interact with several other medications applied to the skin or vagina. The combined effect may cause severe skin irritation or disorders of the labia or vagina.

Storage

This medicine should be stored cool, but Do not freeze. Store away from heat and direct light. Keep out of reach of children. Do not use on other members of the family without consulting your doctor. Do not store in the bathroom medicine cabinet because the heat or moisture may cause the medicine to break down. Do not keep outdated medicine or medicine no longer needed. Flush the contents down the toilet, unless otherwise directed.

Nycopren

A y preparation of naproxen. It is used to relieve and pain of rheumatic diseases.

Nylax Tablets

A compound preparation of bisacodyl, phenolphthalein and senna. It is used to treat constipation.

Nystadermal

A proprietary, prescription-only compound preparation of nystatin and triamcinolone. It is used to treat serious fungal infections.

Nystaform

A compound preparation of nystatin and chlorhexidine. It is used to treat Candida fungal infections.

Nystaform-HC

A compound preparation of nystatin and hydrocortisone. It is used to treat infections with inflammation of the skin.

Nystatin

A proprietary, prescription-only antifungal and antibacterial drug. It is used to treat Candida fungal infections.

Nystatin-Dome

A proprietary, prescription-only compound preparation of nystatin and hydrocortisone. It is used to treat infections with inflammation of the skin.

O

Occlusal
A proprietary, non-prescription preparation of salicylic acid. It can be used to remove warts and hard skin.

Octoxinol
A spermicidal drug that is used to assist barrier methods of contraception.

Octreotide
A proprietary, prescription-only analogue of somatostatin. It can be used as an anticancer drug.

Ocufen
A proprietary, prescription-only preparation of flurbiprofen. It can be used by topical application to inhibit constriction of the pupil.

Ocusert Pilo
A preparation of pilocarpine. It can be used to constrict the pupil and treat glaucoma.

Odrik
A proprietary, prescription-only preparation of trandolapril. It can be used to treat raised blood pressure.

Oestradiol
A main female sex hormone. It can be used therapeutically to make up hormonal deficiencies.

Oestradiol Implants
A proprietary, prescription-only preparation of oestradiol. It can be used therapeutically to make up hormonal deficiencies.

Oestrifen
A proprietary, prescription-only preparation of tamoxifen. It can be used to treat estrogen-dependent cancers.

Oestriol
A main female sex hormone. It can be used therapeutically to make up hormonal deficiencies.

estrogen
Name for a group of steroid sex hormones that promote the growth and functioning of the female sex organs.

Omega-3 marine triglycerides
Lipids derived from fish oil and used as lipid-lowing drugs.

Omeprazole
A proprietary, prescription-only ulcer-healing drug. It can be used to treat benign gastric and duodenal ulcers.

Omnopon
A proprietary, prescription-only preparation of papaveretum. It can be used to treat severe pain.

Oncovin
A proprietary, prescription-only preparation of the cytotoxic drug vincristine sulphate. It can be used to treat nausea and vomiting, especially in patients receiving radiotherapy or chemotherapy.

Ondansetron
A proprietary, prescription-only antiemetic and antinauseant drug. It can be used to treat vomiting and nausea.

One-Alpha
A proprietary, prescription-only preparation of alfacalcidol. It can be used to treat a deficiency of vitamin D.

Operidine
A proprietary, prescription-only preparation of phenoperidine hydrochloride. It can be used during surgery for the relief of pain.

Ophthaine
A proprietary, prescription-only preparation of proximetracaine. It can be used during ophthalmic procedures.

Opilon
A proprietary, prescription-only preparation of thymoxamine. It can be used to treat peripheral vascular disease.

Opticrom
A proprietary, prescription-only preparation of sodium cromoglycate. It can be used to treat allergic conjunctivitis.

Opticrom Allergy Eye Drops
A proprietary, prescription-only preparation of sodium cromoglycate. It can be used to treat allergic conjunctivitis.

Optimax
A proprietary, prescription-only preparation of tryptophan. It can be used to treat long-standing depressive illness.

Optimine
A proprietary, non-prescription preparation of azatadine maleate. It can be used to relieve the symptoms of allergic reactions, such as hay fever.

Oralcer
A preparation of clioquinol. It can be used to treat infections and ulcers in the mouth.

Oraldene
A proprietary, non-prescription preparation of hexetidine. It can be used to treat minor mouth infection, including thrush.

Oramorph
A proprietary, prescription-only preparation of morphine sulphate. It can be used to relieve pain following surgery.

Orap
A proprietary, prescription-only preparation of pimozide. It can be used to treat and tranquillize patients with psychotic disorders.

Orbenin
A proprietary, prescription-only preparation of the antibacterial and antibiotic drug cloxacillin. It can be used to treat bacterial infections.

Orciprenaline sulphate
A proprietary, prescription-only beta-receptor stimulant drug. It can be used as a bronchodilator in reversible obstructive airways disorders.

Orelox
A proprietary, prescription-only preparation of the antibacterial and antibiotic drug cefprodoxime. It can be used to treat infections of the upper respiratory tract.

Optimine

Properties
This medicine contains azatadine as active ingredient; it is used to treat or prevent symptoms of allergy. This medication belongs to a group known as antihistamines. Antihistamines block the action of histamine, a chemical that is released by the body during an allergic reaction. Some of the antihistamines are also used to prevent motion sickness, nausea, vomiting, and dizziness.

Before using this medicine
Before you use this medicine check with your doctor, or pharmacist:
- if you ever had any unusual or allergic reaction to antihistamines.
- if you are on a low-salt, low-sugar, or any other special diet, or if you are allergic to any substance, such as sulfites or other preservatives or dyes.
- if you are pregnant or intending to become pregnant while using this medicine.
- if you are breast-feeding an infant. Small amounts of antihistamines pass into the breast milk. Use is not recommended since the chances are greater for most antihistamines to cause side effects, such as unusual excitement or irritability in the infant.
- if you have any of the following medical problems:
  Asthma attack
  Enlarged prostate
  Glaucoma
  Urinary tract blockage
  Difficult urination

Treatment
This medication is used to relieve or prevent the symptoms of your medical problem. Take them as directed. Do not take more of them and do not take them more often than recommended on the label, unless otherwise directed by your doctor. To do so may increase the chance of side effects.

Side effects
The following minor side effects may occur:
- Blurred vision
- Confusion
- Constipation
- Diarrhea
- Difficult or painful urination
- Dizziness
- Dry mouth, throat, or nose
- Headache
- Irritability
- Loss of appetite
- Nausea or stomach upset
- Ringing or buzzing in the ears
- Unusual increase in sweating.

These side effects should disappear as your body adjusts to the medication.

Tell your doctor about any side effects that are persistent or particularly bothersome. It is especially important to tell your doctor about a change in menstruation, clumsiness, feeling faint, flushing of the face, hallucinations, rash, palpitations, seizures, shortness of breath, fever, sleeping disorders, sore throat, tightness in the chest, unusual bleeding or bruising, or unusual tiredness or weakness.

Interactions
This medicine interacts with several other drugs such as central nervous system depressants and it can decrease the activity of oral anticoagulants.
Be sure to tell your doctor about any medications you are currently taking.

Storage
Tablets, elixir, etc. should be stored at room temperature in tightly closed containers. Sore away from heat and direct light. Keep out of reach of children, since overdose may be very dangerous in children. Do not keep outdated medicine or medicine no longer needed. Flush the contents of the container down the toilet, unless otherwise directed.

Orgafol
A proprietary, prescription-only preparation of urofollitrophin. It can be used to treat infertility in women.

Orgaran
A proprietary, prescription-only preparation of danaparoid sodium. It can be used to prevent deep vein thrombosis.

Original Andrews Salts
A proprietary, non-prescription compound preparation of bicarbonate, magnesium sulphate and citric acid. It can be used to treat upset stomach, indigestion and dyspepsia.

Orimeten
A proprietary, prescription-only preparation of aminoglutethimide. It can be used to treat various types of cancer.

Orlept
A proprietary, prescription-only preparation of sodium valproate. It can be used to treat all forms of epilepsy.

Orphenadrine citrate
A proprietary, prescription-only anticholinergic drug. It can be used for the symptomatic relief of skeletal muscle spasm.

Orphenadrine hydrochloride
A proprietary, prescription-only anticholinergic drug. It can be used for

Oral contraceptives

These are prophylactic (preventive) sex hormone preparations, which are taken by women to prevent conception following sexual intercourse and are commonly referred to as the pill. The majority of oral contraceptives contain both an estrogen and a progestogen.

The estrogen inhibits the release of follicle-stimulating hormone (FSH) and prevents the development, the progestogen inhibits release of luteinizing hormone (LH), prevents ovulation and makes the cervix mucus unsuitable for sperm.

Their combined action is to alter the uterine lining (endometrium) and prevent any fertilized egg from implanting. This type of preparation is known as the combined oral contraception, or combined pill, and is taken daily for three weeks and stopped for one week during which menstruation occurs.

Two forms of the combined pill (the phased formulation) are the biphasic and triphasic pills. In these the hormonal content varies according to the time of the month at which each pill is to be taken (and are produced in a "calendar pack") and the dose is reduced to the bare minimum.

Another type of pill is the progestogen-only pill and this is though to work by making the cervical mucus inhospitable to sperm and by preventing implantation. This form has the advantage that is can be used by breast-feeding women.

the symptomatic relief of symptoms of parkinsonism.

Ortho-Creme
A proprietary, non-prescription spermicidal contraceptive for use in combination with barrier methods of contraception.

Ortho Dienoestrol
A proprietary, prescription-only preparation of dienoestrol. It can be used to treat infection and irritation of the membranous surface of the vagina.

Ortho-Gynest
A proprietary, prescription-only preparation of oestriol. It can be used to treat infection and irritation of the membranous surface of the vagina.

Ortho-Gynol
A proprietary, non-prescription spermicidal contraceptive for use in combination with barrier methods of contraception.

Ortho Novin 1/50
A proprietary, prescription-only preparation of an estrogen and a progestogen. It can be used to treat menstrual disorders and as an oral contraceptive.

Orudis
A proprietary, prescription-only preparation of ketoprofen. It can be used to treat pain and inflammation of rheumatic disorders.

Oruvail Gel 2.5 %
A proprietary, prescription-only preparation of ketoprofen. It can be used to treat pain and inflammation of rheumatic disorders.

Osmolax
A proprietary, non-prescription preparation of lactulose. It can be used to treat constipation.

Ossopan
A proprietary, non-prescription preparation of calcium carbonate. It can be used as a mineral supplement.

Otex
A proprietary, non-prescription com-

bined preparation of hydrogen peroxide and urea. It can be used to dissolve and wash out earwax.

Otomize
A proprietary, prescription-only compound preparation of dexamethasone and neomycin sulphate. It can be used to treat bacterial infections in the outer ear.

Otosporin
A proprietary, prescription-only compound preparation of hydrocortisone and neomycin sulphate. It can be used to treat bacterial infections in the outer ear.

Otrivine Adult Formula Drops
A proprietary, non-prescription preparation of xylometazoline hydrochloride. It can be used as a nasal congestant.

Otrivine Adult Formula Spray
A proprietary, non-prescription preparation of xylometazoline hydrochloride. It can be used as a nasal congestant, rhinitis and sinusitis.

Otrivine-Antistin
A compound preparation of xylometazoline hydrochloride and antazoline sulphate. It can be used for the relief of allergic conjunctivitis.

Otrivine Children's Formula Spray
A proprietary, non-prescription preparation of xylometazoline hydrochloride. It can be used as a nasal congestant, rhinitis and sinusitis.

Otrivine-Antistin
A proprietary, non-prescription compound preparation of xylometazoline hydrochloride and antazoline sulphate. It can be used for the relief of allergic conjunctivitis.

Otrivine Children's Formula Drops
A proprietary, non-prescription preparation of xylometazoline hydrochloride. It can be used for the relief of nasal congestion and rhinitis.

Ovestin
A proprietary, prescription-only pre-

paration of oestril. It can be used in hormone replacement therapy.

Ovex Tablets
A proprietary, non-prescription preparation of mebendazole. It can be used to treat infection by threadworms.

Ovran
A proprietary, prescription-only compound preparation of an estrogen and a progestogen. It can be used to treat menstrual problems and as an oral contraceptive.

Ovran 30
A proprietary, prescription-only compound preparation of an estrogen and a progestogen. It can be used to treat menstrual problems and as an oral contraceptive.

Ovranette
A proprietary, prescription-only compound preparation of an estrogen and a progestogen. It can be used to treat menstrual problems and as an oral contraceptive.

Ovysmen
A proprietary, prescription-only compound preparation of an estrogen and a progestogen. It can be used to treat menstrual problems and as an oral contraceptive.

Owbridge's for Dry Tickly and Allergy Coughs
A proprietary, non-prescription preparation of dextromethorphan hydrobromide and glycerine. It can be used for the symptomatic relief of dry, ticklish unproductive coughs.

Oxatomide
A proprietary, prescription-only antihistamine drug. It can be used to relieve the symptoms of hay fever, urticaria and food allergy.

Oxazepam
A proprietary, prescription-only benzodiazepine drug. It can be used to treat anxiety.

Oxerutins
A mixture of rutosides that are thought to reduce the fragility and the permeability of capillary blood vessels. It can be used to treat disorders of the veins.

Oxethazaine
A proprietary, prescription-only local anesthetic drug. It can be used for the relief of local pain.

Oxitropium bromide
A proprietary, prescription-only anticholinergic drug. It can be used to treat chronic bronchitis.

Oxivent
A proprietary, prescription-only preparation of oxitropium bromide. It can be used to treat chronic bronchitis.

Oxpentifylline
A proprietary, prescription-only vasodilator drug. It can be used to treat peripheral vascular disease.

Oxprenolol hydrochloride
A beta-blocker drug. It can be used to treat and prevent angina pectoris and to regularize heartbeat.

Oxy 5 Lotion
A proprietary, non-prescription preparation of benzoyl peroxide. It can be used to treat acne.

Oxy 10 Lotion
A proprietary, non-prescription preparation of benzoyl peroxide. It can be used to treat acne.

Oxybuprocaine hydrochloride
A proprietary, prescription-only local anesthetic drug. It can be used by topical application in ophthalmic procedures.

Oxybutynin hydrochloride
A proprietary, prescription-only anticholinergic drug. It can be used to treat urinary frequency incontinence and bladder spasms.

Oxymetazoline hydrochloride
A proprietary, prescription-only adrenoreceptor stimulant. It can be used to treat nasal congestion.

Oxymetholone
A proprietary, prescription-only anabolic steroid. It can be used to treat aplastic anemia.

Oxymycin
A proprietary, prescription-only preparation of the antibacterial and antibiotic drug oxytetracycline. It can be used to treat a wide range of infections.

Oxypertine
A proprietary, prescription-only antipsychotic drug. It can be used to treat and tranquillize psychotic patients.

Oxyphenisatin
A proprietary, non-prescription stimulant laxative. It can be used to treat constipation.

Oxyphenisatine
A proprietary, non-prescription stimulant laxative. It can be used to treat constipation.

Oxyprenix SR
A proprietary, prescription-only preparation of oxprenolol. It can be used to treat and prevent angina pectoris.

Oxytetracycline
A proprietary, prescription-only antibacterial and antibiotic drug. It can be used to treat many serious infections.

Oxytetramix
A proprietary, prescription-only preparation of the antibacterial and antibiotic drug oxytetracycline. It can be used to treat many serious infections.

Oxytocin
A natural pituitary hormone produced and secreted by the posterior pituitary gland. It can be used to induce or assist labour.

O

P

Pacifene
A proprietary, non-prescription preparation of ibuprofen. It can be used for the relief of pain, including headache, period pain, muscular pain, dental pain and feverishness.

Pacifene Maximum Strength
A proprietary, non-prescription preparation of ibuprofen. It can be used for the relief of pain, including headache, period pain, muscular pain, dental pain and feverishness.

Paclitaxel
A proprietary, prescription-only cytotoxic drug. It can be used tin the treatment of ovarian cancer.

Paldesic
A proprietary, non-prescription preparation of paracetamol. It can be used to reduce fever in infants.

Palfium
A proprietary, prescription-only preparation of dextromoramide. It can be used to treat severe pain.

Paludrine
A proprietary, prescription-only preparation of proguanil. It can be used to treat and prevent malaria.

Pamergan P100
A proprietary, prescription-only compound preparation of pethidine hydrochloride and promethazine hydrochloride. It can be used to relieve pain, especially during childhood.

Pameton
A proprietary, non-prescription compound preparation of paracetamol and methionine. It can be used to provide relief from painful and feverish conditions.

Panadeine Tablets
A proprietary, non-prescription compound preparation of paracetamol and codeine phosphate. It can be used to treat pain, sore throat, period pain, arthritis and rheumatoid pain.

Panadol Capsules
A proprietary, non-prescription preparation of paracetamol. It can be used to treat feverishness and symptoms of colds and flu and musculoskeletal pain.

Panadol Extra Soluble Tablets
A proprietary, non-prescription compound preparation of paracetamol and caffeine. It can be used to treat feverishness, symptoms of colds and flu and musculoskeletal pain.

Panadol Extra Tablets
A proprietary, non-prescription compound preparation of paracetamol and caffeine. It can be used to treat feverishness, symptoms of colds and flu and musculoskeletal pain.

Panadol Junior
A preparation of paracetamol. It can be used to treat feverishness, symptoms of colds and flu and musculoskeletal pain.

Panadol Soluble
A proprietary, non-prescription preparation of paracetamol. It can be used to treat feverishness, symptoms of colds and flu and musculoskeletal pain.

Panadol Tablets
A proprietary, non-prescription preparation of paracetamol. It can be used to treat feverishness, symptoms of colds and flu and musculoskeletal pain.

Panadol Ultra
A proprietary, non-prescription compound preparation of paracetamol and caffeine. It can be used to treat feverishness, symptoms of colds and flu and musculoskeletal pain.

Pancrease
A proprietary, non-prescription preparation of pancreatin. It can be used to treat a deficiency of the digestive juices.

Pancrease HL
A proprietary, non-prescription preparation of pancreatin. It can be used to treat a deficiency of the digestive juices.

Pancreatin
A proprietary, non-prescription extract of the pancreas. It can be used to treat a deficiency of the digestive juices.

Pancrex
A proprietary, non-prescription preparation of pancreatin. It can be used to treat a deficiency of the digestive juices.

Pancrex V
A proprietary, non-prescription preparation of pancreatin. It can be used to treat a deficiency of the digestive juices.

Pancuronium bromide
A proprietary, non-prescription skeletal muscle relaxant drug. It can be used to induce muscle paralysis during surgery.

Panda Baby Cream
A proprietary, non-prescription compound preparation of zinc oxide, castor oil and wool fat. It can be used as a barrier cream for nappy rash.

Panoxyl 5 Gel
A proprietary, non-prescription preparation of the keratolytic and antimicrobial drug benzoyl peroxide. It can be used to treat acne.

Panoxyl 10 Gel
A proprietary, non-prescription preparation of the keratolytic and antimicrobial drug benzoyl peroxide. It can be used to treat acne.

Panoxyl Aquagel 10
A proprietary, non-prescription preparation of the keratolytic and antimicrobial drug benzoyl peroxide. It can be used to treat acne.

Panoxyl Aquagel 25
A proprietary, non-prescription preparation of the keratolytic and antimicrobial drug benzoyl peroxide. It can be used to treat acne.

Panoxyl Wash
A proprietary, non-prescription preparation of the keratolytic and antimicrobial drug benzoyl peroxide. It can be used to treat acne.

Fever
Pain
Infection

Panadol

Properties
This medicine contains as active ingredient acetaminophen, a medicine used to relieve pain and reduce fever. Buffered acetaminophen is used only to relieve pain, especially when an antacid is also needed to relieve an upset stomach.

Before using this medicine
Before you use this medicine check with your doctor, or pharmacist:
- if you ever had any unusual or allergic reaction to acetaminophen or related compounds.
- if you are on a low-salt, low-sugar, or any other special diet, or if you are allergic to any substance, such as sulfites or other preservatives or dyes.
- if you are pregnant or intending to become pregnant while using this medicine. Studies on birth defects have not been done in humans.
- if you are breast-feeding an infant. Although this medicine has not been shown to cause problems in humans, it passes into the breast milk in small amounts.
- if you have any of the following medical problems:
  Virus infection of the liver
  Alcohol abuse
  Kidney disease
  Liver disease
- if you are now taking any of the following medicines:
  Anticoagulants
  Antihistamines
  Antineoplastics
  Barbiturates
  Contraceptives
  Corticosteroids
  Estrogens
  Sulfapreparations

Treatment
This medication is used to relieve pain and reduce fever. Unlike aspirin, it does not relieve the redness, stiffness, or swelling caused by rheumatoid arthritis.
Unless otherwise directed by your doctor or pharmacist take this as directed. Do not take more of them and do not take them more often than recommended on the label.
Children up to 12 years of age should not take this medicine more than 3 times a day or for more than 5 days in a row.

Side effects
Along with the needed effects, a medicine may cause some unwanted effects. Although the following side effects occur very rarely when this medicine is taken as recommended, they may be more likely to occur if:
- too much medicine is taken;
- it is taken in large doses;
- it is taken for a long period of time;
- it is taken by patients with kidney disease.
This drug is relatively free from side effects.
Check with your doctor immediately if any of the following side effects occur: yellowing of eyes or skin; bloody or cloudy urine; difficult or painful urination; skin rash, hives, or itching; sudden decrease in amount of urine; unexplained sore throat and fever; unusual bleeding or bruising; unusual tiredness or weakness.

Interactions
This medicine may interact with several other drugs such as adrenocorticosteroids, aspirin, caffeine-containing medications; theophylline, antibiotics, sulfonamides, etc.
Be sure to tell your doctor about any medications you are currently taking.

Storage
Tablets, elixir, suppository etc. should be stored at room temperature and away from direct light. Keep out of reach of children, since overdose may be very dangerous in children. Do not store in the bathroom medicine cabinet because the heat or moisture may cause the medicine to break down. Do not keep outdated medicine.

P

Panzytrat 25.000
A preparation of pancreatin. It can be used to treat a deficiency of the digestive juices.

Papavereton
A preparation of alkaloids of opium. It can be used to treat pain during or following surgery.

Papaverine
A prescription-only smooth muscle relaxant. It can be used to treat pain.

Paracetamol
A proprietary, non-prescription non-narcotic analgesic drug. It can be used to treat all forms of mild to moderate pain. (see page 726)

Paracets
A proprietary, non-prescription preparation of the non-narcotic analgesic drug paracetamol. It can be used to treat all forms of mild to moderate pain.

Paracets Capsules
A proprietary, non-prescription preparation of the non-narcotic analgesic drug paracetamol. It can be used to treat all forms of mild to moderate pain.

Paraclear
A proprietary, non-prescription preparation of the non-narcotic analgesic drug paracetamol. It can be used to treat all forms of mild to moderate pain.

Fever
Pain
Infection

Paracetamol

Properties
This medicine contains as active ingredient acetaminophen, a medicine used to relieve pain and reduce fever. Buffered acetaminophen is used only to relieve pain, especially when an antacid is also needed to relieve an upset stomach.

Before using this medicine
Before you use this medicine check with your doctor, or pharmacist:
- if you ever had any unusual or allergic reaction to acetaminophen or related compounds.
- if you are on a low-salt, low-sugar, or any other special diet, or if you are allergic to any substance, such as sulfites or other preservatives or dyes.
- if you are pregnant or intending to become pregnant while using this medicine. Studies on birth defects have not been done in humans.
- if you are breast-feeding an infant. Although this medicine has not been shown to cause problems in humans, it passes into the breast milk in small amounts.
- if you have any of the following medical problems:
  Virus infection of the liver.
  Alcohol abuse.
  Kidney disease.
  Liver disease.
- if you are now taking any of the following medicines:
  Anticoagulants
  Antihistamines
  Antineoplastics
  Barbiturates
  Contraceptives
  Corticosteroids
  Estrogens
  Sulfapreparations

Treatment
This medication is used to relieve pain and reduce fever. Unlike aspirin, it does not relieve the redness, stiffness, or swelling caused by rheumatoid arthritis.
Unless otherwise directed by your doctor or pharmacist take this as directed. Do not take more of them and do not take them more often than recommended on the label.
Children up to 12 years of age should not take this medicine more than 3 times a day or for more than 5 days in a row.

Side effects
Along with the needed effects, a medicine may cause some unwanted effects. Although the following side effects occur very rarely when this medicine is taken as recommended, they may be more likely to occur if:
- too much medicine is taken;
- it is taken in large doses;
- it is taken for a long period of time;
- it is taken by patients with kidney disease.
This drug is relatively free from side effects.
Check with your doctor immediately if any of the following side effects occur: yellowing of eyes or skin; bloody or cloudy urine; difficult or painful urination; skin rash, hives, or itching; sudden decrease in amount of urine; unexplained sore throat and fever; unusual bleeding or bruising; unusual tiredness or weakness.

Interactions
This medicine may interact with several other drugs such as adrenocorticosteroids, aspirin, caffeine-containing medications; theophylline, antibiotics, sulfonamides, etc.
Be sure to tell your doctor about any medications you are currently taking.

Storage
Tablets, elixir, suppository etc. should be stored at room temperature and away from direct light. Keep out of reach of children, since overdose may be very dangerous in children. Do not store in the bathroom medicine cabinet because the heat or moisture may cause the medicine to break down. Do not keep outdated medicine.

Paraclear Extra Strength
A proprietary, non-prescription preparation of the non-narcotic analgesic drug paracetamol and caffeine. It can be used to treat all forms of mild to moderate pain.

Paraclear Junior
A proprietary, non-prescription preparation of the non-narcotic analgesic drug paracetamol. It can be used to treat all forms of mild to moderate pain.

Paracodol Capsules/ Tablets
A proprietary, non-prescription compound preparation of the non-narcotic analgesic drug paracetamol and codeine phosphate. It can be used to treat all forms of mild to moderate pain and to reduce high body temperature.

Paraffin
A hydrocarbon derived from petroleum. It can be used to treat constipation.

Parake
A proprietary, non-prescription compound preparation of the non-narcotic analgesic drug paracetamol and codeine phosphate. It can be used to treat all forms of mild to moderate pain and to reduce high body temperature.

Paraldehyde
A proprietary, prescription-only anticonvulsant. It can be used in the treatment of status epilepticus.

Paramax

A proprietary, prescription-only preparation of metoclopramide hydrochloride and paracetamol. It can be used to treat migraine.

Paramol Tablets

A proprietary, prescription-only preparation of dihydrocodeine tartrate and paracetamol. It can be used for general pain relief.

Paraplatin

A proprietary, prescription-only preparation of carboplatin. It can be used to treat ovarian cancer.

Parlodel

A proprietary, prescription-only preparation of bromocriptine. It can be used to treat symptoms of parkinsonisme.

Parmid

A proprietary, prescription-only preparation of metoclopramide. It can be used to treat nausea and vomiting.

Parnate

A proprietary, prescription-only monoamine-oxidase inhibitor drug. It can be used to treat depressive illness.

Paroven

A proprietary, prescription-only preparation of oxerutins. It can be used to treat cramp and other manifestations of poor circulation.

Paoxetine

A proprietary, prescription-only antidepressant drug. It can be used to treat depressive illness.

Parstelin

A proprietary, prescription-only compound preparation of tranylcypromine and trifluoperazine. It can be used to treat depressive illness.

Partobulin

A proprietary, prescription-only preparation of an anti-immunoglobulin. It can be used to prevent rhesus-negative mothers from making antibodies against foetal rhesus-positive cells.

Parvolex

A proprietary, prescription-only preparation of acetylcysteine. It can be used to treat overdose poisoning by paracetamol.

Pavadol

A proprietary, non-prescription preparation of pholcodine. It can be used to treat painful coughs.

Pavulon

A proprietary, prescription-only preparation of pancuronium bromide. It can be used to induce muscle paralysis during surgery.

Pecram

A proprietary, non-prescription preparation of aminophylline. It can be used in the treatment of asthma and bronchitis.

Pemoline

A proprietary, prescription-only amphetamine preparation. It can be used to treat hyperactivity (ADHD) in children.

Penbritin

A proprietary, prescription-only preparation of the antibacterial and antibiotic drug ampicillin. It can be used to treat systemic bacterial infections.

Pendramine

A proprietary, prescription-only preparation of penicillamine. It can be used as an antidote to copper or lead poisoning.

Penetrol Inhalant

A proprietary, non-prescription compound preparation of the aromatic oils peppermint and menthol. It can be used for the symptomatic relief of nasal congestion associated with catarrh, hay fever and colds.

Penicillamine

A proprietary, prescription-only derivative of penicillin. It can be used as an antidote to various types of metallic poisoning.

Penicillin

A proprietary, prescription-only antibiotic and antibacterial drug. It can

Penicillin

This is an antibacterial and antibiotic drug that works by interfering with the synthesis of bacterial cell walls. The early penicillins were mainly effective against Gram-positive bacteria, though they could be used against Gram-negative organisms that caused gonorrhoea and meningitis, as well as the organisms causing syphilis.

Later penicillins (for example ampicillin and piperacillin) expanded the spectrum to include an greater range of Gram-negative microorganisms. The are absorbed rapidly by most (but not all) body tissues and fluids and are excreted in the urine.

One great disadvantage of penicillins is that many patients are allergic to them - allergy to one, means allergy to all of them - and may have reactions that range from a minor rash right up to anaphylactic shock, which occasionally can be fatal. Otherwise they are remarkably non-toxic.

Rarely, very high dosage may cause convulsions, hemolytic anemia, or abnormally high levels of sodium or potassium in the body with consequent symptoms. Those taken orally tend to cause diarrhea and there is also a risk with broad-spectrum penicillins of allowing a superinfection to develop.

be used to treat various types of infections.

PenMix 10/90

A proprietary, prescription-only preparation of human biphasic isophane insulin. It can be used as a diabetic therapy to treat and maintain diabetic patients.

PenMix 20/80
A proprietary, prescription-only preparation of human biphasic isophane insulin. It can be used as a diabetic therapy to treat and maintain diabetic patients.

PenMix 30/70
A proprietary, prescription-only preparation of human biphasic isophane insulin. It can be used as a diabetic therapy to treat and maintain diabetic patients.

PenMix 40/60
A proprietary, prescription-only preparation of human biphasic isophane insulin. It can be used as a diabetic therapy to treat and maintain diabetic patients.

PenMix 50/50
A proprietary, prescription-only preparation of human biphasic isophane insulin. It can be used as a diabetic therapy to treat and maintain diabetic patients.

Pentacarinat
A proprietary, prescription-only preparation of the antiprotozoal drug pentamidine isothionate. It can be used to treat pneumonia caused by Pneumocystis carinii.

Pentaerythritol tetranitrate
A proprietary, prescription-only vasodilator drug. It can be used to treat angina pectoris.

Pentamidine isothionate
A proprietary, prescription-only antiprotozoal drug. It can be used to treat pneumonia caused by Pneumocystis carinii.

Pentamidine isotionate
A proprietary, prescription-only antiprotozoal drug. It can be used to treat pneumonia caused by Pneumocystis carinii.

Pentasa
A proprietary, prescription-only preparation of mesalazine. It can be used to treat ulcerative colitis.

Pentazocine
A proprietary, prescription-only narcotic analgesic drug. It can be used to treat moderate to severe pain.

Pentostam
A proprietary, prescription-only preparation of stibogluconate. It can be used to treat skin infections by protozoal organisms.

Pentran
A proprietary, prescription-only preparation of phenytoin. It can be used to treat all forms of seizures and trigeminal neuralgia.

Pentrax
A proprietary, non-prescription preparation of coal tar. It can be used to treat skin conditions such as dandruff.

Pepcid
A proprietary, prescription-only preparation of the ulcer-healing drug famotidine. It can be used to treat benign peptic ulcers.

Pepcid AC
A proprietary, prescription-only preparation of the ulcer-healing drug famotidine. It can be used to treat benign peptic ulcers.

Peptimax
A proprietary, prescription-only preparation of the ulcer-healing drug cimetidine. It can be used to treat benign peptic ulcers.

Percutol
A proprietary, prescription-only preparation of glyceryl trinitrate. It can be used to treat and prevent angina pectoris.

Perfan
A proprietary, prescription-only preparation of enoximone. It can be used to treat heart failure disorders.

Pergolide
A proprietary, prescription-only ergot-derivative. It can be used to treat symptoms of parkinsonism.

Pergolal
A proprietary, prescription-only preparation of human menopausal gonadotrophin. It can be used to treat infertility in women.

Periactin
A proprietary, non-prescription preparation of cyprohepatine hydrochloride. It can be used for the symptomatic relief of allergic disorders.

Pericyazine
A proprietary, prescription-only phenothiazine derivative. It can be used to treat schizophrenia and other psychoses.

Perinal
A proprietary, prescription-only compound preparation of hydrocortisone and lignocaine. It can be used to treat hemorrhoids and inflammation in the anal region.

Perindopril
A proprietary, prescription-only ACE inhibitor drug. It can be used to treat raised blood pressure and heart failure conditions.

Permitabs
A proprietary, non-prescription preparation of potassium permanganate. It can be used for cleaning of wounds.

Perphenazine
A proprietary, prescription-only phenothiazine derivative. It can be used to treat schizophrenia and other psychoses.

Persantin
A proprietary, prescription-only preparation of dipyridamole. It can be used to prevent thrombosis.

Pertofran
A proprietary, prescription-only preparation of desipramine. It can be used to treat depressive illness.

Pethidine hydrochloride
A proprietary, prescription-only narcotic analgesic drug. It can be used to treat moderate to severe pain.

Pevaryl
A proprietary, non-prescription preparation of econazole nitrate. It can be used to treat fungal infections on the skin.

Phenindamine

Properties
This medicine contains phenindamine as active ingredient; it is used to treat or prevent symptoms of allergy. This medication belongs to a group known as antihistamines. Antihistamines block the action of histamine, a chemical that is released by the body during an allergic reaction. Some of the antihistamines are also used to prevent motion sickness, nausea, vomiting, and dizziness.

Before using this medicine
Before you use this medicine check with your doctor, or pharmacist:
- if you ever had any unusual or allergic reaction to antihistamines.
- if you are on a low-salt, low-sugar, or any other special diet, or if you are allergic to any substance, such as sulfites or other preservatives or dyes.
- if you are pregnant or intending to become pregnant while using this medicine.
- if you are breast-feeding an infant. Small amounts of antihistamines pass into the breast milk. Use is not recommended since the chances are greater for most antihistamines to cause side effects, such as unusual excitement or irritability in the infant.
- if you have any of the following medical problems:
  Asthma attack
  Enlarged prostate
  Urinary tract blockage
  Difficult urination

Treatment
This medication is used to relieve or prevent the symptoms of your medical problem. Take them as directed. Do not take more of them and do not take them more often than recommended on the label, unless otherwise directed by your doctor. To do so may increase the chance of side effects.

Side effects
The following minor side effects may occur:
- Blurred vision
- Confusion
- Constipation
- Diarrhea
- Difficult or painful urination
- Dizziness
- Dry mouth, throat, or nose
- Headache
- Loss of appetite
- Nausea or stomach upset
- Unusual increase in sweating.

These side effects should disappear as your body adjusts to the medication.
Tell your doctor about any side effects that are persistent or particularly bothersome. It is especially important to tell your doctor about a change in menstruation, clumsiness, feeling faint, flushing of the face, hallucinations, rash, palpitations, seizures, shortness of breath, fever, sleeping disorders, sore throat, tightness in the chest, unusual bleeding or bruising, or unusual tiredness or weakness.

Interactions
This medicine interacts with several other drugs such as central nervous system depressants and it can decrease the activity of oral anticoagulants.
Be sure to tell your doctor about any medications you are currently taking.

Storage
Tablets, elixir, etc. should be stored at room temperature in tightly closed containers. Store away from heat and direct light. Keep out of reach of children, since overdose may be very dangerous in children. Do not keep outdated medicine or medicine no longer needed. Flush the contents of the container down the toilet, unless otherwise directed.

Pevaryl TC
A proprietary, non-prescription compound preparation of econazole nitrate and triamcinolone. It can be used to treat fungal infections on the skin.

Phasal
A preparation of lithium. It can be used to treat acute mania, manic-depressive bouts and recurrent depression.

Phenazocine hydrobromide
A proprietary, prescription-only narcotic analgesic drug. It can be used for the relief of severe pain.

Phenelzine
A proprietary, prescription-only anti-depressant drug. It can be used to treat depressive illness.

Phenergan
A preparation of promethazine. It can be used to treat allergic disorders of the upper respiratory tract.

Phenindamine tartrate
A proprietary, non-prescription anti-histamine drug. It can be used for the symptomatic relief of allergic symptoms.

Phenindione
A anticoagulant drug. It can be used in the treatment and prevention of thrombosis.

Pheniramine maleate
A proprietary, prescription-only anti-histamine drug. It can be used for the relief of allergic symptoms.

Phenobarbital
A proprietary, prescription-only barbiturate drug. It can be used to treat and prevent most types of recurrent epileptic seizures.

Phenobarbitone

A proprietary, prescription-only barbiturate drug. It can be used to treat and prevent most types of recurrent epileptic seizures.

Phenolphthalein

A proprietary, non-prescription stimulant laxative. It can be used to treat constipation.

Phenoperidine hydrochloride

A proprietary, prescription-only narcotic analgesic drug. It can be used to relieve pain during surgery.

Phenoxybenzamine

A proprietary, prescription-only adrenoreceptor blocker drug. It can be used to treat raised blood pressure and hypertensive crisis.

Phensedyl Plus

A proprietary, non-prescription compound preparation of promethazine hydrochloride and pseudoephedrine hydrochloride. It can be used for the symptomatic relief of coughs and colds.

Phensic

A proprietary, non-prescription-only preparation of aspirin and caffeine. It can be used to treat mild to moderate pain, and to relieve the symptoms of colds and coughs.

Phentermine

A proprietary, prescription-only appetite suppressant drug. It can be used to treat obesity.

Phentolamine mesylate

A proprietary, prescription-only adrenoceptor blocker drug. It can be used to treat raised blood pressure and hypertensive crisis.

Phenylbutazone

A proprietary, prescription-only non-narcotic analgesic and antirheumatic drug. It can be used in the treatment of ankylosing spondylitis.

Phenylephrine hydrochloride

A proprietary, prescription-only vasoconstrictor drug. It can be used to treat low blood pressure.

Phenytoin

A proprietary, prescription-only anticonvulsant drug. It can be used to treat most forms of epilepsy.

Phimetin

A proprietary, prescription-only preparation of cimetidine. It can be used to treat benign peptic ulcers.

Phiso-med

A preparation of chlorhexidine. It can be used to treat ance and seborrhoeic conditions.

Pholcodine

A proprietary, prescription-only weak opioid drug. It can be used as a cough suppressant.

Pholcomed

A proprietary, prescription-only preparation of the weak opioid drug pholcodine. It can be used as a cough suppressant.

PhorPain

A proprietary, prescription-only preparation of ibuprofen. It can be used to treat headache, backache, muscular pain, dental pain and cold and flu symptoms.

Phyllocontin Continus

A proprietary, non-prescription preparation of aminophylline. It can be used to treat asthma and bronchitis.

Physostigmine sulphate

A proprietary, prescription-only anticholinesterase drug. It can be used to stimulate the pupil of the eye.

Phytex

A proprietary, non-prescription compound preparation of salicylic acid, tannic acid and boric acid. It can be used to treat fungal infections of the skin.

Picolax

A proprietary, non-prescription compound preparation of sodium picosulphate and magnesium citrate. It can be used to treat in pre-surgical procedures.

Pilocarpine

A proprietary, prescription-only parasympathicomimetic drug. It can be used to dilate the pupil for ophthalmological procedures.

Pimozide

A proprietary, prescription-only antipsychotic drug. It can be used to treat schizophrenia and other psychoses.

Pindolol

A beta-blocker drug. It can be used to treat raised blood pressure and angina pectoris.

Pipenzolate bromide

A proprietary, prescription-only anticholinergic drug. It can be used to treat gastrointestinal spasms.

Piperacillin

A proprietary, prescription-only antibacterial and antibiotic drug. It can be used to treat many serious bacterial infections.

Piperazine

A proprietary, prescription-only phenothiazine derivative. It can be used to treat infestation by roundworm or threadworm.

Piportil Depot

A proprietary, prescription-only preparation of pipothiazine. It can be used to treat chronic schizophrenia and other psychotic disorders.

Pipothiazine palmitate

A proprietary, prescription-only antipsychotic drug. It can be used to treat chronic schizophrenia and other psychotic disorders.

Pipotiazine palmitate

A proprietary, prescription-only antipsychotic drug. It can be used to treat chronic schizophrenia and other psychotic disorders.

Pipril

A proprietary, prescription-only preparation of the antibacterial and antibiotic drug piperacillin. It can be used to treat many serious bacterial infections.

Piptalin

A proprietary, prescription-only com-

Fever
Pain
Infection

Piroxicam

Properties
This medicine contains as active ingredient piroxicam. It belongs to the group of medicines called non-steroidal anti-inflammatory drugs (NSAIDs). These drugs are taken by mouth to relieve some symptoms caused by arthritis or rheumatism, such as inflammation, swelling, stiffness, and joint pain. However, these medicines do not cure arthritis and will help you only as long as you continue to take them. Some of these medicines are also used to relieve other kinds of pain or to treat other painful conditions, such as gout attacks, bursitis, tendinitis, sprains, strains, menstrual cramps. The drug reduces the tissue concentration of prostaglandins.

Before using this medicine
Before you use this medicine check with your doctor, or pharmacist:
- if you ever had any unusual or allergic reaction, such as skin rash, hives, or itching or breathing problems, to any of the anti-inflammatory analgesics.
- if you are on a low-salt, low-sugar, or any other special diet, or if you are allergic to any substance, such as sulfites or other preservatives or dyes.
- if you are pregnant or intending to become pregnant while using this medicine. Studies on birth defects have not been done in humans. However, if taken regularly during the last months of pregnancy, there is a chance that these medicines may cause unwanted effects on the heart or blood flow in the fetus or newborn infant.
- if you are breast-feeding an infant. Although this medicine has not been shown to cause problems in humans, it passes into the breast milk in small amounts.
- if you have any of the following medical problems:
Asthma
Bleeding problems
Colitis, or other intestinal problems
Stomach ulcer
Heart disease
High blood pressure
Kidney or liver disease

Treatment
This medication is used to relieve pain or other symptoms caused by arthritis. For safe and effective use of this medicine, do not take more of it, do not take it more often, and do not take it for a longer period of time than ordered by your physician or directed by the package label.
If you are taking this medication on a regular schedule and you miss a dose, take the missed dose as soon as possible, unless it is almost time for your next dose. In that case do not take the missed dose at all.
To lessen stomach upset, anti-inflammatory analgesics may be taken with food or antacids.

Side effects
Along with the needed effects, a medicine may cause some unwanted effects. These side effects may go away during treatment as your body adjusts to the medicine. Such minor side effects are: dizziness; nausea; pain; headache; drowsiness; swollen feet, face or leg; constipation or diarrhea; vomiting; dry mouth.
Check with your doctor immediately if any of the following side effects occur:
- *Muscle cramps*
- *Numbness or tingling*
- *Mouth ulcers*
- *Convulsions or confusion*
- *Rash, hives, or itch*
- *Tightness in chest*

Interactions
This medicine may interact with several other drugs.
Be sure to tell your doctor about any medications you are currently taking.

Storage
The medicine should be stored at room temperature in a tightly closed, light-resistant container. Store away from heat and direct light. Keep out of reach of children.

P

---

pound preparation of pipenzolate and dimethicone. It can be used for the relief of stomach muscle spasm.

Piracetam
A proprietary, prescription-only antispasmodic drug. It n be used to treat myoclonus.

Pirbuterol
A proprietary, prescription-only sympathicomimetic drug. It can be used

as a bronchodilator in various disorders of the upper respiratory tract.

Pirenzepine
A proprietary, prescription-only anticholinergic drug. It can be used to reduce the production of gastric acid.

Piretanide
A proprietary, prescription-only diuretic drug. It can be used to treat raised blood pressure.

Piriton
A proprietary, non-prescription preparation of chlorpheniramine. It can be used to treat allergic conditions.

Piroxicam
A proprietary, prescription-only nonnarcotic analgesic drug. It can be used to treat the pain and inflammation of rheumatic diseases.

Pirozip

A proprietary, prescription-only preparation of the non-narcotic analgesic drug piroxicam. It can be used to treat the pain and inflammation of rheumatic diseases.

Pitressin

A proprietary, prescription-only preparation of vasopressin. It can be used to treat diabetes insipidus.

Pivampicillin

A proprietary, prescription-only preparation of the antibacterial and antibiotic drug ampicillin. It can be used to treat a wide variety of infections.

Pizotifen

A proprietary, prescription-only antihistamine and serotonin antagonist drug. It can be used to treat migraine.

Plaquenil

A proprietary, prescription-only preparation of hydrochloroquine sulphate. It can be used to treat rheumatoid arthritis and lupus erythematosus.

Plavix

A proprietary, prescription-only preparation of clopidogrel. is used for the prevention of heart attacks or stroke.

Plendil

A proprietary, prescription-only preparation of felodipine. It can be used to treat raised blood pressure.

Plesmet

A proprietary, non-prescription preparation of ferrous glycine sulphate. It can be used to treat certain types of anemia.

Plicamycin

A proprietary, prescription-only cytotoxic drug. It can be used to treat excessive levels of calcium in the bloodstream.

Podophyllum

A keratolytic and caustic agent. It can be used to treat and dissolve warts.

Poldine methylsulphate

A proprietary, prescription-only anticholinergic drug. It can be used for the symptomatic relief of smooth muscle spasm.

Poldine metilsulfate

A proprietary, prescription-only anticholinergic drug. It can be used for the symptomatic relief of smooth muscle spasm.

Pollon-Eze

A proprietary, non-prescription preparation of astemizole. It can be used to treat the symptoms of allergic disorders.

Polyestradiol phosphate

A proprietary, prescription-only analogue of estrogen. It can be used to treat cancer of the prostate gland.

Polyfax

A proprietary, prescription-only preparation of the antibacterial and antibiotic drug polymyxin B. It can be used to treat infections of the skin and eye.

Polymyxin

A proprietary, prescription-only antibacterial and antibiotic drug. It can be used to treat a wide variety of infections.

Polymyxin B sulphate

A proprietary, prescription-only antibacterial and antibiotic drug. It can be used to treat a wide variety of infections.

Polynoxylin

A proprietary, prescription-only antifungal and antibacterial drug. It can be used to treat minor skin infection.

Polystar Emollient

A proprietary, non-prescription preparation of coal tar. It can be used to treat psoriasis, eczema and dermatitis.

Polythiazide

A proprietary, prescription-only diuretic drug. It can be used to treat oedema associated with congestive heart failure,

Polytrim

A proprietary, prescription-only compound preparation of the antibacterial and antibiotic drugs polymyxin B and trimethoprim. It can be used to treat infections in the eye.

Ponderax

A proprietary, prescription-only preparation of fenfluramine. It can be used to treat obesity.

Pondocillin

A proprietary, prescription-only preparation of the antibacterial and antibiotic drug pivemcillin. It can be sued to treat a wide variety of infections.

Ponstan

A proprietary, prescription-only preparation of mefenamic acid. It can be used to treat pain in rheumatic diseases.

Posalfilin

A proprietary, non-prescription compound preparation of salicylic acid and podophyllum. It can be used to treat and remove warts.

Posiject

A proprietary, prescription-only preparation of dobutamine hydrochloride. It can be used to treat serious heart disorders.

Potaba

A proprietary, non-prescription preparation of potassium aminobenzoate. It can be used to treat scleroderma and related skin disorders.

Potassium aminobenzoate

A proprietary, non-prescription preparation of potassium and benzoate. It can be used to treat disorders associated with excess fibrous tissue, such as scleroderma.

Potassium canrenoate

A proprietary, prescription-only mild diuretic drug. It can be used to treat oedema associated with aldosteronism.

Potassium permanganate

A proprietary, non-prescription antiseptic agent. It can be used for cleaning burns and abrasions.

Fever
Pain
Infection

Ponstan

Properties
This medicine contains as active ingredient mefenamic acid. It belongs to the group of medicines called non-steroidal anti-inflammatory drugs (NSAIDs). These drugs are taken by mouth to relieve some symptoms caused by arthritis or rheumatism, such as inflammation, swelling, stiffness, and joint pain. However, these medicines do not cure arthritis and will help you only as long as you continue to take them. Some of these medicines are also used to relieve other kinds of pain or to treat other painful conditions, such as gout attacks, bursitis, tendinitis, sprains, strains, menstrual cramps. The drug reduces the tissue concentration of prostaglandins (hormones which produce inflammation and pain).

Before using this medicine
Before you use this medicine check with your doctor, or pharmacist:
- if you ever had any unusual or allergic reaction, such as skin rash, hives, or itching or breathing problems, to any of the anti-inflammatory analgesics.
- if you are on a low-salt, low-sugar, or any other special diet, or if you are allergic to any substance, such as sulfites or other preservatives or dyes.
- if you are pregnant or intending to become pregnant while using this medicine. Studies on birth defects have not been done in humans. However, if taken regularly during the last months of pregnancy, there is a chance that these medicines may cause unwanted effects on the heart or blood flow in the fetus or newborn infant.
- if you are breast-feeding an infant. Although this medicine has not been shown to cause problems in humans, it passes into the breast milk in small amounts.
- if you have any of the following medical problems:
  Asthma
  Bleeding problems
  Colitis
  Stomach ulcer
  Heart disease
  Kidney or liver disease

Treatment
This medication is used to relieve pain or other symptoms caused by arthritis. For safe and effective use of this medicine, do not take more of it, do not take it more often, and do not take it for a longer period of time than ordered by your physician or directed by the package label.
If you are taking this medication on a regular schedule and you miss a dose, take the missed dose as soon as possible, unless it is almost time for your next dose. In that case do not take the missed dose at all.
To lessen stomach upset, anti-inflammatory analgesics may be taken with food or antacids.

Side effects
Along with the needed effects, a medicine may cause some unwanted effects. These side effects may go away during treatment as your body adjusts to the medicine. Such minor side effects are: dizziness; nausea; pain; headache; drowsiness; swollen feet, face or leg; constipation or diarrhea; vomiting; dry mouth.
Check with your doctor immediately if any of the following side effects occur:
- *Muscle cramps*
- *Numbness or tingling*
- *Mouth ulcers*
- *Convulsions or confusion*
- *Rash, hives, or itch*
- *Tightness in chest*

Interactions
This medicine may interact with several other drugs.
Be sure to tell your doctor about any medications you are currently taking.

Storage
The medicine should be stored at room temperature in a tightly closed, light-resistant container. Store away from heat and direct light. Keep out of reach of children.

Povidone-iodine
A proprietary, non-prescription antiseptic agent. It can be used for cleaning burns and abrasions.

Powerin Analgesic Tablets
A compound preparation of aspirin, paracetamol and caffeine. It can be used to treat mild to moderate pain.

Pragmatar
A proprietary, non-prescription compound preparation of coal tar, salicylic acid and sulphur. It can be used to treat psoriasis and eczema.

Paralidoxine mesylate
An antidote used to treat poisoning by organophosphorous compounds.

Pramoxine hydrochloride
A proprietary, prescription-only local anesthetic drug. It can be used to treat hemorrhoids.

Pravastatin
A proprietary, prescription-only lipid-lowering drug. It can be used to treat high levels of lipids in the bloodstream.

Praxilene
A proprietary, prescription-only preparation of neftidrofuryl oxalate. It can be used to help improve blood circulation to the hands and feet.

P

Praziquantal

A proprietary, prescription-only anthelminthic drug. It can be used to treat schistosomiasis.

Prazosin hydrochloride

A proprietary, prescription-only adrenoreceptor blocker drug. It can be used to treat heart failure, urinary retention and benign prostatic hypertrophy.

Precortisyl

A proprietary, prescription-only preparation of prednisolone. It can be used to treat allergic and rheumatic disorders.

Predenema

A proprietary, prescription-only preparation of prednisolone. It can be used to treat rectal inflammation.

Predfoam

A proprietary, prescription-only preparation of prednisolone. It can be used to treat rectal inflammation.

Pred Forte

A proprietary, prescription-only preparation of prednisolone. It can be used to treat inflammatory conditions of the eye.

Prednesol

A proprietary, prescription-only preparation of prednisolone. It can be used to treat allergic and rheumatic conditions.

Prednisolone

A proprietary, prescription-only corticosteroid drug. It can be used to treat allergic and rheumatic conditions.

Prednisone

A proprietary, prescription-only corticosteroid drug. It can be used to treat allergic and rheumatic conditions.

Predsol

A proprietary, prescription-only corticosteroid drug. It can be used to treat rectal inflammation.

Predsol-N

A proprietary, prescription-only compound preparation of prednisolone and neomycin sulphate. It can be used to treat inflammatory conditions of the eye.

Preferid

A proprietary, prescription-only preparation of the corticosteroid budesonide. It can be used to treat inflammatory conditions.

Prefil

A proprietary, non-prescription preparation of the laxative drug sterculia. It can be used in the medical treatment of obesity.

Pregaday

A proprietary, non-prescription compound preparation of ferrous fumarate and folic acid. It can be used as iron and folic acid supplement during pregnancy.

Pregnyl

A proprietary, prescription-only preparation of human chorionic gonadotrophin. It can be used to treat infertility in women.

Premarin

A proprietary, prescription-only preparation of conjugated estrogens. It can be used in hormone replacement therapy.

Prempak-C

A proprietary, prescription-only compound preparation of conjugated estrogens and progestogen. It can be used in hormone replacement therapy.

Prepadine

A proprietary, prescription-only preparation of dothiepin hydrochloride. It can be used to treat depressive illness.

Prepidil

A proprietary, prescription-only preparation of dinoprostone. It can be used to induce labour.

Prepuilsid

A proprietary, prescription-only motility stimulant drug. It can be used to stimulate stomach and intestine.

Prescal

A preparation of isradipine. It can be used to treat raised blood pressure.

Prestim

A proprietary, prescription-only compound preparation of timolol maleate and bendrofluazide. It can be used to treat raised blood pressure.

Prestim Forte

A proprietary, prescription-only compound preparation of timolol maleate and bendrofluazide. It can be used to treat raised blood pressure.

Priadel

A proprietary, prescription-only preparation of lithium. It can be used to treat acute mania, manic-depressive bouts and recurrent depression.

Prilosec

A proprietary, prescription-only preparation of omeprazole. It is used to for the symptomatic treatment of heartburn.

Primacor

A proprietary, prescription-only preparation of milrinone. It can be used to treat heart failure.

Primalan

A proprietary, prescription-only preparation of mequitadine. It can be used to treat symptoms of allergic disorders.

Primaquine

A proprietary, prescription-only antimalarian drug. It can be used in malaria treatment.

Primaxin

A proprietary, prescription-only compound preparation of imipenem and cilastin. It can be used to treat infections of the urogenital tract.

Primidone

A proprietary, prescription-only anticonvulsant drug. It can be used to treat all forms of epilepsy.

Primolut N

A proprietary, prescription-only preparation of norethisterone. It can be used to treat uterine bleeding and other menstrual problems.

Primoteston Depot
A proprietary, prescription-only preparation of testosterone enanthate. It can be used to treat hormonal deficiency in men.

Primperan
A proprietary, prescription-only preparation of metroclopramide. It can be used to treat nausea and vomiting.

Prioderm
A proprietary, non-prescription preparation of malathion. It can be used to treat lice infestations of the scalp and pubic region.

Pripsen Mebendazole
A proprietary, non-prescription preparation of mebendazole. It can be used to treat infestations by threadworm and roundworm.

Pripsen Powder
A proprietary, non-prescription preparation of mebendazole. It can be used to treat infestations by threadworm and roundworm.

Pripsen Worm Elixir
A proprietary, non-prescription preparation of mebendazole. It can be used to treat infestations by threadworm and roundworm.

Pro-Actidil
A proprietary, non-prescription preparation of triprolidine. It can be used to treat the symptoms of various allergic disorders.

Pro-Bantine
A proprietary, prescription-only preparation of probanthidine. It can be used to treat spasmodic conditions of the gastrointestinal tract.

Probenecid
A proprietary, prescription-only cellular transport drug. It can be used to stimulate urine secretion and to prevent attacks of gout.

Probucol
A proprietary, prescription-only lipid-lowering drug. It can be used to treat high levels of lipids in the blood.

Procainamide Durules
A proprietary, prescription-only preparation of procainamide hydrochloride. It can be used to treat irregularities of the heartbeat.

Procaine
A proprietary, prescription-only local anesthetic drug. It can be used to treat regional anesthesia.

Procaine penicillin
A proprietary, prescription-only antibacterial and antibiotic drug. It can be used to treat a wide variety of infections.

Procarbazine
A proprietary, prescription-only cytotoxic drug. It can be used to treat Hodgkin's disease.

Prochlorperazine
A proprietary, prescription-only phenothiazine derivative. It can be used to treat psychotic disorders and anxiety.

Proctofibe
A proprietary, non-prescription preparation of the laxative bran. It can be used to treat constipation.

Proctofoam HC
A proprietary, prescription-only compound preparation of hydrocortisone and promaxine hydrochloride. It can be used to treat various painful conditions of the anus and rectum.

Proctosedyl
A proprietary, prescription-only compound preparation of hydrocortisone and cinchocaine hydrochloride. It can be used to treat various painful conditions of the anus and rectum.

Procyclidine hydrochloride
A proprietary, prescription-only anticholinergic drug. It can be used to treat symptoms of parkinsonism.

Profasi
A proprietary, prescription-only preparation of human chorionic gonadotrophin. It can be used to treat undescended testicles and delayed puberty in men and hormonal deficiency in women.

Proflex
A proprietary, non-prescription preparation of ibuprofen. It can be used for the symptomatic relief of rheumatic and muscular pain, headache, sprains, strains, and lumbago.

Proflex Sustained Relief Capsules
A proprietary, non-prescription preparation of ibuprofen. It can be used for the symptomatic relief of rheumatic and muscular pain, headache, sprains, strains, and lumbago.

Proflex Tablets
A proprietary, non-prescription preparation of ibuprofen. It can be used for the symptomatic relief of rheumatic and muscular pain, headache, sprains, strains, and lumbago.

Progesic
A proprietary, non-prescription preparation of fenoprofen. It can be used for the symptomatic relief of rheumatic and muscular pain, headache, sprains, strains, and lumbago.

Progesterone
A proprietary, prescription-only progestogen. It can be used to treat various menstrual and gynaecological disorders.

Prograf
A proprietary, prescription-only preparation of tacrolimus. It can be used to prevent tissue rejection in transplant patients.

Proguanil hydrochloride
A proprietary, prescription-only antimalarial drug. It can be used to prevent the contraction of malaria by visitors to tropical countries.

Progynova
A proprietary, prescription-only preparation of oestradiol. It can be used in hormone replacement therapy.

Prolactin
A hormone secreted into the blood-

stream by the anterior pituitary gland. It can be used to prevent or suppress lactation.

Proleukin
A proprietary, prescription-only preparation of aldesleukin. It can be used to treat metastatic renal cell carcinoma.

Proluton Depot
A proprietary, prescription-only preparation of hydroprogesterone. It can be used to treat recurrent (habitual) abortion.

Promazine hydrochloride
A proprietary, prescription-only phenothiazine derivative. It can be used to tranquillize agitated and restless patients.

Promethazine hydrochloride
A proprietary, prescription-only antihistamine drug. It can be used to treat symptoms of allergic conditions.

Promethazine teoclate
A proprietary, prescription-only phenothiazine derivative. It can be used to treat nausea and vomiting.

Promethazine theoclate
A proprietary, prescription-only phenothiazine derivative. It can be used to treat nausea and vomiting.

Prominal
A proprietary, prescription-only preparation of methylphenobarbitone. It can be used to treat most forms of epilepsy.

Pronestyl
A proprietary, prescription-only preparation of procainamide hydrochloride. It can be used to treat irregularities of the heartbeat.

Propaderm
A proprietary, prescription-only preparation of beclomathasone diproprionate. It can be used to treat severe skin disorders such as eczema.

Propafenone hydrochloride
A proprietary, prescription-only cardiac drug. It can be used to treat and prevent irregularities of the heartbeat.

Propain Tablets
A proprietary, non-prescription compound preparation of codeine phosphate, diphenhydramine, paracetamol and caffeine. It can be used to relieve pain, including headache, migraine, muscular pain and period pain and to relieve cold and flu symptoms.

Propamidine isothionate
A proprietary, prescription-only antibacterial drug. It can be used to treat infections of the eyelids.

Propanix
A proprietary, prescription-only preparation of the beta-blocker drug propranolol. It can be used to treat and prevent raised blood pressure and angina pectoris.

Propantheline bromide
A proprietary, prescription-only anticholinergic drug. It can be used to treat spasms of the gastrointestinal tract.

Propine
A proprietary, prescription-only preparation of dipivefrine hydrochloride. It can be used to treat glaucoma.

Propofol
A proprietary, prescription-only general anesthetic drug. It can be used in the induction and maintenance of general anesthesia.

Propranolol hydrochloride
A proprietary, prescription-only beta-blocker drug It can be used to treat and prevent raised blood pressure and angina pectoris.

Propylthiouracil
A proprietary, prescription-only antagonist of thyroid hormones. It can be used to treat an excess of thyroid hormones.

Prosaid
A preparation of naproxen. It can be used to relieve pain and inflammation, particularly rheumatic and arthritic pain.

Proscar
A proprietary, prescription-only pre-

paration of finasteride. It can be used to treat benign prostatic hyperplasia.

Prostap SR
A proprietary, prescription-only preparation of leucoprorelin acetate. It can be used to treat cancer of the prostate gland.

Prostigmin
A proprietary, prescription-only preparation of neostigmin. It can be used to treat myasthenia gravis.

Prostin E2
A proprietary, prescription-only preparation of a prostaglandin. It can be used to induce labour or to cause therapeutic abortion.

Prostin F2 alpha
A proprietary, prescription-only preparation of a prostaglandin. It can be used to induce therapeutic abortion.

Prostin F2 alpha
A proprietary, prescription-only preparation of a prostaglandin. It can be used to assist newborns with heart defects.

Prosulf
A proprietary, prescription-only preparation of protamine sulphate. It can be used to counteract heparin overdose.

Protamine sulfate
A proprietary, prescription-only drug used to treat an overdose of heparin.

Protamine sulphate
A proprietary, prescription-only drug used to treat an overdose of heparin.

Protamine zinc insulin
A proprietary, prescription-only form of purified insulin. It is used to treat diabetes.

Prothiaden
A proprietary, prescription-only preparation of dothiepin. It can be used to treat depressive illness.

Protirelin
A proprietary, prescription-only nat-

Propaderm

Properties
This medicine belongs to the family of topical (applied to the skin) corticosteroids, containing an adrenocorticoid as active ingredient. It is used to relieve the symptoms of any itching, rash, or inflammation of the skin; it does not treat the underlying cause of the skin problem. It also relieves redness, swelling and itching caused by insect bites, poison ivy, poison oak, poison sumach, soaps, cosmetics, sunburn, and numerous skin rashes.
Topical adrenocorticosteroids are absorbed through the skin and may rarely affect growth in children. Before using this medicine in children you should discuss the use of it with your doctor.

Before using this medicine
Before you use this medicine check with your doctor, or pharmacist:
- if you ever had any unusual or allergic reaction to adrenocorticoids or corticosteroids in general.
- if you are on a low-salt, low-sugar, or any other special diet, or if you are allergic to any substance, such as certain preservatives or dyes.
- if you have diabetes, stomach ulcer, or infection at the treatment site.
- if you are pregnant, intending to become pregnant or breast-feeding an infant while using this medicine.
- if you have any of the following medical problems:
Diabetes mellitus (sugar diabetes)
Infection at the place of treatment
Ulceration at the place of treatment
Tuberculosis

Treatment
This medication is used to relieve or prevent the symptoms of your medical problem. Take them as directed. Do not take more of them and do not take them more often than recommended on the label.
To do so may increase the chance of absorption through the skin and the chance of side effects. In addition, too much use, especially on thin skin areas (for example, armpits, face, groin), may result in thinning of the skin and stretch marks.

Side effects
The following side effects may occur:
- Acne or oily skin
- Blistering
- Burning sensations
- Itching
- Dryness of the skin
- Secondary infection
- Thinning of skin
- Unusual hair growth
- Unusual loss of hair

These side effects should disappear as your body adjusts to the medication. Tell your doctor about any side effects that are persistent or particularly bothersome.
The above side effects are more likely to occur in children and elderly patients, who are usually more sensitive to the effects of this medicine.
When the gel, solution, lotion, or aerosol from this medicine is applied, a mild, temporary stinging may be expected.

Interactions
This medicine interacts with several other drugs such as antibiotics (causing a decreased antibiotic effect) and antifungals (causing a decreased antifungal effect).
Be sure to tell your doctor about any medications you are currently taking.

Storage
This medicine should be stored at room temperature in closed containers. Store away from heat and direct light. Keep out of reach of children, since overdose may be dangerous in children. Do not store in the bathroom medicine cabinet because the heat or moisture may cause the medicine to break down. Keep the medicine from freezing. Do not keep outdated medicine.

---

ural hypothalamic hormone. It can be used to treat assess thyroid function in clinical conditions.

Protriptyline hydrochloride
A proprietary, prescription-only antidepressant drug. It can be used to treat depressive illness.

Provera
A preparation of medroxyprogesterone acetate. It can be used to treat endometriosis and cancer of the female genital organs.

Pro-Viron
A preparation of mesterolone. It can be used to treat hormonal deficiencies.

Proxymetacaine
A proprietary, prescription-only local anesthetic drug. It can be used in ophthalmic treatments.

Prozac
A preparation of fluoxetine hydrochloride. It can be used to treat depressive illness and bulimia nervosa.

Pseudoephedrine hydrochloride
A proprietary, prescription-only vasoconstrictor drug. It can be used to treat obstructive airways disease.

Psoradrate
A proprietary, non-prescription compound preparation of dibranol and urea. It can be used to treat psoriasis, eczema and dandruff.

Psoriderm
A proprietary, non-prescription compound preparation of coal tar and

lecithin. It can be used to treat psoriasis, eczema and dandruff.

Psorigel

A proprietary, non-prescription preparation of coal tar. It can be used to treat psoriasis, eczema and dandruff.

Psorin

A proprietary, non-prescription preparation of dithranol, salicylic acid and coal tar. It can be used to treat psoriasis, eczema and dandruff.

Pulmadil

A proprietary, prescription-only preparation of the beta-blocker drug rimiterol hydrobromide. It can be used to treat and prevent asthma and chronic bronchitis.   .

Pulmicort Inhaler

A preparation of the corticosteroid drug budesonide. It can be used to treat and prevent asthmatic attacks and chronic bronchitis.

Pulmicort Respules

A proprietary, prescription-only preparation of the corticosteroid drug budesonide. It can be used to treat and prevent asthmatic attacks and chronic bronchitis.

Pulmicort Turbohaler

A proprietary, prescription-only preparation of the corticosteroid drug budesonide. It can be used to treat and prevent asthmatic attacks and chronic bronchitis.

Pur-in Mix 15/85

A proprietary, non-prescription preparation of purified human biphasic isophase insulin. It can be used to treat diabetes.

Pur-in Mix 25/75

A proprietary, non-prescription preparation of purified human biphasic isophase insulin. It can be used to treat diabetes.

Pur-in Mix 50/50

A proprietary, non-prescription preparation of purified human biphasic isophase insulin. It can be used to treat diabetes.

Puri-Nethol

A proprietary, prescription-only preparation of mercaptopurine. It can be used to treat acute leukaemia.

Pur-in Neutral

A proprietary, non-prescription preparation of purified human neutral soluble insulin. It can be used to treat diabetes.

Pyopen

A proprietary, prescription-only preparation of the antibacterial and antibiotic drug carbenicillin. It can be used to treat serious pseudomonas infections.

Pyralvex

A proprietary, non-prescription preparation of salicylic acid and rhubarb extract. It can be used for the symptomatic relief of mouth ulcers.

Pyrantel

A proprietary, prescription-only anthelminthic drug. It can be used to treat infections by roundworm, threadworm and hookworm.

Pyrazinamide

A proprietary, prescription-only antibacterial drug. It can be used in the treatment of tuberculosis.

Pyridostigmine

A proprietary, prescription-only anticholinesterase drug. It can be used to treat myasthenia gravis.

Pyrimethamine

A proprietary, prescription-only antimalarial drug. It can be used to treat and prevent malaria.

Pyrogastrone

A proprietary, prescription-only compound preparation of carbenoxolone hydroxide, magnesium trisilicate, alginic acid and sodium bicarbonate. It can be used as an ulcer-healing drug in benign peptic ulcer.

Q

Q-Mazine Syrup

A proprietary, non-prescription preparation of promethazine hydrochloride. It can be used to treat nausea and motion sickness.

Questran/A

A proprietary, prescription-only preparation of cholestyramine. It can be used to reduce high levels of lipids in the bloodstream.

Quinagolide

A proprietary, prescription-only analogue of bromocriptine. It can be used to treat hormone disorders.

Quinapril

A proprietary, prescription-only ACE inhibitor. It can be used to treat raised blood pressure and angina pectoris.

Quinidine

A cinchona alkaloid chemically related to quinine. It can be used to treat irregularities of the heartbeat.

Quinine

A cinchona alkaloid chemically related to quinidine. It can be used to treat malaria.

Quinocort

A proprietary, prescription-only preparation of the antifungal and antibacterial drug hydroxyquinoline sulphate. It can be used to treat inflammation, particularly associated with fungal infections.

Quinoderm Cream/Lotio-Gel

A proprietary, non-prescription compound preparation of the keratolytic and antimicrobial drug benzoyl peroxide and hydroquinoline sulphate. It can be used to treat acne.

Quinoped

A proprietary, non-prescription compound preparation of the keratolytic and antimicrobial drug benzoyl peroxide and potassium hydroquinoline. It can be used to treat fungal skin infections.

R

Radian B Heat Spray
A proprietary, non-prescription compound preparation of camphor, menthol, salicylic acid and ammonium salicylate. It can be applied to the skin for symptomatic relief of muscle and rheumatic pain, sciatica, lumbago, fibrosis and muscle stiffness.

Radian B Muscle Lotion
A proprietary, non-prescription compound preparation of camphor, menthol, salicylic acid and ammonium salicylate. It can be applied to the skin for symptomatic relief of muscle and rheumatic pain, sciatica, lumbago, fibrosis and muscle stiffness.

Radian B Muscle Rub
A proprietary, non-prescription compound preparation of camphor, menthol, salicylic acid and capsicum oleoresin. It can be applied to the skin for symptomatic relief of muscle and rheumatic pain, sciatica, lumbago, fibrosis and muscle stiffness.

Ralgex Cream
A proprietary, non-prescription compound preparation of capsicum oleoresin, glycol salicylate and methyl nicotinate. It can be applied to the skin for symptomatic relief of muscle and rheumatic pain, sciatica, lumbago, fibrosis and muscle stiffness.

Ralgex Stick
A proprietary, non-prescription compound preparation of glycol salicylate, capsicum oleoresin, menthol and ethyl salicylate. It can be applied to the skin for symptomatic relief of muscle and rheumatic pain, sciatica, lumbago, fibrosis and muscle stiffness.

Ramipril
A proprietary, prescription-only vasodilator and ACE inhibitor. It is used to treat raised blood pressure and heart failure.

Ramysin
A proprietary, prescription-only preparation of the antibacterial and antibiotic drug doxycycline. It can be used to treat infections of many kinds.

Ranitidine
A proprietary, prescription-only ulcer-healing drug. It is used to treat benign peptic ulcers, reflux esophagitis, heartburn and other gastric disorders.

Rapifen
A proprietary, prescription-only preparation of alfentanil. It is used to treat moderate to severe pain.

Rapitard
A proprietary, prescription-only preparation of biphasic insulin. It is used to treat diabetes.

Rastinon
A proprietary, prescription-only preparation of tolbutamide. It is used in diabetic treatment for Type II diabetes.

Razoxane
A proprietary, prescription-only cytotoxic drug. It is used to treat some forms of cancer, including leukaemia.

Razoxin
A proprietary, prescription-only preparation of the cytotoxic drug razoxane. It is used to treat some forms of cancer, including leukaemia.

Recormon
A proprietary, prescription-only preparation of epoetin beta. It is used to treat anemia.

Redeptin
A proprietary, prescription-only preparation of fluspirilene. It is used to treat psychoses, including schizophrenia.

Redoxon
A proprietary, non-prescription preparation of vitamin C. It is used to treat symptoms of vitamin C deficiency.

Refolinon
A proprietary, prescription-only preparation of folinic acid. It is used to treat the toxic effects of certain anti-cancer drugs.

Regaine
A proprietary, prescription-only preparation of minoxidil. It is used to treat male-pattern baldness.

Regulan
A proprietary, non-prescription preparation of the laxative ispagluha husk. It is used to treat constipation and a number of gastrointestinal disorders, including irritable bowel syndrome.

Reguletts
A proprietary, non-prescription preparation of phenolphthaleine. It is used to treat constipation.

Regulose
A proprietary, non-prescription preparation of lactulose. It is used to treat constipation.

Relaxit Micro-enema
A proprietary, non-prescription compound preparation of sodium citrate, sorbic acid, sorbitol and glycerol. It is used to treat constipation.

Relenza
A proprietary, prescription-only preparation of zanamivir. It is used for the prevention and treatment of influenza.

Relifex
A proprietary, prescription-only preparation of nabumetone. It is used to treat and relieve pain and inflammation, particularly arthritic and rheumatic pain.

Relpax
A proprietary, prescription-only preparation of eletriptan. It is used for the prevention and treatment of migraine.

Remedeine
A proprietary, prescription-only compound preparation of paracetamol and dihydrocodeine tartrate. It is used to treat severe to moderate pain.

Remegel Original
A proprietary, non-prescription pre-

R

paration of calcium carbonate. It is used for the relief of heartburn, acid indigestion and upset stomach.

Remnos
A proprietary, prescription-only preparation of the benzodiazepine drug nitrazepam. It is used to treat insomnia.

Rennie Gold
A proprietary, non-prescription preparation of calcium carbonate. It is used for the relief of acid indigestion, heartburn, upset stomach and dyspepsia.

Rennie Tablets
A proprietary, non-prescription compound preparation of calcium carbonate and magnesium carbonate. It is used for the relief of acid indigestion, heartburn, upset stomach and dyspepsia.

Replenine
A proprietary, prescription-only preparation of factor IC fraction. It is used to treat patients with a deficiency in factor IX.

Reproterol hydrochloride
A proprietary, prescription-only betablocker drug. It is used as a bronchodilator to treat reversible obstructive airways disorders.

Requib
A proprietary, prescription-only preparation of ropinirole. It is used for the relive of symptoms of restless leg syndrome.

Resolve
A proprietary, non-prescription compound preparation of paracetamol, vitamin C and various antacid salts. It is used to treat headache with stomach upset or with nausea.

Resonium
A proprietary, non-prescription preparation of sodium polystyrene sulphonatc. It is used to treat high blood potassium levels.

Resorcinol
A proprietary, non-prescription keratolytic preparation. It is used in ointments and lotions for the treatment of acne.

Respacal
A proprietary, prescription-only preparation of tulobuterol. It is used as bronchodilator to treat reversible obstructive airways disease.

Restandol
A proprietary, prescription-only preparation of testosterone. It is used to treat deficiency in men and for breast cancer in women.

Restasis
A proprietary, prescription-only preparation of cyclosporne. It is used to increase the eye's ability to produce tears which may be suppressed by inflammation.

Retrovir
A proprietary, prescription-only preparation of the antiviral drug zidovudine. It is used in the treatment of AIDS.

Revanil
A proprietary, prescription-only preparation of the antiparkinsonism drug lysuride maleate. It is used to treat symptoms of Parkinson disease.

Rezulin
A proprietary, prescription-only preparation of troglitazone. It is used in diabetes to control blood sugar levels.

Rheumacin LA
A proprietary, prescription-only preparation of indomethacin. It is used to relieve pain and inflammation, particularly rheumatic and arthritis pain and to treat other musculoskeletal disorders.

Rheumox
A proprietary, prescription-only preparation of azopropazone. It is used to relieve pain and inflammation of severe rheumatoid arthritis, ankylosing spondylitis and acute gout.

Rhinocort
A proprietary, prescription-only preparation of the corticosteroid drug budenoside. It is used to treat nasal rhinitis.

Rhinocort Aqua Nasal Aerosol
A proprietary, prescription-only preparation of the corticosteroid drug budenoside. It is used to treat nasal rhinitis.

Rhinocort Aqua Nasal Spray
A proprietary, prescription-only preparation of the corticosteroid drug budenoside. It is used to treat nasal rhinitis.

Rhuska Herbal Syrup
A proprietary, non-prescription preparation of the laxatives senna, rhubarb and cascara. It is used to relieve constipation.

Rhumalgan
A preparation of diclofenac sodium. It is used to treat arthritic and rheumatic pain and other musculoskeletal disorders.

Ridaura
A proprietary, prescription-only preparation of auranofin. It is used to treat rheumatoid arthritis.

Rideril
A proprietary, prescription-only preparation of the antipsychotic drug thioridazine. It is used to treat and tranquillize psychotic patients, particularly manic forms of behavioral disturbance.

Rifabutin
A proprietary, prescription-only preparation of the antibacterial and antibiotic drug of the rifamycin family of antibiotics. It is used to treat and to prevent tuberculosis.

Rifadin
A proprietary, prescription-only preparation of the antibacterial and antibiotic drug rifamycin. It is used to treat leprosy.

Rifampicin
A proprietary, prescription-only antibacterial and antibiotic drug. It is used to treat tuberculosis, leprosy, brucellosis, legionnaires' disease and serious staphylococcal infections.

Rifater
A proprietary, prescription-only com-

Resorcinol
(Topical)

Properties

This medicine belongs to the family of topical (applied to the skin) anti-acne preparations, usually containing tretinoin as active ingredient. It is used in the treatment for acne and other skin conditions such as psoriasis (common skin condition characterized by patches of red, thickened and scaling skin), ichthyosis (skin disease which causes the epidermis to become dry and horny like fish scales), keratosis (skin condition characterized by an increase of horny substance), folliculitis (inflammation of a hair follicle), and flat warts.

This medication works by decreasing the cohesiveness of skin cells, causing the skin to peel, which is helpful in the treatment of mild acne and other skin conditions. This drug is usually not effective in treating severe acne.

Drug may work in 2 to 3 weeks.

Before using this medicine

Before you use this medicine check with your doctor, or pharmacist:

- if you ever had any unusual or allergic reaction to tretinoin.
- if you are on a low-salt, low-sugar, or any other special diet, or if you are allergic to any substance, such as certain preservatives or dyes.
- if you are sunburned, or have an open skin wound.
- if you are pregnant, intending to become pregnant or breast-feeding an infant while using this medicine.

Tretinoin has been shown to cause abnormal skull formation in animal fetuses. Birth defects in animals have also been caused by Tretinoin, but studies with humans have not been conducted. Pregnant women should avoid this drug.

Treatment

This medication is used to relieve or prevent the symptoms of your medical problem. Take them as directed. Do not take more of them and do not take them more often than recommended on the label. To do so may increase the chance of absorption through the skin and the chance of side effects.

Wash skin with non-medicated soap, pat dry, wait 20 minutes before applying.

SOLUTION: Apply to affected areas with gauze pad or cotton swab. Avoid getting too wet so medicine does not drip into eyes, lips or inside nose.

CREAM/GEL: Apply to affected areas with finger tips and rub in gently.

Keep this drug away from your eyes, nose, mouth, and mucous membranes. Avoid exposure to sunlight and sunlamp. Consult your doctor if you have eczema.

Side effects

The following side effects may occur:
- Pigment change in treated area
- Warmth or stinging of skin
- Peeling of skin
- Redness and swelling

These side effects should disappear as your body adjusts to the medication. Tell your doctor about any side effects that are persistent or particularly bothersome.

You should discontinue the use of the drug when the following side effects occur:
- *Blistering*
- *Crusting*
- *Severe burning*
- *Swelling*

Interactions

This medicine interacts with several other medications such as anti-acne topical preparations, medicated cosmetics, skin preparations with alcohol, and also with soaps or cleansers. The combined effect may cause severe skin irritation.

Storage

This medicine should be stored at room temperature in closed containers. Store away from heat and direct light.
Keep out of reach of children.

---

pound preparation of the antibacterial drugs rifampicin, isoniazid and pyrazinamide. It is used to treat tuberculosis.

Rifna

A compound preparation of the antibacterial drugs rifampicin and isoniazid. It is used to treat tuberculosis.

Rimacid

A proprietary, prescription-only preparation of indomethacin. It is used to treat pain and inflammation of rheumatic disease and other musculoskeletal disorders.

Rimacillin

A preparation of the antibacterial and antibiotic drug ampicillin. It is used to treat systemic bacterial infections, infections of the upper respiratory tract, of the ear, nose and throat and the urogenital tract.

Rimactane

A proprietary, prescription-only preparation of the antibacterial and antibiotic drug rifampicin. It is used to treat systemic bacterial infections and tuberculosis.

Rimactazid

A compound preparation of the antibacterial and antibiotic drugs rifampicin and isoniazid. It is used to treat tuberculosis.

Rimafen

A proprietary, prescription-only preparation of ibuprofen. It is used to relieve pain, particularly the pain of rheumatic disease and other musculoskeletal disorders.

Rimapam

A proprietary, prescription-only preparation of the benzodiazepine drug diazepam. It is used to treat anxiety, insomnia, convulsions and as skeletal muscle relaxant.

Rimapurinol

A proprietary, prescription-only preparation of allopurinol. It is used to treat excess uric acid and to prevent kidney stones and attacks of gout.

Rimifon

A proprietary, prescription-only preparation of the antibacterial drug isoniazid. It is used to treat tuberculosis.

Rimiterol hydrobromide

A proprietary, prescription-only beta-receptor stimulant drug. It is used as bronchodilator to treat reversible obstructive airways disease.

Rimoxallin

A proprietary, prescription-only preparation of the antibacterial and antibiotic drug amoxycillin. It is used to treat bacterial infections.

Rinatec

A proprietary, prescription-only preparation of ipratropium bromide. It is used to treat watery rhinitis.

Risperal

A proprietary, prescription-only preparation of the antipsychotic drug risperidone. It is used to tranquillize patients suffering from schizophrenia and other psychotic disorders.

Risperidone

A antipsychotic drug. It is used to tranquillize patients suffering from schizophrenia and other psychotic disorders.

Ritodrine hydrochloride

A proprietary, prescription-only beta-receptor stimulant drug. It is used to prevent of delay premature labour.

Rivotril

A proprietary, prescription-only preparation of the benzodiazepine drug clonazepam. It is used to treat epilepsy.

Roaccutane

A proprietary, prescription-only preparation of isotretinoin. It is used to treat severe acne.

Robaxin

A proprietary, prescription-only preparation of methocarbamol. It is used to relieve acute muscle spasm.

Robaxical Forte

A proprietary, prescription-only compound preparation of methocarbamol and aspirin. It is used to treat rheumatic pain and other musculoskeletal disorders.

Robinul

A proprietary, prescription-only preparation of glycopyrronium bromide. It can be used before operations for drying up saliva and other secretions.

Robinul-Neostigmine

A proprietary, prescription-only compound preparation of glycopyrronium bromide and neostigmine. It can be used after operations to reverse the actions of competitive neuromuscular blocking agents.

Robitussin Chesty Cough

A proprietary, non-prescription compound preparation of guaiphenesin and pseudoephedrine hydrochloride. It is used to treat chesty cough and nasal congestion.

Robitussin Dry Cough

A proprietary, non-prescription preparation of dextromethorphan hydrobromide. It is used to treat dry, irritant cough.

Rocaltrol

A proprietary, prescription-only preparation of calcitrol. It is used to treat vitamin D deficiency.

Roccal

A proprietary, non-prescription preparation of benzalkonium chloride. It is used to cleanse wounds and the skin before operations.

Roccal Concentrate

A proprietary, non-prescription preparation of benzalkonium chloride. It is used to cleanse wounds and the skin before operations.

Rocephin

A proprietary, prescription-only preparation of the antibacterial and antibiotic drug cephalosporin. It is used to treat bacterial infections and to prevent infection arising during and after surgery.

Rocuronium bromide

A proprietary, prescription-only skeletal muscle relaxant drug. It is used to induce muscle paralysis during surgery.

Roferon-A

A proprietary, prescription-only preparation of interferon. It is used as an anticancer drug.

Rogitine

A proprietary, prescription-only preparation of phentolamine mesylate. It is used to treat raised blood pressure.

Rohypnol

A proprietary, prescription-only preparation of the benzodiazpine drug flunitrazepam. It is used to treat insomnia.

Rommix

A proprietary, prescription-only preparation of the antibacterial and antibiotic drug erythromycin. It can be used to treat and to prevent many forms of infection.

Ronicol

A proprietary, prescription-only preparation of the vasodilator drug nicotinyl alcohol. It can be used to improve blood circulation to the hands and feet.

Rowachol

A proprietary, prescription-only pre-

R

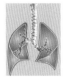

Robitussin

Properties

This medicine contains guaifenesin as active ingredient; it is used to treat severe cough symptoms. This medication is taken by mouth to relieve coughs due to colds or influenza. Guaifenesin works by loosening the mucus or phlegm in the lungs. It increases production of watery fluids to thin mucus so it can be coughed out or absorbed. *Regular use for 5 to 7 days is necessary for maximum benefit.*

Before using this medicine

This medicine is not to be used for the chronic cough that occurs with smoking, asthma, or emphysema or when there is an unusually large amount of mucus or phlegm with the cough. Before you use this medicine, check with your doctor or pharmacist:
- if you ever had any unusual or allergic reaction to any of the compounds of this medicine.
- if you are on a low-salt, low-sugar, or any other special diet, or if you are allergic to any substance, such as sulfites or other preservatives or dyes.
- if you are pregnant, intending to become pregnant or breast-feeding an infant while using this medicine.

Do not take this drug with other medicine without consulting your doctor or pharmacist.

Treatment

This medication is used to relieve or prevent the symptoms of your medical problem. Take them as directed. Do not take more of them and do not take them more often than recommended on the label.

If you must take this medicine regularly and you miss a dose, take it as soon as possible. However, if it is almost time for your next dose, skip the missed dose and go back to your regular dosing schedule. Do not double doses.

Side effects

Along with its needed effects, a medicine may cause some unwanted effects. Although not all of these side effects appear very often, when they do occur they may require medical attention. The following minor side effects may occur:
- Diarrhea
- Drowsiness
- Nausea
- Skin rash
- Stomach pain
- Vomiting

Symptoms of overdose include the following:
- Drowsiness
- Mild weakness
- Nausea and vomiting

An overdose is unlikely to threaten life. If a person takes much larger doses than prescribed, call a doctor, poison control center or hospital emergency room for instructions. The side effects should disappear as your body adjusts to the medication. Tell your doctor about any side effects that are persistent or particularly bothersome. Adverse reactions and side effects may be more frequent and severe in people over 60 years than in younger persons.

Driving, piloting or hazardous work should be avoided if you feel drowsy.

Interactions

This medicine interacts with several other drugs such as anticoagulants. There exists a possible risk of bleeding.

Storage

This medicine should be stored at room temperature in tightly closed containers. Store away from heat and direct light. Keep out of reach of children, since overdose may be dangerous in children. Do not store in the bathroom medicine cabinet because the heat or moisture may cause the medicine to break down. Do not refrigerate the syrup form of this medicine. Do not keep outdated medicine or medicine no longer needed.

---

paration of plant oils, including terpenes, camphene, cineole, mendone, menthol and pipene. It is used to treat gallstones and liver disorders.

Rowatinex

A proprietary, prescription-only preparation of plant oils, including terpenes, camphene, cineole, mendone, menthol and pipene. It is used to treat gallstones and liver disorders.

Rusyde

A proprietary, prescription-only pre-

paration of diuretic drug frusemide. It is used to treat oedema, particularly pulmonary oedema in patients with chronic heart failure.

Rynacrom

A proprietary, non-prescription preparation of sodium chromoglycate. It is used in the prevention of allergic rhinitis.

Rynacrom Compound

A proprietary, non-prescription compound preparation of sodium chro-

moglycate and xylometazoline hydrochloride. It is used in the prevention of allergic rhinitis.

Rythmodan

A proprietary, prescription-only preparation of disopyramide. It is used to treat disorders of the heart beat.

Rythmodan Retard

A proprietary, prescription-only preparation of disopyramide. It is used to treat disorders of the heart beat.

R

S

Sabril
A proprietary, prescription-only preparation of vigabatrin. It can be used to assist in the control of seizures.

Salactol
A proprietary, non-prescription preparation of salicylic acid. It can be used to remove hard skin and warts.

Salagen
A proprietary, prescription-only preparation of pilocarpine. It is used for the stimulation of salivary glands in Sjogren's syndrome.

Salamol
A proprietary, prescription-only preparation of salbutamol. It can be used to treat as a bronchodilator in reversible obstructive airways disease.

Salatac
A proprietary, non-prescription preparation of salicylic acid. It can be used to remove warts and hard skin.

Salazopyrin
A proprietary, prescription-only preparation of sulphasalazine. It can be used to treat active rheumatoid arthritis, ulcerative colitis and Crohn's disease.

Salazopyrin EN-Tabs
A proprietary, prescription-only preparation of sulphasalazine. It can be used to treat active rheumatoid arthritis, ulcerative colitis and Crohn's disease.

Salbulin
A proprietary, prescription-only preparation of salbutamol. It can be used as bronchodilator to treat reversible obstructive airways disease and severe asthma.

Salbutamol/ Cyclocaps
A proprietary, prescription-only beta-receptor stimulant drug. It can be used as bronchodilator to treat reversible obstructive airways disease and severe asthma.

Salcatonin
A proprietary, prescription-only preparation of calcitonin. It can be used to lower the levels of calcium and phosphate in the blood.

Salicylate
A term used to describe a group of drugs that are chemically related to salicylic acid used to treat inflammation, pain symptoms and to reduce fever.

Salivace
A proprietary, non-prescription compound preparation of carmellose and various other salts and constituents. It can be used as a form of synthetic saliva.

Salmeterol
A proprietary, prescription-only beta-receptor stimulant. It can be used as a bronchodilator to treat reversible obstruction airways disease and severe asthma.

Salofalk
A proprietary, prescription-only preparation of mesalazine. It can be used to treat ulcerative colitis.

Saluric
A proprietary, prescription-only preparation of the diuretic drug chlorothiazide. It can be used to treat oedema and raised blood pressure.

Salzone
A proprietary, non-prescription preparation of paracetamol. It can be used to relieve mild to moderate pain and to reduce temperature in fever.

Sandocal
A proprietary, non-prescription compound preparation of calcium carbonate, calcium lactate gluconate and citric acid. It can be used to treat calcium deficiency.

Sando-K
A proprietary, non-prescription compound preparation of potassium chloride and potassium bicarbonate. It can be used to treat potassium deficiency.

Sandostatin
A proprietary, prescription-only preparation of ostreotide. It can be used to treat in certain types of cancer.

Sandomigran
A proprietary, prescription-only preparation of pizotifen. It can be used to treat headache, particularly migraine and cluster headache.

Sarafem
A proprietary, prescription-only preparation of fluoxetine. It is used for the symptomatic treatment of premenstrual dysphoric disorder.

Saventrine
A proprietary, prescription-only preparation of isoprenaline hydrochloride. It can be used to treat low heart rate or heart block.

Schering PC4
A proprietary, prescription-only oral contraceptive that contains a estrogen and a progestogen. It can be used to after sexual intercourse has taken place.

Scheriproct
A proprietary, prescription-only compound preparation of prenisolone and cinchocaine. It can be used by topical application to treat hemorrhoids.

Scoline
A preparation of suxamethonium chloride. It can be used to induce muscle paralysis during surgery.

Scopoderm TTS
A proprietary, prescription-only preparation of hyoscine. It can be used to treat motion sickness.

Scopolamine hydrobromide
A preparation of hyoscine. It can be used to treat motion sickness.

Secaderm
A proprietary, non-prescription compound preparation of phenol, turpentine oil and terebene. It can be used to treat chilblains and varicose veins.

Secadrex
A proprietary, prescription-only compound preparation of acebutolol and

Seldane

Properties
This medicine contains terfenadine as active ingredient; it is used to treat or prevent symptoms of allergy. This medication belongs to a group known as antihistamines. Antihistamines block the action of histamine, a chemical that is released by the body during an allergic reaction. Some of the antihistamines are also used to prevent motion sickness, nausea, vomiting, and dizziness.

Before using this medicine
Before you use this medicine check with your doctor, or pharmacist:
- if you ever had any unusual or allergic reaction to antihistamines.
- if you are on a low-salt, low-sugar, or any other special diet, or if you are allergic to any substance, such as sulfites or other preservatives or dyes.
- if you are pregnant or intending to become pregnant while using this medicine.
- if you are breast-feeding an infant. Small amounts of antihistamines pass into the breast milk. Use is not recommended since the chances are greater for most antihistamines to cause side effects, such as unusual excitement or irritability in the infant.
- if you have any of the following medical problems:
  Asthma attack
  Enlarged prostate
  Glaucoma
  Urinary tract blockage
  Difficult urination

Treatment
This medication is used to relieve or prevent the symptoms of your medical problem. Take them as directed. Do not take more of them and do not take them more often than recommended on the label, unless otherwise directed by your doctor. To do so may increase the chance of side effects.

Side effects
The following minor side effects may occur:
- Blurred vision
- Confusion
- Constipation
- Diarrhea
- Difficult or painful urination
- Dizziness
- Dry mouth, throat, or nose
- Headache
- Irritability
- Loss of appetite
- Nausea or stomach upset
- Ringing or buzzing in the ears
- Unusual increase in sweating

These side effects should disappear as your body adjusts to the medication.
Tell your doctor about any side effects that are persistent or particularly bothersome. It is especially important to tell your doctor about a change in menstruation, clumsiness, feeling faint, flushing of the face, hallucinations, rash, palpitations, seizures, shortness of breath, fever, sleeping disorders, sore throat, tightness in the chest, unusual bleeding or bruising, or unusual tiredness or weakness.

Interactions
This medicine interacts with several other drugs such as central nervous system depressants and it can decrease the activity of oral anticoagulants.
Be sure to tell your doctor about any medications you are currently taking.

Storage
Tablets, elixir, etc. should be stored at room temperature in tightly closed containers. Store away from heat and direct light. Keep out of reach of children, since overdose may be very dangerous in children. Do not keep outdated medicine or medicine no longer needed. Flush the contents of the container down the toilet, unless otherwise directed.

---

hydrochlorothiazide. It can be used to treat raised blood pressure.

Seconal Sodium
A proprietary, prescription-only preparation of quinalbarbitone. It can be used to treat persistent and intractable insomnia.

Sectral
A proprietary, prescription-only preparation of acebutolol. It can be used to treat raised blood pressure and angina pectoris and to regularize heartbeat.

Securon/ SR
A proprietary, prescription-only preparation of verapamil. It can be used to treat raised blood pressure, angina pectoris and to regularize heartbeat.

Securopen
A proprietary, prescription-only preparation of the antibacterial and antibiotic drug azlocillin. It can be used to treat pseudomonas infections of the urinary tract, upper respiratory tract and septicaemia.

Seldane
A proprietary, non-prescription preparation of terfenadine. It can be used to treat symptoms of allergic disorders such as hay fever and allergic skin conditions.

Select-A-Jet Dopamine
A proprietary, prescription-only pre-

paration of dopamine. It can be used to treat cardiogenic shock following a heart attack.

Seligiline
A proprietary, prescription-only enzyme inhibitor. It can be used to treat symptoms of parkinsonism.

Selsun
A proprietary, non-prescription preparation of selenium sulphide. It can be used to treat dandruff.

Semi-Daonil
A proprietary, prescription-only preparation of glibenclamide. It can be used in the treatment of Type II diabetes.

Semprex
A proprietary, prescription-only preparation of acrivastine. It can be used to treat symptoms of allergic disorders such as hay fever and urticaria.

Senlax
A proprietary, non-prescription preparation of senna. It can be used to treat constipation.

Senna
A proprietary, non-prescription stimulant laxative. It can be used to treat constipation.

Senokot Granules
A proprietary, non-prescription preparation of the laxative senna. It can be used to treat obstipation.

Senokot Syrup
A proprietary, non-prescription preparation of the laxative senna. It can be used to treat obstipation.

Senokot Tablets
A proprietary, non-prescription preparation of the laxative senna. It can be used to treat obstipation.

Septrin
A proprietary, prescription-only compound preparation of the antibacterial drugs sulphamethoxazole and trimethoprin. It can be used to treat bacterial infections, especially infections of the urinary tract, prostatitis and bronchitis.

Serc
A proprietary, prescription-only preparation of betahistine hydrochloride. It can be used to treat nausea associated with vertigo, tinnitus and hearing loss in Ménière's disease.

Serenace
A proprietary, prescription-only preparation of haloperidol. It can be used to treat psychotic disorders, especially schizophrenia.

Serevent
A proprietary, prescription-only preparation of salmeterol. It can be used as bronchodilator to treat reversible obstructive airways disease and asthma.

Sermorelin
An analogue of growth hormone releasing-hormone. It is used therapeutically to assess the secretion of growth hormone.

Serophene
A proprietary, prescription-only preparation of clomiphene citrate. It can be used as an infertility treatment.

Seroxat
A proprietary, prescription-only preparation of paroxetine. It can be used to treat depressive disorders.

Sertraline
A proprietary, prescription-only antidepressant drug. It can be used to treat depressive disorders.

Setlers Tablets
A proprietary, non-prescription preparation of calcium carbonate. It can be used to relief heartburn, indigestion, dyspepsia, nausea and flatulence.

Setlers Tums-Assorted
A proprietary, non-prescription preparation of calcium carbonate. It can be used to relief heartburn, indigestion, dyspepsia, nausea and flatulence.

Sevredol
A proprietary, prescription-only preparation of morphine sulphate. It can be used to relieve pain following surgery.

Silver sulphadiazine
A proprietary, prescription-only compound preparation of the antibacterial drug sulphadiazine and silver. It can be used to treat a broadspectrum of bacterial infections.

Simplene
A proprietary, prescription-only preparation of adrenaline. It can be used to treat glaucoma, but not closed-angle glaucoma.

Simvastatin
A proprietary, prescription-only lipid-lowering drug. It can be used to reduce the levels of various lipids in the bloodstream.

Sinemet
A proprietary, prescription-only compound preparation of levodopa and carbidopa. It can be used to treat the symptoms of parkinsonism.

Sinemet CR
A proprietary, prescription-only compound preparation of levodopa and carbidopa. It can be used to treat the symptoms of parkinsonism.

Sinemet LS
A proprietary, prescription-only compound preparation of levodopa and carbidopa. It can be used to treat the symptoms of parkinsonism.

Sinemet-Plus
A proprietary, prescription-only compound preparation of levodopa and carbidopa. It can be used to treat the symptoms of parkinsonism.

Sinequan
A proprietary, prescription-only preparation of the antidepressant drug doxepin. It can be used to treat depressive illness.

Siopel
A proprietary, non-prescription compound preparation of cetrimide and dimethicone. It can be used as a barrier cream to treat and dress itching or infected skin, nappy rash and bedsores.

Skinoren
A proprietary, prescription-only pre-

Senna

Properties

This medicine contains as active ingredient senna, a stimulant laxative. Stimulant laxatives (also known as contact laxatives) are medicines taken by mouth to encourage bowel movements by acting on the intestinal wall. They increase the muscle contractions that move along the stool mass.

Before using this medicine

Before you use this medicine check with your doctor, or pharmacist:
- if you ever had any unusual or allergic reaction to laxatives.
- if you are on a low-salt, low-sugar, or any other special diet, or if you are allergic to any substance, such as sulfites or other preservatives or dyes.
- if you are pregnant. Stimulant laxatives may cause unwanted effects in the expectant mother if improperly used. Some of the stimulant laxatives may cause contractions of the womb.
- if you are breast-feeding an infant. Some stimulant laxatives may pass into the breast milk. Although the amount of laxative in the milk is generally thought to be too small to cause problems in the child, your doctor should be told that you plan to use such laxatives.
- if you have any of the following medical problems:
  Appendicitis (or signs of)
  Colostomy
  Diabetes (sugar disease)
  Heart disease
  Hypertension
  Ileostomy
  Intestinal blockage
  Laxative habit
  Rectal bleeding

Treatment

For safe and effective use of bulk-forming laxatives:
Follow your doctor's orders if this laxative was prescribed.
Follow the manufacturer's package directions if you are treating yourself.
At least six to eight 8-ounce glasses of liquids should be taken each day.
Stimulant laxatives are usually taken on an empty stomach for rapid effect. Results are slowed if taken with food.
Laxatives should not be given to young children (up to 6 years of age) unless prescribed by their doctor. Since children cannot usually describe their symptoms very well, a doctor should check the child before giving this medicine.

Side effects

Along with the needed effects, a medicine may cause some unwanted effects.
Side effects that should be reported to your doctor: breathing difficulty; burning on urination; confusion; headache; irregular heartbeat; irritability; mood or mental changes; muscle cramps; skin rash; unusual tiredness.

Laxative habit

Laxatives are to be used to provide short-term relief only, unless otherwise directed by your doctor. Laxatives are overused by many people. Such a practice often leads to dependence on the laxative action to produce a bowel movement. In some cases, overuse of some laxatives has caused damage to the nerves, muscles, and tissues of the intestines and bowel.

Interactions

This medicine may interact with several other drugs, such as amiloride, antacids, other laxatives, potassium supplements, tetracycline antibiotics and triamterene.
Be sure to tell your doctor about any medications you are currently taking.

Storage

Store away from heat and direct light. Keep out of the reach of children. Do not store in the bathroom medicine cabinet because the heat or moisture may cause the medicine to break down.

S

---

paration of azelaric. It can be used to treat severe acne.

Slo-Indo

A proprietary, prescription-only preparation of indomethacin. It can be used to relieve pain and inflammation of rheumatic disease, acute gout and other inflammatory musculoskeletal disorders.

Slo-Phyllin

A proprietary, prescription-only pre-

paration of theophylline. It can be used as bronchodilator to treat chronic bronchitis and asthma.

Sloprolol

A proprietary, prescription-only preparation of propanolol hydrochloride. It can be used to treat raised blood pressure and angina pectoris and to regularize heartbeat.

Slow-Fe

A proprietary, non-prescription pre-

paration of ferrous sulphate. It can be used to treat iron deficiency.

Slow-Fe Folic

A proprietary, compound preparation of ferrous sulphate and folic acid. It can be used as a supplement during pregnancy.

Slow-K

A proprietary, non-prescription preparation of potassium chloride. It can be used to treat deficiency of potassium in the blood.

Slow-Trasicor

A proprietary, prescription-only preparation of oxprenolol hydrochloride. It can be used to treat raised blood pressure and angina pectoris and to regularize heartbeat.

Slozem

A proprietary, prescription-only preparation of diltiazem hydrochloride. It can be used to treat raised blood pressure and angina pectoris.

Sno Phenicol

A proprietary, preparation of the antibacterial and antibiotic drug chloramphenicol. It can be used to treat bacterial infections in the eye.

Sno Pilo

A proprietary, prescription-only preparation of pilocarpine. It can be used to treat glaucoma and to facilitate inspection of the eye.

Sno Tears

A proprietary, non-prescription of polyvinyl alcohol. It can be used as artificial tears where there is dryness of the eyes.

Sodium acid phosphate

A mineral which is mainly used as a phosphorous supplement.

Sodium amytal

A proprietary, prescription-only preparation of the barbiturate drug amylobarbitone. It can be used to treat sleeping disorders.

Sodium aurothiomalate

A proprietary, prescription-only preparation of gold. It can be used to treat severe conditions of active rheumatoid arthritis and juvenile arthritis.

Sodium bicarbonate

A proprietary, non-prescription-only antacid preparation. It can be used to relieve hyperacidity, dyspepsia and for the symptomatic relief of heartburn.

Sodium bicarbonate BP

A proprietary, non-prescription-only antacid preparation. It can be used to relieve hyperacidity, dyspepsia and for the symptomatic relief of heartburn.

Sodium calciumedetate

A proprietary, prescription-only chelating agent. It can be used as an antidote to poisoning by heavy metals.

Sodium cellulose phosphate

A proprietary, non-prescription preparation used to reduce high calcium levels in the bloodstream.

Sodium chlodronate

A drug that affects calcium metabolism and is used to treat high calcium levels associated with malignant tumors and bone lesions.

Sodium citrate

An alkaline compound, which is used to treat mild infections of the urinary tract in which the urine is acid.

Sodium cromoglicate

A proprietary, prescription-only anti-allergic drug. It can be used to prevent recurrent asthma attacks (but not to treat acute attacks) and allergic symptoms in the eye and elsewhere.

Sodium cromoglycate

A proprietary, prescription-only anti-allergic drug. It can be used to prevent recurrent asthma attacks (but not to treat acute attacks) and allergic symptoms in the eye and elsewhere.

Sodium hypochlorite

A powerful oxidizing agent, which can be used in solution as an antiseptic for cleansing abrasions.

Sodium nitroprusside

A proprietary, prescription-only vasodilator drug. It can be used to treat raised blood pressure.

Sodium perborate

An antiseptic agent used in solution as a mouthwash.

Sodium picosulphate

A proprietary, stimulant laxative. It can be used to treat constipation.

Sodium salicylate

A proprietary, non-prescription analgesic and antirheumatic drug. It can be used to treat rheumatic diseases and other musculoskeletal disorders.

Sodium stibogluconate

A proprietary, prescription-only antiprotozoal drug. It can be used to treat various forms of the tropical disease leishmaniasis.

Sodium thiosulphate

A compound that is used in the emergency treatment of cyanide poisoning.

Sodium valproate

A proprietary, prescription-only anticonvulsant and anti-epileptic drug. It can be used to treat all forms of epilepsy.

Sofradex

A proprietary, prescription-only compound preparation of the antibacterial and antibiotic drug framycetin and dexamethasone. It can be used to treat inflammation and infection of the eye or outer ear.

Sofradex

A proprietary, prescription-only preparation of the antibacterial and antibiotic drug framycetin. It can be used to treat inflammation and infection of the eye or skin.

Solatrcaine

A proprietary, non-prescription preparation of benzocaine and triclosan. It can be used to treat local pain and skin irritation.

Solpadeine Capsules

A proprietary, non-prescription compound preparation of paracetamol and codeine phosphate. It can be used to relieve headache, period pain and rheumatic and musculoskeletal pain.

Solpadeine Soluble Tablets

A proprietary, non-prescription compound preparation of paracetamol, caffeine and codeine phosphate. It can be used to relieve headache, period pain and rheumatic and musculoskeletal pain.

Solpadeine Tablets

A proprietary, compound preparation of paracetamol, caffeine and codeine phosphate. It can be used to relieve headache, period pain and rheumatic and musculoskeletal pain.

Solpadol
A proprietary, non-prescription compound preparation of paracetamol and codeine phosphate. It can be used to relieve headache, period pain and rheumatic and musculoskeletal pain.

Solu-Cortef
A proprietary, prescription-only preparation of the corticosteroid hydrocortisone. It can be used to treat inflammation, allergic symptoms and shock.

Solu-Medrone
A proprietary, prescription-only preparation of the corticosteroid methylprednisolone. It can be used to treat inflammation, allergic symptoms, cerebral oedema and shock.

Somatropin
A name for the pituitary human growth hormone. It can be used to treat short stature.

Sominex
A proprietary, non-prescription preparation of promethazine. It can be used to treat sleep disorders.

Somnite
A proprietary, preparation of the benzodiazepine drug nitrazepam. It can be used to treat sleep disorders.

Soneryl
A proprietary, prescription-only preparation of butobarbitone. It can be used to treat persistent and intractable insomnia.

Soni-Slo
A proprietary, prescription-only preparation of isosorbide dinitrate. It can be used to treat heart failure and to prevent and treat angina pectoris.

Sootheye
A proprietary, non-prescription preparation of zinc sulphate. It can be used for the symptomatic relief of minor eye irritation.

Sorbichew
A proprietary, prescription-only preparation of isosorbide dinitrate. It can be used to treat heart failure and to prevent and treat angina pectoris.

Sorbid SA
A proprietary, prescription-only preparation of isosorbide dinitrate. It can be used to treat heart failure and to prevent and treat angina pectoris.

Sorbitol
A sweet-tasting carbohydrate, which is used as sugar-substitute.

Sorbitrate
A proprietary, prescription-only preparation of isosorbide dinitrate. It can be used to treat heart failure and to prevent and treat angina pectoris.

Sotacor
A proprietary, prescription-only preparation of sotalol hydrochloride. It can be used to treat raised blood pressure, to prevent and treat angina pectoris and tom regularize heartbeat.

Sotalol hydrochloride
A proprietary, prescription-only cardiovascular drug. It can be used to treat raised blood pressure, to prevent and treat angina pectoris and tom regularize heartbeat.

Sotazide
A proprietary, prescription-only compound preparation of sotalol and hydrochlorothiazide. It can be used to treat raised blood pressure.

Sparine
A proprietary, prescription-only preparation of promazine. It can be used to soothe agitated and restless patients, particularly elderly patients.

Spasmonal
A proprietary, non-prescription preparation of alverine citrate. It can be used to treat muscle spasm of the gastrointestinal tract.

Spectinomycin
A proprietary, prescription-only preparation antibacterial and antibiotic drug. It can be used to treat infections in patients who are allergic to penicillin.

Spectraban Lotion
A proprietary, non-prescription sunscreen lotion. It can be used for skin protection.

Spectraban Ultra
A proprietary, non-prescription sunscreen lotion. It can be used for skin protection.

Spiro-Co/ 50
A proprietary, prescription-only compound preparation of spironolactone and hydroflumethiazide. It can be used to treat congestive heart failure.

Spiroctan/M
A preparation of spironolactone. It can be used to treat congestive heart failure and oedema.

Spirolone
A proprietary, prescription-only compound preparation of spironolactone and hydroflumethiazide. It can be used to treat congestive heart failure.

Spirolactone
A proprietary, prescription-only diuretic drug. It can be used in conjunction with other types of diuretics and is used to treat oedema associated with aldosteronism.

Spirospare
A proprietary, prescription-only preparation of the diuretic drug spirolactone. It can be used in conjunction with other types of diuretics and is used to treat oedema associated with aldosteronism.

Sporanox
A proprietary, prescription-only preparation of itraconazole. It can be used to treat candidiasis infections of the vagina, vulva and oropharynx and ringworm infections of the skin.

Stafoxil
A proprietary, prescription-only preparation of the antibacterial and antibiotic drug flucloxacillin. It can be used to treat bacterial infections.

Stanozalol
A proprietary, prescription-only anabolic steroid drug. It can be used to assist the metabolic synthesis of protein and to treat hereditary angiooedema.

Staril
A proprietary, prescription-only pre-

paration of fosinopril. It can be used to treat raised blood pressure.

STD
A proprietary, prescription-only preparation of sodium tetradecyl sulphate. It can be used in scleropathy to treat varicose veins.

Stelazine
A proprietary, prescription-only preparation of trifluoperazine. It can be used to treat and tranquillize psychotic patients.

Stemetil
A proprietary, prescription-only preparation of prochlorperazine. It can be used to relieve the symptoms of nausea.

Steri-Neb Ipratropium
A proprietary, prescription-only preparation of ipratropium bromide. It can be used to treat the symptoms of chronic bronchitis.

Steri-Neb Salamol
A proprietary, prescription-only preparation of salbutamol. It can be used as bronchodilator to treat reversible obstructive airways disease.

Steripod Chlorhexidine
A proprietary, non-prescription preparation of chlorhexidine. It can be used for swabbing and cleaning wounds.

Stesolid
A proprietary, prescription-only preparation of the benzodiazepine drug diazepam.
It can be used to treat anxiety and insomnia.

Stiedex
A proprietary, prescription-only preparation of the corticosteroid drug desoxymethasone. It can be used to treat severe acute inflammation and chronic skin disorders.

Stiemycin
A proprietary, prescription-only preparation of the antibacterial and antibiotic drug erythromycin. It can be used to treat severe acne.

Stilboestrol
A synthetic sex hormone with estrogen activity. It can be used in hormone replacement therapy.

Stilnoct
A proprietary, non-prescription preparation of zolpidem tartrate. It can be used to treat insomnia.

Streptase
A proprietary, prescription-only preparation of streptokinase. It can be used to treat thrombosis and embolism.

Streptokinase
A proprietary, prescription-only preparation fibrinolytic drug. It can be used to treat thrombosis and embolism.

Streptomycin
A proprietary, prescription-only preparation of antibacterial and antibiotic drug of the aminoglycoside family. It can be used to treat tuberculosis.

Stromba
A proprietary, prescription-only preparation of the anabolic steroid stanozolol. It can be used to treat angio-oedema.

Stugeron
A proprietary, non-prescription preparation of cinnarizine.
It can be used to treat nausea and vertigo.

Stugeron Forte
A proprietary, non-prescription preparation of cinnarizine. It can be used to treat nausea and vertigo. It is also used as peripheral vasodilator.

Sublimaze
A proprietary, prescription-only preparation of fentanyl. It can be used to treat moderate to severe pain.

Sucralfate
A proprietary, non-prescription compound preparation of aluminium hydroxide and sulphated sucrose. It can be used to treat gastric and duodenal ulcers.

Sudafed Elixir
A proprietary, non-prescription preparation of pseudoephedrine hydrochloride. It can be used for the symptomatic relief of allergic and vasomotor rhinitis and colds and flu.

Sudafed Expectorant
A proprietary, non-prescription compound preparation of pseudoephedrine hydrochloride and guaiphenesin. It can be used for the symptomatic relief of upper respiratory tract disorders.

Sudafed Expectorant
A proprietary, non-prescription compound preparation of pseudoephedrine hydrochloride and dextromethorphan. It can be used for the symptomatic relief of upper respiratory tract disorders and dry cough.

Sudafed-Co Tablets
A proprietary, non-prescription compound preparation of pseudoephedrine hydrochloride and paracetamol. It can be used for the symptomatic relief of upper respiratory tract disorders and colds and flu.

Sudafed Nasal Spray
A proprietary, non-prescription preparation of oxymetazoline hydrochloride. It can be used for the symptomatic relief of nasal congestion.

Sudafed Tablets
A proprietary, non-prescription preparation of pseudoephedrine hydrochloride. It can be used for the symptomatic relief of upper respiratory tract disorders and colds and flu.

Sudocrem Antiseptic Cream
A proprietary, non-prescription compound preparation of zinc oxide, benzyl alcohol, benzyl benzoate and lanolin. It can be used to treat nappy rash and incontinence dermatitis.

Sulconazole nitrate
A proprietary, prescription-only antifungal preparation. It can be used to treat skin infections, particularly those caused by tinea.

Suleo-C/M
A proprietary, non-prescription pre-

paration of carbaryl. It can be used to treat infestations of the scalp and pubic hair by lice.

Sulfadoxine
A proprietary, prescription-only sulphonamide drug. It can be used to treat and prevent malaria.

Sulfametopyrazine
A proprietary, prescription-only sulphonamide drug. It can be used to treat and prevent malaria.

Sulindac
A proprietary, prescription-only analgesic and antirheumatic drug. It can be used to treat pain and inflammation in rheumatic disease and other musculoskeletal disorders.

Sulphabenzamide
A sulphonamide drug. It can be used to treat bacterial infections of the vagina.

Sulphacetamide
A proprietary, prescription-only sulphonamide antibacterial drug. It can be used to treat bacterial infections of the vagina and cervix.

Sulphadiazine
A proprietary, prescription-only sulphonamide antibacterial drug. It can be used to treat serious bacterial infections.

Sulphadimethoxine
A proprietary, prescription-only sulphonamide antibacterial drug. It can be used to treat the eye disorder trachoma.

Sulphadimidine
A proprietary, prescription-only sulphonamide antibacterial drug. It can be used to treat serious bacterial infections.

Sulphamethoxazole
A proprietary, sulphonamide antibacterial drug. It can be used to treat a wide range of infections.

Sulphasalazine
A aminosalicylate drug. It can be used to treat Crohn's disease and ulcerative colitis.

Sulphonamides

Sulpha drugs of sulphonamides are derivatives of a red dye called sulphanilamide and have the property of preventing the growth of bacteria. They were the first group of drugs suitable for antimicrobial use as relatively save antibacterial agents.

Today, along with other similar synthetic classes of chemotherapeutic drugs, are commonly referred to as antibiotics, although, strictly speaking, they are not antibiotics (in the literal sense of agents produced by, or obtained from, microorganisms, that inhibit the growth of, or destroy, other microorganisms).

Their antibacterial action stems from their chemical similarity to a compound required by bacteria to generate the essential growth factor, folic acid. This similarity inhibits the production of folic acid by bacteria (and therefore growth), while the human host is able to utilize folic acid in the diet.

Most sulphonamides are administered orally and are rapidly absorbed into the blood. They are short-acting and may have to be taken several times a day. Their quick progress through the body and excretion in the urine makes them particularly suited for the treatment of urinary infections.

One or two sulphonamides are long-acting and may be used to treat diseases such as malaria or leprosy.

Sulphathiazole
A proprietary, prescription-only sulphonamide antibacterial drug. It can be used to treat a wide range of infections.

Sulphinpyrazone
A proprietary, prescription-only drug. It can be used to treat and prevent gout and renal hyperurea.

Sulpride
A proprietary, prescription-only antipsychotic drug. It can be used to treat the symptoms of schizophrenia and other psychotic disorders.

Sulpitil
A preparation of the antipsychotic drug sulpride. It can be used to treat the symptoms of schizophrenia and other psychotic disorders.

Sultrin
A proprietary, prescription-only compound preparation of sulphacetamide, sulphabenzamide and sulphathiaziode. It can be used to treat bacterial infections of the vagina and cervix.

Sumatriptan
A proprietary, prescription-only antimigraine drug. It can be used to treat acute migraine attacks.

Suprane
A proprietary, prescription-only preparation of desflurane. It can be used for the induction and maintenance of general anesthesia.

Suprax
A proprietary, prescription-only preparation of the antibacterial and antibiotic drug cefixime. It can be used to treat acute bacterial infections, particularly infections of the urinary tract.

Suprecur
A preparation of the hormone buserelin. It can be used to treat endometriosis in women and some forms of cancer in men.

S

Suprefact

A proprietary, prescription-only preparation of the hormone buserelin. It can be used to treat endometriosis in women and some forms of cancer in men

Surgam

A proprietary, prescription-only preparation of tiaprofenic acid. It can be used to treat the pain of rheumatic disease and other musculoskeletal disorders.

Surmontil

A proprietary, prescription-only preparation of trimipramine. It can be used to treat depressive illness, especially in cases where there is a need for sedation.

Suscard

A proprietary, prescription-only preparation of glyceryl trinitrate. It can be used to treat and prevent angina pectoris.

Sustac

A proprietary, prescription-only preparation of glyceryl trinitrate. It can be used to treat and prevent angina pectoris.

Sustamycin

A proprietary, prescription-only preparation of the antibacterial and antibiotic drug tetracycline. It can be used to treat infections of many kinds.

Sustenon 100

A proprietary, prescription-only preparation of the androgen hormone testosterone. It can be used to treat testosterone deficiency.

Sustenon 250

A proprietary, prescription-only preparation of the androgen hormone testosterone. It can be used to treat testosterone deficiency.

Suxamethonium chloride

A proprietary, prescription-only skeletal muscle relaxant drug. It can be used to induce muscle paralysis during surgery.

Symmetrel

A proprietary, prescription-only preparation of amantadine hydrochloride. It can be used to treat the symptoms of parkinsonism.

Synacthen

A proprietary, prescription-only preparation of tetracosatrin. It can be used to stimulate the adrenal glands of to test the function of the adrenal glands.

Synacthen Depot

A proprietary, prescription-only preparation of tetracosatrin. It can be used to stimulate the adrenal glands of to test the function of the adrenal glands.

Synalar

A proprietary, prescription-only preparation of fluocinolone acetonide. It can be used to treat severe, acute inflammatory skin disorders.

Synalar C

A proprietary, prescription-only compound preparation of fluocinolone acetonide and clioquinol. It can be used to treat severe, acute inflammatory skin disorders.

Synalar N

A proprietary, prescription-only compound preparation of fluocinolone acetonide and neomycin. It can be used to treat severe, acute inflammatory skin disorders.

Synarel

A proprietary, prescription-only preparation of nafarelin. It can be used to treat endometriosis.

Syndol

A proprietary, prescription-only compound preparation of codeine phosphate, doxylamine succinate and caffeine. It can be used to treat mild to moderate pain, including tension headache, toothache, period pain, muscle pain, neuralgia and pain following surgery.

Synflex

A proprietary, prescription-only preparation of naproxen. It can be used to relieve pain and inflammation, particularly rheumatic and arthritis pain.

Synkavit

A proprietary, non-prescription preparation of menadiol sodium phosphate. It can be used to treat certain types of vitamin K deficiency.

Synphase

A proprietary, prescription-only compound hormonal preparation. It can be used as a triphasic oral contraceptive or to treat certain menstrual disorders.

Syntaris

A proprietary, prescription-only preparation of the corticosteroid drug flunisolide. It can be used to treat nasal allergy, such as hay fever.

Syntex Menopause

A proprietary, prescription-only preparation of the female sex hormones mestranol and norethisterone. It can be used in hormone replacement therapy.

Syntocinon

A proprietary, prescription-only preparation of the natural pituitary hormone oxytocin. It can be used to assist or induce labour.

Syntometrine

A proprietary, prescription-only preparation of ergometrine and oxytocin. It can be used to assist the third and final stage of labour.

Syntopressin

A proprietary, prescription-only preparation of lypressin. It can be used to treat pituitary-originated diabetes insipidus.

Synvisc

A proprietary, prescription-only preparation of hylan. It is used to relieve the pain of osteoarthritis knees.

T

Tagamet
A proprietary, prescription-only preparation of cimetidine. It can be used to treat benign peptic ulcer, gastroesophageal reflux, dyspepsia and associated conditions.

Tambocor
A proprietary, prescription-only preparation of flecainide acetate. It can be used to treat irregularities of the heartbeat.

Tamiflu
A proprietary, prescription-only preparation of oseltamivir. It is used for the prevention and treatment of influenza.

Tamofen
A proprietary, prescription-only preparation of the sex hormone antagonist tamoxifen. It can be used as an anticancer drug for cancers that depend on the presence of estrogens.

Tamoxifen
A sex hormone antagonist, an anti-estrogen. It antagonizes the natural estrogen present in the body and can be useful in treating infertility in women. A second and major use, is an anticancer drug in the treatment of existing estrogen-dependent breast cancer.

Tampovagan
A proprietary, prescription-only preparation of stilboestrol, a sex hormone analogue with estrogen activity. It can be used to treat conditions of the vagina caused by hormonal deficiency.

Tancolin
A proprietary, non-prescription preparation of dextromethorphan hydrobromide. It can be used for the symptomatic relief of coughs, particularly those associated with infection in the upper respiratory tract.

Tarcortin
A proprietary, prescription-only compound preparation of the corticosteroid hydrocortisone and coal tar. It can be used to treat eczema and psoriasis.

Targocid
A proprietary, prescription-only preparation of the antibacterial and antibiotic drug teicoplanin. It can be used to treat infections, such as endocarditis and peritonitis and infections due to Staphylococcus aureus.

Tarivid
A proprietary, prescription-only preparation of the antibacterial and antibiotic drug ofloxacin. It can be used to treat complicated infections of the urinary tract, septicaemia and gonorrhoea.

Tavegil
A proprietary, non-prescription preparation of clemastine. It can be used to treat the symptoms of allergic disorders such as hay fever and urticaria.

Taxol
A proprietary, prescription-only preparation of the anticancer drug paclitaxel. It can be used to treat ovarian cancer.

Tazocin
A proprietary, prescription-only compound preparation of the broad-spectrum antibacterial and antibiotic drug piperacillin and the enzyme inhibitor tazobactam. It can be used to treat serious or compound forms of bacterial infections.

TCT Antiseptic Throat Pastilles
A proprietary, non-prescription preparation of phenol. It can be used for the relief of minor sore throats.

TCT Liquid Antiseptic
A proprietary, non-prescription preparation of phenol. It can be used for the relief of sore throat including those associated with colds and flu.

Teejel Gel
A proprietary, non-prescription compound preparation of cetalkonium chloride and choline salicylate. It can be applied to the mouth for the symptomatic relief of pain from mouth ulcers.

Tegretol
A proprietary, prescription-only preparation of carbamazepine. It can be used in the preventive treatment of most forms of epilepsy, for trigeminal neuralgia and in the management of manic-depressive illness.

Teicoplanin
An antibacterial and antibiotic drug belonging to the glycopeptide family.It can be used to treat serious infections, including endocarditis and peritonitis.

Temazepam
A proprietary, prescription-only benzodiazepine preparation. It can be used to treat insomnia.

Temgesic
A proprietary, prescription-only preparation of the narcotic analgesic drug buprenorphine. It can be used to treat all forms of pain.

Temocillin
A proprietary, prescription-only antibiotic and antibacterial drug. It can be used to treat infections that other penicillins are incapable of countering, due to the production of penicillinase by the bacteria concerned.

Temopen
A proprietary, prescription-only preparation of the antibiotic and antibacterial drug temocillin. It can be used to treat infections that other penicillins are incapable of countering, due to the production of penicillinase by the bacteria concerned.

Tenchlor
A proprietary, prescription-only compound preparation of atenolol and chlorthalidone. It can be used to treat raised blood pressure.

Tenif
A proprietary, prescription-only compound preparation of atenolol and nifedipine. It can be used to treat raised blood pressure.

Tenoret 50
A proprietary, prescription-only compound preparation of atenolol and chlorthalidone. It can be used to treat raised blood pressure.

Tenoretic
A proprietary, prescription-only compound preparation of atenolol and chlorthalidone. It can be used to treat raised blood pressure.

Tenormin
A proprietary, prescription-only preparation of atenolol. It can be used to treat raised blood pressure and as an anti-angina treatment to relieve the symptoms and improve excessive tolerance and to regularize heartbeat.

Tenoxicam
A proprietary, prescription-only non-narcotic and analgesic antirheumatic drug. It can be used to treat pain and inflammation in rheumatic disease and other musculoskeletal disorders.

Tensium
A proprietary, prescription-only preparation of the benzodiazepine drug diazepam. It can be used to treat anxiety, insomnia and certain forms of epilepsy.

Tenuate Dospan
A proprietary, prescription-only preparation of diethylpropion hydrochloride. It can be used in the medical treatment of obesity.

Teoptic
A proprietary, prescription-only preparation of carteol hydrochloride. It can be used to treat glaucoma.

Terazosin
A proprietary, prescription-only alpha-adrenoreceptor blocker drug. It can be used to treat raised blood pressure and urinary retention.

Terbinafine
A proprietary, prescription-only antifungal drug. It can be used to treat ringworm infections of the skin and fungal infections of the nails.

Terbutaline sulphate
A proprietary, prescription-only sym-pathicomimetic stimulant. It can be used as a bronchodilator in reversible obstructive airways disease.

Terfenadine
A proprietary, prescription-only antihistamine drug. It can be used for the symptomatic relief of allergic symptoms.

Tertipressin
A proprietary, prescription-only preparation of vasopressin. It can be used as a vasoconstrictor to treat bleeding from varices in the esophagus.

Terra-Cortril
A proprietary, prescription-only compound preparation of the anti-inflammatory and corticosteroid drug hydrocortisone and the antibacterial and antibiotic drug oxytetracycline. It can be used to treat skin disorders in which bacterial or other infection is also implicated.

Terra-Cortril Nystatin
A proprietary, prescription-only compound preparation of the anti-inflammatory and corticosteroid drug hydrocortisone and the antibacterial and antibiotic drug oxytetracycline and the antifungal drug nystatin. It can be used to treat skin disorders caused by fungal or bacterial infection.

Terramycin
A proprietary, prescription-only preparation of the antibacterial and antibiotic drug oxytetracycline. It can be used to treat a wide range of infections.

Tertroxin
A proprietary, prescription-only preparation of liothyronine, a form of the thyroid hormone triiodothyronine. It can be used to treat hormonal deficiency (hypothyroidism).

Testosterone
A proprietary, prescription-only male sex hormone (androgen). It can be used to treat testosterone deficiency and maintenance of the male sex organs.

Tetrabenazine
A proprietary, prescription-only psychoactive drug. It can be used to assist a patient to regain voluntary control of movement, or at least to lessen die extent of involuntary movements, in Huntington's chorea and related disorders.

Tetrabid-Organon
A proprietary, prescription-only preparation of the antibacterial and antibiotic drug tetracycline. It can be used to treat infections of many kinds.

Tetrachel
A preparation of the antibacterial and antibiotic drug tetracycline. It can be used to treat infections of many kinds.

Tetracosactrin
A proprietary, prescription-only synthetic hormone, an analogue of the pituitary hormone corticotrophin. It can be used to test adrenal function.

Tetracycline
A proprietary, prescription-only broad-spectrum antibacterial and antibiotic drug. It can be used to treat many forms of infection.

Tetralysal 300
A proprietary, prescription-only preparation of the antibacterial and antibiotic drug lymercycline. It can be used to treat many forms of infection.

Theo-Dur
A preparation of the bronchodilator drug theophylline. It can be used to treat chronic bronchitis and asthma.

Theophylline
A proprietary, prescription-only bronchodilator drug. It can be used to treat chronic bronchitis and asthma.

Theophorin
A proprietary, non-prescription preparation of the antihistamine drug phenindamine. It can be used to treat the symptoms of allergic disorders.

Thiabendazole
A proprietary, non-prescription-only azole drug. It can be used to treat in-

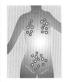

Terfenadine

Properties
This medicine contains terfenadine as active ingredient; it is used to treat or prevent symptoms of allergy. This medication belongs to a group known as antihistamines. Antihistamines block the action of histamine, a chemical that is released by the body during an allergic reaction. Some of the antihistamines are also used to prevent motion sickness, nausea, vomiting, and dizziness.

Before using this medicine
Before you use this medicine check with your doctor, or pharmacist:
- if you ever had any unusual or allergic reaction to antihistamines.
- if you are on a low-salt, low-sugar, or any other special diet, or if you are allergic to any substance, such as sulfites or other preservatives or dyes.
- if you are pregnant or intending to become pregnant while using this medicine.
- if you are breast-feeding an infant. Small amounts of antihistamines pass into the breast milk. Use is not recommended since the chances are greater for most antihistamines to cause side effects, such as unusual excitement or irritability in the infant.
- if you have any of the following medical problems:
  Asthma attack
  Enlarged prostate
  Glaucoma
  Urinary tract blockage
  Difficult urination

Treatment
This medication is used to relieve or prevent the symptoms of your medical problem. Take them as directed. Do not take more of them and do not take them more often than recommended on the label, unless otherwise directed by your doctor. To do so may increase the chance of side effects.

Side effects
The following minor side effects may occur:
- blurred vision
- confusion
- constipation
- diarrhea
- difficult or painful urination
- dizziness
- dry mouth, throat, or nose
- headache
- irritability
- loss of appetite
- nausea or stomach upset
- ringing or buzzing in the ears
- unusual increase in sweating.
These side effects should disappear as your body adjusts to the medication.
Tell your doctor about any side effects that are persistent or particularly bothersome. It is especially important to tell your doctor about a change in menstruation, clumsiness, feeling faint, flushing of the face, hallucinations, rash, palpitations, seizures, shortness of breath, fever, sleeping disorders, sore throat, tightness in the chest, unusual bleeding or bruising, or unusual tiredness or weakness.

Interactions
This medicine interacts with several other drugs such as central nervous system depressants and it can decrease the activity of oral anticoagulants.
Be sure to tell your doctor about any medications you are currently taking.

Storage
Tablets, elixir, etc. should be stored at room temperature in tightly closed containers. Store away from heat and direct light. Keep out of reach of children, since overdose may be very dangerous in children. Do not keep outdated medicine or medicine no longer needed. Flush the contents of the container down the toilet, unless otherwise directed.

festations by worm parasites, particularly those of the Strongyloides species.

Thioguanine
A proprietary, prescription-only cytotoxic drug. It can be used to treat acute leukaemia.

Thiopentone Sodium
A proprietary, prescription-only general anesthetic drug. It can be used for the induction of anesthesia.

Thioridazine
A proprietary, prescription-only antipsychotic drug. It can be used to treat and tranquillize psychotic patients (such as schizophrenics), particularly those experiencing behavioral disturbances.

Thiotepa
A proprietary, prescription-only cytotoxic drug. It can be used to treat tumors in the bladder or other body cavities.

Thymoxamine
A proprietary, prescription-only alpha-adrenoreceptor blocker drug. It can be used to treat peripheral vascular disease.

Thyrotrophin
A proprietary, prescription-only anterior pituitary hormone. It can be used to test certain clinical disorders.

Thyroxine sodium
A   proprietary,   prescription-only

preparation of thyroxine, which is one of the two main natural thyroid hormones. It can be used to treat hormonal deficiency (hypothyroidism).

Thiaprofenic acid
A proprietary, prescription-only non-narcotic analgesic and antirheumatic drug. It can be used to treat pain and inflammation in rheumatic disease and other musculoskeletal disorders.

Tibolone
A proprietary, prescription-only hormonal preparation with estrogen and progestogen activity. It can be used to treat menopausal problems in hormone replacement therapy.

Ticar
A proprietary, prescription-only preparation of the antibacterial and antibiotic drug ticarcillin. It can be used to treat serious infections such as septicaemia, peritonitis and infections of the respiratory and urinary tract.

Ticarcillin
A proprietary, prescription-only preparation antibacterial and antibiotic drug. It can be used to treat serious infections such as septicaemia, peritonitis and infections of the respiratory and urinary tract.

Tilade
A proprietary, prescription-only preparation of the anti-asthma drug nedocromil sodium. It can be used to treat recurrent attacks of asthma.

Tildiem/LA/Retard
A proprietary, prescription-only preparation of the calcium-channel blocker drug tildiazem hydrochloride. It can be used to treat raised blood pressure and to prevent and treat attacks of angina pectoris.

Timecef
A preparation of the antibacterial and antibiotic drug cefodizime. It can be used to treat infections of the lower respiratory tract and of the urinary tract.

Timentin
A proprietary, prescription-only compound preparation of the antibacterial and antibiotic drug ticarcillin and the enzyme inhibitor clavulanic acid. It can be used to treat serious infections that occur in patients whose immune systems are undermined by disease or drugs.

Timodine
A proprietary, prescription-only compound preparation of the corticosteroid drug hydrocortisone, the antifungal drug nystatin and the antiseptic drug benzylalkonium chloride. It can be used to treat fungal infections.

Timolol maleate
A proprietary, prescription-only beta-blocker drug. It can be used to treat raised blood pressure, and as an anti-angina treatment to relieve symptoms and improve exercise tolerance and to regularize heartbeat.

Timoptol
A proprietary, prescription-only beta-blocker drug. It can be used to treat glaucoma.

Timpron
A proprietary, prescription-only preparation of the non-narcotic analgesic and antirheumatic drug naproxen. It can be used to relieve pain of musculoskeletal disorders.

Tinaderm Cream
A proprietary, non-prescription preparation of the antifungal drug tolnaftate. It can be used to treat athlete's foot.

Tinaderm-M
A proprietary, prescription-only compound preparation of the antifungal drug tolnaftate and the antifungal and antibiotic drug nystatin. It can be used to treat Candida fungal infections of the skin and nails.

Tinaderm Plus Powder
A proprietary, non-prescription preparation of the antifungal drug tolnaftate. It can be used to treat athlete's foot.

Tinaderm Plus Powder Aerosol
A proprietary, non-prescription preparation of the antifungal drug tol-

naftate. It can be used to treat athlete's foot.

Tinidazole
A proprietary, prescription-only azole drug with antibacterial and antiprotozoal properties. It can be used to treat anaerobic infections such as bacterial vaginitis and protozoal infections.

Tinset
A proprietary, non-prescription preparation of the antihistamine drug oxatomide. It can be used to treat the symptoms of allergic conditions.

Tioconazole
A proprietary, prescription-only azole antifungal drug. It can be used to treat fungal infections of the nails.

Tisept
A proprietary, non-prescription compound preparation of the antiseptic agents chlorhexidine and cetrimide. It can be used as a general skin disinfectant.

Tixylix Cough and Cold
A compound preparation of the antitussive drug pholcodine, the antihistamine drug chlorpheniramine and the decongestant drug pseudo-ephedrine. It can be used for the relief of dry, thickly coughs, runny nose and congestion.

Tobralex
A proprietary, prescription-only preparation of the antibacterial and antibiotic drug tobramycin. It can be used to treat bacterial infections of the eye.

Tobramycin
A proprietary, prescription-only antibacterial and antibiotic drug. It can be used to treat serious Gram-negative infections caused by Pseudomonas aeruginosa.

Tocainide hydrochloride
A proprietary, prescription-only anti-arrhythmic drug. It can be used to treat heartbeat irregularities.

Tofranil
A proprietary, prescription-only pre-

**Fever
Pain
Infection**

Tolectin

Properties
This medicine contains as active ingredient tolmetin. It belongs to the group of medicines called non-steroidal anti-inflammatory drugs (NSAIDs). These drugs are taken by mouth to relieve some symptoms caused by arthritis or rheumatism, such as inflammation, swelling, stiffness, and joint pain. However, these medicines do not cure arthritis and will help you only as long as you continue to take them. Some of these medicines are also used to relieve other kinds of pain or to treat other painful conditions, such as gout attacks, bursitis, tendinitis, sprains, strains, menstrual cramps. The drug reduces the tissue concentration of prostaglandins.

Before using this medicine
Before you use this medicine check with your doctor, or pharmacist:
- if you ever had any unusual or allergic reaction, such as skin rash, hives, or itching or breathing problems, to any of the anti-inflammatory analgesics.
- if you are on a low-salt, low-sugar, or any other special diet, or if you are allergic to any substance, such as sulfites or other preservatives or dyes.
- if you are pregnant or intending to become pregnant while using this medicine. Studies on birth defects have not been done in humans. However, if taken regularly during the last months of pregnancy, there is a chance that these medicines may cause unwanted effects on the heart or blood flow in the fetus or newborn infant.
- if you are breast-feeding an infant. Although this medicine has not been shown to cause problems in humans, it passes into the breast milk in small amounts.
- if you have any of the following medical problems:
  Asthma
  Bleeding problems
  Colitis, or other intestinal problems
  Stomach ulcer
  Heart disease
  High blood pressure
  Kidney or liver disease

Treatment
This medication is used to relieve pain or other symptoms caused by arthritis. For safe and effective use of this medicine, do not take more of it, do not take it more often, and do not take it for a longer period of time than ordered by your physician or directed by the package label.
If you are taking this medication on a regular schedule and you miss a dose, take the missed dose as soon as possible, unless it is almost time for your next dose. In that case do not take the missed dose at all.
To lessen stomach upset, anti-inflammatory analgesics may be taken with food or antacids.

Side effects
Along with the needed effects, a medicine may cause some unwanted effects. These side effects may go away during treatment as your body adjusts to the medicine. Such minor side effects are: dizziness; nausea; pain; headache; drowsiness; swollen feet, face or leg; constipation or diarrhea; vomiting; dry mouth.
Check with your doctor immediately if any of the following side effects occur:
- *Muscle cramps*
- *Numbness or tingling*
- *Mouth ulcers*
- *Convulsions or confusion*
- *Rash, hives, or itch*
- *Tightness in chest*

Interactions
This medicine may interact with several other drugs.
Be sure to tell your doctor about any medications you are currently taking.

Storage
The medicine should be stored at room temperature in a tightly closed, light-resistant container. Store away from heat and direct light. Keep out of reach of children.

---

paration of imipramine. It can be used to treat depressive illness, particularly in patients who are withdrawn and apathic.

Tolanase
A proprietary, prescription-only preparation of tolazamide. It can be used in diabetic treatment for Type 2 diabetes (non-insulin-dependent diabetes).

Tolazamide
A proprietary, prescription-only sulphonylurea drug. It can be used in diabetic treatment for Type 2 diabetes (non-insulin-dependent diabetes).

Tolbutamide
A proprietary, prescription-only sulphonylurea drug. It can be used in diabetic treatment for Type 2 diabetes (non-insulin-dependent diabetes).

Tolectin
A preparation of tolmetin. It can be used to treat the pain and inflammation of rheumatic disease and other musculoskeletal disorders.

Tolerzide
A proprietary, prescription-only compound preparation of sotalol hydrochloride and hydrochlorothiazide. It can be used to treat raised blood pressure.

Tolmetin

A proprietary, prescription-only antirheumatic drug. It can be used to treat the pain and inflammation of rheumatic disease and other musculoskeletal disorders.

Tolnaftate

A proprietary, non-prescription antifungal drug. It can be used to treat infections caused by the tinea species.

Tonocard

A proprietary, prescription-only preparation of the anti-arrhythmic drug tocainide hydrochloride. It can be used to treat heart irregularities.

Topal

A proprietary, non-prescription compound preparation of the antacids aluminium hydrochloride and magnesium carbonate and the demulcent agent alginic acid. It can be used to treat heartburn, severe indigestion and the symptoms of hiatus hernia.

Topicycline

A proprietary, prescription-only preparation of the antibacterial and antibiotic drug tetracycline. It can be used to treat acne.

Toprol

A proprietary, prescription-only preparation of metoprolol. It is to treat high blood pressure. Il works to help manage high blood pressure throughout the day.

Toradol

A proprietary, prescription-only preparation of the non-narcotic analgesic drug ketorolac trometamol. It can be used to treat acute postoperative pain.

Torasemide

A proprietary, prescription-only diuretic drug. It can be used to treat oedema in patients with chronic heart failure and to treat raised blood pressure.

Torem

A proprietary, prescription-only preparation of the diuretic drug torasemide. It can be used to treat oedema in patients with chronic heart failure and to treat raised blood pressure.

Totamol

A proprietary, prescription-only preparation of the beta-blocker drug atenolol. It can be used to treat raised blood pressure and to relieve symptoms of angina pectoris.

Tracrium

A proprietary, prescription-only preparation of the skeletal muscle relaxant drug atracurium besylate. It can be used to induce muscle paralysis during surgery.

Tramadol hydrochloride

A proprietary, prescription-only narcotic analgesic drug, which is similar to morphine in relieving pain. It can be used to treat severe pain conditions.

Tramazoline hydrochloride

A proprietary, non-prescription sympathicomimetic and vasoconstrictor drug. It can be used as a nasal decongestant to treat allergic rhinitis.

Tramil 500 Analgesic Capsules

A proprietary, non-prescription preparation of paracetamol. It can be used to treat many forms of pain, including headache, migraine, muscular pain and period pain.

Trancopal

A proprietary, prescription-only preparation of the anxiolytic drug chlormezanone. It can be used to treat anxiety and insomnia.

Trandate

A preparation of lebatalol hydrochloride. It can be used to treat raised blood pressure.

Tramdolapril

A proprietary, prescription-only ACE inhibitor and vasodilator drug. It can be used to treat raised blood pressure.

Tranexamic acid

A proprietary, prescription-only antifibrinolytic preparation. It can be used to treat bleeding conditions such as dental extractions and excessive period bleeding.

Transiderm-Nitro

A proprietary, prescription-only preparation of glycerol trinitrate. It can be used to treat and prevent angina pectoris and to prevent phlebitis.

Transvasin Heat Rub

A proprietary, non-prescription compound preparation of tetrahydrofurfuryl salicylate, hexyl nicotinate and ethyl salicylate. It can be used for the symptomatic relief of muscular aches and pains.

Tranxene

A proprietary, prescription-only preparation of the anxiolytic drug clorazepam dipotassium. It can be used to treat anxiety.

Tranylcypromine

A proprietary, prescription-only antidepressant drug of the MAO class. It can be used to treat depressive illness.

Trasicor

A proprietary, prescription-only preparation of oxprenolol hydrochloride. It can be used to treat raised blood pressure, as an anti-angina treatment to relieve symptoms and as an anti-arrhythmic to regulate heartbeat.

Trasidrex

A proprietary, prescription-only preparation of oxprenolol hydrochloride. It can be used to treat raised blood pressure, as an anti-angina treatment to relieve symptoms and as an anti-arrhythmic to regulate heartbeat.

Trasylol

A proprietary, prescription-only preparation of aprotinin. It can be used to prevent life-threatening clot formation.

Tavasept 100

A proprietary, non-prescription compound preparation of cetrimide and chlorhexedine. It can be used for cleaning wounds and burns.

Travogyn

A proprietary, prescription-only preparation of the antifungal drug isoconazole. It can be used to treat fungal infections of the vagina.

Traxam
A proprietary, prescription-only preparation of felbinac. It can be used for the symptomatic relief of underlying muscle or joint pain.

Trazodone hydrochloride
A proprietary, prescription-only tricyclic-related antidepressant drug. It can be used to treat depressive illness.

Trental
A proprietary, non-prescription preparation of the vasodilator drug oxpentifylline. It can be used to help improve blood circulation to the hands and feet.

Treosulfan
A proprietary, prescription-only preparation of the cytotoxic drug treosulfan. It can be used to treat ovarian cancer.

Tretinoin
A proprietary, non-prescription retinoid, a derivative of vitamin A. It can be used to treat acne.

TRH-Cambridge
A proprietary, prescription-only preparation of the natural pituitary thyrotropin-releasing hormone. It can be used to test thyroid function.

Tri-Adcortyl
A proprietary, prescription-only compound preparation of the corticosteroid drug triamcinolone and the antibacterial and antibiotic drugs gramicidin and nystatin. It can be used to treat severe infective skin inflammation.

Tri-Adcortyl Otic
A proprietary, prescription-only compound preparation of the corticosteroid drug triamcinolone and the antibacterial and antibiotic drugs gramicidin and neomycin and the antifungal drug nystatin. It can be used to treat severe infective skin inflammation, such as eczema and psoriasis.

Triadene
A proprietary, prescription-only compound preparation of ethinyloestradiol and gestodene. It can be used as an contraceptive and certain menstrual problems.

Triamcinolone
A proprietary, prescription-only synthetic corticosteroid. It can be used to treat the symptoms of inflammation, when it is caused by allergic disorders.

Triamcinolone acetonide
A proprietary, prescription-only synthetic corticosteroid. It can be used to treat the symptoms of inflammation, when it is caused by allergic disorders.

Triamcinolone hexacetonide
A proprietary, prescription-only synthetic corticosteroid. It can be used to treat the symptoms of inflammation, when it is caused by allergic disorders.

Triam-Co
A proprietary, prescription-only compound preparation of hydrochlorthiazide and triamterine. It can be used to treat raised blood pressure and oedema.

Triamterene
A proprietary, prescription-only diuretic drug of the potassium-sparing type. It can be used to treat oedema, raised blood pressure and congestive heart failure.

Triazole
A proprietary, prescription-only antifungal drug. It can be used to treat fungal infections.

Tribavirin
A proprietary, prescription-only antiviral drug that inhibits a wide range of DNA and RNA viruses. It can be used to treat various viral diseases such as lassa fever.

Tribiotic
A proprietary, prescription-only compound preparation of neomycin sulphate, polymyxin B sulphate and bacitracin. It can be used to treat infections of the skin.

Triclofos oral solution
A non-proprietary, prescription-only preparation of the hypnotic drug tri-

Tranquillizers
These medicines calm, soothe and relieve anxiety and may also cause some degree of sedation. Although somewhat misleading, they are often classified in two groups: major and minor tranquillizers.

The major tranquillizers, which are also called neuroleptics or antipsychotic medicines, are used primarily to treat severe mental disorders such as psychoses (including schizophrenia and mania).

They are extremely effective in restoring a patient to a calmer, less-disturbed state of mind. The hallucinations, both auditory and visual, the gross disturbance of logical thinking and to some extent the delusions typical of psychotic states are generally well controlled by these medicines.

Violent, aggressive behavior that presents a danger to the patients themselves and to those that look after them, is also effectively treated by major tranquillizers. For this reason they are often used in the management of difficult, aggressive, antisocial individuals.

Minor tranquillizers are also calming drugs, but they are ineffective in the treatment of psychotic states. Their principal applications are as anxiolytic, hypnotic and sedative drugs. The best-known and most-used minor tranquillizers are undoutedly the benzodiazepines. However, prolonged treatment with minor tranquillizers can lead to dependence (addiction).

clofos sodium. It can be used to treat insomnia in children.

Triclofos sodium
A non-proprietary, prescription-only preparation of the hypnotic drug triclofos sodium. It can be used to treat insomnia.

Triclosan
A proprietary, non-prescription antiseptic agent. It can be used to prevent the spread of infections of the skin.

Tridil
A proprietary, prescription-only preparation of glyceryl trinitrate. It can be used to treat and prevent angina pectoris. It can also be used in the treatment of heart failure.

Trientine dihydrochloride
A chelating agent that is used to reduce the abnormally high levels of copper in the body that occur in Wilson's disease.

Trifluoperazine
A proprietary, prescription-only phenothiazine derivative. It can be used to treat psychotic conditions and to tranquillize psychotic patients.

Trifluoperidol
A proprietary, prescription-only phenothiazine derivative. It can be used to treat psychotic conditions and to tranquillize psychotic patients.

Trifyba
A proprietary, non-prescription preparation of the natural laxative bran. It can be used to treat obstipation.

Triiodothyronine
A proprietary, prescription-only preparation of liothyronine sodium, which is a form of the thyroid hormone triiodothyronine. It can be used to treat hormonal deficiency (hypothyroidism).

Trilostane
A proprietary, prescription-only enzyme inhibitor. It can be used to treat conditions that result from the excessive secretion of corticosteroids in the bloodstream.

Triludan
A proprietary, non-prescription preparation of terfenadine. It can be used to treat the symptoms of allergic conditions.

TrimaxCo
A proprietary, prescription-only compound preparation of triamterine and hydrochlorthiazide. It can be used to treat oedema and raised blood pressure.

Trimeprazine tartrate
A proprietary, prescription-only phenothiazine derivative. It can be used to treat the symptoms of allergic disorders.

Trimetaphan camsylate
A proprietary, prescription-only ganglion blocker drug. It can be used to treat raised blood pressure.

Trimethoprim
A proprietary, prescription-only antibacterial drug which is similar to the sulphonamides. It can be used to treat and prevent the spread of many forms of bacterial infections, but particularly infections of the respiratory and urinary tract.

Tri-Minulet
A proprietary, prescription-only compound preparation of ethinyloestradiol and gestodene. It can be used as a contraceptive and to treat certain menstrual problems.

Trimipramine
A proprietary, prescription-only antidepressant drug of the tricyclic class. It can be used to treat depressive illness

Trimogal
A proprietary, prescription-only preparation of the antibacterial drug trimethoprim. It can be used to treat infections of the upper respiratory tract and the urinary tract.

Trimovate
A proprietary, prescription-only compound preparation of the corticosteroid drug clobetasone butyrate, the antibacterial and antibiotic drug tetracycline and the antifungal drug nystatin. It can be used to treat skin infections.

Trinordiol
A proprietary, prescription-only preparation of ethinyloestradiol and levonorgestrel. It can be used as a contraceptive and to treat certain menstrual problems.

TriNovum
A proprietary, prescription-only preparation of ethinyloestradiol and norethisterone. It can be used as a contraceptive and to treat certain menstrual problems.

TriNovum ED
A proprietary, prescription-only preparation of ethinyloestradiol and norethisterone. It can be used as a contraceptive and to treat certain menstrual problems.

Triogesic Tablets
A preparation of paracetamol and phenylpropanolamine. It can be used to treat nasal and sinus congestion and associated pain.

Triominic
A proprietary, non-prescription compound preparation of phenylpropanolamine hydrochloride and pheniramine maleate. It can be used as a nasal congestant for the relief of allergic rhinitis.

Triperidol
A proprietary, prescription-only preparation of the antipsychotic drug trifluperidol. It can be used to treat psychoses (including schizophrenia).

Triprimix
A proprietary, prescription-only preparation of the antibacterial drug trimethoprim. It can be used to treat infections of the upper respiratory tract and urinary tract.

Tripolidine hydrochloride
A proprietary, non-prescription antihistamine drug. It can be used for the symptomatic relief of allergic symptoms such as hay fever and urticaria.

Triptafen
A proprietary, prescription-only com-

pound preparation of the antidepressant drug amitriptyline and the antipsychotic drug perphenazine. It can be used to treat depressive illness, particularly in association with anxiety.

Trisequens
A proprietary, prescription-only compound preparation of the female sex hormones oestriol, oestradiol and norethisterone. It can be used to treat menopausal problems.

Trisodium edetate
A chelating agent that binds calcium and forms an inactive compound. It can be used as an antidote to treat conditions in which there is excessive calcium in the bloodstream.

Tritace
A proprietary, prescription-only preparation of the ACE inhibitor ramipril. It can be used to treat raised blood pressure and in heart failure treatment.

Trobicin
A proprietary, prescription-only preparation of the antibacterial and antibiotic drug spectinomycin. It can be used to treat gonorrhoea in patients who are allergic to penicillin.

Tropicamide
A proprietary, prescription-only anticholinergic preparation. It can be used to dilate the pupil and paralyse the focusing of the eye for ophthalmic conditions.

Tropisetron
A proprietary, prescription-only antiemetic and antinauseant drug. It can be used to treat nausea and vomiting, especially in patients receiving radiotherapy or chemotherapy.

Tropium
A proprietary, prescription-only preparation of the benzodiazepine drug chlordiazepoxide. It can be used for the short-term treatment of anxiety.

Trosyl
A proprietary, prescription-only preparation of the antifungal drug tio-

conazole. It can be used to treat fungal infections of the nails.

Tryptizol
A proprietary, prescription-only preparation of the antidepressant drug amitriptyline. It can be used in the treatment of depressive illness, especially in cases where sedation is required.

Tubocurarine chloride
A proprietary, prescription-only skeletal muscle relaxant. It can be used to induce muscle paralysis during surgery.

Tuinal
A proprietary, prescription-only compound preparation of the barbiturate drugs amylbarbitone and quinalbarbitone. It can be used to treat persistent and intractable insomnia.

Tolubuterol hydrochloride
A proprietary, prescription-only beta-receptor stimulant drug. It can be used as a bronchodilator in reversible obstructive airways disease.

Tylex
A proprietary, prescription-only compound preparation of codeine sulphate and paracetamol. It can be used to treat a painkiller.

Tyrocane Throat Lozenges
A proprietary, non-prescription compound preparation of the antiseptic agent cetylpyridinium chloride and the local anesthetic drug benzocaine. It can be used for the relief of minor infections of the mouth and throat.

Tyrothricin
A proprietary, non-prescription antiseptic agent. It can be used to treat sore throat.

Tyrozets
A proprietary, non-prescription compound preparation of the antiseptic agent tyrothricin and the local anesthetic drug benzocaine. It can be used for the relief of minor mouth and throat irritations.

U

Ubretid
A proprietary, prescription-only preparation of the anticholinesterase and parasympathomimetic drug distigmine bromide. It can be used to treat bladder and intestinal activity.

Ulcerax
A proprietary, prescription-only preparation of the antihistamine drug hydroxyzine hydrochloride. It can be used for the relief of allergic symptoms.

Ukidan
A proprietary, prescription-only preparation of the fibrinolytic drug urokinase. It can be used to treat venous thrombi, pulmonary embolism and peripheral vascular occlusion.

Ultec
A proprietary, prescription-only preparation of cimetidine. It can be used to treat benign peptic ulcers in the stomach or duodenum.

Ultra Clearasil Maximum Strength
A proprietary, non-prescription preparation of benzoyl peroxide (10 %). It can be used to treat acne, spots and pimples.

Ultra Clearasil Regular Strength
A proprietary, non-prescription preparation of benzoyl peroxide (5 %). It can be used to treat acne, spots and pimples.

Ultradil Plain
A proprietary, prescription-only preparation of the corticosteroid and anti-inflammatory drug fluocortolone. It can be used to treat inflammatory skin infections.

Ultralanum Plain
A proprietary, prescription-only preparation of the corticosteroid and anti-inflammatory drug fluocortolone. It can be used to treat inflammatory skin infections.

Ultraproct

A proprietary, prescription-only compound preparation of the corticosteroid and anti-inflammatory drug fluocortolone and the local anesthetic cinchocaine. It can be used to treat hemorrhoids.

Unguentum Merck

A proprietary, non-prescription compound preparation of liquid paraffin, white soft paraffin and several other constituents. It can be used as an emollient for dry skin.

Unihep

A proprietary, prescription-only preparation of the anticoagulant drug heparin. It can be used to treat various forms of thrombosis.

Uniparin

A proprietary, prescription-only preparation of the anticoagulant drug heparin. It can be used to treat various forms of thrombosis.

Uniparin Calcium

A preparation of the anticoagulant drug heparin. It can be used to treat various forms of thrombosis.

Uniphyllin Continus

A proprietary, non-prescription preparation of the bronchodilator drug theophylline. It can be used to treat asthma and bronchitis.

Uniroid-HC

A proprietary, prescription-only compound preparation of the corticosteroid hydrocortisone and the local anesthetic cinchocaine. It can be used to treat hemorrhoids.

Unisept

A proprietary, non-prescription preparation of chlorhexidine gluconate. It can be used to clean wounds.

Unisomnia

A proprietary, prescription-only preparation of the benzodiazepine drug nitrazepam. It can be used to treat insomnia.

Univer

A proprietary, prescription-only preparation of the calcium-channel blocker drug verapamil. It can be used to treat raised blood pressure and to prevent attacks of angina pectoris.

Uriben

A proprietary, prescription-only preparation of the antibacterial and antibiotic drug nalidixic. It can be used to treat infections of the urinary tract.

Urispas

A proprietary, prescription-only preparation of the anticholinergic drug flavoxate hydrochloride. It can be used to treat urinary frequency and incontinence.

Urofolitrophin

A pituitary follicle-stimulating hormone, used in the treatment of infertility due to abnormal pituitary gland function.

Urokinase

A proprietary, prescription-only preparation of the fibrinolytic drug urokinase. It can be used in the treatment of venous thrombi, pulmonary embolism and peripheral vascular occlusion.

Uromitexan

A proprietary, prescription-only preparation of the drug mesna. It can be used to treat hemorrhagic cystitis.

Ursofalk

A proprietary, prescription-only preparation of ursodeoxycholic acid. It can be used to dissolve gallstones.

Utinor

A proprietary, prescription-only preparation of the antibacterial and antibiotic drug norfloxacin. It can be used to treat infections of the urinary tract.

Utovlan

A proprietary, prescription-only preparation of the progestogen norethisterone. It can be used to treat uterine bleeding, endometriosis, premenstrual tension syndrome and abnormally heavy menstruation.

V

Vagifem

A proprietary, prescription-only preparation of estradiol. It is a local estrogen therapy designed to relieve vaginal symptoms of menopause.

Vaginyl

A proprietary, prescription-only preparation of the antibacterial and antiprotozoal drug nitrodinazole. It can be used to treat infections of many kinds.

Valclair

A proprietary, prescription-only preparation of the benzodiazepine drug diazepam. It can be used to treat anxiety and insomnia.

Valenac

A proprietary, prescription-only preparation of declofenac sodium. It can be used to treat arthritic and rheumatic pain and other musculoskeletal disorders.

Valium

A proprietary, prescription-only preparation of the benzodiazepine drug diazepam. It can be used to treat anxiety, insomnia, certain forms of epilepsy. It can also be used as a muscle relaxant and to help alleviate alcohol withdrawal syndrome.

Vallergan

A proprietary, prescription-only preparation of the antihistamine drug trimeprazine tartrate. It can be used to treat the symptoms of allergic disorders.

Valoid

A proprietary, non-prescription preparation of cyclizine. It can be used to treat nausea, vomiting, vertigo, motion sickness and disorders of the balance function of the inner ear.

Valrox

A proprietary, prescription-only preparation of naproxen. It can be used to treat arthritic and rheumatic pain and other musculoskeletal disorders.

Valtrex

A proprietary, prescription-only

Vaginyl

Properties

This medicine belongs to the family of topical (applied to the skin) antifungal preparations. It is used in the treatment of fungus infections on the skin and in the vagina. The medication fights infections such as ringworm of the scalp, athlete's foot, jockey itch, sun fungus, nail fungus and fungus infections of the vagina.

Fungal diseases may develop especially in people with disorders of immunity or diabetes and those on certain drugs (steroid, immunosuppressives, antibiotics). Thrush is common in the mouth and vagina but rarely causes systemic disease.

The drug kills fungi by damaging the fungal wall; it causes loss of essential elements to sustain fungus cell life.

Before using this medicine

Before you use this medicine check with your doctor, or pharmacist:
- if you ever had any unusual or allergic reaction to topical antifungal preparations.
- if you are on a low-salt, low-sugar, or any other special diet, or if you are allergic to any substance, such as certain preservatives or dyes.
- if you are sunburned, or have an open skin wound.
- if you are pregnant, intending to become pregnant or breast-feeding an infant while using this medicine.

Pregnant women should avoid using the vaginal cream during the first three months of pregnancy. They should use it during the next six months only if it is absolutely necessary.

Treatment

This medication is used to relieve or prevent the symptoms of your medical problem. Take them as directed. Do not take more of them and do not take them more often than recommended on the label. To do so may increase the chance of absorption through the skin and the chance of side effects. If you forget to take a dose of this drug, take it as soon as you remember. If it is almost time for your next regularly scheduled application, skip the forgotten application and continue with your regular schedule.

CREAM, LOTION, OINTMENT, GEL: Bathe and dry area before use. Apply small amount and rub gently.

POWDER: Apply lightly to the skin.

VAGINAL CREAM & TABLETS: Insert into vagina with applicator as illustrated in instructions.

The treatment may require a period of 6 to 8 weeks for a complete cure. The usual schedule calls for an application twice a day, morning and evening, unless otherwise directed by your doctor or pharmacist. Be sure to complete the full course of treatment prescribed for you.

Side effects

The following side effects may occur:
- Itching
- Swelling of treated skin
- Redness of skin
- Vaginal burning and itching
- Irritation of vagina
- Increased discharge

You should discontinue the use of the drug when these side effects occur. Call your doctor right away.

Interactions

This medicine may interact with several other medications applied to the skin or vagina. The combined effect may cause severe skin irritation or disorders of the labia or vagina.

Storage

This medicine should be stored cool, but Do not freeze. Store away from heat and direct light. Keep out of reach of children. Do not use on other members of the family without consulting your doctor. Do not store in the bathroom medicine cabinet because the heat or moisture may cause the medicine to break down. Do not keep outdated medicine or medicine no longer needed. Flush the contents down the toilet, unless otherwise directed.

---

preparation of valacyclovir. It is used to for the treatment of viral infections such as herpes.

Vancocin

A proprietary, prescription-only preparation of the antibacterial and antibiotic drug vancomycin. It can be used to treat infections such as pseudomembranous colitis and endocarditis.

Vancomycin

A proprietary, prescription-only antibacterial and antibiotic drug. It can be used to treat infections such as pseudomembranous colitis and endocarditis.

Varidase Topical

A proprietary, prescription-only preparation of the enzymes streptokinase and streptodornase. It can be used to cleanse and soothe skin ulcers.

Vascase

A proprietary, prescription-only preparation of the ACE inhibitor cilazapril. It can be used to treat raised blood pressure.

Vasogen Cream

A proprietary, non-prescription compound preparation of zinc oxide, dimeticone and calamine. It can be used for nappy rash, bedsores and the skin around a stoma.

Vasopressin

A pituitary hormone secreted by the posterior lobe of the hypophysis. It can be used to treat pituitary-originated diabetes insipidus.

Vasoxine

A proprietary, prescription-only preparation of methoxamine hydrochloride. It can be used to treat cases of acute hypotension.

Vecuronium bromide

A proprietary, non-prescription skeletal muscle relaxant drug. It can be used to induce muscle paralysis during surgery.

Veganin Tablets

A proprietary, non-prescription compound preparation of aspirin, paracetamol and codeine phosphate. It can be used to treat the symptoms of flu, headache, rheumatism, toothache and period pain.

Velbe

A proprietary, prescription-only preparation of the cytotoxic drug vinblastine sulphate. It can be used to treat lymphoma, acute leukaemia and some solid tumors.

Velosef

A proprietary, prescription-only preparation of the antibacterial and antibiotic drug cephradine. It can be used to treat a wide range of bacterial infections.

Velosulin

A proprietary, prescription-only insulin preparation. It can be used in diabetic treatment.

Venlafaxine

A proprietary, prescription-only antidepressant drug. It can be used to treat depressive disorders.

Veno's Cough Mixture

A proprietary, non-prescription compound preparation of glucose and treacle. It can be used to treat the symptoms of cough.

Veno's Expectorant

A proprietary, non-prescription compound preparation of glucose, guaiphenesin and treacle. It can be used to treat the symptoms of cough.

Veno's Honey and Lemon

A proprietary, non-prescription compound preparation of glucose, honey and lemon juice.

Ventide

A proprietary, prescription-only compound preparation of beclomethasone and salbutamol. It can be used for the symptomatic relief of obstructive airways disease and asthma.

Ventodisks

A proprietary, prescription-only preparation of the beta-receptor stimulant drug salbutamol. It can be used as a bronchodilator in reversible obstructive airways disease and asthma.

Ventolin

A proprietary, prescription-only preparation of the beta-receptor stimulant drug salbutamol. It can be used as a bronchodilator in reversible obstructive airways disease and asthma.

Vepesid

A proprietary, prescription-only preparation of the cytotoxic drug etoposide. It can be used to treat cancers, particularly lymphoma, testicular carcinoma and some other malignant tumors.

Veracur

A proprietary, non-prescription preparation of formaldehyde. It can be used to treat warts.

Verapamil hydrochloride

A proprietary, prescription-only calcium-channel blocker. It can be used to treat and prevent angina attacks and rhythmic disorders of the heart,

Veripaque

A proprietary, non-prescription preparation of the laxative oxyphenisatin. It can be used to treat constipation.

Vermox

A proprietary, prescription-only preparation of mebendazole. It can be used to treat infections by roundworm, threadworm, whipworm and hookworm.

Verrugon

A proprietary, non-prescription preparation of the keratolytic agent salicylic acid. It can be used to treat warts and hard skin.

Verucasep

A proprietary, non-prescription pre-

paration of the keratolytic agent glutaraldehyde. It can be used to treat warts and hard skin.

Viagra

A proprietary, prescription-only preparation of sildenafil. It is indicated for the treatment of erectile dysfunction.

Vibramycin

A proprietary, prescription-only preparation of the antibacterial and antibiotic drug doxycycline. It can be used to treat infections of many kinds.

Vicks Children's Vaposyrup

A proprietary, non-prescription preparation of dextromethorphan hydrobromide. It can be used for relieving and calming coughs.

Vicks Vaposyrup

A proprietary, non-prescription preparation of guaiphenesin. It can be used for relieving a productive cough.

Videne

A proprietary, non-prescription preparation of povidone-iodine. It can be used for disinfecting the skin.

Vidopen

A proprietary, prescription-only preparation of the antibacterial and antibiotic drug ampicillin. It can be used to treat infections of many kinds.

Vindesine sulphate

A proprietary, prescription-only cytotoxic drug. It can be used to treat acute leukaemias, lymphomas and some solid malignant tumors.

Vioform-Hydrocortisone

A proprietary, prescription-only compound preparation of hydrocortisone and clioquinol. It can be used to treat inflammatory skin disorders.

Vioxx

A proprietary, prescription-only preparation believed to fight pain and inflammation by inhibiting the effect of a natural enzyme called COX-2.

Viraferon

A proprietary, prescription-only preparation of interferon (alpha-2b). It

V

can be used in the treatment of chronic hepatitis.

Virudox

A preparation of the antiviral drug idoxuridine. It can be used to treat skin infections caused by herpes simplex or herpes zoster.

Visken

A proprietary, prescription-only preparation of the beta-blocker drug pindolol. It can be used to treat raised blood pressure and to relieve symptoms of angina pectoris.

Visudyne

A proprietary, prescription-only preparation of verteporfin. It is used for the symptomatic treatment of age-related macular degeneration.

Vivalan

A proprietary, prescription-only preparation of the tricyclic-related antidepressant drug viloxazine. It can be used to treat depressive illness.

Volital

A proprietary, prescription-only preparation of pemoline. It can be used to treat hyperkinesis in children.

Volraman

A proprietary, prescription-only preparation of diclofenac sodium. It can be used to treat arthritic and rheumatic pain and other musculoskeletal disorders.

Voltarol

A proprietary, prescription-only preparation of diclofenac sodium. It can be used to treat arthritic and rheumatic pain and other musculoskeletal disorders.

Voltarol Emulgel

A proprietary, prescription-only preparation of diclofenac sodium. It can be used topically for the symptomatic relief of underlying muscle or joint pain.

Vytorin

A proprietary, prescription-only preparation of cezetimibe/simvastatin. It is used to lower levels of total cholesterol, and fatty substances in the blood.

W

Warfarin sodium

A proprietary, prescription-only anticoagulant drug. It can be used to prevent the formation of clots in heart disease, venous thrombosis and pulmonary embolism.

Warfarin WPF

A proprietary, prescription-only anticoagulant drug. It can be used to prevent the formation of clots in heart disease, venous thrombosis and pulmonary embolism.

Warticon

A proprietary, prescription-only preparation of podophyllotoxin. It can be used to treat and remove penil warts.

Warticon Fem

A proprietary, prescription-only preparation of podophyllotoxin. It can be used to treat and remove warts on the external genital organs of women.

Waxol

A proprietary, non-prescription preparation of docusate sodium. It can be used for the dissolution and removal of earwax.

Wellbutrin

A proprietary, prescription-only preparation of ezetimide. It is used to treat symptoms of certain depressive illnesses.

Welldorm

A proprietary, prescription-only preparation of chloral hydrate. It can be used to treat short-term insomnia.

Wellferon

A proprietary, non-prescription preparation of interferon (alpha-N1) It can be used in the treatment of hairy cell leukaemia and chronic active hepatitis.

X Y

Xamoterol

A proprietary, prescription-only beta-receptor stimulant drug. It can be used as a cardiac stimulant in the treatment of certain heart conditions.

Xanax

A preparation of the benzodiazepine drug alprazolam. It can be used in the treatment of anxiety conditions.

Xanthomax

A proprietary, prescription-only preparation of the enzyme inhibitor allopurinol. It can be used to treat excess uric acid in the blood and so prevent renal stones and attacks of gout

Xatral

A proprietary, prescription-only preparation of the alpha-adrenoreceptor blocker drug alfuosin. It can be used to treat urinary retention, for instance in benign prostatic hyperplasia.

Xipamide

A proprietary, prescription-only diuretic drug. It can be used to treat raised blood pressure and congestive heart failure.

Xuret

A proprietary, prescription-only preparation of metolazone. It can be used for the treatment of raised blood pressure.

Xylocaine

A proprietary, prescription-only preparation of the local anesthetic drug lignocaine. It can be used as local anesthetic and for the relief of pain.

Yomesan

A proprietary, non-prescription preparation of niclosamide. It can be used to treat infestation by tapeworm.

Yutopar

A proprietary, prescription-only preparation of the beta-adrenoceptor stimulant drug ritodrine hydrochloride. It can be used to prevent or delay premature labour.

Z

Zaditen
A proprietary, prescription-only preparation of keftotifen. It can be used in the treatment of asthma.

Zadstat
A proprietary, prescription-only preparation of metrodinazole. It can be used to treat anaerobic infections.

Zalcitabine
A proprietary, prescription-only antiviral drug. It can be used in the treatment of AIDS.

Zantac
A proprietary, prescription-only preparation of the ulcer-healing drug ranitidine. It can be used to treat benign peptic ulcers, gastro-esophageal reflux, dyspepsia and associated conditions.

Zarontin
A proprietary, prescription-only preparation of ethosuximide. It can be used to treat absence, myoclonic and some types of seizure.

Zestoretic
A proprietary, prescription-only compound preparation of the ACE inhibitor lisinopril and hydrochlorothiazide. It can be used to treat raised blood pressure.

Zetia
A proprietary, prescription-only preparation of bandronate sodium. It is used to treat or prevent osteoporosis in women after menopause.

Zidovudine
A proprietary, prescription-only antiviral drug. It can be used in the treatment of AIDS.

Zimovane
A proprietary, prescription-only preparation of zoplicone. It can be used to treat insomnia.

Zinamide
A proprietary, prescription-only preparation of the antibacterial drug pyrazinamide. It can be used to treat tuberculosis.

Zinc oxide
A mild astringent agent, which is used primarily to treat skin disorders such as nappy rash, urinary rash and eczema.

Zineryt
A proprietary, prescription-only preparation of the antibacterial and antibiotic drug erythromycin. It can be used to treat infections of many kinds.

Zirtek
A proprietary, prescription-only preparation of citirizine. It can be used to treat the symptoms of allergic disorders.

Zita
A proprietary, prescription-only preparation of the ulcer-healing drug cimetidine. It can be used to treat benign peptic ulcers, gastro-esophageal reflux, dyspepsia and associated conditions.

Zithromax
A proprietary, prescription-only preparation of the antibacterial and antibiotic drug azithromycin. It can be used to treat infections of many kinds.

Zocor
A proprietary, prescription-only preparation of the lipid-lowering drug simvastatin. It can be used to treat high blood levels of lipids.

Zofran
A proprietary, prescription-only preparation of the drug ondansetron. It can be used to treat nausea and vomiting.

Zoladex
A proprietary, prescription-only preparation of the drug goserelin. It can be used in the treatment of cancer of the prostate gland, breast and for uterine endometriosis.

Zoloft
A proprietary, prescription-only preparation of sertraline. It is used for the relief of the symptoms of depression.

Zolpedem tartrate
A proprietary, prescription-only hypnotic drug. It can be used for the treatment of short-term insomnia.

Zonulysin
A proprietary, prescription-only preparation of the enzyme chymotrypsin. It can be used to dissolve a suspensory ligament of the lens of the eye in certain ophthalmic operations.

Zopiclone
A proprietary, non-prescription preparation of the zopiclone. It can be used in the short-term treatment of insomnia.

Zoton
A proprietary, prescription-only preparation of lansoprazole. It can be used as an ulcer-healing drugs.

Zovirax
A proprietary, prescription-only preparation of the antiviral drug acyclovir. It can be used to treat infections by herpes simplex and herpes zoster viruses.

Zuclopenthixol acetate
A proprietary, prescription-only antipsychotic drug. It can be used for the short-term management of acute psychotic and mania disorders.

Zyloric
A proprietary, prescription-only preparation of the enzyme inhibitor allopurinol. It can be used to treat excess uric acid in the blood and to prevent renal stones and attacks of gout.

Index

A

M

M

955